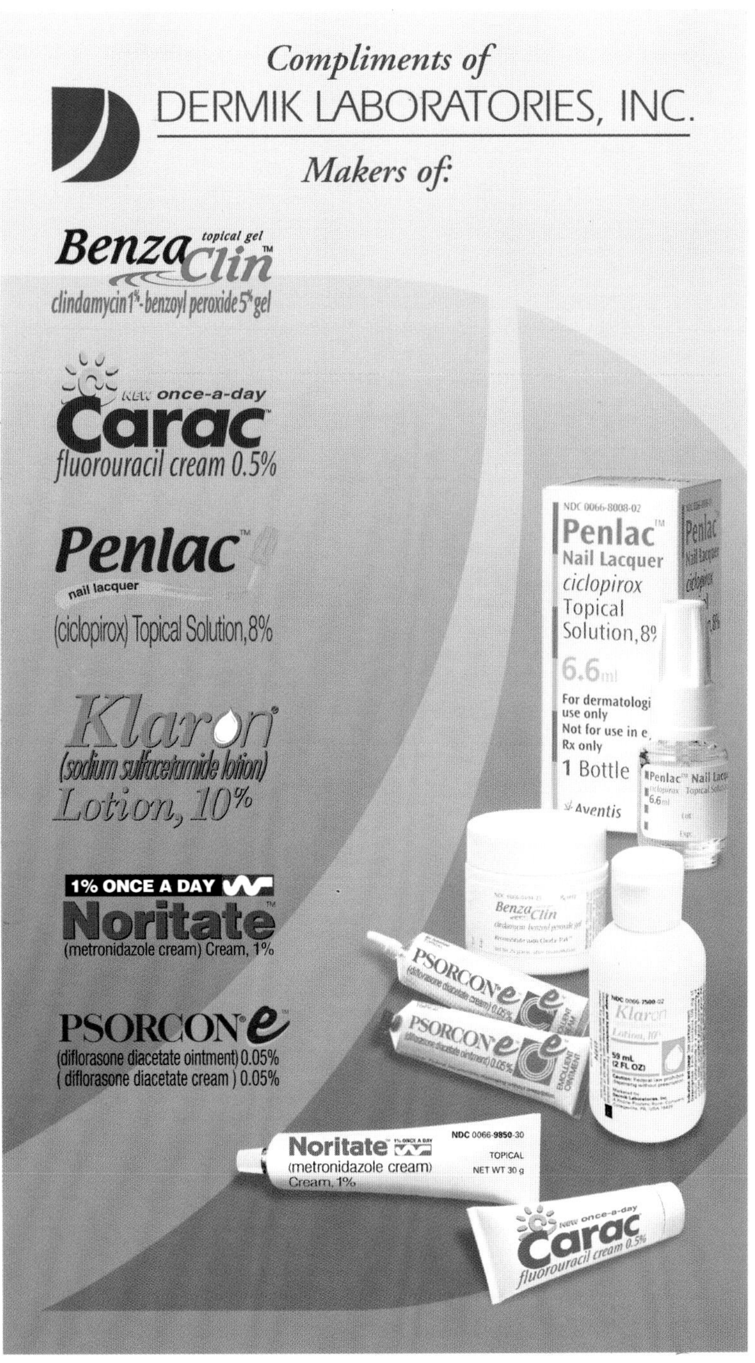
Compliments of
DERMIK LABORATORIES, INC.
Makers of:
BenzaClin topical gel
clindamycin 1%-benzoyl peroxide 5% gel
NEW once-a-day
Carac
fluorouracil cream 0.5%
Penlac
nail lacquer
(ciclopirox) Topical Solution, 8%
Klaron
(sodium sulfacetamide lotion)
Lotion, 10%
1% ONCE A DAY
Noritate
(metronidazole cream) Cream, 1%
PSORCON e
(diflorasone diacetate ointment) 0.05%
( diflorasone diacetate cream ) 0.05%

# DRUG ERUPTION

## REFERENCE MANUAL

*with CD-ROM*

## 9th EDITION

# DRUG ERUPTION REFERENCE MANUAL

*with CD-ROM*

## 9th EDITION

Jerome Z. Litt, MD

*Assistant Clinical Professor of Dermatology*
*Case Western Reserve University School of Medicine*
*Cleveland, Ohio, USA*

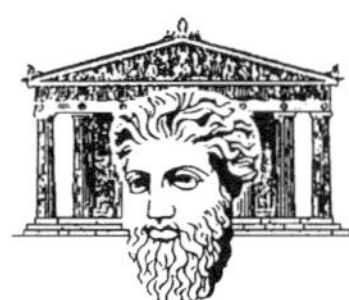

**The Parthenon Publishing Group**
International Publishers in Medicine, Science & Technology

A CRC PRESS COMPANY
BOCA RATON LONDON NEW YORK WASHINGTON, D.C.

Published in the USA by
The Parthenon Publishing Group Inc.
345 Park Avenue South, 10th Floor
New York, NY 10010, USA

Published in the UK and Europe by
The Parthenon Publishing Group Ltd.
23-25 Blades Court, Deodar Road,
London SW15 2NU, UK

**Library of Congress Cataloging-in-Publication Data**

Data available on application

**British Library Cataloguing in Publication Data**

Litt, Jerome Z.
Drug eruption reference manual with CD-ROM : DERM. – 9th ed.
1. Dermatopharmacology – Handbooks, manuals, etc.
2. Drugs – Side effects – Handbooks, manuals etc.
I. Title
615.7′04



ISBN 1-84214-204-6



Typeset by AMA DataSet Limited, Preston, UK
Printed and bound in the USA

# Contents

**To Vel – my Muse**

# INTRODUCTION

Any drug can cause any rash.

According to the World Health Organization, an adverse reaction (ADR) – or an adverse event (ADE) – to a drug has been defined as any noxious or unintended reaction to a drug that has been administered in standard doses by the proper route for the purposes of prophylaxis, diagnosis, or treatment. This definition does not include abuse, overdose, withdrawal, or error of administration. It appears that most ADRs are related to the dose. Death is the ultimate adverse drug event, and has now been incorporated into the manual.

ADRs are underreported and thus are an underestimated cause of morbidity and mortality. The incidence and severity of ADRs can be influenced by age, sex, disease, genetic factors, type of drug, route of administration, duration of therapy, dosage, and bioavailability, as well as interactions with other drugs. It has been estimated that fatal ADRs are the third or fourth leading cause of death in the US.

Adverse drug reactions have been arbitrarily classified into six types:

1. Dose-related (e.g. Digoxin toxicity)
2. Non-dose-related (e.g. Immunological reactions)
3. Dose-related and Time-related (e.g. Corticosteroids)
4. Time-related (e.g. Tardive dyskinesia)
5. Withdrawal (e.g. Opiate or beta-blocker withdrawal)
6. Unexpected failure of therapy (e.g. Inadequate dosage of an oral contraceptive)

Cutaneous drug eruptions can mimic almost any inflammatory dermatosis. While most eruptions are mild and self-limited, severe and life-threatening eruptions do occur, as seen in Stevens–Johnson Syndrome and Toxic Epidermal Necrolysis.

More and more people – primarily the older population – are taking more and more prescription and over-the-counter medications. New drugs are appearing in the medical marketplace on an almost daily basis. More and more drug reactions – in the form of cutaneous eruptions – are developing from all drugs. It has been reported that more than 100,000 hospitalized people in the United States alone died in 1999 as a result of medications.

Dermatologists and general physicians are often perplexed by the nature of some of these problems. The few sources that are available to identify the causes of many of these side effects cannot be accessed by proprietary (trade, brand) names.

This Manual is a Drug Eruption Reference guide that describes and catalogs the adverse cutaneous side effects of **884** commonly prescribed and over-the-counter generic drugs. The drugs have been listed and indexed by both their **Generic** and **Trade (Brand)** names for easy accessibility.

Some of the more than fifty newer generic drugs in the past year that have been catalogued for this latest edition include (the **Trade/Brand** name drugs are in bold):

Anagrelide (**Agrylin**), Anastrozole (**Arimidex**), Anisindione (**Miradon**), Anthrax Vaccine, Arbutamine (**GenESA**), Basiliximab (**Simulect**), Bimatoprost (**Lumigan**), Bivalirudin (**Angiomax**), Bosentan (**Tracleer**), Caspofungin (**Cancidas**), Cistatracurium (**Nimbex**), Desloratadine (**Clarinex**), Fondaparinux (**Arixtra**), Formoterol (**Foradil**), Frovatriptan (**Frova**), Galantamine (**Reminyl**), Imiquimod (**Aldara**), Interferon Beta 1-A (**Avonex**), Levalbuterol (**Xopenex**), Midodrine (**Pro-Amatine**), Nesiritide (**Natrecor**), Olmesartan (**Benicar**), Pancuronium (**Pavulon**), Paromomycin (**Humatin**), PEG-Interferon (**PEG-Intron**), Pemirolast (**Alamast**), Phenylpropanolamine, Pimecrolimus (**Elidel**), Tenofovir (**Viread**), Trastuzumab (**Herceptin**), Travoprost (**Travatan**), Valdecoxib (**Bextra**), Valganciclovir (**Valcyte**), Zoledronic Acid (**Zometa**), and others. The number of herbals and supplements has also increased, and vaccines have been added.

In addition to adverse cutaneous reactions, there are many severe, hazardous interactions between two or more drugs. Unlike the voluminous interaction details in previous editions of the Manual, some of which were either moderate or mild, I have incorporated only the highly, clinically significant drug interactions that can trigger potential harm, and could be life-threatening. These interactions are predictable and well documented in controlled studies; they should be avoided. The section denoting hazardous interactions has been omitted from those drugs where no such interactions have been reported.

Since the last edition, many generic drugs have been withdrawn from the marketplace. These are: Astemizole, Bromfenac, Cerivastatin, Cisapride, Dexfenfluramine, Fenfluramine, Mibefradil, Terfenadine, and Troglitazone and, therefore, have been deleted from this edition.

For each drug, I have listed all the known adverse side effects – in the form of drug reactions – that can develop from the use of the corresponding drug. These side effects include those that primarily involve the skin, the hair, the nails and the mucous membranes. The section entitled 'other' has been expanded to include such reactions as tinnitus, serotonin syndrome and death.

Appropriate references (author, journal or book, volume, date and page) for each side effect for every drug have been cited. Where there is more than one reference to a particular side effect, I have employed the most illustrative and most recent citation(s) in the literature.

In this new, 2003 state-of-the-art ninth edition, I have cited more than **22,500** references and sources from journals articles, books and observations from dermatologists all over the world, via the Internet and from personal communications.

The first part of the Manual lists, in alphabetical order, all the listed **800+ Generic** and **Trade** drugs with their corresponding names for easy access to the **A–Z** section – main body of the Manual.

Next comes a listing of the various **Classes** of drugs, and those **Generic** drugs that belong to each class.

The major portion of the Manual – the body of the work – lists the 884 Generic drugs, herbals and supplements in alphabetical order and the adverse reactions that can arise from their use, along with the appropriate references.

The last parts of the Manual include a description of the 31 most common **Reaction Patterns**; a listing of those drugs that can occasion more than **100** different reaction patterns, including, among others, **Acne, Acute Exanthematous Pustulosis, Alopecia, Aphthous Stomatitis, Bullous Eruptions, Bullous Pemphigoid, Erythema Multiforme, Erythema Nodosum, Exanthems, Exfoliative Dermatitis, Fixed Eruptions, Lichenoid Eruptions, Lupus Erythematosus, Onycholysis, Pemphigus, Photosensitivity, Pityriasis Rosea, Pruritus, Psoriasis, Purpura, Pustular Eruptions, Stevens-Johnson Syndrome, Toxic Epidermal Necrolysis, Urticaria,** and **Vasculitis**. This is followed by color photographs of some of these reactions.

## USAGE, STYLE & CONVENTIONS EMPLOYED IN THIS MANUAL

The **Generic Drug** name is at the top of each page.

The **Trade (Brand) Name(s)** are then listed alphabetically. When there are many **Trade Names**, the ten (or so) most commonly recognized ones are listed. This compilation lists and cross-references both the **Trade *and* Generic** names of all the cataloged drugs. Following the more common **Trade Name** drugs are recorded – in parentheses – the latest name of the pharmaceutical company that is marketing the drug. As a result of acquisitions, mergers, and other factors in the pharmaceutical industry, many of the names of the companies have changed from earlier editions of this Manual.

Beneath the **Trade Name** listing is a list of **Other Common Trade Names**, those drugs from other countries. Then appears the **Indication(s)**, the **Category** in which the drug belongs, and the **Half-Life** of each drug, when known. On occasion, an important or pertinent **Note** will follow.

**Reactions**: These are the **Adverse Reactions** to the particular **Generic** drug. They are classified in four **Categories: Skin, Hair, Nails,** and **Other**. (**Other** refers to **Mucous Membrane, Teeth, Muscle** and various other forms of **Reactions**.) **Reactions** are listed alphabetically in each **Category**.

Under each **Reaction Pattern** are listed the **References** (the sources of the information). These are arranged in reverse chronological order – the most recent reference appearing first on the list.

In the case of herbals and supplements, the format is slightly different. The herbals give the scientific species and genus, purported indications and other uses. Then follows the same format as the generic drugs.

References in the English language predominate. For the few foreign references, we have resorted to the summary or abstract. The majority of the citations come from the *J Am Acad Dermatol*, *Arch Dermatol*, *Cutis*, *Int J Dermatol*, *Contact Dermatitis*, *Br J Dermatol*, *JAMA*, *Lancet*, *BMJ*, *Aust J Dermatol*, *N Engl J Med*, *Ann Intern Med*, and other prominent and easily accessible journals.

Many reference works have been consulted in the course of compiling this manual. These include:

(1998): Kauppinen K et al, SKIN REACTIONS TO DRUGS, CRC Press, Boca Raton etc.

(1996): Bruinsma W, A GUIDE TO DRUG ERUPTIONS, The File of Medicines, PO Box 21, 1474 HJ Oosthuizen, Netherlands.

(1994): Goldstein S & Wintroub BU, ADVERSE CUTANEOUS REACTIONS TO MEDICATION, CoMedica, New York.

(1992): Zürcher K & Krebs A, CUTANEOUS DRUG REACTIONS, Karger, Basel.

(1992): Breathnach SM & Hintner H, ADVERSE DRUG REACTIONS and the SKIN, Blackwell, Oxford.

(1988): Bork K, CUTANEOUS SIDE EFFECTS OF DRUGS, WB Saunders, Philadelphia.

Other references, based on package inserts, have been obtained from:

(2002): LEXI-COMP'S CLINICAL REFERENCE LIBRARY, Hudson, Ohio

(2002): DRUG FACTS & COMPARISONS, St. Louis, Missouri.

(2002): PDR GENERICS, Montvale, New Jersey.

There are occasions when there are very few adverse reactions to a specific drug. These drugs are still included in the Manual since there is often a positive significance in negative findings.

As a departure from the official, conventional and established style guide, and as a function of space constraints, the order of each Reference will appear as follows:

* The year in parentheses. The most recent citation appearing first.

* Last name and initial(s) of the principal author.

* A plus sign (+) after the author's name denotes one or more co-authors.

* Journal name (standard abbreviation where possible), in italics.

* Volume number (often followed by a parenthetical Part or Supplemental number).

* First page of the article

* Books when cited are italicized in UPPER CASE followed by the publisher and page number.

Other notes:

* (sic) means just so. This is how the authors designated the REACTION.
For example, Rash (sic); Dermatitis (sic); Skin Rash (sic)*

* I have used the term passim to mean 'in passing.' Forgive me.

There are occasional allusions to the incidence of many of the listed Reactions. Percentages – which for the most part are essentially vague and meaningless – are obtained from articles, from Zürcher & Krebs, and from Bork.

I have simplified the references to the many Reaction Patterns by eliminating, for the most part, tags such as '-like' as in Psoriasis-Like, '-reactivation,' '-syndrome,' '-dissemination,' '-iform,' etc.

'Observation' means just that. Observations (read: Anecdotes) are derived from information obtained from reliable dermatologists from the Internet and from personal correspondence. And if you send me your observations, they will be cataloged and you will be given appropriate attribution and recognition in the next Edition.

Enjoy!

Jerome Z. Litt, MD
January, 2003

* The term **skin rash** is a deplorable and reprehensible idiotism adored by non-dermatologists and the writers of the PDR (read package inserts). Can you have a **rash** on any other organ?

# INDEX OF GENERIC AND TRADE NAMES

Generic drug names are in **bold**

# INDEX OF HERBALS

Herbal drug names are in **bold**

# Classes of Drugs

**ACE inhibitors**

benazepril
candesartan*
captopril
cilazapril
enalapril
eprosartan*
fosinopril
irbesartan*
lisinopril
losartan*
moexipril
olmesartan
perindopril
quinapril
ramipril
spirapril
telmisartan*
trandolapril
valsartan*

*Angiotenin II receptor antagonist

**Alpha adrenergic receptor inhibitors**

brimonidine
doxazosin
phenoxybenzamine
phentolamine
prazosin
tamsulosin
terazosin

**Alpha adrenoreceptor agonists**

apraclonide
clonidine
guanabenz
guanethidine
guanfacine
tizanidine

**Aminoglycoside antibiotics**

amikacin
ceftazidime
gentamicin
kanamycin
neomycin
netilmicin
paromomycin
streptomycin
tobramycin

**Amphetamines**

amphetamine sulfate
dextroamphetamine
diethylpropion
mazindol
methamphetamine
methylphenidate
phendimetrazine
phentermine

**Antiarrhythmic agents and class**

adenosine
amiodarone III
atropine
belladonna
beta-blockers II
bretylium III
chlorothiazide
digoxin
diltiazem IV
disopyramide IV
dofetilide III
edrophonium
esmolol II
flecainide IC
ibutilide III
indecainide IC
isoproterenol
lidocaine IB
magnesium sulfate
metoprolol
mexiletine IB
minoxidil
moricizine IA
phenytoin IB
procainamide IA
propafenone IC
propranolol II
quinidine IA
sotalol III
tocainide IB
verapamil IV

**Anticholinergic agents**

albuterol
amantadine
atropine
belladonna
benztropine
biperiden
bromocriptine
carbidopa
clidinium
dicyclomine
diphenhydramine
glycopyrrolate
homatropine
hyoscyamine
ipratropium
levodopa
methantheline
orphenadrine
pergolide
physostigmine
procyclidine
propantheline
scopolamine
selegiline
tacrine
tolterodine
trihexiphenidyl

**Anticoagulants [1]**
**Antiplatelets [2]**
**Thrombolytics [3]**

abciximab [2]
alteplase [3]
anagrelide [2]
anisindione [1]
anistreplase [3]
ardeparin [1]
argatroban [1]
aspirin [2]
bivalirudin [1]
cilostazol [2]
clopidogrel [2]
dalteparin [1]
danaparoid [1]
dicumarol [1]
dipyridamole [2]
enoxaparin [1]
heparin [1]
reteplase [3]
streptokinase [3]
tenecteplase [3]
ticlopidine [2]
tinzaparin [1]
torsemide [1]
urokinase [3]
warfarin [1]

**Anticonvulsants**

acetazolamide
amobarbital
carbamazepine
chlorpromazine
clonazepam
clorazepate
diazepam
divalproex
ethosuximide
ethotoin
felbamate
fosphenytoin
gabapentin
hydroxyzine
lamotrigine
levetiracetam

lorazepam
mephenytoin
mephobarbital
methsuximide
oxazepam
oxcarbazepine
paraldehyde
paramethadione
pentobarbital
phenobarbital
phensuximide
phenytoin
primidone
thiopental
tiagabine
topiramate
trimethadione
valproic acid
vigabatrin
zonisamide

**Antidepressants**

Tricyclics I = 1st generation
Tricyclics II = 2nd generation
Tricyclics III = 3rd generation

amitriptyline I
amoxapine II
benactyzine
bupropion II
citalopram III
clomipramine I
desipramine I
divalproex
doxepin I
fluoxetine III
fluvoxamine III
imipramine I
isocarboxazid
lithium
loxapine
maprotiline II
methylphenidate
mirtazapine III
nefazodone III
nortriptyline I
paroxetine III
perphenazine
phenelzine
protriptyline I
sertraline III
thioridazine
tranylcypromine
trazodone II
trimipramine I
venlafaxine III

**Antidiabetic agents**

acarbose
acetohexamide
chlorpropamide
glimepiride
glipizide
glucagon
glyburide
insulin
metformin
miglitol
nateglinide
pioglitazone
repaglinide
rosiglitazone
tolazamide
tolbutamide
troglitazone

**Antifungals**

amphotericin B
caspofungin
clotrimazole
fluconazole
flucytosine
griseofulvin
itraconazole
ketoconazole
metronidazole
miconazole
nystatin
terbinafine
vorinconazole

**Antihypertensives**

acebutolol
amiloride
amlodipine
atenolol
benazepril
bendroflumethiazide
benzthiazide
betaxolol
bisoprolol
bumetanide
candesartan
captopril
carteolol
carvedilol
chlorothiazide
chlorthalidone
clonidine
cyclothiazide
diazoxide
diltiazem
doxazosin
enalapril
eprosartan
esmolol
ethacrynic acid
felodipine
fosinopril
furosemide
guanabenz
guanethidine
guanfacine
hydralazine
hydrochlorothiazide
hydroflumethiazide
indapamide
isradipine
labetalol
lisinopril
losartan
meclofenamate
methyclothiazide
methyldopa
methylphenidate
metolazone
metoprolol
minoxidil
moexipril
nadolol
nicardipine
nifedipine
nimodipine
nisoldipine
nitroglycerin
penbutolol
phentolamine
pindolol
polythiazide
prazosin
propantheline
propranolol
quinapril
quinethazone
ramipril
reserpine
spironolactone
terazosin
timolol
torsemide
triamterene
trichlormethiazide
valsartan
verapamil
yohimbine

**Antimalarial agents**

chloroquine
hydroxychloroquine
mefloquine
primaquine
pyrimethamine
quinacrine
quinine

**Antimigraine drugs**

5-HT, receptor agonists

almotriptan
frovatriptan
naritriptan
rizatriptan
sumatritan
zolmitriptan

**Antimycobacterial agents**

aminosalicylic acid
capreomycin

clofazimine
cycloserine
dapsone
ethambutol
ethionamide
isoniazid
kanamycin
pyrazinamide
rifampin
rifapentine
streptomycin

**Antineoplastics**

aldesleukin
alemtuzumab
altretamine
anastrazole
azathioprine
asparaginase
bleomycin
busulfan
carboplatin
carmustine
chlorambucil
chlorotrianisene
cisplatin
clomiphene
cyclophosphamide
cyclosporine
cytarabine
dacarbazine
dactinomycin
danazol
daunorubicin
diethylstilbestrol
docetaxel
doxorubicin
estradiol
estramustine
etoposide
exemestane
fluorouracil
fluoxymesterone
flutamide
fluvestrant
gemcitabine
hydroxyprogesterone
hydroxyurea
ibritumomab
idarubicin
ifosfamide
imatinib
interferon
leucovorin
leuprolide
levamisole
lomustine
masoprocol
mechlorethamine
medroxyprogesterone
megestrol
melphalan
mercaptopurine
mesna
methotrexate
methyltestosterone
mitomycin
mitotane
mitoxantrone
nafarelin
octreotide
paclitaxel
pentostatin
plicamycin
procarbazine
progesterone
somastatin
streptozocin
tamoxifen
taxol
testosterone
thioguanine
thiotepa
topotecan
trimetrexate
triptorelin
vinblastine
vincristine
vinorelbine

**Antiparkinsonian agents**

amantadine
benztropine
biperiden
bromocriptine
cabergoline
carbidopa
entacapone
levodopa/carbidopa
pergolide
pramipexole
procyclidine
ropinirole
selegiline
tolcapone
trihexyphenidyl

**Antipsychotic agents**

acetophenazine
chlorpromazine
chlorprothixene
clozapine
droperidol
fluphenazine
haloperidol
lithium
loxapine
mesoridazine
molindone
olanzapine
perphenazine
prochlorperazine
pimozide
promazine
quetiapine
riluzole
risperidone
sertindole
thioridazine
thiothixene
trifluoperazine
ziprasidone

**Antiretroviral agents**

Nucleoside analog reverse transcriptase inhibitors (NRTIs)

abacavir
didanosine
lamivudine
stavudine
tenofovir
zalcitabine
zidovudine

Non-nucleoside reverse transcriptase inhibitors (NNRTIs)

delavirdine
efavirenz
nevirapine

Protease inhibitors

amprenavir
indinavir
lopinavir
nelfinavir
ritonavir
saquinavir
valacyclovir

**Anxiolytics, sedatives and hypnotics**

alprazolam
amobarbital
aprobarbital
buspirone
butabarbital
chloral hydrate
chlordiazepoxide
chlormezanone
chlorzoxazone
clonazepam
clorazepate
diazepam
droperidol
estazolam
ethchlorvynol
fentanyl
flurazepam
glutethimide
hydroxyzine
ketamine
lorazepam
mephobarbital
meprobamate
methohexital
midazolam
opium alkaloids
oxazepam
paraldehyde

paroxetine
pentobarbital
phenobarbital
prazepam
prochlorperazine
promethazine
propofol
quazepam
secobarbital
sertraline
temazepam
thiopental
triazolam
trifluoperazine
zaleplon
zolpidem

**Benzodiazepines**
alprazolam
amitriptyline
chlordiazepoxide
clonazepam
clorazepate
diazepam
estazolam
flurazepam
halazepam
lorazepam
midazolam
olanzapine
oxazepam
prazepam
quazepam
temazepam
triazolam

**Beta-blockers**
acebutolol
atenolol
betaxolol
bisoprolol
carteolol
carvedilol
esmolol
labetalol
levobetaxolol
levobunolol
metipranolol
metoprolol
nadolol
penbutolol
pindolol
propranolol
sotalol
timolol

**Beta-lactam antibiotics**
aztreonam
cefixime
cefoxitin
imipenen/cilastin
loracarbef
meropenem
moxalactam
tazobactam

**Bronchodilators**
albuterol
aminophylline
atropine
bitolterol
ephedrine
epinephrine
ipratropium
isoetharine
isoproterenol
levalbuterol
metaproterenol
montelukast
pirbuterol
salmeterol
terbutaline
theophylline
zafirlukast
zileuton

**Calcium channel blockers**
amlodipine
bepridil
diltiazem
enalapril
felodipine
isradipine
nicardipine
nifedipine
nimodipine
nisoldipine
trandolapril
verapamil

**Cephalosporin antibiotics**
By generation
First generation
cefadroxil
cefazolin
cephalexin
cephalothin
cephapirin
cephradine
Second generation
cefaclor
cefamandole
cefmetazole
cefonicid
ceforanide
cefotetan
cefoxitin
cefprozil
cefuroxime
loracarbef
Third generation
cefdinir
cefixime
cefoperazone
cefotaxime
cefpodoxime
ceftazidime
ceftibuten
ceftizoxime
ceftriaxone
Fourth generation
cefepime

**Diuretics**
acetazolamide
amiloride
bendroflumethiazide
benzthiazide
bumetanide
chlorthalidone
chorothiazide
cyclothiazide
ethacrynic acid
furosemide
hydrochlorothiazide
hydroflumethiazide
indapamide
isosorbide
mannitol
methyclothiazide
metolazone
polythiazide
potassium chloride
quinethazone
spironolactone
torsemide
triamterene
trichlormethiazide
urea

**Diuretics, loop**
bumetanide
ethacrynic acid
furosemide
torsemide

**Fluoroquinolones + Quinolones**
alatrofloxacin
cinoxacin
ciprofloxacin
enoxacin
gatifloxacin
grepafloxacin
levofloxacin
lomefloxacin
moxifloxacin
norfloxacin
ofloxacin
sparfloxacin
trovafloxacin

**$H_2$ antagonists**
cimetidine
famotidne
nizatidine

ranitidine
roxatidine

**Hypnotics**
aprobarbital
ethchlorvynol
flurazepam
glutethimide
L-tryptophan
methohexital
opium alkaloids
pentobarbital
phenobarbital
propofol
quazepam
secobarbital
temazepam
thiopental
triazolam
zolpidem

**Hypolipidemic agents HMG-CoA reductase inhibitors (statins)**
atorvastatin
cerivastatin
cholestyramine
clofibrate
colesevelam
colestipol
dextrothyroxine
fenofibrate
fluvastatin
gemfibrozil
lovastatin
niacin
pravastatin
probucol
simvastatin

**Macrolide antibiotics**
azithromycin
clarithromycin
dirithromycin
erythromycin
lincomycin
troleandomycin

**Monamine oxidase inhibitors**
isocarboxazid
pargyline
phenelzine
tranylcypromine

**Narcotic agonists**
alfentanil
buprenorphine
butorphanol
codeine
fentanyl
hydrocodone
hydromorphone
levorphanol
meperidine
methadone
morphine
nalbuphine
oxycodone
pentazocine
propoxyphene
remifentanil
sufentanil

**Neuroleptics**
amitriptyline
chlorpromazine
fluphenazine
haloperidol
lithium
loxapine
molindone
prochlorperazine
thioridazine
thiothixene
tranylcypromine
trifluoperazine

**Neuromuscular blocking agents**
atracurium
cisatracurium
doxacurium
gallimine
metocurine
mivacurium
pancuronium
pipecuronium
rapacuronium
rocuronium
succinylcholine
tubocurarine
vecuronium

**NSAIDs**
aspirin
bromfenac
celecoxib
choline salicylate
diclofenac
diflunisal
etodolac
fenoprofen
flurbiprofen
ibuprofen
indomethacin
ketoprofen
ketorolac
magnesium salicylate
meclofenamate
mefenamic acid
meloxicam
mesalamine
methotrexate
nabumetone
naproxen
olsalazine
oxaprozin
oxyphenbutazone
phenylbutazone
piroxicam
rofecoxib
salsalate
sodium salicylate
sulindac
tolmetin
valdecoxib

**Penicillin antibiotics**
amoxicillin
ampicillin
carbenicillin
cloxacillin
dicloxacillin
methicillin
mezlocillin
nafcillin
oxacillin
penicillin
piperacillin
ticarcillin

**Selective serotonin reuptake inhibitors (SSRIs)**
almotriptan
citalopram
eletriptan
fluoxetine
fluvoxamine
nefazodone
paroxetine
sertraline
trazodone
venlafaxine

**Sulfonamide derivatives**
Antimicrobial agents
mafenide acetate
silver sulfadiazine
sodium sulfacetamide
sulfadiazine
sulfamethiazole
sulfamethoxazole
sulfisoxazole
Diuretic, carbonic anhydrase inhibitor
acetazolamide
dichlorphenamide
methazolamide
Diuretics, loop
bumetanide
furosemide
torsemide
Diuretics, thiazide
bendroflumethiazide
benzthiazide
chlorothiazide
chlorthalidone
cyclothiazide

- hydrochlorothiazide
- hydroflumethiazide
- indapamide
- methyclothiazide
- metolazone
- polythiazide
- quinethazone
- trichlormethiazide

Hypoglycemic agents, oral

- acetohexamide
- chlorpropamide
- glipizide
- glyburide
- tolazamide
- tolbutamide

Other agents

- cyclamate
- dorzolamide
- saccharin
- sulfasalazine

**Tranquilizers**

- amitriptyline
- buspirone
- chlordiazepoxide
- chlormezanone
- chlorpromazine
- clorazepate
- diazepam
- doxepin
- droperidol
- fluphenazine
- haloperidol
- hydroxyzine
- lorazepam
- loxapine
- meprobamate
- mesoridazine
- molindone
- oxazepam
- perphenazine
- pimozide
- prochlorperazine
- promazine
- promethazine
- reserpine
- risperidone
- thioridazine
- thiothixene
- trifluoperazine

**Tetracycline antibiotics**

- demeclocycline
- doxycycline
- minocycline
- oxytetracycline
- tetracycline

**Vasodilators**

- hydralazine
- isoxusprine
- minoxidil
- nesiritide
- nitroglycerin
- nitroprusside
- papaverine
- tolazoline

## ABACAVIR

**Trade name:** Ziagen (GSK)
**Indications:** HIV infections in combination with other antiretrovirals
**Category:** Antiretroviral; nucleoside reverse transcriptase inhibitor
**Half-life:** 1.5 hours

### *Reactions*

#### Skin

Chills
(1999): Escaut L+, *AIDS* 13, 1419
Edema
(1999): Spruance SL, *Skin and Allergy News* October, 37
Erythroderma
(2001): Shapiro M+, *The AIDS Reader* 11, 222
Exanthems
(1999): Nathanson N (from Internet ) (observation) (generalized)
(1999): Spruance SL, *Skin and Allergy News* October, 37
(1998): Saag M+, *AIDS* 12, F203
Kawasaki syndrome
(2002): Toerner JG+, *Clin Infect Dis* 34(1), 131
Perioral Parasthesias
(2001): McMahon D+, *Antivir Ther* 6(2), 105
Pruritus
(1998): Saag M+, *AIDS* 12, F203
Rash (sic) (10%)
(2002): Kessler HA+, *Clin Infect Dis* 34(4), 535
(2001): Hetherington S+, *Clin Ther* 23(10), 1603
(2000): Hervey PS+, *Drugs* 60, 447 (5%)
(1999): Hughes W+, *Antimicrob Agents Chemother* 43, 609 (9%)
(1999): Spruance SL, *Skin and Allergy News* October, 37 (69%)
(1998): Foster RH+, *Drugs* 55, 729
(1998): Kessler H+, *36th Meeting of the Infectious Disease Society of America, Denver* Abstract 453 (10–15%)
(1998): Saag M+, *AIDS* 12, F203 (10–15%)
(1998): Staszewski S+, *AIDS* 12, F197 (10–15%)

#### Other

Anaphylactoid reactions
(2001): Frissen PH+, *AIDS* 15, 289
(1999): Spruance SL, *Skin and Allergy News* October, 37 (3–4%)
(1999): Walensky RP+, *AIDS* 13, 999
Cough
(2001): Hetherington S+, *Clin Ther* 23(10), 1603 (10%)
Death
Hypersensitivity (5%)
(2002): Hetherington S+, *Lancet* 359(9312), 1121
(2002): Hewitt RG, *Clin Infect Dis* 34(8), 1137 (3.7%)
(2002): Kessler HA+, *Clin Infect Dis* 34(4), 535
(2002): Mallal S+, *Lancet* 359, 727 (5%)
(2001): Cutrell A+, *International AIDS Society Conference on HIV Buenos Aires* Abstract 527
(2001): Frissen PH+, *AIDS* 15, 289
(2001): Hetherington S, *AIDS Read* 11(12), 620
(2001): Hetherington S+, *Clin Ther* 23(10), 1603 (4.3%)
(2001): Keiser P+, *8th Conferences on Retroviruses* (Chicago) Abstract 622
(2001): Loeliger AE+, *AIDS* 15(10), 1325
(2001): Peyrieere H+, *Ann Pharmacother* 35(10), 1291
(2001): Shapiro M+, *The AIDS Reader* 11, 222
(2001): Wit FW+, *AIDS* 15(18), 2423
(2000): Clay PG+, *Ann Pharmacother* 34, 247
(2000): GlaxoWellcome, *Important Drug Warning* July (severe or fatal)
(2000): Hervey PS+, *Drugs* 60, 447 (3–5%)
(2000): *AIDS Read* 10, 525
(2000): *AIDS Treat News* 337, 7
(2000): *Prescrire Int* 9, 67
(2000): Keiser P+, *Conference on Retroviruses & Opportunistic Infections* (Chicago) Abstract 622
(1999): Escaut L+, *AIDS* 13, 1419
(1999): Miller JL, *Am J Health Syst Pharm* 56, 304
(1998): Foster RH+, *Drugs* 55, 729 (2–3%)
(1998): *AIDS Patient Care SDS* 12, 405
(1998): *Newsline People AIDS Coalit N Y* Feb, 35
(1998): Saag M+, *AIDS* 12, F203 (2–5%)
(1998): Staszewski S+, *AIDS* 12, F197
(1997): James JS, *AIDS Treat News* 285, 1, 5
Myalgia
(1999): Escaut L+, *AIDS* 13, 1419
(1999): Spruance SL, *Skin and Allergy News* October, 37
Oral ulceration
(1999): Spruance SL, *Skin and Allergy News* October, 37
Paresthesias

## ABCIXIMAB

**Synonym:** C7E3
**Trade name:** Reopro (Lilly)
**Indications:** Thrombotic arterial disease
**Category:** Non-nucleoside reverse transcriptase inhibitor; platelet aggregation inhibitor
**Half-life:** 10–30 minutes – given intravenously
**Clinically important, potentially hazardous interactions with:** fondaparinux, reteplase

### *Reactions*

#### Skin

Cellulitis (0.3%)
Peripheral edema (1.6%)
Petechiae (0.3%)
Pruritus (0.3%)

#### Other

Anaphylactoid reactions
(2001): Iakovou Y+, *Cardiology* 95(4), 215
(1999): Guzzo JA+, *Catheter Cardiovasc Interv* 48, 71
Hypesthesia (1%)
Injection-site reactions (3.6%)
Myalgia (0.3%)
Myopathy (0.3%)

## ACARBOSE

**Trade name:** Precose (Bayer)
**Other common trade names:** *Glucobay; Glumida; Prandase*
**Indications:** Non-insulin dependent diabetes type II
**Category:** Oral antidiabetic (alpha-glucosidase inhibitor)
**Half-life:** 2.7–9 hours

### *Reactions*

#### Skin

Erythema (<1%)
(2000): Schmutz JL+, *Ann Dermatol Venereol* 127, 869 (polymorphous)

Erythema multiforme
(1999): Kono T+, *Lancet* 354, 396 (generalized)
Rash (sic)
Urticaria (<1%)

### Other

Ageusia
(1996): Martin Bun N+, *Med Clin (Barc)* (Spanish) 28, 399

## ACEBUTOLOL

**Trade name:** Sectral (Wyeth)
**Other common trade names:** *Acecor; Acetanol; Alol; Apo-Acebutolol; Monitan; Neptal; Novo-Acebutolol; Nu-Acebutolol; Prent; Rhodiasectral; Rhotral*
**Indications:** Hypertension, angina, ventricular arrhythmias
**Category:** Cardioselective beta-adrenergic blocker; antiarrhythmic; antihypertensive
**Half-life:** 3–7 hours
**Clinically important, potentially hazardous interactions with:** clonidine, verapamil

**Note:** Cutaneous side effects of beta-receptor blockaders are clinically polymorphous. They apparently appear after several months of continuous therapy. Atypical psoriasiform, lichen planus-like, and eczematous chronic rashes are mainly observed. (1983): Hödl St, *Z Hautkr* (German) 1:58, 17

### *Reactions*

### Skin

Dermatitis (sic)
Diaphoresis
(1995): Schmutz JL+, *Dermatology* 190, 86
Edema (1–10%)
Erythema multiforme (<1%)
Exanthems (4%)
(1985): Singh BN+, *Drugs* 29, 531
Exfoliative dermatitis
Facial edema (<1%)
Hyperkeratosis (palms and soles)
Lichenoid eruption
(1982): Taylor AEM+, *Clin Exp Dermatol* 7, 219
(1978): Savage RL+, *BMJ* 1, 987
Lupus erythematosus (<1%)
(1997): Burlingame RW, *Clin Lab Med* 17, 367
(1992): Rubin RL+, *J Clin Invest* 90, 165
(1992): Stevens MB, *Hosp Pract* 27, 27
(1987): Doktor D, *Rev Fr Allergol Immunol* (French) 27, 77
(1985): Hourdebaight-Larrusse P+, *Ann Cardiol Angeiol* (Paris) (French) 34, 421
(1985): Singh BN+, *Drugs* 29, 531
(1984): Bigot MC+, *Therapie* (French) 39, 571
(1984): Meyer O+, *Rev Rhum Mal Osteoartic* (French) 51, 303
(1983): Homberg JC+, *J Pharmacol* (French) 14, 61
(1982): Taylor AE+, *Clin Exp Dermatol* 7, 219
(1981): Record NB, *Ann Intern Med* 95, 326
(1981): Simon P+, *Nouv Presse Med* (French) 10, 105
Pigmentation
Pityriasis rubra pilaris
(1978): Finlay AY+, *BMJ* 1, 987
Pruritus (<2%)
Psoriasis
(1986): Czernielewski J+, *Lancet* 1, 808
(1984): Arntzen N+, *Acta Derm Venereol* (Stockh) 64, 346
Rash (sic) (1–10%)
Raynaud's phenomenon
(1984): Eliasson K+, *Acta Med Scand* 215, 333
(1976): Marshall AJ+, *BMJ* 1, 1498
Toxic epidermal necrolysis
Urticaria
(1977): Ashford R+, *Lancet* 2, 462
Vasculitis
(1988): Bonnefoy M+, *Ann Dermatol Venereol* (French) 115, 27
(1977): Ashford R+, *Lancet* 2, 462
Xerosis

### Hair

Hair – alopecia

### Nails

Nails – bluish
Nails – dystrophy
Nails – onycholysis
Nails – pincer (reverse transverse curvature of the nails)
(1998): Greiner D+, *J Am Acad Dermatol* 39, 486

### Other

Dysgeusia
Hyperesthesia (<2%)
Hypesthesia (<2%)
Myalgia (1–10%)
Oculo-mucocutaneous syndrome
(1982): Cocco G+, *Curr Ther Res* 31, 362
Oral lichenoid eruption
Peyronie's disease
(1979): Pryor JP+, *Lancet* 1, 331
Xerostomia (<1%)

## ACETAMINOPHEN

**Synonyms:** APAP; paracetamol
**Trade names:** Anacin-3 (Wyeth); Bromo-Seltzer; Darvocet-N; Datril; Dristan (Wyeth); Excedrin; Liquiprin; Lorcet (Forest); Mapap; Neopap; Panadol (GSK); Percogesic; Percoset; Phenaphen; Sinutab; Tylenol; Valadol; Vicodin
**Other common trade names:** *Abenol; Anaflon; Ben-U-Ron; Doliprane; Geluprane; Panadol*
**Indications:** Pain, fever
**Category:** Non-narcotic antipyretic analgesic
**Half-life:** 1–3 hours
**Clinically important, potentially hazardous interactions with: alcohol**, cholestyramine

**Note:** Acetaminophen is the active metabolite of phenacetin

### *Reactions*

### Skin

Acute generalized exanthematous pustulosis (AGEP)
(1998): Leger F+, *Acta Derm Venereol* 78, 222
(1996): DeConinck AL+, *Dermatology* 193, 338
(1995): Moreau A+, *Int J Dermatol* 34, 263 (passim)
(1991): Roujeau J-C+, *Arch Dermatol* 127, 1333
Angioedema (<1%)
(2002): Litt JZ, Beachwood, OH (personal case) (observation) (patient inadvertently re-challenged herself)
(1997): de Almeida MA+, *Allergy Asthma Proc* 18, 313
(1990): Van Diem L+, *Eur J Clin Pharmacol* 38, 389
(1986): Idoko JA+, *Trans R Soc Trop Med Hyg* 80, 175
(1985): Stricker BH+, *BMJ* 291, 938
(1970): Henriques CC, *JAMA* 214, 2336

Contact dermatitis
(1997): Mathelier-Fusada P+, *Contact Dermatitis* 36, 267
(1996): Szczurko C+, *Contact Dermatitis* 35, 299
Dermatitis (sic)
(1995): Barbaud A+, *Lancet* 346, 902
Diaphoresis
Erythema (sic)
(1985): Stricker BH+, *BMJ* 291, 938
Erythema multiforme
(1995): Dubey NK+, *Indian Pediatr* 32, 1117
(1984): Hurvitz H+, *Isr J Med Sci* 20, 145
Erythema nodosum (<1%)
Exanthems
(1997): Foong H, Malaysia (from Internet) (observation)
(1985): Matheson I+, *Pediatrics* 76, 651
(1985): Stricker BH+, *BMJ* 291, 938
(1975): Michelson PA, *Ann Intern Med* 83, 374
(1970): Henriques CC, *JAMA* 214, 2336
Exfoliative dermatitis
(1984): Guerin C+, *Therapie* (French) 39, 47
Fixed eruption (<1%)
(2001): Silva A+, *Pediatr Dermatol* 18(2), 163
(2000): Bernand S+, *Dermatology* 201, 184 (similar to ondansetron)
(2000): Galindo PA+, *J Investig Allergol Clin Immunol* 9, 399
(2000): Ko R+, *Clin Exp Dermatol* 25, 96
(2000): Ozkaya-Bayazit E+, *Eur J Dermatol* 10, 288
(1999): Sehgal VN, *Pediatr Dermatology* 16, 165 (multiple)
(1998): Hern S+, *Br J Dermatol* 139, 1129,
(1998): Litt JZ, Beachwood, OH (personal case) (observation)
(1998): Mahboob A+, *Int J Dermatol* 37, 833
(1996): Gomez-Martinez M+, *J Investig Allergol Clin Immunol* 6, 131
(1996): Kawada A+, *Int J Dermatol* 35, 148
(1996): Laude TA, *Cosmetic Dermatology* 9, 7
(1995): Harris A+, *Br J Dermatol* 133, 790
(1994): Rademaker M+, *N Z Med J* 107, 295
(1992): Cohen HA+, *Ann Pharmacother* 26, 1596
(1992): Zemtsov A+, *Cutis* 50, 281
(1991): Thankappen TP+, *Int J Dermatol* 30, 867
(1990): Duhra P+, *Clin Exp Dermatol* 15, 293
(1990): Gaffoor PMA+, *Cutis* 45, 242 (passim)
(1989): Valsecchi R, *Dermatologica* 179, 51
(1988): Guin J+, *Cutis* 41, 107
(1987): Bharija SC+, *Australas J Dermatol* 28, 85
(1987): Guin J+, *J Am Acad Dermatol* 17, 399
(1986): Meyrick-Thomas RH+, *Br J Dermatol* 115, 357
(1985): Verbov J, *Dermatologica* 171, 60 (with chlormezanone)
(1975): Wilson HTH, *Br J Dermatol* 92, 213
(1970): Henriques CC, *JAMA* 214, 2336
(1965): Fitzpatrick TB, *Arch Dermatol* 92(4), 484 (phenacetin)
Flushing
(1985): Stricker BH+, *BMJ* 291, 938
Neutrophilic eccrine hidradenitis
(1988): Kuttner BJ+, *Cutis* 41, 403
Pemphigus
(1990): Brenner S+, *Acta Derm Venereol* 70, 357
Penile edema
(1997): Cabanes Higuero N+, *Med Clin (Barc)* (Spanish) 109, 685
Photosensitivity
(1999): Popescu C, Bucharest, Romania (from Internet) (observation)
Pityriasis rosea
(1993): Yosipovitch G+, *Harefuah* (Israel) 124, 198; 247
Progressive pigmentary purpura (Schamberg's disease)
(1992): Abeck D+, *J Am Acad Dermatol* 27, 123
Pruritus
(1985): Stricker BH+, *BMJ* 291, 938
Purpura
(1998): Kwon SJ+, *J Dermatol* 25, 756
(1993): Guccione JL+, *Arch Dermatol* 129, 1267
(1992): Abeck D+, *J Am Acad Dermatol* 27, 123
(1980): Miescher PA+, *Clin Haematol* 9, 505
(1977): Ameer B+, *Ann Intern Med* 87, 202
(1973): Skokan JD+, *Cleve Clin Quart* 40, 89
Purpura fulminans
(1993): Guccione JL+, *Arch Dermatol* 129, 1267
Rash (sic) (<1%)
Sensitivity (sic)
(1998): Mendizabal SL+, *Allergy* 53, 457
Stevens–Johnson syndrome
(1995): Kuper K+, *Ophthalmologue* (German) 92, 823
(1985): Ting HC+, *Int J Dermatol* 24, 587
Toxic epidermal necrolysis
(2002): Cordova M, (Lima) (Peru) March AAD Poster
(2002): Thakker J+, *World Congress Dermatol* Poster, 0129 (with nimesulide)
(2000): Halevi A+, *Ann Pharmacother* 34, 32
(1991): Sakellariou G+, *Int J Artif Organs* 14, 634
(1986): Roupe G+, *Int Arch Allergy Appl Immunol* 80, 145
Urticaria
(2002): Litt JZ, Beachwood, OH (personal case) (observation) (patient inadvertently re-challenged herself)
(2000): Samanta BB, *J Assoc Physicians India* 47, 464
(1997): de Almeida MA+, *Allergy Asthma Proc* 18, 313
(1997): Ownby DR, *J Allergy Clin Immunol* 99, 151
(1985): Cole TO, *Clin Exp Dermatol* 10, 404
(1985): Stricker BH+, *BMJ* 291, 938
(1975): Michelson PA, *Ann Intern Med* 83, 374
(1970): Henriques CC, *JAMA* 214, 2336
Vasculitis
(1995): Harris A+, *Br J Dermatol* 133, 790
(1988): Dussarat GV+, *Presse Med* (French) 17, 1587

## Hair

Hair – alopecia
(1998): Litt JZ, Beachwood, OH (personal case) (observation)

## Nails

Nails – disorder (sic)
(1975): Michelson PA, *Ann Intern Med* 83, 374

## Other

Anaphylactoid reactions
(2001): Verma S, Baroda, India (from Internet)(observation) (with ibuprofen)
(2000): Ayonrinde OT+, *Postgrad Med J.* 76, 501
(2000): de Paramo BJ+, *Ann Allergy Asthma Immunol* 85, 508 (4 patients)
(2000): Stephenson I+, *Postgrad Med* 76, 503
(1999): Kumar RK+, *Hosp Med* 60, 66
(1999): Spitz E, *Ann Allergy Asthma Immunol* 82, 591
(1998): Galindo PA+, *Allergol Immunopathol (Madr)* (Spanish) 26, 199
(1998): Huitema AD+, *Hum Exp Toxicol* 17, 406
(1990): Van Diem L+, *Eur J Clin Pharmacol* 38, 389
(1988): *Allergy Observer* (Janssen Pharmaceutica) 5(7), 1
(1985): Stricker BH+, *BMJ* 291, 938
Dysgeusia
(1976): Rollin H, *Laryngol Rhinol Otol* (Stuttgart) (German) 55, 873
Hypersensitivity (<1%)
(1999): Kivity S+, *Allergy* 54, 187
(1997): Vidal C+, *Ann Allergy Asthma Immunol* 79, 320
(1996): Ibanez MD+, *Allergy* 51, 121
(1993): Martin JA+, *Med Clin (Barc)* (Spanish) 100, 158
Rhabdomyolysis
(1999): Moneret-Vautrin DA+, *Allergy* 54(10), 1115
(1996): Riggs JE+, *Mil Med* 161(11), 708 (with alcohol)

# ACETAZOLAMIDE

**Trade name:** Diamox (Storz)
**Other common trade names:** *Acetazolam; Ak-Zol; Dazamide; Defiltran; Diuramid; Novo-Zolamide*
**Indications:** Epilepsy, glaucoma
**Category:** Anticonvulsant; carbonic anhydrase inhibitor; sulfonamide* diuretic
**Half-life:** 2–6 hours
**Clinically important, potentially hazardous interactions with:** lithium

### *Reactions*

#### Skin

Acute generalized exanthematous pustulosis (AGEP)
(1995): Moreau A+, *Int J Dermatol* 34, 263 (passim)
(1992): Ogoshi M+, *Dermatology* 184, 142
Bullous eruption (<1%)
(1957): Ellis FA, *Arch Dermatol* 75, 836
Erythema multiforme
(1961): Baer RL+, *Year Book of Dermatology*, Year Book Medical Publishers, 9
(1956): Spring M, *Ann Allergy* Jan/Feb, 41
Exanthems
(1967): Lockey SD, *Med Sci* 18, 43
(1956): Spring M, *Ann Allergy* Jan/Feb, 41
Frostbite
(2001): Laemmle T, *Wilderness Environ Med* 12(4), 290
Lupus erythematosus
(1966): Cohen P+, *JAMA* 197, 817
Photosensitivity
Pruritus
Purpura
(1976): Underwood LC, *JAMA* 161, 1477
Pustular eruption
(1992): Ogoshi M+, *Dermatology* 184, 142
Pustular psoriasis
(1995): Kuroda K+, *J Dermatol* 22, 784
Rash (sic) (<1%)
Rosacea
(1993): Shah P+, *Br J Dermatol* 129, 647
Stevens–Johnson syndrome
Toxic epidermal necrolysis (<1%)
(1957): Ellis FA, *Arch Dermatol* 75, 836
Urticaria

#### Hair

Hair – hirsutism
(1974): Weiss IS, *Am J Ophthalmol* 78, 327

#### Other

Ageusia
Anaphylactoid reactions
(2000): Gerhards LJ+, *Ned Tijdschr Geneeskd* (Dutch) 144, 1228
(1998): Tzanakis N+, *Br J Ophthalmol* 82, 588
Anosmia
Dysgeusia (>10%) (metallic taste)
(1997): Martinez-Mir I+, *Ann Pharmacother* 31, 373
(1990): Miller LG+, *J Fam Pract* 31, 199
(1981): Lichter PR, *Ophthalmol* 88, 266
Extravasation
(1994): Callear A+, *Br J Ophthalmol* 78, 731
Paresthesias (<1%)
(1981): Lichter PR, *Ophthalmol* 88, 266
Tinnitus
Xerostomia (<1%)

***Note:** Acetazolamide is a sulfonamide and can be absorbed systemically. Sulfonamides can produce severe, possibly fatal, reactions such as toxic epidermal necrolysis and Stevens–Johnson syndrome

# ACETOHEXAMIDE

**Trade name:** Dymelor (Lilly)
**Other common trade names:** *Dimelin; Dimelor*
**Indications:** non-insulin dependent diabetes type II
**Category:** Sulfonylurea* antidiabetic; oral hypoglycemic
**Half-life:** 1–6 hours
**Clinically important, potentially hazardous interactions with:** phenylbutazones

### *Reactions*

#### Skin

Diaphoresis
Eczema (sic)
Erythema (<1%)
Exanthems (<1%)
Lichenoid eruption
Photosensitivity (1–10%)
Pruritus (<1%)
Rash (sic) (1–10%)
Urticaria (1–10%)

#### Hair

Hair – alopecia
(1962): Boshell BR+, *Clin Pharmacol Ther* 3, 750

#### Other

Paresthesias
Porphyria cutanea tarda

***Note:** Acetohexamide is a sulfonamide and can be absorbed systemically. Sulfonamides can produce severe, possibly fatal, reactions such as toxic epidermal necrolysis and Stevens–Johnson syndrome

# ACITRETIN

**Trade name:** Soriatane (Roche)
**Other common trade name:** *Neotigason*
**Indications:** Psoriasis
**Category:** Antipsoriatic retinoid
**Half-life:** 49 hours
**Clinically important, potentially hazardous interactions with: alcohol**, chloroquine, cholestyramine, corticosteroids, danazol, ethanolamine, isotretinoin, lithium, medroxyprogesterone, methotrexate, minocycline, progestins, tetracycline, vitamin A

### *Reactions*

#### Skin

Atrophy (10–25%)
Bullous eruption (1–10%)
Cheilitis (>75%)
(2001): Berbis P, *Ann Dermatol Venereol* 128(6), 737
(1999): Katz HI+, *J Am Acad Dermatol* 41, S7 (>75%)

(1997): Buccheri L+, *Arch Dermatol* 133, 711 (100%)
(1996): Lacour M+, *Br J Dermatol* 134, 1023
(1991): Murray HE+, *J Am Acad Dermatol* 24, 598 (49%)
(1990): Ruzicka T+, *Arch Dermatol* 126, 482 (80%)
(1989): Gupta AK+, *J Am Acad Dermatol* 21, 1088 (100%)
(1988): Geiger J-M+, *Dermatologica* 176, 182 (82%)

Chills
(2001): Liss WA, Pleasanton, CA (from Internet) (observation)

Cold/clammy skin (1–10%)

Dermatitis (sic) (1–10%)

Diaphoresis (1–10%)
(1997): Buccheri L+, *Arch Dermatol* 133, 711 (18.2%)
(1988): Geiger J-M+, *Dermatologica* 176, 182 (9%)

Edema
(2001): Liss WA, Pleasanton, CA (from Internet) (observation)

Erythema (sic)
(1997): Buccheri L+, *Arch Dermatol* 133, 711 (18.2%)

Erythroderma
(2001): Liss WA, Pleasanton, CA (from Internet) (observation)

Exanthems (10–25%)
(1999): Katz HI+, *J Am Acad Dermatol* 41, S7
(1990): Ruzicka T+, *Arch Dermatol* 126, 482 (2%)

Exfoliation
(1999): Katz HI+, *J Am Acad Dermatol* 41, S7 (25–50%)
(1997): Buccheri L+, *Arch Dermatol* 133, 711 (36.4%)

Exfoliative dermatitis
(2001): Blumenthal HL, Beachwood, OH (observation)

Fissures (1–10%)

Milia
(1993): Chang A+, *Acta Derm Venereol* 73, 235

Palmar–plantar desquamation
(1991): Murray HE+, *J Am Acad Dermatol* 24, 598 (29%)
(1990): Ruzicka T+, *Arch Dermatol* 126, 482 (20–25%)
(1989): Gupta AK+, *J Am Acad Dermatol* 21, 1088 (50–80%)
(1988): Geiger J-M+, *Dermatologica* 176, 182 (26%)

Palmar–plantar peeling
(2001): Berbis P, *Ann Dermatol Venereol* 128(6), 737
(2001): *Ami* (from Internet) (observation) (severe)

Phototoxicity
(1999): Katz HI+, *J Am Acad Dermatol* 41, S7

Pruritus (25–50%)
(1999): Katz HI+, *J Am Acad Dermatol* 41, S7
(1997): Buccheri L+, *Arch Dermatol* 133, 711 (54.5%)
(1996): Lacour M+, *Br J Dermatol* 134, 1023
(1991): Murray HE+, *J Am Acad Dermatol* 24, 598 (32%)
(1990): Ruzicka T+, *Arch Dermatol* 126, 482 (37%)
(1989): Gupta AK+, *J Am Acad Dermatol* 21, 1088 (10–20%)
(1988): Geiger J-M+, *Dermatologica* 176, 182 (16%)

Psoriasis (1–10%)

Purpura (1–10%)

Pyogenic granuloma (1–10%)
(2002): Diederen PVMM+, *World Congress Dermatol* Poster, 0099

Rash (sic) (>10%)

Seborrhea (1–10%)

Shaking (sic)

Stickiness (10–25%%)
(1999): Katz HI+, *J Am Acad Dermatol* 41, S7
(1997): Buccheri L+, *Arch Dermatol* 133, 711 (18%)
(1991): Murray HE+, *J Am Acad Dermatol* 24, 598 (8%)
(1989): Schröder K+, *Acta Derm Venereol* (Stockh) 69, 111 (3%)
(1988): Geiger J-M+, *Dermatologica* 176, 182 (2.5%)

Sunburn (1–10%)

Ulceration (1–10%)

Urticaria

Xerosis (25–50%)
(2001): Berbis P, *Ann Dermatol Venereol* 128(6), 737
(1999): Katz HI+, *J Am Acad Dermatol* 41, S7 (15–25%)
(1997): Buccheri L+, *Arch Dermatol* 133, 711 (45.5%)
(1991): Murray HE+, *J Am Acad Dermatol* 24, 598 (24%)
(1990): Ruzicka T+, *Arch Dermatol* 126, 482 (48%)
(1989): Gupta AK+, *J Am Acad Dermatol* 21, 1088 (10–20%)
(1989): Schröder K+, *Acta Derm Venereol* (Stockh) 69, 111 (65%)
(1988): Geiger J-M+, *Dermatologica* 176, 182 (30%)

## Hair

Hair – alopecia (50–75%)
(2001): Berbis P, *Ann Dermatol Venereol* 128(6), 737
(2001): Popescu C, Bucharest, Romania (from Internet) (observation)
(2001): Thaler D, Monona, WI (from Internet) (observation) (diffuse)
(2001): Vedamurthy V, Chennai, India (from Internet) (observation) (scalp, mustache, eyebrows & beard)
(1999): Katz HI+, *J Am Acad Dermatol* 41, S7 (10–25%)
(1997): Buccheri L+, *Arch Dermatol* 133, 711 (45.5%)
(1991): Murray HE+, *J Am Acad Dermatol* 24, 598 (33%)
(1990): Ruzicka T+, *Arch Dermatol* 126, 482 (12%)
(1989): Gupta AK+, *J Am Acad Dermatol* 21, 1088 (30–70%)
(1989): Schröder K+, *Acta Derm Venereol* (Stockh) 69, 111 (13%)
(1988): Geiger J-M+, *Dermatologica* 176, 182 (20%)

Hair – alopecia (total)
(2002): Chave TA+, *World Congress Dermatol* Poster 0092 (regrowth in 6 months)

Hair – alopecia universalis
(1998): Haycox CL, Seattle, WA (from Internet) (observation)
(1998): Nadel RS, Springfield, MA (from Internet) (observation)

Hair – pili torti
(2001): Davidson DM, Groton, CT (from Internet) (observation)

## Nails

Nails – disorder (sic) (25–50%)

Nails – fragility (sic)
(1991): Murray HE+, *J Am Acad Dermatol* 24, 598 (27%)
(1990): Ruzicka T+, *Arch Dermatol* 126, 482
(1988): Geiger J-M+, *Dermatologica* 176, 182 (10%)

Nails – paronychia (10–25%)
(2002): Hirsch R, Brooklyn, NY (from Internet) (observation)
(1999): Katz HI+, *J Am Acad Dermatol* 41, S7
(1997): Buccheri L+, *Arch Dermatol* 133, 711 (18.2%)
(1991): Murray HE+, *J Am Acad Dermatol* 24, 598 (7%)

Nails – periungual granuloma
(1997): Buccheri L+, *Arch Dermatol* 133, 711 (9.1%)

Nails – pyogenic granulomas
(1999): Guzick N, Houston, TX (from Internet) (observation)

## Other

Bromhidrosis (1–10%)
(2001): Liss WA, Pleasanton, CA (from Internet) (observation)
(2000): Liss WA, Pleasanton, CA (from Internet) (observation)

Dry mucosae
(2001): Berbis P, *Ann Dermatol Venereol* 128(6), 737

Gingival bleeding (1–10%)

Gingivitis (1–10%)

Gouty tophi
(1998): Vanhooteghem O+, *Clin Exp Dermatol* 23, 274

Hyperesthesia (10–25%)
(1999): Katz HI+, *J Am Acad Dermatol* 41, S7

Myopathy
(1996): Lister RK+, *Br J Dermatol* 134, 989

Oral mucosal lesions
(1988): Geiger J-M+, *Dermatologica* 176, 182 (6%)

Paresthesias (10–25%)
(1999): Katz HI+, *J Am Acad Dermatol* 41, S7

Pseudotumor cerebri
(1999): Katz HI+, *J Am Acad Dermatol* 41, S7

Sialorrhea (1–10%)
Stomatitis (1–10%)
Ulcerative stomatitis (1–10%)
Vulvovaginal candidiasis
(1995): Sturkenboom MC+, *J Clin Epidemiol* 48, 991
Xerostomia (10–25%)
(1999): Katz HI+, *J Am Acad Dermatol* 41, S7
(1997): Buccheri L+, *Arch Dermatol* 133, 711 (63.6%)
(1989): Schröder K+, *Acta Derm Venereol* (Stockh) 69, 111 (60%)
(1988): Geiger J-M+, *Dermatologica* 176, 182 (30%)

# ACTINOMYCIN-D

(See DACTINOMYCIN)

# ACYCLOVIR

**Synonyms:** aciclovir; ACV; acycloguanosine
**Trade name:** Zovirax (GSK)
**Other common trade names:** *Acifur; Acyclo-V; Acyvir; Avirax; Herpefug; Zyclir*
**Indications:** Herpes simplex, herpes zoster
**Category:** Antiviral; antiherpes drug (oral, parenteral and topical)
**Half-life:** 3 hours (adults)
**Clinically important, potentially hazardous interactions with:** meperidine

### *Reactions*

## Skin

Acne (<3%)
Contact dermatitis
(2001): Lammintausta K+, *Contact Dermatitis* 45(3), 181
(2000): Serpentier-Daude A+, *Ann Dermatol Venereol* 127, 191
(1996): Bourezane Y+, *Allergy* 51, 755
(1995): Koch P, *Contact Dermatitis* 33, 255
(1991): Goday J+, *Contact Dermatitis* 24, 381
(1990): Baes H+, *Contact Dermatitis* 23, 200
(1990): Valsecchi R+, *Contact Dermatitis* 23, 372
(1989): Gola M+, *Contact Dermatitis* 20, 394
(1988): Camarasa JG+, *Contact Dermatitis* 19, 235
Dermatitis (sic)
(1989): O'Brien JJ+, *Drugs* 37, 233 (vesicular)
(1985): Robinson GE+, *Genitourin Med* 61, 62 (palms and soles)
Diaphoresis
Edema
(1991): Medina S+, *Int J Dermatol* 30, 305
Erythema
(2002): Carrasco L+, *Clin Exp Dermatol* 27(2), 132
Erythema nodosum
(1983): Richards DM+, *Drugs* 26, 378
Exanthems (1–5%)
(1991): Whitley R+, *N Engl J Med* 324, 444
(1985): Robinson GE+, *Genitourin Med* 61, 62
(1984): Strauss SE+, *N Engl J Med* 301, 1545
(1983): Balfour HH+, *N Engl J Med* 308, 1448
(1983): Richards DM+, *Drugs* 26, 378
Facial edema (3–5%)
(2000): Colin J+, *Ophthalmology* 107, 1507
Fixed eruption
(1997): Montoro J+, *Contact Dermatitis* 36, 225
Herpes zoster (recurrent)
(1993): Murphy F, *The Schoch Letter* 43, 28, #104 (observation)
Lichenoid eruption
(1985): Robinson GE+, *Genitourin Med* 61, 62
Periorbital edema (3–5%)
(2000): Colin J+, *Ophthalmology* 107, 1507
Peripheral edema
(1991): Medina S+, *Int J Dermatol* 30, 305
(1988): Hisler BM+, *J Am Acad Dermatol* 18, 1142
Photoreactions
(2001): Schmutz JL+, *Ann Dermatol Venereol* 128, 184
Pruritus (1–10%)
(1993): Goldberg LH+, *Arch Dermatol* 129, 582 (passim)
Rash (sic) (<3%)
(1985): Lundgren G+, *Scand J Infect Dis* Suppl 47, 137
(1983): Balfour HH+, *N Engl J Med* 308, 1448
(1983): Masaoka T+, *Gan To Kagaku Ryoho* (Japanese) 10, 944
Recall dermatitis
(2002): Carrasco L+, *Clin Exp Dermatol* 27(2), 132
(2001): *Ann Dermatol Venereol* 128(2), 184
Stevens–Johnson syndrome
(1995): Fazal BA+, *Clin Infect Dis* 21, 1038
Urticaria (1–5%)
(1985): Robinson GE+, *Genitourin Med* 61, 62
(1983): Richards DM+, *Drugs* 26, 378
(1982): Smith CI+, *Am J Med* 73, 267
(1981): Balfour HH+, *Minn Med* 64, 739
Vasculitis
(1983): Richards DM+, *Drugs* 26, 378
Vesicular eruptions
(1993): Buck ML+, *Ann Pharmacother* 27, 1458

## Hair

Hair – alopecia (<3%)

## Other

Anaphylactoid reactions (<1%)
Dysgeusia (0.3%)
Hypersensitivity
(2001): Kawsar M+, *Sex Transm Infect* 77(3), 204
Injection-site inflammation (>10%)
(1989): O'Brien JJ+, *Drugs* 37, 233
Injection-site necrosis
(1987): Fayol J+, *Therapie* (French) 42(2), 249
Injection-site thrombophlebitis (9%)
(1988): Arndt KA, *J Am Acad Dermatol* 18, 188
Injection-site vesicular eruption
(1986): Sylvester RK+, *JAMA* 255, 385
Paresthesias (<1%)
(1993): Goldberg LH+, *Arch Dermatol* 129, 582 (passim)
Tremors
Vaginitis (candidal)
(1993): Goldberg LH+, *Arch Dermatol* 129, 582 (passim)

# ADAPALENE

**Trade names:** Adaferin; Differin (Galderma)
**Indications:** Acne vulgaris
**Category:** Retinoid (topical)
**Half-life:** N/A
**Clinically important, potentially hazardous interactions with:** resorcinol, salicylates

### *Reactions*

## Skin

Acne (<1%)
Burning (<1%)

(2001): Nyirady J+, *J Dermatolog Treat* 12(3), 149
(2001): Tu P+, *J Eur Acad Dermatol Venereol* 15 (Suppl 3), 31
(1998): Ellis CN+, *Br J Dermatol* 139, Suppl 52:41
Contact dermatitis (<1%)
Dermatitis (sic) (<1%)
Eczema (<1%)
Erythema (<1%)
(2001): Leyden J+, *Cutis* 67(6 Suppl), 17
(2001): Nyirady J+, *J Dermatolog Treat* 12(3), 149
(2001): Tu P+, *J Eur Acad Dermatol Venereol* 15, (Suppl 3) 31
(1998): Ellis CN+, *Br J Dermatol* 139, Suppl 52:41
Eyelid edema (<1%)
Irritation (sic) (<1%)
(2001): Queille-Roussel C+, *Clin Ther* 23(2), 205
(1998): Bonardeaux C+, *Rev Med Liege* 53(2), 109 (mild)
Pruritus (<1%)
(2001): Nyirady J+, *J Dermatolog Treat* 12(3), 149
(2001): Tu P+, *J Eur Acad Dermatol Venereol* 15 (Suppl 3), 31
(1998): Ellis CN+, *Br J Dermatol* 139, Suppl 52:41
Rash (sic) (<1%)
Scaling (<1%)
(2001): Tu P+, *J Eur Acad Dermatol Venereol* 15 (Suppl 3), 31
(1998): Ellis CN+, *Br J Dermatol* 139, Suppl 52:41
Xerosis (<1%)
(2001): Leyden J+, *Cutis* 67(6 Suppl), 17
(2001): Tu P+, *J Eur Acad Dermaol Venereol* 15 (Suppl 3), 31
(1998): Dunlap FE+, *Br J Dermatol* 139 (Suppl 52), 17 (3 cases)
(1998): Ellis CN+, *Br J Dermatol* 139, Suppl 52:41

### Other
Conjunctivitis

# ALBENDAZOLE

**Trade name:** Albenza (GSK)
**Other common trade names:** *ABZ; Albezole; Alzol; Bendex; Eskazole; Vermin; Zentel*
**Indications:** Nematode infections, hydatid cyst disease
**Category:** Anthelmintic
**Half-life:** 8–12 hours

## *Reactions*

### Skin
Allergic reactions (sic) (<1%)
Contact dermatitis
(1991): Macedo NA+, *Contact Dermatitis* 25, 73
Fixed eruption
(1998): Mahboob A+, *Int J Dermatol* 37, 833
(1998): Mahboob A+, *JPMA J Pak Med Assoc* 48, 316
Pruritus (<1%)
Rash (sic) (<1%)
Stevens–Johnson syndrome
(1997): Dewardt S+, *Acta Derm Venereol* 77, 411
Urticaria (<1%)
(1991): Macedo NA+, *Contact Dermatitis* 25, 73

### Hair
Hair – alopecia (<1%)
(1993): Tomas S+, *Enferm Infecc Microbiol Clin* (Spanish) 11, 113
(1990): Pilar-Garcia-Muret M+, *Int J Dermatol* 29, 669

### Other
Xerostomia (<1%)

# ALBUTEROL

**Synonym:** salbutamol
**Trade names:** AccuNeb; Airet (Medeva); Combivent (Boehringer Ingelheim); Duoneb (Muro); Proventil (Key); Ventolin (GSK); Volmax (Muro)
**Other common trade names:** *Asmaven; Broncho-Spray; Cobutolin; Salbulin; Ventoline*
**Indications:** Bronchospasm associated with asthma
**Category:** Beta$_2$ adrenergic agonist; bronchodilator (sympathomimetic)
**Half-life:** 3–6 hours
**Clinically important, potentially hazardous interactions with:** epinephrine

Combivent is albuterol and ipratropium

## *Reactions*

### Skin
Angioedema
Chills
Contact dermatitis
(1994): Smeenk G+, *Contact Dermatitis* 31, 123
Diaphoresis (1–10%)
(1989): Price AH+, *Drugs* 38, 77
Erythema (palmar) (with infusion)
(1992): Lebre C+, *Ann Dermatol Venereol* (French) 119, 293
(1990): Morin Leport LRM+, *Br J Dermatol* 122, 116
Exanthems
Flushing (1–10%)
Lupus erythematosus (pseudo-lupus)
(1987): Lacour JP+, *Presse Med* (French) 16, 1599
Pallor
Pruritus
(1991): Hatton MQ+, *Lancet* 337, 1169
Shakiness (sic)
Urticaria
(1991): Hatton MQ+, *Lancet* 337, 1169

### Other
Dysgeusia (1–10%)
Tinnitus
Tremors
Xerostomia (1–10%)

# ALDESLEUKIN

**Synonyms:** IL-2; interleukin-2
**Trade name:** Proleukin (Chiron)
**Other common trade names:** *Aerovent; Atem; Atronase; Narilet; Tropium*
**Indications:** Metastatic renal cell carcinoma
**Category:** Antineoplastic; biological response modulator (parenteral)
**Half-life:** 6–85 minutes
**Clinically important, potentially hazardous interactions with:** altretamine, amikacin, aminoglycosides, antineoplastics, bleomycin, busulfan, carboplatin, carmustine, chlorambucil, cisplatin, corticosteroids, cyclophosphamide, cytarabine, dacarbazine, dactinomycin, daunorubicin, docetaxel, doxorubicin, estramustine, etoposide, fludarabine, fluorouracil, gemcitabine, gentamicin, hydroxyurea, idarubicin, ifosfamide, indomethacin, kanamycin, levamisole, lomustine, mechlorethamine, melphalan, mercaptopurine, methotrexate, mitomycin, mitotane, mitoxantrone, neomycin, pentostatin, plicamycin, procarbazine, streptomycin, streptozocin, thioguanine, thiotepa, tobramycin, tretinoin, uracil, vinblastine, vincristine, vinorelbine

## *Reactions*

### Skin

Allergic granulomatous angiitis (Churg–Strauss syndrome)
(1997): Shiota Y+, *Inren Med* 36, 709
Allergic reactions (sic) (<1%)
Angioedema
(1992): Baars JW+, *Ann Oncol* 3, 243
Bullous eruption
(1991): Staunton MR, *J Natl Cancer Inst* 83, 56
Bullous pemphigoid
(1993): Fellner MJ, *Clin Dermatol* 11, 515
Dermatitis (sic)
(1989): Kerker BJ+, *Semin Dermatol* 8, 173
(1987): Gaspari AA+, *JAMA* 258, 1624 (1–5%)
Desquamation
(2001): Chi KH+, *Oncology* 60, 110
Eczema reactivation
(1997): Cork MJ+, *Br J Dermatol* 136, 644
Edema (47%)
(1994): Rosenberg SA+, *JAMA* 271, 907
(1990): Chien CH+, *Pediatrics* 86, 937
Erythema (sic) (41%)
(1993): Wolkenstein P+, *J Am Acad Dermatol* 28, 66
(1992): Blessing K+, *J Pathol* 167, 313
(1988): Lee RE+, *Arch Dermatol* 124, 1811
(1987): Gaspari AA+, *JAMA* 258, 1624
Erythema nodosum
(1989): Kerker BJ+, *Semin Dermatol* 8, 173
(1987): Weinstein A+, *JAMA* 258, 3120
Erythroderma
(1992): Blessing K+, *J Pathol* 167, 313
(1991): Siegel JP+, *J Clin Oncol* 9, 694 (>5%)
(1989): Kerker BJ+, *Semin Dermatol* 8, 173
(1987): Gaspari AA+, *JAMA* 258, 1624
Exanthems
(1991): Dummer R+, *Dermatologica* 183, 95
(1991): Siegel JP+, *J Clin Oncol* 9, 694 (>5%)
(1989): Jost LM+, *Schweiz Med Wochenschr* (German) 119, 137
(1987): Gaspari AA+, *JAMA* 258, 1624
Exfoliative dermatitis (14%)
(1993): Larbre B+, *Ann Dermatol Venereol* (French) 120, 528
Graft-versus-host reaction
(1995): Costello R+, *Bone Marrow Transplant* 16, 199
Intertriginous cutaneous eruption (sic)
(1996): Prussick R+, *J Am Acad Dermatol* 35, 705
Kaposi's sarcoma
(1989): Krigel RL+, *J Biol Response Mod* 8, 359
Linear IgA bullous dermatosis
(2002): Cohen LM+, *J Am Acad Dermatol* 46, S32 (passim)
(1996): Tranvan A+, *J Am Acad Dermatol* 35, 865
(1993): Oeda E+, *Am J Hematol* 44, 213
(1990): Guillaume JC+, *Ann Dermatol Venereol* (French) 117, 899
Pemphigus
(1995): Wolkenstein P+, *Arch Dermatol* 130, 890
(1994): Prussick R+, *Arch Dermatol* 130, 890
(1989): Ramseur WL+, *Cancer* 63, 2005 (fatal)
Peripheral edema (1–10%)
Petechiae (4%)
Photosensitivity
(1992): Blessing K+, *J Pathol* 167, 313
Pruritus (48%)
(2001): Chi KH+, *Oncology* 60, 60
(1995): Wahlgren CF+, *Arch Dermatol Res* 287, 572
(1994): Rosenberg SA+, *JAMA* 271, 907
(1993): Wolkenstein P+, *J Am Acad Dermatol* 28, 66
(1988): Lee RE+, *Arch Dermatol* 124, 1811
(1987): Gaspari AA+, *JAMA* 258, 1624
Psoriasis
(1991): Siegel JP+, *J Clin Oncol* 9, 694 (>5%)
(1989): Kerker BJ+, *Semin Dermatol* 8, 173
(1988): Lee RE+, *Arch Dermatol* 124, 1811 (exacerbation)
(1987): Gaspari AA+, *JAMA* 258, 1624
Purpura (4%)
(1989): Kerker BJ+, *Semin Dermatol* 8, 173
Rash (sic) (26%)
Sarcoidosis
(2000): Blanche P+, *Clin Infect Dis* 31, 1493
Scleroderma
(1994): Boni R, *Dermatology* 189, 330
(1994): Puett DW+, *J Rheumatol* 21, 752
Toxic epidermal necrolysis
(1992): Wiener JS+, *South Med J* 85, 656
Urticaria (2%)
(1993): Wolkenstein P+, *J Am Acad Dermatol* 28, 66
(1992): Baars JW+, *Ann Oncol* 3, 243
Vitiligo
(1996): Rosenberg SA+, *J Immunother Emphasis Tumor Immunol* 19, 81
(1995): Wolkenstein P+, *Arch Dermatol* 130, 890
(1994): Scheibenbogen C+, *Eur J Cancer* (30A) 8, 1209
Xerosis (15%)

### Hair

Hair – alopecia (<1%)
(1989): Jost LM+, *Schweiz Med Wochenschr* (German) 119, 137
(1987): Gaspari AA+, *JAMA* 258, 1624 (10%)

### Other

Aphthous stomatitis
(1987): Gaspari AA+, *JAMA* 258, 1624 (5%)
Death
Depression
(2001): Maes M+, *Mol Psychiatry* 6(4), 475
Dysgeusia (7%)
Glossitis
(1987): Gaspari AA+, *JAMA* 258, 1624 (30%)
Injection-site inflammation
(1999): Asadullah K+, *Arch Dermatol* 135, 187
Injection-site nodules (sic)
(1993): Klapholtz L+, *Bone Marrow Transplant* 11, 443

Injection-site panniculitis
(1992): Baars JW+, *Br J Cancer* 66, 698
Injection-site reactions (sic) (3%)
Myalgia (6%)
Necrosis
(1993): Wolkenstein P+, *J Am Acad Dermatol* 28, 66
(1988): Rosenberg SA+, *Ann Intern Med* 108, 853 (3%)
Oral mucosal eruption
(1989): Kerker BJ+, *Semin Dermatol* 8, 173
(1987): Gaspari AA+, *JAMA* 258, 1624
Oral ulceration
(1990): Chien CH+, *Pediatrics* 86, 937
Rhabdomyolysis
(1995): Anderlini P+, *Cancer* 76(4), 678
Stomatitis (32%)
Xerostomia
(2001): Chi KH+, *Oncology* 60, 110

## ALEMTUZUMAB

**Synonyms:** Campath-1H; DNA-derived Humanized Monoclonal Antibody; Humanized IgG1 Anti-CD52 Monoclonal Antiobdy
**Trade names:** Campath (Berlex); MabCampath (Schering)
**Indications:** B-cell chronic lymphotic leukemia, non-Hodgkin's lymphoma
**Category:** Antineoplastic agent; monoclonol anitbody; recombinant DNA-derived humanized monoclonal antibidy
**Half-life:** 12 days

**Note:** Prophylactic therapy against PCP pneumonia and herpes viral infections is recommended upon initiation of therapy and for at least 2 months following last dose

### *Reactions*

#### Skin

Allergic reactions (sic) (<1%)
Angioedema (<1%)
Bullous eruption (<1%)
Cellulitis (<1%)
Chills
(2000): Flynn JM+, *Curr Opin Oncol* 12(6), 574
Facial edema (<1%)
Flushing
(2000): Tang SC+, *Leuk Lymphoma* 24(1-2), 93
Hematomas (<1%)
Infections (sic)
(2002): Keating MJ+, *J Clin Oncol* 20(1), 205
(2001): Khorana A+, *Leuk Lymphoma* 41(1), 77
(2000): Tang SC+, *Leuk Lymphoma* 24(1-2), 93
(1998): Lundin J+, *J Clin Oncol* 16(10), 3257
Malignant lymphoma (<1%)
Peripheral edema (13%)
Purpura (8%)
Squamous cell carcinoma (<1%)
Urticaria
(2000): Tang SC+, *Leuk Lymphoma* 24(1-2), 93

#### Other

Anaphylactoid reactions (<1%)
Death
(2002): Keating MJ+, *J Clin Oncol* 20(1), 205 (2 cases)
(1998): Lundin J+, *J Clin Oncol* 16(10), 3257
Depression (7%)
Dysesthesia (15%)
Dysgeusia (<1%)
Gingivitis (<1%)
Infusion-site pruritus (30–40%)
Infusion-site rash (14–24%)
Infusion-site reactions
(2002): Keating MJ+, *Blood* 99(10), 3554
(2002): Keating MJ+, *J Clin Oncol* 20(1), 205
(2001): Khorana A+, *Leuk Lymphoma* 41(1), 77
Infusion-site urticaria (22–30%)
Lymphoproliferative disease (64% to 70%)
Myalgia (11%)
Myositis (<1%)
Phlebitis (<1%)
Polymyositis (<1%)
Stomatitis (14%)
Stomatodynia
Thrombophlebitis (<1%)

## ALENDRONATE

**Trade name:** Fosamax (Merck)
**Other common trade name:** *Fosalan*
**Indications:** Osteoporosis in postmenopausal women, Paget's disease
**Category:** Inhibitor of bone resorption; biphosphonate
**Half-life:** >10 years

### *Reactions*

#### Skin

Erythema (<1%)
(1996): Keen RW+, *Br J Clin Pract* 50, 211
Erythema multiforme
(2000): Madnani N, Mumbai, India (from Internet) (observation)
Exanthems
(2000): Madnani N, Mumbai, India (from Internet) (observation)
Fixed eruption
(1998): McCarthy J, Ft. Worth, TX (from Internet) (observation)
Peripheral edema
Petechiae
(1997): Berger R, St. George, UT (from Internet) (observation)
Pruritus (0.6%)
(2000): Madnani N, Mumbai, India (from Internet) (observation)
(1997): Kyriakidou-Himonas M+, *Advances in Therapy* 14, 281
Rash (sic) (<1%)
(1997): Berger R, St. George, UT (from Internet) (observation)
(1996): Freedholm D+, *Osteoporosis Int* 6, 261
(1996): Keen RW+, *Br J Clin Pract* 50, 211
(1996): Selby PL, *Osteoporosis Int* 6, S21
(1995): Chestnut CH+, *Am J Med* 99, 144

#### Other

Dysgeusia (0.6%)
(1997): Kyriakidou-Himonas M+, *Advances in Therapy* 14, 281
Hypersensitivity
(1996): Kirk JK+, *Am Fam Physician* 54, 2053
Ocular inflammation
(1999): Mbekeani JN+, *Arch Ophthalmol* 117, 837
Oral ulceration
(1999): Demerjian N+, *Clin Rheumatol* 18, 349

## ALFENTANIL

**Trade name:** Alfenta (Taylor)
**Other common trade name:** *Rapifen*
**Indications:** General anesthesia, post-operative pain
**Category:** Narcotic agonist analgesic
**Half-life:** 83–97 minutes (adults)
**Clinically important, potentially hazardous interactions with:** erythromycin, ranitidine, ritonavir

### *Reactions*

#### Skin

Clammy skin (<1%)
Pruritus (<1%)
 (1999): Kyriakides K+, *Br J Anaesth* 82, 439
Rash (sic) (<1%)
Shivering (sic) (3–9%)
Urticaria (<1%)

#### Other

Dysesthesia

## ALITRETINOIN

**Trade name:** Panretin (Ligand)
**Indications:** Kaposi's sarcoma cutaneous lesions
**Category:** Antineoplastic retinoic acid derivative (topical)
**Half-life:** no data

### *Reactions*

#### Skin

Abrasion
Bullous eruption
Burning
 (2002): Morganroth GS, *Arch Dermatol* 138, 542
Edema (3–8%)
 (2000): Duvic M+, *Arch Dermatol* 136, 1461 (3%)
Exfoliative dermatitis (3–9%)
Flushing
Pain (0–34%)
 (2000): Duvic M+, *Arch Dermatol* 136, 1461 (18%)
Photosensitivity
Pigmentation (3%)
 (2000): Duvic M+, *Arch Dermatol* 136, 1461 (3%)
Pruritus (8–11%)
Rash (sic) (25–77%)
 (2000): Duvic M+, *Arch Dermatol* 136, 1461 (69%)
Skin disorder (sic) (0–8%) (17%)
 (2000): Duvic M+, *Arch Dermatol* 136, 1461 (17%)
Skin toxicity (sic)
 (2002): Miles SA+, *AIDS* 16(3), 421
Ulceration (2%)
 (2000): Duvic M+, *Arch Dermatol* 136, 1461
Xerosis (10%)
 (2000): Duvic M+, *Arch Dermatol* 136, 1461 (10%)

#### Hair

Hair – alopecia

#### Other

Application-site dermatitis
 (2002): Morganroth GS, *Arch Dermatol* 138, 542
Application-site reactions
 (1999): Walmsley S+, *J Acquir Immune Defic Syndr* 22, 325
Myalgia
Paresthesias (3–22%)

## ALLOPURINOL

**Trade name:** Zyloprim (Faro)
**Other common trade names:** *Allo 300; Allo-Puren; Alloprin; Atisuril; Bleminol; Caplenal; Hamarin; Novo-Purol; Purinol; Unizuric; Zyloric*
**Indications:** Gouty arthritis
**Category:** Uricosuric; anti-gout
**Half-life:** 1–3 hours
**Clinically important, potentially hazardous interactions with:** amoxicillin, ampicillin, azathioprine, dicumarol, mercaptopurine

### *Reactions*

#### Skin

Acute generalized exanthematous pustulosis (AGEP)
 (1995): Moreau A+, *Int J Dermatol* 34, 263 (passim)
Angiitis (<1%)
Angioedema
 (1996): Yale SH+, *Hosp Pract Off Ed* 31, 92
Chills (1–10%)
Cutaneous reactions (sic) (severe)
 (1999): Tanna SB+, *Ann Pharmacother* 33 1180
Diaphoresis (<1%)
Ecchymoses (<1%)
Edema (periorbital)
 (1981): McInnes GT+, *Ann Rheum Dis* 40, 245
Erythema multiforme (<1%)
 (2001): Perez A+, *Contact Dermatitis* 44, 113 (with amoxicillin)
 (1999): Fonseka MM+, *Ceylon Med J* 44, 190
 (1996): Kumar A+, *BMJ* 312, 173
 (1984): Pennell DJ+, *Lancet* 1, 463
 (1979): Lupton GP+, *J Am Acad Dermatol* 1, 365
Exanthems (1–5%)
 (2001): Fam AG+, *Arthritis Rheum* 44, 231
 (1998): Dintiman B, Fairfax, VA (from Internet) (observation)
 (1992): Fam AG+, *Am J Med* 93, 299
 (1989): Chan SH+, *Dermatologica* 179, 32
 (1987): Hoigné R+, *N Engl J Med* 316, 1217
 (1984): Hande KR+, *Am J Med* 76, 47
 (1981): Jick H+, *J Clin Pharmacol* 21, 456 (with ampicillin 14%)
 (1981): McInnes GT+, *Ann Rheum Dis* 40, 245
 (1979): Lang GP+, *South Med J* 72, 1361
 (1979): Lupton GP+, *J Am Acad Dermatol* 1, 365
 (1976): Lockard O+, *Ann Intern Med* 85, 333
 (1976): Utsinger PD+, *Am J Med* 61, 287
 (1971): Mills RM, *JAMA* 216, 799
Exfoliative dermatitis (>10%)
 (2001): Dominguez Ortega J+, *An Med Intern* 18(1), 27
 (1996): Emmerson BT, *N Engl J Med* 334, 445
 (1996): Sigurdsson V+, *J Am Acad Dermatol* 35, 53
 (1989): Chan SH+, *Dermatologica* 179, 32
 (1984): Vinciullo C, *Aust J Dermatol* 25, 59
 (1979): Lang GP+, *South Med J* 72, 1361
 (1979): Lupton GP+, *J Am Acad Dermatol* 1, 365
 (1977): Boyer TD+, *West J Med* 126, 143
 (1976): McMenamin RA+, *Aust N Z J Med* 6, 583
 (1975): Sisca TS, *J Clin Pharmacol* 15, 566
 (1973): Feuerman EJ+, *Br J Dermatol* 89, 83
 (1966): Rundles RW+, *Ann Intern Med* 64, 229

Fixed eruption (<1%)
(2001): Dominguez Ortega J+, *An Med Intern* 18(1), 27
(1999): Sehgal VN+, *J Dermatol* 26, 198 (transitory giant)
(1998): Mahboob A+, *Int J Dermatol* 37, 833
(1998): Umpierrez A+, *J Allergy Clin Immunol* 101, 286
(1996): Gimbel Moral LF+, *Med Clin (Barc)* (Spanish) 106, 119
(1996): Kelso JM+, *J Allergy Clin Immunol* 97, 1171
(1990): Audicana M+, *Clin Exp Allergy* 20(Supp 1), 121
Graft-versus-host reaction
(1998): Jappe U+, *Hautarzt* (German) 49, 126
Granuloma annulare (disseminated)
(1995): Becker D+, *Hautarzt* (German) 46, 343
Ichthyosis
(1968): Auerbach R+, *Arch Dermatol* 98, 104
Lichen planus (<1%)
Lupus erythematosus
(1978): Pereyo-Torrellas N, *Arch Dermatol* 114, 1097
(1975): Lee SL+, *Semin Arthritis Rheum* 5, 83
Lymphocytoma cutis
(1988): Raymond JZ+, *Cutis* 41, 323
Necrotizing angiitis
Perforating foot ulceration
(1997): Bouloc A+, *Clin Exp Dermatol* 21, 351
Petechiae
(1977): Chan HL+, *Aust N Z J Med* 7, 518
Photosensitivity
(1986): Lerman S, *Ophthalmology* 93, 304
Pruritus (<1%)
(2001): Dominguez Ortega J+, *An Med Intern* 18(1), 27
(2001): Fam AG+, *Arthritis Rheum* 44, 231
(1998): Dintiman B, Fairfax, VA (from Internet) (observation)
(1979): Lang GP+, *South Med J* 72, 1361
(1979): Lupton GP+, *J Am Acad Dermatol* 1, 365
(1965): Klinenberg JR+, *Ann Intern Med* 62, 639
Purpura (>10%)
(1979): Lang GP+, *South Med J* 72, 1361
(1977): Boyer TD+, *West J Med* 126, 143
Pustular eruption
(2002): Lun K+, *Australas J Dermatol* 43(2), 140
Pustuloderma
(1994): Fitzgerald DA+, *Clin Exp Dermatol* 19, 243
Rash (sic) (>10%)
(2001): Dominguez Ortega J+, *An Med Intern* 18(1), 27
(1996): Yale SH+, *Hosp Pract Off Ed* 31, 92
Sensitivity (sic)
(1979): Haughey DB+, *Am J Hosp Pharm* 36, 1377
Stevens–Johnson syndrome (>10%)
(1995): Roujeau JC+, *N Engl J Med* 333, 1600
(1993): Leenutaphong V+, *Int J Dermatol* 32, 428
(1992): Goodglick TA+, *Ophthalmic Surg* 23, 557
(1989): Chan SH+, *Dermatologica* 179, 32
(1985): Edwards R+, *Dimens Crit Care Nurs* 4, 335
(1985): Renwick IG, *BMJ* 291, 485
(1985): Ting HC+, *Int J Dermatol* 24, 587
(1984): Pennell DJ+, *Lancet* 1, 463 (fatal)
(1979): Lupton GP+, *J Am Acad Dermatol* 1, 365
(1978): Assaad D+, *Can Med Assoc* 118, 154
(1977): Chan HL+, *Aust N Z J Med* 7, 518
Toxic epidermal necrolysis
(2002): Correia O+, *Arch Dermatol* 138, 29 (2 cases)
(2001): Hammer B+, *Dtsch Med Wochenschr* 126(47), 1331
(1999): Sorkin MJ, Denver, CO (from Internet) (observation)
(1995): Roujeau JC+, *N Engl J Med* 333, 1600
(1995): Wolkenstein P+, *Arch Dermatol* 131, 544
(1994): Alfandari S+, *Infection* 22, 365
(1993): Correia O+, *Dermatology* 186, 32
(1993): Leenutaphong V+, *Int J Dermatol* 32, 428
(1991): Sakellariou G+, *Int J Artif Organs* 14, 634
(1987): Guillaume JC+, *Arch Dermatol* 123, 1166
(1986): Kumar L, *Indian J Dermatol* 31, 53
(1985): Auboeck J+, *BMJ* 290, 1969
(1985): Renwick IG, *BMJ* 291, 485
(1985): Zakraoui L+, *Tunis Med* (French) 63, 167
(1984): Chan HL, *J Am Acad Dermatol* 10, 973
(1984): Dan M+, *Int J Dermatol* 23, 142
(1979): Lang GP+, *South Med J* 72, 1361
(1979): Lupton GP+, *J Am Acad Dermatol* 1, 365
(1978): Assaad D+, *Can Med Assoc* 118, 154
(1977): Bennett TO+, *Arch Ophthalmol* 95, 1362 (ocular)
(1977): Chan HL+, *Aust N Z J Med* 7, 518
(1976): Fellner MJ, *Arch Dermatol* 112, 1327
(1975): Ellman MH+, *Arch Dermatol* 111, 986
(1975): Sisca TS, *J Clin Pharmacol* 15, 566
(1975): Trentham DE+, *N Engl J Med* 292, 870
(1972): Stratigos JD+, *Br J Dermatol* 86, 564
(1970): Kantor GL, *JAMA* 212, 478 (fatal)
Toxic erythema
(1995): Rademaker M, *N Z Med J* 108, 165
Toxic pustuloderma
(1994): Boffa MJ+, *Br J Dermatol* 131, 447
(1994): Fitzgerald DA+, *Clin Exp Dermatol* 19, 243
(1993): Yu RC+, *Br J Dermatol* 128, 95
Urticaria (>10%)
(2001): Dominguez Ortega J+, *An Med Interna* 18(1), 27
(1999): Litt JZ, Beachwood, OH (personal case) (observation)
(1992): Breathnach SM+, *Adverse Drug Reactions and the Skin* Blackwell, Oxford, 193 (passim)
(1991): Anderson MH+, *Ann Allergy* 66, 207
Vasculitis (<1%)
(2001): Dominguez Ortega J+, *An Med Intern* 18(1), 27
(1998): Choi HK+, *Clin Exp Rheumatol* 16, 743
(1996): Emmerson BT, *N Engl J Med* 334, 445
(1977): Boyer TD+, *West J Med* 126, 143
(1976): Bailey RR+, *Lancet* 2, 907
(1971): Mills RM, *JAMA* 216, 799

## Hair

Hair – alopecia (1–10%)
(1974): Lovatt GE, *Br J Dermatol* 91, 115
(1968): Auerbach R+, *Arch Dermatol* 98, 104

## Nails

Nails – onycholysis (<1%)

## Other

Death
(2002): Correia O+, *Arch Dermatol* 138, 29 (one case)
(2001): Hammer B+, *Dtsch Med Wochenschr* 126(47), 1331
DRESS syndrome
(2001): Descamps V+, *Arch Dermatol* 137, 301 (passim)
Dysgeusia
Hypersensitivity*
(2002): Sommers LM+, *Arch Intern Med* 162(10), 1190
(2001): Arakawa M+, *Intern Med* 40(4), 331
(2001): Benito-Leon J+, *Eur Neurol* 45, 186
(2001): Dominguez Ortega J+, *An Med Interna* 18(1), 27
(2001): Hammer B+, *Dtsch Med Wochenschr* 126(47), 1331
(2001): Rivas Gonzalez P+, *Rev Clin Esp* 201(8), 493
(1999): Gillott TJ+, *Rheumatology* (Oxford) 38, 85
(1999): Melsom RD, *Rheumatology* 38, 1301 (familial)
(1999): Morel D+, *Nephrol Dial Transplant* 14, 780
(1998): Kluger E, *Ugeskr Laeger* (Danish) 160, 1179
(1998): Pluim HJ+, *Neth J Med* 52, 107
(1997): Carpenter C, *Tenn Med* 90, 151
(1996): Kumar A+, *BMJ* 312, 173
(1995): Elasy T+, *West J Med* 162, 360
(1994): Lee SS+, *Chung Hua Min Kuo Wei Sheng Wu Chi Mien I Hsueh Tsa Chih* 27, 140
(1994): Salinas Martin A+, *Aten Primaria* (Spanish) 14, 694

(1989): Puig JG+, *J Rheumatol* 16, 842
(1988): McDonald J+, *J Rheumatol* 15, 865
(1985): Stein CM, *S Afr Med J* 67, 935
(1984): Vinciullo C, *Aust J Dermatol* 25, 59
(1984): Vinciullo C, *Med J Aust 141, 449*
(1979): Lupton GP+, *J Am Acad Dermatol* 1, 365
(1976): Utsinger PD+, *Am J Med* 61, 287

Mucocutaneous eruption

Myalgia
(2002): Terawaki H+, *Nippon Jinzo Gakkai Shi* 44, 50
(1996): Ghanem BM+, *J Egypt Soc Parasitol* 26, 619

Myopathy (<1%)

Oral ulceration
(1984): Chau NY+, *Oral Surg Oral Med Oral Pathol* 58, 397 (lichenoid)
(1979): Lang GP+, *South Med J* 72, 1361

Paresthesias (<1%)

Polyarteritis nodosa
(1976): Bailey RR+, *Lancet* 2, 907
(1974): Young JL+, *Arch Intern Med* 134, 553
(1970): Jarzobski J+, *Am Heart J* 79, 116

Stomatitis
(1981): McInnes GT+, *Ann Rheum Dis* 40, 245
(1977): Chan HL+, *Aust N Z J Med* 7, 518 (ulcerative)

Thrombophlebitis (<1%)

Tinnitus

Tongue edema (<1%)

***Note:** The antiepileptic drug hypersensitivity syndrome is a severe, occasionally fatal, disorder characterized by any or all of the following: pruritic exanthem, toxic epidermal necrolysis, Stevens–Johnson syndrome, exfoliative dermatitis, fever, hepatic abnormalities, eosinophilia, and renal failure

## ALMOTRIPTAN

**Trade name:** Axert (Pharmacia & Upjohn)
**Indications:** Migraine headaches
**Category:** Serotonin 5-Ht1d receptor agonist
**Half-life:** 3-4 hours
**Clinically important, potentially hazardous interactions with:** dihydroergotamine, ergotamines, ketoconazole, methysergide

### *Reactions*

#### Skin

Chills (<1%)

Dermatitis (sic)

Diaphoresis (<1%)

Erythema (<1%)

Flu-like syndrome (12%)
(2001): Cabarrocas X+, *Headache* 41, 57 (5.62%)

Photosensitivity (<1%)

Pruritus (<1%)

Rash (sic) (<1%)

Upper respiratory infection (20%)

#### Other

Arthralgia (<1%)

Depression (<1%)

Dysgeusia (<1%)

Hyperesthesia (<1%)

Injection-site irritation
(2001): Cabarrocas X, *Clin Ther* 23(11), 1867

Myalgia (<1%)

Myopathy (<1%)

Paresthesias (1%)
(2002): Keam SJ+, *Drugs* 62(2), 387
(2001): Dodick DW, *Headache* 41(5), 449

Parosmia (<1%)

Sialorrhea (<1%)

Skeletal pain
(2002): Keam SJ+, *Drugs* 62(2), 387

Tinnitus (<1%)

Xerostomia (1%)

## ALOE VERA (GEL, JUICE, LEAF)

**Scientific names:** *Aloë africana; Aloë barbadensis; Aloë ferox; Aloë spicata*
**Other common names:** Aloë; *Aloe capensis*; Aloe leaf gel; Barbados aloe; Curacau aloe; Kumari (Sanskrit); Lu Hui (Chinese); Salvia
**Family:** Liliaceae
**Purported indications:** Orally: General tonic (cleanser, anesthetic, antiseptic, antipyretic, antipruritic, vasodilator, anti-inflammatory agent, promoter of cell proliferation). Vermifuge, antifungal. Gastroduodenal ulcers, diabetes, asthma. Topically: To promote healing of burns or wounds, cold sores, ulcerations, radiations injuries, psoriasis, frostbite. Also used for its moisturizing and emollient properties
**Other uses:** Used in non-laxative drugs and cosmetic products

### *Reactions*

#### Skin

Allergic reactions (sic)
(1999): Reynolds T+, *J Ethnopharmacol* 68(1–3), 3
(1974): Diba SA, *Zh Ushn Nos Gorl Bolezn* Mar-Apr 0(2), 108 (from juice)

Contact dermatitis

#### Other

Anaphylactoid reactions
(1970): Trakhtenberg SB, *Klin Med* (Mosk) (following injection)

Hypersensitivity
(1980): Morrow DM+, *Arch Dermatol* 116, 1064

**Note:** *"I have perfumed my bed with myrrh, aloes and cinnamon" (Proverbs 7:17)
* Cleopatra regarded the gel as a fountain of youth and used it to preserve her skin against the ravages of the Egyptian sun.
* Alexander the Great is said to have acquired Madagascar so that he could utilize the *Aloë vera* growing there to treat soldiers' wounds.
* One blade of aloe can be used for weeks. The severed end of the blade is self healing.
* Many of the so-called aloe preparations on the market contain watered-down and very little of the actual plant, and therefore are not very beneficial

## ALOSETRON

**Trade name:** Lotronex (GSK)
**Indications:** Irritable bowel syndrome
**Category:** 5-$HT_3$ receptor antagonist
**Half-life:** 1.5 hours

### *Reactions*

#### Skin
Acne (<1%)
Allergic reactions (sic) (<1%)
Bacterial infections
Folliculitis (<1%)
Hematomas (<1%)

#### Other
Dysgeusia (<1%)
Parosmia (<1%)

## ALPRAZOLAM

**Trade name:** Xanax (Pharmacia & Upjohn)
**Other common trade names:** *Alprox; APO-Alpraz; Cassadan; Kalma; Nu-Alprax; Ralozam; Tafil*
**Indications:** Anxiety, depression, panic attacks
**Category:** Benzodiazepine anxiolytic tranquilizer
**Half-life:** 11–16 hours
**Clinically important, potentially hazardous interactions with: alcohol**, clarithromycin, CNS depressants, delavirdine, digoxin, efavirenz, fluconazole, fluoxetine, fluvoxamine, **grapefruit juice**, indinavir, itraconazole, ivermectin, **kava**, ketoconazole, propoxyphene, ritonavir, saquinavir

### *Reactions*

#### Skin
Acne
(1985): Levy MH+, *Semin Oncol* 12, 411
Allergic reactions (sic)
(1996): Bhatia MS, *Indian J Med Sci* 50, 285 (to the tartrazine dye)
Dermatitis (sic) (3.8%)
(1984): Elie R+, *J Clin Psychopharmacol* 4, 125
(1982): Fawcett JA+, *Pharmacotherapy* 2, 243
(1981): Evans RL, *Drug Intell Clin Pharm* 15, 633
(1981): Kolin IS+, *J Clin Psychiatry* 42, 169
(1976): Fabre LF, *Curr Ther Res* 19, 661
Diaphoresis (15.8%)
Edema (4.9%)
Exanthems
(1988): Warnock JK+, *Am J Psychiatry* 145, 425
Photosensitivity
(1999): Watanabe Y+, *J Am Acad Dermatol* 40, 832
(1998): Pazzagli L+, *Pharm World Sci* 20, 136 (with fluoxetine)
(1994): Shelley WB+, *Cutis* 54, 70 (observation)
(1990): Kanwar AJ+, *Dermatologica* 181, 75
Phototoxicity
(1993): Litt JZ, Beachwood, OH (personal case) (observation)
(1991): Shelley WB+, *Cutis* 48, 187 (observation)
Pruritus
(1988): Islas JA+, *Curr Ther Res* 43, 384
(1982): Chouinard G+, *Psychopharmacol* 77, 229
Purpura
Rash (sic) (10.8%)
(1987): Fyer AJ+, *Am J Psychiatry* 144, 303
(1985): Jerram TC, *Side Eff Drugs Annu* 9, 39
(1985): Rush AJ+, *Arch Gen Psychiatry* 42, 1154
(1983): Davison K+, *Psychopharmacol* 80, 308
Urticaria
Xerosis
(1982): Chouinard G+, *Psychopharmacol* 77, 229

#### Other
Dysgeusia (<1%)
(1982): Chouinard G+, *Psychopharmacol* 77, 229
Galactorrhea
Gynecomastia
Oral ulceration
Paresthesias (2.4%)
Pseudolymphoma
(1995): Magro CM+, *J Am Acad Dermatol* 32, 419
Sialopenia (32.8%)
Sialorrhea (4.2%)
Tinnitus
Xerostomia (14.7%)
(1988): Islas JA+, *Curr Ther Res* 43, 384
(1984): Elie R+, *J Clin Psychopharmacol* 4, 125
(1982): Chouinard G+, *Psychopharmacol* 77, 229
(1982): Fawcett JA+, *Pharmacotherapy* 2, 243
(1981): Evans RL, *Drug Intell Clin Pharm* 15, 633

## ALPROSTADIL

**Synonyms:** PGE; prostaglandin $E_1$
**Trade names:** Caverject (Pharmacia & Upjohn); Edex (Schwarz); Muse (Vivus); Prostin VR (Pharmacia & Upjohn)
**Other common trade names:** *Lyple; Minprog; Palux; Prostine VR; Prostivas*
**Indications:** Impotence, to maintain patent ductus arteriosus
**Category:** Prostaglandin; erectile dysfunction agent
**Half-life:** 5–10 minutes

### *Reactions*

#### Skin
Balanitis (<1%)
Diaphoresis (<1%)
Ecchymoses
(1996): Linet OI+, *N Engl J Med* 334, 873 (8%)
Edema (1%)
Flushing (>10%)
Lichen sclerosus (penile shaft hypopigmentation)
(1998): English JC+, *J Am Acad Dermatol* 39, 801
Penile edema (1%)
Penile pain (37%)
(1997): Padma-Nathan H+, *N Engl J Med* 336, 1 (32.7%)
(1996): Linet OI+, *N Engl J Med* 334, 873 (50%)
Penile pruritus (<1%)
Penile rash (1–10%)
Rash (sic) (<1%)
Toxic epidermal necrolysis
(1996): Lecorvaisier-Pieto C+, *J Am Acad Dermatol* 35, 112
Urticaria
(2000): Carter EL+, *Pediatr Dermatol* 17, 58

#### Other
Hypesthesia (<1%)
Injection-site ecchymoses (1–10%)

(1996): Linet OI+, *N Engl J Med* 334, 873 (8%)
Injection-site hematoma (3%)
Injection-site inflammation (<1%)
Injection-site pain (2%)
(1996): Hellstrom WJG, *Urology* 48, 851
Injection-site pruritus (<1%)
Priapism (4%)
(1999): Lue TF, *J Urol* 161, 725
(1998): Bettocchi C+, *Br J Urol* 81, 926
(1997): *Med Lett Drugs Ther* 39, 32
(1996): Hellstrom WJG, *Urology* 48, 851
(1996): Linet OI+, *N Engl J Med* 334, 873 (1%)
Xerostomia (<1%)

# ALTEPLASE

**Trade name:** Activase (Genentech)
**Other common trade names:** *Actilyse; Activacin; Lysatec-rt-PA*
**Indications:** Acute myocardial infarction, acute pulmonary embolism
**Category:** Thrombolytic (tissue plasminogen activator)
**Half-life:** 30–45 minutes
**Clinically important, potentially hazardous interactions with:** nitroglycerin, ticlopidine

## *Reactions*

### Skin

Angioedema
(2001): Pechlaner C+, *Blood Coagul Fibrinolysis* 12(6), 491
(2000): Hill MD+, *CMAJ* 162, 1281
(2000): Rudolf J+, *Neurology* 55, 599
Ecchymoses (1–10%)
Purpura (<1%)
(1990): De Trana+, *Arch Dermatol* 126, 690 (painful) (<1%)
Rash (sic) (<0.02%)
Urticaria (<1%)
(1989): Collen D+, *Drugs* 38, 346

### Other

Anaphylactoid reactions (<0.02%)
(2001): Pechlaner C+, *Blood Coagul Fibrinolysis* 12(6), 491
(2000): Hill MD+, *CMAJ* 162, 1281 (fatal)
(1999): Rudolf J+, *Stroke* 30, 1142
Death
Gingival bleeding (<1%)
Hypersensitivity
(2001): Pechlaner C+, *Blood Coagul Fibrinolysis* 12(6), 491

# ALTRETAMINE

**Synonym:** hexamethylmelamine
**Trade name:** Hexalen (US Bioscience)
**Other common trade names:** *Hexamethylmelamin; Hexastat; Hexinawas*
**Indications:** Palliative treatment of recurrent ovarian cancer
**Category:** Antineoplastic
**Half-life:** 13 hours
**Clinically important, potentially hazardous interactions with:** aldesleukin

## *Reactions*

### Skin

Dermatitis (sic)
Exanthems
Pruritus (<1%)
Rash (sic) (<1%)

### Hair

Hair – alopecia (<1%)

### Other

Mucocutaneous side effects (sic)
(1978): Levine LR, *Cancer Treat Rev* 5, 67
Paresthesias
(2001): Rothenberg ML+, *Gynecol Oncol* 82(2), 317
Tremors (<1%)

# AMANTADINE

**Trade name:** Symmetrel (Endo Lab)
**Other common trade names:** *Amixx; Endantadine; Grippin-Merz; Mantadix; PK-Merz; Protexin; Tregor*
**Indications:** Parkinsonism, influenza A viral infection
**Category:** Antiviral; antidyskinetic and antifatigue; antiparkinsonian
**Half-life:** 10–28 hours

**Note:** Fifty to 90% of patients receiving amantadine for Parkinsonism develop "a more or less livedo reticularis"

## *Reactions*

### Skin

Ankle edema
(1972): Calne DB+, *Drugs* 4, 49
(1972): Schwab RS+, *JAMA* 222, 792
(1971): Parkes JD+, *Lancet* 1, 1085
(1971): Vollum DI+, *BMJ* 2, 628
Contact dermatitis
(1997): Jauregui I+, *J Invest Allergol Clin Immunol* 7, 260
(1990): Patruno C+, *Contact Dermatitis* 22, 187
(1988): van Ketel WG, *Derm Beruf Umwelt* (German) 36, 23
(1987): Angelini G+, *Contact Dermatitis* 15, 114
(1987): Miranda A+, *Contact Dermatitis* 17, 55
(1987): van Joost T+, *Ned Tijdschr Geneeskd* (Dutch) 131, 21
(1987): van Ketel WG, *Ned Tijdschr Geneeskd* (Dutch) 131, 461
(1985): Tosti A+, *Contact Dermatitis* 13, 339
(1985): Valsecchi R+, *Contact Dermatitis* 13, 341
(1984): Agathos M+, *Derm Beruf Umwelt* (German) 32, 157
(1984): Lembo G+, *Contact Dermatitis* 10, 317
(1984): Santucci B+, *Contact Dermatitis* 10, 317
(1983): Przybilla B, *J Am Acad Dermatol* 9, 165

(1982): Brandao FM+, *Contact Dermatitis* 8, 140
(1982): van der Walle HB+, *Ned Tijdschr Geneeskd* (Dutch) 126, 1033
(1982): van Ketel WG, *Contact Dermatitis* 8, 71
(1980): Przybilla B+, *MMW Munch Med Wochenschr* (German) 122, 1195
(1978): Miescher P+, *Hautarzt* (German) 29, 337
(1976): Fanta D+, *Contact Dermatitis* 2, 282

Dermatitis (sic) (0.1%)
(1972): Schwab RS+, *JAMA* 222, 792

Discoloration (sic)
(1971): Parkes JD+, *Lancet* 1, 1083

Eczematous eruption (sic)
(1983): Hellgren L+, *Dermatologica* 167, 267

Edema
(1975): Butzer JF+, *Neurology* 25, 603

Erythema multiforme
(2000): Mitchell D, Thomasville, GA (from Internet) (observation)

Exanthems
(1971): Vollum DI+, *BMJ* 2, 627

Eyelid edema

Leg edema
(2002): Litt JZ, Beachwood, OH (observation)

Livedo reticularis (50–90%)
(2002): Litt JZ, Beachwood, OH (observation)
(2001): Vaughn K, (from Internet) (observation)
(2000): Litt JZ, Beachwood, OH (personal case) (observation)
(1998): Loffler H+, *Hautarzt* (German) 49, 224
(1996): Eisner J, Mount Vernon, WA (from Internet) (observation)
(1995): Paulson GW+, *Clin Neuropharmacol* 18, 466
(1975): Butzer JF+, *Neurology* 25, 603 (25%)
(1974): Kalsbeek GL+, *Ned Tijdschr Geneeskd* (Dutch) 118, 66
(1972): Schwab RS+, *JAMA* 222, 792
(1972): Silver DE+, *Neurology* 22, 665
(1971): Marchoul JC+, *Bull Soc Fr Dermatol Syphiligr* (French) 78, 236
(1971): Parkes JD+, *Lancet* 1, 1083 (90%)
(1971): Vollum DI+, *BMJ* 2, 627
(1970): Shealy CN+, *JAMA* 212, 1522 (55%)

Peripheral edema (1–10%)

Photosensitivity
(1983): van den Berg WH+, *Contact Dermatitis* 9, 165
(1974): van Ketel WG+, *Dermatologica* 148, 124

Pruritus (<1%)
(2002): Litt JZ, Beachwood, OH (observation)
(1972): Schwab RS+, *JAMA* 222, 792

Rash (sic) (<1%)

Urticaria

### Hair

Hair – alopecia
(1975): Butzer JF+, *Neurology* 25, 603 (8%)

Hair – hypertrichosis
(1975): Butzer JF+, *Neurology* 25, 603

### Nails

Nails – increased growth
(1975): Butzer JF+, *Neurology* 25, 603

### Other

Xerostomia (1–10%)
(1972): Schwab RS+, *JAMA* 222, 792
(1971): Parkes JD+, *Lancet* 1, 1085

# AMIFOSTINE

**Synonyms:** ethiofos; gammaphos
**Trade name:** Ethyol (Alza)
**Other common trade name:** *Ethyol 500*
**Indications:** Nephrotoxicity prophylaxis
**Category:** Antidote (cisplatin); cytoprotective
**Half-life:** 9 minutes

## *Reactions*

### Skin

Allergic reactions (sic)

Chills (sic) (>10%)
(2000): Sriswasdi C+, *J Med Assoc Thai* 83, 374

Flushing (>10%)
(2001): Awasthy BS+, *J Assoc Physicians India* 49, 236 (19%)
(2001): Genvresse I+, *Anticancer Drugs* 12(4), 345
(2000): Sriswasdi C+, *J Med Assoc Thai* 83, 374

Rash (sic) (<1%)
(1998): Buresh CM+, *J Pediatr Hematol Oncol* 20, 361

### Other

Dysgeusia
(2001): Genvresse I+, *Anticancer Drugs* 12(4), 345
(2000): Sriswasdi C+, *J Med Assoc Thai* 83, 374

Xerostomia
(2002): Anne PR+, *Semin Radiat Oncol* 12(1), 18
(2001): Genvresse I+, *Anticancer Drugs* 12(4), 345

# AMIKACIN

**Trade name:** Amikacin Sulfate (Elkins-Sinn)
**Other common trade names:** *Amicacina; Amicasil; Amikan; Biclin; Biklin; Gamikal; Kanbine; Lukadin; Miacin; Yectamid*
**Indications:** Short-term treatment of serious infections due to gram-negative bacteria
**Category:** Aminoglycoside antibiotic (parenteral)
**Half-life:** 1.5–2.5 hours (adults)
**Clinically important, potentially hazardous interactions with:** aldesleukin, aminoglycosides, atracurium, bumetanide, cephalexin, doxacurium, ethacrynic acid, furosemide, succinylcholine, torsemide

## *Reactions*

### Skin

Dermatitis (sic)
(1989): Rudzki E+, *Contact Dermatitis* 20, 391
(1985): Holdiness MR, *Int J Dermatol* 24, 280

Exanthems
(1977): Pollack AA+, *JAMA* 237, 562 (3.7%)
(1977): Yu VL+, *JAMA* 238, 943 (3.7%)

Pruritus
(1985): Holdiness MR, *Int J Dermatol* 24, 280

Rash (sic) (<1%)
(1995): Rodriguez-Noriega E+, *J Chemother* 7, 155

Urticaria

### Other

Injection-site induration

Injection-site necrosis
(1993): Plantin P+, *Presse Med* (French) 22, 1366

Injection-site pain

Paresthesias (<1%)

Tremors (<1%)

# AMILORIDE

**Trade names:** Midamor (Merck); Moduretic (Merck)
**Other common trade names:** *Amikal; Kaluril; Medamor; Midoride; Modamide; Nirulid; Ride*
**Indications:** Prevention of hypokalemia associated with kaliuretic diuretics and management of edema in hypertension
**Category:** Potassium-sparing antihypertensive diuretic
**Half-life:** 6–9 hours
**Clinically important, potentially hazardous interactions with:** ACE inhibitors, benazepril, captopril, cyclosporine, enalapril, fosinopril, lisinopril, moexipril, potassium salts, quinapril, quinidine, ramipril, spironolactone, trandolapril

Moduretic is amiloride and hydrochlorothiazide

### *Reactions*

#### Skin
Diaphoresis
Exanthems
(1972): *Drug Ther Bull*
Flushing (>1%)
Photosensitivity
(1981): *Aust Prescriber* 5, 23
Pruritus (<1%)
Purpura
Rash (sic) (<1%)
Urticaria
Vasculitis
Xerosis (<1%)

#### Hair
Hair – alopecia (<1%)

#### Other
Anaphylactoid reactions
Dysgeusia (<1%)
Gynecomastia (1–10%)
Paresthesias (<1%)
Tinnitus
Tremors
Xerostomia (<1%)

# AMINOCAPROIC ACID

**Trade name:** Amicar (Immunex)
**Other common trade names:** *Capramol; Caproamin; Caprolisin; Ipron; Ipsilon; Resplamin*
**Indications:** To provide hemostasis in the treatment of fibrinolysis
**Category:** Antifibrinolytic; hemostatic
**Half-life:** 1–2 hours

### *Reactions*

#### Skin
Bullous eruption
(1992): Brooke CP+, *J Am Acad Dermatol* 27, 880
Contact dermatitis
(2000): Miyamoto H+, *Contact Dermatitis* 42, 50
(1989): Shono M, *Contact Dermatitis* 21, 106
Dermatitis (sic) (systemic)
(1999): Villarreal O, *Contact Dermatitis* 40, 114
Eczematous eruption (sic)
(1989): Shono M, *Contact Dermatitis* 21, 106
Edema
Exanthems
(1995): Gonzalez-Gutierrez ML+, *Allergy* 50, 745
Kaposi's sarcoma
Pruritus
Purpura
(1985): Verstraete M, *Drugs* 29, 236
(1980): Chakrabarti A+, *BMJ* 281, 197
Rash (sic) (1–10%)
Urticaria

#### Other
Anaphylactoid reactions
Death
(2001): Fanashawe MP+, *Anesthesiology* 95(6), 1525 (2 cases)
Injection-site erythema
Injection-site phlebitis
Injection-site reactions (sic)
Muscle necrosis
Myalgia
Myopathy (1–10%)
(1988): Kane MJ+, *Am J Med* 85, 861
Rhabdomyolysis
(1997): Seymour BD+, *Ann Pharmacother* 31(1), 56
(1983): Luliri P+, *Haematologica* 68(5), 664 (2 cases)
(1983): Morris CD+, *S Afr Med J* 64(10), 363
(1982): Brown JA+, *J Neurosurg* 57(1), 130
(1982): Vanneste JA+, *Eur Neurol* 21(4), 242
(1980): Britt CW+, *Arch Neurol* 37(3), 187
(1980): Le Porrier M+, *Nouv Presse Med* 9(33), 2347
(1978): Griffin JD+, *Semin Thromb Hemost* 5(1), 27
(1969): Korsan-Bengtsen K+, *Acta Med Scand* 185(4), 341
Thrombophlebitis
Tinnitus

# AMINOGLUTETHIMIDE

**Trade name:** Cytadren (Novartis)
**Other common trade names:** *Orimeten; Orimetene; Rodazol*
**Indications:** Suppression of adrenal function, metastatic carcinoma
**Category:** Antiadrenal and antineoplastic
**Half-life:** 7–15 hours

### *Reactions*

#### Skin
Angioedema
(1967): Horky K+, *Schweiz Med Wochenschr* (German) 98, 1843
Erythema
(1987): Williams DS+, *Br J Radiology* 60, 1226
Exanthems
(1990): Vanek N+, *Med Pediatr Oncol* 18, 162
(1987): Williams DS+, *Br J Radiology* 60, 1226
(1986): Leloire O+, *Presse Med* (French) 15, 34
(1984): Coltart RS, *Br J Radiol* 57, 531
(1982): Naysmith A+, *N Engl J Med* 306, 45 (26%)
(1982): Santen RJ+, *Ann Intern Med* 96, 94 (29%)
(1980): Savaraj N+, *Med Pediatr Oncol* 8, 251
(1967): Horky K+, *Schweiz Med Wochenschr* (German) 98, 1843 (4–30%)
Exfoliative dermatitis
(1967): Horky K+, *Schweiz Med Wochenschr* (German) 98, 1843

Lupus erythematosus (>10%)
(1980): McCraken M+, *BMJ* 281, 1254
Pruritus (5%)
Purpura
(1994): Stratakis CA+, *Am J Hosp Pharm* 51, 2589
Pustular psoriasis
(1984): Coltart RS, *Br J Radiol* 57, 531
Rash (sic) (>10%)
Urticaria

### Hair

Hair – hirsutism (1–10%)

### Other

Anaphylactoid reactions
(1986): Leloire O+, *Presse Med* (French) 15, 34
Myalgia (3%)
Oral mucosal eruption
(1984): Coltart RS, *Br J Radiol* 57, 531
(1967): Horky K+, *Schweiz Med Wochenschr* (German) 98, 1843
Oral ulceration
(1984): Coltart RS, *Br J Radiol* 57, 531

## AMINOLEVULINIC ACID

**Trade name:** Levulan Kerastick* (Dusa)
**Indications:** Non-hyperkeratotic actinic keratoses of face & scalp
**Category:** Photosensitizing agent; porphyrin
**Half-life:** 30 ± 10 hours

### *Reactions*

### Skin

Burning (>50%)
(1997): Jeffes EW+, *Arch Dermatol* 133, 727
(1996): Stender IM+, *Br J Dermatol* 135, 454
Contact dermatitis
(1998): Gnaizdowska B+, *Contact Dermatitis* 38, 348
Crusting (64–71%)
(2000): Hongcharu W+, *J Invest Dermatol* 115, 183
(1995): Lang S+, *Laryngorhinootologie* (German) 74, 85
Edema (35%)
(1997): Jeffes EW+, *Arch Dermatol* 133, 727
(1995): Lang S+, *Laryngorhinootologie* (German) 74, 85
Erosion (14%)
Erythema (99%)
(1997): Jeffes EW+, *Arch Dermatol* 133, 727
(1995): Lang S+, *Laryngorhinootologie* 74, 85
Exfoliation (when treated for acne)
(2000): Hongcharu W+, *J Invest Dermatol* 115, 183
(1996): Stender IM+, *Br J Dermatol* 135(3), 454
Hypopigmentation (22%)
Koebner phenomenon (psoriasis)
(1996): Stender IM+, *Acta Derm Venereol* 76, 392
Melanoma
(1997): Wolf P+, *Dermatology* 194, 53 (on scalp)
Photosensitivity
Pigmentation (when treated for acne) (22%)
(2000): Hongcharu W+, *J Invest Dermatol* 115, 183
Pruritus (25%)
Pustular eruption (<4%)
Scaling (64–71%)
Stinging (>50%)
(1997): Jeffes EW+, *Arch Dermatol* 133, 727
Ulceration (4%)
Vesiculation (4%)

### Other

Dysesthesia (2%)

***Note:** To be used in conjunction with the Blue Light Photodynamic Therapy Illuminator

## AMINOPHYLLINE

**Synonym:** theophylline ethylenediamine
**Trade names:** Aerolate; Aminophyllin; Bronkodyl; Choledyl; Elixophyllin; Norphyl; Phyllocontin; Quibron; Slo-Bid; Somophyllin; Theo-Dur; Truphylline
**Other common trade names:** *Corophyllin; Euphyllin; Palaron; Phyllotemp; Planphylline; Tefamin*
**Indications:** Prevention or treatment of reversible bronchospasm
**Category:** Xanthine bronchodilator
**Half-life:** 3–15 hours (in adult nonsmokers)
**Clinically important, potentially hazardous interactions with:** cimetidine, erythromycin, halothane

### *Reactions*

### Skin

Allergic reactions (sic) (<1%)
(1986): Cusano F+, *G Ital Dermatol Venereol* (Italian) 121, 443
(1985): Editorial, *Lancet* 1, 289
(1983): Gibb W+, *Br Med J (Clin Res Ed)* 13, 501
(1983): Hardy C+, *Br Med J (Clin Res Ed)* 286, 2051
Baboon syndrome
(1999): Guin JD+, *Contact Dermatitis* 40, 170
Contact dermatitis
(1994): Corazza M+, *Contact Dermatitis* 31, 328
(1984): Editorial, *Lancet* 2, 1192
(1983): Berman BA+, *Cutis* 31, 594
(1983): van den Berg WH+, *Ned Tijdschr Geneeskd* (Dutch) 127, 1801
(1980): Vazquez Botet M, *Bol Asoc Med P R* (Spanish) 72, 14
(1959): Baer RL+, *Arch Dermatol* 79, 647
Cutaneous side effects (sic)
(1995): Simon PA+, *JAMA* 273, 1737
Dermatitis (sic)
(1985): Editorial, *Lancet* 2, 1192
(1978): Tsyrkunova LP+, *Gig Tr Prof Zabol* (Russian) October, 52
Diaphoresis
Exanthems
(1985): Editorial, *Lancet* 2, 1192
(1984): Thompson PJ+, *Thorax* 39, 600
(1983): Hardy C+, *BMJ* 286, 2051
(1981): de Shazo RD+, *Ann Allergy* 46, 152
(1980): Lawyer CH+, *J Allergy Clin Immunol* 65, 353
Exfoliative dermatitis
(1984): Thompson PJ+, *Thorax* 39, 600
(1982): Nierenberg DW+, *West J Med* 137, 328
(1981): Elias JA+, *Am Rev Respir Dis* 123, 550
(1979): Bernstein JE+, *Arch Dermatol* 115, 360
(1976): Petrozzi JW+, *Arch Dermatol* 112, 525
(1958): Tas J+, *Acta Allergologica* 12, 39
Flushing
Pruritus
(1980): Lawyer CH+, *J Allergy Clin Immunol* 65, 353
(1971): Davidson MB, *N Engl J Med* 285, 689
(1971): Wong D+, *J Allergy* 48, 165
Rash (sic) (<1%)

(1983): Hardy C+, *BMJ* 286, 2051
Shakiness (sic)
Stevens–Johnson syndrome
(1989): Hidalgo HA, *Pediatr Pulmonol* 6, 209 (theophylline)
Urticaria
(1994): Urbani CE, *Contact Dermatitis* 31, 198
(1985): Editorial, *Lancet* 2, 1192
(1984): Thompson PJ+, *Thorax* 39, 600
(1982): Neumann H, *Dtsch Med Wochenschr* (German) 107, 116
(1979): Booth BH+, *Ann Allergy* 43, 289
(1971): Wong D+, *J Allergy* 48, 165

### Hair

Hair – alopecia

### Other

Hypersensitivity
(1999): Yoshizawa A+, *Arerugi* (Japanese) 48, 1206 (from ethylenediamine)
(1985): Gibb WR, *Lancet* 1, 49
(1981): Elias JA+, *Am Rev Respir Dis* 123, 550
(1970): Foussereau J+, *Bull Soc Fr Dermatol Syphiligr* (French) 77, 415
(1967): Sonnischen N, *Allerg Asthma Leipz* (German) 13, 215
(1967): Sonnischen N, *Allerg Asthma Leipz* (German) 13, 259
Parosmia
Rhabdomyolysis
(1991): Aoshima M+, *Nihon Kyobu Shikkan Gakki Zasshi* 29(8), 1064

## AMINOSALICYLATE SODIUM

**Synonyms:** para-aminosalicylate sodium; PAS
**Trade names:** Paser Granules (Jacobus); Sodium P.A.S. (Lannett); Tubasal
**Other common trade names:** *Aminox; Eupasal; Nemasol*
**Indications:** Tuberculosis
**Category:** Antimycobacterial; anti-inflammatory
**Half-life:** 45–60 minutes

***Reactions***

### Skin

Allergic reactions (sic)
(1988): Fardy JM+, *J Clin Gastroenterol* 10, 635
Angioedema
(1964): Lajouanine P+, *Ann Pédiatr* (Paris) (French) 40, 620
(1959): Bereston ES, *J Invest Dermatol* 33, 427
Bullous eruption
(1964): Lajouanine P+, *Ann Pédiatr* (Paris) (French) 40, 620
(1959): Bereston ES, *J Invest Dermatol* 33, 427
Eczematous eruption (sic) (<1%)
Erythema multiforme
(1963): Van Ketel WG, *Ned Tijdschr Geneeskd* (Dutch) 107, 952
Exanthems
(1988): Gron I+, *Ugeskr Laeger* (Danish) 150, 32
(1982): Nagaratnam N, *Postgrad Med J* 58, 729
(1968): Sarkany I, *Proc R Soc Med* 61, 891
(1964): Duncan JT, *Am Rev Respir Dis* 89, 103
(1964): Lajouanine P+, *Ann Pédiatr* (Paris) (French) 40, 620
(1963): Filoz-Diaz JA+, *Archos Méd Panama* (Spanish) 12, 68
(1960): Simpson DG+, *Am J Med* 29, 297 (1–5%)
(1959): Bereston ES, *J Invest Dermatol* 33, 427 (1–5%)
(1950): Cuthbert J, *Lancet* 2, 209
Exfoliative dermatitis
(1972): Kauppinen K, *Acta Derm Venereol* (Stockh) 52 (suppl), 68
(1967): Coleman WP, *Med Clin North Am* 51, 1073
(1965): Griffiths HED+, *J Bone Joint Surg* (Edinburgh) 47, 86
(1964): Bower G, *Am Rev Respir Dis* 89, 440
(1964): Lajouanine P+, *Ann Pédiatr* (Paris) (French) 40, 620
(1961): Gupta SK, *Indian J Dermatol* 6, 115
Fixed eruption
(1972): Levantine A+, *Br J Dermatol* 86, 604
(1965): Laszczka C, *Gruzlica* (Polish) 33, 935
(1965): Snelling MRJ+, *Tubercle* 46, 284
(1961): Welch AL+, *Arch Dermatol* 84, 1004
(1952): Warring FC+, *Am Rev Tuberc Pulm Dis* 65, 235
(1949): Kierland RR+, *Proc Staff Meet Mayo Clin* 24, 539
Lichenoid eruption
(1971): Almeyda J+, *Br J Dermatol* 95, 604
(1964): Baker H+, *Br J Dermatol* 76, 186
(1953): Shatin H+, *J Invest Dermatol* 21, 135
Lupus erythematosus
(1985): Holdiness MR, *Int J Dermatol* 24, 280
(1961): Bickers JN+, *N Engl J Med* 265, 131
Lymphoma (benign)
(1982): Nagaratnam N, *Postgrad Med J* 58, 729
Photosensitivity
(1972): Kuokkanen K, *Acta Allergol* 27, 407
(1971): Girard JP, *Helv Med Acta* 36, 3
(1964): Lajouanine P+, *Ann Pédiatr* (Paris) (French) 40, 620
Pruritus
(1968): No Author, *BMJ* 3, 664
(1964): Berté SJ+, *Am Rev Respir Dis* 90, 598
(1960): Simpson DG+, *Am J Med* 29, 297
Purpura
(1980): Miescher PA+, *Clin Haematol* 9, 505
(1963): Filoz-Diaz JA+, *Archos Méd Panama* (Spanish) 12, 68
(1959): Bereston ES, *J Invest Dermatol* 33, 427
(1952): Warring FC+, *Am Rev Tuberc Pulm Dis* 65, 235
Toxic epidermal necrolysis
(1963): Filoz-Diaz JA+, *Archos Méd Panama* (Spanish) 12, 68
Urticaria
(1964): Lajouanine P+, *Ann Pédiatr* (Paris) (French) 40, 620
(1961): Gupta SK, *Indian J Dermatol* 6, 115
(1960): Simpson DG+, *Am J Med* 29, 297
(1959): Bereston ES, *J Invest Dermatol* 33, 427
(1952): Warring FC+, *Am Rev Tuberc Pulm Dis* 65, 235
Vasculitis (<1%)
(1972): Levantine A+, *Br J Dermatol* 87, 646

### Hair

Hair – alopecia
(1982): Kutty PK+, *Ann Intern Med* 97, 785
(1965): Griffiths HED+, *J Bone Joint Surg* (Edinburgh) 47, 86
(1960): Simpson DG+, *Am J Med* 29, 297
(1951): Grandjean LC, *Acta Derm Venereol* (Stockh) 31, 615

### Other

Hypersensitivity
Oral lichenoid eruption
Oral mucosal eruption
(1964): Lajouanine P+, *Ann Pédiatr* (Paris) (French) 40, 620
(1960): Simpson DG+, *Am J Med* 29, 297

# AMIODARONE

**Trade names:** Cordarone (Wyeth); Pacerone (Upsher-Smith)
**Other common trade names:** *Aratac; Corbionax; Cordarex; Cordarone X; Tachydaron*
**Indications:** Ventricular fibrillation, ventricular tachycardia
**Category:** Class III antiarrhythmic
**Half-life:** 26–107 days
**Clinically important, potentially hazardous interactions with:** amprenavir, anisindione, anticoagulants, arsenic, ciprofloxacin, dicumarol, digoxin, diltiazem, enoxacin, fentanyl, gatifloxacin, lomefloxacin, methotrexate, moxifloxacin, norfloxacin, ofloxacin, quinidine, quinolones, rifabutin, rifampin, rifapentine, ritonavir, sparfloxacin, verapamil, warfarin

## *Reactions*

### Skin

Allergic reactions (sic)
(1989): Reingardene DI, *Klin Med Mosk* (Russian) 67, 128
Angioedema
(2000): Burches E+, *Allergy* 55, 1199
Basal cell carcinoma
(1995): Monk BE, *Br J Dermatol* 133, 148
Cutaneous side effects (sic)
(1994): Shukla R+, *Postgrad Med J* 70, 492
Diaphoresis
(1985): Raeder EA+, *Am Heart J* 109, 979 (0.5%)
(1983): McGovern B+, *BMJ* 287, 175 (2.5%)
Ecchymoses (<1%)
Edema (1–10%)
Erythema multiforme
(2002): Yung A+, *Australas J Dermatol* 43(1), 35
Erythema nodosum (<1%)
(1983): Fogoros RN+, *Circulation* 68, 88 (1%)
(1976): Rosenbaum MB+, *Am J Cardiol* 38, 934
Exanthems
(1985): Raeder EA+, *Am Heart J* 109, 975 (0.9%)
(1984): Rotmensch HH+, *Ann Intern Med* 101, 462 (0.7%)
(1983): Fogoros RN+, *Circulation* 68, 88 (2%)
(1983): Harris L+, *Circulation* 67, 45
(1969): Kappart A, *Z Ther* (German) #8, 474
Exfoliative dermatitis
(1988): Moots RJ+, *BMJ* 296, 1332
Facial erythema (3.1%)
(1984): Rotmensch HH+, *Ann Intern Med* 101, 462
(1983): Harris L+, *Circulation* 67, 45
Flushing (1–10%)
Iododerma
(1997): Ricci C+, *Ann Dermatol Venereol* (French) 124, 260
(1975): Porters JE+, *Arch Dermatol* 111, 1656
(1975): Zantkuyl CF+, *Dermatologica* 151, 311
Keratosis pilaris
(1999): Capper N, Mobile, AL (from Internet) (observation)
Linear IgA bullous dermatosis
(2002): Cohen LM+, *J Am Acad Dermatol* 46, S32 (passim)
(1996): Primka EJ+, *J Cutan Pathol* 23, 58
(1996): Tranvan A+, *J Am Acad Dermatol* 35, 865
(1994): Primka EJ+, *J Am Acad Dermatol* 31, 809
(1990): Espagne E+, *Ann Dermatol Venereol* (French) 117, 898
Lupus erythematosus
(2002): Sheikhzadeh A+, *Arch Intern Med* 162(7), 834
(1999): Susano R+, *Ann Rheum Dis* 58, 655
(1985): Raeder EA+, *Am Heart J* 109, 979 (4.6%)
Photosensitivity (10–30%)
(2000): Burns KE+, *Can Respir* 7, 193 (passim)
(1997): O'Reilly FM+, American Academy of Dermatology Meeting, Poster #14
(1995): Collins P+, *Br J Dermatol* 132, 956
(1995): Tisdale JE+, *J Clin Pharmacol* 35, 351
(1995): Zehender M, *Circulation* 92, 1665
(1993): Allen JE, *Clin Pharm* 12, 580
(1993): Ettler K+, *Sb Ved Pr Lek Fak Karlovy Univerzity Hradci KraloveD Suppl (Czech) 36, 305* (9.4%)
(1992): Editorial, *JAMA* 267, 3322
(1992): Gosselink AT+, *JAMA* 267, 3289
(1990): Monk B, *Clin Exp Dermatol* 15, 319
(1989): Rappersberger K+, *J Invest Dermatol* 93, 201
(1988): Hyatt RH+, *Age Aging* 17, 116 (10%)
(1988): Parodi A, *Photodermatology* 5, 146
(1987): Roupe G+, *Acta Derm Venereol* (Stockh) 67, 76
(1987): Waitzer S+, *J Am Acad Dermatol* 16, 779
(1986): Boyle J, *Br J Dermatol* 115, 253
(1986): Ferguson J, *Br J Clin Pract Symp* Suppl 44, 63
(1986): Ljunggren B+, *Photodermatol* 3, 26
(1986): Toback AC+, *Dermatol Clin* 4, 223
(1986): Török L+, *Hautarzt* (German) 37, 507 (24%)
(1985): Ferguson J+, *Br J Dermatol* 113, 537
(1985): Mulrow JP+, *Ann Int Med* 103, 68
(1985): Raeder EA+, *Am Heart J* 109, 979 (4.6%)
(1985): Stäubli M, *Postgrad Med J* 61, 245
(1985): Vila Serra MD+, *Med Clin (Barc)* (Spanish) 84, 379
(1984): Diffey BL+, *Clin Exp Dermatol* 9, 248
(1984): Ferguson J+, *Lancet* 2, 414
(1984): Guerciolini R+, *Lancet* 1, 962
(1984): Kaufmann G, *Lancet* 1, 51
(1984): Walter JF+, *Arch Dermatol* 120, 1591
(1984): Zachary CB+, *Br J Dermatol* 110, 451
(1983): Fogoros RN+, *Circulation* 68, 88 (11%)
(1983): Harris L+, *Circulation* 67, 45 (57%)
(1983): McGovern B+, *BMJ* 287, 175 (8.75%)
(1983): Nadamanee K+, *Ann Intern Med* 98, 577 (5.3%)
(1982): Chalmers RJ+, *Br Med J Clin Res Ed* 285, 341
Pigmentation
(2001): Dereure O, *Am J Clin Dermatol* 2(4), 253
(2001): Haas N+, *Arch Dermatol* 137, 313 (blue-gray)
(2001): High WA+, *N Engl J Med* 345, 1464
(2001): Rubegni P+, *Am Fam Physician* 63, 1409
(2000): Burns KE+, *Can Respir* 7, 193 (passim)
(2000): Gutknecht DR, *Cutis* 66, 294 (blue-gray)
(1999): Karrer S+, *Arch Dermatol* 135, 251
(1997): Sivaram CA+, *N Engl J Med* 337, 1813
(1996): Ammann R+, *Hautarzt* (German) 47, 930
(1996): Kounis NG+, *Clin Cardiol* 19, 592
(1995): Tisdale JE+, *J Clin Pharmacol* 35, 351 (blue-gray)
(1993): Balslev E+, *Ugeskr Laeger* (Danish) 155, 4014 (blue-gray)
(1993): Colquhoun JP, *Aust Fam Physician* 22, 2168
(1993): Ettler K+, *Sb Ved Pr Lek Fak Karlovy Univerzity Hradci Kralove* Suppl *(Czech) 36, 305* (9.4%)
(1992): Editorial, *JAMA* 267, 3322
(1992): Fitzpatrick JE, *Derm Clinics* 10, 19
(1992): Son En Ai+, *Klin Med Mosk* (Russian) 70, 46
(1991): Blackshear JL+, *Mayo Clin Proc* 66, 721
(1991): Fazekas T+, *Szent Gyorgyi Albert Orvostudomanyi Egyetem* (Hungarian) 132, 2157
(1990): Brazzelli V+, *G Ital Dermatol Venereol* (Italian) 125, 521
(1989): Klein AD+, *Arch Dermatol* 125, 417
(1989): Rappersberger K+, *J Invest Dermatol* 93, 201
(1989): Reingardene DI, *Kardiologiia* (Russian) 29, 112
(1988): Beukema WP+, *Am J Cardiol* 62, 1146
(1988): Zadionchenko VS+, *Klin Med Mosk* (Russian) 66, 126
(1987): Goldstein GD+, *Chest* 91, 772
(1987): Waitzer S+, *J Am Acad Dermatol* 16, 779
(1986): Dowson JH+, *Arch Dermatol* 122, 244
(1986): Rappersberger K+, *Br J Dermatol* 114, 189
(1986): Török L+, *Hautarzt* (German) 37, 507

(1985): Alinovi A+, *J Am Acad Dermatol* 12, 563
(1985): Lakatos A, *Orv Hetil* (Hungarian) 126, 1343
(1985): Varotti C+, *G Ital Dermatol Venereol* (Italian) 120, 183
(1984): Miller RAW+, *Arch Dermatol* 120, 646
(1984): Onofrey BE+, *J Am Optom Assoc* 55, 337
(1984): Rotmensch HH+, *Ann Intern Med* 101, 462 (4.6%)
(1984): Weiss SR+, *J Am Acad Dermatol* 11, 898
(1984): Zachary CB+, *Br J Dermatol* 110, 451
(1983): Harris L+, *Circulation* 67, 45 (1.4%)
(1983): McGovern B+, *BMJ* 287, 175
(1983): Trimble JW+, *Arch Dermatol* 119, 914
(1982): Ferrer I+, *Med Clin (Barc)* (Spanish) 79, 355
(1982): Quintanilla E+, *Med Cutan Ibero Lat Am* (Spanish) 10, 177
(1981): Granstein RD+, *J Am Acad Dermatol* 5, 1 (blue-gray)
(1981): Korting HC+, *Hautarzt* (German) *32, 301*
(1979): Nageli U+, *Schweiz Med Wochenschr* (German) 109, 1708
(1978): Cassilas-Ruiz JA+, *Rev Esp Cardiol* (Spanish) 31, 617
(1975): Delage C+, Can Med Assoc J 112(10), 1205
(1975): Lambert D+, *Ann Dermatol Syphiligr Paris* (French) 102, 277
(1974): Olmos L+, *Med Cutan Ibero Lat Am* (Spanish) 2, 447
(1972): Balouet G+, *Arch Anat Pathol* (Paris) (French) 20, 265
(1971): Labouche F+, *Bull Soc Fr Dermatol Syphiligr* (French) 78, 27
(1971): Thiers H+, *Bull Soc Fr Dermatol Syphiligr* (French) 78, 548

Pruritus (1–5%)
(1969): Kappart A, *Z Ther* (German) #8, 474 (4.1%)
(1968): Leutenegger A+, *Schweiz Med Wochenschr* (German) 98, 2020 (4.1%)

Psoriasis
(1986): Abel EA+, *J Am Acad Dermatol* 15, 1007
(1982): Muir AD, *N Z Med J* 95, 711

Purpura (2%)
(1983): Fogoros RN+, *Circulation* 68, 88

Pustular psoriasis
(1982): Muir AD, *N Z Med J* 95, 711

Rash (sic) (<1%)

Rosacea
(1987): Reifler DM+, *Am J Ophthalmol* 103, 594

Stevens–Johnson syndrome (<1%)

Toxic epidermal necrolysis
(2002): Yung A+, *Australas J Dermatol* 43(1), 35 (fatal)
(2000): Danby WF, Manchester, NH (from Internet) (observation)
(1985): Bencini PL+, *Arch Dermatol* 121, 838

Urticaria
(1983): McGovern B+, *BMJ* 287, 175 (1.25%)

Vasculitis (<1%)
(2001): Scharf C+, *Lancet* 358, 2045
(1994): Dootson G+, *Clin Exp Dermatol* 19, 422
(1994): Gutierrez R+, *Ann Pharmacother* 28, 537
(1985): Starke ID+, *BMJ* 291, 940
(1985): Stäubli M, *Postgrad Med J* 61, 245

### Hair

Hair – alopecia (<1%)
(2000): Litt JZ, Beachwood, OH (personal case) (observation) (after 2 weeks of therapy)
(1995): Ahmad S, *Arch Intern Med* 155, 1106
(1992): Samuel LM+, *Postgrad Med J* 68, 771
(1985): Raeder EA+, *Am Heart J* 109, 979 (4.1%)
(1984): Rotmensch HH+, *Ann Intern Med* 101, 462 (0.7%)
(1983): McGovern B+, *BMJ* 287, 175 (2.5%)

Hair – hypertrichosis
(1985): Ferguson J+, *Br J Dermatol* 113, 537

### Other

Death
(2002): Kharabsheh S+, *Am J Cardiol* 89(7), 896
(2002): Yung A+, *Australas J Dermatol* 43(1), 35

Dyschromatopsia
(2002): Ikaheimo K+, *Acta Ophthalmol Scand* 80(1), 59

Dysgeusia (1–10%)
(1983): McGovern B+, *BMJ* 287, 175

Paresthesias (4–9%)

Parosmia (1–10%)

Pseudoporphyria
(1988): Parodi A, *Photodermatology* 5, 146

Pseudotumor cerebri (<1%)

Sialorrhea (1–3%)

Tremors

## AMITRIPTYLINE

**Trade names:** Elavil (AstraZeneca); Limbitrol (ICN)
**Other common trade names:** *Amineurin; Domical; Laroxyl; Lentizol; Levate; Novotriptyn; Saroten; Tryptanol; Tryptizol*
**Indications:** Depression
**Category:** Tricyclic antidepressant; antimigraine
**Half-life:** 10–25 hours
**Clinically important, potentially hazardous interactions with:** amprenavir, clonidine, epinephrine, guanethidine, isocarboxazid, linezolid, MAO inhibitors, phenelzine, quinolones, sparfloxacin, tranylcypromine

Limbitrol is amitriptyline and chlordiazepoxide

### *Reactions*

### Skin

Acne

Allergic reactions (sic) (<1%)

Angioedema
(1999): Garcia-Doval I+, *Cutis* 63, 35 (passim)

Bullous eruption (<1%)
(1979): Herschthal D+, *Arch Dermatol* 115, 499

Dermatitis (sic)
(1966): Hollister LE+, *J Nerv Ment Dis* 142, 460

Dermatitis herpetiformis
(1969): Rhyner K, *Diss Zürich* (German)

Diaphoresis (1–10%)
(1995): Feder R, *J Clin Psychiatry* 56, 35

Erythema

Erythema annulare centrifugum
(1999): Garcia-Doval I+, *Cutis* 63, 35

Erythroderma
(1999): Garcia-Doval I+, *Cutis* 63, 35 (passim)

Exanthems

Exfoliative dermatitis

Facial edema

Fixed eruption
(1998): McCarthy J, Ft. Worth, TX (from Internet) (observation)

Flushing

Lichen planus
(1999): Garcia-Doval I+, *Cutis* 63, 35 (passim)

Lupus erythematosus
(1993): Dove FB, *Hosp Pract Off Ed* 28, 14

Necrosis
(1999): Fogarty BJ+, *Burns* 25, 768

Petechiae

Photosensitivity (<1%)
(1999): Garcia-Doval I+, *Cutis* 63, 35 (passim)
(1996): Taniguchi S+, *Am J Hematol* 53, 49
(1966): Hollister LE+, *J Nerv Ment Dis* 142, 460
Pigmentation
(1999): Garcia-Doval I+, *Cutis* 63, 35 (passim)
(1988): Warnock JK+, *Am J Psychiatry* 145, 425
(1985): Basler RS+, *J Am Acad Dermatol* 12, 577
Pruritus
(1999): Garcia-Doval I+, *Cutis* 63, 35 (passim)
(1988): Larrey D+, *Gastroenterology* 94, 200
(1966): Hollister LE+, *J Nerv Ment Dis* 142, 460
Purpura
(1999): Garcia-Doval I+, *Cutis* 63, 35 (passim)
(1971): Kozakova M, *Cesk Dermatol* (Czech) 46, 158
Rash (sic)
Urticaria
Vasculitis
(1969): Gisslén H+, *Dermatol Monatsschr* (German) 155, 783

## Hair

Hair – alopecia (<1%)
(1992): Breathnach SM+, *Adverse Drug Reactions and the Skin* Blackwell, Oxford, 196 (passim)

## Other

Ageusia
Anaphylactoid reactions
Black tongue
Bromhidrosis
Dysgeusia (>10%)
Galactorrhea (<1%)
Glossitis
Gynecomastia (<1%)
Hypersensitivity
(2000): Milionis HJ, *Postgrad Med J* 76, 361
Lymphoid hyperplasia
(1995): Crowson AN+, *Arch Dermatol* 131, 925
Oral mucosal eruption
(1964): Pollack B+, *Am J Psychiatry* 121, 384
Paresthesias
Parkinsonism
Pseudolymphoma
(1995): Crowson AN+, *Arch Dermatol* 131, 925
(1995): Magro CM+, *J Am Acad Dermatol* 32, 419
Rhabdomyolysis
(1983): Caruana RJ+, *N C Med* 44(1), 18 (with lorazepam and perphenazine)
Sialopenia
(1995): Loesche WJ+, *J Am Geriatr Soc* 43, 401
Sialorrhea
Stomatitis
(1988): Larrey D+, *Gastroenterology* 94, 200
Stomatopyrosis
Tinnitus
Tongue edema
Tremors
Vaginitis
Xerostomia (>10%)
(1996): Rani PU+, *Anesth Analg* 83, 371
(1995): Loesche WJ+, *J Am Geriatr Soc* 43, 401
(1966): Hollister LE+, *J Nerv Ment Dis* 142, 467

# AMLODIPINE

**Trade names:** Lotrel (Novartis); Norvasc (Pfizer)
**Other common trade names:** *Amdepin; Amlodin; Amlogard; Amlopin; Amlor; Istin; Norvas*
**Indications:** Hypertension, angina
**Category:** Calcium channel blocker; antianginal; antihypertensive
**Half-life:** 30–50 hours
**Clinically important, potentially hazardous interactions with:** epirubicin, imatinib

Lotrel is amlodipine and benazepril

### *Reactions*

## Skin

Ankle edema
(2001): Zanchetti A+, *J Cardiovasc Pharmacol* 38(4), 642
Dermatitis (sic) (1–10%)
Diaphoresis (<1%)
Discoloration (sic) (<1%)
Edema (5–14%)
(2001): Chugh SK+, *J Cardiovasc Pharmacol* 38(3), 356
(1996): Corea L+, *Clin Pharmacol Ther* 60, 341
(1992): DiBianco R+, *Clin Cardiol* 15, 519
(1992): Johnson BF+, *Am J Hypertens* 5, 727
(1991): Elliott HL+, *Postgrad Med J* 67, S20
(1991): Murdoch D+, *Drugs* 41, 478
(1989): Chahine RA+, *Am Heart J* 118, 1128
(1989): Doyle GD+, *Eur J Clin Pharmacol* 36, 205 (ankle)
(1989): Estrada JN+, *Am Heart J* 118, 1130
(1989): Osterloh I, *Am Heart J* 118, 1114
(1988): Glasser SP+, *Am J Cardiol* 62, 518
Erythema multiforme
(1993): Bewley AP+, *BMJ* 307, 241
Exanthems (2–4%)
(1989): Doyle GD+, *Eur J Clin Pharmacol* 36, 205
Flushing (1–10%)
(1992): *Med Lett Drugs Ther* 34, 99
(1992): Johnson BF+, *Am J Hypertens* 5, 727
(1991): Murdoch D+, *Drugs* 41, 478
(1989): Osterloh I, *Am Heart J* 118, 1114
Granuloma annulare
(2002): Lim AC+, *Australas J Dermatol* 43(1), 24
Lichen planus
(2001): Swale VJ+, *Br J Dermatol* 144, 920
Lichenoid eruption
(1998): Silver B, Deerfield, IL (from Internet) (observation)
Lupus erythematosus
(2002): Boye T+, *World Congress Dermatol* Poster 0088
Peripheral edema (>10%)
(2002): Litt JZ, Beachwood, OH (personal case) (observation)
(2001): Lenz TL+, *Pharmacotherapy* 21(8), 898 (4 cases) (with nisoldipine)
(1994): Clavijo GA+, *Am J Hosp Pharm* 51, 59
(1993): Ellis JS+, *Lancet* 341, 1102
Petechiae (<1%)
Pruritus (2–4%)
(1998): Litt JZ, Beachwood, OH (personal case) (observation)
(1997): Orme S+, *BMJ* 315, 463
(1994): Baker BA+, *Ann Pharmacother* 28, 118
(1993): Ellis JS+, *Lancet 341*, 1102
Purpura (<1%)
(1994): Dacosta A+, *Therapie* (French) 49, 515
Rash (sic) (1–10%)
Telangiectases (facial)
(2000): Grabczynska SA+, *Br J Dermatol* 142, 1255

(1999): van der Vleuten CJ+, *Acta Derm Venereol* 79, 323
(1997): Basarab T+, *Br J Dermatol* 136, 974 (photo-induced)
Urticaria (<1%)
Vasculitis
(1995): del Rio Fermandez MC+, *Rev Clin Esp* (Spanish) 195, 738
Xerosis (<0.1%)

### Hair

Hair – alopecia (<1%)

### Other

Acute intermittent porphyria
(1997): Kepple A+, *Ann Pharmacother* 31, 253
Dysgeusia (<1%)
Gingival hyperplasia
(2001): Morisaki I+, *Spec Care Dentist* 21(2), 60
(2000): James JA+, *J Clin Periodontol* 27, 109 (with cyclosporine)
(1999): Ellis JS+, *J Periodontol* 70, 63 (3.3%)
(1999): van der Vleuten CJ+, *Acta Derm Venereol* 79, 323
(1997): Infante-Cossio P+, *An Med Interna* (Spanish) 14, 83
(1997): Jorgensen MG, *J Periodontol* 68, 676
(1995): Salerno L+, *Clin Ter* (Italian) 146, 275
(1995): Wynn RL, *Gen Dent* 43, 218
(1994): Juncadella Garcia E+, *Med Clin (Barc)* (Spanish) 103, 358
(1994): Seymour RA+, *J Clin Periodontol* 21, 281
(1993): Ellis JS+, *Lancet* 341, 1102
(1993): Smith RG, *Br Dent J* 175, 279
(1991): Wynn RL, *Gen Dent* 39, 240
Gynecomastia
(1994): Zochling J+, *Med J Aust* 160, 807
Hypesthesia (<1%)
Paresthesias (<1%)
Parosmia (<0.1%)
Tendinitis
(1999): Zambanini A+, *J Hum Hypertens* 13, 565 (Achilles)
Tinnitus
Tremors
Xerostomia (<1%)

## AMOBARBITAL

**Trade name:** Amytal (Lilly)
**Other common trade names:** *Amytal Sodium; Isoamitil Sedante; Neur-Amyl; Novambarb; Sodium Amytal*
**Indications:** Insomnia, sedation
**Category:** Intermediate-acting barbiturate; anticonvulsant; hypnotic; sedative
**Half-life:** initial: 40 minutes; terminal: 20 hours
**Clinically important, potentially hazardous interactions with: alcohol**, dicumarol, ethanolamine, warfarin

#### *Reactions*

### Skin

Acne
Angioedema
Bullous eruption
Erythema
(1979): Rudzki E, *Przegl Dermatol* (Polish) 66, 415
Exanthems
Exfoliative dermatitis (<1%)
Photosensitivity
Purpura
Rash (sic) (<1%)
Stevens–Johnson syndrome (<1%)
Toxic epidermal necrolysis
(1969): Strom J, *Scand J Infect Dis* 1, 209
Urticaria (<1%)

### Other

Hypersensitivity
Injection-site pain (>10%)
Rhabdomyolysis
(1990): Larpin R+, *Presse Med* 19(30), 1403
Serum sickness
Thrombophlebitis (<1%)

## AMOXAPINE

**Trade name:** Amoxapine (Watson)
**Other common trade names:** *Amoxan; Asendis; Defanyl; Demolox*
**Indications:** Depression
**Category:** Tricyclic antidepressant
**Half-life:** 11–30 hours
**Clinically important, potentially hazardous interactions with:** amprenavir, clonidine, epinephrine, guanethidine, isocarboxazid, linezolid, MAO inhibitors, phenelzine, quinolones, sparfloxacin, tranylcypromine

#### *Reactions*

### Skin

Acne
Acute generalized exanthematous pustulosis (AGEP)
(1998): Loche F+, *Acta Derm Venereol* 78, 224
(1994): Larbre B+, *Ann Dermatol Venereol* (French) 121, 40
Allergic reactions (sic) (<1%)
Cutaneous side effects (sic) (5.1%)
(1982): Jue SG+, *Drugs* 24, 1
Dermatitis (sic)
Diaphoresis (1–10%)
Edema (>1%)
Erythema multiforme (observation)
(1982): Bishop L, *ADRRS* oral communication
Exanthems
(1996): Nagayama H+, *J Dermatol* 23, 899
(1982): Jue SG+, *Drugs* 24, 1
Flushing
Petechiae
Photosensitivity (<1%)
Pruritus (<1%)
(1988): Warnock JK+, *Am J Psychiatry* 145, 425
Pseudoparkinsonism (sic)
Purpura
Rash (sic) (>1%)
Toxic epidermal necrolysis
(1988): Warnock JK+, *Am J Psychiatry* 145, 425
(1983): Camisa C+, *Arch Dermatol* 119, 709
Urticaria (<1%)
Vasculitis (<1%)
(1988): Warnock JK+, *Am J Psychiatry* 145, 425
Xerosis

### Hair

Hair – alopecia (<1%)

### Other

Black tongue
Bromhidrosis

Dysgeusia (>10%)
Galactorrhea (<1%)
(1979): Gelenberg AJ+, *JAMA* 242, 1900
(1978): Jaffe K, *J Clin Psychiatry* 39, 821
Glossitis
Gynecomastia (<1%)
Paresthesias (<1%)
Sialorrhea
Stomatitis
Tinnitus
Tremors
Vaginitis
Xerostomia (14%)
(1982): Jue SG+, *Drugs* 24, 1

# AMOXICILLIN

**Synonym:** amoxycillin
**Trade names:** Amoxil (GSK); Augmentin (GSK); Prevpac (TAP)
**Other common trade names:** *A-Gram; Acimox; Almodan; Amodex; Apo-Amoxi; Clamoxyl; Eupen; Fisamox; Lin-Amnox; Novamoxin; Nu-Amoxi; Pro-Amox*
**Indications:** Infections of the respiratory tract, skin and urinary tract
**Category:** Aminopenicillin antibiotic
**Half-life:** 0.7–1.4 hours
**Clinically important, potentially hazardous interactions with:** allopurinol, chloramphenicol, demeclocycline, doxycycline, erythromycin, methotrexate, minocycline, oxytetracycline, sulfonamides, tetracyclines

Augmentin is amoxicillin and clavulanate

## *Reactions*

### Skin

Acute generalized exanthematous pustulosis (AGEP)
(2002): Pattee SF+, *Arch Dermatol* 138(8), 1091
(2001): de Thier F+, *Contact Dermatitis* 44, 114
(2000): Meadows KP+, *Pediatric Dermatology* 17, 399
(1997): Gibert-Agullo A+, *An Esp Pediatr* (Spanish) 46, 285
(1997): Zabawski, E, Dallas, TX (from Internet) (observation)
(1996): Wolkenstein P+, *Contact Dermatitis* 35, 234
(1995): Moreau A+, *Int J Dermatol* 34, 263 (passim)
(1991): Roujeau J-C+, *Arch Dermatol* 127, 1333
(1989): Epelbaum S+, *Pediatrie* (French) 44, 387
Angioedema (1–10%)
(1998): Minguez MA+, *Allergol Immunopathol (Madr)* (Spanish) 26, 43
(1994): Galindo-Bonilla PA+, *Contact Dermatitis* 31, 319
(1994): Vega JM+, *Allergy* 49, 317
(1989): Chopra R+, *Can Med Assoc J* 140, 921 (in children)
Baboon syndrome
(2002): Strub C+, *Schweiz Rundsch Med Prax* 91(6), 232
(2000): Kick G+, *Contact Dermatitis* 43, 366
(1996): Kohler LD+, *Int J Dermatol* 35, 502
(1994): Duve S+, *Acta Derm Venereol* 74, 480
(1993): Herfs H+, *Hautarzt* (German) 44, 466
Bullous pemphigoid
(1997): Miralles J+, *Int J Dermatol* 36, 42
(1988): Alcalay J+, *J Am Acad Dermatol* 18, 345
Contact dermatitis
(2001): Petavy-Catala C+, *Contact Dermatitis* 44, 251 (consort)
(1996): Garcia R+, *Contact Dermatitis* 35, 116
(1995): Gamboa P+, *Contact Dermatitis* 32, 48 (occupational)
Cutaneous side effects (sic)
(1994): Paparello SF+, *AIDS* 8, 276
Diaper rash
(1988): Honig PJ+, *J Am Acad Dermatol* 19, 275
Ecchymoses
Edema
(1993): Echeverria-Arellano A+, *An Esp Pediatr* (Spanish) 39, 448
Erythema multiforme
(2001): Perez A+, *Contact Dermatitis* 44, 113 (with allopurinol)
(1999): Benjamin S+, *Ann Pharmacother* 33, 109
(1999): Wakelin SH+, *Clin Exp Dermatol* 24, 71
(1996): Webster GF, Philadelphia, PA (from Internet) (observation)
(1995): Wolkenstein P+, *Arch Dermatol* 131, 544
(1992): Gross AS+, *J Am Acad Dermatol* 27, 781
(1990): Chan HL+, *Arch Dermatol* 126, 43
(1990): Escallier F+, *Rev Med Interne* (French) 11, 73
(1989): Chopra R+, *Can Med Assoc J* 140, 921 (in children)
(1988): Massullo RE+, *J Am Acad Dermatol* 19, 358
(1988): Platt R, *J Infect Dis* 158, 474
(1986): Davidson NJ+, *BMJ* 292, 380
(1986): Dikland WJ+, *Pediatr Dermatol* 3, 135
(1982): Freeman T, *Can Med Assoc J* 127, 818
Exanthems (>5%)
(1999): Wakelin SH+, *Clin Exp Dermatol* 24, 71 (flexural)
(1997): Barbaud AM+, *Arch Dermatol* 133, 481
(1997): Blumenthal HL, Beachwood, OH (personal case) (observation)
(1995): Romano A+, *Allergy* 50, 113
(1995): Wolkenstein P+, *Arch Dermatol* 131, 544
(1994): Litt JZ, Beachwood, OH (personal case) (observation)
(1993): Fellner MJ, *Int J Dermatol* 32, 308
(1993): Romano A+, *J Invest Allergol Clin Immunol* 3, 53
(1990): Pauszek ME, *Indiana Med* 83, 330
(1989): Battegay M+, *Lancet* 2, 1100
(1989): Chopra R+, *Can Med Assoc J* 140, 921 (in children)
(1989): Kennedy C+, *Contact Dermatitis* 20, 313
(1986): Bigby M+, *JAMA* 256, 3358 (5.14%)
(1986): de Haan P+, *Allergy* 41, 75
(1986): Sonntag MR+, *Schweiz Med Wochenschr* (German) 116, 142 (7%)
(1985): Levine LR, *Pediatr Infect Dis* 4, 358
(1981): Odegaard OR, *Tidsskr Nor Laegeforen* (Norwegian) 101, 1973
(1977): Taylor B+, *BMJ* 2, 552 (3.7%)
(1975): Brogden RN+, *Drugs* 9, 88 (1–22%)
(1974): Wise PJ+, *J Infect Dis* 129 (Suppl), s266
(1973): Dubb S, *S A Med J* 47, 1218
Exfoliative dermatitis
Fixed eruption
(2001): Agnew KL+, *Australas J Dermatol* 42(3), 200 (reproducible)
(2000): Brabek E+, *Dtsch Med Wochenschr* 125(42), 1260
(1998): Mahboob A+, *Int J Dermatol* 37, 833
(1997): Jimenez I+, *Allergol Immunopathol (Madr)* 25, 247 (glans penis)
(1997): Zabawski E, Dallas, TX (from Internet) (observation)
(1995): Arias J+, *Clin Exp Dermatol* 20, 339
(1995): Dhar S+, *Pediatr Dermatol* 12, 51 (tongue)
(1994): Gil-Garcia JF+, *Med Clin (Barc)* (Spanish) 102, 438
(1989): Shuttleworth D, *Clin Exp Dermatol* 14, 367 (pustular)
(1982): Chowdhury FH, *Practitioner* 226, 1450 (penile)
Fixed eruption (neutrophilic)
(2001): Agnew KI+, *Aust J Dermatol* 42, 200
Hematomas
Intertrigo
(1992): Wolf B+, *Acta Derm Venereol* (Stockh) 72, 441
Jarisch–Herxheimer reaction
(1998): Maloy AL+, *J Emerg Med* 16, 437
Keratosis pilaris

(1997): Kay M, North Hollywood, CA (from Internet) (observation)
Pemphigus
(1997): Brenner S+, *J Am Acad Dermatol* 36, 919
(1997): Landau M+, *Am J Dermatopathol* 19, 411
(1991): Escallier F+, *Ann Dermatol Venereol* (French) 118, 381
(1983): Toan ND+, *Ann Dermatol Venereol* (French) 110, 917
Perleche
(1982): Arata J+, *Jpn J Antibiot* (Japanese) 35, 394
Petechiae (Rumpel–Leede sign)
(1992): Gross AS+, *J Am Acad Dermatol* 27, 781
Pruritus
(2000): Blumenthal HL, Beachwood, OH (personal case) (observation)
(1996): Drouet M+, *Allerg Immunol Paris* (French) 28, 311
(1995): Shelley WB+, *Cutis* 55, 202 (observation)
(1993): Fellner MJ, *Int J Dermatol* 32, 308
(1989): Battegay M+, *Lancet* 2, 1100
Psoriasis
(1993): Litt JZ, Beachwood, OH (personal case) (observation)
Purpura
Pustular eruption
(2000): Whittam LR+, *Clin Exp Dermatol* 25, 122
(1995): Wolkenstein P+, *Arch Dermatol* 131, 544
(1992): Trueb R+, *Hautarzt* (German) 43, 595
(1991): Armster H+, *Hautarzt* (German) 42, 713
(1991): Roujeau J-C+, *Arch Dermatol* 127, 1333
(1990): Guy C+, *Nouv Dermatol* (French) 9, 540
(1989): Epelbaum S+, *Pédiatrie* (French) 44, 387
(1989): Shuttleworth D, *Clin Exp Dermatol* 14, 367
Pustular psoriasis
(1987): Katz M, *J Am Acad Dermatol* 17, 918
Rash (sic) (1–10%)
(1997): Van Buchem FL+, *Lancet* 349, 683
(1989): Battegay M+, *Lancet* 2, 1100
(1982): Arata J+, *Jpn J Antibiot* (Japanese) 35, 394
(1982): Millard G, *Scott Med J* 27, S35
(1980): Porter J+, *Lancet* 1, 1037
Stevens–Johnson syndrome
(1999): Limauro DL+, *Ann Pharmacother* 33, 560
(1996): Cullimore KC, Westminster, CO (from Internet) (observation)
(1992): Martin Mateos MA+, *J Investig Allergol Clin Immunol* 2, 278
(1988): Platt R, *J Infect Dis* 158, 474
Toxic epidermal necrolysis
(2001): Spies M+, *Pediatrics* 108, 1162
(1996): Blum L+, *J Am Acad Dermatol* 34, 1088
(1996): Surbled M+, *Ann Fr Anesth Reanim* (French) 15, 1095
(1993): Correia O+, *Dermatology* 186, 32
(1993): Romano A+, *J Invest Allergol Clin Immunol* 3, 53
(1988): Massullo RE+, *J Am Acad Dermatol* 19, 358
(1984): Herman TE+, *Pediatr Radiol* 14, 439
Toxic pustuloderma
(1992): Trueb R+, *Hautarzt* (German) 43, 595
(1991): Armster H+, *Hautarzt* (German) 42, 713
Urticaria (1–5%)
(2001): Torres MJ+, *Allergy* 56(9), 850
(2000): Blumenthal HL, Beachwood, OH (personal case) (observation)
(1998): Minguez MA+, *Allergol Immunopathol (Madr)* (Spanish) 26, 43
(1997): Delpre G+, *Dig Dis Sci* 42, 728
(1997): Thaler D, Monona, WI (from internet) (observation)
(1995): Litt JZ, Beachwood, OH (personal case) (observation)
(1994): Vega JM+, *Allergy* 49, 317
(1990): Fraj J+, *Clin Exp Allergy* 20, 121
(1989): Battegay M+, *Lancet* 2, 1100
(1989): Chopra R+, *Can Med Assoc J* 140, 921 (in children)
(1985): Goolamali SK, *Postgrad Med J* 61, 925
Vasculitis
(1999): Garcia-Porrua C+, *J Rheumatol* 26, 1942
Vesicular eruptions

## Other

Anaphylactoid reactions
(2001): Torres MJ+, *Allergy* 56(9), 850
(1999): Salgado Fernandez J+, *Rev Esp Cardiol* (Spanish) 52, 622
(1998): Rich MW, *Tex Heart Inst J* 25, 194
(1994): Vega JM+, *Allergy* 49, 317
(1993): van der Klauw MM+, *Br J Clin Pharmacol* 35, 400
(1990): Fraj J+, *Clin Exp Allergy* 20, 121
(1988): Blanca M+, *Allergy* 43, 508
Black tongue
Dysgeusia
Glossitis
Glossodynia
Hypersensitivity
(2000): da Fonseca MA, *Pediatr Dent* 22(5), 401
(1995): Mokry C, *N Engl J Med* 333, 1151
(1993): Romano A+, *Contact Dermatitis* 28, 190
(1989): Kennedy C+, *Contact Dermatitis* 20, 313
Injection-site pain
Oral candidiasis
Serum sickness (1–10%)
(1995): Martin J+, *N Z Med J* 108, 123
(1992): Stricker BH+, *J Clin Epidemiol* 45, 1177
(1990): Heckbert SR+, *Am J Epidemiol* 132, 336
(1989): Chopra R+, *Can Med Assoc J* 140, 921 (in children)
(1988): Platt R+, *J Infect Dis* 158, 474
Stomatitis
(1996): Drouet M+, *Allerg Immunol Paris* (French) 28, 311
Stomatodynia
Tooth discoloration
(2001): Garcia-Lopez M+, *Pediatrics* 108(3), 819
Vaginitis (1%)
(1996): Drouet M+, *Allerg Immunol Paris* (French) 28, 311
(1978): Fang LST+, *N Engl J Med* 298, 413
Xerostomia

# AMPHOTERICIN B

**Trade names:** Abelcet; AmBisome (Fujisawa); Amphocin (Pharmacia & Upjohn); Fungizone (Apothecon)
**Other common trade names:** *Ampho-Moronal; Fungilin; Fungizone*
**Indications:** Potentially life-threatening fungal infections
**Category:** Antifungal; antiprotozoal (parenteral)
**Half-life:** initial: 15–48 hours; terminal: 15 days
**Clinically important, potentially hazardous interactions with:** aminoglycosides, cephalothin, cidofovir, cyclosporine, digoxin, fluconazole, ganciclovir, itraconazole, ketoconazole, probenecid

### *Reactions*

## Skin

Angioedema
Burning (sic) (from topical)
Chills
Contact dermatitis
Diaphoresis
Erythema
Erythema multiforme

Exanthems (<1%)
(1999): Cesaro S+, *Support Care Cancer* 7, 284
(1976): Lorber B+, *Ann Intern Med* 84, 54
(1966): Beaty HN+, *Ann Intern Med* 65, 641
Exfoliative dermatitis
(1961): Sternberg TH+, *Med Clin North Am* 45, 781
Fixed eruption
(1969): Kandil E, *Dermatologica* 139, 37
Flushing (1–10%)
(1964): Martin WJ, *Med Clin North Am* 48, 255
(1961): Sternberg TH+, *Med Clin North Am* 45, 781
Pigmentation
Pruritus
(1999): Cesaro S+, *Support Care Cancer* 7, 284
(1966): Beaty HN+, *Ann Intern Med* 65, 641
Purpura
(1971): Costello MJ, *Arch Dermatol* 79, 184
(1966): Beaty HN+, *Ann Intern Med* 65, 641
(1961): Sternberg TH+, *Med Clin North Am* 45, 781
Rash (sic)
(1995): Oppenheim BA+, *Clin Infect Dis* 21, 1145
Raynaud's phenomenon (cyanotic)
(1997): Zernikow B+, *Mycoses* 40, 359
Red man syndrome
(1990): Ellis ME+, *BMJ* 300, 1468
Ulceration
Urticaria
Vesicular eruptions
Xerosis

## Hair

Hair – alopecia

## Other

Anaphylactoid reactions
(2001): Bishara J+, *Ann Pharmacother* 35, 308
(1999): Cronin JE+, *Clin Infect Dis* 28, 1342
(1998): Schneider P+, *Br J Haematol* 102, 1108
Death
(2001): Collazos J+, *Clin Infect Dis* 33(7), E75
Infusion-site pain
Infusion-site thrombophlebitis
(1995): Goodwin SD+, *Clin Infect Dis* 20, 755
Infusion-site toxicity
(2000): Karthaus M+. *Chemotherapy* 46, 293
Myalgia
Paresthesias (1–10%)
Rhabdomyolysis
(1970): Drutz DJ+, *JAMA* 211(5), 824
Stomatitis
Thrombophlebitis (1–10%)
(1993): Dietze R+, *Clin Infect Dis* 17, 981
Tinnitus
Xerostomia

# AMPICILLIN

**Trade names:** D-Amp; Marcillin; Omnipen (Wyeth); Polycillin (Mead Johnson); Principen (Bristol-Myers Squibb); Totacillin (GSK)
**Other common trade names:** *Amfipen; Ampicin; Binotal; Penbritin; Penstabil; Pro-Ampi; Sinaplin; Taro-Ampicillin Trihydrate; Totapen; Vidopen*
**Indications:** Susceptible strains of gram-negative and gram-positive bacterial infections
**Category:** Aminopenicillin antibiotic
**Half-life:** 1–1.5 hours
**Clinically important, potentially hazardous interactions with:** allopurinol, anticoagulants, chloramphenicol, cyclosporine, demeclocycline, doxycycline, erythromycin, methotrexate, minocycline, oxytetracycline, sulfonamides, tetracyclines

**Note:** Five to 10% of people taking ampicillin develop eruptions between the 5th and 14th day following initiation of therapy. Also, there is a 95% incidence of exanthematous eruptions in patients who are treated for infectious mononucleosis with ampicillin. The allergenicity of ampicillin appears to be enhanced by allopurinol or by hyperuricemia. Ampicillin is clearly the more allergenic of the two drugs when given alone

### *Reactions*

## Skin

Acute generalized exanthematous pustulosis (AGEP)
(1995): Moreau A+, *Int J Dermatol* 34, 263 (passim)
(1994): Manders SM+, *Cutis* 54, 194
(1991): Roujeau J-C+, *Arch Dermatol* 127, 1333
Allergic reactions (sic) (1–10%)
(1993): Grover JK+, *Indian J Physiol Pharmacol* 37, 247 (2.9%)
(1974): Revuz J+, *Nouv Presse Med* (French) *3, 1169*
Angioedema (<1%)
(1982): Valsecchi R+, *Contact Dermatitis* 8, 278
(1980): Kraemer MJ+, *Pediatrics in Review* 1, 197
Baboon syndrome
(1993): Herfs H+, *Hautarzt* (German) 44, 466
(1985): Rasmussen LP+, *Ugeskr Laeger* (Danish) 147, 1341
(1984): Andersen KE+, *Contact Dermatitis* 10, 97
Bullous eruption (<1%)
(1982): Stepien B+, *Przegl Dermatol* (Polish) 69, 65
Bullous pemphigoid
(1990): Hodak E+, *Clin Exp Dermatol* 15, 50
Candidiasis
(1973): Bass JW+, *J Pediatrics* 83, 106
Contact dermatitis
(1997): Romano A+, *Clin Exp Allergy* 27, 1425
(1995): Gamboa P+, *Contact Dermatitis* 32, 48
(1988): Andersen KE, *Acta Derm Venereol* Suppl (Stockh) 135, 62 (systemic)
(1986): Pigatto PD+, *Contact Dermatitis* 14, 196
(1978): Bruevich TS+, *Vest Dermatol Venerol* (Russian) March, 74
(1970): Schulz KH+, *Berufsdermatosen* (German) 18, 132
(1969): Braun W+, *Ther Ggw* (German) 108, 250
Diaper rash
(1973): Bass JW+, *J Pediatrics* 83, 106 (4.5–13%)
Erythema annulare centrifugum
(1975): Gupta HL+, *J Indian Med Assoc* 65, 307
Erythema multiforme (<1%)
(1995): Dhar S+, *Dermatology* 191, 76
(1994): Garty BZ+, *Ann Pharmacother* 28, 730
(1990): Chan HL+, *Arch Dermatol* 126, 43
(1985): Konstantinidis AB+, *J Oral Med* 40, 168
(1984): Gebel K+, *Dermatologica* 168, 35

(1979): Gupta HL+, *J Indian Med Assoc* 72, 188
(1975): Böttiger LE+, *Acta Med Scand* 198, 229
(1972): Kauppinen K, *Acta Derm Venereol* (Stockh) 52, 68
(1970): Crow KD, *Trans A Rep St John's Hosp Dermatol Soc* 56, 35

Exanthems (>10%)
(1997): Romano A+, *Clin Exp Allergy* 27, 1425
(1996): Adcock BB+, *Arch Fam Med* 5, 301
(1996): Marra CA+, *Ann Pharacother* 30, 401
(1995): Romano A+, *Allergy* 50, 113
(1994): Grayson ML+, *Clin Infect Dis* 18, 683
(1994): Shelley WB+, *Cutis* 53, 40 (observation)
(1993): Romano A+, *J Invest Allergol Clin Immunol* 3, 53
(1993): Warrington RJ+, *J Allergy Clin Immunol* 92, 626
(1988): Hou SR, *Chung Hua Nei Ko Tsa Chih* (Chinese) 27, 36
(1987): Pavithran K, *Indian J Lepr* 59, 309
(1986): Cabo HA+, *Med Cutan Ibero Lat Am* (Spanish) 14, 177
(1986): de Haan P+, *Allergy* 41, 75
(1986): Sonntag MR+, *Schweiz Med Wochenschr* (German) 116, 142 (8%)
(1985): Bruynzeel DP+, *Dermatologica* 171, 429
(1985): Hefelfinger DC, *Ala Med* 55, 16
(1983): Bianchi C+, *Med Cutan Ibero Lat Am* (Spanish) 11, 113
(1983): Scioli C+, *Boll Ist Sieroter Milan* (Italian) 62, 287
(1982): Dourmischev AL+, *Dermatol Monatsschr* (German) 168, 469
(1982): Gatter KC+, *Clin Allergy* 12, 279
(1981): Jick H+, *J Clin Pharmacol* 21, 456 (5.9%)
(1981): Lin CS+, *Arch Dermatol* 117, 282
(1980): Kraemer MJ+, *Pediatrics in Review* 1, 197
(1980): Porter D+, *Lancet* 1, 1037
(1980): Scherzer W+, *Derm Beruf Umwelt* (German) 28, 175
(1979): Murphy TF, *Ann Intern Med* 91, 324
(1978): Geyman JP+, *J Fam Pract* 7, 493
(1978): Kouba K+, *Cesk Pediatr* (Czech) 33, 487
(1978): Pollowitz JA, *Am J Dis Child* 132, 819
(1977): Campbell AB+, *Pediatrics* 59, 638
(1977): Gupta HL+, *J Indian Med Assoc* 68, 33
(1977): Sokoloff B, *Pediatrics* 59, 637
(1976): Arndt KA+, *JAMA* 235, 918 (5.2%)
(1976): Fellner MJ+, *N Y State J Med* 76, 101
(1976): Morris J, *Lancet* 1, 423
(1976): Wuthrich B, *Dtsch Med Wochenschr* (German) 101, 470
(1975): Editorial, *BMJ* 2, 708
(1975): Esten H+, *Med Welt* (German) 26, 296
(1975): Gleckman RA, *JAMA* 233, 427 (2.5%)
(1975): Krsic B+, *Lijec Vjesn* (Serbo-Croatian-Roman) 97, 339
(1975): Lehnhoff B, *Monatsschr Kinderheilkd* (German) 123, 548
(1974): Spitzy KH, *Acta Med Austriaca* (German) 2, 46
(1974): Webster AW+, *Clin Exp Immunol* 18, 553
(1973): Bass JW+, *J Pediatrics* 83, 106 (4.75%)
(1973): Boston Collaborative Drug Surveillance Program, *Arch Dermatol* 107, 74 (9.7%)
(1973): Gregg I, *BMJ* 1, 295
(1973): *BMJ* 1, 7
(1973): *N Z Med J* 77, 105
(1973): Kerns DL+, *Am J Dis Child* 125, 187
(1973): Wemmer U, *Fortschr Med* (German) 91, 1232
(1973): Zürcher K+, *Dermatologica* (German) 147, 1
(1972): Almeyda J+, *Br J Dermatol* 87, 293
(1972): Balfour HH+, *Clin Pediatr Phila* 11, 417
(1972): Bierman CW+, *JAMA* 220, 1098
(1972): Harris JR+, *BMJ* 1, 687
(1972): *BMJ* 1, 195
(1972): *BMJ* 1, 505
(1972): *N Engl J Med* 286, 1217
(1972): Kuokkanen K, *Acta Allergol* 27, 407
(1972): Potter JPL, *BMJ* 1, 749
(1972): Schulz KH, *Arch Dermatol Forsch* (German) 244, 309
(1972): Steiniger U, *Dtsch Gesundheitsw* (German) 27, 1164
(1972): Weuta H, *Arzneimittelforschung* (German) 22, 1300
(1971): Beckmann H, *Munch Med Wochenschr* (German) 113, 1423
(1971): Bronsert U, *Med Klin* (German) 66, 352
(1971): Kroidon EaP, *Antibiotiki* (Russian) 16, 549
(1971): Pullen H, *BMJ* 2, 653
(1971): Speck WT, *Clin Pediatr Phila* 10, 59
(1970): Corless JD+, *South Med J* 63, 1341
(1970): Crow KD, *Trans St Johns Hosp Dermatol Soc* 56, 35
(1970): Fournier A+, *J Sci Med Lille* (French) 88, 529
(1970): Jaffe IA, *Lancet* 1, 245
(1970): Kerrebijn KF, *Lancet* 1, 245
(1970): Knudsen ET+, *BMJ* 1, 469
(1970): Kronig B+, *Arzneimittelforschung* (German) 20, 1930
(1970): Shapiro S+, *Lancet* 1, 194 (9.5%)
(1970): Weary PE+, *Arch Dermatol* 101, 86
(1969): Hurwitz N+, *BMJ* 1, 531 (7.8%)
(1969): No Author, *Lancet* 2, 993
(1969): Sanders DY, *Clin Pediatr Phila* 8, 47
(1969): Shapiro S+, *Lancet* 2, 969 (7.7%)
(1968): Gabbert WR+, *J Ky Med Assoc* 66, 967
(1968): Levene G+, *Br J Dermatol* 80, 417
(1968): Loffler H+, *Med Welt* (German) 32, 1736
(1966): Stevenson J+, *BMJ* 1, 1359

Exfoliative dermatitis
(1985): Fong PH+, *Ann Acad Med Singapore* 14, 693
(1974): Tay C, *Asian J Med* 10, 223

Fixed eruption
(2000): Brabek E+, *Dtsch Med Wochenschr* 125(42), 1260
(1998): Mahboob A+, *Int J Dermatol* 37, 833
(1990): Bharija SC+, *Dermatologica* 181, 237
(1990): Gaffoor PMA+, *Cutis* 45, 242
(1987): Sharma SN, *J Assoc Physicians India* 35, 608
(1986): Kanwar AJ+, *Dermatologica* 172, 315
(1986): Panagariya A, *J Ass Physicians India* 34, 458
(1984): Chan H-L, *Arch Dermatol* 120, 542
(1983): Chan H-L, *Int J Dermatol* 23, 607
(1970): Savin JA, *Br J Dermatol* 83, 546

Linear IgA bullous dermatosis
(2002): Cohen LM+, *J Am Acad Dermatol* 46, S32 (passim)
(1996): Tranvan A+, *J Am Acad Dermatol* 35, 865
(1981): Boffety B+, *Journées Dermatologiques de Paris* (French), 53–53a

Pemphigus
(1997): Brenner S+, *J Am Acad Dermatol* 36, 919
(1996): Takizawa H+, *Am J Gastroenterol* 91, 1654
(1993): Brenner S+, *Isr J Med Sci* 29, 44
(1986): Brenner S+, *J Am Acad Dermatol* 14, 453
(1986): Wilson JP+, *Drug Intell Clin Pharm* 20, 219
(1980): Fellner MJ+, *Int J Dermatol* 19, 392

Pityriasis rosea
(1987): Olumide Y, *Int J Dermatol* 26, 234

Pruritus (1–5%)
(1996): Adcock BB+, *Arch Fam Med* 5, 301
(1982): Bernhard JD+, *Cutis* 29, 158
(1980): Kraemer MJ+, *Pediatrics in Review* 1, 197
(1973): Bass JW+, *J Pediatrics* 83, 106 (0.75%)

Psoriasis
(1993): Litt JZ, Beachwood, OH (personal case) (observation)
(1992): Breathnach SM+, *Adverse Drug Reactions and the Skin* Blackwell, Oxford, 141 (passim)
(1990): Saito S+, *J Dermatol* 17, 677
(1988): Tsankov N+, *J Am Acad Dermatol* 19, 629

Purpura
(1993): Pang BK+, *Ann Acad Med Singapore* 22, 870
(1990): Hannedouche T+, *J Antimicrob Chemother* 20, 3
(1982): Beeching NL+, *J Antimicrob Chemother* 10, 479
(1981): Valman HB, *Br Med J Clin Res Ed* 283, 970
(1973): Croydon EAP+, *BMJ* 1, 7
(1971): Parker JC+, *Arch Intern Med* 127, 474

Pustular eruption

(1995): Lim JT+, *Cutis* 56, 163
(1994): Jay S+, *Arch Dermatol* 130, 787 (localized)
(1991): Roujeau J-C+, *Arch Dermatol* 127, 1333
(1990): Guy C+, *Nouv Dermatol* (French) 9, 540

Pustular psoriasis
(1987): Katz M+, *J Am Acad Dermatol* 17, 918
(1986): Verner E+, *Harefuah* (Hebrew) 110, 132

Rash (sic) (1–10%)

Stevens–Johnson syndrome
(1990): Cavanzo FJ+, *Gastroenterology* 99, 854
(1990): Chan HL+, *Arch Dermatol* 126, 43
(1987): Howell CG+, *J Pediatr Surg* 22, 994
(1985): Ting HC+, *Int J Dermatol* 24, 587
(1985): Turck M, *Hosp Pract Off Ed* 20, 49
(1979): Gupta HL+, *J Indian Med Assoc* 72, 188
(1978): Assaad D+, *Can Med Assoc* 118, 154
(1975): McArthur JE+, *N Z Med J* 81, 390
(1972): Kauppinen K, *Acta Derm Venereol* (Stockh) 52, 68

Toxic epidermal necrolysis (<1%)
(2002): Zelenkova H+, *World Congress Dermatol* Poster, 0136
(1997): Rodrigues-Ares MT+, *Int Ophthalmol* 21, 39
(1993): Romano A+, *J Invest Allergol Clin Immunol* 3, 53
(1991): Heng MC+, *J Am Acad Dermatol* 25, 778
(1985): Robbens EJ+, *Acta Clin Belg* 40, 115
(1983): Tagami H+, *Arch Dermatol* 119, 910
(1981): Berkel AI+, *Turk J Pediatr* 23, 37
(1980): Giuffre L+, *Minerva Pediatr* (Italian) 32, 633
(1979): Rosenthal AL+, *Cutis* 24, 437
(1978): Assaad D+, *Can Med Assoc* 118, 154
(1975): Böttiger LE+, *Acta Med Scand* 198, 229
(1975): McArthur JE+, *N Z Med J* 81, 390
(1975): Schopf E+, *Z Haut* (German) 50, 865
(1972): Carli-Basset C+, *Sem Hop* (French) 48, 497

Urticaria
(1997): Romano A+, *Clin Exp Allergy* 27, 1425
(1996): Adcock BB+, *Arch Fam Med* 5, 301
(1985): Goolamali SK, *Postgrad Med J* 61, 925
(1982): Valsecchi R+, *Contact Dermatitis* 8, 278
(1980): Kraemer MJ+, *Pediatrics in Review* 1, 197
(1977): Gupta HL+, *J Indian Med Assoc* 68, 33
(1975): Gleckman RA, *JAMA* 233, 427 (0.8%)
(1973): Croydon EAP+, *BMJ* 1, 7
(1972): Bierman CW+, *JAMA* 220, 1098
(1969): Coskey RJ+, *Arch Dermatol* 100, 717
(1969): Knudsen ET, *BMJ* 1, 846
(1969): Pullen H, *BMJ* 2, 247
(1963): Kennedy WPU+, *BMJ* 2, 962 (10%)

Vasculitis
(1991): Estrada-Rodriguez JL+, *J Investig Allergol Clin Immunol* 1, 69
(1990): Hannedouche T+, *J Antimicrob Chemother* 20, 3
(1975): Pevny I+, *MMW Munch Med Wochenschr* (German) 117, 9
(1974): Tay C, *Asian J Med* 10, 223

## Other

Anaphylactoid reactions
(1998): Rich MW, *Tex Heart Inst J* 25, 194
(1997): Romano A+, *Clin Exp Allergy* 27, 1425
(1996): Adcock BB+, *Arch Fam Med* 5, 301
(1976): Fellner MJ, *Int J Dermatol* 15, 497
(1975): Pietzcker F+, *Z Hautkr* (German) 50, 437
(1973): Weck AL de, *Munch Med Wochenschr* (German) 115, 1650
(1972): Ohela K+, *Duodecim* (Finnish) 88, 1177

Black tongue
(1966): Meyler L (ed), *Side Effects of Drugs* 5th ed. Amsterdam, Excerpta Medica

Glossitis

Hypersensitivity
(1996): Torricelli R+, *Hautarzt* (German) 47, 392
(1993): Romano A+, *Contact Dermatitis* 28, 190
(1987): Ackerman Z+, *Postgrad Med J* 63, 55
(1970): Klemola E, *Scand J Infect Dis* 2, 29

Injection-site pain (>10%)

Oral candidiasis

Oral mucosal eruption
(1984): Gebel K+, *Dermatologica* 168, 35

Phlebitis

Serum sickness
(1974): Caldwell JR+, *JAMA* 230, 77

Stomatitis

Thrombophlebitis

Vaginal candidiasis

# AMPRENAVIR

**Trade name:** Agenerase (GSK)
**Indications:** HIV infection
**Category:** Protease inhibitor*; sulfonamide**
**Half-life:** no data
**Clinically important, potentially hazardous interactions with:** amiodarone, amitriptyline, amoxapine, benzodiazepines, bepridil, clomipramine, clonazepam, clorazepate, desipramine, diazepam, dihydroergotamine, doxepin, ergotamine, fentanyl, flurazepam, imipramine, lidocaine, lorazepam, methysergide, midazolam, nortriptyline, oxazepam, phenytoin, protriptyline, quazepam, quinidine, rifampin, sildenafil, **St John's wort**, temazepam, tricyclic antidepressants, trimipramine, vitamin E

### *Reactions*

## Skin

Exanthems

Pruritus

Rash (sic) (25%)
(2001): Scott T+, *Clin Ther* 23(2), 252 (8%)
(2000): Noble S+, *Drugs* 60(6), 1383
(2000): Pedneault L+, *Clin Ther* 22(12), 1378 (3%)

Stevens–Johnson syndrome (4%)

## Other

Buffalo hump

Dysgeusia (10%)

Gynecomastia

Hypesthesia
(1999): Sadler BM+, *Antimicrob Agents Chemother* 14, 1686

Paresthesias (perioral) (26%)
(2001): *Prescrire Int* 10(53), 70
(2001): McMahon D+, *Antivir Ther* 6(2), 105
(2000): Pedneault L+, *Clin Ther* 22(12), 1378

***Note:** Protease inhibitors cause dyslipidemia which includes elevated triglycerides and cholesterol and redistribution of body fat centrally to produce the so-called "protease paunch," breast enlargement, facial atrophy, and "buffalo hump"

****Note:** Amprenavir is a sulfonamide and can be absorbed systemically. Sulfonamides can produce severe, possibly fatal, reactions such as toxic epidermal necrolysis and Stevens–Johnson syndrome

## AMYL NITRITE

**Synonym:** isoamyl nitrite
**Trade name:** Amyl Nitrite (Lilly)
**Other common trade name:** *Nitrit*
**Indications:** Angina pectoris
**Category:** Antianginal; coronary vasodilator
**Half-life:** no data

### *Reactions*

#### Skin

Allergic reactions (sic)
(1989): Dax EM+, *Am J Med* 86, 732
Contact dermatitis
(1985): Bos JD+, *Contact Dermatitis* 12, 109
(1982): Romaguera C+, *Contact Dermatitis* 8, 266
Dermatitis (sic)
(1984): Fisher AA, *Cutis* 34, 118
Diaphoresis
Edema
Flushing (1–10%)
Pallor
Rash (sic) (<1%)

## ANAGRELIDE

**Trade name:** Agrylin (Roberts)
**Indications:** Essential thrombocytopenia. To reduce elevated platelet count and the risk of thrombosis
**Category:** Phospholipase A2 inhibitor; platelet inhibitor
**Half-life:** ~3 Days
**Clinically important, potentially hazardous interactions with:** fondaparinux

### *Reactions*

#### Skin

Chills (<5%)
Ecchymoses (<5%)
Edema (19.8%)
(2002): Kornblihtt LI+, *Medicina (B Aires)* 62(3), 231
(1998): Oertel MD, *Am J Health Syst Pharm* 55(19), 1979
Flu-like syndrome (<5%)
Peripheral edema (7.1%)
(1992): Mazzucconi MG+, *Haematologica* 77(4), 315
Photosensitivity (<5%)
Pruritus (<5%)
Rash (sic) (7.8%)
Skin disease (sic) (<5%)
Urticaria (7.8%)

#### Hair

Hair – alopecia (<5%)

#### Other

Aphthous stomatitis (<5%)
Arthralgia (<5%)
Back pain (6.4%)
Depression (<5%)
Leg cramps (<5%)
Myalgia (<5%)
Paresthesias (7.3%)
Tinnitus (<5%)

## ANASTROZOLE

**Trade name:** Arimidex (AstraZeneca)
**Indications:** Breast carcinoma (localized-advanced or metastatic)
**Category:** Antineoplastic; aromatase inhibitor
**Half-life:** 50 hours

### *Reactions*

#### Skin

Chills
Diaphoresis
(1997): Jonat W, *Oncology* 54 (Suppl 2), 15
Flu-like syndrome (6.9%)
Flushing (>5%)
Hot flashes (26.5%)
(1998): Higa GM+, *Am J Health* 55(5), 445
Infections (sic) (2–5%)
Pain (13.8%)
(1998): Higa GM+, *Am J Health* 55(5), 445
Peripheral edema (10.1%)
Pruritus (2–5%)
Rash (sic) (7.5%)
Shivering

#### Hair

Hair – alopecia (2–5%)

#### Other

Arthralgia (2–5%)
Bone pain (10.7%)
Cough (10.9%)
Depression (4.5%)
Mastodynia (2–5%)
Myalgia (2–5%)
Paresthesias
Thrombophlebitis (2–5%)
Tumor pain (>5%)
Vaginal dryness (1.7%)
Xerostomia

## ANDROSTENEDIONE

**Scientific names:** *4-androstene-3,17-dione; Androst-4-ene-3,17-dione*
**Other common names:** Andro; Androstene
**Family:** N/A
**Purported indications:** Enhanced athletic performance, increased energy, to keep red blood cells healthy
**Other uses:** Heightened sexual arousal & function

### *Reactions*

#### Skin

Acne
(1999): Pheatt N, *Sports Supplements. Pharmacist's Letter* 99, 1
(1998): *Med Lett Drugs Ther* 40, 105
Coarsening of skin (sic)
(1998): *Med Lett Drugs Ther* 40, 105

#### Hair

Hair – alopecia
(1998): *Med Lett Drugs Ther* 40, 105
Hair – hirsutism (in women)
(1999): Pheatt N, *Sports Supplements. Pharmacist's Letter* 99, 1

### Other

Gynecomastia
Priapism
(2000): Kachhi PN+, *Ann Emerg Med* 35, 391

**Note:** Androstenedione gained popularity as the supplement used by homerun-hitter, Mark McGuire

## ANISINDIONE

**Trade name:** Miradon (Schering)
**Indications:** Adjunct in treatment of coronary occlusion, Atrial fibrillation
**Category:** Indanedione oral anticoagulant
**Half-life:** 3–5 days
**Clinically important, potentially hazardous interactions with:** amiodarone, anabolic steroids, antihyroid agents, barbiturates, bivalirudin, cimetidine, clofibrate, clopidogrel, cyclosporine, delavirdine, dextrothyroxine, disulfiram, fluconazole, glutethimide, imatinib, itraconazole, ketoconazole, metronidazole, miconazole, penicillins, phenylbutazone, pipericillin, quinidine, quinine, rifabutin, rifampin, rifapentine, rofecoxib, salicylates, sulfinpyrazone, sulfonamides, testosterone, thyroids, zileuton

#### *Reactions*

### Skin

Chills
Dermatitis (sic)
Ecchymoses
Erythema
Erythema multiforme
Exanthems
Exfoliative dermatitis
Necrosis
Petechiae
Purple toe syndrome
Urticaria

### Hair

Hair – alopecia

### Other

Death
Hypersensitivity
Oral ulceration
Priapism
Stomatitis
Stomatodynia

## ANISTREPLASE

**Synonym:** APSAC
**Trade name:** Eminase (Roberts)
**Other common trade name:** *Iminase*
**Indications:** Acute myocardial infarction
**Category:** Thrombolytic enzyme
**Half-life:** 70–120 minutes

#### *Reactions*

### Skin

Allergic reactions (sic)
Angioedema
Chills (<1%)
Diaphoresis (<1%)
Ecchymoses
Exanthems
(1995): Dykewicz MS+, *J Allergy Clin Immunol* 95, 1020
Flushing
Livedo reticularis
(1994): Gianni R+, *Ann Ital Med Int* (Italian) 9, 105
Purpura
Rash (sic)
Ulcer
(1994): Gianni R+, *Ann Ital Med Int* (Italian) 9, 105
Urticaria
(1995): Dykewicz MS+, *J Allergy Clin Immunol* 95, 1020
Vasculitis
(1994): Gianni R+, *Ann Ital Med Int* (Italian) 9, 105
(1992): Burrows N+, *J Am Acad Dermatol* 26, 508
(1990): Burrows N+, *Br Heart J* 64, 289
(1988): Bucknall C+, *Br Heart J* 59, 9
(1988): Gemmill JD+, *Br Heart J* 60, 361

### Other

Anaphylactoid reactions (1–10%)
(1997): Cannas S+, *G Ital Cardiol* (Italian) 27, 278
Gingival hemorrhage
Hypersensitivity
(1993): Lee HS+, *Eur Heart J* 14, 1640
Myalgia
(1994): Gianni R+, *Ann Ital Med Int* (Italian) 9, 105
Serum sickness
(1993): Lee HS+, *Eur Heart J* 14, 1640

## ANTHRAX VACCINE

**Trade names:** Anthrax Vaccine Adsorbed [AVA] (BioPort); Carbosap
**Indications:** Anthrax prophylaxis
**Category:** Aluminum hydroxide-adsorbed supernatant material from fermentor cultutres of toxigenic; nonencapsulated strains of *Bacillus anthracis*
**Half-life:** Requires 1 month to achieve immunity (92.5% efficient)

#### *Reactions*

### Skin

Allergic reactions (sic)
(2000): Captain James Bishop, *Citizen Airman* (0,002%)
(1999): Ellenberg SS, *Center for Biologics Evaluation & Research, FDA Statement* (widespread)

Angioedema
(2000): *MMWR* 49(RR15), 1
Cellulitis
(2000): *MMWR* 49(RR15), 1
Chills (<0.06%)
(2000): *MMWR* 49(RR15), 1
Diaphoresis
(2001): Swanson-Biearman B+, *J Toxicol Clin Toxicol* 39(1), 81
(1999): Dr. Sue Bailey, *Asst Sec Defense Health Affairs – Service Member #16* 21
Edema (3%)
(2000): *MMWR* 49(RR15), 1
Erythema
(2000): *MMWR* 49(RR15), 1
Eyelid edema
(1999): Dr. Sue Bailey, *Asst Sec Defense Health Affairs – Service Member #16* 21
Flu-like syndrome (<0.2%)
(2001): Swanson-Biearman B+, *J Toxicol Clin Toxicol* 39(1), 81
(2000): Captain James Bishop, *Citizen Airman* (0.0006%)
(1999): Dr. Sue Bailey, *Asst Sec Defense Health Affairs – Service Member #1*
Hot flashes
(1999): Dr. Sue Bailey, *Asst Sec Defense Health Affairs – Service Member #31* 34, 37
Lupus erythematosus
(2000): *MMWR* 49(RR15), 1
(1999): Ellenberg SS, *Center for Biologics Evaluation & Research, FDA Statement*
Photosensitivity
(1999): Dr. Sue Bailey, *Asst Sec Defense Health Affairs – Service Member #1*
Pruritus
(2000): *MMWR* 49(RR15), 1
(1999): Dr. Sue Bailey, *Asst Sec Defense Health Affairs – Service Member #5*
Rash (sic)
(1999): Dr. Sue Bailey, *Asst Sec Defense Health Affairs – Service Members #5, 9, 14, 25, 44*
(1999): Ellenberg SS, *Center for Biologics Evaluation & Research, FDA Statement*
Urticaria
(2001): Swanson-Biearman B+, *J Toxicol Clin Toxicol* 39(1), 81

## Hair

Hair – alopecia

## Other

Anaphylactoid reactions
(2000): *MMWR* 49(RR15), 1
(1999): Dr. Sue Bailey, *Asst Sec Defense Health Affairs – Service Member #29*
Arthralgia
(2000): *MMWR* 49(RR15), 1
(1999): Dr. Sue Bailey, *Asst Sec Defense Health Affairs – Service Member #46*
Asthenia
(2000): *MMWR* 49(RR15), 1
Chronic fatigue syndrome
(1999): Dr. Sue Bailey, *Asst Sec Defense Health Affairs – Service Member #39*
Depression
(1999): Dr. Sue Bailey, *Asst Sec Defense Health Affairs – Service Member #23*
Fever (<1%)
(2000): *MMWR* 49(RR15), 1
Gingival bleeding
(1999): Dr. Sue Bailey, *Asst Sec Defense Health Affairs – Service Member #32*
Guillain–Barré syndrome
(2000): *MMWR* 49(RR15), 1
(1999): Ellenberg SS, *Center for Biologics Evaluation & Research, FDA Statement* (2 cases)
Hypersensitivity
(2001): Swanson-Biearman B+, *J Toxicol Clin Toxicol* 39(1), 81
(1999): Ellenberg SS, *Center for Biologics Evaluation & Research, FDA Statement* (2 cases)
(1996): Shlyakhov E+, *Med Trop (Mars)* 56(2), 148
(1996): Uhr JW, *Physiol Rev.* 46:359
(1994): Shlyakhov E+, *Med Trop (Mars)* 54(1):33
Injection-site burning
(1999): Dr. Sue Bailey, *Asst Sec Defense Health Affairs – Service Member #12,27*
Injection-site edema
(2000): *MMWR* 49(RR15), 1
(1999): Dr. Sue Bailey, *Asst Sec Defense Health Affairs – Service Member #4, 12, 32*
(1999): Ellenberg SS, *Center for Biologics Evaluation & Research, FDA Statement*
(1962): Brachman PS+, *Am J Pub Health* 52, 632 (up to 48 hours)
(1954): Wright GG+, *J Immunol* 73, 387 (2.4%)
Injection-site erythema
(1999): Dr. Sue Bailey, *Asst Sec Defense Health Affairs – Service Member #21, 27, 47*
(1962): Brachman PS+, *Am J Pub Health* 52, 632
Injection-site hematoma
(1999): Dr. Sue Bailey, *Asst Sec Defense Health Affairs – Service Member #12*
Injection-site hypersensitivity
(2000): *MMWR* 49(RR15), 1
Injection-site induration
(1962): Brachman PS+, *Am J Pub Health* 52, 632
Injection-site inflammation
Injection-site local reaction (sic)
(2001): Swanson-Biearman B+, *J Toxicol Clin Toxicol* 39(1), 81 (30%)
(2000): Hayes SC+, *J R Army Med Corps* 146(3), 191 (47%)
(2000): *MMWR* 49(RR15), 1
(1999): Ellenberg SS, *Center for Biologics Evaluation & Research, FDA Statement* (severe)
(1963): Puziss M+, *J. Bacteriol* 85, 230
(1956): Darlow HM+, *Lancet* 2, 476
Injection-site nodules (sic)
(1999): Dr. Sue Bailey, *Asst Sec Defense Health Affairs – Service Members #2, 24, 28, 37, 40, 47*
(1962): Brachman PS+, *Am J Pub Health* 52, 632 lasting up to several weeks
Injection-site numbness
(1999): Dr. Sue Bailey, *Asst Sec Defense Health Affairs – Service Members #6, 13, 15, 22, 26, 31, 39, 43*
Injection-site pain
(2001): Swanson-Biearman B+, *J Toxicol Clin Toxicol* 39(1), 81
(2000): *MMWR* 49(RR15), 1
(1999): Bailey S MD, *Asst Sec Defense Health Affairs – Service Members #1, 4, 8, 13, 18, 19, 20, 42, 45, 47, 49*
Injection-site pain and itching
Injection-site pruritus
(1962): Brachman PS+, *Am J Pub Health* 52, 632
(1954): Wright GG+, *J Immunol* 73, 387 (2.4%)
Injection-site tenderness
(1962): Brachman PS+, *Am J Pub Health* 52, 632 (24–48 hours)
Joint pains
(1999): Dr. Sue Bailey, *Asst Sec Defense Health Affairs – Service Members #6, 13, 15, 22, 26, 31, 39, 43*
Myalgia
(2000): *MMWR* 49(RR15), 1
(1999): Dr. Sue Bailey, *Asst Sec Defense Health Affairs – Service Members #1, 6, 12, 22, 40, 41*

(1954): Wright GG+, *J Immunol* 73, 387 (0.7%)

Paresthesias

(1999): Dr. Sue Bailey, *Asst Sec Defense Health Affairs – Service Members #3, 4, 11, 17, 28, 31, 34, 36, 37, 49*

Scrotal edema

(1999): Dr. Sue Bailey, *Asst Sec Defense Health Affairs – Service Members #9*

Systemic reactions (sic)

(2000): Hayes SC+, *J R Army Med Corps* 146(3), 191 (47%)

Tinnitus

(1999): Dr. Sue Bailey, *Asst Sec Defense Health Affairs – Service Members #1, 6, 7, 10, 11, 13, 14, 23, 24, 28, 29, 48, 49*

Tremors

(1999): Dr. Sue Bailey, *Asst Sec Defense Health Affairs – Service Members #1*

**Note:** Dr. Sue Bailey, Assistant Secretary for Health Affairs, released a statement on June 29, 1999 that 'almost one million shots given, the anthrax immunization is proving to be one of the safest vaccination programs on record.' The above reports occurred for '50 service members at one installation alone.' Note that no number of military personnel were mentioned at this installation, nor did it give any percentages of the above reation patterns

# ANTIRETROVIRAL AGENTS

(Please refer to individual generic drugs for reaction patterns)

**PROTEASE INHIBITORS***

**Generic names:**

**Amprenavir**
Trade name: Agenerase (GSK)

**Indinavir**
Trade name: Crixivan (Merck)

**lopinavir (ABT-378/r)**
Trade name: Kaletra

**Nelfinavir**
Trade name: Viracept (Agouron)

**Ritonavir**
Trade name: Norvir (Abbott)

**Saquinavir**
Trade names: Invirase; Fortovase (Roche)

***Note:** Protease inhibitors cause dyslipidemia which includes elevated triglycerides and cholesterol and redistribution of body fat centrally to produce the so-called "protease paunch," breast enlargement, facial atrophy, and "buffalo hump."

**NUCLEOSIDE ANALOG REVERSE TRANSCRIPTASE INHIBITORS (NRTIs)**

**Generic names:**

**Abacavir (ABC)**
Trade name: Ziagen (GSK

**Didanosine (ddI)**
Trade name: Videx (Bristol-Myers Squibb)

**Lamivudine (3TC)**
Trade names: Epivir, Combivir (GSK)

**Stavudine (d4T)**
Trade name: Zerit (Bristol-Myers Squibb)

**Zalcitabine (ddc)**
Trade names: ddC; Hivid (Roche)

**Zidovudine (AZT)**
Trade names: AZT; Retrovir (GSK)

**NON-NUCLEOSIDE REVERSE TRANSCRIPTASE INHIBITORS (NNRTIs)**

**Generic names:**

**Delavirdine**
Trade name: Rescriptor (Pharmacia & Upjohn)

**Efavirenz**
Trade name: Sustiva (Dupont)

**Nevirapine**
Trade name: Viramune (Roxane)

**NUCLEOSIDE REVERSE TRANSCRIPTASE INHIBITORS (NRTIs)**

**Tenofovir**
Trade name: Viread (Gilead)

Combivir is a combination of lamivudine and zidovudine

# APRACLONIDINE

**Trade name:** Iopidine (Alcon)
**Indications:** Postsurgical intraocular pressure elevation
**Category:** Alpha$_2$ adrenergic agonist; sympathomimetic ophthalmic solution; vasoconstrictor
**Half-life:** 8 hours

### *Reactions*

## Skin

Allergic reactions (sic) (<1%)

(2000): Geyer O+, *Graefes Arch Clin Exp Ophthalmol* 238, 149
(1999): Britt MT+, *Br J Ophthalmol* 83, 992 (progressing to ectropion)
(1998): Gordon RN+, *Eye* 12, 697
(1995): Butler P+, *Arch Ophthalmol* 113, 293
(1995): Feibel RM, *Arch Ophthalmol* 113, 1579

Burning

(1996): Stewart WC, *Klin Monatsbl Augenheilkd* (German) 209, A7

Contact dermatitis (<1%)

(2001): Holdiness MR, *Am J Contact Dermat* 12(4), 217
(2001): Silvestre JF+, *Contact Dermatitis* 45(4), 251
(1998): Armisen M+, *Contact Dermatitis* 39, 193

Dermatitis (sic) (<1%)

Edema (eyelids) (<3%)

Facial edema (<1%)

Pruritus (10%)

(1996): Stewart WC, *Klin Monatsbl Augenheilkd* (German) 209, A7

Xerosis

## Other

Dysgeusia (3%)

Myalgia (0.2%)

Ocular inflammation

(1999): Shin DH+, *Am J Ophthalmol* 127, 511

Paresthesias (<1%)

Parosmia (0.2%)

Periocular dermatitis

(2000): Williams GC+, *Glaucoma* 9, 235

Xerostomia (1–10%)

(1987): Abrams DA+, *Arch Ophthalmol* 105, 1205 (52%)

## APROBARBITAL

**Trade name:** Alurate (Roche)
**Indications:** Short-term sedation, sleep induction
**Category:** Intermediate-acting barbiturate
**Half-life:** 14–34 hours
**Clinically important, potentially hazardous interactions with: alcohol**, brompheniramine, buclizine, dicumarol, ethanolamine, warfarin

### *Reactions*

#### Skin
Angioedema
Exanthems
Exfoliative dermatitis
Purpura
Rash (sic)
Stevens–Johnson syndrome
Urticaria

#### Other
Rhabdomyolysis
(1990): Larpin R+, *Presse Med* 19(30), 1403
Serum sickness

## APROTININ

**Trade name:** Trasylol (Bayer)
**Indications:** For prophylactic use to reduce blood loss in patients undergoing coronary artery bypass surgery
**Category:** Hemostatic agent (a natural protease inhibitor)
**Half-life:** 150 minutes

### *Reactions*

#### Skin
Allergic reactions (sic) (0.5%)
(1994): Bayo M+, *Rev Esp Anestesiol Reanim* (Spanish) 41, 123
(1983): Freeman JG+, *Curr Med Res Opin* 8, 559 (2 cases)
Angioedema
Erythema
Exanthems
(2000): Beierlein W+, *Transfusion* 40, 302 (generalized)
Pruritus
Rash (sic)
Urticaria

#### Other
Anaphylactoid reactions (0.5%)
(2001): Dietrich W+, *Anesthesiology* 95(1), 64
(2000): Beierlein W, *Ann Thorac Surg* 69, 1298
(2000): Laxenaire MC+, *Ann Fr Anesth Reanim* (French) 19, 96
(2000): Pecquet C+, *Ann Fr Anesth* 19(10), 755
(1999): Cohen DM+, *Ann Thorac Surg* 67, 837
(1999): Laxenaire MC, *Ann Fr Anesth Reanim* (French) 18, 796 (4 cases)
(1999): Ong BC+, *Anaesth Intensive Care* 27, 538
(1999): Ryckwaert Y+, *Ann Fr Anesth Reanim* (French) 18, 904
(1998): Scheule AM+, *Gastrointest Endosc* 48, 83
(1997): Dietrich W+, *J Thorac Cardiovasc Surg* 113, 194
(1997): Orsel I+, *Ann Fr Anesth Reanim* (French) 16, 292
(1997): Scheule AM+, *Ann Thorac Surg* 63, 242
(1996): Martinelli L+, *Ann Thorac Surg* 61, 1288
(1995): Ceriana P+, *J Cardiothorac Vasc Anesth* 9, 477
(1995): Diefenbach C+, *Anesth Analg* 80, 830
(1994): Kon NF+, *Masui* (Japanese) 43, 1606
(1993): Cottineau C+, *Ann Fr Anesth Reanim* (French) 12, 590
(1993): Schulze K+, *Eur J Cardiothorac Surg* 7, 495 (2 patients)
(1984): *BMJ* 289, 1696
(1984): LaFerla GA+, *BMJ* 289, 1176
(1976): Proud G+, *Lancet* 2, 48
(1971): Bauer J+, *Am J Gastroenterol* 56, 542
Hypersensitivity
(2000): Beierlein W+, *Transfusion* 40, 302
(1998): Dietrich W, *Ann Thoracic Surg* 65, S60 (1.8%)
(1975): Ariani G+, *Minerva Anestesiol* (Italian) 41, 138
Lipohypertrophy
(1985): Boag F+, *N Engl J Med* 312, 245 (in a diabetic)
(1985): Dandona P+, *Diabetes Res* 2, 213 (in a diabetic)
Phlebitis (1–10%)
Shock (sic)
(1971): Vashchuk VV, *Klin Med (Mosk)* (Russian) 49, 128

## ARBUTAMINE

**Trade name:** GenESA (Gensia)
**Indications:** Diagnostic aid for coronary artery disease
**Category:** Adrenergic agonist; nonradioactive diagnostic; synthetic catecholamine
**Half-life:** 1.8 hours
**Clinically important, potentially hazardous interactions with:** clidinium, clomipramine, desipramine, dicyclomine, digoxin, doxepin, flavoxate, glycopyrrolate, hyoscyamine, imipramine, nortriptyline, oxybutynin, procyclidine, propantheline, protriptyline, scopolamine, trihexyphenidyl, trimipramine

### *Reactions*

#### Skin
Diaphoresis (1.5%)
Flushing (3%)
(2001): Wright DJ+, *Nucl Med Commun* 22(12), 1305 (35%)
Hot flashes (3%)
Rash (sic)

#### Other
Application-site reaction (0.1%)
Back pain (0.1%)
Cough (0.2%)
Dysgeusia (1.3%)
(2001): Wright DJ+, *Nucl Med Commun* 22(12), 1305 (23%)
Hyperesthesia (1.0%)
Pain (1.8%)
Paresthesias (2%)
Tremors (15%)
(1997): Cohen A+, *Am J Cardiol* 79(6), 713 (5.6%)
Twitching (0.3%)
Xerostomia (1.1%)

## ARGATROBAN

**Trade name:** Acova (GSK)
**Indications:** Heparin-induced thrombocytopenia
**Category:** Anticoagulant; thrombin inhibitor
**Half-life:** 40-50 minutes
**Clinically important, potentially hazardous interactions with:** butabarbital

### *Reactions*

#### Skin
Allergic reactions (sic)
Bullous eruption (<1%)
Infections (sic) (4%)
Rash (sic) (<1%)

#### Other
Injection-site bleeding (2–5%)

## ARISTOLOCHIA*

**Scientific names:** *Aristolochia auricularia; Aristolochia clematitis; Aristolochia fangchi; Aristolochia heterophylla; Aristolochia kwangsiensis; Aristolochia moupinensis; Aristolochia reticulata; Aristolochia serpentaria; Aristolochia* species
**Other common names:** Birthwort; Long Birthwort; Pelican Flower; Red River Snakeroot; Sangree Root; Sangrel; Serpentaria; Snakeroot; Snakeweed; Texas Snakeroot; Virginia Serpentary; Virginia Snakeroot
**Family:** Aristolochiaceae
**Purported indications:** Aphrodisiac, anticonvulsant, immune stimulant and to promote menstruation
**Other uses:** To treat allergic gastrointestinal colic and gallbladder colic

### *Reactions*

#### Skin
None

***Note:** While there are no reported dermatologic adverse side effects, it's worthy to note that aristolochia has been reported to cause severe kidney damage and death. Reported as "Chinese herb nephropathy," many of these cases progressed to end stage renal failure requiring dialysis or transplantation. Eighteen patients developed carcinomas of the bladder, ureter and/or renal pelvis

****Note:** Aristolochia is banned in Austria, France, Germany, Britain, Japan, and Belgium

## ARNICA

**Scientific names:** *Arnica fulgens; Arnica montana; Arnica sororia*
**Other common names:** Arnica Flos; Arnica Flower; Leopard's Bane; Wolf's Bane
**Family:** Asteraceae; compositae
**Purported indications:** Inflammation and immune system stimulation associated with bruises, aches and sprains, insect bites, superficial phlebitis. Diuretic (Historically used as an abortifacient.)
**Other uses:** Flavoring agent, candy, puddings; found in hair tonics, anti-dandruff shampoos

### *Reactions*

#### Skin
Acute febrile neutrophilic dermatosis (Sweet's syndrome)
Contact dermatitis
Dermal irritation (sic)

#### Other
Mucous membrane irritation (sic)

## ARSENIC

**Trade names:** Trisonex (Cell Therapeutics); Fowler's Solution (rarely employed); found in pesticides and herbal medicines
**Indications:** Acute promyelocytic leukemia, psoriasis (in the early 1900s), devitalization of pulp in dental procedures
**Category:** Trace metal
**Half-life:** no data
**Clinically important, potentially hazardous interactions with:** amiodarone, bretylium, chlorpromazine, ciprofloxacin, disopyramide, enoxacin, fluphenazine, gatifloxacin, lomefloxacin, mesoridazine, moxifloxacin, norfloxacin, ofloxacin, phenothiazines, procainamide, prochlorperazine, promethazine, quinidine, quinolones, sotalol, sparfloxacin, thioridazine, trifluoperazine

### *Reactions*

#### Skin
Acrocyanosis
(2002): Hall AH, *Toxicol Lett* 128(1), 69
Basal cell carcinoma
(2001): Guo HR+, *Cancer Causes Control* 12(10), 909
Bullous eruption
(1993): Alain G+, *Int J Dermatol* 32, 899 (passim)
(1992): Breathnach SM+, *Adverse Drug Reactions and the Skin* Blackwell, Oxford, 236 (passim)
(1988): Bork K, *Cutaneous Side Effects of Drugs* WB Saunders, 114
(1968): Privat Y+, *Bull Soc Med Afr Noire Lang Fr* (French) 13, 195
(1955): Alexander HL, *Reactions with Drug Therapy* Philadelphia, WB Saunders
Cancer (sic)
(1997): Schwartz RA, *Int J Dermatol* 36, 241
(1995): Fawell J, *Hum Exp Toxicol* 14, 464
(1995): Hsueh YM+, *Br J Cancer* 71, 109
(1993): Urbach F, *Recent Results Cancer Res* 128, 243
(1992): Wong O+, *Int Arch Occup Environ Health* 64, 235
(1989): Bickley LK+, *N J Med* 86, 377
(1988): Chen CJ+, *Lancet* 1, 414

(1988): Durocher LP+, *Union Med Can* (French) 117, 345
(1976): Spoor HJ, *Cutis* 18, 631
(1970): Thivolet J+, *Lyon Med* (French) 223, 457
(1969): Thivolet J+, *Bull Soc Fr Dermatol Syphiligr* (French) 76, 892

Carcinoma
(2002): Hall AH, *Toxicol Lett* 128(1), 69
(2002): Liu J+, *Environ Health Perspect* 110(2), 119
(2001): Guo HR+, *Cancer Causes Control* 12(10), 909
(2001): Rahman MM+, *J Toxicol Clin Toxicol* 39(7), 683
(2001): Yu HS+, *J Dermatol* 28(11), 628

Contact dermatitis
(1995): Barbaud A+, *Contact Dermatitis* 33, 272
(1986): Wahlberg JE+, *Derm Beruf Umwelt* (German) 34, 10
(1964): Gaffi A, *Gazz Int Med Chir* (Italian) 69, 3363

Dermatitis (sic)
(2001): Guo X+, *Mol Cell Biochem* 222(1), 137
(1955): Alexander HL, *Reactions with Drug Therapy* Philadelphia, WB Saunders

Dermatofibrosarcoma protuberans
(1986): Shneidman D+, *Cancer* 58, 1585

Erythema multiforme
(1990): Vassileva S+, *Int J Dermatol* 29, 381
(1988): Bork K, *Cutaneous Side Effects of Drugs* WB Saunders, 145
(1967): Coleman WP, *Med Clin North Am* 51, 1073
(1955): Alexander HL, *Reactions with Drug Therapy* Philadelphia, WB Saunders
(1945): Fletcher MWC+, *J Pediatr* 27, 465

Erythema nodosum
(1988): Bork K, *Cutaneous Side Effects of Drugs* WB Saunders, 148

Exanthems
(1993): Alain G+, *Int J Dermatol* 32, 899 (passim)
(1974): *Med Lett* 16, 11
(1974): Tay CH, *Aust J Dermatol* 15, 121 (16%)
(1955): Alexander HL, *Reactions with Drug Therapy* Philadelphia, WB Saunders
(1952): Sulzberger MB+, *Postgrad Med* 11, 549

Exfoliative dermatitis
(1993): Alain G+, *Int J Dermatol* 32, 899 (passim)
(1992): Breathnach SM+, *Adverse Drug Reactions and the Skin* Blackwell, Oxford, 236 (passim)
(1973): Nicolis GD+, *Arch Dermatol* 108, 788
(1967): Coleman WP, *Med Clin North Am* 51, 1073
(1967): Lockey SD, *Med Sci* 18, 43
(1965): Fellner MJ+, *Med Clin North Am* 49, 709
(1963): Abrahams I+, *Arch Dermatol* 87, 96
(1955): Alexander HL, *Reactions with Drug Therapy* Philadelphia, WB Saunders

Fixed eruption
(1988): Bork K, *Cutaneous Side Effects of Drugs* WB Saunders, 108
(1964): Browne SG, *BMJ* 2, 1041
(1961): Welsh AL, *The Fixed Drug Eruption*, Thomas, Springfield
(1955): Alexander HL, *Reactions with Drug Therapy* Philadelphia, WB Saunders

Follicular keratosis (sic)
(1952): Sulzberger MB+, *Postgrad Med* 11, 549

Freckles
(1995): Gritiyarangsan P+, *Photodermatol Photoimmunol Photomed* 11, 174

Hyperhidrosis
(1993): Alain G+, *Int J Dermatol* 32, 899 (passim)

Hyperkeratosis (palms and soles) (40%)
(2001): Kurokawa M+, *Arch Dermatol* 137, 102
(1996): Maloney ME, *Dermatol Surg* 22, 301 (passim)
(1965): Fierz U, *Dermatologica* 131, 41

Keratoses
(2002): Liu J+, *Environ Health Perspect* 110(2), 119
(2001): Rahman MM+, *J Toxicol Clin Toxicol* 39(7), 683
(2001): Yu HS+, *J Dermatol* 28(11), 628
(1999): Tondel M+, *Environmental Health Perspectives* 107, 727
(1998): Guha Mazumder DN+, *Int J Epidemiol* 27, 871
(1993): Alain G+, *Int J Dermatol* 32, 899 (passim)
(1992): Breathnach SM+, *Adverse Drug Reactions and the Skin* Blackwell, Oxford, 236 (passim)
(1988): Bork K, *Cutaneous Side Effects of Drugs* WB Saunders, 232
(1978): Reymann F+, *Arch Dermatol* 114, 378
(1969): Bartruff JK, *Arch Dermatol* 100, 382
(1965): Dobson RL+, *Arch Dermatol* 92, 553

Leukomelanoderma (sic)
(1999): Tondel M+, *Environmental Health Perspectives* 107, 727
(1993): Sass U+, *Dermatology* 186, 303
(1974): Tay CH, *Aust J Dermatol* 15, 121 (31%)
(1952): Sulzberger MB+, *Postgrad Med* 11, 549

Leukomelanosis (sic)
(2001): Kurokawa M+, *Arch Dermatol* 137, 102
(2001): Rahman MM+, *J Toxicol Clin Toxicol* 39(7), 683

Lichen planus (bullous)
(1970): Aguilera-Diaz LF, *Ann Dermatol Syphiligr Paris* (French) 97, 39

Livedo reticularis
(1974): Nagy G+, *Z Hautkr* (German) 25, 534

Melanoderma
(1992): Breathnach SM+, *Adverse Drug Reactions and the Skin* Blackwell, Oxford, 236 (passim)

Melanoma
(1984): Philipp R+, *Br Med J Clin Res Ed* 288, 237
(1980): Clough P, *BMJ* 280, 112
(1980): Evans S, *BMJ* 280, 403
(1976): Grobe JW, *Berufsdermatosen* (German) 24, 167

Melanosis
(2001): Rahman MM+, *J Toxicol Clin Toxicol* 39(7), 683

Merkel cell carcinoma
(1999): Huang-Chun L+, *J Am Acad Dermatol* 41, 641
(1998): Tsuruta D+, *Br J Dermatol* 139, 291
(1997): Ohnishi Y+, *J Dermatol* 24, 310
(1991): Huang HP+, *J Formos Med Assoc* 90, 900

Morphea
(1952): Sulzberger MB+, *Postgrad Med* 11, 549

Palmar–plantar erythema
(1952): Sulzberger MB+, *Postgrad Med* 11, 549

Palmar–plantar hyperhidrosis
(2000): Gerdssn R+, *Acta Derm Venereol* 80, 292
(1974): Tay CH, *Aust J Dermatol* 15, 121 (31%)

Palmar–plantar hyperkeratosis
(2002): Hall AH, *Toxicol Lett* 128(1), 69
(2000): Gerdsen R+, *Acta Derm Venereol* 80, 292
(1998): Tsuruta D+, *Br J Dermatol* 139, 291
(1997): Ohnishi Y+, *J Dermatol* 24, 310
(1996): Maloney ME, *Dermatol Surg* 22, 301 (passim)
(1996): Person JR, *Cutis* 58, 65
(1994): Hsieh LL+, *Cancer Lett* 86, 59
(1993): Alain G+, *Int J Dermatol* 32, 899 (passim)
(1992): Breathnach SM+, *Adverse Drug Reactions and the Skin* Blackwell, Oxford, 236 (passim)
(1989): Koh E+, *Eur Urol* 16, 398
(1989): Shannon RL+, *Hum Toxicol* 8, 99
(1988): Ismail R+, *J Dermatol* 15, 65
(1983): Heddle R+, *Chest* 84, 776
(1982): Ohyama K, *Dermatologica* 164, 161
(1982): Rosen T+, *J Am Acad Dermatol* 7, 364
(1979): Allen RB+, *Cutis* 23, 805
(1974): Tay CH, *Aust J Dermatol* 15, 121
(1973): Yeh S, *Human Path* 4, 469

Palmar–plantar keratoderma

(1996): Maloney ME, *Dermatol Surg* 22, 301 (passim)
(1996): Matsumura Y+, *Int J Cancer* 65, 778
(1994): McNutt NS+, *Arch Dermatol* 130, 225
(1993): Alain G+, *Int J Dermatol* 32, 899 (passim)
(1993): Sass U+, *Dermatology* 186, 303
(1993): Ziegler A+, *Proc Natl Acad*
(1992): Breathnach SM+, *Adverse Drug Reactions and the Skin* Blackwell, Oxford, 236 (passim)
(1987): Chakraborty AK+, *Indian J Med Res* 85, 326
(1986): Munzberger H+, *Z Arztl Fortbild Jena* (German) 80, 985
(1985): Kastl J+, *Dermatol Monatsschr* (German) 171, 158
(1984): Schroeder P+, *Fortschr Med* (German) 102, 1128
(1980): Weiss J+, *Hautarzt* (German) 31, 654
(1974): Tay CH, *Aust J Dermatol* 15, 121 (6%)
(1973): Yeh S, *Human Path* 4, 469
(1972): Hadida E+, *Bull Soc Fr Dermatol Syphiligr* (French) 79, 287
(1967): Schulz EJ *S Afr Med J* 41, 819
(1965): Fierz U, *Dermatologica* 131, 41

Palmar–plantar punctate keratoses
(1996): Maloney ME, *Dermatol Surg* 22, 301 (passim)
(1992): Breathnach SM+, *Adverse Drug Reactions and the Skin* Blackwell, Oxford, 236 (passim)

Parapsoriasis
(1952): Sulzberger MB+, *Postgrad Med* 11, 549

Photosensitivity
(1992): Breathnach SM+, *Adverse Drug Reactions and the Skin* Blackwell, Oxford, 236 (passim)

Pigmentation
(2002): Hall AH, *Toxicol Lett* 128(1), 69
(2002): Liu J+, *Environ Health Perspect* 110(2), 119
(2001): Kurokawa M+, *Arch Dermatol* 137, 102
(2001): Yu HS+, *J Dermatol* 28(11), 628
(1999): Tondel M+, *Environmental Health Perspectives* 107, 727
(1998): Guha Mazumder DN+, *Int J Epidemiol* 27, 871
(1996): Maloney ME, *Dermatol Surg* 22, 301 (passim)
(1993): Alain G+, *Int J Dermatol* 32, 899 (passim)
(1992): Breathnach SM+, *Adverse Drug Reactions and the Skin* Blackwell, Oxford, 236 (passim)
(1989): Shannon RL+, *Hum Toxicol* 8, 99
(1981): Granstein RD+, *J Am Acad Dermatol* 5, 1 (bronze)
(1974): Tay CH, *Aust J Dermatol* 15, 121 (85%)
(1973): Levantine A+, *Br J Dermatol* 89, 105

Pityriasis rosea (from organic arsenic)
(1988): Bork K, *Cutaneous Side Effects of Drugs* WB Saunders, 169
(1952): Sulzberger MB+, *Postgrad Med* 11, 549

Pruritus
(1967): Young AW, *J Am Geriatr Soc* 15, 750

Psoriasis
(1952): Sulzberger MB+, *Postgrad Med* 11, 549

Purpura
(1988): Bork K, *Cutaneous Side Effects of Drugs* WB Saunders, 191
(1955): Alexander HL, *Reactions with Drug Therapy* Philadelphia, WB Saunders

Raynaud's phenomenon
(2002): Hall AH, *Toxicol Lett* 128(1), 69

Squamous cell carcinoma
(2001): Guo HR+, *Cancer Causes Control* 12(10), 909
(1996): Maloney ME, *Dermatol Surg* 22, 301 (passim)
(1993): Alain G+, *Int J Dermatol* 32, 899 (passim)
(1992): Breathnach SM+, *Adverse Drug Reactions and the Skin* Blackwell, Oxford, 236 (passim)
(1989): Shannon RL+, *Hum Toxicol* 8, 99
(1988): Ismail R+, *J Dermatol* 15, 65
(1988): Scholz S+, *Z Arztl Fortbild Jena* (German) 82, 1201
(1979): Brownstein MH+, *Int J Dermatol* 18, 1
(1979): Southwick GJ+, *J Surg Oncol* 12, 115
(1974): Tay CH, *Aust J Dermatol* 15, 121
(1973): Yeh S, *Human Path* 4, 469

Stevens–Johnson syndrome
(1990): Vassileva S+, *Int J Dermatol* 29, 381
(1967): Coleman WP, *Med Clin North Am* 51, 1073
(1945): Fletcher MWC+, *J Pediatr* 27, 465

Ulceration
(2002): Liu J+, *Environ Health Perspect* 110(2), 119

Urticaria
(1955): Alexander HL, *Reactions with Drug Therapy* Philadelphia, WB Saunders

Vitiligo
(1989): Bickley LK+, *N J Med* 86, 377

## Hair

Hair – alopecia
(1993): Alain G+, *Int J Dermatol* 32, 899 (passim)
(1992): Breathnach SM+, *Adverse Drug Reactions and the Skin* Blackwell, Oxford, 236 (passim)
(1988): Bork K, *Cutaneous Side Effects of Drugs* WB Saunders, 249
(1974): Tay CH, *Aust J Dermatol* 15, 121 (5%)

## Nails

Nails – leukonychia
(1988): Bork K, *Cutaneous Side Effects of Drugs* WB Saunders, 262

Nails – pigmentation
(1988): Bork K, *Cutaneous Side Effects of Drugs* WB Saunders, 261
(1978): Shah PC+, *Br J Dermatol* 98, 675 (passim)

Nails – transverse white bands
(1993): Alain G+, *Int J Dermatol* 32, 899 (passim)
(1993): Sass U+, *Dermatology* 186, 303

## Other

Dysgeusia
(2002): Hall AH, *Toxicol Lett* 128(1), 69

Foetor ex ore (halitosis)
(1988): Bork K, *Cutaneous Side Effects of Drugs* WB Saunders, 310

Gangrene
(1952): Sulzberger MB+, *Postgrad Med* 11, 549

Gynecomastia
(1992): Breathnach SM+, *Adverse Drug Reactions and the Skin* Blackwell, Oxford, 237 (passim)

Oral mucosal eruption (8%)
(1974): Tay CH, *Aust J Dermatol* 15, 121
(1966): Dummett CO, *J Oral Ther Pharmacol* 1, 106
(1952): Sulzberger MB+, *Postgrad Med* 11, 549

Oral mucosal pigmentation
(1988): Bork K, *Cutaneous Side Effects of Drugs* WB Saunders, 288

Stomatitis
(1966): Dummett CO, *J Oral Ther Pharmacol* 1, 106

Tumors (malignant)
(2001): Kurokawa M+, *Arch Dermatol* 137, 102

## ASCORBIC ACID

**Synonym:** vitamin C
**Trade names:** Ascorbicap; Cebid; Cecon; Cemill; Cetane; Cevalin (Lilly); Cevi-Bid; Dull-C; Sunkist; Vita-C
**Other common trade names:** *Apo-C; Ce-Vi-Sol; Cebion; Cetebe; Laroscorbine; Potent C; Pro-C; Redoxon*
**Indications:** Prevention of scurvy
**Category:** Water-soluble nutritional supplement
**Half-life:** no data
**Clinically important, potentially hazardous interactions with:** deferoxamine, penicillamine

#### *Reactions*

### Skin
Angioedema
(1980): Bilyk MA+, *Vrach Delo* (Russian) May, 81
Cutaneous side effects (sic)
(1992): Breathnach SM+, *Adverse Drug Reactions and the Skin* Blackwell, Oxford, 265 (passim)
(1980): Bilyk MA+, *Vrach Delo* (Russian) May, 81
Eczema (sic)
(1980): Metz J+, *Contact Dermatitis* 6, 172
Erythema
Flushing (<1%)

### Other
Injection-site irritation

## ASPARAGINASE

**Synonym:** L-asparaginase
**Trade name:** Elspar (Merck)
**Other common trade names:** *Crasnitin; Erwinase; Kidrolase; Laspar; Leunase*
**Indications:** Acute lymphocytic leukemia, lymphoma
**Category:** Antineoplastic; protein synthesis inhibitor (parenteral)
**Half-life:** 8–30 hours (IV); 39–49 hours (IM)

#### *Reactions*

### Skin
Angioedema
(1983): Bronner AK+, *J Am Acad Dermatol* 9, 645 (15%)
(1981): Weiss RB+, *Ann Intern Med* 94, 66
(1971): Jacquillat C+, *Med Welt* (German) 22, 503 (<1.0%)
Chills
Diaphoresis
Edema
Exanthems
Flushing
(1983): Bronner AK+, *J Am Acad Dermatol* 9, 645 (15%)
Pruritus (<1%)
(1981): Weiss RB+, *Ann Intern Med* 94, 66
Rash (sic) (<1%)
Toxic epidermal necrolysis
(1989): Stern RS+, *J Am Acad Dermatol* 21, 317
(1980): Rodriguez AR, *J Med Assoc Ga* 69, 355
Urticaria (<1%)
(1983): Bronner AK+, *J Am Acad Dermatol* 9, 645 (15%)
(1981): Weiss RB+, *Ann Intern Med* 94, 66
(1979): Ertel IJ+, *Cancer Res* 39, 3893
(1971): Jacquillat C+, *Med Welt* (German) 22, 503 (<0.5%)

### Hair
Hair – alopecia

### Other
Anaphylactoid reactions (10–40%)
(1983): Bronner AK+, *J Am Acad Dermatol* 9, 645 (15%)
(1982): Dunagin WG, *Semin Oncol* 9, 14 (3%)
(1979): Ertel IJ+, *Cancer Res* 39, 3893
Aphthous stomatitis (1–10%)
Hypersensitivity (10–40%)
(2001): Bryant R, *J Intraven Nurs* 24(3), 169
(1998): Bonno M+, *J Allergy Clin Immunol* 101, 571
(1998): Larson RA+, *Leukemia* 12, 660
(1992): Weiss RB, *Semin Oncol* 19, 458
(1982): Dunagin WG, *Semin Oncol* 9, 14 (33%)
(1981): Weiss RB+, *Ann Intern Med* 94, 66 (6–43%)
(1978): Levine N+, *Cancer Treat Res* 5, 67 (5–20%)
(1974): Levantine A+, *Br J Dermatol* 90, 239
Injection-site erythema
Oral mucosal lesions (26%)
Serum sickness
(1983): Bronner AK+, *J Am Acad Dermatol* 9, 645 (15%)

## ASPARTAME

**Trade names:** Equal; Nutrasweet*
**Indications:** No data
**Category:** Low-calorie artificial sweetener
**Half-life:** no data

#### *Reactions*

### Skin
Allergic reactions (sic)
(1998): Garriga MM+, *Ann Allergy* 61, 63
(1996): Roberts HJ, *Arch Intern Med* 156, 1027
Angioedema
(1992): Downham TF, *Clin Cases in Dermatol* 4, 12 (observation)
(1988): Metcalfe DD, *Skin and Allergy News* 19, 52 (observation)
Dermatitis (sic)
(1992): Downham TF, *Clin Cases in Dermatol* 4, 12 (observation)
Exanthems
(1986): *Arzneimittelinformation ATI Berlin GmbH* (German) 12, 121
Pruritus
(1994): Shelley WB+, *Cutis* 53, 77 (observation)
(1988): Metcalfe DD, *Skin and Allergy News* 19, 52 (observation)
Pruritus ani
(1994): Shelley WB+, *Cutis* 53, 237 (observation)
Purpura
(1999): Leal G, Fortaleza, Brazil (from Internet) (observation)
(1992): Downham TF, *Clin Cases in Dermatol* 4, 12 (observation)
Rash (sic)
(1988): Metcalfe DD, *Skin and Allergy News* 19, 52 (observation)
Urticaria
(1995): Kulczycki A, *J Allergy Clin Immunol* 95, 639
(1992): Downham TF, *Clin Cases in Dermatol* 4, 12 (observation)
(1988): Metcalfe DD, *Skin and Allergy News* 19, 52 (observation)
(1986): Kulczycki A, *Ann Intern Med* 104, 207
Vasculitis
(1992): Downham TF, *Clin Cases in Dermatol* 4, 12 (observation)

### Other
Anaphylactoid reactions
(1996): Roberts HJ, *Arch Intern Med* 156, 1027
Panniculitis

(1992): Geha RS, *J Am Acad Dermatol* 26, 277 (lobular)
(1991): McCauliffe DP+, *J Am Acad Dermatol* 24, 298 (lobular)
(1985): Novick NL, *Ann Intern Med* 102, 206 (granulomatous)

***Note:** Aspartame can be found in instant breakfasts, breath mints, cereals, sugar-free chewing gum, cocoa mixes, coffee beverages, frozen desserts, gelatin desserts, juice beverages, laxatives, multivitamins, milk drinks, pharmaceuticals and supplements, shake mixes, soft drinks, tabletop sweeteners, tea beverages, instant teas and coffees, topping mixes, wine coolers, yogurt

# ASPIRIN

**Synonyms:** acetylsalicylic acid; ASA
**Trade names:** Aggrenox (Boehringer Ingelheim); Alka-Seltzer; Anacin (Wyeth); Ascriptin (Novartis); Aspergum; Bufferin; Coricidin D; Darvon Compound; Ecotrin (GSK); Empirin; Equagesic; Excedrin; Fiorinal; Gelprin; Halfprin; Measurin; Norgesic; Percodan; Robaxisal; Soma Compound; Talwin Compound (Sanofi); Vanquish
**Other common trade names:** *ASA; Aspro; ASS; Bex; Caprin; Claragine; Disprin; Ecotrin; etc; Novasen; Rhonal*
**Indications:** Pain, fever, inflammation
**Category:** Nonsteroidal anti-inflammatory (NSAID) analgesic; salicylate
**Half-life:** 15–20 minutes
**Clinically important, potentially hazardous interactions with:** anticoagulants, bismuth, cholestyramine, dicumarol, etodolac, **ginkgo biloba**, **ginseng**, heparin, ibuprofen, indomethacin, ketoprofen, ketorolac, methotrexate, NSAIDs, reteplase, tirofiban, urokinase, valdecoxib, valproic acid, verapamil, warfarin

Aggrenox is aspirin and dipyridamole

## *Reactions*

### Skin

Acute generalized exanthematous pustulosis (AGEP)
(1993): Ballmer-Weber BK+, *Schweiz Med Wochenschr (German)* 123, 542
Allergic reactions (sic) (<1%) (with dipyridamole)
(1991): VanArsdel PP Jr, *JAMA* 266, 3343
Angioedema (1–5%)
(2000): Ghislain PD+, *Ann Med Interne* (Paris) 151, 227 (Nuchal scalp)
(2000): Pradalier A+, *Rev Med Interne* (French) 21, 75
(2000): Wong JT+, *J Allergy Clin Immunol* 105, 997
(1998): Grzelewska-Rzymowska I, *Pol Merkuriusz Lek* (Polish) 4, 233
(1998): Quiralte J, *Ann Allergy Asthma Immunol* 81, 459 (periorbital)
(1997): Tomaz EM+, *Allergy Asthma Proc* 18, 319
(1996): Chan TY, *Br J Clin Pract* 50, 412
(1993): Grzelewska-Rzymowska I+, *Pneumonol Alergol Pol* (Polish) 61, 29
(1988): Botey J+, *Allergol Immunopathol Madr* (Spanish) 16, 43
(1984): Botey J+, *Ann Allergy* 53, 265
(1981): Juhlin L, *Br J Dermatol* 104, 369
(1977): Abrishami MA+, *Ann Allergy* 39, 28
(1977): Szczeklik A+, *J Allergy Clin Immunol* 60, 276
(1974): Schlumberger HD+, *Acta Med Scand* 196, 451
(1972): Kauppinen K, *Acta Derm Venereol* (Stockh) 52 (Suppl), 68
(1970): Baker H+, *Br J Dermatol* 82, 319
(1969): Girard JP+, *Helv Med Acta* 35, 86
(1967): Moore-Robinson M+, *BMJ* 4, 263
Bullous eruption (<1%)
(1989): Sfar Z +, *Tunis Med* 67, 805
(1979): Odinokova VA+, *Arkh Patol* (Russian) 41, 37
(1972): Kauppinen K, *Acta Derm Venereol* (Stockh) 52 (Suppl), 68
(1960): Hejier A+, *Acta Derm Venereol* (Stockh) 40, 35
Dermatitis herpetiformis
(1966): Brannen M+, *Tex State J Med* 62, 58
Dermatomyositis
(1964): Shelley WB, *JAMA* 189, 986
Diaphoresis
Erythema multiforme (<1%)
(1998): Lee SG+, *Eur J Dermatol* 8, 280
(1985): Laurberg G+, *Ugeskr Laeger* 147, 1853
(1985): Ting HC+, *Int J Dermatol* 24, 587
(1982): Bailin PL+, *Clin Rheum Dis* 8, 493 (passim)
(1977): Davis JD+, *Clin Pharm Ther* 21, 52
(1975): Bottiger LE+, *Acta Med Scand* 198, 229
(1968): Bianchine JR+, *Am Med J* 44, 390
(1966): Brannen M+, *Tex State J Med* 62, 58
(1960): Hejier A+, *Acta Derm Venereol* (Stockh) 40, 35
Erythema nodosum (<1%)
(1996): Buckshee K+, *Int J Gynaecol Obstet* 55, 293
(1996): Durden FM+, *Int J Dermatol* 35, 39
(1994): Fernandes NC+, *Rev Inst Med Trop Sao Paulo* (Portuguese) 36, 507
(1987): Blasetti P, *Clin Ter* 123(4), 303
(1982): Bailin PL+, *Clin Rheum Dis* 8, 493 (passim)
(1982): Ubogy Z+, *Acta Derm Venereol* 62, 265
(1970): Baker H+, *Br J Dermatol* 82, 319
(1966): Brannen M+, *Tex State J Med* 62, 58
(1964): Shelley WB, *JAMA* 189, 985
Erythroderma
(1974): Tay C, *Asian J Med* 10, 223
Exanthems
(1993): Ballmer-Weber BK+, *Schweiz Med Wochenschr* 123, 542
(1989): Hass WK+, *N Engl J Med* 321, 501 (5.2%)
(1987): Castles JJ+, *Arch Intern Med* 138, 362 (2.8%)
(1982): Morley PA+, *Drugs* 23, 250 (5%)
(1980): Goerz G+, *Fortschr Med* 98, 726
(1977): Chalem F+, *Curr Ther Res* 22, 769
(1977): Davis JD+, *Clin Pharm Ther* 21, 52 (1–5%)
(1975): Blechman WJ+, *JAMA* 233, 336 (2.5%)
(1975): Bowers DE+, *Ann Intern Med* 83, 470 (18%)
(1972): Kauppinen K, *Acta Derm Venereol* (Stockh) 52 (Suppl), 68
(1960): Hejier A+, *Acta Derm Venereol* (Stockh) 40, 35
Exfoliative dermatitis
(1969): Girard JP+, *Helv Med Acta* 35, 86
Fixed eruption (<1%)
(1999): Galindo PA+, *J Investig Allergol Clin Immunol* 9, 399
(1998): Mahboob A+, *Int J Dermatol* 37, 833
(1997): Bhargava P+, *Int J Dermatol* 36, 236
(1992): Hatzis J+, *Cutis* 50, 50
(1991): Thankappen TP+, *Int J Dermatol* 30, 867 (1.7%)
(1990): Bharija SC+, *Dermatologica* 181, 237
(1990): Gaffoor PMA+, *Cutis* 45, 242
(1989): Shiohara T+, *Arch Dermatol* 125, 1371
(1986): Kanwar AJ, *Dermatologica* 172, 315
(1986): Kanwar AJ+, *J Dermatol* 11, 383
(1985): Gomez B+, *Allergol Immunopathol Madr* (Spanish) 13, 87
(1985): Kauppinen K+, *Br J Dermatol* 112, 575
(1984): Boyle J+, *Br Med J Clin Res Ed* 289, 802
(1984): Chan HL, *Int J Dermatol* 23, 607
(1984): Pandhi RK+, *Sex Transm Dis* 11, 164
(1982): Bailin PL+, *Clin Rheum Dis* 8, 493 (passim)
(1981): Shukla SR, *Dermatologica* 163, 160
(1975): Gimenez-Camarasa JM+, *N Engl J Med* 292, 819
(1974): Kuokkanen K, *Int J Dermatol* 13, 4
(1972): Kauppinen K, *Acta Derm Venereol* (Stockh) 52 (Suppl), 68
(1970): Savin JA, *Br J Dermatol* 83, 546
Flushing

(1964): Shelley WB, *JAMA* 189, 986
Genital herpes
(1964): Shelley WB, *JAMA* 189, 986
Graft-versus-host reaction
(1998): Jappe U+, *Hautarzt* (German) 49, 126 (passim)
Herpes simplex
(1984): Boyle J, Moul B, *Br Med J (Clin Res Ed)* 289, 802
Jitters (sic)
Lichenoid eruption
(1988): Bharija SC+, *Dermatologica* 177, 19
(1966): Brannen M+, *Tex State J Med* 62, 58
Parapsoriasis
(1966): Brannen M+, *Tex State J Med* 62, 58
Pemphigus
(1986): Pisani M+, *G Ital Dermatol Venereol* (Italian) 121, 39
Periorbital edema
(1997): Price KS+, *Ann Allergy Asthma Immunol* 79, 420
(1993): Katz Y+, *Allergy* 48, 366
Petechiae
(1997): Blumenthal HL, Beachwood, OH (personal case) (observation)
Photo-recall
(1998): Lee SG+, *Eur J Dermatol* 8, 280
Pigmented purpuric eruption
(1999): Lipsker D+, *Ann Dermatol Venereol* (French) 126, 321
Pityriasis rosea
(1993): Yosipovitch G+, *Harefuah* (Hebrew) 124, 198; 247
(1966): Brannen M+, *Tex State J Med* 62, 58
Pruritus
(1981): Settipane GA, *Arch Intern Med* 141, 328
(1977): Chalem F+, *Curr Ther Res* 22, 769 (1–5%)
(1977): Davis JD+, *Clin Pharm Ther* 21, 52 (>5%)
(1975): Blechman WJ+, *JAMA* 233, 336 (2%)
(1969): Girard JP+, *Helv Med Acta* 35, 86
(1967): Moore-Robinson M+, *BMJ* 4, 263
Psoriasis
(1966): Brannen M+, *Tex State J Med* 62, 58
(1964): Shelley WB, *JAMA* 189, 986
Purpura
(2001): Tsuda T+, *J Int Med Res* 29(4), 374
(1997): Sola-Alberich R+, *Ann Intern Med* 126, 665
(1989): Hass WK+, *N Engl J Med* 321, 501 (2%)
(1980): Miescher PA+, *Clin Haematol* 9, 505
(1976): Karchmer AW+, *N Engl J Med* 295, 451
(1972): Kauppinen K, *Acta Derm Venereol* (Stockh) 52 (Suppl), 68
(1971): Davis SL+, *Nebraska St Med J* 56, 432
Pustular psoriasis
(1976): Lindgren S+, *Acta Derm Venereol* (Stockh) 56, 139
(1964): Shelley WB, *JAMA* 189, 985
Rash (sic) (1–10%)
Stevens–Johnson syndrome
(1993): Leenutaphong V+, *Int J Dermatol* 32, 428
(1972): Monnat A, *Schweiz Med Wochenschr* (French) 102, 1876
(1968): Bianchine JR+, *Am Med J* 44, 390
(1966): Brannen M+, *Tex State J Med* 62, 58
Toxic epidermal necrolysis (<1%)
(2002): Correia O+, *Arch Dermatol* 138, 29
(1993): Leenutaphong V+, *Int J Dermatol* 32, 428
(1988): Dahle MG, *Tidsskr Nor Laegeforen* (Norwegian) 108, 1917
(1987): Guillaume JC+, *Arch Dermatol* 123, 1166
(1979): Hunziker N, *Schweiz Rundsch Med Prax* (French) 68, 283
(1972): Spahr A+, *Rev Med Suisse Romande* (French) 92, 935
(1970): Ocheret'ko MP, *Pediatriia* (Russian) 49, 86
(1967): Lowney ED+, *Arch Dermatol* 95, 359
(1967): Lyell A, *Br J Dermatol* 79, 662
Ulceration (<1%) (with dipyridamole)
Urticaria (1–10%)
(2001): Cousin F+, *Ann Dermatol Venereol* 128(10), 1166
(2001): Harada S+, *Br J Dermatol* 145(2), 336
(2000): Pradalier A+, *Rev Med Interne* (French) 21, 75
(2000): Wong JT+, *J Allergy Clin Immunol* 105, 997
(1999): Eseverri JL+, *Allergol Immunopathol (Madr)* (Spanish) 27, 104
(1998): Grzelewska-Rzymowska I, *Pol Merkuriusz Lek* (Polish) 4, 233
(1998): Ohnishi-Inoue Y+, *Br J Dermatol* 138, 483
(1997): Tomaz EM+, *Allergy Asthma Proc* 18, 319
(1995): Gebhardt M+, *Z Rheumatol* (German) 54, 405
(1995): Grzelewska-Rzymowska I+, *J Invest Allergol Clin Immunol* 5, 272
(1994): Paul E+, *Hautarzt* (German) 45, 12
(1994): Smith RJ+, *Br J Dermatol* 131, 583
(1993): Grzelewska-Rzymowska I+, *Pneumonol Alergol Pol* (Polish) 61, 29
(1992): Grzelewska-Rzymowska I+, *J Invest Alergol Clin Immunol* 2, 39
(1989): Alanko K+, *Acta Derm Venereol* (Stockh) 69, 223 (1–5%)
(1989): Grzelewska-Rzymowska I, *Allergol Immunopathol Madr* (Spanish) 16, 231
(1989): Hass WK+, *N Engl J Med* 321, 501 (0.3%)
(1988): Botey J+, *Allergol Immunopathol Madr* (Spanish) 16, 43
(1987): Asad SI+, *Ann Allergy* 59, 219
(1986): Dupont C, *Int J Dermatol* 25, 334
(1986): Finzi AF+, *Minerva Med* (Italian) 77, 1401
(1986): Nagy G+, *Dermatol Monatsschr* 72, 594
(1986): Wojnerowicz-*Grajewska M+, Przegl Dermatol* (Polish) 73, 115
(1984): Botey J+, *Ann Allergy* 53, 265
(1984): Kauppinen K+, *Allergy* 39, 469
(1983): Kaplan AP, *Postgrad Med* 74, 209
(1982): Kirchhof B+, *Dermatol Monatsschr* (German) 168, 513
(1981): Juhlin L, *Br J Dermatol* 104, 369
(1981): Settipane GA, *Arch Intern Med* 141, 328
(1980): Settipane RA+, *Allergy* 35, 149
(1980): Wuthrich B+, *Z Hautkr* (German) 55, 102
(1978): Hofmann C+, *Munch Med Wochenschr* (German) 120, 65
(1978): Oshima K+, *Nippon Hifuka Gakkai Zasshi* (Japanese) 88, 459
(1977): Abrishami MA+, *Ann Allergy* 39, 28
(1977): Chalem F+, *Curr Ther Res* 22, 769
(1977): Doeglas HM, *Dermatologica* 154, 308
(1977): Rudzki E, *Przegl Dermatol* (Polish) 64, 163
(1977): Szczeklik A+, *J Allergy Clin Immunol* 60, 276
(1976): Erlings M+, *Ned Tijdschr Geneeskd* (Dutch) 120, 1565
(1976): Ros AM+, *Br J Dermatol* 95, 19
(1976): Stubb S, *Acta Derm Venereol* (Stockh) 56 (Suppl 76), 16
(1975): Blechman WJ+, *JAMA* 233, 336 (0.5%)
(1975): Doeglas HM, *Br J Dermatol* 93, 135
(1974): Schlumberger HD+, *Acta Med Scand* 196, 451
(1973): Samter M, *Hosp Pract* 8, 85
(1972): Kauppinen K, *Acta Derm Venereol* (Stockh) 52 (Suppl), 68
(1972): Sheffer AL, *N Y State J Med* 72, 922
(1971): Davis SL+, *Nebraska St Med J* 56, 432
(1970): Baker H+, *Br J Dermatol* 82, 319
(1970): James J+, *Br J Dermatol* 82, 204
(1970): Naess K, *Tidsskr Nor Laegeforen* (Norwegian) 90, 112
(1969): Champion RH+, *Br J Dermatol* 81, 588
(1969): Girard JP+, *Helv Med Acta* 35, 86
(1967): Moore-Robinson M+, *BMJ* 4, 262
(1966): Brannen M+, *Tex State J Med* 62, 58
(1960): Hejier A+, *Acta Derm Venereol* (Stockh) 40, 35
(1960): Warin RP, *Br J Dermatol* 72, 350
Vasculitis
(1999): Crutchfield CE+, *Skin and Aging* May, 84 (leukocytoclastic)
(1984): Ekenstam E+, *Arch Dermatol* 120, 484
(1971): Meszaros C, *Börgyogy Vener Sz* (Hungarian) 47, 20

### Hair

Hair – alopecia
(1968): Rawnsley HM+, *Lancet* 1, 561

### Other

Ageusia (<1%) (with dipyridamole)
Anaphylactoid reactions (1–10%)
(2001): Harada S+, *Br J Dermatol* 145(2), 336
(1999): Kubota Y+, *Eur J Dermatol* 9, 559
(1984): Stevenson DD, *J Allergy Clin Immunol* 74, 617
(1972): Ohela K+, *Duodecim* (Finnish) 88, 1177
Aphthous stomatitis
(2001): Vincent L+, *Ann Dermatol Venereol* 128, 57
(1982): Bailin PL+, *Clin Rheum Dis* 8, 493 (passim)
(1966): Brannen M+, *Tex State J Med* 62, 58
Dysgeusia
Gingival bleeding (<1%) (with dipyridamole)
Granulomata
(1982): Cozzutto C+, *Virchows Arch A Pathol Anat Histol* 397, 61
Hypersensitivity
(2001): Hinrichs R+, *Allergy* 56(8), 789
(2001): Rueff F+, *Allergy* 56, 258
Myalgia (1.2%) (with dipyridamole)
Oral burn (sic)
(1998): Dellinger TM+, *Ann Pharmacother* 32, 1107
Oral lichen planus
(1989): Espana-Alonso A+, *An Med Interna* (Spanish) 6, 219
Oral mucosal eruption
(1988): Bork K, *Cutaneous Side Effects of Drugs* WB Saunders, 283
(1966): Brannen M+, *Tex State J Med* 62, 58
(1964): Shelley WB, *JAMA* 189, 986
Oral ulceration
(1975): Kawashima Z+, *JAMA* 91, 130
(1974): Glick GL+, *N Y St Dent J* 40, 475
(1970): Baker H+, *Br J Dermatol* 82, 319
(1967): Claman HN, *JAMA* 202, 651
Paresthesias (<1%) (with dipyridamole)
Pseudolymphoma
(1980): Olmos L+, *Rev Clin Esp* 157, 67
Pseudoporphyria
(1994): Hazen PG, *J Am Acad Dermatol* 31, 500
Tinnitus

## ATENOLOL

**Trade names:** Tenoretic (AstraZeneca); Tenormin (AstraZeneca)
**Other common trade names:** *Antipressan; Apo-Atenol; AteHexal; Atendol; Evitocor; Noten; Novo-Atenol; Nu-Atenol; Taro-Atenol; Tenolin; Tenormine*
**Indications:** Angina, hypertension, acute myocardial infarction
**Category:** Beta-adrenergic blocker; antianginal; antihypertensive
**Half-life:** 6–7 hours (adults)
**Clinically important, potentially hazardous interactions with:** clonidine, epinephrine, verapamil

Tenoretic is atenolol and chlorthalidone

### *Reactions*

### Skin

Acrocyanosis
(1987): Naeyaert JM+, *Br J Dermatol* 117, 371
Dermatitis (sic)
(1979): Harrison PV+, *Clin Exp Dermatol* 4, 547
Diaphoresis
Edema
Erythema multiforme
Exanthems
Facial edema
Fixed eruption
(1999): Palungwachira P+, *J Med Assoc Thai* 82, 1158
Grinspan's syndrome*
(1990): Lamey PJ+, *Oral Surg Oral Med Oral Pathol* 70, 184
Hyperkeratosis (palms and soles)
Lichenoid eruption
(1978): Savage RL+, *BMJ* 1, 987
Lupus erythematosus
(1997): McGuiness M+, *J Am Acad Dermatol* 37, 298
(1986): Gouet D+, *J Rheumatol* 13, 446
Necrosis
(1979): Gokal R+, *BMJ* 1, 721
(1979): Rees PJ, *BMJ* 1, 955
(1977): Simpson WT, *Postgrad Med J* 53, 162
Papular and nodular eruption
(1992): Shelley WB+, *Cutis* 50, 87 (observation)
Photosensitivity
Pityriasis rubra pilaris
(1978): Finlay AY+, *BMJ* 1, 987
Pruritus (1–5%)
Psoriasis
(1990): Wakefield PL+, *Arch Dermatol* 126, 968 (exacerbation)
(1990): Wolf R, *Dermatologica* 181, 51
(1988): Gold MH+, *J Am Acad Dermatol* 19, 837
(1988): Heng MCY+, *Int J Dermatol* 27, 619
(1986): Abel EA+, *J Am Acad Dermatol* 15, 1007
(1984): Gawkrodger DJ+, *Clin Exp Dermatol* 9, 92
Purpura
Pustular psoriasis
(1990): Wakefield PE+, *Arch Dermatol* 126, 968
Rash (sic)
(1987): Bolzano K+, *J Cardiovasc Pharmacol* 9 (Suppl 3), S43
Raynaud's phenomenon
(1976): Marshall AJ+, *BMJ* 1, 1498 (35%)
Toxic epidermal necrolysis
Urticaria
(1989): Wolf R+, *Cutis* 43, 231
(1988): Howard PJ+, *Scott Med J* 33, 344
Vasculitis
(1989): Wolf R+, *Cutis* 43, 231
Vitiligo
Xerosis

### Hair

Hair – alopecia
(1991): Shelley WB+, *Cutis* 48, 368 (observation)

### Nails

Nails – bluish
Nails – dystrophy
Nails – onycholysis
Nails – splinter hemorrhages
(1987): Naeyaert JM+, *Br J Dermatol* 117, 371

### Other

Anaphylactoid reactions
(1988): Howard PJ+, *Scott Med J* 33, 344
Death
(2001): Briggs GG+, *Ann Pharmacother* 35(7), 859
Oculo-mucocutaneous syndrome
(1982): Cocco G+, *Curr Ther Res* 31, 362
Oral lichenoid eruption
(1990): Lamey PJ+, *Oral Surg Oral Med Oral Pathol* 70, 184

Peyronie's disease
Pseudolymphoma
(1990): Henderson CA+, *Clin Exp Dermatol* 15, 119

***Note:** Grinspan's syndrome: the triad of oral lichen planus, diabetes mellitus, and hypertension

# ATORVASTATIN

**Trade name:** Lipitor (Parke-Davis)
**Indications:** Hypercholesterolemia
**Category:** HMG-CoA reductase inhibitor; antihyperlipidemic
**Half-life:** 14 hours
**Clinically important, potentially hazardous interactions with:** azithromycin, bosentan, clarithromycin, cyclosporine, erythromycin, gemfibrozil, imatinib, itraconazole, niacin, verapamil

### *Reactions*

## Skin

Acne (<2%)
Allergic reactions (sic) (<2%)
Cheilitis (<2%)
Contact dermatitis (<2%)
Dermatomyositis
(2001): Noel B+, *Am J Med* 110, 670
Dermographism
(2001): Adcock BB+, *J Am Board Fam Prac* 14, 148
Diaphoresis (<2%)
Ecchymoses (<2%)
Eczema (sic) (<2%)
Edema (<2%)
Exanthems
Facial edema (<2%)
Flu-like syndrome (sic)
Lichenoid eruption
(1998): Silver B, Deerfield, IL (from Internet) (observation)
Linear IgA bullous dermatosis
(2001): König C+, *J Am Acad Dermatol* 44, 689
Lymphocytic infiltration
(2001): Faivre M+, *Ann Dermatol Venereol* 128, 67
Petechiae (<2%)
Photosensitivity (<2%)
Pruritus (<2%)
Rash (sic) (>3%)
(2001): Coverman M, *The Schoch Letter* 51, 23 (with simvastatin)
Seborrhea (<2%)
Toxic epidermal necrolysis
(1998): Pfeiffer CM+, *JAMA* 279, 1613
Ulceration (<2%)
Urticaria (<2%)
(2002): Anliker MD+, *Allergy* 57(4), 366
Xerosis (<2%)

## Hair

Hair – alopecia (<2%)
(2002): Litt JZ, Beachwood, OH (personal case)
(2001): Altman E, West Orange, NJ (from Internet) (observation)
(1999): Oakley A, Hamilton, New Zealand (from Internet) (observation)
(1997): Litt JZ, Beachwood, OH (personal case) (observation)

## Other

Ageusia (<2%)
Dysgeusia (<2%)
Glossitis (<2%)
Gynecomastia (<2%)
Leg pain
(2001): Wright WL, Castro Valley, CA (from Internet) (observation)
Myalgia (>3%)
(2002): Litt JZ, Beachwood, OH (personal observation)
(2002): Patel DN+, *J Heart Lung Transplant* 21(2), 204
(2001): Litt JZ, Beachwood, OH (2 personal cases)
(2001): Rehbein H, Jacksonville, FL (from Internet) (observation)
(2001): Sorkin M, Denver, CO (from Internet) (observation)
(2001): Wright W, Castro Valley, CA (from Internet) (2 observations)
(1998): Malinowski JM, *Am J Health Syst Pharm* 55, 2253
Myositis
(2002): Patel DN+, *J Heart Lung Transplant* 21(2), 204
Oral ulceration (<2%)
Paresthesias (<2%)
Parosmia (<2%)
Rhabdomyolysis
(2002): Castro JG+, *Am J Med* 112(6), 505 (with delavirdine)
(2002): Patel DN+, *J Heart Lung Transplant* 21(2), 204
(2000): Davidson MH, *Curr Atheroscler Rep* 2(1), 14
(1999): Bottorff M, *Atherosclerosis* 147(Suppl 1), S23
(1999): Maltz HC+, *Ann Pharmacother* 33(11), 1176 (with cyclosporine)
Stomatitis (<2%)
Tendinopathy
(2001): Chazerain P+, *Joint Bone Spine* 68(5), 430

# ATOVAQUONE

**Trade name:** Mepron (GSK)
**Other common trade name:** *Wellvone*
**Indications:** *Pneumocystis carinii infection*
**Category:** Antiprotozoal
**Half-life:** 2.2–2.9 days
**Clinically important, potentially hazardous interactions with:** rifampin

### *Reactions*

## Skin

Diaphoresis (10%)
Erythema multiforme
Exanthems
(1993): Haile LG+, *Ann Pharmacother* 27, 1488
Pruritus (11%)
(1996): Radloff PD+, *Lancet* 347, 1511
Rash (sic) (23%)
(1993): Artymowicz RJ+, *Clin Pharm* 12, 563

## Other

Dysgeusia (3%)
Oral candidiasis (1–10%)

# ATRACURIUM

**Trade name:** Tracrium (GSK)
**Indications:** Neuromuscular blockade, endotracheal intubation
**Category:** Neuromuscular blocking agent; skeletal muscle relaxant
**Half-life:** initial: 2 minutes; terminal: 20 minutes
**Clinically important, potentially hazardous interactions with:** amikacin, aminoglycosides, anesthetics, antibiotics, gentamicin, halothane, kanamycin, neomycin, piperacillin, streptomycin, tobramycin

### *Reactions*

#### Skin

Allergic reactions (sic)
(1985): Aldrete JA, *Br J Anaesth* 57, 929
(1983): Mirakhur RK+, *Anaesthesia* 38, 818
Edema
Erythema (<1%)
Flushing (1–10%)
Pruritus (<1%)
Urticaria (<1%)

#### Other

Injection-site reactions

# ATROPINE SULFATE

**Trade names:** Belladenal*; Bellergal-S; Butibel; Donnagel; Donnatal; Donnazyme; Hycodan; Isopto Atropine; Lofene; Logen; Lomanate; Lomotil; Urised
**Other common trade names:** *Atropine Martinet; Atropt; Chibro-Atropine; Isopto; Tropyn Z; Vitatropine*
**Indications:** Salivation, sinus bradycardia, uveitis, peptic ulcer
**Category:** Anticholinergic and antispasmodic
**Half-life:** 2–3 hours
**Clinically important, potentially hazardous interactions with:** anticholinergics

### *Reactions*

#### Skin

Allergic reactions (sic)
(1997): Moyano P+, *Rev Esp Anestesiol Reanim* (Spanish) 44, 290
Bullous eruption
(1967): Coleman WP, *Med Clin North Am* 51, 1073
Contact allergy
(2001): Decraene T+, *Contact Dermatitis* 45(5), 309
Contact dermatitis
(1988): Gutierrez-Ortega MC+, *Med Cutan Ibero Lat Am* (Spanish) 16, 430
(1987): van der Willigen AH+, *Contact Dermatitis* 17, 56 (periocular)
(1985): Yoshikama K+, *Contact Dermatitis* 12, 56
(1982): Gallasch G+, *Klin Monatsbl Augenheilkd* (German) 181, 96 (periocular)
Eccrine hidrocystomas
(1992): Masri-Fridling GD+, *J Am Acad Dermatol* 26, 780
Erythema multiforme (<1%)
(1979): Guill MA, *Arch Dermatol* 115, 742
(1967): Coleman WP, *Med Clin North Am* 51, 1073
Exanthems
Exfoliative dermatitis
(1955): Alexander HL, *Reactions with Drug Therapy* Saunders, Philadelphia
Eyelid edema
Fixed eruption
(1961): Welsh AL, *The Fixed Eruption*, Thomas, Springfield
Flushing
(1992): Amitai Y+, *JAMA* 268, 630
Hypohidrosis (>10%)
(2001): Sanz-Sanchez T+, *Arch Dermatol* 137, 670 (local)
Photosensitivity (1–10%)
Pruritus
Rash (sic) (<1%)
Sheet-like erythema
Stevens–Johnson syndrome
(1967): Coleman WP, *Med Clin North Am* 51, 1073
Urticaria
(1986): Bigby M+, *JAMA* 256, 3358
Xerosis

#### Other

Dry mucous membranes (sic)
(1992): Amitai Y+, *JAMA* 268, 630
Dysgeusia
Injection-site irritation (>10%)
Tremors
Xerostomia (>10%)

***Note:** Many of the above trade name drugs contain phenobarbital, scopolamine, hyoscyamine, hydrocodone, methenamine, etc

# AURANOFIN

(See GOLD and GOLD COMPOUNDS)

# AUROTHIOGLUCOSE

(See GOLD and GOLD COMPOUNDS)

# AZATADINE

**Trade names:** Rynatan (Wallace); Trinalin (Key)
**Other common trade names:** *Idulamine; Idulian; Lergocil; Nalomet; Verben; Zadine*
**Indications:** Allergic rhinitis, urticaria
**Category:** $H_1$-receptor antihistamine
**Half-life:** 9 hours
**Clinically important, potentially hazardous interactions with:** barbiturates, chloral hydrate, paraldehyde, phenylthiazines, zolpidem

### *Reactions*

#### Skin

Angioedema (<1%)
Diaphoresis
Edema (<1%)
Exanthems
Flushing
Photosensitivity (<1%)
Purpura
Rash (sic) (<1%)
Urticaria

## Other

Myalgia (<1%)
Paresthesias (<1%)
Tinnitus
Xerostomia (1–10%)
(1990): Small P+, *Ann Allergy* 64, 129

# AZATHIOPRINE

**Trade name:** Imuran (Faro)
**Other common trade names:** *Azamedac; Azamune; Azatrilem; Imuprin; Imurek; Imurel; Thioprine*
**Indications:** Lupus nephritis, psoriatic arthritis, rheumatoid arthritis, autoimmune diseases, kidney transplant patients
**Category:** Immunosuppressant and antineoplastic
**Half-life:** 12 minutes
**Clinically important, potentially hazardous interactions with:** allopurinol, chlorambucil, cyclophosphamide, mycophenolate, olsalazine, **vaccines**

### *Reactions*

## Skin

Acanthosis nigricans
(1980): L'Eplattenier JL+, *Schweiz Med Wochenschr* (German) 110, 1307 (0.5%)
(1974): Koranda FC+, *JAMA* 229, 419 (10%)
Acne
(1983): Schmoeckel C+, *Hautarzt* (German) 34, 413
Allergic reactions (sic)
(1996): Parnham AP+, *Lancet* 348, 542
Angioedema
(1988): Saway PA+, *Am J Med* 84, 960 (passim)
Basal cell carcinoma
(2001): Otley CC+, *Arch Dermatol* 137, 459
Cancer (sic)
(1992): Taylor AE+, *Acta Derm Venereol* 72, 115
Chills (>10%)
Contact dermatitis
(2001): Lauerma AI+, *Contact Dermatitis* 44, 129
(1996): Soni BP+, *Am J Contact Dermat* 7, 116
(1992): Burden AD+, *Contact Dermatitis* 27, 329
Cutaneous infections (sic)
(1978): Bergfeld WF+, *Cutis* 22, 169 (62%)
(1974): Koranda FC+, *JAMA* 229, 419 (>5%)
(1973): Haim S+, *Br J Dermatol* 89, 169 (100%)
Erythema multiforme
(1995): Knowles SR+, *Clin Exp Dermatol* 20, 353 (passim)
(1988): Saway PA+, *Am J Med* 84, 960 (passim)
Erythema nodosum
(1995): Knowles SR+, *Clin Exp Dermatol* 20, 353 (passim)
(1988): Saway PA+, *Am J Med* 84, 960 (passim)
Exanthems (<1%)
(1995): Knowles SR+, *Clin Exp Dermatol* 20, 353 (passim)
(1990): Jeurissen ME+, *Ann Rheum Dis* 49, 25 (4%)
(1988): Bergman SM+, *Ann Intern Med* 109, 83
(1988): Saway PA+, *Am J Med* 84, 960
(1978): Franchmont P+, *J Rheumatol* 5 (Suppl 4), 85 (5.4%)
(1972): Decker JL, *Ann Intern Med* 76, 619
(1972): King JO+, *Med J Aust* 2, 939
(1971): Harris J+, *BMJ* 4, 463 (1–5%)
(1969): Mason M+, *BMJ* 1, 420 (1–5%)
(1967): Adams DA+, *JAMA* 199, 459
Exfoliation (sic)
(1997): Hermanns-Le T+, *Dermatology* 194, 175
Fixed eruption
(1990): Black AK+, *Br J Dermatol* 123, 277 (observation)
Formication
(1992): Shelley WB+, *Advanced Dermatologic Diagnosis* WB Saunders, 1042 (passim)
Fungal infection
(1980): L'Eplattenier JL+, *Schweiz Med Wochenschr* (German) 110, 1307 (42%)
Herpes simplex
(1980): L'Eplattenier JL+, *Schweiz Med Wochenschr* (German) 110, 1307 (27%)
(1979): Spencer ES+, *BMJ* 2, 829
(1974): Koranda FC+, *JAMA* 229, 419 (35%)
Herpes zoster
(2001): Vergara M+, *Gastroenterol Hepatol* 24, 47
(1991): Callen JP+, *Arch Dermatol* 127, 515
(1982): Speerstra F+, *Ann Rheum Dis* 41, Suppl 37
(1980): L'Eplattenier JL+, *Schweiz Med Wochenschr* (German) 110, 1307 (27%)
(1974): Koranda FC+, *JAMA* 229, 419 (13%)
(1966): Rifkind D, *J Lab Clin Med* 68, 463 (8%)
Intraepidermal carcinoma
(2001): Austin AS+, *Eur J Gastroenterol Hepatol* 13, 193
Kaposi's sarcoma
(1997): Aebischer MC+, *Dermatology* 195, 91
(1997): Halpern SM+, *Br J Dermatol* 137, 140
(1997): Lesnoni-La-Parola I+, *Dermatology* 194, 229
(1997): Vandercam B+, *Dermatology* 194, 180
(1996): Ozen S+, *Nephrol Dial Transplant* 11, 1162
(1991): Almog Y+, *Clin Exp Dermatol* 9, 285
(1984): Luderschmidt C+, *Klin Wochenschr* (German) 62, 803
(1982): Weiss VC+, *Arch Dermatol* 118, 183
(1980): Iversen OH+, *Scand J Urol Nephrol* 14, 125
(1974): Faye I+, *Bull Soc Fr Dermatol Syphiligr* (French) 81, 379
(1973): Haim S+, *Br J Dermatol* 89, 169
Keratoacanthoma
(1971): Walder BK+, *Lancet* 2, 1282
Lichenoid eruption
(1979): Beaaff D+, *Arch Dermatol* 115, 498
Pellagra
(1996): Oakley A, Hamilton, New Zealand (from Internet) (observation)
Photosensitivity
Pigmentation (sun-exposed skin)
(1974): Koranda FC+, *JAMA* 229, 419 (37%)
Porokeratosis
(1997): Matsushita S+, *J Dermatol* 24, 110 (disseminated superficial actinic)
(1988): Neumann RA+, *Br J Dermatol* 119, 375 (disseminated superficial actinic)
(1987): Tatnall FM+, *J R Soc Med* 80, 180 (Mibelli)
(1974): Macmillan AL+, *Br J Dermatol* 90, 45
Purpura
Pyoderma gangrenosum
(1976): Haim S+, *Dermatologica* 153, 44
Rash (sic) (1–10%)
(1997): Lavaud F+, *Dig Dis Sci* 42, 823
(1990): Jeurissen ME+, *Ann Rheum Dis* 49, 25
(1975): Goldenberg DL+, *J Rheumatol* 2, 346
(1972): King JO+, *Med J Aust* 2, 939
Raynaud's phenomenon
Sarcoma
(1996): Csuka ME+, *Arch Intern Med* 156, 1573
Scabies
(1980): L'Eplattenier JL+, *Schweiz Med Wochenschr* (German) 110, 1307 (1%)
(1978): Bricklin AS+, *Cutis* 22, 81
(1976): Anolik MA+, *Arch Dermatol* 112, 73

(1973): Paterson WD+, *BMJ* 4, 211
Scleroderma
(1993): Choy E+, *Br J Rheumatol* 32, 160
Squamous cell carcinoma
(2001): Otley CC+, *Arch Dermatol* 137, 459
(2001): Werth V, *Dermatology Times* 15
(1995): Bottomley WW+, *Br J Dermatol* 133, 460
(1993): Nachbar F+, *Acta Derm Venereol* 73, 217
(1992): McCain J, *Nurs Pract* 17, 13
(1988): Krickeberg H, *Z Hautkr* (German) 63, 773
(1973): Westburg SP+, *Arch Dermatol* 107, 893
(1971): Walder BK+, *Lancet* 2, 1282
Tinea corporis
(1980): L'Eplattenier JL+, *Schweiz Med Wochenschr* (German) 110, 1307 (3%)
(1974): Koranda FC+, *JAMA* 229, 419 (2%)
Tinea versicolor
(1981): Burkhart CG+, *Cutis* 27, 56
(1974): Koranda FC+, *JAMA* 229, 419 (18%)
Toxic epidermal necrolysis
(1990): Black AK+, *Br J Dermatol* 123, 277
Urticaria
(1995): Knowles SR+, *Clin Exp Dermatol* 20, 353 (passim)
(1990): Wijnands MJ+, *Scand J Rheumatol* 19, 167
(1988): Saway PA+, *Am J Med* 84, 960 (passim)
(1972): Decker JL, *Ann Intern Med* 76, 619
(1970): Drinkard JP+, *Medicine* (Baltimore) 49, 411
Vasculitis
(1995): Blanco R+, *Arthritis Rheum* 39, 1016
(1995): Knowles SR+, *Clin Exp Dermatol* 20, 353 (passim)
(1988): Bergman SM+, *Ann Intern Med* 109, 83
Viral infections
(1980): L'Eplattenier JL+, *Schweiz Med Wochenschr* (German) 110, 1307 (45%)
(1974): Koranda FC+, *JAMA* 229, 419 (43%)
Warts
(1991): Callen JP+, *Arch Dermatol* 127, 515
(1980): L'Eplattenier JL+, *Schweiz Med Wochenschr* (German) 110, 1307 (21%)

### Hair

Hair – alopecia (<1%)
(1982): Bailin PL+, *Clin Rheum Dis* 8, 493 (passim)
(1980): L'Eplattenier JL+, *Schweiz Med Wochenschr* (German) 110, 1307 (27%)
(1974): Koranda FC+, *JAMA* 229, 419 (54%)
Hair – curly
(1996): van der Pijl JW+, *Lancet* 348, 622 (with isotretinoin)

### Nails

Nails – discoloration (red lunulae)
(1974): Koranda FC+, *JAMA* 229, 419 (2%)
Nails – onychomycosis
(1980): L'Eplattenier JL+, *Schweiz Med Wochenschr* (German) 110, 1307 (1%)
(1974): Koranda FC+, *JAMA* 229, 419 (5%)

### Other

Anaphylactoid reactions
(1993): Jones JJ+, *J Am Acad Dermatol* 29, 795
Aphthous stomatitis (<1%)
Cicatricial pemphigoid
(2000): Burgess MJA+, *Arch Dermatol* 136, 1274
Hypersensitivity (<1%)*
(2001): Corbett M+, *Intern Med J* 31(6), 366
(2001): Sofat N+, *Ann Rheum Dis* 60(7), 719
(2001): Werth V, *Dermatology Times* 15
(1999): Korelitz BI+, *J Clin Gastroenterol* 28, 341
(1998): Fields CL+, *South Med J* 91, 471
(1998): Garey KW+, *Ann Pharmacother* 32, 425
(1998): Schlienger RG+, *Epilepsia* 39, S3 (passim)
(1997): Caramaschi P+, *Lupus* 6, 616
(1997): Knowles S+, *Muscle Nerve* 20, 1467
(1996): Compton MR+, *Arch Dermatol* 132, 1254 (with rhabdomyolysis)
(1995): Knowles SR+, *Clin Exp Dermatol* 20, 353
(1982): Mosbech H+, *Ugeskr Laeger* (Danish) 144, 2424
(1975): Goldenberg DL+, *J Rheumatol* 2, 346
(1972): King JO+, *Med J Aust* 2, 939
Lymphoproliferative disease
(1987): Phillips T+, *Clin Exp Dermatol* 12, 444
(1987): Pitt PI+, *J R Soc Med* 80, 428
(1982): Ulreich A+, *Z Rheumatol* (German) 41, 73
Myalgia (<1%)
Non-Hodgkin's lymphoma
(2000): Lewis JD+, *Gastroenterology* 118, 1018
Oral ulceration
(2000): Madinier I+, *Ann Med Interne (Paris)* (French) 151, 248
Rhabdomyolysis
(1996): Compton MR+, *Arch Dermatol* 132, 1254
Rheumatoid nodules (sic)
(1991): Langevitz P+, *Arthritis Rheum* 34, 123
Serum sickness
Stomatitis
(1982): Bailin PL+, *Clin Rheum Dis* 8, 493 (passim)
Tumors (sic)
(1986): Gupta AK+, *Arch Dermatol* 122, 1288 (5.3%) (malignant)
(1982): Bailin PL+, *Clin Rheum Dis* 8, 493 (passim)
(1980): L'Eplattenier JL+, *Schweiz Med Wochenschr* (German) 110, 1307 (2.9%) (benign); (4.3%) (malignant)
(1978): Bergfeld WF+, *Cutis* 22, 169 (4.6%) (malignant)
(1974): Koranda FC+, *JAMA* 229, 419 (3.5%) (malignant)
(1973): Westburg SP+, *Arch Dermatol* 107, 893
(1973): Wishart J, *Arch Dermatol* 108, 563 (reticulosarcoma)
(1971): Walder BK+, *Lancet* 2, 1282 (>5%) (malignant)
Xerostomia

***Note:** The antiepileptic drug hypersensitivity syndrome is a severe, occasionally fatal, disorder characterized by any or all of the following: pruritic exanthems, toxic epidermal necrolysis, Stevens–Johnson syndrome, exfoliative dermatitis, fever, hepatic abnormalities, eosinophilia, and renal failure

## AZELASTINE

**Trade name:** Astelin (Wallace)
**Other common trade names:** *Allergodil; Azeptin*
**Indications:** Allergic rhinitis
**Category:** Antihistamine; intranasal $H_1$-blocker
**Half-life:** 22 hours
**Clinically important, potentially hazardous interactions with:** barbiturates, chloral Hydrate, paraldehyde, phenothiazines, zolpidem

#### *Reactions*

### Skin

Allergic reactions (sic) (<2%)
Contact dermatitis (<2%)
Eczema (sic) (<2%)
Exanthems
(1989): McTavish D+, *Drugs* 38, 19
Flushing (<2%)
Folliculitis (<2%)
Furunculosis (<2%)
Herpes simplex (<2%)

### Other

Ageusia (<2%)
Aphthous stomatitis (<2%)
Dysgeusia (bitter taste) (19.7%)
(1993): Davies RJ+, *Rhinology* 31, 159
(1990): Tinkelman DG+, *Am Rev Respir Dis* 141, 569 (30–52%)
(1988): Weiler JM+, *J Allergy Clin Immunology* 82, 801 (19.7%)
Glossitis (<2%)
Hypesthesia (<2%)
Mastodynia (<2%)
Myalgia (1.5%)
Oral dryness
(1989): McTavish D+, *Drugs* 38, 19
Oral mucosal eruption
(1989): McTavish D+, *Drugs* 38, 19
Stomatitis (ulcerative) (<2%)
Xerostomia (2.8%)
(1990): Tinkelman DG+, *Am Rev Respir Dis* 141, 569 (4–6%)

# AZITHROMYCIN

**Trade name:** Zithromax (Pfizer)
**Other common trade names:** *Azenil; Azitrocin; Azitromax; Zeto; Zitromax*
**Indications:** Infections of the upper and lower respiratory tract, skin infections, sexually-transmitted diseases
**Category:** Macrolide antibiotic
**Half-life:** 68 hours
**Clinically important, potentially hazardous interactions with:** atorvastatin, cyclosporine, fluvastatin, lovastatin, pimozide, pravastatin, simvastatin, warfarin

## *Reactions*

### Skin

Allergic granulomatous angiitis (Churg–Strauss syndrome)
(1998): Dietz A+, *Laryngorhinootologie* (German) 77, 111
(1997): Kranke B+, *Lancet* 350, 1551
Allergic reactions (sic) (<1%)
(1998): Salit IE+, *Infect Med* 15, 773 (0.4%)
Angioedema (<1%)
Contact dermatitis
(2001): Milkovic-Kraus S+, *Contact Dermatitis* 45(3), 184
Cutaneous side effects (sic)
(1993): Hopkins S, *J Antimicrob Chemother* 31 (Suppl E), 111
Diaper rash
(1997): Arguedas A+, *Infections in Medicine* October, 807
Edema
Erythema
(1991): Felstead SJ+, *J Int Med Res* 19, 363
Exanthems
(2000): Schissel DJ+, *Cutis* 65, 123 (in a patient with infectious mononucleosis)
Facial edema
Fixed eruption
(1999): Smith KC, Niagara Falls, Ontario (from Internet) (observation)
Photosensitivity (1%)
Pruritus
(2000): Schissel DJ+, *Cutis* 65, 123 (in a patient with infectious mononucleosis)
Pustular eruption
(1994): Trevis P+, *Clin Exp Dermatol* 19, 280
Rash (sic) (<1%)
(1991): Felstead SJ+, *J Int Med Res* 19, 363
(1991): Hopkins S, *Am J Med* 91, 36s
Stevens–Johnson syndrome
(2001): Brett AS+, *South Med J* 94, 342
(1998): Smith KC, Niagara Falls, Ontario (from Internet) (observation)
Toxic pustuloderma
(1994): Trevisi P+, *Clin Exp Dermatol* 19, 280
Urticaria
(2001): Thaler D, Monana, WI (from Internet) (observation) (2–year-old child 3 hours after initiation of drug)
(1991): Hopkins S, *Am J Med* 91, 36s

### Other

Anaphylactoid reactions
Hypersensitivity (0.6%)
(2001): Cascaval RI+, *Am J Med* 110, 330
(1998): Salit IE+, *Infect Med* 15, 773
Infusion-site erythema
(1997): Luke DR+, *Ann Pharmacother* 31, 965
Infusion-site pain
(2001): Zimmerman T+, *Clin Drug Invest* 21, 527 (58%)
Infusion-site tenderness
(2001): Zimmerman T+, *Clin Drug Invest* 21, 527 (67%)
(1997): Luke DR+, *Ann Pharmacother* 31, 965
Vaginitis (2%)
(1991): Hopkins S, *Am J Med* 91, 36s

# AZTREONAM

**Synonym:** azthreonam
**Trade name:** Azactam (Dura)
**Other common trade names:** *Primbactam; Urobactam*
**Indications:** Aerobic gram-negative bacillary infections
**Category:** Synthetic narrow spectrum antibiotic (monobactam) (parenteral)
**Half-life:** 1.4–2.2 hours

## *Reactions*

### Skin

Angioedema
(1990): Soto Alvarez J+, *Lancet* 335, 1094
Diaphoresis
Erythema multiforme
(1997): Epstein ME+, *J Am Acad Dermatol* 37, 149 (passim)
Exanthems
(1990): Adkinson NF, *Am J Med* 88 (Suppl 3C), 12S (1.6%)
(1990): Fekete T+, *Drug Intell Clin Pharm* 24, 438 (1–5%)
(1988): Pazmiño P, *Am J Nephrol* 8, 68
(1986): Brogden RN+, *Drugs* 18, 241 (1.8%)
Exfoliative dermatitis
(1997): Epstein ME+, *J Am Acad Dermatol* 37, 149 (passim)
Petechiae
(1997): Epstein ME+, *J Am Acad Dermatol* 37, 149 (passim)
Pruritus
(1997): Epstein ME+, *J Am Acad Dermatol* 37, 149 (passim)
(1990): Adkinson NF, *Am J Med* 88 (Suppl 3C), 12S
(1986): Brogden RN+, *Drugs* 18, 241 (1.8%)
Purpura
(1997): Epstein ME+, *J Am Acad Dermatol* 37, 149 (passim)
(1990): Adkinson NF, *Am J Med 88* (Suppl 3C), 12S (0.1%)
Rash (sic) (1–10%)
(1985): Newman TJ+, *Rev Infect Dis* 7, S648
Toxic epidermal necrolysis
(1997): Epstein ME+, *J Am Acad Dermatol* 37, 149 (passim)

(1992): McDonald BJ+, *Ann Pharmacother* 26, 34

Urticaria

(1997): Epstein ME+, *J Am Acad Dermatol* 37, 149 (passim)
(1993): de la Fuente-Prieto R+, *Allergy* 48, 634
(1991): Hantson P+, *BMJ* 302, 294
(1990): Adkinson NF, *Am J Med* 88 (Suppl 3C), 12S (0.2%)
(1990): Soto Alvarez J+, *Lancet* 335, 1094

## Other

Anaphylactoid reactions (<1%)
Aphthous stomatitis (<1%)
Dysgeusia (<1%)
Foetor ex ore (halitosis) (<1%)
Hypersensitivity
Injection-site pain (1–10%)
Injection-site phlebitis (1–10%)
Injection-site reactions (sic)
(1985): Newman TJ+, *Rev Infect Dis* 7, S648
Mastodynia (<1%)
Myalgia (<1%)
Oral ulceration (<1%)
Paresthesias
Thrombophlebitis (1–10%)
Tinnitus
Tongue numb (sic) (<1%)
Vaginal candidiasis
Vaginitis (<1%)

# BACAMPICILLIN

**Synonym:** carampicillin
**Trade name:** Spectrobid (Pfizer)
**Other common trade names:** *Albaxin; Ambacamp; Ambaxin; Bacacil; Bacampicine; Penglobe*
**Indications:** Respiratory tract infections, urinary tract infections, gonorrhea
**Category:** Beta-lactamase-sensitive aminopenicillin
**Half-life:** 65 minutes
**Clinically important, potentially hazardous interactions with:** anticoagulants, cyclosporine, demeclocycline, doxycycline, methotrexate, minocycline, oxytetracycline, tetracycline

### *Reactions*

#### Skin

Acute generalized exanthematous pustulosis (AGEP)
(1990): Guy C+, *Nouv Dermatol* (French) 9, 540
Angioedema
Contact dermatitis
(1986): Stejskal VD+, *J Allergy Clin Immunol* 77, 411
Ecchymoses
Edema
(2002): Liccardi G+, *Lancet* 359, 1700 (lips) ("deep kissing" husband who had taken bacampicillin)
Erythema multiforme
Exanthems
(1989): Alanko K+, *Acta Derm Venereol* (Stockh) 69, 223
(1988): Kohl PK+, *Aktuel Dermatol* 14, 104
(1986): Pauwels R+, *J Int Med Res* 14, 110
Exfoliative dermatitis
Fixed eruption
(1984): Chan HL, *Arch Dermatol* 120, 542
Hematomas
Jarisch–Herxheimer reaction
Pruritus
(2002): Liccardi G+, *Lancet* 359, 1700 (lips) ("deep kissing" husband who had taken bacampicillin)
Pustular eruption
(1998): Isogai Z+, *J Dermatol* 25, 612
Rash (sic) (<1%)
Stevens–Johnson syndrome
Urticaria

#### Other

Anaphylactoid reactions
Black tongue
Dysgeusia
Glossitis
Glossodynia
Hypersensitivity (<1%)
Injection-site pain
Oral candidiasis
Serum sickness
Stomatitis
Stomatodynia
Vaginitis
Xerostomia

# BACLOFEN

**Trade names:** Baclofen (Watson); Lioresal (Watson)
**Other common trade names:** *Alpha-Baclofen; Baclon; Baclosal; Baklofen; Clofen; Dom-Baclofen; Gen-Baclofen; Lebic; Nu-Baclo; Pacifen; PMS-Baclofen; Spinax*
**Indications:** Spasticity resulting from multiple sclerosis
**Category:** Antispastic and analgesic; skeletal muscle relaxant
**Half-life:** 2.5–4 hours

### *Reactions*

#### Skin

Ankle edema
(1993): Albright AL+, *JAMA* 270, 2475
Cutaneous side effects (sic) (1–2%)
(1972): Birkmayer W, *Aspeckte der Muskelspastik Int Symp Wien.* (German) Bern, Huber
Dermatitis (sic)
Diaphoresis
Exanthems
(1983): Lynde CW+, *Ann Neurol* 13, 216
Facial edema
Flushing
Pruritus
Rash (sic) (1–10%)
Urticaria
(1972): Birkmayer W, *Aspeckte der Muskelspastik Int Symp Wien.* (German) Bern, Huber (2%)

#### Other

Dysgeusia (<1%)
(1976): Rollin H, *Laryngol Rhinol Otol* (Stuttgart) (German) 55, 873
Paresthesias (<1%)
Tinnitus
Xerostomia (<1%)

# BALSALAZIDE

**Trade name:** Colazal (Salix)
**Indications:** Mild to moderately active ulcerative colitis
**Category:** 5-Aminosalicylic acid; antiinflammatory
**Half-life:** N/A

### *Reactions*

#### Skin

Flu-like syndrome (1%)
Kawasaki-like syndrome (sic)
Pruritus
Rash (sic)

#### Hair

Hair – alopecia

#### Other

Arthralgia (4%)
Hypersensitivity
(2000): Adhiyaman V+, *BMJ* 320, 613
Myalgia (1%)
Xerostomia (1%)

## BASILIXIMAB

**Trade name:** Simulect (Novartis)
**Indications:** Prophylaxis of organ rejection in renal transplantation
**Category:** A chimeric monoclonal antibody; immunosuppressant
**Half-life:** 7.2 days
**Clinically important, potentially hazardous interactions with:** cyclosporine, mycophenolate

### *Reactions*

#### Skin
- Acne (>10%)
- Candidiasis (>10%)
- Cyst (3–10%)
- Edema (>10%)
- Edema (generalized) (3–10%)
- Facial edema (3–10%)
- Genital edema (sic) (3–10%)
- Hematomas (3–10%)
- Herpes simplex (3–10%)
- Herpes zoster
- Infections (sic) (3–10%)
- Leg edema
- Pain
- Peripheral edema (>10%)
- Pruritus (3–10%)
- Rash (sic) (3–10%)
- Ulceration (3–10%)
- Vascular disorder (sic)
- Viral infection (>10%)

#### Hair
- Hair – hypertrichosis (3–10%)

#### Other
- Anaphylactoid reactions
- Arthralgia (3–10%)
- Depression (3–10%)
- Gingival hyperplasia (3–10%)
- Hypersensitivity (17 cases post-marketing)
- Hypesthesia (3–10%)
- Myalgia (3–10%)
- Paresthesias (3–10%)
- Sneezing
- Stomatitis (3–10%)
- Tremors (>10%)
- Ulcerative stomatitis
- Wound complications (sic) (>10%)

## BENACTYZINE

**Trade name:** Deprol (Wallace)
**Indications:** Depression, anxiety
**Category:** Antidepressant
**Half-life:** no data

Deprol is benactyzine and meprobamate

**Note:** Most of the adverse reactions are due to meprobamate (which see)

### *Reactions*

#### Skin
- Angioedema
- Bullous eruption
- Ecchymoses
- Edema
- Erythema multiforme
- Exanthems
  - (1964): Welsh AL, *Med Clin North Am* 48, 459
- Exfoliative dermatitis
- Fixed eruption
- Petechiae
- Pruritus
- Urticaria

#### Other
- Anaphylactoid reactions
- Paresthesias
- Stomatitis
- Xerostomia

## BENAZEPRIL

**Trade names:** Lotensin (Novartis); Lotensin-HCT (Novartis); Lotrel (Novartis)
**Other common trade names:** *Cibace; Cibacen; Cibacene*
**Indications:** Hypertension
**Category:** Angiotensin-converting enzyme (ACE) inhibitor; antihypertensive and vasodilator
**Half-life:** 11–12 hours
**Clinically important, potentially hazardous interactions with:** amiloride, spironolactone, triamterene

Lotrel is benazepril and amlodipine; Lotensin-HCT is benazepril and hydrochlorothiazide

### *Reactions*

#### Skin
- Angioedema (<1%)
  - (2001): Cohen EG+, *Ann Otol Rhinol Laryngol* 110(8), 701 (64 cases)
  - (1996): O'Mara NB+, *Pharmacotherapy* 16, 675
  - (1992): Kuhn M, *Clin Issues Crit Care Nurs* 3, 461
  - (1991): Anon, *Med Lett Drugs Ther* 33, 83
  - (1991): Balfour JA+, *Drugs* 42, 511
  - (1991): MacNab M+, *Clin Cardiol* 14, IV33
- Ankle edema
  - (1990): Mirvis DM+, *Am J Med Sci* 300, 354
- Dermatitis (sic)
- Diaphoresis (<1%)

(1991): Morant J+ (eds), *Arzneimittel-Kompendium der Schweiz*, Basel (German), Documed, 1990
Exanthems
(1991): Morant J+ (eds), *Arzneimittel-Kompendium der Schweiz*, Basel (German), Documed, 1990
Flushing
(1991): Morant J+ (eds), *Arzneimittel-Kompendium der Schweiz*, Basel (German), Documed, 1990
Lupus erythematosus
(2002): Boye T+, *World Congress Dermatol* Poster 0088
Pemphigus foliaceus
(2000): Ong CS+, *Australas J Dermatol* 41(4), 242
Peripheral edema
Photosensitivity (<1%)
Pruritus
(1991): Morant J+ (eds), *Arzneimittel-Kompendium der Schweiz*, Basel (German), Documed, 1990
Rash (sic) (<1%)
(1991): MacNab M+, *Clin Cardiol* 14, IV33
Urticaria
(1991): Moser M+, *Clin Pharmacol Ther* 49, 322

### Other

Ageusia
Cough
(2001): Adigun AQ+, *West Afr J Med* 20(1), 46–7
(2001): Lee SC+, *Hypertension* 38(2), 166
Dysgeusia
(1991): MacNab M+, *Clin Cardiol* 14, IV33
Hypersensitivity
Myalgia (<1%)
Paresthesias (<1%)
Tinnitus

## BENDROFLUMETHIAZIDE

**Trade name:** Corzide (Bristol-Myers Squibb)
**Other common trade names:** *Aprinox; Berkozide; Centyl; Naturine; Neo-Naclex; Pluryle*
**Indications:** Edema, diabetes insipidus, hypertension
**Category:** Thiazide* diuretic; antihypertensive
**Half-life:** 8.5 hours
**Clinically important, potentially hazardous interactions with:** digoxin, lithium

Corzide is bendroflumethiazide and nadolol

### *Reactions*

### Skin

Allergic reactions (sic)
Contact dermatitis
(1997): Pereira F+, *Contact Dermatitis* 35, 303
Diaphoresis
Exanthems
(1991): Morant J+ (eds), *Arzneimittel-Kompendium der Schweiz*, Basel (German), Documed, 1990
Exfoliative dermatitis
Facial edema
Grinspan's syndrome**
(1990): Lamey PG+, *Oral Surg Oral Med Oral Pathol* 70, 184
Pemphigoid (sic)
Photosensitivity
(1989): Diffey BL+, *Arch Dermatol* 125, 1355
Phototoxicity
(1997): Selvaag E, *Arzneimittelforschung* (German) 47, 97
(1997): Selvaag E+, *In Vivo* 11, 103
Pruritus
(1991): Morant J+ (eds), *Arzneimittel-Kompendium der Schweiz*, Basel (German), Documed, 1990
Purpura
Rash (sic)
Urticaria
Vasculitis

### Hair

Hair – alopecia

### Other

Anaphylactoid reactions
Gynecomastia
Paresthesias
Tinnitus
Xanthopsia
Xerostomia

***Note:** Bendroflumethiazide is a sulfonamide and can be absorbed systemically. Sulfonamides can produce severe, possibly fatal, reactions such as toxic epidermal necrolysis and Stevens–Johnson syndrome

****Note:** Grinspan's syndrome: the triad of oral lichen planus, diabetes mellitus, and hypertension

## BENZTHIAZIDE

**Trade names:** Aquatag; Exna (Robins); Hydrex; Marazide; Proaqua
**Other common trade names:** *Diurin; Fovane; Regulon*
**Indications:** Hypertension
**Category:** Thiazide* diuretic; antihypertensive
**Half-life:** no data
**Clinically important, potentially hazardous interactions with:** digoxin, lithium

### *Reactions*

### Skin

Allergic reactions (sic) (<1%)
Photosensitivity
Purpura
Rash (sic)
Urticaria
Vasculitis

### Other

Dysgeusia
Paresthesias (<1%)
Xanthopsia

***Note:** Benzthiazide is a sulfonamide and can be absorbed systemically. Sulfonamides can produce severe, possibly fatal, reactions such as toxic epidermal necrolysis and Stevens–Johnson syndrome

# BENZTROPINE

**Trade name:** Cogentin (Merck)
**Other common trade names:** *Akitan; Apo-Benzthioprine; Cogentine; Cogentinol; Phatropine; PMS-Benztropine*
**Indications:** Parkinsonism
**Category:** Antidyskinetic and anticholinergic; antiparkinsonian
**Half-life:** 6–48 hours
**Clinically important, potentially hazardous interactions with:** anticholinergics

### *Reactions*

#### Skin
Exanthems
Hypohidrosis (>10%)
Photosensitivity (1–10%)
Pruritus
Rash (sic) (<1%)
Urticaria
Xerosis (>10%)

#### Other
Black tongue
(2000): Heymann WR, *Cutis* 66, 25
Death
(2001): Lynch MJ+, *Med Sci Law* 41(2), 155
Dysgeusia
(2000): Heymann WR, *Cutis* 66, 25
Glossodynia
Paresthesias
Stomatodynia
Tinnitus
Xerostomia (>10%)
(2000): Heymann WR, *Cutis* 66, 25
(1989): Gelenberg AJ+, *J Clin Psychopharmacol* 9, 180

# BEPRIDIL

**Trade name:** Vascor (McNeil)
**Other common trade names:** *Bapadin; Bepricol; Cordium; Cruor*
**Indications:** Angina pectoris
**Category:** Calcium channel blocker; antianginal
**Half-life:** 24 hours
**Clinically important, potentially hazardous interactions with:** amprenavir, ciprofloxacin, enoxacin, epirubicin, gatifloxacin, lomefloxacin, **mistletoe**, moxifloxacin, norfloxacin, ofloxacin, qunolones, ritonavir, sparfloxacin

### *Reactions*

#### Skin
Diaphoresis (<2%)
Edema (1–10%)
Irritation (sic)
Peripheral edema (<1%)
Rash (sic) (<2%)
(1988): Sharma MK+, *Am J Cardiol* 61, 1210

#### Other
Dysgeusia (<1%)
Myalgia (<1%)
Paresthesias (2.5%)
Tinnitus
Tremors (<9%)
Xerostomia (1–10%)
(1988): Hasegawa GR, *Clin Pharm* 7, 97
(1988): Krusell LR+, *Eur J Clin Pharmacol* 34, 221

# BETA-CAROTENE

**Trade name:** Solatene (Merck)
**Other common trade names:** *B-Tene; Betavin; Carotaben; Solvin*
**Indications:** Photosensitivity reactions
**Category:** Fat-soluble vitamin supplement; photosensitivity reaction suppressant
**Half-life:** no data
**Clinically important, potentially hazardous interactions with:** bexarotene

### *Reactions*

#### Skin
Carotenemia (>10%)
(2000): Frieling UM+, *Arch Dermatol* 136, 179 (15.9%)
Dermatitis (sic)
(1992): Zürcher K and Krebs A, *Cutaneous Drug Reactions* Karger, 280
Ecchymoses (<1%)
Purpura (<1%)

# BETAXOLOL

**Trade names:** Betoptic [Ophthalmic] (Alcon); Kerlone (Searle)
**Other common trade names:** *Betoptic S; Betoptima; Kerlon; Optipres*
**Indications:** Open-angle glaucoma, hypertension
**Category:** Beta-adrenergic blocker; antihypertensive
**Half-life:** 14–22 hours
**Clinically important, potentially hazardous interactions with:** clonidine, verapamil

**Note:** Cutaneous side effects of beta-receptor blockaders are clinically polymorphous. They apparently appear after several months of continuous therapy. Atypical psoriasiform, lichen planus-like, and eczematous chronic rashes are mainly observed. (1983): Hödl St, *Z Hautkr* 1:58, 17

### *Reactions*

#### Skin
Acne
Allergy (sic) (<2%)
Angioedema
Cold extremities (sic)
Contact dermatitis
(2001): Holdiness MR, *Am J Contact Dermat* 12(4), 217
(1993): O'Donnell BF+, *Contact Dermatitis* 28, 121
Diaphoresis (<2%)
Edema (1.3%)
Erythema (1–10%)
Exanthems
Exfoliative dermatitis
Facial edema
Flushing (<2%)

Lupus erythematosus
(1997): Hardee JT+, *West J Med* 167, 106
Photosensitivity
Pigmentation (palms)
(1997): Adams DR+, *Am J Contact Dermat* 8, 183
Pruritus (1–10%)
Psoriasis
Purpura
Rash (sic) (1.2%)
(1989): Burris JF+, *Arch Intern Med* 149, 2437
Raynaud's phenomenon
Toxic epidermal necrolysis
Urticaria
Xerosis

### Hair

Hair – alopecia (following topical use) (<2%)
(1990): Buckley MMT+, *Drugs* 40, 75
Hair – hypertrichosis (<2%)

### Nails

Nails – pigmentation (bluish)

### Other

Ageusia (<2%)
Anaphylactoid reactions
Depression
(2001): Schweitzer I+, *Aust NZ J Psychiatry* 35(5), 569
Dysgeusia (<2%)
Glossitis (following topical use)
Mastodynia (<2%)
Myalgia (3.2%)
Myasthenia gravis
(1997): Khella SL+, *Muscle Nerve* 20, 631
Oral ulceration (<2%)
Paresthesias (1.9%)
Peyronie's disease (<2%)
Sialorrhea (<2%)
Tinnitus
Xerostomia (<2%)

## BETHANECHOL

**Trade name:** Urecholine (Merck)
**Other common trade names:** *Muscaran; Myocholine-Glenwood; Myotonine Chloride; Urocarb*
**Indications:** Nonobstructive urinary retention
**Category:** Urinary tract cholinergic stimulant
**Duration of action:** up to 6 hours
**Clinically important, potentially hazardous interactions with:** galantamine

#### *Reactions*

### Skin

Diaphoresis (1–10%)
Flushing (<1%)
Miliaria
(1967): Rochmis PG+, *Arch Dermatol* 95, 499

### Other

Sialorrhea (<1%)

## BEXAROTENE

**Trade name:** Targretin (Ligand)
**Indications:** Cutaneous T-cell lymphoma (CTCL), (mycosis fungoides)
**Category:** Retinoid (rexinoid)
**Half-life:** 7 hours
**Clinically important, potentially hazardous interactions with:** acetretin, beta-carotene, gemfibrozil, isotretinoin, tretinoin, vitamin A

#### *Reactions*

### Skin

Acne (<10%)
Bacterial infection (1.2–13.2%)
Cellulitis
Cheilitis (<10%)
Chills (9.5%)
(2001): Duvic M+, *Arch Dermatol* 137, 581
Cold hands and feet
(2000): Bedikian AY+, *Oncol Rep* 7, 883
Erythema
(2002): Breneman D+, *Arch Dermatol* 138, 352
(2002): Liu HL+, *Arch Dermatol* 138, 398
Exanthems (<10%)
Exfoliative dermatitis (10–28%)
(2001): Duvic M+, *Arch Dermatol* 137, 581 (7%)
Facial edema
(2002): Breneman D+, *Arch Dermatol* 138, 325
Flu-like syndrome (sic) (3.6–13.2%)
Necrosis
(2002): Breneman D+, *Arch Dermatol* 138, 325
Nodule (sic) (<10%)
Peripheral edema (13.1%)
Photosensitivity
Pruritus (20–30%)
(2002): Breneman D+, *Arch Dermatol* 138, 325
(2001): Duvic M+, *Arch Dermatol* 137, 581 (20%)
(2000): Duvic M, *Dermatology Times*, August, 3 (25%)
Pustular eruption
Rash (sic) (16.7%)
(2001): Duvic M+, *Arch Dermatol* 137, 581
Skin disorder (sic)
(2001): Duvic M+, *Arch Dermatol* 137, 581 (13%)
Ulceration (<10%)
(2002): Breneman D+, *Arch Dermatol* 138, 325
Vasculitis
(2002): Breneman D+, *Arch Dermatol* 138, 325
Vesiculobullous eruption (<10%)
(2002): Breneman D+, *Arch Dermatol* 138, 325
Xerosis (10.7%)

### Hair

Hair – alopecia (4–11%)

### Other

Gingivitis (<10%)
Hyperesthesia (<10%)
Hypesthesia
Mastodynia (<10%)
Myalgia (<10%)
(2000): Bedikian AY+, *Oncol Rep* 7, 883
Pain
(2002): Breneman D+, *Arch Dermatol* 138, 325
Xerostomia (<10%)

## BICALUTAMIDE

**Trade name:** Casodex (AstraZeneca)
**Indications:** Metastatic prostatic carcinoma
**Category:** Antiandrogen antineoplastic
**Half-life:** up to 10 days

### *Reactions*

#### Skin

Diaphoresis (6%)
Edema (2–5%)
Exanthems (<1%)
Hot flashes (49%)
(2001): Kucuk O+, *Urology* 58(1), 53 (23%)
(1996): Bales GT+, *Urology* 47, 38
(1995): Lunglmayr G, *Anticancer Drugs* 6, 508
(1994): Eri LM+, *Eur Urol* 26, 219
(1990): Mahler C+, *J Steroid Biochem Mol Biol* 37, 921
Peripheral edema (8%)
Pruritus (2–5%)
Rash (sic) (6%)
Xerosis (2–5%)

#### Hair

Hair – alopecia (2–5%)

#### Other

Gynecomastia (38%)
(2001): Wirth M+, *Urology* 58(2), 146 (17.4%)
(1998): Goa KL+, *Drugs Aging* 12, 401
(1996): Bales GT+, *Urology* 47, 38
(1996): Kotake T+, *Hinyokika Kiyo* (Japanese) 42, 157
(1995): Lunglmayr G, *Anticancer Drugs* 6, 508
(1994): Eri LM+, *Eur Urol* 26, 219
(1990): Mahler C+, *J Steroid Biochem Mol Biol* 37, 921
Injection-site reactions (2–5%)
Mastodynia (39%)
(2001): Wirth M+, *Urology* 58(2), 146 (17.6%)
(1998): Goa KL+, *Drugs Aging* 12, 401
(1996): Bales GT+, *Urology* 47, 38
(1996): Kotake T+, *Hinyokika Kiyo* (Japanese) 42, 157
(1995): Lunglmayr G, *Anticancer Drugs* 6, 508
(1994): Eri LM+, *Eur Urol* 26, 219
(1990): Mahler C+, *J Steroid Biochem Mol Biol* 37, 921
Myalgia (2–5%)
Paresthesias (6%)
Xerostomia (2–5%)

## BIMATOPROST

**Trade name:** Lumigan (Allergan)
**Indications:** Open-angle glaucoma, ocular hypertension
**Category:** Ophthalmic agent; prostamide
**Half-life:** 45 minutes

### *Reactions*

#### Skin

Ocular pruritus (>10%)
Pigmentation of eyelid skin
Upper respiratory infection (10%)

#### Hair

Eyelashes – change in color
Eyelashes – growth (>10%)
Hirsutism (1–5%)

#### Other

Blepharitis (3–10%)
Conjuctival hyperemia (>10%)
(2001): DuBiner H+, *Surv Ophthalmol* 45(Suppl 4), S353–60
(2001): Gandolfi S+, *Adv Ther* 18(3), 110
(2001): Laibovitz RA+, *Arch Ophthalmol* 119(7), 994
(2001): Sherwood M+, *Surv Ophthalmol* 45(Suppl 4), S361–8
Eyelid erythema (3–10%)
Eyelid irritation (3–10%)
Eyelid pain (3–10%)
Eyelid pigmentation (3–10%)
Eyelid xerosis (3–10%)
Iris pigmentation (1–3%)
(2001): Sherwood M+, *Surv Ophthalmol* 45(suppl 4), S361–8 (1.1%)
Pigmentation – eye color

## BIPERIDEN

**Trade name:** Akineton (Abbott)
**Other common trade names:** *Biperen; Bipiden; Dekinet; Desiperiden; Dyskinon*
**Indications:** Parkinsonism
**Category:** Anticholinergic; antiparkinsonian
**Half-life:** 18–24 hours
**Clinically important, potentially hazardous interactions with:** anticholinergics

### *Reactions*

#### Skin

Contact dermatitis
(1995): Torinuki W, *Tohoku J Exp Med* 176, 249
Diaphoresis
(2001): Richardson C+, *Am J Psychiatry* 158(8), 1329
Exanthems
Flushing
Rash (sic)
Urticaria

#### Other

Glossodynia
Paresthesias
Stomatodynia
Xerostomia

## BISACODYL

**Trade names:** Biscolax; Carter's Little Pills; Dacodyl; Dulcagen; Dulcolax (Novartis); Fleet Laxative (Fleet)
**Other common trade names:** *Apo-Bisacodyl; Dulcolan; Laxit*
**Indications:** Constipation
**Category:** Irritant/stimulant laxative
**Onset of action:** 6–10 hours

### *Reactions*

#### Skin

Diaphoresis
Exanthems

Fixed eruption
(1997): Burrow WH, Jackson, MS (from Internet) (observation)
(1961): Welsh AL+, *Arch Dermatol* 84, 1004
Urticaria

# BISMUTH

**Trade names:** Bismuth salicylate; Bismuth subcitrate; Bismuth subgallate (colostomy deodorant); Bismuth subnitrate and Bismuth idoform paraffin paste (BIPP); Bismuth subsalicylate; Bismuth sucralfate
**Other common trade names:** *Bismatrol; Caved-S; Colo-Fresh; De-Nol; Devrom (Parthenon); Diotame; Pepto-Bismol (Procter & Gamble); Pink Bismuth*
**Indications:** As part of 'triple therapy' (antibiotics + bismuth) for eradication of *H.pylori*. Bismuth subgallate initiates clotting via activation of factor XII, and is used for bleeding during tonsillectomy and adenoidectomy. BIPP impregnated ribbon gauze is used for packing following ear surgery. Bismuth subsalicylate is in OTC products for gastrointestinal complaints and peptic ulcer disease.
**Category:** Antidiarrheal
**Half-life:** 21–72 days
**Clinically important, potentially hazardous interactions with:** aspirin, ciprofloxacin, doxycycline, hypoglycemics, lomefloxacin, methotrexate, minocycline, tetracycline, warfarin

### *Reactions*

## Skin

Adverse effects (sic) (triple therapy)
(2001): Danese S+, *Hepatogastroenterology* 48(38), 465
(2001): Sotudehmanesh R+, *J Gastroenterol Hepatol* 16(3), 264
(2000): de Boer WA+, *Am J Gastroenterol* 95(3), 641
(2000): Malekzadeh R+, *Aliment Pharmacol Ther* 14(3), 299
(2000): Spinzi GC+, *Aliment Pharmacol Ther* 14(3), 325
(1999): Monkemuller KE+, *Aliment Pharmacol Ther* 13(5), 661
(1999): Olafsson S+, *Aliment Pharmacol Ther* 13(5), 651
(1999): Xiao SD+, *Aliment Pharmacol Ther* 13(3), 311
(1998): Cammarota G+, *Aliment Pharmacol Ther* 12(6), 539
(1998): Cestari R, *Aliment Pharmacol Ther* 12(10), 991
(1998): Dobrucali A+, *Wien Med Wochenschr* (German) 148(20), 464
(1998): Lerang F+, *Am J Gastroenterol* 93(2), 212
(1998): Ricciardiello L+, *Aliment Pharmacol Ther* 12(6), 533
(1998): Spadaccini A+, *Aliment Pharmacol Ther* 12(10), 997
(1998): van der Wouden EJ+, *Am J Gastroenterol* 93(8), 1228
(1997): Henriksen M+, *Am J Gastroenterol* 92, 653
(1997): Huang JQ+, *J Gastroenterol Hepatol* 12(8), 590
(1997): Kolkman JJ+, *Aliment Pharmacol Ther* 11(6), 1123
(1997): Kung NN+, *Am J Gastroenterol* 92(3), 438
(1997): Laine L+, *Am J Gastroenterol* 92(12), 2213
(1996): Thijs JC+, *Am J Gastroenterol* 91(1), 93
(1996): van der Hulst RW+, *Helicobacter* 1(1), 6
(1996): Weldon MJ+, *Aliment Pharmacol Ther* 10(3), 279
(1995): al-Assi MT+, *Am J Gastroenterol* 90(3), 403
(1995): Hoffenberg P+, *Rev Med Chil* 123(2), 185
(1995): Rauws EA+, *Drugs* 50(6), 984
(1995): Webb DD+, *Am J Gastroenterol* 90(8), 1273
(1994): Borody TJ+, *Am J Gastroenterol* 89(1), 33
(1994): Hentschel E, *Wien Klin Wochenschr* (German) 106(17), 543
(1994): Park KN+, *Eur J Gastroenterol Hepatol* 6 (Suppl 1), S103
(1994): Reijers MH+, *Aliment Pharmacol Ther* 8(3), 351 (sucralfate)
(1994): Wilhelmsen I+, *Hepatogastroenterol* 41(1), 43
(1993): Malfertheiner P, *Scand J Gastroenterol* Suppl 196, 34
(1992): Berstad K+, *Scand J Gastroenterol* 27(12), 1006
(1992): Burgess E+, *Drug Saf* 7(4), 282
(1992): Wilhelmsen I+, *Tidsskr Nor Laegeforen* (Norwegian) 112(25), 3197
(1990): Steffen R, *Rev Infect Dis* 12(Suppl1), S80 (subsalicylate)
(1989): Bradley B+, *J Clin Pharm Ther* 14(6), 423 (subsalicylate and subcitrate)
(1988): Borsch G, *Med Klin* (German) 83(18), 605
(1988): Dipalma JR, *Am Fam Physician* 38(5), 244
(1988): Eskens GT, *Postgrad Med J* 64(755), 724
(1980): Fournier PE, *Therapie* (French) 35(3), 319
(1980): Henderson IW, *Can Med Assoc J* 123(9), 848
(1977): Glozman VN+, *Vestn Dermatol Venerol* (Russian) 4, 88
(1976): Martin-Bouyer G, *Therapie* (French) 31(6), 683
(1976): Rebattu JP+, *JFORL J Fr Otorhinolaryngol Audidphonol Chir Maxillofac* 25(9), 627 (suppositories)
(1974): Lowe DJ, *Med J Aust* 2(18), 664
Allergy (sic)
(1985): Jones PH, *J Laryngol Otol* 99(4), 389
(1981): Anchupane IS+, *Vestn Dermatol Venerol* (Russian) 11, 63
Angioedema (subcitrate)
(1994): Ottervanger JP+, *Ned Tijdschr Geneeskd* (Dutch) 138(3), 152
Black granules on skin (subsalicylate)
(1997): Ruiz-Maldonado R+, *J Am Acad Dermatol* 37(3), 489
Contact dermatitis
(2001): Wictorin A+, *Contact Dermatitis* 45(5), 318 (ointment)
(1987): Goh CL+, *Contact Dermatitis* 16(2), 109 (subnitrate)
Erythema (subcitrate)
(1994): Ottervanger JP+, *Ned Tijdschr Geneeskd* (Dutch) 138(3), 152
Exanthems (subcitrate)
(1994): Ottervanger JP+, *Ned Tijdschr Geneeskd* (Dutch) 138(3), 152
Exfoliative dermatitis
(1969): Singh R, *Indian J Dermatol* 15(1), 13
Fixed eruption
(1981): Granstein RD+, *J Am Acad Dermatol* 5, 1
Pigmentation
(1993): Zala L+, *Dermatology* 187(4), 288
(1981): Granstein RD+, *J Am Acad* 5(1), 1
(1973): Levantine A+, *Br J Dermatol* 89(1), 105
(1970): Plisek V+, *Vnitr Lek* (Czech) 16(11), 1085
Prurigo pigmentosa
(1987): Dijkstra JW+, *Int J Dermatol* 26(6), 379
Pruritus (triple therapy)
(1998): Pozzato P+, *Aliment Pharmacol Ther* 12(5), 447
Rash (sic)
(1990): Burnett JW, *Cutis* 45(4), 220
Vasculitis

## Hair

Hair – alopecia
(1990): Gollnick H+, *Z Haut* (German) 65, 1128

## Other

Arthopathy
(1993): Kendel K+, *Dtsch Med Wochenschr* (German) 118(7), 221 (sub-gallate)
(1981): Emile J+, *Clin Toxicol* 18(11), 1285
(1980): Gaucher A+, *Rev Rhum Mal* 47(1), 31
(1979): Emile J+, *Ann Med Interne* 130(2), 75
(1979): Gaucher A+, *Med J Aust* 1(4), 129
(1979): Murray JR, *Med J Aust* 1(11), 522
(1979): Netter P+, *Pathol Biol* (Paris) (French) 27(5), 300
(1978): Sany J+, *Rev Rhum Mal Osteosrtic* 45(12), 729
(1976): Monseu G+, *Acta Neurol Belg* 76(5), 301
(1975): Buge A+, *Rev Rhum Mal Osteoartic* 42(12), 721
Body pains (10%) (triple therapy)

(1998): Scott BB, *Aliment Pharmacol Ther* 12(3), 277 (10%)
Death
(1991): Sainsbury SJ, *West J Med* 155(6), 637 (subsalicylate)
(1990): Jones JA, *Oral Surg Oral Med Oral Pathol* 69(6), 668 (BIPP)
(1989): Hudson M+, *BMJ* 299(6692), 159 (subcitrate)
(1985): Sanz Gallen P+, *Med Clin* (Barc) (Spanish) 84(13), 538
(1980): Allain P+, *Therapie* (French) 35(3), 303
(1978): Lhermitte F+, *Nouv Presse Med* (French) 7(24), 2170
(1978): Martin-Bouyer G, *Gastroenterol Clin Biol* 2(4), 349
(1978): Rouzaud P+, *Toxicol Eur Res* 1(4), 273
(1977): Robert JF, *Infirm Fr* 780(188), 24
(1976): Loiseau P+, *J Neurol Sci* 27(2), 133
Depression
Dysgeusia (46%) (triple therapy)
(2001): Gisbert JP+, *Helicobacter* 6(2), 157
(2001): Kaviani MJ+, *Eur J Gastroenterol Hepatol* 13(8), 915
(1998): Scott BB, *Aliment Pharmacol Ther* 12(3), 277 (10%)
(1997): Chey WD+, *Am J Gastroenterol* 92(9), 1483 (39%)
(1993): Ateshkadi A+, *Clin Pharm* 12(1), 34
(1993): Friedland RP+, *Clin Neuropharmacol* 16(2), 173 (subgallate)
Gingivitis
(1989): Slikkerveer A+, *Med Toxicol Adverse Drug Exp* 4(5), 303 (subnitrate, subcarbonate and subgallate)
Hypersensitivity
(1998): Lim PV+, *J Laryngol Otol* 112(4), 335 (impregnated tape)
(1981): Anchupane IS+, *Vestn Dermatol Venerol* (Russian) Nov 11, 63
Injection-site lymphoma
(1984): Krivitzky A+, *Ann Med Interne* (Paris) (French) 135(3), 205
Oral mucosal pigmentation
(1984): Sutak J+, *Prakt Zuban Lek* (Czech) 32(6), 166
(1983): Dayan D+, *Clin Prev Dent* 5(3), 25 (after root canal filling with AH-26)
(1971): Dummett CO, *Postgrad Med* 49(1), 78
Porphyria cutanea tarda
(1966): Bielicky T, *Dermatol Wochenschr* (German) 152(30), 761
Stomatitis
(1990): Burnett JW, *Cutis* 45(4), 220
(1989): Slikkerveer A+, *Med Toxicol Adverse rug Exp* 4(5), 303 (subnitrate, subcarbonate and subgallate)
(1966): Jackson JA, *Oral Surg Oral Med Oral Pathol* 21(2), 154
(1955): Nagel V, *Hautarzt* (German) 6, 232
Tinnitus
(1987): DuPont HL+, *JAMA* 257(10), 1347 (subsalicylate)
Tongue discoloration (>10%)
(2001): Ioffreda MD+, *Arch Dermatol* 137(7), 968 (black)
(1987): DuPont HL+, *JAMA* 257(10), 1347 (black)
Tooth discoloration
(1990): Burnett JW, *Cutis* 45(4), 220
Tremors
(1993): Kendel K+, *Dtsch Med Wochenschr* (German) 118(7), 221 (sub-gallate)
(1975): Aimard G+, *Nouv Presse Med* (French) 4(39), 2816
Xerostomia (41%) (triple therapy)
(2001): Kaviani MJ+, *Eur J Gastroenterol Hepatol* 13(8), 915

# BISOPROLOL

**Trade names:** Zebeta (Lederle); Ziac (Lederle)
**Other common trade names:** *Concor; Cordalin; Detensiel; Emcor; Fondril; Monocor; Soprol*
**Indications:** Hypertension
**Category:** Beta-adrenergic blocker
**Half-life:** 9–12 hours

Ziac is bisoprolol and hydrochlorothiazide

## *Reactions*

### Skin
Acne
Angioedema
Ankle edema (1–10%)
Diaphoresis (1%)
Eczema (sic)
Edema (3%)
Exanthems
Exfoliative dermatitis
Facial edema
Flushing
Lupus erythematosus
Photosensitivity
Pigmentation
Pruritus
Psoriasis
Purpura
Rash (sic) (1–10%)
Raynaud's phenomenon (1–10%)
Urticaria
Xerosis

### Hair
Hair – alopecia

### Nails
Nails – bluish

### Other
Anaphylactoid reactions
Dysgeusia
Hypesthesia (1.5%)
Myalgia (1–10%)
Paresthesias
Peyronie's disease
Tinnitus
Xerostomia (1.3%)

# BIVALIRUDIN

**Synonym:** Hirulog
**Trade name:** Angiomax (The Medicines Company)
**Indications:** Angioplasty adjunct
**Category:** Anticoagulant; thrombin inhibitor
**Half-life:** 25 minutes
**Clinically important, potentially hazardous interactions with:** anisindione, heparin, reteplase, streptokinase, tenecteplase, urokinase

### *Reactions*

#### Skin
Infections (sic)

#### Other
Back pain (42%)
Injection-site pain (8%)
Pain (15%)

# BLACK COHOSH

**Scientific names:** *Actaea macrotys; Actaea racemosa; Cimicifuga racemosa*
**Other common names:** Baneberry; Black Snakeroot; Bugbane; Cimifuga; Rattle Root; Rattle Snakeroot; Rattleweed; Squawroot
**Family:** Ranunculaceae
**Purported indications:** Hormone replacement therapy, dysmenorrhea, hot flashes
**Other uses:** Dyspepsia, rheumatism, fever, sore throat, cough, insect repellent. Fresh root applied topically for rattlesnake bites

### *Reactions*

#### Skin
Diaphoresis
Toxic reactions (sic)

**Note:** Black cohosh was also used as an ingredient in Lydia Pinkham's Vegetable Compound

# BLEOMYCIN

**Synonyms:** bleo; BLM
**Trade name:** Blenoxane (Bristol-Myers Squibb)
**Other common trade names:** *Bleo; Bleocin; Bleomycine; Bleomycinum; BLM*
**Indications:** Melanomas, sarcomas, lymphomas, testicular carcinoma
**Category:** Antineoplastic antibiotic
**Half-life:** 1.3–9 hours
**Clinically important, potentially hazardous interactions with:** aldesleukin

### *Reactions*

#### Skin
Acral erythema
(1982): Burgdorf WHC+, *Ann Intern Med* 97, 61
Acral gangrene
(1998): Reiser M+, *Eur J Clin Microbiol Infect Dis* 17, 58
(1997): Hladunewich M+, *J Rheumatol* 24, 2371
Acral sclerosis
(1984): Snauwaert J+, *Dermatologica* 169, 172
Acrocyanosis
(1983): Bork K+, *Hautarzt* (German) 34, 10
Angioedema
(1984): Khansur T+, *Arch Intern Med* 144, 2267
Bullous eruption (1–5%)
Chills (>10%)
Cutaneous toxicity (sic)
(1998): Mullai N+, *J Clin Oncol* 16, 1625
(1998): Yeo W+, *J Clin Oncol* 16, 1626
Dermatitis (sic)
Digital necrosis
(1997): Emmerich J, *Presse Med* (French) 26, 1580
(1997): Sibilia J+, *Presse Med* (French) 26, 1564
Erythema
(2001): Robinson JB+, *Gynecol Oncol* 82(3), 550
Exanthems
(1993): Haerslev T+, *Cutis* 52, 45 (linear and symmetrical)
(1980): Lincke-Plewig H, *Hautarzt* (German) 31, 616
(1976): Werner Y+, *Acta Derm Venereol* (Stockh) 56, 155
Flagellate erythema
(1999): Rubeiz NG+, *Int J Dermatol* 38, 140 (urticarial)
(1998): Yamamoto T+, *Dermatology* 197, 399
(1997): Polsky D+, New York, American Academy of Dermatology Meeting (SF), (gross and microscopic)
(1995): Watanabe T+, *Dermatology* 190, 230
(1994): Mowad CM+, *Br J Dermatol* 131, 700
(1994): Zaki I+, *Clin Exp Dermatol* 19, 366
(1992): Barduagni O+, *Dermatol Clin* (Italian) 3, 169
(1992): Jolin-Garijo L+, *An Med Interna* (Spanish) 9, 520
(1991): Duhra P+, *Clin Exp Dermatol* 16, 216
(1990): Cortina P+, *Dermatologica* 180, 106
(1990): Miori L+, *Am J Dermatopathol* 12, 598
(1990): Miori L+, *Dermatologica* 181, 238
(1987): Lindae ML+, *Arch Dermatol* 123, 395
Flagellate pigmentation
(2001): Nigro MG+, *Cutis* 68, 285
(1993): Lincke-Plewig H, *Hautarzt* (German) 44, 331
(1993): Tsuji T+, *J Am Acad Dermatol* 28, 503
(1992): Albig J+, *Hautarzt* (German) 43, 376
(1990): Vicente MA+, *Med Cutan Ibero Lat Am* (Spanish) 18, 148
(1986): Polla BS+, *J Am Acad Dermatol* 14, 690
(1985): Fernandez-Obregon AC+, *J Am Acad Dermatol* 13, 464
(1972): Yagoda A+, *Ann Intern Med* 77, 861
(1970): Moulin G+, *Bull Soc Fr Dermatol Syphiligr* 77, 293
Flushing
(2001): Robinson JB+, *Gynecol Oncol* 82(3), 550
Hyperkeratosis (palms and soles)
(1976): Werner Y+, *Acta Derm Venereol* (Stockh) 56, 155
(1971): de Bast C+, *Arch Dermatol* 104, 509
Ichthyosis
(1971): de Bast C+, *Arch Dermatol* 104, 509
Intertrigo
(1971): de Bast C+, *Arch Dermatol* 104, 509
Linear streaking (sic)
(1989): Vignini M+, *Clin Exp Dermatol* 14, 261
(1988): Lazar A+, *Cutis* 42, 397
(1987): Rademaker M+, *Clin Exp Dermatol* 12, 457
(1975): Lowitz BB, *N Engl J Med* 292, 1300
Lymphangitis
(1998): Allen AL+, *J Am Acad Dermatol* 39, 295
Neutrophilic eccrine hidradenitis
(1988): Scallan PJ+, *Cancer* 62, 2532
Nodular eruption
(1997): Polsky D+, New York, American Academy of Dermatology Meeting (SF), (gross and microscopic)

Painful erythema (elbows, knees, palms)
(1980): Lincke-Plewig H, *Hautarzt* (German) 31, 616
(1976): Werner Y+, *Acta Derm Venereol* (Stockh) 56, 155
Palmar nodules (sic)
(1993): Haerslev T+, *Cutis* 52, 45
Palmar–plantar erythema
(1990): Pagliuca A+, *Postgrad Med J* 66, 242
Pigmentation (~50%)
(2001): Mutafoglu-Uysal K+, *Turk J Pediatr* 43(2), 172
(1998): Behrens S+, *Hautarzt* (German) 49, 725
(1993): Tsuji T+, *J Am Acad Dermatol* 28, 503 (in striae distensae)
(1992): Gallais V+, *Ann Dermatol Venereol* (French) 119, 471
(1990): Wright AL+, *Dermatologica* 181, 255 (reticulate)
(1988): Massone L+, *G Ital Dermatol Venereol* (Italian) 123, 225 (striae)
(1986): Guillet G+, *Arch Dermatol* 122, 381 (in stripes)
(1985): Polla L+, *Ann Dermatol Venereol* (French) 112, 821
(1984): Schuler G+, *Hautarzt* (German) 35, 383 (linear)
(1983): Bork K+, *Hautarzt* (German) 34, 10
(1982): Kukla LJ+, *Cancer* 50, 2283
(1981): Granstein RD+, *J Am Acad Dermatol* 5, 1 (brown-black)
(1981): Nixon DW+, *Cutis* 27, 181
(1978): Perrot H+, *Arch Dermatol Res* 261, 245
(1973): Cohen IS+, *Arch Dermatol* 107, 553
(1973): Kiefer O, *Dermatologica* 146, 229
Pruritus (>5%)
(2001): Robinson JB+, *Gynecol Oncol* 82(3), 550
(1990): Caumes E+, *Lancet* 336, 1593
Radiation recall
(1993): Stelzer KJ+, *Cancer* 71, 1322
Raynaud's phenomenon (>10%)
(2001): Vanhooteghem O+, *Pediatr Dermatol* 18(3), 249
(1998): Reiser M+, *Eur J Clin Microbiol Infect Dis* 17, 58
(1997): Emmerich J, *Presse Med* (French) 26, 1580
(1997): Hladunewich M+, *J Rheumatol* 24, 2371
(1997): Sibilia J+, *Presse Med* (French) 26, 1564 (12.6%)
(1996): Epstein E, *The Schoch Letter* 46, 34 (observation)
(1996): Munn SE+, *Br J Dermatol* 135, 969
(1993): von Gunten CF+, *Cancer* 72, 2004
(1992): de Pablo P+, *Acta Derm Venereol* (Stockh) 72, 465
(1992): Doll DC+, *Semin Oncol* 19(5), 580
(1992): Gregg LJ, *J Am Acad Dermatol* 26, 279
(1991): Epstein E, *J Am Acad Dermatol* 24, 785
(1985): Adoue D+, *Ann Dermatol Venereol* (French) 112, 151
(1985): Bovenmyer DA, *J Am Acad Dermatol* 13, 470
(1985): Epstein E, *J Am Acad Dermatol* 13, 468
(1984): Adoue D+, *Ann Intern Med* 100, 770
(1984): Snauwaert J+, *Dermatologica* 169, 172
(1981): Kukla LJ+, *Arch Dermatol* 117, 604
Scleroderma
(2000): D'Cruz D, *Toxicol Lett* 112 and 421
(1999): Passiu G+, *Clin Rheumatol* 18, 422
(1998): Behrens S+, *Hautarzt* (German) 49, 725 (pseudoscleroderma)
(1997): Komosinska K+, *Postepy Hig Med Dosw* (Polish) 51, 285
(1994): Marck Y+, *Ann Dermatol Venereol* (French) 121, 712,
(1992): Kerr LD+, *J Rheumatol* 19, 294
(1991): Bourgeois P+, *Baillieres Clin Rheumatol* 5, 13
(1991): Guseva NG, *Revmatologiia Mosk* (Russian) 1, 33
(1985): Haustein UF+, *Int J Dermatol* 24, 147
(1984): Rush PJ+, *J Rheumatol* 11, 262
(1983): Bork K+, *Hautarzt* (German) 34, 10
(1980): Finch WR+, *J Rheumatol* 7, 651
(1973): Cohen IS+, *Arch Dermatol* 107, 533
(1971): de Bast C+, *Arch Dermatol* 104, 509
Stevens–Johnson syndrome
(1989): Brodsky A+, *J Clin Pharmacol* 29, 821
(1986): Giaccone G+, *Tumori* 72, 331
Thickening (sic)
Urticaria
Xerosis
(1973): Cohen IS+, *Arch Dermatol* 107, 555, 556

## Hair

Hair – alopecia (~50%)
(1992): Breathnach SM+, *Adverse Drug Reactions and the Skin* Blackwell, Oxford, 292 (passim)
(1990): Siegel RD+, *Chest* 98, 507
(1982): Kukla LJ+, *Cancer* 50, 2283
(1973): Cohen IS+, *Arch Dermatol* 107, 553
(1973): Kiefer O, *Dermatologica* 146, 229
(1971): de Bast C+, *Arch Dermatol* 104, 509
Hair – gray

## Nails

Nails – Beau's lines (transverse nail bands)
(1994): Ben-Dyan D+, *Acta Haematol* 91, 89
Nails – dystrophy
(1984): Miller RAW, *Arch Dermatol* 120, 963
Nails – growth reduced
(1971): de Bast C+, *Arch Dermatol* 104, 509
Nails – loss
(1986): Gonzalez FU+, *Arch Dermatol* 122, 974
Nails – onychodystrophy
(1985): Baran R, *Ann Dermatol Venereol* (French) 112, 463
Nails – onycholysis
(1998): Roussou P+, *Acta Derm Venereol* 78, 303
(1984): Snauwaert J+, *Dermatologica* 169, 172
Nails – pigmentation (banding)
(1977): Shetty MR, *Cancer Treatment Reports* 61, 501
Nails – shedding
(1973): Cohen IS+, *Arch Dermatol* 107, 553

## Other

Anaphylactoid reactions (<1%)
Calcinosis
(1983): Bork K+, *Hautarzt* (German) 34, 10
(1975): Ihde DC+, *Cancer Chemother* 59, 1039 (penis)
Gangrene (digital)
(1998): Reiser M+, *Eur J Clin Microbiol Infect Dis* 17, 58
(1998): Surville-Barland J+, *Eur J Dermatol* 8, 221
(1993): Vayssairat M+, *J Rheumatol* 20, 921
Glossitis
(1992): Breathnach SM+, *Adverse Drug Reactions and the Skin* Blackwell, Oxford, 292 (passim)
Hyperesthesia
Hypersensitivity (1–10%)
(2001): Mutafoglu-Uysal K+, *Turk J Pediatr* 43(2), 172
(2001): Robinson JB+, *Gynecol Oncol* 82(3), 550
(1992): Weiss RB, *Semin Oncol* 19, 458
Injection-site phlebitis (1–10%)
Oral papillomatosis
(1978): Hagedorn M+, *Hautarzt* (German) 29, 425
Oral ulceration
(1992): Breathnach SM+, *Adverse Drug Reactions and the Skin* Blackwell, Oxford, 292 (passim)
(1971): de Bast C+, *Arch Dermatol* 104, 509
Paresthesias
Stomatitis (>10%)
(1993): Haerslev T+, *Cutis* 52, 45
(1990): Siegel RD+, *Chest* 98, 507
(1983): Bronner AK+, *J Am Acad Dermatol* 9, 645
(1976): Werner Y+, *Acta Derm Venereol* (Stockh) 56, 176
(1975): Khlebnov AV+, *Klin Med Mosk* (Russian) 52, 78
(1973): Cohen IS+, *Arch Dermatol* 107, 553
(1973): Kiefer O, *Dermatologica* 146, 229
Tongue erosions
(1973): Cohen IS+, *Arch Dermatol* 107, 553

# BLOODROOT

**Scientific name:** *Sanguinaria canadensis*
**Other common names:** Blood Root; Coon Root; Indian Plant; Indian Red Paint; Red Puccoon; Red Root; Sanguinaria; Snakebite; Sweet Slumber; Tetterwort
**Family:** Papaveraceae
**Purported indications:** Orally, used as an emetic, cathartic, expectorant and antispasmodic. Topically, used as an irritant and debriding agent and, in dentistry, to remove plaque
**Other uses:** Bronchitis, asthma, croup, laryngitis, pharyngitis, scabies, eczema, athlete's foot, nasal polyps, rheumatism, cancer, dental analgesia, fever, anemia and general tonic

### *Reactions*

## Skin

Contact dermatitis
(1998): Brinker F, *Contraindications and Drug Interactions*, Eclectic Medical Publications
Irritation (sic)

# BOSENTAN

**Trade name:** Tracleer (Actelion)
**Indications:** Pulmonary arterial hypertension
**Category:** Endothelial receptor antagonist
**Half-life:** ~5 hours
**Clinically important, potentially hazardous interactions with:** atorvastatin, cyclosporine, fluvastatin, glyburide, itraconazole, ketoconazole, lovastatin, simvastatin, **St John's wort**, warfarin

### *Reactions*

## Skin

Edema (8%)
Flushing (9%)
Peripheral edema (8%)
Pruritus (4%)

# BOTULINUM TOXIN (A & B)

**Trade names:** Botox (Allergan); Dysport (Speywood); Myobloc (Elan)
**Indications:** Blepharospasm, hemifacial spasm, spasmodic torticollis, sialorrhea, hyperhidrosis, strabismus, oromandibular dystonia, cervical dystonia, spasmodic dysphonia. cosmetic application for wrinkles
**Category:** Neuromuscular blocking agent; toxin
**Half-life:** 3–6 months

### *Reactions*

## Skin

Acne
Allergic reactions (sic)
Depigmentation
(1999): Roehm PC+, *J Neuroophthalmol* 19(1), 7
Erythema multiforme
Eyelid edema
(1990): NIH Consensus Statement 8(8), 1
Flu-like syndrome (2–10%)
(2002): Molloy F, *eMedicine Journal* 3(2)
(1990): NIH Consensus Statement 8(8), 1
Hematomas
(1997): Heinen F+, *Neuropediatrics* 28(6), 307 (local)
(1997): Nussgens Z+, *Graefes Arch Clin Exp Opthalmol* 235(4), 197
Infections (sic) (13–19%)
Peripheral edema (1–10%)
Pruritus (1–10%)
Psoriasis
Purpura (1–10%)
Rash (sic)
Urticaria

## Other

Anaphylactoid reactions
(1997): LeWitt PA+, *Mov Disord* 12(6), 1064 (localized)
Arthralgia (<7%)
Death
Depression
(1999): Brenner R+, *South Med J* 92(7), 738
Dry eyes (6.3%)
Dysgeusia (1–10%)
Ectropion
(1990): *NIH Consensus Statement* 8(8), 1
Entropion
Hyperesthesia (1–10%)
Injection-site bruising
(2002): Molloy F, *eMedicine Journal* 3(2)
(1998): Goodman G, *Australas J Dermatol* 39(3), 158
Injection-site burning
(2000): Karamfilov T+, *Arch Dermatol* 136(4), 487
Injection-site ecchymoses
(1997): Guerrissi J+, *Ann Plast Surg* 39(5), 447
(1990): NIH, *Consensus Statement* 8(8), 1
Injection-site edema
(2000): Ahn KY+, *Plast Reconstr Surg* 105(2), 778
(2000): Wissel J+, *J Pain Symptom Manage* 20(1), 44
(1997): Guerrissi J+, *Ann Plast Surg* 39(5), 447
Injection-site pain (2–10%)
(2002): Molloy F, *eMedicine Journal* 3(2)
(2001): de Almeida+, *Dermatol Surg* 27(1), 34
(2000): Karamfilov T+, *Arch Dermatol* 136(4), 487
(2000): Wissel J+, *J Pain Symptom Manage* 20(1), 44
(1990): *NIH Consensus Statement* 8(8), 1
Injection-site rash (sic)
(1997): LeWitt PA+, *Mov Disord* 12(6), 1064
Leg pain
Pain (6–13%)
(1997): Truong DD+, *Mov Disord* 12(5), 772
Ptosis (14–20%)
(2002): Molloy F, *eMedicine Journal* 3(2) (10%)
(1997): Nussgens Z+, *Graefes Arch Clin Exp Ophthalmol* 235(4), 197
(1990): *NIH Consensus Statement* 8(8), 1
Stomatitis (1–10%)
Tinnitus (1–10%)
Tremors (1–10%)
(1997): Truong DD+, *Mov Disord* 12(5), 772
Vaginal candidiasis (1–10%)
Xerostomia (3–34%)

**Note:** An antitoxin is available in the event of overdose or misinjection

## BRETYLIUM

**Trade name:** Bretylol (Abbott)
**Other common trade names:** *Bretylate; Critifib*
**Indications:** Ventricular tachycardia and fibrillation
**Category:** Antiarrhythmic class III
**Half-life:** 4–17 hours
**Clinically important, potentially hazardous interactions with:** arsenic, ciprofloxacin, enoxacin, gatifloxacin, lomefloxacin, moxifloxacin, norfloxacin, ofloxacin, quinolones, sparfloxacin

### *Reactions*

#### Skin
Diaphoresis (<1%)
Flushing (<1%)
Rash (sic) (<1%)

#### Other
Injection-site atrophy (<1%)
Injection-site necrosis (<1%)

## BRIMONIDINE

**Trade name:** Alphagan (Allergan)
**Indications:** Open-angle glaucoma, ocular hypertension
**Category:** Alpha-2 adrenergic receptor agonist
**Half-life:** 12 hours

### *Reactions*

#### Skin
Allergic reactions (sic) (<1%)
(1999): thoe Schwartzenberg GW+, *Ophthalmology* 106, 1616
(1998): Gordon RN+, *Eye* 12, 697
Blepharitis (1–10%)
Eyelid crusting (1–10%)
Eyelid edema (1–10%)
Eyelid erythema (1–10%)
Ocular erythema
(2001): Stewart WC+, *Am J Opthalmol* 131(5), 631
Periocular dermatitis
(2000): Williams GC+, *Glaucoma* 9, 235
Upper respiratory infection (1–10%)

#### Other
Depression
Dysgeusia (1–10%)
Ocular allergy (sic) (4.2%)
(2000): Melamed S+, *Clin Ther* 22, 103
(1999): Shin DH+, *Am J Ophthalmol* 127, 511
(1998): LeBlanc RP, *Ophthalmology* 105, 1960
(1996): Schuman JS, *Surv Ophthalmol* 41, Suppl 1:S27
Ocular burning (<10%)
(1998): LeBlanc RP, *Ophthalmology* 105, 1960
(1997): Schuman JS+, *Arch Ophthalmol* 115, 847 (28.1%)
(1996): Schuman JS, *Surv Ophthalmol* 41, Suppl 1:S27
Ocular pruritus (<10%)
Ocular stinging (<10%)
(1998): LeBlanc RP, *Ophthalmology* 105, 1960
(1997): Schuman JS+, *Arch Ophthalmol* 115, 847 (28.1%)
(1996): Schuman JS, *Surv Ophthalmol* 41, Suppl 1:S27
Teardrop sign*
(2000): Scruggs JT+, *Br J Ophthalmol* 84, 671
Xerostomia (<10%)
(2000): Detry-Morel M+, *J Fr Ophtalmol* 23, 763
(1998): LeBlanc RP, *Ophthalmology* 105, 1960
(1997): Derick RJ+, *Ophthalmology* 104, 131
(1997): Schuman JS+, *Arch Ophthalmol* 115, 847 (33%)
(1996): Schuman JS, *Surv Ophthalmol* 41, Suppl 1:S27
(1996): Walters TR, , *Surv Ophthalmol* 41, Suppl 1:S19

***Note:** The Teardrop sign is a laceration or deformity of the limbus of the eye

## BROMOCRIPTINE

**Trade name:** Parlodel (Novartis)
**Other common trade names:** *Apo-Bromocriptine; Bromed; Cryocriptina; Kripton; Parilac; Pravidel; Serocryptin*
**Indications:** Amenorrhea, parkinsonism, infertility
**Category:** Dopamine agonist; antihyperprolactinemic; infertility therapy adjunct; lactation inhibitor; antidyskinetic; growth hormone suppressant; ergot alkaloid; antiparkinsonian
**Half-life:** initial: 6–8 hours; terminal: 50 hours
**Clinically important, potentially hazardous interactions with:** erythromycin, pseudoephedrine, sympathomimetics

### *Reactions*

#### Skin
Erythromelalgia
(1983): Dupont E+, *Neurology* 33, 670
(1981): Eisler T+, *Neurology* 31, 1368
(1979): Eisler T+, *Neurology* 29, 571
(1978): Calne DB+, *Lancet* 1, 735 (11%)
Exanthems
Flushing
(1992): Shelley WB+, *Advanced Dermatologic Diagnosis* WB Saunders, 582 (passim)
Livedo reticularis
(1985): Hoehn MMM+, *Neurology* 35, 199
(1978): Calne DB+, *Lancet* 1, 735
(1978): Lees AJ+, *Arch Neurol* 35, 503 (2%)
Morphea
(1989): Leshin B+, *Int J Dermatol* 28, 177
Pedal edema
Purpura
Rash (sic)
Raynaud's phenomenon (1–10%)
(1987): Quagliarello J+, *Fertility and Sterility* 48, 877
(1978): Lees AJ+, *Arch Neurol* 35, 503 (5%)
(1978): Pearce I+, *BMJ* 1, 1402
(1976): Duvoisin RC, *Lancet* 2, 204
(1976): Wass JAH+, *Lancet* 1, 1135
Scleroderma
(1989): Leshin B+, *Int J Dermatol* 28, 177
(1983): Dupont E+, *Neurology* 33, 670
Urticaria
Vasculitis
(1978): Lees AJ+, *Arch Neurol* 35, 503

#### Hair
Hair – alopecia
(1993): Fabre N+, *Clin Neuropharmacol* 16, 266
(1980): Blum I+, *N Engl J Med* 303, 1418

#### Other
Anaphylactoid reactions
(1980): Parkes S, *N Engl J Med* 302, 750
Dysgeusia (metallic taste)

Paresthesias
(1985): Hoehn MMM+, *Neurology* 35, 199
Priapism (clitoral)
Stomatopyrosis
(1985): Hoehn MMM+, *Neurology* 35, 199
Xerostomia (4–10%)
(1985): Hoehn MMM+, *Neurology* 35, 199
(1982): Gauthier G+, *Eur Neurol* 21, 217

## BROMPHENIRAMINE

**Trade name:** Dimetane (Robins)
**Other common trade names:** *Bromine; Brommine; Bromphen; Dimegan; Ilvin; Kinmedon; Nasahist; ND-Stat; Neo-Meton*
**Indications:** Allergic rhinitis, urticaria
**Category:** Antihistamine; $H_1$ blocker
**Half-life:** 12–48 hours
**Clinically important, potentially hazardous interactions with:** aprobarbital, butabarbital, chloral hydrate, ethchlorvynol, mephobarbital, pentobarbital, phenobarbital, phenothiazines, primidone, secobarbital, zolpidem

### *Reactions*

#### Skin
Angioedema (< 1%)
Exanthems (< 1%)
Photosensitivity (< 1%)
Rash (sic) (< 1%)

#### Other
Myalgia (< 1%)
Paresthesias (< 1%)
Xerostomia (1–10%)

## BUCLIZINE

**Trade names:** Bucladin-S (Stuart); Vibazine
**Other common trade names:** *Aphilan; Buclixin; Longifene; Odetin; Postafeno; Vibazina*
**Indications:** Motion sickness, nausea/vomiting
**Category:** Antihistamine; anticholinergic; antiemetic/antivertigo
**Half-life:** no data
**Clinically important, potentially hazardous interactions with:** aprobarbital, butabarbital, chloral hydrate, ethchlorvynol, mephobarbital, pentobarbital, phenobarbital, phenothiazines, primidone, secobarbital, zolpidem

### *Reactions*

#### Other
Tremors
Xerostomia

## BUMETANIDE

**Trade name:** Bumetanide (Baxter)
**Other common trade names:** *Bumedyl; Burinex; Fondiuran; Fontego; Lunetoron; Miccil; Primex*
**Indications:** Edema associated with congestive heart failure
**Category:** Sulfonamide* loop diuretic; antihypertensive
**Half-life:** 1–1.5 hours
**Clinically important, potentially hazardous interactions with:** amikacin, aminoglycosides, digoxin, gentamicin, kanamycin, neomycin, streptomycin, tobramycin

### *Reactions*

#### Skin
Allergic reactions (sic)
Bullous eruption
(1990): Leitao EA+, *J Am Acad Dermatol* 23, 129
Bullous pemphigoid
(1998): Boulinguez S+, *Br J Dermatol* 138, 549
Contact dermatitis
(1989): Moller NE+, *Contact Dermatitis* 20, 393
Cutaneous side effects (sic) (1.1%)
(1984): Ward A+, *Drugs* 28, 426 (1–5%)
Diaphoresis (0.1%)
Edema (periorbital)
(1981): Handler B+, *J Clin Pharmacol* 21, 691
Erythema multiforme (< 1%)
(1975): Ring-Larsen H, *Acta Med Scand* 195, 411
Exanthems
Exfoliative dermatitis
(1981): Handler B+, *J Clin Pharmacol* 21, 691
Photosensitivity
(1990): Leitao EA+, *J Am Acad Dermatol* 23, 129
Pruritus (< 1%)
(1992): Shelley WB+, *Cutis* 50, 17 (observation)
(1984): Ward A+, *Drugs* 28, 426 (1–5%)
Purpura
Rash (sic) (0.2%)
Urticaria (0.2%)
(1981): Handler B+, *J Clin Pharmacol* 21, 691
Vasculitis

#### Other
Nipple tenderness (0.1%)
Pseudoporphyria
(1990): Leitao EA+, *J Am Acad Dermatol* 23, 129
Xerostomia (0.1%)

***Note:** Bumetanide is a sulfonamide and can be absorbed systemically. Sulfonamides can produce severe, possibly fatal, reactions such as toxic epidermal necrolysis and Stevens–Johnson syndrome

## BUPROPION

**Trade names:** Wellbutrin (GSK); Zyban (GSK)
**Indications:** Depression, aid to smoking cessation
**Category:** Heterocyclic antidepressant; aid to smoking cessation
**Half-life:** 14 hours
**Clinically important, potentially hazardous interactions with:** isocarboxazid, phenelzine, ritonavir, tranylcypromine, trimipramine

### *Reactions*

---

#### Skin

Acne (1–10%)
Angioedema
Diaphoresis (5%)
 (1983): Feighner JP, *J Clin Psychiatry* 44, 49
 (1981): Halaris AE+, *Psychopharmacol Bull* 17, 140
Ecchymoses (<0.1%)
Edema (>1%)
 (1999): Peloso PM+, *JAMA* 282, 1817
Erythema multiforme
 (2002): Drago F+, *Arch Intern Med* 162(7), 843
 (2001): Carrillo-Jimenez R+, *Arch Intern Med* 161(12), 1556
 (2001): Lineberry TW+, *Mayo Clin Proc* 76, 664
Exanthems (<0.1%)
 (1983): Fabre LF+, *J Clin Psychiatry* 44, 88
 (1981): Halaris AE+, *Psychopharmacol Bull* 17, 140
Exfoliative dermatitis
Flushing (4%)
Hot flashes
Lupus panniculitis
 (1986): Ottuso P, *The Schoch Letter*, 46, 37 (observation)
Peripheral edema
 (1999): Peloso PM+, *JAMA* 282, 1817
Photosensitivity (<0.1%)
Pruritus (4%)
 (1983): Cato AE+, *J Clin Psychiatry* 44, 187
Rash (sic) (4%)
 (2000): McCollom RA+*Ann Pharmacother* 34, 471
 (1985): Golden RN+, *Am J Psychiatry* 142, 1459 (vascular)
Stevens–Johnson syndrome
Urticaria
 (1999): Peloso PM+, *JAMA* 282, 1817
 (1983): Cato AE+, *J Clin Psychiatry* 44, 187
 (1983): Fabre LF+, *J Clin Psychiatry* 44, 88
 (1983): Feighner JP, *J Clin Psychiatry* 44, 49
 (1983): Mendels J+, *J Clin Psychiatry* 44, 118
 (1978): Fann WE+, *Curr Ther Res* 23, 222
Xerosis (1–10%)

#### Hair

Hair – alopecia (<1%)
 (2002): Klein AD, Statesboro, GA (from Internet) (observation)
Hair – color change (sic) (<1%)
Hair – hirsutism (1–10%)

#### Other

Anaphylactoid reactions
Bromhidrosis
Bruxism (<0.1%)
Death
 (2002): Wooltorton E, *CMAJ* 166(1), 68
Dry mouth
 (2002): Zwar N+, *Aust Fam Physician* 31(5), 443
Dysgeusia (4%)
 (1999): Berigan TR, *JAMA* 281, 233 (letter)
Gingivitis
Glossitis
Gynecomastia (<1%)
Hypersensitivity
 (2002): *Prescrire Int* 11(58), 49
 (2002): Zwar N+, *Aust Fam Physician* 31(5), 443
 (2001): Benson E, *Med J Aust* 174(12), 650
Hypesthesia (<0.1%)
Myalgia (6%)
 (1999): Peloso PM+, *JAMA* 282, 1817
Oral edema (<1%)
Painful erection
Paresthesias (2%)
Parkinsonism
 (2001): Jerome L, *Can J Psychiatry* 46(6), 560
Priapism
 (1995): Levenson JL, *Am J Psychiatry* 152, 813
Rhabdomyolysis
 (1999): David D+, *J Clin Psychopharmacol* 19(2), 185
Seizures
 (2002): Wooltorton E, *CMAJ* 166(1), 68
 (2002): Zwar N+, *Aust Fam Physician* 31(5), 443
 (2001): Enns MW, *J Clin Psychiatry* 62(6), 476 (with trimipramine)
Serum sickness
 (2002): Wooltorton E, *CMAJ* 166(1), 68
 (2001): Davis JS+, *Med J Aust* 174, 479
 (2000): McCollom RA+*Ann Pharmacother* 34, 471
 (1999): Peloso PM+, *JAMA* 282, 1817
 (1999): Tripathi A+, *Ann Allergy Asthma Immunol* 83, 165
 (1999): Yolles JC+, *Ann Pharmacother* 33, 931
Sialorrhea
Stomatitis (>1%)
Tinnitus
Tongue edema (0.1%)
 (2000): McCollom RA+*Ann Pharmacother* 34, 471
Tremors (>10%)
Twitching (2%)
Vaginitis
Xerostomia (up to 64%)
 (1999): Settle EC+, *Clin Ther* 21, 454
 (1997): Hurd RD+, *N Engl J Med* 337, 1195
 (1991): James WA+, *South Med J* 84, 222
 (1986): Feighner JP+, *J Clin Psychopharmacol* 6, 27
 (1983): Chouinard G, *J Clin Psychiatry* 44, 121
 (1983): Feighner JP, *J Clin Psychiatry* 44, 49
 (1981): Halaris AE+, *Psychopharmacol Bull* 17, 140

## BUSPIRONE

**Trade name:** BuSpar (Bristol-Myers Squibb)
**Other common trade names:** *Ansail; Apo-Buspirone; Bespar; Biron; Busirone; Bustab; Kallmiren; Narol; Neurosine; Nu-Buspirone*
**Indications:** Anxiety
**Category:** Nonbenzodiazepine anxiolytic tranquilizer; serotonin antagonist
**Half-life:** 2–3 hours
**Clinically important, potentially hazardous interactions with:** nefazodone

### *Reactions*

---

#### Skin

Acne (<0.1%)
Bullous eruption (<1%)

Diaphoresis
(1986): Newton RE+, *Am J Med* 3B:80, 17
Ecchymoses
Edema
Exanthems
Facial edema (1%)
Flushing
Hypopigmentation
(2002): Chapman MS+, *Am J Contact Dermat* 13(1), 46
Pruritus (1%)
Purpura (1%)
Radiation recall
(1989): Vassal G+, *Cancer Chemother Pharmacol* 23, 117
Rash (sic) (<1%)
Seborrheic dermatitis
(1993): Litt JZ, Beachwood, OH (personal case) (observation)
Sicca syndrome
(1977): Sidi Y+, *JAMA* 238, 1951
Urticaria (<1%)
Xerosis (1%)

### Hair

Hair – alopecia (1%)
(2000): Mercke Y+, *Ann Clin Psychiatry* 12, 35
(1995): Ljungman P+, *Bone Marrow Transplant* 15, 869

### Nails

Nails – thinning (<0.1%)

### Other

Dysgeusia (<1%)
Galactorrhea (<0.1%)
Glossodynia
Glossopyrosis
Myalgia
Paresthesias (1%)
(1986): Newton RE+, *Am J Med* 3B:80, 17
Parosmia (1%)
Serotonin syndrome
(2000): Manos GH, *Ann Pharmacother* 34(7–8), 871 (with fluoxetine)
Sialorrhea
Tinnitus
Xerostomia (3%)

## BUSULFAN

**Trade name:** Myleran (GSK)
**Other common trade names:** *Citosulfan; Leukosulfan; Mablin; Misulban*
**Indications:** Chronic myelogenous leukemia, bone marrow disorders
**Category:** Antineoplastic
**Half-life:** 3.4 hours (after first dose)
**Clinically important, potentially hazardous interactions with:** aldesleukin

***Reactions***

### Skin

Bullous eruption
(1970): Dosik H+, *Blood* 35, 543
Cheilitis
(1980): Wintroub B+, *Clinical Cancer Medicine*, GK Hall and Company, 206
(1961): Haut A+, *Blood* 17, 1
Eccrine squamous syringometaplasia
(1997): Valks R+, *Arch Dermatol* 133, 873
Erythema (macular) (>10%)
(1985): Hymes SR+, *J Cutan Pathol* 12, 125
Erythema multiforme (<1%)
(1981): Weiss RB+, *Ann Intern Med* 94, 66
(1980): Adrian RM+, *CA* 30, 143
(1978): Levine N+, *Cancer Treat Rev* 5, 67
(1974): Levantine A+, *Br J Dermatol* 90, 239
(1970): Dosik H+, *Blood* 35, 543
Erythema nodosum (<1%)
(1978): Levine N+, *Cancer Treat Rev* 5, 67
(1961): Kyle BA+, *Blood* 18, 497
(1956): Marinko HM+, *Arq Brasil Med* (Portuguese) 46, 161
Exanthems
(1992): Fitzpatrick JE, *Derm Clinics* 10, 19 (passim)
(1978): Leyden MJ+, *Lancet* 2, 797
Granulomatous dermatitis
(2002): Longo M+, *World Congress Dermatol* Poster, 0110
Kaposi's sarcoma
(1998): Roszkiewicz A+, *Cutis* 61, 137
Pigmentation (1–10%) ("busulfan tan")
(1999): Simonart T+, *Ann Dermatol Venereol* (French) 126, 439
(1992): Fitzpatrick JE, *Derm Clinics* 10, 19 (passim)
(1985): Hymes SR+, *J Cutan Pathol* 12, 125
(1983): Bronner AK+, *J Am Acad Dermatol* 9, 645
(1981): Granstein RD+, *J Am Acad Dermatol* 5, 1 (brown-black)
(1980): Adam BA+, *J Dermatol* 7, 405
(1971): Burns WA+, *Med Ann DC* 40, 567
(1966): Harrold BP, *BMJ* 1, 463
(1966): Sprunt JG+, *BMJ* 5489, 736
(1965): Desai RG, *N Engl J Med* 272, 808
(1963): Marchal G+, *Sem Ther* (French) 39, 565
(1961): Haut A+, *Blood* 17, 1
(1961): Kyle RA+, *Blood* 18, 497
Purpura
(2001): Chuang C+, *Movement Disorders* 16, 990 (with cyclophosphamide)
Urticaria (>10%)
(1981): Spiegel RJ, *Cancer Treat Rev* 8, 197
(1981): Weiss RB+, *Ann Intern Med* 94, 66
(1978): Levine N+, *Cancer Treat Rev* 5, 67
(1961): Kyle BA+, *Blood* 18, 497
(1960): Ducach C+, *Rev Med Chile* (Spanish) 88, 36
Vasculitis
(1992): Breathnach SM+, *Adverse Drug Reactions and the Skin* Blackwell, Oxford, 288 (passim)
(1982): Weiss RB, *Sem Oncology* 9, 5
(1967): Coleman WP, *Med Clin North Am* 51, 1073
Xerosis
(1961): Haut A+, *Blood* 17, 1

### Hair

Hair – alopecia (>10%)
(2000): Tran D+, *Australas J Dermatology* 41, 106
(1995): Ljungman P+, *Bone Marrow Transplant* 15, 869
(1993): Vowels M+, *Bone Marrow Transplant* 12, 347
(1977): Moschella S, *Cutis* 19, 603
(1975): Dreizen S+, *Postgrad Med* 58, 150
(1961): Haut A+, *Blood* 17, 1

### Nails

Nails – pigmentation

### Other

Anhidrosis
(1961): Haut A+, *Blood* 17, 1
Dysgeusia
(1961): Haut A+, *Blood* 17, 1

Gynecomastia (<1%)
(1979): Harrington WJ, *Adv Intern Med* 24, 141
(1979): White DR+, *N C Med J* 40, 73
(1977): Moschella SL, *Cutis* 19, 603
Oral mucosal pigmentation
(1965): Desai RG, *N Engl J Med* 272, 808
Oral mucositis
(2000): Wardley AM+, *Br J Haematol* 110, 292
Parkinsonism
Porphyria cutanea tarda
(1983): Bronner AK+, *J Am Acad Dermatol* 9, 645
(1964): Kyle BA+, *Blood* 23, 776
Stomatitis

# BUTABARBITAL

**Trade names:** Butalan; Buticaps; Butisol (Wallace)
**Other common trade name:** *Day-Barb*
**Indications:** Sedation
**Category:** Sedative-hypnotic barbiturate
**Half-life:** 40–140 hours
**Clinically important, potentially hazardous interactions with: alcohol**, antihistamines, ardeparin, argatroban, brompheniramine, buclizine, chlorpheniramine, dalteparin, danaparoid, dicumarol, enoxaparin, ethanolamine, heparin, imatinib, tinzaparin, warfarin

## *Reactions*

### Skin
Acneform eruption
Angioedema (<1%)
Bullous eruption
(1970): Groeschel D+, *N Engl J Med* 283, 409
Erythema multiforme
(1975): Böttiger LE, *Acta Med Scand* 198, 229
Exanthems
(1943): Davison TC, *Curr Res Anesth Analg* 22, 52
Exfoliative dermatitis (<1%)
(1944): Potter JK+, *Ann Intern Med* 21, 1041
Fixed eruption
(1970): Savin JA, *Br J Dermatol* 83, 546
Herpes simplex
Lupus erythematosus
(1967): Williams DI, *Proc R Soc Med* 60, 299
(1951): Grant Peterkin GA, *Edinb Med J* 58, 41
Necrosis
(1972): Almeyda J+, *Br J Dermatol* 86, 313
Photosensitivity
(1939): Stryker GV, *J Mo Med Assn* 36, 484
Pruritus
Purpura
(1946): Grant Peterkin GA, *BMJ* 2, 52
Rash (sic) (<1%)
Stevens–Johnson syndrome (<1%)
Toxic epidermal necrolysis
(1973): Stüttgen G, *Br J Dermatol* 88, 291
Urticaria
Vasculitis

### Other
Oral ulceration
Porphyria variegata
Rhabdomyolysis
(1990): Larpin R+, *Presse Med* 19(30), 1403
Thrombophlebitis (<1%)

# BUTALBITAL

**Trade name:** Fiorinal (Novartis)
**Other common trade names:** *Amaphen; Anoquan; Axotal; Butace; Fioricet; Marnal; Medigesic; Phrenilin; Tecnal*
**Other Trade names:** Amaphen; Anoquan; Axotal; Butace; Fioricet; Marnal; Medigesic; Phrenilin; Tecnal
**Indications:** Tension headaches
**Category:** Sedative and analgesic barbiturate
**Half-life:** 35 hours
**Clinically important, potentially hazardous interactions with: alcohol**, dicumarol

## *Reactions*

### Skin
Bullous eruption
(1970): Groeschel D+, *N Engl J Med* 283, 409
Erythema multiforme
(1984): Gebel K+, *Dermatologica* 168, 35
(1975): Böttiger LE, *Acta Med Scand* 198, 229
Exanthems
(1943): Davison TC, *Curr Res Anesth Analg* 22, 52
Exfoliative dermatitis (<1%)
(1944): Potter JK+, *Ann Intern Med* 21, 1041
Fixed eruption
(1970): Savin JA, *Br J Dermatol* 83, 546
Herpes simplex
Lupus erythematosus
(1967): Williams DI, *Proc R Soc Med* 60, 299
(1951): Grant Peterkin GA, *Edinb Med J* 58, 41
Necrosis
(1972): Almeyda J+, *Br J Dermatol* 86, 313
Photosensitivity
(1939): Stryker GV, *J Mo Med Assn* 36, 484
Pruritus
Purpura
(1946): Grant Peterkin GA, *BMJ* 2, 52
Rash (sic) (1–10%)
Stevens–Johnson syndrome (<1%)
Toxic epidermal necrolysis
(1973): Stüttgen G, *Br J Dermatol* 88, 291
Urticaria
(1993): Litt JZ, Beachwood, OH (personal case) (observation)
Vasculitis

### Other
Anaphylactoid reactions (1–10%)
Oral erythema multiforme
(1984): Gebel K+, *Dermatologica* 168, 35
Oral ulceration
Porphyria variegata
Rhabdomyolysis
(1990): Larpin R+, *Presse Med* 19(30), 1403

# BUTORPHANOL

**Trade name:** Stadol (Bristol-Myers Squibb)
**Other common trade names:** *Biforal; Busphen; Stadol NS*
**Indications:** Pain, migraine
**Category:** Narcotic; analgesic
**Half-life:** 2.5–4 hours
**Clinically important, potentially hazardous interactions with:** cimetidine

## *Reactions*

### Skin

Clammy skin (sic)
Diaphoresis (1–10%)
Edema (<1%)
Exanthems
Flushing (1–10%)
Gooseflesh (sic)
Pruritus (1–10%)
(1989): Ackerman WE+, *Can J Anaesth* 36, 388
(1981): Bernstein JE+, *J Am Acad Dermatol* 5, 227
Rash (sic) (<1%)
Urticaria (<1%)

### Other

Dysgeusia (3–9%)
Injection-site reactions
Paresthesias
Tinnitus
Xerostomia (3–9%)

# BUTTERBUR

**Scientific names:** *Petasites hybridus; Petasites officinalis*
**Other common names:** Blatterdock; bog rhubarb; bogshorn; butterdock; butterfly dock; capdockin; flapperdock; langwort; Petadolex* (Weber & Weber); umbrella leaves
**Family:** Asteraceae (Compositae)
**Purported indications:** Allergic rhinitis, asthma, bronchitis, chills, cough, dysmenorrhea, hay fever, headache, heart tonic, migraine, peptic ulcer
**Other uses:** Anodyne, anti-inflammatory, antispasmodic, appetite stimulant, preventing gastric ulcers, irratable bladder and urinary tract spasm, poultice over wounds or skin ulcerations

***Note:** Petadolex formulation has had the potentially carcinogenic pyrrolizidine alkaloids removed

## *Reactions*

### Skin

Edema (<0.1%)
(2000): Grossmann WM+, *Int J Clin Pharmacol Ther* 38(9), 430
(1996): Grossman W, *Der Freie Arzt* (German) 3, 44
Erythema (<0.1%)
(2000): Grossmann WM+, *Int J Clin Pharmacol Ther* 38(9), 430
(1996): Grossman W, *Der Freie Arzt* (German) 3, 44
Ocular pruritus (<1%)
(2002): Schapowal A, *Br Med J* 324(733), 144
Pruritus (<1%)
(2002): Schapowal A, *Br Med J* 324(7330), 144
Rash (sic)
(2000): Grossmann WM+, *Int J Clin Pharmacol Ther* 38(9), 430
(1996): Grossman W, *Der Freie Arzt* (German) 3, 44

### Other

Hypersensitivity (<0.1%)
(2000): Grossmann WM+, *Int J Clin Pharmacol Ther* 38(9), 430
(1996): Grossman W, *Der Freie Arzt* (German) 3, 44

## CABERGOLINE

**Trade name:** Dostinex (Pharmacia & Upjohn)
**Indications:** Hyperprolactinemia, parkinsonism
**Category:** Dopamine receptor agonist; ergot alkaloid
**Half-life:** 63–69 hours

### *Reactions*

#### Skin

Acne (1%)
(1997): Rademaker M, New Zealand (from Internet) (observation)
Ankle edema (1%)
Facial edema (1%)
Fixed eruption
(1997): Rademaker M, New Zealand (from Internet) (observation)
Flu-like syndrome (sic) (1%)
Hot flashes (3%)
Periorbital edema (1%)
Peripheral edema (1%)
Pruritus (1%)

#### Other

Mastodynia (2%)
Paresthesias (5%)
Toothache (1%)
Xerostomia (2%)

## CAFFEINE

**Scientific names:** *black tea (Thea sinensis); Coffea arabica; Coffea canephora (robusta); Cola acuminata; guarana (Paullinia cupana); Theobroma cacao*
**Other common names:** 1, 3, 7 trimethylxanthine; Also in dozens of cola soft drinks; Anacin; Aqua-Ban; Cafergot; Coryban-D; Darvon Compound; Dexatrim; Dristan; Elsinore; Endolor; Esgic; Excedrin; Fioricet; Fiorinal; ingredient in: Adipokinetix; Midol; Migralam; NoDoz; Norgesic; Norgesic Forte; Percodan; Prolamine; Synalgos-DC; Synalgos-DC-A; Triaminicin; Vanquish; Vivarin (GSK)
**Family:** Rubiales
**Purported indications:** mild central nervous system stimulant
**Other uses:** In combination with ergotamine for migraine headaches and with NSAIDs in analgesics. Somnolytic, headache, respiratory depresssion in neonates, postprandial hypotension and obesity, and to enhance seizure duration in electroconvulsive therapy. Ingredient in cough and cold remedies. Enhances athletic performance
**Half Life:** 2–7 hours
**Clinically important, potentially hazardous interactions with:** ciprofloxacin

**Note:** Caffeine is an addictive psychoactive substance. Spontaneous abortion and low birthweight babies have occurred in pregnant women consuming 150 mg caffeine per day. Abuse can lead to cardiac damage or death*

***Note:** A typical lethal dose of caffeine is 10 grams. A shot of espresso has 100 mg. It would take 100 shots of espresso or 50 double cappuccinos to get that 'big cafe in the sky.'

Physical Dependence & Withdrawal of Caffeine

Common symptoms of caffeine withdrawal are headache; drowsiness; yawning, impaired concentration; lassitude; irritability; decreased contentedness, well-being and self-confidence; decreased sociability; flu-like symptoms; muscle aches and stiffness; hot or cold spells; nausea or vomiting; and blurred vision

### *Reactions*

#### Skin

Angioedema
Bullous eruption
Burning (feet)
(1982): Young JJ+, *Drug Intell Clin Pharm* 16(10), 779
Chills
(1988): Mattila M+, *Int Clin Psychopharmacol* 3(3), 215
Ecchymoses
Exfoliation
Facial edema
Pemphigus
(1990): Brenner S+, *Acta Derm Venereol* 70(4), 357 (+paracetamol, chlorpheniramine, phenylephrine)
Pruritus
Purpura
Rash (sic)
Rosacea
(2001): Goldman D, *J Am Acad Dermatol* 44(6), 995
Urticaria
(1999): Kubota Y+, *Eur J Dermatol* 9(7), 559 (+aspirin)
(1993): Caballero T+, *J Investig Allergol Clin Immunol* 3(3), 160
(1991): Quirce Gancedo+, *J Allergy Clin Immunol* 88(4), 680
(1988): Pola J+, *Ann Allergy* 60(3), 207
Xanthoderma

#### Other

Anaphylactoid reactions
(1999): Kubota Y+, *Eur J Dermatol* 9(7), 559 (+aspirin)
(1983): Przybilla B+, *Hautarzt* (German) 34(2), 73
Death (from abuse/overdose)
(2001): Ahrendt DM, *Am Fam Physician* 63(5), 913
(2000): Le Coz, *Presse Med* (French) 29(1), 33
(2000): Tanskanen A+, *Eur J Epidemiol* 16(9), 789
(2000): Zivkovic R, *Acta Med Croatica* 54(1), 33
(1999): Zahn KA+, *J Emerg Med* 17(2), 289 (herbal ecstasy)
(1998): Ferslew KE+, *J Forensic Sci* 43(5), 1082 (+clozapine, fluoxetine)
(1997): Shum S+, *Vet Hum Toxicol* 39(4), 228
(1990): Lake CR+, *Int J Obes* 14(7), 575 (+phenylpropanolamine)
(1989): Mrvos RM+, *Vet Hum Toxicol* 31(6), 571 (diet pills)
(1986): Hanzlick R+, *J Anal Toxicol* 10(3), 126
(1985): Garriott JC+, *J Anal Toxicol* 9(3), 141
(1985): Winek CL+, *Forensic Sci Int* 29(3–4), 207
(1985): Zimmerman PM+, *Ann Emerg Med* 14(12), 1227
(1981): Bryant J, *Arch Pathol Lab Med* 105, 685
(1980): McGee MB, *J Forensic Sci* 25(1), 29
(1977): Turner JE+, *Clin Toxicol* 10(3), 341
(1974): Dimaio VJ+, *Forensic Sci* 3(3), 275
(1973): Alstott RL+, *J Forensic Sci* 18(2), 135
(1959): Jokela S+, *Acta Pharmacologica et Toxilogica* 15, 331
Depression
(1996): Rapoport A+, *Headache* 36(1), 14 (+migraine medication)
Paresthesias
(2000): Yates KM+, *N Z Med* 113(1114), 315 (herbal ecstasy)
Rhabdomyolysis
(1999): Kamijo Y+, *Vet Hum Toxicol* 41(6), 381 (oolong tea)
(1998): Kasamatsu Y+, *Intern Med* 37(2), 169 (cold remedy)

(1995): Dawson JK+, *J Accid Emerg Med* 12(1), 49 (+ephedrine, theophylline)
(1991): Michaelis HC+, *J Toxicol Clin Toxicol* 29(4), 521 (overdose, +acetaminophen, phenazone)
(1989): Wrenn KD+, *Ann Emerg Med* 18(1), 94 (overdose)

Tic disorder
(1998): Davis RE+, *Pediatrics* 101(6), E4

Tremors
(1992): Astrup A+, *Int J Obes Relat Metab Disord* 16(4), 269 (+ephedrine)
(1991): Hughes JR+, *Arch Gen Psychiatry* 48(7), 611
(1988): Mattila M+, *Int Clin Psychopharmacol* 3(3), 215 (+yohimbine)
(1981): Malchow-Moller A+, *Int J Obes* 5(2), 183 (Elsinore[ephedrine])

# CALCITONIN

(HUMAN and SALMON)
**Trade names:** Calcimar (Aventis); Miacalcin (Novartis)
**Other common trade names:** *Caltine; Cibacalcine; Clasynar; Miacalcic*
**Indications:** Paget's disease of bone
**Category:** Calcium regulator; osteoporosis therapy adjunct; bone resorption inhibitor
**Half-life:** 70–90 minutes

### *Reactions*

---

## Skin

Allergy (sic)
(2001): Rodriguez A+, *Allergy* 56(8), 801
Edema of feet
Exanthems
Flushing (>10%)
(1995): Kobayashi T+, *J Endocrinol* 146, 431
(1975): Goldsmith RS, *JAMA* 232, 1156
(1975): *Med Lett* 17, 97
Granuloma annulare
(1993): Goihman YM, *Int J Dermatol* 32, 150
Pruritus
Rash (sic) (<1%)
Tender palms and soles (sic)
Urticaria (<1%)
(1975): *Med Lett* 17, 97

## Other

Anaphylactoid reactions
Dysgeusia (metallic or salty)
Hypersensitivity
Injection-site edema (>10%)
Injection-site inflammation (>10%)
(1975): Goldsmith RS, *JAMA* 232, 1156
(1975): *Med Lett* 17, 97
Injection-site pain
(1988): Warrell RP+, *Ann Intern Med* 108, 669 (62%)
Paresthesias (<1%)

# CALFACTANT

**Trade name:** Infasurf (Forest)
**Indications:** Prevention of respiratory distress syndrome
**Category:** Lung surfactant (intratracheal)
**Half-life:** no data

### *Reactions*

---

## Other

None

# CANDESARTAN

**Trade name:** Atacand (AstraZeneca)
**Other common trade name:** *Amias*
**Indications:** Hypertension
**Category:** Angiotensin II receptor antagonist; antihypertensive
**Half-life:** 9 hours

### *Reactions*

---

## Skin

Angioedema
Diaphoresis (>0.5%)
Edema
Exanthems (<1%)
Peripheral edema (>1%)
Rash (sic) (>0.5%)

## Other

Myalgia (>0.5%)
Paresthesias (>0.5%)

# CAPECITABINE

**Trade name:** Xeloda (Roche)
**Indications:** Metastatic breast cancer
**Category:** Antineoplastic; antimetabolite (a prodrug of 5-FU)
**Half-life:** 0.5–1 hour

### *Reactions*

---

## Skin

Acral erythema
Blistering
Dermatitis (sic) (37%)
(1999): Dooley M+, *Drugs* 58, 69
Diaphoresis (0.2%)
Edema (9%)
(1996): Bajetta E+, *Tumori* 82, 450
Erythema
Exfoliative dermatitis (31–37%)
Infections (sic) (<1%)
Palmar–plantar erythrodysesthesia (57%)
(2002): Abushullaih S+, *Cancer Invest* 20(1), 3 (68.3%)
(2002): Liu X+, *Zhonghua Zhong Liu Za Zhi* 24(1), 71
(2002): Wenzel C+, *Am J Kidney Dis* 39(1), 48 (7.7%)
(2001): Elasmar SA+, *Jpn J Clin Oncol* 31(4), 172 (passim)
(2001): McGavin JK+, *Drugs* 61(15), 2309
(2001): Oshaughnessy JA+, *Ann Oncol* 12(9), 1247
(2001): Seitz JF, *Semin Oncol* 28(1 Suppl 1), 41

(1999): Blum JL+, *J Clin Oncol* 17, 485 (10%)
(1999): Blum JL, *Oncology* 57, 16
(1999): Dooley M+, *Drugs* 58, 69
(1999): Mrozek-Orlowski ME+, *Oncol Nurs Forum* 26, 753
(1998): Budman DR+, *J Clin Oncol* 16, 1795

Photosensitivity (<1%)

Pigmentation
(2002): Liu X+, *Zhonghua Zhong Liu Za Zhi* 24(1), 71

Pruritus

Purpura (0.2%)

Radiation recall (<1%)

Repigmentation (of vitiligo)
(2001): Schmid-Wendtner M-H+, *Lancet* 358, 1575

Vitiligo
(2001): Schmid-Wendtner MH+, *Lancet* 358(9293), 1575

Xerosis

## Hair

Hair – alopecia (<1%)
(2001): Hoff PM+, *J Clin Oncol* 19(8), 2282
(2001): McGavin JK+, *Drugs* 61(15), 2309
(2001): Oshaughnessy JA+, *Ann Oncol* 12(9), 1247

## Nails

Nail – disorder (sic) (7%)

Nails – onycholysis
(2001): Chen G-Y+, *Br J Dermatol* 145(3), 521

Nails – onychomadesis
(2001): Chen G-Y+, *Br J Dermatol* 145(3), 521

## Other

Hypersensitivity (<1%)

Mucositis
(2001): Bell KA+, *J Am Acad Dermatol* 45(5), 790

Myalgia (9%)

Oral candidiasis (0.2%)

Oral ulceration

Paresthesias (21%)

Stomatitis (24%)
(2002): Liu X+, *Zhonghua Zhong Liu Za Zhi* 24(1), 71
(2001): Hoff PM+, *J Clin Oncol* 19(8), 2282
(2001): McGavin JK+, *Drugs* 61(15), 2309

Thrombophlebitis (0.2%)

# CAPTOPRIL

**Synonym:** ACE
**Trade names:** Capoten (Bristol-Myers Squibb); Capozide (Bristol-Myers Squibb)
**Other common trade names:** *Acenorm; Acepril; Adocor; APO-Capto; Captolane; Captoril; Lopirin; Lopril; Nu-Capto; Precaptil*
**Indications:** Hypertension
**Category:** Angiotensin-converting enzyme (ACE) inhibitor; antihypertensive and vasodilator
**Half-life:** <3 hours
**Clinically important, potentially hazardous interactions with:** amiloride, spironolactone, triamterene

Capozide is captopril and hydrochlorothiazide

### *Reactions*

## Skin

Angioedema (<1%)
(2001): Cohen EG+, *Ann Otol Rhinol Laryngol* 110(8), 701 (64 cases)
(1998): Smoger SH+, *South Med J* 91, 1060
(1997): Brown NJ+, *JAMA* 278, 232
(1997): Tisch M+, *Anaesthesiol Intensivmed Notfallmed Schmerzther* (German) 32, 122
(1996): Ekborn A+, *Lakartidningen* (Swedish) 93, 468
(1996): Pillans PI+, *Eur J Clin Pharmacol* 51, 123
(1995): Bauwens LJ+, *Ned Tijdschr Geneeskd* (Dutch) 139, 674
(1995): Kozel MM+, *Clin Exp Dermatol* 20, 60
(1993): Chu TJ+, *Ann Intern Med* 118, 314
(1993): Thompson T+, *Laryngoscope* 103, 10
(1992): Diehl KL+, *Dtsch Med Wochenschr* (German)117, 727
(1992): Dobroschke B+, *Anasthesiol Intensivmed Notfallmed Schmerzther* (German) 27, 510
(1992): Hedner T+, *BMJ* 304, 941
(1992): Jason DR, *J Forensic Sci* 37, 1418 (fatal)
(1992): Sanchez-Hernandez J+, *An Med Interna* (Spanish) 9, 572
(1991): Pek F, *HNO* (German) 39, 410
(1991): Roberts JR+, *Ann Emerg Med* 20, 555
(1990): Cameron DI, *Can J Cardiol* 6, 265
(1990): DiNardo LJ+, *Trans Pa Acad Ophthalmol Otolaryngol* 42, 998
(1990): Gannon TH+, *Laryngoscope* 100, 1156
(1990): McAreavey D+, *Drugs* 40, 326
(1990): Motel PJ, *J Am Acad Dermatol* 23, 124
(1990): Seidman MD+, *Otolaryngol Head Neck Surg* 102, 727
(1990): Zech J+, *HNO* (German) 38, 143
(1989): Barna JS+, *Va Med* 116, 147
(1989): Werber JL+, *Otolaryngol Head Neck Surg* 101, 96
(1988): Brogden RN+, *Drugs* 36, 540
(1988): Slater EE+, *JAMA* 260, 967 (0.1%)
(1988): Wernze H, *Z Kardiol* (German) 77, 61
(1987): Edwards IR+, *Br J Clin Pharmacol* 23, 529
(1987): Ferner RE+, *BMJ* 294, 1119
(1987): No Author, *Am J Med* 82, 576
(1987): Wood SM+, *BMJ* 294, 91
(1986): Suarez M+, *Am J Med* 81, 336
(1984): Jett GK, *Ann Emerg Med* 13, 489
(1984): Materson BJ+, *Ann Intern Med* 144, 1947 (2.1%)
(1984): Smit AJ+, *Clin Allergy* 14, 413 (2%)
(1982): Vidt DG+, *N Engl J Med* 306, 214 (passim)
(1980): Wilkin JK+, *Arch Dermatol* 116, 903 (15%)

Bullous eruption
(1989): Klein LE+, *Cutis* 44, 393

Bullous pemphigoid
(2000): Popescu C, Bucharest, Romania (from Internet) (observation)
(1993): Fitzgerald DA, *Clin Exp Dermatol* 18, 196
(1989): Mallet L+, *Drug Intell Clin Pharm* 23, 63

Contact dermatitis
(1990): Cnudde F+, *Contact Dermatitis* 23, 375

Cutaneous reactions (sic)
(2001): Martinez JC+, *Allergol Immunopathol* (Madr) 29(6), 279
(1998): Lluch-Bernal M+, *Contact Dermatitis* 39, 316

Dermatitis (sic)
(2001): Martinez JC+, *Allergol Immunopathol* (Madr) 29(6), 279 (positive patch test)

Erythroderma
(1989): Allegue F+, *Rev Clin Esp* (Spanish) 184, 210
(1985): Goodfield MJ+, *BMJ* 290, 1111

Exanthems (4–7%)
(1993): Fitzgerald DA, *Clin Exp Dermatol* 18, 196 (passim)
(1990): Cnudde F+, *Contact Dermatitis* 23, 375
(1990): McAreavey D+, *Drugs* 40, 326 (0.5–4%)
(1990): Motel PJ, *J Am Acad Dermatol* 23, 124
(1989): Clemens G+, *Verh Dtsch Ges Inn Med* (German) 95, 721
(1989): Gomez-Martino-Arroyo JR+, *Rev Clin Esp* (Spanish) 184, 497
(1988): Bretin N+, *Dermatologica* 177, 11
(1988): Brogden RN+, *Drugs* 36, 540 (0.5–4%)
(1988): Warner NJ+, *Drugs* 35 (Suppl 5) 89 (4–7%)

(1985): Goodfield MJ+, *BMJ* 290, 1111
(1985): Todd PA+, *Drugs* 31, 198
(1984): Smit AJ+, *Clin Allergy* 14, 413 (7%)
(1983): Romankiewicz JA+, *Drugs* 25, 6 (4.6%)
(1983): Steinman TI+, *Am J Med* 75, 154
(1982): Luderer JR+, *J Clin Pharm* 22, 151
(1982): Vidt DG+, *N Engl J Med* 306, 214 (passim)
(1980): Heel RC+, *Drugs* 20, 409 (8–14%)
(1980): Wilkin JK+, *Arch Dermatol* 116, 903
(1978): Gavras H+, *N Engl J Med* 298, 991 (10%)

Exfoliative dermatitis (<2%)
(1990): Motel PJ, *J Am Acad Dermatol* 23, 124
(1989): O'Neill PG+, *Tex Med* 85, 40
(1988): Lai KN+, *Singapore Med J* 29, 526
(1982): Solinger AM, *Cutis* 29, 437

Flushing (<1%)
(1989): Healy LA+, *N Engl J Med* 321, 763
(1987): Ferner RE+, *Br Med J Clin Res Ed* 294, 1119

Graft-versus-host reaction
(1998): Jappe U+, *Hautarzt* (German) 49, 126 (passim)

Kaposi's sarcoma
(1991): Larbre JP, *J Rheumatol* 18, 476
(1990): Puppin D+, *Lancet* 336, 1251

Lichen planus (pemphigoides)
(1986): Flageul B+, *Dermatologica* 173, 248

Lichenoid eruption
(2002): Feijoo A+, *World Congress Dermatol* Poster, 0100 (generalized)
(1996): Revenga-Arranz F+, *Rev Clin Esp* (Spanish) 196, 412
(1994): Phillips WG+, *Clin Exp Dermatol* 19, 317
(1992): Perez-Roldan E+, *Rev Clin Esp* (Spanish) 191, 501
(1992): Wong SS+, *Acta Derm Venereol* (Stockh) 72, 358
(1990): Pascual J+, *Nephron* 56, 110
(1989): Cox NH+, *Br J Dermatol* 120, 319
(1989): Rotstein E+, *Australas J Dermatol* 30, 9
(1988): Bretin N+, *Dermatologica* 177, 11
(1984): Smit AJ+, *Clin Allergy* 14, 413 (1%)
(1983): Bravard P+, *Ann Dermatol Venereol* (French) 110, 433
(1983): Bravard P+, *Presse Med* (French) 12, 577
(1983): Reinhardt LA+, *Cutis* 31, 98

Linear IgA bullous dermatosis
(2002): Cohen LM+, *J Am Acad Dermatol* 138, 29 (two cases)
(1998): Friedman IS+, *Int J Dermatol* 37, 608
(1994): Kuechle MK+, *J Am Acad Dermatol* 30, 187
(1989): Klein LE+, *Cutis* 44, 393

Lupus erythematosus
(1995): Fernandez-Diaz ML+, *Lancet* 345, 398
(1993): Bertin P+, *Clin Exp Rheumatol* 11, 695
(1993): Pelayo M+, *Ann Pharmacother* 27, 1541
(1990): Sieber C+, *BMJ* 301, 669
(1985): Patri P+, *Acta Derm Venereol* (Stockh) 65, 447

Mycosis fungoides
(1995): Carroll J+, *Cutis* 56, 276 (pustular)
(1986): Furness PN+, *J Clin Pathol* 39, 902

Palmar–plantar pustulosis
(1995): Eriksen JG+, *Ugeskr Laeger* (Danish) 157, 3335

Pemphigus (<2%)
(1995): Butt A+, *Br J Dermatol* 132, 315
(1994): Kuechle MK+, *Mayo Clin Proc* 69, 1166
(1994): Trinidad-Paz JM+, *Rev Clin Esp* (Spanish) 194, 999
(1992): Kaplan RP+, *J Am Acad Dermatol* 26, 364
(1992): Pinto GM+, *J Am Acad Dermatol* 27, 281 (vegetans)
(1992): Ruocco V+, *Int J Dermatol* 31, 33
(1991): Beaulieu P+, *Ann Dermatol Venereol* (French) 118, 547
(1991): Korman NJ+, *J Invest Dermatol* 96, 273
(1990): Black AK+, *Br J Dermatol* 123, 277
(1990): Motel PJ, *J Am Acad Dermatol* 23, 124
(1990): Ruocco V+, *Arch Dermatol* 126, 965
(1988): Blanken R+, *Acta Derm Venereol* (Stockh) 68, 456
(1988): Bretin N+, *Dermatologica* 177, 11
(1987): Arnoux D+, *Ann Dermatol Venereol* (French) 114, 1241
(1987): Katz RA+, *Arch Dermatol* 123, 20
(1986): Ricci G+, *Recenti Prog Med* (Italian) 77, 321
(1985): Bernard P+, *Ann Dermatol Venereol* (French) 112, 661
(1982): Christeler A+, *Schweiz Med Wochenschr* (German) 112, 1483
(1982): Ruocco V+, *Arch Dermatol Res* 274, 123
(1981): Clement MI, *Arch Dermatol* 117, 525
(1980): Parfrey PS+, *BMJ* 281, 194

Pemphigus foliaceus
(2000): Ong CS+, *Australas J Dermatol* 41(4), 242

Penile ulcers
(1983): Romankiewicz JA+, *Drugs* 25, 6 (4.6%)
(1981): Nicholls MG+, *Ann Intern Med* 94, 695

Photosensitivity
(1994): Shelley WB+, *Cutis* 54, 70 (observation)
(1990): Motel PJ, *J Am Acad Dermatol* 23, 124
(1988): Mauduit G+, *Ann Dermatol Venereol* (French) 115, 167

Phototoxicity (<2%)

Pigmentation
(1990): Black AK+, *Br J Dermatol* 123, 277
(1987): O'Neill MB+, *BMJ* 295, 33

Pityriasis rosea (<2%)
(1990): Ghersetich I+, *G Ital Dermatol Venereol* (Italian) 125, 457
(1990): Motel PJ, *J Am Acad Dermatol* 23, 124
(1990): Wolf R+, *Dermatologica* 181, 51
(1988): Bretin N+, *Dermatologica* 177, 11
(1983): Reinhardt LA+, *Cutis* 31, 98
(1982): Wilkin JK+, *Arch Dermatol* 118, 186

Pruritus (4–7%)
(1992): Shelley WB+, *Cutis* 49, 391 (observation)
(1990): Motel PJ, *J Am Acad Dermatol* 23, 124
(1984): Materson BJ+, *Ann Intern Med* 144, 1947 (0.2%)
(1983): Daniel F+, *Ann Dermatol Venereol* (French) 110, 441 (10%)
(1983): Romankiewicz JA+, *Drugs* 25, 6 (4%)
(1983): Steinman TI+, *Am J Med* 75, 154
(1982): Liebau G, *Klin Wochenschr* (German) 60, 107
(1982): Vidt DG+, *N Engl J Med* 306, 214 (passim)
(1980): Luderer JR+, *Clin Res* 28, 589A

Psoriasis
(1995): Ikai K, *J Am Acad Dermatol* 32, 819
(1993): Coulter DM+, *N Z Med J* 106, 392
(1992): Shelley WB+, *Cutis* 50, 87 (observation)
(1990): Sieber C+, *BMJ* 301, 669
(1990): Wolf R+, *Dermatologica* 181, 51
(1987): Hamlet DW+, *BMJ* 295, 1352
(1987): Wolf R+, *Cutis* 40, 162
(1986): Hauschild TT+, *Hautarzt* (German) 37, 274

Purpura
(1989): Grosbois B+, *BMJ* 298, 189

Rash (sic) (4–7%)
(1990): Kahan A+, *Clin Pharmacol Ther* 47, 483
(1985): Jenkins AC+, *J Cardiovasc Pharmacol* 7, S96
(1984): Kubo SH+, *Ann Intern Med* 100, 616
(1984): Martin MF+, *Lancet* 1, 1325
(1983): Romankiewicz JA+, *Drugs* 25, 6
(1983): Rotmensch HH+, *Pharmacotherapy* 3, 131
(1983): Steinman TI+, *Am J Med* 75, 154
(1982): Liebau G, *Klin Wochenschr* (German) 60, 107
(1982): Rosendorff C, *S Afr Med J* 62, 593
(1981): Luderer JR+, *Am J Med* 71, 493

Stevens–Johnson syndrome
(1984): Pennell DJ+, *Lancet* 1, 463 (fatal)

Toxic epidermal necrolysis
(1999): Winfred RI+, *South Med J* 92, 918
(1983): Sala F+, *G Ital Dermatol Venereol* (Italian) 118, 89

Urticaria

(1996): Pillans PI+, *Eur J Clin Pharmacol* 51, 123
(1993): Fitzgerald DA, *Clin Exp Dermatol* 18, 196 (passim)
(1988): Bretin N+, *Dermatologica* 177, 11
(1988): Slater EE+, *JAMA* 260, 967
(1987): Wood SM+, *BMJ* 294, 91
(1985): Goodfield MJD+, *BMJ* 290, 1111
(1984): Materson BJ+, *Ann Intern Med* 144, 1947 (1.4%)
(1984): Smit AJ+, *Clin Allergy* 14, 413 (7%)
(1980): Wilkin JK+, *Arch Dermatol* 116, 902

Vasculitis
(1994): Dorman RL+, *AJR Am J Roentgenol* 163, 840
(1990): Black AK+, *Br J Dermatol* 123, 277 (fatal)
(1988): Lotti T+, *G Ital Dermatol Venereol* (Italian) 123, 657
(1988): Miralles R+, *Ann Intern Med* 109, 514
(1987): Laaban J+, *European Heart J* 8, 319
(1984): Goodfield MJD+, *Lancet* 2, 517
(1984): Smit AJ+, *Clin Allergy* 14, 413

Xerosis
(1983): Smit AJ+, *Nephron* 34, 196

## Hair

Hair – alopecia (<2%)
(1994): Shelley WB+, *Cutis* 52, 264 (observation)
(1990): Motel PJ, *J Am Acad Dermatol* 23, 124
(1984): Leaker B+, *Aust N Z J Med* 14, 866
(1984): Smit AJ+, *Clin Allergy* 14, 413 (3%)
(1983): Smit AJ+, *Nephron* 34, 196

## Nails

Nails – dystrophy
(1984): Brueggemeyer CD+, *Lancet* 1, 1352
(1983): Smit AJ+, *Nephron* 34, 196

Nails – onycholysis
(1986): Borders JV, *Ann Intern Med* 105, 305
(1984): Brueggemeyer CD+, *Lancet* 1, 1352

## Other

Ageusia (2–4%)
(1997): Acanfora D+, *Am J Ther* 4, 181
(1993): Fitzgerald DA, *Clin Exp Dermatol* 18, 196 (passim)
(1988): Rumboldt Z+, *Int J Clin* 8(3), 181
(1987): Edwards IR+, *Br J Clin Pharmacol* 23, 529
(1987): O'Connor DT+, *J Clin Hypertens* 3(4), 405
(1984): Martin MF+, *Lancet* 1, 1325
(1983): Smit AJ+, *Nephron* 34, 196
(1982): Liebau G, *Klin Wochenschr* (German) 60, 107
(1982): Vidt DG+, *N Engl J Med* 306, 214 (passim)
(1979): McNeil JJ+, *BMJ* 6204, 1555
(1979): Vlasses PH+, *Lancet* 2, 526

Anaphylactoid reactions (during hemodialysis)

Aphthous stomatitis (<2%)
(1983): Daniel F+, *Ann Dermatol Venereol* (French) 110, 441
(1982): Vidt DG+, *N Engl J Med* 306, 214 (passim)
(1980): Heel RC+, *Drugs* 20, 409
(1979): Seedat YK, *Lancet* 2, 1297

Cough
(2001): Adigun AQ+, *West Afr J Med* 20(1), 46–7
(2001): Lee SC+, *Hypertension* 38(2), 166

Death

Dysgeusia (2–4%) (metallic or salty taste)
(2000): Zervakis J+, *Physiol Behav* 68, 405
(1993): Boyd I, *Lancet* 342, 304
(1993): Zazgornik J+, *Lancet* 341, 1542
(1990): Kahan A+, *Clin Pharmacol Ther* 47, 483
(1985): Jenkins AC+, *J Cardiovasc Pharmacol* 7, S96
(1985): Mauersberger H+, *Lancet* 1, 517
(1983): Kayanakis JG+, *Arch Mal Coeur Vaiss* (French) 76, 1065
(1983): Romankiewicz JA+, *Drugs* 25, 6
(1979): McNeil JJ+, *BMJ* 6204, 1555

Glossitis
(1989): Drucker CR+, *Arch Dermatol* 125, 1437 (atrophic)
(1983): Romankiewicz JA+, *Drugs* 25, 6
(1981): Nicholls MG+, *Ann Intern Med* 94, 659

Glossopyrosis
(1989): Drucker CR+, *Arch Dermatol* 125, 1437

Gynecomastia
(2000): Hugues FC+, *Ann Med Interne (Paris)* (French) 151, 10 (passim)
(1990): Nakamura Y+, *BMJ* 300, 541
(1988): Markusse HM+, *BMJ* 296, 1262

Lymphadenopathy
(1981): Aberg H+, *BMJ* 283, 1297

Myalgia

Oral mucosal eruption
(1989): Firth NA+, *Oral Surg Oral Med Oral Pathol* 67, 41 (lichenoid)
(1985): Todd PA+, *Drugs* 31, 198
(1980): Heel RC+, *Drugs* 20, 409

Oral ulceration
(2000): Madinier I+, *Ann Med Interne (Paris)* (French) 151, 248
(1993): Fitzgerald DA, *Clin Exp Dermatol* 18, 196 (passim)
(1982): Viraben R+, *Arch Dermatol* 118, 959

Paresthesias (<2%)

Scalded mouth (sic)
(1982): Vlasses PH+, *BMJ* 284, 1672

Tongue ulceration
(1982): Viraben R+, *Arch Dermatol* 118, 959
(1982): Vlasses PH+, *BMJ* 284, 1672 (passim)
(1981): Nicholls MG+, *Ann Intern Med* 94, 659

Xerostomia (<2%)

# CARBAMAZEPINE

**Trade names:** Carbatrol (Shire Richwood); Tegretol (Novartis)
**Other common trade names:** *Apo-Carbamazepine; Atreol; Foxsalepsin; Kodapan; Lexin; Mazepine; Sirtal; Tegretol XR; Teril; Timonil*
**Indications:** Epilepsy, pain or trigeminal neuralgia
**Category:** Anticonvulsant; antineuralgic; antimanic; antidiuretic and antipsychotic
**Half-life:** 18–55 hours
**Clinically important, potentially hazardous interactions with:** charcoal, clarithromycin, clorazepate, clozapine, diltiazem, doxacurium, erythromycin, felodipine, imatinib, midazolam, troleandomycin, verapamil, voriconazole

### *Reactions*

---

## Skin

Acne keloid
(1990): Grunwald MH+, *Int J Dermatol* 29, 559

Acute generalized exanthematous pustulosis (AGEP)
(1999): Lachgar T, *Allerg Immunol* (Paris) (French) 31, 151
(1999): Poster Exhibit #163, AAD Meeting, March 1999 (Reported by ED and WB Shelley)
(1996): Wolkenstein P+, *Contact Dermatitis* 35, 234
(1995): Moreau A+, *Int J Dermatol* 34, 263 (passim)
(1991): Roujeau J-C+, *Arch Dermatol* 127, 1333

Allergic reactions (sic)
(1999): Pasmans SG+, *Allergy* 54, 649
(1995): Tijhuis GJ+, *Ned Tijdschr Geneeskd* (Dutch) 139, 2265 (42 cases)
(1993): Beran RG, *Epilepsia* 34, 163
(1992): Dzianott A+, *Wiad Lek* (Polish) 45, 465
(1985): Moore NC+, *Am J Psychiatry* 142, 974

Angioedema (<1%)
(2001): Grieco A+, *Eur J Gastroenterol Hepatol* 13(8), 973
(1977): Houwerzijl J+, *Clin Exp Immunol* 29, 272
(1971): Virolainen M, *Clin Exp Immunol* 9, 429
(1967): Livingston S+, *JAMA* 200, 204
Ankle edema
Anticonvulsant hypersensitivity syndrome
(2002): Metin A+, *World Congress Dermatol* Poster, 0116
(2000): Moore, SJ+, *J Med Genet* 37, 489
(2000): Popescu C, Bucharest, Romania (from Internet) (observation)
Bullous eruption (<1%)
(2001): Grieco A+, *Eur J Gastroenterol Hepatol* 13(8), 973
(1990): Gebauer K+, *Australas J Dermatol* 31, 89 (passim)
(1988): Warnock JK+, *Am J Psychiatry* 145, 425
(1983): Godden DJ+, *Postgrad Med J* 59, 336
Collagen disease (sic)
(1966): Simpson JR, *BMJ* 2, 1434
Contact dermatitis
(1992): Duhra P+, *Contact Dermatitis* 27, 325
(1991): Ljunggren B+, *Contact Dermatitis* 24, 259
(1991): Rodriguez-Mosquera M+, *Contact Dermatitis* 25, 137
Cutaneous side effects (sic)
(1994): Jones M+, *Dermatology* 188, 18 (4%)
(1967): Livingston S+, *JAMA* 200, 204 (4.5%)
Dermatitis (sic)
(1992): Duhra P+, *Contact Dermatitis* 27, 325
(1989): Malanin G+, *Duodecim* (Finnish) 105, 784
(1989): Terui T+, *Contact Dermatitis* 20, 260
(1981): Roberts DL+, *Arch Dermatol* 117, 273
(1967): Arieff AJ+, *Dis Nerv Syst* 28, 820
Diaphoresis (1–10%)
Eczematous eruption (sic)
(1999): Ozkaya-Bayazit E+, *J Eur Acad Dermatol Venereol* 12, 182
(1992): Duhra P+, *Contact Dermatitis* 27, 325
Edema
Eosinophilic pustular folliculitis (Ofuji's disease)
(1998): Mizoguchi S+, *J Am Acad Dermatol* 38, 641
Epidermolysis bullosa
(1992): Kong LN, *Chung Hua Hu Li Tsa Chih* (Chinese) 27, 495
Erythema
(2001): Gaida-Hommernick B+, *Epilepsia* 42(6), 793
Erythema multiforme
(1999): Frederickson K, (from Internet) (observation)
(1994): Friedmann PS+, *Arch Dermatol* 130, 598
(1993): Alanko K, *Contact Dermatitis* 29, 254
(1993): Bruynzeel I+, *Br J Dermatol* 129, 45
(1992): Chevenet C+, *Ann Dermatol Venereol* (French) 119, 929
(1989): Alanko K+, *Acta Derm Venereol* (Stockh) 69, 223
(1989): Busch RL, *N Engl J Med* 321, 692
(1988): McDanal CE, *J Clin Psychiatr* 49, 369
(1988): Warnock JK+, *Am J Psychiatry* 145, 425
(1987): Fawcett RG, *J Clin Psychiatry* 48, 416
(1986): Green ST, *Clin Neuropharmacol* 9, 561
(1985): Delafuente JC, *Drug Intell Clin Pharm* 19, 114
(1985): Patterson JF, *J Clin Psychopharmacol* 5, 185
(1984): Meisel S+, *Clin Pharm* 3, 15
(1975): Böttiger LE+, *Acta Med Scand* 198, 229
Erythema nodosum (<1%)
Erythroderma
(2000): Bugatti L (Italy) (from Internet) (observation)
(1998): Tayoro J+, *Therapie* 53, 513
(1996): Okuyama R+, *J Dermatol* 23, 489
(1995): Koga T+, *Contact Dermatitis* 33, 275
(1993): Blasco-Sarramian A+, *An Med Interna* (Spanish) 10, 341
(1990): Ruiz-Ezquerro JJ+, *An Med Interna* (Spanish) 31, 89
(1989): Romaguera C+, *Contact Dermatitis* 20, 304
(1987): Granier F+, *Rev Med Interne* (French) 8, 206
(1986): Silva R+, *Contact Dermatitis* 15, 254
(1982): Chennebault JM+, *Therapie* (French) 37, 106
(1980): Gaulier A+, *Nouv Presse Med* (French) 9, 1388
Exanthems (>5%)
(2002): Maradeix S+, *World Congress Dermatol* Poster, 0112
(2000): Thaler D, Monona, WI (from Internet) (observation)
(1999): Lombardi SM+, *Ann Pharmacother* 33, 571
(1998): Nathan D+, *J Am Acad Dermatol* 38, 806
(1997): Hyson C+, *Can J Neurol Sci* 24, 245
(1995): Wolkenstein P+, *Arch Dermatol* 131, 544
(1993): Alanko K, *Contact Dermatitis* 29, 254
(1993): Hermle L+, *Nervenarzt* (German) 64, 208 (generalized)
(1993): Konishi T+, *Eur J Pediatr* 152, 605
(1990): Garavelli PL+, *Minerva Med* (Italian) 81, 115
(1990): Gebauer K+, *Australas J Dermatol* 31, 89 (passim)
(1989): Eames P, *Lancet* 1, 509
(1988): Shear NH+, *J Clin Invest* 82, 1826
(1988): Warnock JK+, *Am J Psychiatry* 145, 425
(1984): Chadwick D+, *J Neurol Neurosurg Psychiatry* 47, 642 (17%)
(1982): Breathnach SM+, *Clin Exp Dermatol* 7, 585 (4%)
(1981): Sillanpää M, *Acta Neurol Scand* 64 (Suppl 88), 145
(1981): Taylor MW+, *Practitioner* 225, 219
(1977): Houwerzijl J+, *Clin Exp Immunol* 29, 272
(1974): Livingston S+, *Dis Nerv Syst* 35, 103 (2.7%)
(1972): Levantine A+, *Br J Dermatol* 87, 646 (3–4%)
(1971): Virolainen M, *Clin Exp Immunol* 9, 429
Exfoliative dermatitis
(2001): Dintiman B, Fairfax, VA (from Internet)
(1999): Lombardi SM+, *Ann Pharmacother* 33, 571
(1996): Sigurdsson V+, *J Am Acad Dermatol* 35, 53
(1996): Troost RJ+, *Pediatr Dermatol* 13, 316
(1995): Bahamdan KA+, *Int J Dermatol* 34, 661
(1995): Corazza M+, *Contact Dermatitis* 33, 447
(1995): Koga T+, *Contact Dermatitis* 32, 181
(1993): Alanko K, *Contact Dermatitis* 29, 254
(1991): Blin O+, *Therapie* (French) 46, 91
(1990): Gebauer K+, *Australas J Dermatol* 31, 89 (passim)
(1989): Alanko K+, *Acta Derm Venereol* (Stockh) 69, 223
(1989): Romaguera C+, *Contact Dermatitis* 20, 304
(1989): Vaillant L+, *Arch Dermatol* 125, 299
(1988): Cox NH+, *Postgrad Med J* 64, 249
(1987): Gimenez Garcia RM+, *Rev Clin Esp* (Spanish) 181, 542
(1987): Granier F+, *Rev Med Interne* 8, 206
(1985): Camarasa JG, *Contact Dermatitis* 12, 49
(1984): Shuttleworth D+, *Clin Exp Dermatol* 9, 421
(1982): Reed MD+, *Clin Pharm* 1, 78
(1981): Roberts DL+, *Arch Dermatol* 117, 273
(1977): Houwerzijl J+, *Clin Exp Immunol* 29, 272
(1968): Ford GR+, *N Z Med J* 68, 386
Facial edema
Fixed eruption (<1%)
(1997): Chan HL+, *J Am Acad Dermatol* 36, 259
(1997): de Argila D+, *Allergy* 52, 1039
(1993): Alanko K, *Contact Dermatitis* 29, 254
(1990): Gaffoor PMA+, *Cutis* 45, 242 (passim)
(1989): Stubb S+, *Br J Dermatol* 120, 583
(1988): Bhariga JC+, *Sex Transm Dis* 15, 177
(1988): Warnock JK+, *Am J Psychiatry* 145, 425
(1985): Kauppinen K+, *Br J Dermatol* 112, 575
(1984): Shuttleworth D+, *Clin Exp Dermatol* 9, 424
Lichenoid eruption
(1994): Thompson DF+, *Pharmacotherapy* 14, 561
(1990): Atkin SL+, *Clin Exp Dermatol* 15, 382
(1990): Gebauer K+, *Australas J Dermatol* 31, 89 (passim)
(1989): Ohtsuyama M+, *Nishinihon J Dermatol* (Japanese) 51, 958
(1988): Yasuda S+, *Photodermatology* 5, 206 (photosensitive)
(1981): Roberts DL+, *Arch Dermatol* 117, 273
Linear IgA bullous dermatosis
(2002): Cohen LM+, *J Am Acad Dermatol* 46(2), S32

Lupus erythematosus
(1998): Bachmeyer C+, *Presse Med* (French) 27, 966
(1998): Toepfer M+, *Eur J Clin Pharmacol* 54, 193 (late onset)
(1997): Milesi-Lecat AM+, *Mayo Clin Proc* 72, 1145
(1997): Reiffers-Mettelock J+, *Dermatology* 195, 306
(1996): Ghorayeb I+, *Rev Med Interne* (French) 17, 503
(1993): Drory VE+, *Clin Neuropharmacol* 16, 19 (passim)
(1993): Ohashi T+, *Rinsho Shinkeigaku* (Japanese) 33, 1094
(1992): Boon DM+, *Ned Tijdschr Geneeskd* (Dutch) 136, 2085 (disseminated)
(1992): Kanno T+, *Intern Med* 31, 1303
(1992): Schmidt S+, *Br J Psychiatry* 161, 560
(1992): Yust I+, *Intern Med* 31, 1303
(1991): De Giorgio CM+, *Epilepsia* 32, 128
(1991): Jain KK, *Drug Saf* 6, 350
(1990): Gebauer K+, *Australas J Dermatol* 31, 89 (passim)
(1990): Oner A+, *Clin Neurol Neurosurg* 92, 261
(1989): Drory VE+, *Clin Neuropharmacol* 12, 115
(1987): Alballa S+, *J Rheumatol* 14, 599
(1986): Leyh F+, *Z Haut* (German) 61, 611
(1985): Bateman DE, *Br Med J Clin Res Ed* 291, 632
(1985): *Br Med J Clin Res Ed* 291, 1125
(1985): Lovisetto P+, *Recenti Prog Med* (Italian) 76, 84
(1985): McNicholl B, *BMJ* 291, 1126
(1983): Kolstee HJ, *Ned Tijdschr Geneeskd* (Dutch) 127, 1588
(1976): Takigawa M+, *Arch Dermatol* 112, 845
(1974): Livingston S+, *Dis Nerv Syst* 35, 103 (2.7%)
(1969): Gayford JJ+, *Proc R Soc Med* 62, 615
(1967): Livingston S+, *JAMA* 200, 204
(1966): Simpson JR, *BMJ* 2, 1434

Lymphoma
(2001): Di Lernia V+, *Arch Dermatol* 137, 675

Mucocutaneous lymph node syndrome (Kawasaki syndrome)
(1990): Gebauer K+, *Australas J Dermatol* 31, 89 (passim)
(1987): Hicks RA+, *Pediatr Infect Dis J* 7, 525

Mycosis fungoides
(1991): Rijlaarsdam U+, *J Am Acad Dermatol* 24(2 Pt 1), 219 (with phenytoin)
(1991): Rijlaarsdam U+, *J Am Acad Dermatol* 24, 216
(1990): Welykyi S+, *J Cutan Pathol* 17, 111

Pellagra
(2002): Valikhani M+, *World Congress Dermatol* Poster, 0131
(1998): Heyer G+, *Hautarzt* (German) 49, 123

Periorbital edema
(2001): Dintiman B, Fairfax, VA (from Internet) (observation)

Petechiae
(1993): Konishi T+, *Eur J Pediatr* 152, 605

Photosensitivity
(2001): Hebert AA+, *J Clin Psychiatry* 62(suppl 14), 22
(1991): Ljunggren B+, *Contact Dermatitis* 24, 259
(1990): Gebauer K+, *Australas J Dermatol* 31, 89 (passim)
(1989): Terui T+, *Contact Dermatitis* 20, 260
(1988): Warnock JK+, *Am J Psychiatry* 145, 425
(1988): Yasuda S+, *Photodermatology* 5, 206
(1986): Silva R+, *Contact Dermatitis* 15, 54
(1981): Sillanpää M, *Acta Neurol Scand* 64 (Suppl 88), 145
(1972): Levantine A+, *Br J Dermatol* 87, 646

Pigmentation

Pruritus (<1%)
(2001): Gaida-Hommernick B+, *Epilepsia* 42(6), 793
(1969): Davis EH, *Headache* 9, 77
(1967): Livingston S+, *JAMA* 200, 204
(1964): Spillane D, *Practitioner* 192, 71

Psoriasis
(1994): Brenner S+, *Isr J Med Sci* 30, 283

Purpura
(2001): Hebert AA+, *J Clin Psychiatry* 62(suppl 14), 22
(1988): Warnock JK+, *Am J Psychiatry* 145, 425
(1984): Staughton RCD+, *J R Soc Med* 77 (Suppl 4), 6
(1972): Levantine A+, *Br J Dermatol* 87, 646
(1969): Peterkin GAG+, *Practitioner* 202, 117
(1967): Harman RRM, *Br J Dermatol* 79, 500
(1967): Livingston S+, *JAMA* 200, 204
(1964): Spillane D, *Practitioner* 192, 71

Pustular eruption
(1991): Kleier RS+, *Arch Dermatol* 127, 1361
(1990): Gebauer K+, *Australas J Dermatol* 31, 89 (passim)
(1988): Commens CA+, *Arch Dermatol* 124, 178
(1984): Staughton RCD+, *J R Soc Med* 77 (Suppl 4), 6

Rash (sic) (>10%)
(1999): van Ginneken EE+, *Neth Med J* 54, 158
(1998): Cates M+, *Ann Pharmacother* 32, 884
(1996): Boyle N+, *Am J Psychiatry* 152, 1234
(1996): Puig L+, *Contact Dermatitis* 34, 435
(1994): Kramlinger KG+, *J Clin Psychopharmacol* 14, 408 (12%)
(1993): Hosoda N+, *Jpn J Psychiatry Neurol* 47, 300
(1993): Konishi T+, *Eur J Pediatr* 152, 605
(1991): Frederick TE, *Neurology* 41, 1328
(1991): Murphy JM+, *Neurology* 41, 144
(1990): Garavelli PL+, *Minerva Med* (Italian) 81, 115
(1983): Ponte CD, *Drug Intell Clin Pharm* 17, 642
(1983): Vick NA, *N Engl J Med* 309, 1193

Schamberg's disease

Sheet-like erythema

Stevens–Johnson syndrome (1–10%)
(2002): Garcia M+, *Dig Dis Sci* 47(1), 177
(2001): Duggal HS+, *J Assoc Physicians India* 49, 591
(2001): Hebert AA+, *J Clin Psychiatry* 62(suppl14), 22
(2000): Straussberg R+, *Pediatr Neurol* 22, 231
(2000): Suarez Moro R+, *An Med Interna* (Spanish) 17, 105
(1999): Dhar S+, *Dermatology* 199, 194
(1999): Petter G+, *Hautarzt* (German) 50, 884
(1999): Ruble R+, *CNS Drugs* 12, 215
(1999): Rzany B+, *Lancet* 353, 2190
(1995): Huang SC+, *Gen Hosp Psychiatry* 17, 458
(1995): Hughes-Davies L, *N Engl J Med* 332, 959
(1995): Keating A+, *Ann Pharmacother* 29, 538
(1995): Wolkenstein P+, *Arch Dermatol* 131, 544
(1993): Konishi T+, *Eur J Pediatr* 152, 605
(1993): Leenutaphong V+, *Int J Dermatol* 32, 428
(1993): Pagliaro LA+, *Hosp Community Psychiatry* 44, 999
(1993): Server Climent M, *Aten Primaria* (Spanish) 11, 377
(1992): Chevenet C+, *Ann Dermatol Venereol* (French) 119, 929 (with brain irradiation)
(1990): Gebauer K+, *Australas J Dermatol* 31, 89 (passim)
(1990): Hoang-Xuan K+, *Neurology* 40, 1144 (with cranial irradiation)
(1990): Khe HX+, *Neurology* 40, 1144
(1990): Roustan G+, *Actas Dermosifiliogr* (Spanish) 81, 775
(1990): Wong KE, *Singapore Med J* 31, 432
(1989): Alanko K+, *Acta Derm Venereol* (Stockh) 69, 223
(1988): McDanal CE, *J Clin Psychiatr* 49, 369
(1988): Warnock JK+, *Am J Psychiatry* 145, 425
(1987): Fawcett RG, *J Clin Psychiatry* 48, 416
(1975): Böttiger LE+, *Acta Med Scand* 198, 229 (4 of 77 cases)
(1965): Coombs BW, *Med J Aust* 1, 895
(1965): Inglis W, *Med J Aust* 2, 94

Toxic epidermal necrolysis (1–10%)
(2002): Correia O+, *Arch Dermatol* 138, 29 (two cases)
(2001): Udawat H+, *J Assoc Physicians India* 49, 918
(1999): Dhar S+, *Dermatology* 199, 194
(1999): Egan CA+, *J Am Acad Dermatol* 40, 458
(1999): Petter G+, *Hautarzt* (German) 50, 884
(1999): Ruble R+, *CNS Drugs* 12, 215
(1999): Rzany B+, *Lancet* 353, 2190
(1997): Belgodere X+, *Arch Pediatr* (French) 4, 1020
(1997): Jarrett P+, *Clin Exp Dermatol* 22, 146
(1996): Blum L+, *J Am Acad Dermatol* 34, 1088
(1995): Sterker M+, *Int J Clin Pharmacol Ther* 33, 595

(1995): Urbanowski S+, *Wiad Lek* (Polish) 48, 154
(1995): Wolkenstein P+, *Arch Dermatol* 131, 544
(1994): Friedmann PS+, *Arch Dermatol* 130, 598
(1993): Correia O+, *Dermatology* 186, 32
(1993): Leenutaphong V+, *Int J Dermatol* 32, 428
(1993): Pagliaro LA+, *Hospital and Community Psychiatry* 44, 999
(1992): Park BK+, *Br J Clin Pharmacol* 34. 377
(1992): Weller M+, *Am J Psychiatry* 149, 1114
(1992): Weller M+, *Nervenarzt* (German) 63, 308
(1991): Sakellariou G+, *Int J Artif Organs* 14, 634
(1990): Gebauer K+, *Australas J Dermatol* 31, 89 (passim)
(1990): Roujeau JC+, *Arch Dermatol* 126, 37
(1988): Shear NH+, *J Clin Invest* 82, 1826
(1987): Guillaume JC+, *Arch Dermatol* 123, 1166
(1986): Rusciani L+, *G Ital Dermatol Venereol* (Italian) 121, 149
(1984): Husegaard HC+, *Ugeskr Laeger* (Danish) 146, 2784
(1984): Staughton RCD+, *J R Soc Med* 77 (Suppl 4), 6
(1982): Breathnach SM+, *Clin Exp Dermatol* 7, 585
(1977): Houwerzijl J+, *Clin Exp Immunol* 29, 272
(1976): Mutina ES+, *Klin Med Mosk* (Russian) 54, 124
(1972): Carli-Basset C+, *Sem Hop* (French) 48, 497

Toxic pustuloderma (sic) (probably AGEP [ed])
(1990): Gebauer K+, *Australas J Dermatol* 31, 89
(1988): Commens CA+, *Arch Dermatol* 124, 178
(1984): Staughton RCD+, *J R Soc Med* 77 (Suppl 4), 6

Toxic-allergic shock (sic)
(1979): Rummel GL, *ZFA (Stuttgart)* 55, 627

Toxicoderma (sic)
(1983): Rozov VD+, *Vestn Dermatol Venerol* (Russian) September, 48

Urticaria
(2001): Hebert AA+, *J Clin Psychiatry* 62(suppl 14), 22
(1993): Alanko K, *Contact Dermatitis* 29, 254
(1993): Konishi T+, *Eur J Pediatr* 152, 605
(1990): Gebauer K+, *Australas J Dermatol* 31, 89 (passim)
(1988): Warnock JK+, *Am J Psychiatry* 145, 425
(1987): Johannessen AC+, *Ugeskr Laeger* (Danish) 149, 376
(1984): Staughton RCD+, *J R Soc Med* 77 (Suppl 4), 6
(1977): Houwerzijl J+, *Clin Exp Immunol* 29, 272
(1976): Al-Ubaidy SS+, *Br J Oral Surg* 13, 289 (4.2%)
(1969): Rull JA+, *Diabetologia* 5, 215 (6.6%)
(1967): Arieff AJ+, *Dis Nerv Syst* 28, 820
(1964): Spillane D, *Practitioner* 192, 71

Vasculitis
(1993): Drory VE+, *Clin Neuropharmacol* 16, 19 (passim)
(1990): Gebauer K+, *Australas J Dermatol* 31, 89 (passim)
(1987): Harats N+, *J Neurol Neurosurg Psychiatry* 50, 1241
(1978): Nieme KM+, *Acta Derm Venereol* (Stockh) 58, 337
(1967): Harman RRM, *Br J Dermatol* 79, 500

## Hair

Hair – alopecia
(2000): Mercke Y+, *Ann Clin Psychiatry* 12, 35 (~6%)
(1997): Ikeda A+, *J Neurol Neurosurg Psychiatry* 63, 549
(1996): McKinney PA+, *Ann Clin Psychiatry* 8, 183
(1988): Warnock JK+, *Am J Psychiatry* 145, 425
(1985): Shuper A+, *Drug Intell Clin Pharm* 19, 924
(1982): Breathnach SM+, *Clin Exp Dermatol* 7, 585

## Nails

Nails – discoloration (bluish-black)
(1989): Mishra D+, *Int J Dermatol* 28, 460

Nails – hypoplasia
(1985): Niesen M+, *Neuropediatrics* 16, 167

Nails – lichen planus
(1989): Ohtsuyama M+, *Nishinihon J Dermatol* (Japanese) 51, 958

Nails – loss (sic)
(1982): Breathnach SM+, *Clin Exp Dermatol* 7, 585

Nails – onychomadesis
(1989): Mishra D+, *Int J Dermatol* 28, 460

## Other

Acute intermittent porphyria
(1984): Doss M+, *Lancet* 1, 1026
(1983): Liawah AC+, *Lancet* 1, 1442
(1983): Rideout JM+, *Lancet* 2, 464
(1983): Shanley BC, *Lancet* 1, 1229
(1983): Yeung Laiwah AACY+, *Lancet* 1, 790

Death
(2002): Correia O+, *Arch Dermatol* 138, 29

DRESS syndrome
(2002): Maradeix S+, *World Congress Dermatol* Poster, 0112
(2001): Descamps V+, *Arch Dermatol* 137, 301 (5 patients)
(2001): Queyrel V+, *Rev Med Interne* 22(6), 582

Dyschromatopsia
(2000): Nousiainen I+, *Ophthalmology* 107, 884

Dysgeusia
(1976): Rollin H, *Laryngol Rhinol Otol* (Stuttgart) (German) 55, 873

Fetal anticonvulsant syndrome
(2000): Moore SJ+, *J Med Genet* 37, 489

Glossitis

Hypersensitivity*
(2001): Bessmertny O+, *Ann Pharmacother* 35(5), 533
(2001): Nashed MH+, *Pharmacotherapy* 21(4), 502
(2001): Sekine N+, *JAMA* 285(9), 1153
(2000): Bugatti L, Italy (from Internet) (observation)
(2000): Elstner S+, *Fortschr Neurol Psychiatr* (German) 68, 188
(2000): Ivry S+, *Harefuah* (Hebrew) 138, 545
(2000): Straussberg R+, *Pediatr Neurol* 22, 231
(1999): Balasubrananian S+, *Indian Pediatr* 36, 98
(1999): Brown KL+, *Dev Med Child Neurol* 41, 267
(1999): Hamer HM+, *Seizure* 8, 190
(1999): Lombardi SM+, *Ann Pharmacother* 33, 571
(1999): Mesec A+, *J Neurol Neurosurg Psychiatry* 66, 249
(1999): Moss DM+, *J Emerg Med* 17, 503
(1998): Dertinger S+, *J Hepatol* 28, 356
(1998): Schlienger RG+, *Epilepsia* 39, S3 (passim)
(1997): Morkunas AR+, *Crit Care Clin* 13, 727
(1997): Pichler WJ+, *New Engl J Med* 336, 377
(1997): Stein J+, *Dtsch Med Wochenschr* (German) 122, 314
(1997): Tennis P+, *Neurology* 49, 542
(1997): Waagner DC, *New Engl J Med* 336, 376
(1996): Callot V+, *Arch Dermatol* 132, 1315
(1996): *New Engl J Med* 335, 577
(1996): Knowles SR+, *J Clin Psychopharmacol* 16, 263
(1996): Koopman R, Enschede, The Netherlands (from Internet) (observation)
(1996): Oakley A, Hamilton, New Zealand (from Internet) (observation)
(1995): Bellman B+, *J Am Acad Child Adolesc Psychiatry* 34, 1405
(1995): De Vriese AS+, *Medicine Baltimore* 74, 144
(1995): Periole B+, *Ann Dermatol Venereol (French)* 122, 121
(1994): Alldredge BK+, *Pediatr Neurol* 10, 169
(1994): Gall H+, *Hautarzt* (German) 45, 494
(1994): Naranjo CA+, *Clin Pharmacol Ther* 56, 564
(1993): Handfield-Jones SE+, *Br J Dermatol* 129, 175
(1993): Parha S+, *Eur J Pediatr* 152, 1040
(1993): Scerri L+, *Clin Exp Dermatol* 18, 540
(1991): Baguena F+, *Med Clin (Barc)* (Spanish) 96, 237
(1991): Hosoda N+, *Arch Dis Child* 66, 722
(1989): Malanin G+, *Duodecim* (Finnish) 105, 784
(1983): Bernstein DI+, *Clin Pediatr* (Phila) *22, 524*
(1978): Stephan WC+, *Chest* 74, 463 (pneumonitis)
(1977): Houwerzijl J+, *Clin Exp Immunol* 29, 272

Lymphoproliferative disease
(1992): Schlaifer D+, *Eur J Dermatol* 48, 274
(1992): Sigal-Nahum M+, *Br J Dermatol* 127, 545
(1990): Katzin WE+, *Arch Pathol Lab Med* 114, 1244
(1987): Severson GS+, *Am J Med* 83, 597

(1984): Shuttleworth D+, *Clin Exp Dermatol* 9, 421
Mucocutaneous eruption
(1999): Edwards SG+, *Postgrad Med J* 75, 680
(1993): Konishi T+, *Eur J Pediatr* 152, 605
(1979): Pollack MA+, *Ann Neurol* 5, 262
(1975): Böttiger LE+, *Acta Med Scand* 198, 229
Oral lichenoid eruption
(1989): Ohtsuyama M+, *Nishinihon J Dermatol* (Japanese) 51, 958
Oral mucosal eruption
(1964): Spillane D, *Practitioner* 192, 71
Oral ulceration
(2001): Hebert AA+, *J Clin Psychiatry* 62(suppl 14), 22
Porphyria cutanea tarda
(1996): Leo RJ+, *Am J Psychiatry* 153, 443
Porphyria variegata
(2001): Grieco A+, *Eur J Gastroenterol Hepatol* 13(8), 973
Pseudolymphoma
(2001): Cogrel O+, *Br J Dermatol* 144, 1235
(1999): Saeki H+, *J Dermatol* 26, 329
(1998): d'Incan M+, *Ann Dermatol Venereol* 125, 52
(1998): Nathan D+, *J Am Acad Dermatol* 38, 806
(1997): Kim ST+, Korea, American Academy of Dermatology Meeting (SF), Poster #82
(1997): Paramesh H+, *Indian Pediatr* 34, 829
(1996): Callot V+, *Arch Dermatol* 132, 1315
(1995): Magro CM+, *J Am Acad Dermatol* 32, 419
(1993): Rondas AA+, *Ned Tijdschr Geneeskd* (Dutch) 137, 1258
(1993): Sigal M+, *Ann Dermatol Venereol* (French) 120, 175
(1990): Sinnige HAM+, *J Intern Med* 227, 355
(1986): Yates P+, *J Clin Pathol* 39, 1224
(1984): Shuttleworth D+, *Clin Exp Dermatol* 9, 424
Rhabdomyolysis
(1992): Zele I+, *Minerva Med* 83(12), 847
Serum sickness
(1993): Igarashi M+, *Int Arch Allergy Immunol* 100, 378
Stomatitis
Thrombophlebitis
Tinnitus
Tongue ulceration
(1998): Melgarejo Moreno PJ+, *An Otorrinolaringol Ibero Am* (Spanish) 25, 167
(1964): Spillane D, *Practitioner* 192, 71
Xerostomia

***Note:** The antiepileptic drug hypersensitivity syndrome is a severe, occasionally fatal, disorder characterized by any or all of the following: pruritic exanthems, toxic epidermal necrolysis, Stevens–Johnson syndrome, exfoliative dermatitis, fever, hepatic abnormalities, eosinophilia, and renal failure

# CARBENICILLIN

**Trade name:** Geocillin (Pfizer)
**Other common trade names:** *Carbecin; Carbelin; Geopen; Pyopen*
**Indications:** Urinary tract infections
**Category:** Penicillinase-sensitive penicillin
**Half-life:** 1.0–1.5 hours
**Clinically important, potentially hazardous interactions with:** anticoagulants, cyclosporine, demeclocycline, doxycycline, gentamicin, methotrexate, minocycline, oxytetracycline, tetracyclines

### *Reactions*

## Skin

Allergic reactions (sic)
(1994): Pleasants RA+, *Chest* 106, 1124 (in patients with cystic fibrosis)
Angioedema
Bullous eruption
Ecchymoses
Edema
Erythema multiforme
Erythema nodosum
Exanthems
Exfoliative dermatitis
Hematomas
Jarisch–Herxheimer reaction
Pruritus
Purpura
(1976): Karchmer AW+, *N Engl J Med* 295, 451
(1970): McClure PD+, *Lancet* 2, 1307
Rash (sic) (<1%)
Stevens–Johnson syndrome
Toxic epidermal necrolysis
(1984): Westly ED+, *Arch Dermatol* 120, 721
Urticaria (<1%)
Vasculitis
Vesicular eruptions

## Other

Anaphylactoid reactions
Black tongue
Dysgeusia (1–10%)
Glossitis (1–10%)
Glossodynia
Hypersensitivity
Injection-site pain
Oral candidiasis
Serum sickness
Stomatitis
Stomatodynia
Thrombophlebitis (<1%)
Tongue, furry
Vaginitis (<1%)
Xerostomia

# CARBIDOPA

(See LEVODOPA)

# CARBOPLATIN

**Trade name:** Paraplatin (Bristol-Myers Squibb)
**Other common trade names:** *Carboplat; Carbosin; Ercar; Oncocarbin; Paraplatine*
**Indications:** Various carcinomas and sarcomas
**Category:** Antineoplastic
**Half-life:** terminal: 22–40 hours
**Clinically important, potentially hazardous interactions with:** aldesleukin

### *Reactions*

#### Skin

Allergic reactions (sic)
(2001): Yu DY+, *J Pediatr Hematol Oncol* 23(6), 349 (11.1%)
Depigmentation
(1990): Costello SA+, *Clin Oncol R Coll Radiol* 2, 182
Erosion of body folds (sic)
(1996): Prussick R+, *J Am Acad Dermatol* 35, 705
Erythema (2%)
(2001): Robinson JB+, *Gynecol Oncol* 82(3), 550
(1995): Inbar M+, *Anticancer Drugs* 6, 775
Exanthems
(1995): Inbar M+, *Anticancer Drugs* 6, 775
(1992): Beyer J+, *Bone Marrow Transplant* 10, 491
(1989): Wagstaff AJ+, *Drugs* 37, 162
Facial edema
(1992): Beyer J+, *Bone Marrow Transplant* 10, 491
Flushing
(2001): Robinson JB+, *Gynecol Oncol* 82(3), 550
Pigmentation
(1992): Beyer J+, *Bone Marrow Transplant* 10, 491
(1991): Singal R+, *Pediatr Dermatology* 8, 231
Pruritus (2%)
(2001): Robinson JB+, *Gynecol Oncol* 82(3), 550
Rash (sic) (2%)
Urticaria (2%)
(1996): Broome CB+, *Med Pediatr Oncol* 26, 105
(1995): Sredni B+, *J Clin Oncol* 13, 2342

#### Hair

Hair – alopecia (3%)
(2002): Sehouli J+, *Gynecol Oncol* 85(2), 321 (with paclitaxel)
(1989): Wagstaff AJ+, *Drugs* 37, 162

#### Other

Anaphylactoid reactions (<1%)
Hypersensitivity (2%)
(2002): Markman M, *Gynecol Oncol* 84(2), 353
(2001): Robinson JB+, *Gynecol Oncol* 82(3), 550 (with paclitaxel)
(1999): Menczer J+, *Eur J Gynaecol Oncol* 20, 214 (4 patients)
(1999): Schiavetti A+, *Med Pediatr Oncol* 32, 183 (9.2%)
(1999): Shukunami K+, *Gynecol Oncol* 72, 431
(1998): Kook H+, *Bone Marrow Transplant* 21, 727
(1996): Broome CB+, *Med Pediatr Oncol* 26, 105
Injection-site pain (>10%)
Oral mucosal lesions
(1989): Wagstaff AJ+, *Drugs* 37, 162
Parkinsonism
(2001): Chuang C+, *Movement Disorders* 16, 990 (with paclitaxel)
Stomatitis (>10%)

# CARISOPRODOL

**Synonyms:** carisoprodate; isobamate
**Trade name:** Soma (Wallace)
**Other common trade names:** *Artifar; Carisoma; Myolax; Sanoma; Sodol; Somadril; Soridol*
**Indications:** Painful musculoskeletal disorders
**Category:** Skeletal muscle relaxant
**Half-life:** 4–6 hours

### *Reactions*

#### Skin

Angioedema (1–10%)
Diaphoresis
(1983): Rollings HE+, *Curr Ther Res* 34, 926
Edema
(1983): Rollings HE+, *Curr Ther Res* 34, 926
Erythema multiforme (<1%)
Exanthems
(1962): Honeycutt WM+, *JAMA* 180, 691 (passim)
Fixed eruption (<1%)
(1965): Gore HC, *Arch Dermatol* 91, 627
(1962): Honeycutt WM+, *JAMA* 180, 691
Flushing (1–10%)
Photosensitivity
(1994): Hazen PG, *J Am Acad Dermatol* 31, 498
Pruritus (<1%)
Rash (sic) (<1%)
Urticaria (<1%)
(1962): Honeycutt WM+, *JAMA* 180, 691 (passim)

#### Other

Anaphylactoid reactions
Paresthesias
(1983): Rollings HE+, *Curr Ther Res* 34, 926
Pseudoporphyria
(1994): Hazen PG, *J Am Acad Dermatol* 31, 498
Tinnitus
Trembling (sic) (1–10%)
Xerostomia
(1983): Rollings HE+, *Curr Ther Res* 34, 926

# CARMUSTINE

**Synonym:** BCNU
**Trade names:** BiCNU (Bristol-Myers Squibb); Gliadel Wafer (Aventis)
**Other common trade names:** *Becenun; Carmubris; Nitrumon*
**Indications:** Brain tumors, Hodgkin's disease, multiple myeloma
**Category:** Antineoplastic
**Half-life:** initial: 1.4 minutes; secondary: 20 minutes
**Clinically important, potentially hazardous interactions with:** aldesleukin, cimetidine, clorazepate

### *Reactions*

#### Skin

Contact dermatitis
(1994): Zackheim HS, *Semin Dermatol* 13, 202
(1990): Zackheim HS+, *J Am Acad Dermatol* 22, 802
Dermatitis (sic) (<1%)
Eccrine squamous syringometaplasia
(1997): Valks R+, *Arch Dermatol* 133, 873

Erythema
(1992): Breathnach SM+, *Adverse Drug Reactions and the Skin* Blackwell, Oxford, 292
Exanthems
(1978): Levine N+, *Cancer Treat Rev* 5, 67
Flushing (1–10%)
(1978): Levine N+, *Cancer Treat Rev* 5, 67
(1971): Young RC+, *N Engl J Med* 285, 475
Pigmentation (on accidental contact)
(1982): Dunagin WG, *Semin Oncol* 9, 14
(1966): Frost P+, *Arch Dermatol* 94, 265
Skin tenderness (sic)
(1992): Breathnach SM+, *Adverse Drug Reactions and the Skin* Blackwell, Oxford, 292
Telangiectases
(1994): Zackheim HS, *Semin Dermatol* 13, 202
(1992): Breathnach SM+, *Adverse Drug Reactions and the Skin* Blackwell, Oxford, 292

### Hair
Hair – alopecia (1–10%)

### Other
Gynecomastia
Injection-site burning (>10%)
Injection-site necrosis
(1987): Dufresne RG, *Cutis* 39, 197
Injection-site pain
Oral mucositis
(2000): Wardley AM+, *Br J Haematol* 110, 292
Stomatitis (1–10%)

## CARTEOLOL

**Trade names:** Cartrol (Abbott); Ocupress (ophthalmic) (Otsuka)
**Other common trade names:** *Arteolol; Arteoptic; Calte; Carteol; Endak; Mikelan; Teoptic*
**Indications:** Glaucoma, hypertension
**Category:** Beta-adrenergic blocker
**Half-life:** 6 hours
**Clinically important, potentially hazardous interactions with:** clonidine, epinephrine, verapamil

**Note:** Cutaneous side effects of beta-receptor blockaders are clinically polymorphous. They apparently appear after several months of continuous therapy. Atypical psoriasiform, lichen planus-like, and eczematous chronic rashes are mainly observed. (1983): Hödl St, *Z Hautkr* (German) 1:58, 17

### *Reactions*

### Skin
Acne
Angioedema
Ankle edema (<1%)
Cold extremities (sic)
Contact dermatitis (eye-drops)
(2001): Holdiness MR, *Am J Contact Dermat* 12(4), 217
(2000): Quiralte J+, *Contact Dermatitis* 42, 245
Dermatitis (sic)
Diaphoresis (<1%)
(1997): Schmutz JL+, *Dermatology* 194, 197 (from topical)
Edema
Exanthems
Exfoliative dermatitis
Facial edema
Flushing
Lupus erythematosus
Peripheral edema (1.7%)
Photosensitivity
Pigmentation
Pruritus
Psoriasis
Purpura (<1%)
Rash (sic) (2.5%)
Raynaud's phenomenon (<1%)
Vesiculobullous eruption
Xerosis

### Hair
Hair – alopecia

### Nails
Nails – discoloration (bluish)

### Other
Anaphylactoid reactions
Dysgeusia (from topical application)
Myalgia
Paresthesias (2%)
Peyronie's disease
Tinnitus
Xerostomia

## CARVEDILOL

**Trade name:** Coreg (GSK)
**Other common trade names:** *Dibloc; Dilatrend; Dimitone; Kredex; Querto*
**Indications:** Hypertension
**Category:** Beta-adrenergic blocker; antihypertensive
**Half-life:** 7–10 hours

### *Reactions*

### Skin
Allergy (sic) (<1%)
Angioedema
(1988): Ogihara G+, *Drugs* 36, 75 (<1%)
Cutaneous reactions (sic)
(1998): Simpson SH+, *Can J Cardiol* 14, 1277
Diaphoresis (2.9%)
Edema (generalized) (5.1%)
Exanthems (<1%)
(2000): Litt JZ, Beachwood, OH (personal case) (observation)
(1988): Ogihara G+, *Drugs* 36, 75 (2%)
Exfoliative dermatitis (<1%)
Infections (sic) (2.2%)
Pain (8.6%)
Peripheral edema (1.4%)
Photosensitivity (<1%)
Pruritus (<1%)
(2000): Litt JZ, Beachwood, OH (personal case) (observation)
Psoriasis (<1%)
Purpura (1–10%)
Rash (sic) (<1%)
Stevens–Johnson syndrome
(1997): Kowalski BJ+, *Am J Cardiol* 80, 669

### Hair

Hair – alopecia (<0.1%)

### Other

Anaphylactoid reactions (<1%)
Hypesthesia (<1%)
Myalgia (3.4%)
Paresthesias (2%)
Xerostomia (<1%)

## CASPOFUNGIN

**Trade name:** Cancidas (Merck)
**Indications:** Invasive Aspergillus infection
**Category:** Antifungal (parenteral) (Glucan synthesis inhibitor)
**Half-life:** Beta phase: 9–11 hours; terminal: 40–50 hours
**Clinically important, potentially hazardous interactions with:** cyclosporine

***Reactions***

### Skin

Chills (~3%)
Diaphoresis (<1%)
Edema (~3%)
Erythema (1–2%)
Facial edema (3%)
Flu-like syndrome (3%)
Flushing (3%)
Pain (1–5%)
Pruritus (2–3%)
Rash (sic) (1–4%)
Vasculitis (2%)

### Other

Anaphylactoid reactions (<2%)
Infusion-site induration (~3%)
Infusion-site reactions (2–12%)
(2001): Keating GM+, *Drugs* 61(8), 1121
Myalgia (~3%)
Paresthesias (1–3%)
Phlebitis (~16%)
Tremors (<2%)

## CEFACLOR

**Trade name:** Ceclor (Lilly)
**Other common trade names:** *Alfatil; Apo-Cefaclor; CEC 500; Cefabiocin; Distaclor; Kefolor; Panoral; Sigacefal*
**Indications:** Various infections caused by susceptible organisms
**Category:** Second generation cephalosporin
**Half-life:** 0.6–0.9 hours

**Note:** Penicillin and cephalosporins share a common beta-lactam structure. People who are allergic to penicillin are approximately 4 times more likely to develop an allergic reaction to a cephalosporin than those people who have no penicillin allergy. (From 5 to 16% of patients allergic to penicillin develop reactions to cephalosporins)

***Reactions***

### Skin

Acute generalized exanthematous pustulosis (AGEP)
(1995): Moreau A+, *Int J Dermatol* 34, 263 (passim)
(1992): Ogoshi M+, *Dermatology* 184, 142
Angioedema (<1%)
(1998): Litt JZ, Beachwood, OH (personal case) (observation)
Candidiasis (vaginal)
(1992): Stotka JL+, *Postgrad Med J* 68, S73
Dermatitis (sic)
(1986): Hirata M+, *Kokyu To Junkan* (Japanese) 34, 791
Edema
(1995): Dark DS+, *Infections in Medicine* October, 551
Erythema multiforme
(2000): Ibia EO+, *Arch Dermatol* 136, 849
(1999): Joubert GI+, *Can J Clin Pharmacol* 6, 197 (17 cases)
(1988): Platt R+, *J Infect Dis* 158, 474 (0.6%)
(1985): Levine LR, *Ped Infect Dis* 4, 358 (0.6%)
(1982): Lovell SJ+, *Can Med Assoc J* 126, 1032
(1980): Murray DL+, *N Engl J Med* 303, 1003
Exanthems
(2000): Ibia EO+, *Arch Dermatol* 136, 849
(1996): Nagayama H+, *J Dermatol* 23, 899
(1994): Litt JZ, Beachwood, OH (personal case) (observation)
(1994): Shelley WB+, *Cutis* 53, 40 (observation)
(1987): Norrby SR, *Drugs* 34 (Suppl 2), 105 (1–5%)
(1986): Ascher H, *Lakartidningen* (Swedish) 83, 411
(1985): Murray DL+, *Pediatr Infect Dis* 4, 706
(1983): Johnson T, *J Ark Med Soc* 80, 110
(1982): Lovell SJ+, *Can Med Assoc J* 126, 1032
(1981): Ackley AM+, *Southern Med J* 74, 1550
(1980): Murray DL+, *N Engl J Med* 303, 1003
Flushing
Pruritus (<1%)
(1998): Litt JZ, Beachwood, OH (personal case) (observation)
(1988): Platt R+, *J Infect Dis* 158, 474
(1982): Lovell SJ+, *Can Med Assoc J* 126, 1032
(1981): Ackley AM+, *Southern Med J* 74, 1550
(1980): Murray DL+, *N Engl J Med* 303, 1003
Purpura
(1980): Murray DL+, *N Engl J Med* 303, 1003
Pustular eruption
(1992): Ogoshi M+, *Dermatology* 184, 142
Rash (sic) (1–1.5%)
Stevens–Johnson syndrome (<1%)
(1988): Platt R+, *J Infect Dis* 158, 474
Toxic epidermal necrolysis
(1987): Guillaume JC+, *Arch Dermatol* 123, 1166
Urticaria (<1%)
(2000): Ibia EO+, *Arch Dermatol* 136, 849
(1999): Joubert GI+, *Can J Clin Pharmacol* 6, 197 (26 cases)
(1998): Litt JZ, Beachwood, OH (personal case) (observation)
(1995): Blumenthal HL, Beachwood, OH (personal case) (observation)
(1994): Litt JZ, Beachwood, OH (personal case) (observation)
(1993): Litt JZ, Beachwood, OH (2 personal cases) (observation)
(1991): Hebert AA+, *J Am Acad Dermatol* 25, 805
(1985): Levine LR, *Pediatr Infect Dis* 4, 358 (1–5%)
(1982): Lovell SJ+, *Can Med Assoc J* 126, 1032

### Other

Anaphylactoid reactions (<1%)
(1999): Grouhi M+, *Pediatrics* 103, e50
(1986): Nishioka K+, *J Dermatol* 13, 226
Dysgeusia
(1995): Dark DS+, *Infections in Medicine* October, 551
Glossitis
Hypersensitivity
Oral candidiasis
Paresthesias
Serum sickness (<1%)
(2000): Ibia EO+, *Arch Dermatol* 136, 849

(1999): Joubert GI+, *Can J Clin Pharmacol* 6, 197 (31 cases)
(1999): Parshuram CS+, *J Paediatr Child Health* 35, 223
(1999): Phillips R, *Aust Fam Physician* 28, 539
(1998): Boyd IW, *Med J Aust* 169, 443
(1998): Kearns GL+, *Clin Pharmacol Ther* 63, 686 (10 patients)
(1997): Szalai Z+, *Orv Hetil* (Hungarian) 138, 855
(1996): Grammer LC, *JAMA* 275, 1152
(1996): *Can Med Assoc J* 155, 913
(1996): Reynolds RD, *JAMA* 276, 950
(1995): Kearns GL+, *J Pediatr* 125, 805
(1995): Martin J+, *N Z Med J* 108, 123
(1992): Parra FM+, *Allergy* 47, 439
(1992): Stricker BH+, *J Clin Epidemiol* 45, 1177
(1992): Vial T+, *Ann Pharmacother* 26, 910
(1991): Hebert AA+, *J Am Acad Dermatol* 25, 805
(1990): Heckbert SB+, *Am J Epidemiol* 132, 336
(1988): Platt R+, *J Infect Dis* 158, 474
(1987): Norrby SR, *Drugs* 34 (Suppl 2), 105 (1–5%)
(1985): Callahan CW+, *J Am Osteopath Assoc* 85, 450
(1985): Levine LR, *Ped Infect Dis* 4, 358 (0.5%)
(1985): Murray DL+, *Pediatr Inf Dis* 4, 706
(1983): Johnson T+, *J Ark Med Soc* 80, 110
(1982): Lovell SJ+, *Can Med Assoc J* 126, 1032
(1980): Murray DL+, *N Engl J Med* 303, 1003

Vaginitis
(1992): Stotka JL+, *Postgrad Med J* 68, S73 (candidiasis)

# CEFADROXIL

**Trade name:** Duricef (Bristol-Myers Squibb)
**Other common trade names:** *Baxan; Bidocef; Cedrox; Cefamox; Duracef; Moxacef; Oracefal; Sumacef*
**Indications:** Various infections caused by susceptible organisms
**Category:** First generation cephalosporin antibiotic
**Half-life:** 1.2–1.5 hours

**Note:** Penicillin and cephalosporins share a common beta-lactam structure. People who are allergic to penicillin are approximately 4 times more likely to develop an allergic reaction to a cephalosporin than those people who have no penicillin allergy. (From 5 to 16% of patients allergic to penicillin develop allergic reactions to cephalosporins)

## *Reactions*

### Skin

Angioedema (<1%)
Candidiasis
Erythema
(1986): Tanrisever B+, *Drugs* 32(Suppl 3), 1
Erythema multiforme (<1%)
Exanthems (<1%)
(1986): Tanrisever B+, *Drugs* 32(Suppl 3), 1 (0.3%)
Pemphigus
(1986): Wilson JP+, *Drug Intell Clin Pharm* 20, 219
Pruritus (<1%)
(1986): Tanrisever B+, *Drugs* 32(Suppl 3), 1 (0.3%)
Rash (sic) (<1%)
Stevens–Johnson syndrome (<1%)
Toxic epidermal necrolysis
Urticaria (<1%)
(1993): Shelley WB+, *Cutis* 52, 262 (observation)
(1986): Tanrisever B+, *Drugs* 32(Suppl 3), 1 (0.1%)

### Other

Anaphylactoid reactions (<1%)
Glossitis
(1986): Tanrisever B+, *Drugs* 32 (Suppl 3), 1, 21, 43
Hypersensitivity
Oral candidiasis
Oral mucosal eruption
(1986): Tanrisever B+, *Drugs* 32(Suppl 3), 1 (0.1%)
Oral ulceration
(1986): Wilson JP+, *Drug Intell Clin Pharm* 20, 219
Serum sickness (<1%)
Vaginitis (<1%)
(1986): Tanrisever B+, *Drugs* 32(Suppl 3), 1

# CEFAMANDOLE

**Trade name:** Mandol (Lilly)
**Other common trade names:** *Cedol; Cefadol; Kefadol; Kefdole; Mancef; Mandokef*
**Indications:** Various infections caused by susceptible organisms
**Category:** Second generation cephalosporin
**Half-life:** 0.5–1.0 hours

**Note:** Penicillin and cephalosporins share a common beta-lactam structure. People who are allergic to penicillin are approximately 4 times more likely to develop an allergic reaction to a cephalosporin than those people who have no penicillin allergy. (From 5 to 16% of patients allergic to penicillin develop allergic reactions to cephalosporins)

## *Reactions*

### Skin

Acne
Diaper rash
Diaphoresis
Edema
Erythema multiforme
(1987): Argenyi ZB+, *Cleve Clin J Med* 54, 445
Exanthems
(1985): Richards DM+, *Drugs* 29, 281 (1.7%)
(1985): Sanders CV+, *Ann Intern Med* 103, 70 (2%)
Flushing
Linear IgA bullous dermatosis
(1987): Argenyi ZB+, *Cleve Clin J Med* 54, 445
Pruritus (<1%)
Purpura
Rash (sic) (<1%)
Stevens–Johnson syndrome (<1%)
Toxic epidermal necrolysis
(1985): Sanders CV+, *Ann Intern Med* 103, 70 (2%)
(1982): Seifter EJ+, *Johns Hopkins Med J* 151, 326
Toxic erythema
(1995): Rademaker M, *N Z Med J* 108, 165
Urticaria (<1%)

### Other

Anaphylactoid reactions (<1%)
(1992): Lin RY, *Arch Intern Med* 152, 930
Dysgeusia
Glossitis
Hypersensitivity
Injection-site burning
Injection-site cellulitis
Injection-site edema
Injection-site inflammation
Injection-site pain (<1%)
(1985): Sanders CV+, *Ann Intern Med* 103, 70 (7%)

Injection-site thrombophlebitis (1–10%)
(1985): Sanders CV+, *Ann Intern Med* 103, 70 (15%)
Oral candidiasis (<1%)
Paresthesias
Serum sickness (<1%)
Vaginal candidiasis
Vaginitis

# CEFAZOLIN

**Trade names:** Ancef (GSK); Kefzol (Lilly)
**Other common trade names:** *Basocef; Cefacidal; Cefamezin; Elzogram; Gramaxin; Kefarin; Totacef; Zolin*
**Indications:** Various infections caused by susceptible organisms
**Category:** First generation cephalosporin antibiotic
**Half-life:** 1.4–1.8 hours

**Note:** Penicillin and cephalosporins share a common beta-lactam structure. People who are allergic to penicillin are approximately 4 times more likely to develop an allergic reaction to a cephalosporin than those people who have no penicillin allergy. (From 5 to 16% of patients allergic to penicillin develop allergic reactions to cephalosporins)

### *Reactions*

## Skin

Acute generalized exanthematous pustulosis (AGEP)
(1995): Moreau A+, *Int J Dermatol* 34, 263 (passim)
(1994): Manders SM+, *Cutis* 54, 194 (with metronidazole)
Allergic reactions (sic)
(1994): Pleasants RA+, *Chest* 106, 1124 (in patients with cystic fibrosis)
(1993): Faulk D+, *Nurse Anesth* 4, 188 (3–5%)
Contact dermatitis
(2000): Straube MD+, *Contact Dermatitis* 42, 44
Erythema multiforme
Exanthems
(1990): Flax SH+, *Cutis* 46, 59
(1988): Fayol J+, *J Am Acad Dermatol* 19, 571
(1986): Szylit JA+, *Cutis* 37, 390
Fixed eruption (linear)
(1988): Sigal-Nahum M+, *Br J Dermatol* 118, 849
Pemphigus
(1997): Brenner S+, *J Am Acad Dermatol* 36, 919
Photo-recall phenomenon (sic)
(1990): Flax SH+, *Cutis* 46, 59
Photosensitivity
(1990): Flax SH+, *Cutis* 46, 59
Pruritus (<1%)
(1987): Stough D+, *J Am Acad Dermatol* 16, 1051
Pruritus ani
Pustular eruption
(1990): Rustin MHA+, *Br J Dermatol* 123, 119
(1988): Fayol J+, *J Am Acad Dermatol* 19, 571
(1987): Stough D+, *J Am Acad Dermatol* 16, 1051
Rash (sic) (<1%)
Stevens–Johnson syndrome (<1%)
Toxic epidermal necrolysis
(1999): Egan CA+, *J Am Acad Dermatol* 40, 458 (6 cases)
(1994): Julsrud ME, *J Foot Ankle Surg* 33, 255
Urticaria (<1%)

## Other

Anaphylactoid reactions (<1%)
(1996): Warrington RJ+, *J Allergy Clin Immunol* 98, 460
(1995): Konno R+, *J Obstet Gynaecol* 21, 577
(1992): Lin RY, *Arch Intern Med* 152, 930
Hypersensitivity
(2001): Romano AG+, *Allergy Clin Immunol* 107, 134 (delayed)
Injection-site induration
Injection-site pain (<1%)
Injection-site phlebitis (<1%)
Oral candidiasis (<1%)
Phlebitis
Serum sickness (<1%)
Vaginitis (<1%)

# CEFDINIR

**Synonym:** CFDN
**Trade name:** Omnicef (Medicis)
**Indications:** Community-acquired pneumonia and various infections caused by susceptible organisms
**Category:** Third generation cephalosporin
**Half-life:** 1–2 hours

**Note:** Penicillin and cephalosporins share a common beta-lactam structure. People who are allergic to penicillin are approximately 4 times more likely to develop an allergic reaction to a cephalosporin than those people who have no penicillin allergy. (From 5 to 16% of patients allergic to penicillin develop allergic reactions to cephalosporins)

### *Reactions*

## Skin

Candidiasis (1%)
Erythema multiforme
Erythema nodosum
Exanthems (0.2%)
Exfoliative dermatitis
Facial edema
Pruritus (0.2%)
Purpura
Rash (sic) (3%)
Stevens–Johnson syndrome (<1%)
Toxic epidermal necrolysis
Urticaria (<1%)
Vasculitis

## Other

Anaphylactoid reactions
Serum sickness (<1%)
Stomatitis
Vaginal candidiasis (5%)
Vaginitis (1%)

## CEFDITOREN

**Trade name:** Spectracef (TAP)
**Indications:** Various infections caused by susceptible organisms
**Category:** Third generation cephalosporin antibiotic
**Half-life:** ~1.6 hours
**Clinically important, potentially hazardous interactions with:** famotidine

### *Reactions*

#### Skin

Allergic reactions (sic) (<1%)
Diaphoresis (<1%)
Erythema multiforme
Fungal infection (<1%)
Peripheral edema (<1%)
Pruritus (<1%)
Rash (sic) (<1%)
Stevens–Johnson syndrome
Toxic epidermal necrolysis
Urticaria (<1%)

#### Other

Anaphylactoid reactions
Dysgeusia (<1%)
Myalgia (<1%)
Oral candidiasis (<1%)
Oral ulceration (<1%)
Pain (<1%)
Serum sickness
Stomatitis (<1%)
Vaginal candidiasis (3–6%)
(2002): Darkes MJ+ 62, 319
Vaginitis (<1%)
Xerostomia (<1%)

## CEFEPIME

**Trade name:** Maxipime (Dura)
**Other common trade name:** *Maxcef*
**Indications:** Various infections caused by susceptible organisms
**Category:** Fourth generation cephalosporin
**Half-life:** 2–2.3 hours

**Note:** Penicillin and cephalosporins share a common beta-lactam structure. People who are allergic to penicillin are approximately 4 times more likely to develop an allergic reaction to a cephalosporin than those people who have no penicillin allergy. (From 5 to 16% of patients allergic to penicillin develop allergic reactions to cephalosporins)

### *Reactions*

#### Skin

Angioedema
Candidiasis (<1%)
Erythema multiforme
Exanthems (1.8%)
Pruritus (1–10%)
Rash (sic) (51%)
(2000): Sheng WH+, *J Microbiol Immunol Infect* 33, 109
(1996): Holloway WJ+, *Am J Med* 100, 52S
(1994): Okamoto MP+, *Am J Hosp Pharm* 51, 463
Stevens–Johnson syndrome
Toxic epidermal necrolysis
Urticaria (1.8%)

#### Other

Anaphylactoid reactions
Hypersensitivity
Injection-site inflammation (0.6%)
Injection-site pain (0.6%)
Injection-site phlebitis (1.3%)
Injection-site rash (1.1%)
Oral candidiasis
Status epilepticus
(2001): Martinez-Rodriguez JE+, *Am J Med* 111, 115
Vaginitis (<1%)

## CEFIXIME

**Trade name:** Suprax (Lederle)
**Other common trade names:** *Cefspan; Cephoral; Fixime; Oroken; Supran; Uro-cephoral*
**Indications:** Various infections caused by susceptible organisms
**Category:** Third generation cephalosporin antibiotic
**Half-life:** 3–4 hours

**Note:** Penicillin and cephalosporins share a common beta-lactam structure. People who are allergic to penicillin are approximately 4 times more likely to develop an allergic reaction to a cephalosporin than those people who have no penicillin allergy. (From 5 to 16% of patients allergic to penicillin develop allergic reactions to cephalosporins)

### *Reactions*

#### Skin

Candidiasis
Erythema multiforme (<2%)
Pruritus (<2%)
(1987): Tally FP+, *Pediatr Infect Dis J* 6, 976
Pruritus ani
Rash (sic) (<2%)
(2001): Ho MW+, *J Microbiol Immunol Infect* 34(3), 185 (3.2%)
(1987): Tally FP+, *Pediatr Infect Dis J* 6, 976
Stevens–Johnson syndrome (<2%)
Urticaria (<2%)
(1987): Tally FP+, *Pediatr Infect Dis J* 6, 976

#### Other

Anaphylactoid reactions
(1996): Vilas Martinez F+, *Med Clin (Barc)* (Spanish) 106, 439
Hypersensitivity
(1999): Gaig P+, *Allergy* 54(8), 901
Pseudolymphoma
(1998): Jabbar A+, *Br J Haematol* 101, 209
Serum sickness (<2%)
(1987): Tally FP+, *Pediatr Infect Dis J* 6, 976
Vaginal candidiasis
Vaginitis (<2%)
Xerostomia
(1987): Tally FP+, *Pediatr Infect Dis J* 6, 976

# CEFMETAZOLE

**Trade name:** Zefazone (Pharmacia & Upjohn)
**Other common trade names:** *Cefmetazon; Cefotazol; Cemetol; Cetazone; Gomcefa; Metalin*
**Indications:** Various infections caused by susceptible organisms
**Category:** Second generation cephalosporin antibiotic
**Half-life:** 72 minutes

**Note:** Penicillin and cephalosporins share a common beta-lactam structure. People who are allergic to penicillin are approximately 4 times more likely to develop an allergic reaction to a cephalosporin than those people who have no penicillin allergy. (From 5 to 16% of patients allergic to penicillin develop allergic reactions to cephalosporins)

### *Reactions*

#### Skin
Candidiasis (<1%)
Cutaneous reactions (sic)
(1989): Saito A, *J Antimicrob Chemother* 23, 131
Disulfiram-like reaction*
(1989): Saito A, *J Antimicrob Chemother* 23, 131
Hot flashes (<1%)
Periorbital edema
Pruritus (<1%)
Purpura
Rash (sic) (1–10%)
Stevens–Johnson syndrome (<1%)
Toxic epidermal necrolysis
Urticaria (<1%)

#### Other
Anaphylactoid reactions
(1989): Saito A, *J Antimicrob Chemother* 23, 131
Dysgeusia
Hypersensitivity
Injection-site edema
Injection-site induration
Injection-site pain
Injection-site thrombophlebitis (<1%)
Phlebitis (<1%)
Serum sickness (<1%)
Vaginitis (<1%)

***Note:** The disulfiram-like reaction consists of facial flushing, diaphoresis, tachycardia, and pounding headache

# CEFONICID

**Trade name:** Monocid (GSK)
**Other common trade names:** *Dinacid; Monocef; Monocidur*
**Indications:** Various infections caused by susceptible organisms
**Category:** Second generation cephalosporin antibiotic
**Half-life:** 3–6 hours

**Note:** Penicillin and cephalosporins share a common beta-lactam structure. People who are allergic to penicillin are approximately 4 times more likely to develop an allergic reaction to a cephalosporin than those people who have no penicillin allergy. (From 5 to 16% of patients allergic to penicillin develop allergic reactions to cephalosporins)

### *Reactions*

#### Skin
Allergic reactions (sic)
(1994): Martin JA+, *Ann Allergy* 72, 341
Candidiasis (<1%)
Disulfiram-like reaction*
(1990): Marcon G+, *Recenti Prog Med* (Italian) 81, 47
Erythema (<1%)
Erythema multiforme
Pruritus (<1%)
Purpura
Rash (sic) (<1%)
Stevens–Johnson syndrome (<1%)
Toxic epidermal necrolysis
Urticaria (<1%)

#### Other
Anaphylactoid reactions (<1%)
Hypersensitivity
Injection-site edema (>1%)
Injection-site induration (>1%)
Injection-site pain (5.7%)
Injection-site phlebitis (>1%)
Myalgia
Serum sickness (<1%)
(1995): Ortega Calvo M+, *An Med Interna* (Spanish) 12, 289
Vaginitis

***Note:** The disulfiram-like reaction consists of facial flushing, diaphoresis, tachycardia, and pounding headache

# CEFOPERAZONE

**Trade name:** Cefobid (Pfizer)
**Other common trade names:** *Cefobis; Cefogram; Cefozone; CPZ; Mediper; Tomabef; Zoncef*
**Indications:** Various infections caused by susceptible organisms
**Category:** Third generation cephalosporin antibiotic
**Half-life:** 1.6–2.6 hours

**Note:** Penicillin and cephalosporins share a common beta-lactam structure. People who are allergic to penicillin are approximately 4 times more likely to develop an allergic reaction to a cephalosporin than those people who have no penicillin allergy. (From 5 to 16% of patients allergic to penicillin develop allergic reactions to cephalosporins)

### *Reactions*

#### Skin
Candidiasis (<1%)
Disulfiram-like reaction*
(1981): Vonhogen LH+, *Ned Tijdschr Geneeskd* (Dutch) 125, 1610
(1980): Foster TS+, *Am J Hosp Pharm* 37, 858
Erythema multiforme
Exanthems (<1%)
Pruritus (<1%)
Rash (sic) (2%)
(1983): Lyon JA, *Drug Intell Clin Pharm* 17, 7
Stevens–Johnson syndrome (<1%)
Toxic epidermal necrolysis
Urticaria (<1%)
(1983): Lyon JA, *Drug Intell Clin Pharm* 17, 7

#### Other
Hypersensitivity (>2%)
Injection-site induration (<1%)
Injection-site pain (<1%)

(1983): Lyon JA, *Drug Intell Clin Pharm* 17, 7
Phlebitis (<1%)
(1983): Lyon JA, *Drug Intell Clin Pharm* 17, 7
Serum sickness (<1%)
Thrombophlebitis

***Note:** The disulfiram-like reaction consists of facial flushing, diaphoresis, tachycardia, and pounding headache

## CEFOTAXIME

**Trade name:** Claforan (Aventis)
**Other common trade names:** *Alfotax; Benaxima; Biosint; Cefaxim; Cefotax; Molelant; Oritaxim; Primafen; Spirosine; Zariviz*
**Indications:** Various infections caused by susceptible organisms
**Category:** Third generation; broad spectrum; cephalosporin
**Half-life:** adults: 60 minutes

**Note:** Penicillin and cephalosporins share a common beta-lactam structure. People who are allergic to penicillin are approximately 4 times more likely to develop an allergic reaction to a cephalosporin than those people who have no penicillin allergy. (From 5 to 16% of patients allergic to penicillin develop allergic reactions to cephalosporins)

### *Reactions*

#### Skin
Candidiasis
Erythema multiforme
(1990): Todd PA+, *Drugs* 40, 608
(1986): Green ST+, *Postgrad Med J* 62, 415
Exanthems
(1990): Todd PA+, *Drugs* 40, 608
(1984): Smith CR+, *Ann Intern Med* 101, 469 (3.4%)
(1983): Carmine AA+, *Drugs* 25, 223 (2%)
Pruritus (2.4%)
(1990): Todd PA+, *Drugs* 40, 608
(1983): Carmine AA+, *Drugs* 25, 223 (2%)
Rash (sic) (2.4%)
(1982): LeFrock JL+, *Clin Ther* 5, 19
Stevens–Johnson syndrome
Toxic epidermal necrolysis
Urticaria (2.4%)

#### Other
Anaphylactoid reactions (2.4%)
Hypersensitivity
(1993): Papakonstantinou G+, *Clin Investig* 71, 165
Injection-site inflammation (4.3%)
(1983): Carmine AA+, *Drugs* 25, 223 (5%)
Injection-site pain (1–10%)
(1983): Carmine AA+, *Drugs* 25, 223 (32%)
Injection-site thrombophlebitis
Paresthesias
Phlebitis (<1%)
Serum sickness
Vaginitis (<1%)

## CEFOTETAN

**Trade name:** Cefotan (AstraZeneca)
**Other common trade names:** *Apacef; Apatef; Ceftenon; Cepan; Yamatetan*
**Indications:** Various infections caused by susceptible organisms
**Category:** Second generation cephalosporin antibiotic
**Half-life:** 3–5 hours

**Note:** Penicillin and cephalosporins share a common beta-lactam structure. People who are allergic to penicillin are approximately 4 times more likely to develop an allergic reaction to a cephalosporin than those people who have no penicillin allergy. (From 5 to 16% of patients allergic to penicillin develop allergic reactions to cephalosporins)

### *Reactions*

#### Skin
Candidiasis (<1%)
Erythema multiforme
Exanthems
Pruritus (<1%)
Rash (sic) (<1%)
Stevens–Johnson syndrome (<1%)
Toxic epidermal necrolysis
Urticaria (<1%)

#### Other
Anaphylactoid reactions (<1%)
(1990): Faro S+, *Am J Obstet Gynecol* 162, 296
(1988): Bloomberg RJ, *Am J Obstet Gynecol* 159, 125
Hypersensitivity (1.2%)
(2001): Romano A+, *Allergy* 56, 260
Injection-site pain (<1%)
Phlebitis (<1%)
Serum sickness (<1%)
Thrombophlebitis

## CEFOXITIN

**Trade name:** Mefoxin (Merck)
**Other common trade names:** *Cefmore; Cefoxin; Lephocin; Mefoxil; Mefoxitin*
**Indications:** Various infections caused by susceptible organisms
**Category:** Second generation, broad spectrum cephalosporin
**Half-life:** 40–60 minutes

**Note:** Penicillin and cephalosporins share a common beta-lactam structure. People who are allergic to penicillin are approximately 4 times more likely to develop an allergic reaction to a cephalosporin than those people who have no penicillin allergy. (From 5 to 16% of patients allergic to penicillin develop allergic reactions to cephalosporins)

### *Reactions*

#### Skin
Angioedema (<1%)
Candidiasis (<1%)
Exanthems
(1979): Brogden RN+, *Drugs* 17, 1 (2.2%)
Exfoliative dermatitis (<1%)
(1987): Norrby SR, *Drugs* 34 (Suppl 2) 105
(1985): Sanders CV+, *Ann Intern Med* 103, 70 (2%)

(1983): Tietze KJ+, *Clin Pharmacy* 2, 582
(1982): Kannangara DW+, *Arch Intern Med* 142, 1031
Flushing
(1985): Sanders CV+, *Ann Intern Med* 103, 70
Pruritus (<1%)
(1983): Tietze KJ+, *Clin Pharmacy* 2, 582
(1979): Brogden RN+, *Drugs* 17, 1
Purpura
(1990): Burstein M+, *Drug Intell Clin Pharm* 24, 206
Pustular eruption
(1994): Spencer JM+, *Br J Dermatol* 130, 514
Rash (sic) (<1%)
Stevens–Johnson syndrome (<1%)
Toxic epidermal necrolysis (<1%)
Urticaria

### Other

Anaphylactoid reactions (<1%)
(1992): Lin RY, *Arch Intern Med* 152, 930 (11 cases)
Injection-site induration
Injection-site pain
(1985): Sanders CV+, *Ann Intern Med* 103, 70 (10%)
(1979): Brogden RN+, *Drugs* 17, 1 (>5%)
Injection-site tenderness
Serum sickness (<1%)
(1986): Panwalker AP+, *Drug Intell Clin Pharm* 20, 953
Thrombophlebitis

## CEFPODOXIME

**Trade name:** Vantin (Pharmacia & Upjohn)
**Other common trade names:** *Cefodox; Celance; Orelox; Podomexef*
**Indications:** Various infections caused by susceptible organisms
**Category:** Third generation cephalosporin
**Half-life:** 2.1–2.8 hours

**Note:** Penicillin and cephalosporins share a common beta-lactam structure. People who are allergic to penicillin are approximately 4 times more likely to develop an allergic reaction to a cephalosporin than those people who have no penicillin allergy. (From 5 to 16% of patients allergic to penicillin develop allergic reactions to cephalosporins)

#### *Reactions*

### Skin

Acne
Candidiasis (<1%)
Diaper rash (12.1%)
Diaphoresis
Edema
Erythema multiforme
Exfoliation (sic) (<1%)
Flushing (<1%)
Pruritus (<1%)
Rash (sic) (1.4%)
(2001): Fulton B+, *Paediatr Drugs* 3(2), 137
Stevens–Johnson syndrome (<1%)
Toxic epidermal necrolysis
Urticaria (<1%)

### Other

Anaphylactoid reactions (<1%)
Dysgeusia (<1%)
Glossitis
Hypersensitivity
Injection-site burning
Injection-site cellulitis
Injection-site edema
Injection-site inflammation
Injection-site thrombophlebitis
Oral candidiasis
Paresthesias
Serum sickness (<1%)
Sialopenia (<1%)
Tinnitus
Vaginal candidiasis (<1%)
Vaginitis
(1991): Tack KJ+, *Drugs* 42, 51

## CEFPROZIL

**Trade name:** Cefzil (Bristol-Myers Squibb)
**Indications:** Various infections caused by susceptible organisms
**Category:** Second generation cephalosporin antibiotic
**Half-life:** 1.3 hours

**Note:** Penicillin and cephalosporins share a common beta-lactam structure. People who are allergic to penicillin are approximately 4 times more likely to develop an allergic reaction to a cephalosporin than those people who have no penicillin allergy. (From 5 to 16% of patients allergic to penicillin develop allergic reactions to cephalosporins)

#### *Reactions*

### Skin

Angioedema (<1%)
Candidiasis
Diaper rash (1.5%)
Erythema multiforme (<1%)
Exanthems
Pruritus
Rash (sic) (<1%)
Stevens–Johnson syndrome (<1%)
Toxic epidermal necrolysis
Urticaria (<1%)

### Other

Anaphylactoid reactions (<1%)
Genital pruritus (1.6%)
Glossitis
Hypersensitivity
Oral candidiasis
Paresthesias
Serum sickness (<1%)
(1994): Lowery N+, *J Pediatr* 125, 325
Vaginitis (1.6%)

## CEFTAZIDIME

**Trade names:** Ceptaz (GSK); Fortaz (GSK); Tazicef (GSK); Tazidime (Lilly)
**Other common trade names:** *Ceftazim; Fortum; Tagal; Taloken; Waytrax*
**Indications:** Various infections caused by susceptible organisms
**Category:** Third generation cephalosporin
**Half-life:** 1–2 hours

**Note:** Penicillin and cephalosporins share a common beta-lactam structure. People who are allergic to penicillin are approximately 4 times more likely to develop an allergic reaction to a cephalosporin than those people who have no penicillin allergy. (From 5 to 16% of patients allergic to penicillin develop allergic reactions to cephalosporins)

### *Reactions*

#### Skin

Acne
Allergic reactions (sic)
(1994): Pleasants RA+, *Chest* 106, 1124 (in patients with cystic fibrosis)
Angioedema (2%)
Candidiasis (<1%)
Diaper rash
Diaphoresis
Edema
Erythema multiforme (2%)
(1983): Pierce TH+, *J Antimicrob Chemother* 12 (Suppl A), 21
Exanthems
(1985): Richards DM+, *Drugs* 29, 105 (1.6%)
Flushing
Pemphigus erythematosus (sic)
(1993): Iannantuono M+, *Int J Dermatol* 32, 675
(1993): Pellicano R+, *Int J Dermatol* 32, 675
Photosensitivity
(1993): Vinks SA+, *Lancet* 341, 1221
Pruritus (2%)
(1996): Holloway WJ+, *Am J Med* 100, 52S
(1985): Richards DM+, *Drugs* 29, 105
Rash (sic) (2%)
(1996): Holloway WJ+, *Am J Med* 100, 52S
Stevens–Johnson syndrome (2%)
Toxic epidermal necrolysis (2%)
Toxic erythema
(1995): Rademaker M, *N Z Med J* 108, 165
Toxic pustuloderma
(1990): Rustin MHA+, *Br J Dermatol* 123, 119
Urticaria (<1%)

#### Other

Anaphylactoid reactions (2%)
(1985): Richards DM+, *Drugs* 29, 105
Dysgeusia
Glossitis
Hypersensitivity (2%)
(2001): Romano A+, *Allergy* 56, 84
Injection-site burning
Injection-site cellulitis
Injection-site edema
Injection-site inflammation (2%)
Injection-site pain (1.4%)
(1989): Gaut PL+, *Am J Med* 87 (Suppl 5A), 169S
Injection-site thrombophlebitis (2%)
Oral candidiasis
Paresthesias (<1%)
Phlebitis (<1%)
Serum sickness
Vaginal candidiasis
Vaginitis (1%)

## CEFTIBUTEN

**Trade name:** Cedax (Schering)
**Other common trade names:** *Ceten; Cilecef; Keimax; Seftem*
**Indications:** Various infections caused by susceptible organisms
**Category:** Third generation cephalosporin
**Half-life:** 2 hours

**Note:** Penicillin and cephalosporins share a common beta-lactam structure. People who are allergic to penicillin are approximately 4 times more likely to develop an allergic reaction to a cephalosporin than those people who have no penicillin allergy. (From 5 to 16% of patients allergic to penicillin develop allergic reactions to cephalosporins)

### *Reactions*

#### Skin

Candidiasis (<1%)
Diaper rash (<1%)
Pruritus (0.3%)
Rash (sic) (0.3%)
Stevens–Johnson syndrome (<1%)
Toxic epidermal necrolysis
Urticaria (<1%)

#### Other

Dysgeusia (<1%)
Hypersensitivity
Oral candidiasis
Paresthesias (<1%)
Serum sickness (<1%)
Vaginitis (<1%)
Xerostomia (<1%)

## CEFTIZOXIME

**Trade name:** Cefizox (Fujisawa)
**Other common trade names:** *Ceftix; Ceftrax; Epocelin; Lyceft; Rocephin; Tefidox; Ultracef*
**Indications:** Various infections caused by susceptible organisms
**Category:** Third generation cephalosporin antibiotic
**Half-life:** 1.6 hours

**Note:** Penicillin and cephalosporins share a common beta-lactam structure. People who are allergic to penicillin are approximately 4 times more likely to develop an allergic reaction to a cephalosporin than those people who have no penicillin allergy. (From 5 to 16% of patients allergic to penicillin develop allergic reactions to cephalosporins)

### *Reactions*

#### Skin

Candidiasis (<1%)
Pruritus (1–5%)
Rash (sic) (1–5%)

Stevens–Johnson syndrome (<1%)
Toxic epidermal necrolysis
Urticaria (<1%)

### Other

Anaphylactoid reactions (<1%)
Injection-site edema
Injection-site induration
Injection-site pain (1–5%)
Injection-site phlebitis (1–5%)
Oral candidiasis
Paresthesias (1–5%)
Phlebitis (<1%)
Serum sickness (<1%)
Vaginitis (<1%)

## CEFTRIAXONE

**Trade name:** Rocephin (Roche)
**Other common trade names:** *Benaxona; Cefaxona; Cefaxone; Rocefin; Rocephalin; Rocephine; Tacex; Triaken; Zefone*
**Indications:** Various infections caused by susceptible organisms
**Category:** Third generation cephalosporin
**Half-life:** 5–9 hours

**Note:** Penicillin and cephalosporins share a common beta-lactam structure. People who are allergic to penicillin are approximately 4 times more likely to develop an allergic reaction to a cephalosporin than those people who have no penicillin allergy. (From 5 to 16% of patients allergic to penicillin develop allergic reactions to cephalosporins)

### *Reactions*

### Skin

Angioedema
(1984): Richards DM+, *Drugs* 27, 469
Candidiasis (sic) (5%)
(2002): Lamb HM+, *Drugs* 62(7), 1041
(1983): Bittner MJ+, *Antimicrob Agents Chemother* 23, 261 (superficial) (sic)
(1983): Harrison CJ+, *Am J Dis Child* 137, 1048 (superficial) (sic) (5%)
Chills (<1%)
Cutaneous side effects (sic) (3%)
(1984): Richards DM+, *Drugs* 27, 469
Dermatitis (sic)
(1989): Baba S+, *Jap J Antibiotics* 42, 212 (4%)
(1984): Richards DM+, *Drugs* 27, 469 (0.4%)
Diaphoresis (0.2%)
(1984): Moskowitz BL, *Am J Med* 77 (Suppl 4C) 84
Erythema multiforme
(1984): Richards DM+, *Drugs* 27, 469
Exanthems
(1990): Schaad UB+, *N Engl J Med* 322, 141 (4%)
(1988): Richards DM+, *Drugs* 35, 604
(1985): Judson FN+, *JAMA* 253, 1417 (1.2%)
(1984): Moskowitz BL, *Am J Med* 77 (Suppl 4C), 84 (1.74%)
(1984): Richards DM+, *Drugs* 27, 469 (1.4%)
(1983): Eron LJ+, *J Antimicrob Chemother* 12, 65 (6%)
Flushing (<1%)
(1984): Moskowitz BL, *Am J Med* 77 (Suppl 4C), 84 (0.15%)
(1983): Harrison CJ+, *Am J Dis Child* 137, 1048
Jarisch–Herxheimer reaction
(1994): Strominger MB+, *J Neuroophthalmol* 14, 77
Linear IgA bullous dermatosis
(1999): Yawalker N+, *Dermatology* 199, 25
Pemphigus
(1992): Ruocco V+, *Acta Derm Venereol* (Stockh) 72, 48
Pruritus (<1%)
(1984): Moskowitz BL, *Am J Med* 77 (Suppl 4C) 84 (0.34%)
(1984): Richards DM+, *Drugs* 27, 469 (0.3%)
Purpura
Rash (sic) (1.7%)
(2002): Lamb HM+, *Drugs* 62(7), 1041
(1992): Francioli P+, *JAMA* 267, 264
(1983): Eron LJ+, *J Antimicrob Chemother* 12, 65
Status epilepticus
(2001): Martinez-Rodriguez JE+, *Am J Med* 111
Stevens–Johnson syndrome
Toxic epidermal necrolysis
Urticaria (0.1%)
(1984): Richards DM+, *Drugs* 27, 469

### Other

Anaphylactoid reactions
(1999): Romano A+, *J Allergy Clin Immunol* 104, 1113
(1992): Lin RY, *Arch Intern Med* 152, 930 (17 cases)
(1984): Richards DM+, *Drugs* 27, 469
Dysgeusia (<1%)
(1992): Francioli P+, *JAMA* 267, 264
Glossitis
(1984): Moskowitz BL, *Am J Med* 77 (Suppl 4C), 84
(1984): Richards DM+, *Drugs* 27, 469
Hypersensitivity
(2000): Demoly P+, *Allergy* 55, 418 (immediate)
(2000): Romano A+, *Allergy* 55, 415 (immediate)
Injection-site induration
Injection-site pain (1–10%)
(1992): Francioli P+, *JAMA* 267, 264
(1984): Moskowitz BL, *Am J Med* 77 (Suppl 4C), 84 (1%)
(1984): Richards DM+, *Drugs* 27, 469 (1–15%)
Injection-site phlebitis (<1%)
(1984): Moskowitz BL, *Am J Med* 77 (Suppl 4C), 84 (0.95%)
(1984): Richards DM+, *Drugs* 27, 469
Oral mucosal eruption
(1984): Richards DM+, *Drugs* 27, 469
Serum sickness
(1984): Moskowitz BL, *Am J Med* 77 (Suppl 4C), 84 (0.04%)
Vaginitis (<1%)

## CEFUROXIME

**Trade names:** Ceftin (GSK); Kefurox (Lilly); Zinacef (GSK)
**Other common trade names:** *Cefuril; Cepazine; Elobact; Froxal; Zinacet; Zinat; Zinnat; Zoref*
**Indications:** Various infections caused by susceptible organisms
**Category:** Second generation cephalosporin
**Half-life:** 1–2 hours

**Note:** Penicillin and cephalosporins share a common beta-lactam structure. People who are allergic to penicillin are approximately 4 times more likely to develop an allergic reaction to a cephalosporin than those people who have no penicillin allergy. (From 5 to 16% of patients allergic to penicillin develop allergic reactions to cephalosporins)

### *Reactions*

### Skin

Acute generalized exanthematous pustulosis (AGEP)
(2001): Cohen AD+, *Int J Dermatol* 40(7), 458

(1995): Moreau A+, *Int J Dermatol* 34, 263 (passim)
Angioedema (< 1%)
Erythema multiforme (< 1%)
Exanthems
(1997): Litt JZ, Beachwood, OH (personal case) (observation)
(1990): Schaad UB+, *N Engl J Med* 332, 141 (6%)
(1979): Brogden RN+, *Drugs* 17, 233 (4.4–6.7% in penicillin-allergic patients)
Jarisch–Herxheimer reaction
(1992): Nadelman RB+, *Ann Intern Med* 117, 273
Pemphigus
(1997): Brenner S+, *J Am Acad Dermatol* 36, 919
Perianal thrush
(1987): Carson JWK+, *J Antimicrob Chemother* 19, 109
Pruritus (< 1%)
Purpura
Pustular eruption
(1990): Rustin MHA+, *Br J Dermatol* 123, 119
Rash (sic) (< 1%)
(1988): *Med Lett* 30, 57
Stevens–Johnson syndrome (< 1%)
Toxic epidermal necrolysis (< 1%)
(1997): Yossepowitch O+, *Eur J Med Res* 2, 182
(1993): Correia O+, *Dermatology* 186, 32
Urticaria (< 1%)
(1995): Litt JZ, Beachwood, OH (personal case) (observation)
(1987): Parish LC+, *Int J Dermatol* 26, 389

### Other

Anaphylactoid reactions (< 1%)
(2002): Prosser DP+, *Paediatr Anaesth* 12(1), 73
Hypersensitivity
(1998): Romano A+, *J Allergy Clin Immunol* 101, 564
(1992): Romano A+, *Contact Dermatitis* 27, 270
(1991): Powell DA+, *Drug Intell Clin Pharm* 25, 1236
Injection-site pain (< 1%)
Oral candidiasis
(1985): Cooper TJ+, *J Antimicrobial Chemother* 16, 373
Serum sickness (< 1%)
Thrombophlebitis (1–10%)
Vaginitis (< 1%)
(1988): *Med Lett* 30, 57

## CELECOXIB

**Trade name:** Celebrex (Pfizer)
**Indications:** Osteoarthritis, rheumatoid arthritis
**Category:** A benzene-sulfonamide NSAID (Cox-2 inhibitor)*
**Half-life:** 11 hours

### *Reactions*

### Skin

Acute febrile neutrophilic dermatosis (Sweet's syndrome)
(2001): Fye KH+, *J Am Acad Dermatol* 45, 300
Allergic reactions (sic) (<2%)
Angioedema
(2002): Schneider F+, *Lancet* 359, 852
(2001): Kelkar PS+, *J Rheumatol* 28(11), 2553
Bacterial infection (sic) (<2%)
Candidiasis (<2%)
(1999): McClain SA, Bronx, NY (from Internet) (observation)
Dermatitis (sic) (<2%)
Diaphoresis (<2%)
Ecchymoses (<2%)
Erythema multiforme
(1999): Puritz E, Smithtown, NY (from Internet) (observation)
Exanthems (<2%)
(2002): Schneider F+, *Lancet* 359, 852
(2002): Verbeiren S+, *Ann Dermatol Venereol* 129(2), 203
(2000): Valentine MC, Everett, WA (from internet) (observation) (patient was allergic to sulfa)
(1999): Fisher BJ, Toronto, Ontario (from Internet) (observation)
(1999): Graedon J+, *People's Pharmacy* (anecdote from a reader)
(1999): Jaffe PG, Columbia, SC (from Internet) (observation) patient had "trouble" with sulfa years back
(1999): Litt JZ, Beachwood, OH (personal case) (observation)
(1999): Rudolph RI, Wyomissing, PA (from Internet) (observation)
Facial edema (<2%)
Generalized edema (<2%)
Herpes simplex (<2%)
Herpes zoster (<2%)
Hot flashes (<2%)
Peripheral edema (2.1%)
(2000): Fetterman MR, Miami, FL (from Internet) (observation) (leg)
(2000): Panagotacos PJ, San Francisco, CA (from Internet) (observation) (pedal)
(1999): Simon LS+, *JAMA* 282, 1921
Photoreactions
(1999): Zabawski E, Dallas, TX (from Internet) (observation)
Photosensitivity (<2%)
Pruritus (<2%)
(1999): Rudolph RI, Wyomissing, PA (from Internet) (observation)
Psoriasis (palmoplantar)
(2000): Catalano PM, Bradenton, FL (from Internet) (observation)
Rash (sic) (2.2%)
Skin nodule (sic) (<2%)
Soft tissue infection (sic) (<2%)
Stevens–Johnson syndrome
(1999): Puritz E, Smithtown, NY (from Internet) (observation)
Toxic epidermal necrolysis
(2000): Mitchell D, Thomasville, GA (from Internet) (observation)
Urticaria (<2%)
(2002): Schneider F+, *Lancet* 359, 852
(2001): Kelkar PS+, *J Rheumatol* 28(11), 2553
Vasculitis
(2002): Schneider F+, *Lancet* 359, 852
Viral infection (sic) (<2%)
Xerosis (<2%)

### Hair

Hair – alopecia (<2%)

### Nails

Nails – disorder (sic) (<2%)

### Other

Anaphylactoid reactions
(2001): Habki R+, *Ann Med Interne* (Paris) 152(5), 355
(2001): Levy MB+, *Ann Allergy Asthma Immunol* 87, 72
Application site cellulitis (<2%)
Application-site reactions (<2%)
Death
(2002): Schneider F+, *Lancet* 359, 852
(2001): Weaver J+, *Am J Gastroenterol* 96(12), 3449
Dysgeusia (<2%)
Hypesthesia (<2%)
Mastodynia (<2%)

Myalgia (<2%)
Paresthesias (<2%)
Pseudoporphyria
(2000): Cummins R+, *J Rheumatol* 27, 2938
Stomatitis (<2%)
Tendinitis (<2%)
Thrombophlebitis (<0.1%)
Tooth disorder (sic) (<2%)
Vaginal candidiasis (<2%)
Vaginitis (<2%)
Xerostomia (<2%)

***Note:** Celecoxib is a sulfonamide and can be absorbed systemically. Sulfonamides can produce severe, possibly fatal, reactions such as toxic epidermal necrolysis and Stevens–Johnson syndrome

# CEPHALEXIN

**Trade names:** Keflex (Dista); Keftab (DJ Pharma)
**Other common trade names:** *Apo-Cephalex; Biocet; Ceforal; Ceporex; Ceporexine; Kefarol; Novo-Lexin; Ospexin*
**Indications:** Various infections caused by susceptible organisms
**Category:** First generation cephalosporin
**Half-life:** 0.9–1.2 hours
**Clinically important, potentially hazardous interactions with:** amikacin, gentamicin

**Note:** Penicillin and cephalosporins share a common beta-lactam structure. People who are allergic to penicillin are approximately 4 times more likely to develop an allergic reaction to a cephalosporin than those people who have no penicillin allergy. (From 5 to 16% of patients allergic to penicillin develop allergic reactions to cephalosporins)

### *Reactions*

## Skin

Acute generalized exanthematous pustulosis (AGEP)
(1995): Moreau A+, *Int J Dermatol* 34, 263 (passim)
Angioedema (<1%)
(1971): Griffith RS+, *Lancet* 1, 452 (0.7%)
Bullous pemphigoid
(2001): Czechowicz RT, *Australas J Dermatol* 42(2), 132
Contact dermatitis
(1986): Milligan A+, *Contact Dermatitis* 15, 91
Cutaneous side effects (sic) (2%)
(1972): Speight TM+, *Drugs* 3, 9
(1971): Griffith RS+, *Lancet* 1, 452 (0.9%)
Erythema multiforme (<1%)
(1998): Blumenthal HL, Beachwood, OH (personal case) (observation)
(1992): Murray KM+, *Ann Pharmacotherapy* 26, 1230
(1988): Platt R+, *J Infect Dis* 158, 474
(1987): Norrby SR, *Drugs* 34 (Suppl 2), 105
Exanthems
(1999): Litt JZ, Beachwood, OH (personal case) (observation)
(1997): McCloskey GL+, *Cutis* 59, 251
(1995): Litt JZ, Beachwood, OH (personal case) (observation)
(1972): Speight TM+, *Drugs* 3, 9
(1970): 8, 18 (1–5%)
Fixed eruption
(1991): Baran R+, *Br J Dermatol* 125, 592
Pemphigus
(1992): Vaillant L+, *Int J Dermatol* 31, 67
(1991): Wolf R+, *Int J Dermatol* 30, 213
Pruritus
(1999): Litt JZ, Beachwood, OH (personal case) (observation)
(1988): Kumar A+, *Antimicrob Agents Chemother* 32, 882
(1977): Okita K+, *Jpn J Antibiot* (Japanese) 30, 911
(1971): Griffith RS+, *Lancet* 1, 452 (0.7%)
Pruritus ani et vulvae
Purpura
Pustular eruption
(1994): Spencer JM+, *Br J Dermatol* 130, 514
(1988): Jackson H+, *Dermatologica* 177, 292
Rash (sic) (<1%)
Stevens–Johnson syndrome (<1%)
(1992): Murray KM+, *Ann Pharmacother* 26, 1230
(1988): Platt R+, *J Infect Dis* 158, 474
(1975): McArthur JE+, *N Z Med J* 81, 390
Toxic epidermal necrolysis (<1%)
(1995): Jick H+, *Pharmacotherapy* 15, 428
(1991): Dave J+, *J Antimicrob Chemotherapy* 28, 477
(1987): Harnar TJ+, *J Burn Care Rehabil* 8, 554
(1987): Hogan DJ+, *J Am Acad Dermatol* 17, 852
Urticaria (<1%)
(1993): Litt JZ, Beachwood, OH (personal case) (observation)
(1971): Griffith RS+, *Lancet* 1, 452 (0.7%)

## Nails

Nails – paronychia
(1991): Baran R+, *Br J Dermatol* 125, 592

## Other

Anaphylactoid reactions (<1%)
(1999): Nordt SP+, *Am J Emerg Med* 17, 492
(1992): Lin RY, *Arch Intern Med* 152, 930 (17 cases)
(1989): Hoffman DR+, *Ann Allergy* 62, 91 (fatal)
Hypersensitivity
Oral candidiasis
Serum sickness (<1%)
(1988): Platt R+, *J Infect Dis* 158, 474
Vaginitis

# CEPHALOTHIN

**Trade names:** Keflin (Lilly); Kefzol (Lilly)
**Other common trade names:** *Ceftina; Ceporacin; Cepovenin; Keflin Neutral; Keflin Neutro; Keflin-N; Practogen*
**Indications:** Various infections caused by susceptible organisms
**Category:** First generation, broad spectrum cephalosporin
**Half-life:** 30–50 minutes
**Clinically important, potentially hazardous interactions with:** amphotericin B, gentamicin

**Note:** Penicillin and cephalosporins share a common beta-lactam structure. People who are allergic to penicillin are approximately 4 times more likely to develop an allergic reaction to a cephalosporin than those people who have no penicillin allergy. (From 5 to 16% of patients allergic to penicillin develop allergic reactions to cephalosporins)

### *Reactions*

## Skin

Allergic reactions (sic)
(1975): Braun WP, *Contact Dermatitis* 1, 190
(1966): Thoburn R+, *JAMA* 198, 345 (8%)
Candidiasis (<1%)
Erythema multiforme
(1996): Munoz-D+, *Contact Dermatitis* 34, 227
Exanthems (<1%)
(1974): Sanders WE+, *N Engl J Med* 290, 424 (>5%)

(1966): Merrill SL+, *Ann Intern Med* 64, 1 (1–5%)
(1966): Thoburn R+, *JAMA* 198, 345 (5.5%)
(1964): Griffith RS+, *JAMA* 189, 823 (5%)
(1964): Weinstein L+, *JAMA* 189, 829 (1–5%)
Pruritus (<1%)
(1966): Beaty HN+, *Ann Intern Med* 65, 641
Purpura
(1980): Miescher PA+, *Clin Haematol* 9, 505
(1968): Sheiman L+, *JAMA* 203, 601
Rash (sic)
Stevens–Johnson syndrome (<1%)
Toxic epidermal necrolysis
(1988): Dreyfuss DA+, *Ann Plast Surg* 20, 146
Urticaria
(1979): Branch DR+, *JAMA* 241, 495
(1966): Beaty HN+, *Ann Intern Med* 65, 641
(1966): Perkins RL+, *Ann Intern Med* 64, 13 (>5%)
(1966): Thoburn R+, *JAMA* 198, 345 (4%)

### Other

Anaphylactoid reactions
(1987): Norrby SR, *Drugs* 34 (Suppl 2) 105
(1974): Spruill FG+, *JAMA* 229, 440 (2 patients; both fatal)
(1971): Petz LD, *Postgrad Med J* 47 Suppl, 64 (2 cases)
(1966): Rothschild PD+, *JAMA* 196, 372
Injection-site induration (<1%)
Injection-site pain (<1%)
Phlebitis
(1980): Meguro S+, *Jpn J Antibiot* 33, 1163
(1976): Sorrentino AP+, *Am J Hosp Pharm* 33, 642
(1973): Carrizosa J+, *Antimicrob Agents Chemother* 3, 306
(1973): Inagaki J+, *Curr Ther Res Clin Exp* 15, 37
(1973): Lane AZ+, *Antimicrob Agents Chemother* 2, 234
Serum sickness (<1%)
(1974): Sanders WE+, *N Engl J Med* 290, 424

## CEPHAPIRIN

**Trade name:** Cefadyl (Bristol-Myers Squibb)
**Other common trade names:** *Brisfirina; Cefaloject; Cefatrex; Cefatrexyl; Lopitrex; Unipirin*
**Indications:** Various infections caused by susceptible organisms
**Category:** First generation cephalosporin antibiotic
**Half-life:** 36–60 minutes

**Note:** Penicillin and cephalosporins share a common beta-lactam structure. People who are allergic to penicillin are approximately 4 times more likely to develop an allergic reaction to a cephalosporin than those people who have no penicillin allergy. (From 5 to 16% of patients allergic to penicillin develop allergic reactions to cephalosporins)

### *Reactions*

### Skin

Candidiasis (<1%)
Erythema multiforme
Pruritus (1–5%)
Rash (sic) (1–5%)
Stevens–Johnson syndrome (<1%)
Toxic epidermal necrolysis
Urticaria (<1%)

### Other

Anaphylactoid reactions
(1979): Barnett AS+, *Anesth Analg* 58, 337
Hypersensitivity
Injection-site pain (1–5%)
Injection-site phlebitis (1–5%)
Paresthesias (1–5%)
Phlebitis
(1980): Meguro S+, *Jpn J Antibiot* 33, 1163
(1976): Sorrentino AP+, *Am J Hosp Pharm* 33, 642
(1973): Carrizosa J+, *Antimicrob Agents Chemother* 3, 306
(1973): Inagaki J+, *Curr Ther Res Clin Exp* 15, 37
(1973): Lane AZ+, *Antimicrob Agents Chemother* 2, 234
Serum sickness (<1%)
Vaginitis

## CEPHRADINE

**Trade name:** Velosef (Bristol-Myers Squibb)
**Other common trade names:** *Anspor; Cefro; Celex; Doncef; Eskacef; Maxisporin; Opebrin; Sefril; Veracef*
**Indications:** Various infections caused by susceptible organisms
**Category:** First generation cephalosporin
**Half-life:** 1–2 hours

**Note:** Penicillin and cephalosporins share a common beta-lactam structure. People who are allergic to penicillin are approximately 4 times more likely to develop an allergic reaction to a cephalosporin than those people who have no penicillin allergy. (From 5 to 16% of patients allergic to penicillin develop allergic reactions to cephalosporins)

### *Reactions*

### Skin

Acute generalized exanthematous pustulosis (AGEP)
(1995): Moreau A+, *Int J Dermatol* 34, 263 (passim)
Erythema multiforme
Exanthems
(1976): Brillinberg Wurth GH+, *Curr Res Med Opin* 4, 139
Pruritus (<1%)
Purpura
Pustular eruption
(1986): Kalb RE+, *Cutis* 38, 58
Rash (sic) (<1%)
Stevens–Johnson syndrome (<1%)
Toxic epidermal necrolysis
(1990): Balcar-Boron A+, *Wiad Lek* (Polish) 43, 988
Toxic pustuloderma
(1990): Rustin MHA+, *Br J Dermatol* 123, 119
Urticaria (<1%)

### Other

Anaphylactoid reactions
Hypersensitivity
Injection-site pain (<1%)
Injection-site phlebitis (<1%)
Serum sickness
Vaginitis

# CETIRIZINE

**Synonyms:** P-071; UCB-P071
**Trade name:** Zyrtec (Pfizer)
**Other common trade names:** *Alercet; Alerid; Cetrine; Cezin; Reactine; Triz; Virlix; Zirtin*
**Indications:** Allergic rhinitis, urticaria
**Category:** Antihistamine
**Half-life:** 8–11 hours
**Clinically important, potentially hazardous interactions with: alcohol**, CNS depressants

### *Reactions*

**Skin**

Acne (<2%)
Angioedema (<2%)
Bullous eruption (<2%)
Dermatitis (sic) (<2%)
Diaphoresis (<2%)
Edema (periorbital, facial, ankle, generalized, peripheral)
Exanthems (<2%)
(1998): Rehbein H, Jacksonville, FL (generalized) (from Internet) (observation)
(1997): Stingeni L+, *Contact Dermatitis* 37, 249
Facial edema
(2002): Schroer S+, *Clin Exp Dermatol* 27, 185
Fixed eruption
(2000): Kranke B+, *J Allergy Clin Immunol* 106(5), 988 (multilocalized and bullous)
Flushing (<2%)
Furunculosis (<2%)
Hyperkeratosis (<2%)
Photosensitivity (<2%)
Phototoxicity (<2%)
Pruritus (<2%)
(2002): Schroer S+, *Clin Exp Dermatol* 27, 185
Purpura (<2%)
Rash (sic) (<2%)
Seborrhea (<2%)
Urticaria (<2%)
(2002): Schroer S+, *Clin Exp Dermatol* 27, 185
(2001): Calista D+, *Br J Dermatol* 144, 196
(1999): Karamfilov T+, *Br J Dermatol* 140, 979
(1997): Stingeni L+, *Contact Dermatitis* 37, 249
Xerosis (<2%)

**Hair**

Hair – alopecia (<2%)
(1998): Reed BR, Denver, CO (from Internet) (observation)
Hair – hypertrichosis (<2%)

**Other**

Ageusia (<2%)
Anaphylactoid reactions (<2%)
Dysgeusia (<2%)
Hyperesthesia (<2%)
Hypesthesia (<2%)
Mastodynia (<2%)
Myalgia (<2%)
Paresthesias (<2%)
Parosmia (<2%)
Sialorrhea (<2%)
Stomatitis (<2%)
Tongue discoloration (<2%)
Tongue edema (<2%)
Vaginitis (<2%)
Xerostomia (5.7%)
(1995): Breneman D+, *J Am Acad Dermatol* 33, 192

# CETRORELIX

**Trade name:** Cetrotide (Serono)
**Indications:** Inhibition of premature luteinizing hormone surges in women undergoing controlled ovarian stimulation
**Category:** Antigonadotropic
**Half-life:** 5 hours

### *Reactions*

**Skin**

Peripheral edema

**Other**

Anaphylactoid reactions
Injection-site edema
Injection-site erythema
(1994): Leroy I+, *Fertil Steril* 62, 461
Injection-site pruritus
(1994): Leroy I+, *Fertil Steril* 62, 461
Injection-site purpura

# CEVIMELINE

**Trade name:** Exovac (SnowBrand)
**Indications:** Sicca syndrome in patients with Sjøgren's syndrome
**Category:** Muscarinic agonist; cholinergic agent
**Half-life:** 3–4 hours

### *Reactions*

**Skin**

Allergy (sic) (1–10%)
Bullous eruption (<1%)
Dermatitis (sic) (<1%)
Diaphoresis (20%)
Eczema (<1%)
Edema (1–10%)
Exanthems (1–10%)
Flu-like syndrome (sic) (1–10%)
Fungal infection (sic) (1–10%)
Genital pruritus (<1%)
Hot flashes (2%)
Peripheral edema (1–10%)
Photosensitivity (<1%)
Pruritus (1–10%)
Rash (sic) (4%)
Ulceration (<1%)
Vasculitis (<1%)
Xerosis (<1%)

**Hair**

Hair – alopecia (<1%)

**Other**

Dysgeusia (<1%)
Gingival hyperplasia (<1%)
Hypesthesia (1–10%)

Myalgia (1–10%)
Paresthesias (<1%)
Parosmia (<1%)
Sialorrhea (2%)
Stomatitis (<1%)
Tendinitis (<1%)
Thrombophlebitis (<1%)
Tongue discoloration (<1%)
Tongue ulceration (<1%)
Tooth disorder (sic) (1–10%)
Tremors (1–10%)
Ulcerative stomatitis (1–10%)
Vaginitis (1–10%)
Xerostomia (1–10%)

# CHAMOMILE

**Scientific names:** *Chamomilla recutita; Matricaria chamomilla; Matricaria recutita*
**Other common names:** Camomille Allemande; Echte Kamille; Fleur de Camomile; German Chamomile; Manzanilla; Pin Heads; Wild Chamomile
**Family:** Asteraceae; Compositae
**Purported indications:** Flatulence, travel sickness, nervous diarrhea, restlessness, menstrual cramps
**Other uses:** Hemorrhoids, mastitis, leg ulcers, inflammation of the respiratory tract. Used in flavoring, cosmetics, soaps and mouthwashes

### *Reactions*

## Skin
Allergic reactions (sic) (to those allergic to ragweed, marigolds, daisies)
Contact dermatitis
(2000): Foti C+, *Contact Dermatitis* 42(6), 360
(2000): Giordano-Labadie F+, *Contact Dermatitis* 42(4), 247
Irritation

## Other
Anaphylactoid reactions
(2001): Thien FC, *Med J Aust* 175(1), 54 (from enema)
(1989): Subiza J+, *J Allergy Clin Immunol* 84, 353
Hypersensitivity

# CHLORAL HYDRATE

**Synonyms:** chloral; hydrated chloral
**Trade names:** Aquachloral (Alcon); Noctec (Bristol-Myers Squibb)
**Other common trade names:** *Chloraldurat; Medianox; Novochlorhydrate; Somnox; Welldorm*
**Indications:** Insomnia, sedation
**Category:** Sedative hypnotic
**Half-life:** 8–11 hours
**Clinically important, potentially hazardous interactions with:** antihistamines, azatadine, azelastine, brompheniramine, buclizine, chlorpheniramine, clemastine, dexchlorpheniramine, diphenhydramine, meclizine, tripelennamine

### *Reactions*

## Skin
Acne
(1967): Hitch JM, *JAMA* 200, 879
(1956): Christianson HB+, *Arch Dermatol* 74, 232
Angioedema
(1973): Almeyda J+, *Br J Dermatol* 86, 313
(1956): Christianson HB+, *Arch Dermatol* 74, 232
Bullous eruption
(1967): Coleman WP, *Med Clin North Am* 51, 1073
Dermatitis (sic)
(1987): de Groot AC+, *Contact Dermatitis* 16, 229
(1956): Christianson HB+, *Arch Dermatol* 74, 232
Eczematous eruption (sic)
(1956): Christianson HB+, *Arch Dermatol* 74, 232
Erythema
(1956): Christianson HB+, *Arch Dermatol* 74, 232
Erythema multiforme
(1991): Porteous DM+, *Arch Dermatol* 127, 740 (in AIDS)
(1956): Christianson HB+, *Arch Dermatol* 74, 232
Exanthems
(1990): Lindner K+, *Dermatol Monatsschr* (German) 176, 483
(1976): Arndt KA+, *JAMA* 235, 918 (0.02%)
(1956): Christianson HB+, *Arch Dermatol* 74, 232
Fixed eruption
(1973): Almeyda J+, *Br J Dermatol* 86, 313
(1972): Verbov J, *Br J Dermatol* 86, 438
(1966): Miller LH+, *Arch Dermatol* 94, 60
(1961): Welsh AL+, *Arch Dermatol* 84, 1004
(1956): Christianson HB+, *Arch Dermatol* 74, 232
Flushing
(1956): Christianson HB+, *Arch Dermatol* 74, 232
Lichenoid eruption
(1956): Christianson HB+, *Arch Dermatol* 74, 232
Perioral dermatitis
(2001): Caksen H+, *Pediatr Dermatol* 18(5), 454
Pruritus
(1990): Lindner K+, *Dermatol Monatsschr* (German) 176, 483
(1956): Christianson HB+, *Arch Dermatol* 74, 232
Purpura
(1973): Almeyda J+, *Br J Dermatol* 86, 313
(1956): Christianson HB+, *Arch Dermatol* 74, 232
Rash (sic) (1–10%)
Ulceration
(1956): Christianson HB+, *Arch Dermatol* 74, 232
Urticaria (1–10%)
(1973): Almeyda J+, *Br J Dermatol* 86, 313
(1956): Christianson HB+, *Arch Dermatol* 74, 232

## Other
Acute intermittent porphyria

Death
(2001): Gaulier JM+, *J Forensic Sci* 46(6), 1507 (2 cases)
Dysgeusia
Hypersensitivity
Oral mucosal lesions
(2001): Caksen H+, *Pediatr Dermatol* 18(5), 454
(1956): Christianson HB+, *Arch Dermatol* 74, 232
Oral ulceration
(1956): Christianson HB+, *Arch Dermatol* 74, 232
Stomatitis
(1956): Christianson HB+, *Arch Dermatol* 74, 232

# CHLORAMBUCIL

**Trade name:** Leukeran (GSK)
**Other common trade names:** *Chloraminophene; Linfolysin*
**Indications:** Chronic lymphocytic leukemia, lymphomas, carcinomas
**Category:** Antineoplastic
**Half-life:** 1.5 hours
**Clinically important, potentially hazardous interactions with:** aldesleukin, antineoplastics, azathioprine, bone-marrow suppressants, **vaccines**

### *Reactions*

## Skin

Angioedema
(1977): Millard LG+, *Arch Dermatol* 113, 1298
Cutaneous necrosis
(1972): Decker JL, *Ann Intern Med* 76, 619
Cutaneous side effects (sic)
(1968): Moore GE+, *Cancer Chemother Abstr* 52, 661 (20%)
Edema
Erythema multiforme
(1987): Hitchens RN+, *Aust N Z J Med* 17, 600
Exanthems
(1992): Breathnach SM+, *Adverse Drug Reactions and the Skin* Blackwell, Oxford, 289 (passim)
(1987): Hitchens RN+, *Aust N Z J Med* 17, 600
(1986): Peterman A+, *Arch Dermatol* 122, 1358
(1978): Franchimont P+, *J Rheumatol* 5, 85 (1.3%)
(1977): Millard LG+, *Arch Dermatol* 113, 1298
(1971): Knisely RE+, *Arch Dermatol* 104, 77
(1968): Vissian L+, *Bull Soc Fr Dermatol Syphiligr* (French) 75, 570
Exfoliative dermatitis
(1987): Hitchens RN+, *Aust N Z J Med* 17, 600
Facial erythema
(1986): Peterman A+, *Arch Dermatol* 122, 1358
Herpes simplex
(1984): Sahgal SM+, *J R Soc Med* 77, 144
(1971): Degos R+, *Bull Soc Fr Dermatol Syphiligr* (French) 78, 631
Herpes zoster
(2002): Goldstein DA+, *Ophthalmology* 109(2), 370
(1972): Decker JL, *Ann Intern Med* 76, 619 (>5%)
Kaposi's sarcoma
(1974): Faye I+, *Bull Soc Fr Dermatol Syphiligr* (French) 81, 379
Lupus erythematosus
(1986): Peterman A+, *Arch Dermatol* 122, 1358
Pellagra
(1987): Schmutz JL+, *Ann Dermatol Venereol* (French) 114, 569
Periorbital edema
(1992): Breathnach SM+, *Adverse Drug Reactions and the Skin* Blackwell, Oxford, 289 (passim)
(1986): Peterman A+, *Arch Dermatol* 122, 1358
(1977): Millard LG+, *Arch Dermatol* 113, 1298
Photosensitivity
(1987): Schmutz JL+, *Ann Dermatol Venereol* (French) 114, 569
Pruritus
(1971): Knisely RE+, *Arch Dermatol* 104, 77
(1968): Vissian L+, *Bull Soc Fr Dermatol Syphiligr* (French) 75, 570
Psoriasis (exacerbation)
(1968): Vissian L+, *Bull Soc Fr Dermatol Syphiligr* (French) 75, 570
Purpura
(1990): Pietrantonio F+, *Cancer Lett* 54, 109
Rash (sic) (1–10%)
Sezary syndrome
(1981): Ferme F+, *Leuk Res* 5, 169
Stevens–Johnson syndrome
Toxic epidermal necrolysis
(1997): Aydogdu I+, *Anticancer Drugs* 8, 468
(1990): Barone C+, *Eur J Cancer* 26, 1262
(1990): Pietrantonio F+, *Cancer Lett* 54, 109
(1968): Vissian L+, *Bull Soc Fr Dermatol Syphiligr* (French) 75, 570
Urticaria
(1992): Breathnach SM+, *Adverse Drug Reactions and the Skin* Blackwell, Oxford, 289 (passim)
(1977): Millard LG+, *Arch Dermatol* 113, 1298
(1971): Knisely RE+, *Arch Dermatol* 104, 77
(1968): Vissian L+, *Bull Soc Fr Dermatol Syphiligr* (French) 75, 570

## Hair

Hair – alopecia
(1992): Breathnach SM+, *Adverse Drug Reactions and the Skin* Blackwell, Oxford, 289 (passim)
(1978): Franchimont P+, *J Rheumatol* 5, 85 (1.3%)
(1978): Levine N+, *Cancer Treat Rev* 5, 67
(1973): Snaith ML+, *BMJ* 2, 197

## Other

Acute intermittent porphyria
Hypersensitivity (<1%)
(1971): Knisley RE+, *Arch Dermatol* 104, 77
Oral mucosal lesions
(1968): Moore GE+, *Cancer Chemother Abstr* 52, 661 (2%)
Oral ulceration (<1%)
(1987): Hitchens RN+, *Aust N Z J Med* 17, 600
Stomatitis

# CHLORAMPHENICOL

**Trade names:** AK-Chlor (Alcon); Chloromycetin (Parke-Davis); Chloroptic (Allergan); Ophthochlor (Parke-Davis)
**Other common trade names:** *Aquamycetin; Cebenicol; Diochloram; Kloramfenicol; Oleomycetin; Pentamycetin; Sopamycetin; Tifomycine*
**Indications:** Various infections caused by susceptible organisms
**Category:** Broad spectrum antibiotic
**Half-life:** 1.5–3.5 hours
**Clinically important, potentially hazardous interactions with:** amoxicillin, ampicillin, ethotoin, fosphenytoin, mephenytoin, phenytoin

### *Reactions*

## Skin

Acute generalized exanthematous pustulosis (AGEP)
(2000): Lee AY+, *Acta Derm Venereol* 79, 412
(1995): Moreau A+, *Int J Dermatol* 34, 263 (passim)
Angioedema (<1%)
(1985): Schewach-Millet M+, *Arch Dermatol* 121, 587

Bullous eruption
(1963): Ory EM+, *JAMA* 185, 273
Contact dermatitis
(2001): Sachs B+, *Allergy* 56(1), 69
(1998): Le Coz CJ+, *Contact Dermatitis* 38, 108 (face)
(1996): Moyano JC+, *Allergy* 51, 67
(1992): Urrutia I+, *Contact Dermatitis* 26, 66
(1991): Vincenzi C+, *Contact Dermatitis* 25, 64
(1987): Kubo Y+, *Contact Dermatitis* 17, 245
(1987): Raulin C+, *Derm Beruf Umwelt* 35, 64
(1986): Rebandel P+, *Contact Dermatitis* 15, 92
(1986): van Joost T+, *Contact Dermatitis* 14, 176
(1985): Linss G+, *Dermatol Monatsschr* (German) 171, 250
(1978): Blondeel A+, *Contact Dermatitis* 4, 270
(1976): Rudzki E+, *Contact Dermatitis* 2, 181
(1975): Braun WP, *Contact Dermatitis* 1, 241
(1975): Wereide K, *Contact Dermatitis* 1, 271
(1973): Ebner H, *Wien Klin Wochenschr* (German) 85, 203
(1967): Schubert H, *Allerg Asthma Leipz* (German) 13, 25
(1966): Eberhartinger C+, *Arch Klin Exp Dermatol* (German) 224, 463
(1966): Korossy S+, *Z Haut Geschlechtskr* (German) *41, 375*
Dermatitis (sic)
Eczematous eruption (sic)
Erythema multiforme (<1%)
(1996): Lazarov A+, *Cutis* 58, 263 (from eyedrops)
(1986): Fisher AA, *Cutis* 37, 158 (topical application)
(1969): Ting HC+, *Int J Dermatol* 24, 587
(1967): Coleman WP, *Med Clin North Am* 51, 1073
(1965): Mathé P+, *J Med Bordeaux* (French) 42, 1367
(1965): Pieris EV, *Ceylon Med J* 10, 67
Exanthems (1–5%)
(1992): Breathnach SM+, *Adverse Drug Reactions and the Skin* Blackwell, Oxford, 157 (passim)
(1972): Kauppinen K, *Acta Derm Venereol* (Stockh) 52, (Suppl) 68
(1969): Török H, *Dermatol Int* 8, 57
(1951): Altemeier WA+, *JAMA* 145, 489 (1.7%)
(1951): Usndek HE+, *Arch Dermatol* 64, 217
Fixed eruption
(1985): Pandhi RK+, *Australasian J Dermatol* 26, 88
Gray syndrome*
Leucoderma
(1980): Chalfin J+, *Ophthalmic Surg* 11, 194 (eyelid)
Pellagra
Pruritus (<1%)
(1992): Breathnach SM+, *Adverse Drug Reactions and the Skin* Blackwell, Oxford, 157 (passim)
Purpura
(1967): Singh S+, *Indian J Pediatr* 4, 451
(1965): Horowitz HI+, *Semin Hematol* 2, 287
Pustular eruption
(1973): Macmillan AL, *Dermatologica* 146, 285
(1971): Stevanovic DN, *Br J Dermatol* 85, 134
Rash (sic) (<1%)
Sensitization (sic)
(1992): Urrutia I+, *Contact Dermatitis* 26, 66
(1986): van Joost T+, *Contact Dermatitis* 14, 176
Sheet-like erythema
Stevens–Johnson syndrome
(1965): Pieris EV, *Ceylon Med J* 10, 67
Systemic eczematous contact dermatitis
Toxic epidermal necrolysis (<1%)
(1975): Munstermann M+, *Dtsch Med Wochenschr* (German) 100, 2337
(1965): Mathé P+, *J Med Bord* (French) 142, 1367
Urticaria
(1992): Breathnach SM+, *Adverse Drug Reactions and the Skin* Blackwell, Oxford, 157 (passim)
(1987): Perkins JB+, *Drug Intell Clin Pharm* 21, 343
(1985): Schewach-Millet M+, *Arch Dermatol* 121, 587
Vasculitis
(1965): McCombs RP, *JAMA* 194, 1059

### Hair

Hair – alopecia
(1977): Kapp JP+, *Clinical Pediatrics* 16, 64

### Nails

Nails – photo-onycholysis
(1985): Kechijian P, *J Am Acad Dermatol* 12, 552
(1984): Daniel CR+, *J Am Acad Dermatol* 10, 250

### Other

Acute intermittent porphyria
Anaphylactoid reactions
(1976): Kozakova M, *Cesk Dermatol* (Slovak) 51, 82
Black tongue
(1954): Annotations, *Lancet* 2, 179
Glossitis
(1951): Altemeier WA+, *JAMA* 145, 489
Hypersensitivity
(1978): Simon N, *Z Hautkr* (German) 53, 341
(1974): Hegyi E+, *Cesk Dermatol* (Slovak) 49, 96
Oral mucosal eruption
(1951): Altemeier WA+, *JAMA* 145, 489
Oral ulceration
Paresthesias
(1988): Ramilo O+, *Pediatr Infect Dis* 7, 358
Porphyria
(1976): Panica D+, *Folia Med Plovdiv* 18, 161
Stomatitis (<1%)
Xerostomia

***Note:** Gray syndrome: toxic reactions in premature infants and newborns. Signs and symptoms include: abdominal distension, blue-gray skin color, low body temperature, and uneven breathing

## CHLORDIAZEPOXIDE

**Trade names:** Libritabs (ICN); Librium (ICN); Limbitrol (ICN)
**Other common trade names:** *Corax; Huberplex; Medilium; Mitran; Multum; Novopoxide; Psicofar; Reposans-10; Solium; Tropium*
**Indications:** Anxiety
**Category:** Benzodiazepine; antianxiety; sedative-hypnotic; antipanic and antitremor agent
**Half-life:** 6–25 hours
**Clinically important, potentially hazardous interactions with:** chlorpheniramine, clarithromycin, efavirenz, esomeprazole, imatinib, indinavir, ketoconazole, nelfinavir, ritonavir

Limbitrol is amitriptyline and chlordiazepoxide

#### *Reactions*

### Skin

Angioedema (<1%)
(1971): Almeyda J, *Br J Dermatol* 84, 299
(1964): Welsh AL, *Med Clin North Am* 48, 459
Dermatitis (sic) (1–10%)
Diaphoresis (>10%)
Edema (1–10%)
Erythema multiforme (<1%)
(1992): Breathnach SM+, *Adverse Drug Reactions and the Skin* Blackwell, Oxford, 200 (passim)

(1985): Kauppinen K+, *Br J Dermatol* 112, 575
(1981): Edwards JG, *Drugs* 22, 495 (passim)
(1974): Tay C, *Asian J Med* 10, 223
(1971): Almeyda J, *Br J Dermatol* 84, 299

Erythema nodosum (<1%)
(1981): Edwards JG, *Drugs* 22, 495 (passim)
(1971): Almeyda J, *Br J Dermatol* 84, 299

Exanthems
(1976): Arndt KA+, *JAMA* 235, 918 (0.42%)
(1971): Almeyda J, *Br J Dermatol* 84, 299

Fixed eruption (<1%)
(1990): Gaffoor PMA+, *Cutis* 45, 242 (passim)
(1981): Edwards JG, *Drugs* 22, 495 (passim)
(1974): Blair HM, *Arch Dermatol* 109, 914
(1970): Savin JA, *Br J Dermatol* 83, 546
(1964): Welsh AL, *Med Clin North Am* 48, 459
(1961): Gaul LE, *Arch Dermatol* 83, 1010

Lupus erythematosus
(1973): Hicks JH, *Cutis* 11, 33
(1973): McCarthy J, *Arch Dermatol* 108, 733 (discussion)
(1965): Grupper CH+, *Bull Soc Franc Derm Syphiligr* (French) 72, 714

Photosensitivity
(1986): Morliere P, *Biochemie* 68, 849
(1981): Edwards JG, *Drugs* 22, 495 (passim)
(1980): Bjellerup M+, *J Invest Dermatol* 75, 228
(1973): Torre D, *Arch Dermatol* 108, 733 (discussion)
(1971): Almeyda J, *Br J Dermatol* 84, 299
(1965): Luton EF+, *Arch Dermatol* 91, 362

Pigmented purpuric eruption
(1989): Nishioka K+, *J Dermatol* (Tokio) 16, 220

Pruritus
(1977): Ghosh JS, *BMJ* 1, 902

Purpura
(2001): Alexopoulou A+, *Arch Intern Med* 161(14), 1778 (with clidinium)
(1981): Edwards JG, *Drugs* 22, 495 (passim)
(1977): Celada A+, *BMJ* 1, 268
(1971): Almeyda J, *Br J Dermatol* 84, 299
(1967): Copperman IJ, *BMJ* 4, 485

Rash (sic) (>10%)
(1960): Tobin JM, *JAMA* 174, 1242

Urticaria
(1981): Edwards JG, *Drugs* 22, 495 (passim)
(1974): Tay C, *Asian J Med* 10, 223
(1971): Almeyda J, *Br J Dermatol* 84, 299
(1964): Welsh AL, *Med Clin North Am* 48, 459

Vasculitis
(1989): Nishioka K+, *J Dermatol* 16, 220
(1971): Almeyda J, *Br J Dermatol* 84, 299

### Hair

Hair – alopecia
(1977): Celada A+, *BMJ* 1, 268
(1973): Hicks JH, *Cutis* 11, 33
(1965): Luton EF+, *Arch Dermatol* 91, 362

### Other

Acute intermittent porphyria
(1967): de Matteis F, *Pharmacol Rev* 19, 523

Galactorrhea
(1971): Almeyda J, *Br J Dermatol* 84, 299
(1961): Hooper JH+, *JAMA* 178, 506
(1956): Marshall WK+, *Lancet* 1, 152

Gynecomastia
(1965): Vavala V+, *Endocr Metabol* 36, 43

Injection-site phlebitis

Paresthesias

Porphyria
(1983): Eubanks SW+, *Int J Dermatol* 22, 337

Sialopenia (>10%)

Sialorrhea (1–10%)

Xerostomia (>10%)

## CHLORHEXIDINE

**Trade names:** BactoShield; Betasept; Dyna-Hex; Exidine Scrub; Hibiclens; Hibistat; Peridex; PerioChip; Periogard (Various pharmaceutical companies.)
**Other common trade names:** *Alcloxidine; Bactoscrub; Chlorhexamed; Corsodyl; Hexol; Hibident; Hibidil; Hibiscrub; Hibitane; Savlon; Spectro Gram*
**Indications:** Skin antisepsis, gingivitis
**Category:** Topical anti-infective; oral rinse
**Half-life:** no data

### *Reactions*

### Skin

Allergic contact dermatitis (balanitis)
(2001): Barrazza V, *Contact Dermatitis* 45, 42

Allergic reactions (sic)
(2001): Garvey LH+, *Acta Anaesthesiol Scand* 45(10), 1290 (4 cases)
(1995): Yong D+, *Med J Aust* 162, 257
(1992): Ramselaar CG+, *Br J Urol* 70, 451
(1985): Cheung J+, *Anaesth Intensive Care* 13, 429
(1982): Staab W+, *Stomatol DDR* (German) 32, 700

Contact dermatitis
(2001): Barrazza V, *Contact Dermatitis* 45(1), 42
(1998): Ebo DG+, *J Allergy Clin Immunol* 101, 128
(1995): Stingeni L+, *Contact Dermatitis* 33, 172
(1990): Reynolds NJ+, *Contact Dermatitis* 22, 103
(1988): Bergqvist-Karlsson A, *Contact Dermatitis* 18, 84
(1987): Osmundsen PE+, *Ugeskr Laeger* (Danish) 149, 3048
(1985): Lasthein Andersen B+, *Contact Dermatitis* 13, 307 (5.4%)
(1983): Shoji A, *Contact Dermatitis* 9, 156
(1982): Osmundsen PE, *Contact Dermatitis* 8, 81
(1981): Roberts DL+, *Contact Dermatitis* 7, 326
(1972): Ljunggren B+, *Acta Derm Venereol* (Stockh) 52, 308
(1972): Neering H+, *Ned Tijdschr Geneeskd* (Dutch) 116, 1742

Dermatitis (sic)
(1998): Thune P, *Tidsskr Nor Laegeforen* (Norwegian) 118, 3295

Facial edema (<1%)

Fixed eruption
(1991): Moghadam BK+, *Oral Surg Oral Med Oral Pathol* 71, 431

Photosensitivity
(1971): Wahlberg JE+, *Dermatologica* 143, 376

Rash (sic)
(2001): Garvey LH+, *Acta Anaesthesiol Scand* 45(10), 1290 (4 cases)

Urticaria
(1998): Stables GI+, *Br J Urol* 82, 756
(1990): Wong WK+, *Contact Dermatitis* 22, 52 (contact)
(1989): Fisher AA, *Cutis* 43, 17
(1988): Bergqvist-Karlsson A, *Contact Dermatitis* 18, 84

### Other

Anaphylactoid reactions
(2001): Garvey LH+, *Acta Anaesthesiol Scand* 45(10), 1204 (4 cases)
(2001): Knight BA+, *Intern Med J* 31(7), 436
(2001): Lockhart AS+, *Br J Anaesth* 87(6), 940
(2001): Stephens R+, *Br J Anaesth* 87(2), 306 (with sulfadiazine)

(2000): Pham NH+, *Clin Exp Allergy* 30, 1001
(1999): Autegarden JE+, *Contact Dermatitis* 40, 215
(1999): Snellman E+, *J Am Acad Dermatol* 40, 771
(1998): Ebo DG+, *J Allergy Clin Immunol* 101, 128
(1998): Nikaido S+, *Masui* (Japanese) 47, 330
(1998): Olivieri J+, *Schweiz Med Wochenschr* 128, 1508
(1998): Terazawa E+, *Anesthesiology* 89, 1296
(1998): Thune P, *Tidsskr Nor Laegeforen* (Norwegian) 118, 3295
(1997): Chisholm DG+, *BMJ* 315, 785
(1997): Fujita S+, *Masui* (Japanese) 46, 1118 (2 cases)
(1996): Torricelli R, *Clin Exp Allergy* 26, 112
(1995): Parker F+, *Anaesth Intensive Care* 23, 126
(1994): de Groot AC+, *Ned Tijdschr Geneeskd* (Dutch) 138, 1342
(1994): Okuda T+, *Masui* (Japanese) 43, 1352
(1994): Russ BR+, *Anaesth Intensive Care* 22, 611
(1994): Visser LE+, *Ned Tijdschr Geneeskd* (Dutch) 138, 778
(1992): Evans RJ, *BMJ* 304, 686
(1992): Harukuni I+, *Masui* (Japanese) 41, 455
(1992): Peutrell JM, *Anaesthesia* 47, 1013
(1990): Wong WK+, *Contact Dermatitis* 22, 52

Dysgeusia (>10%)
(1978): Schaupp H+, *HNO* (German) 26, 335

Gingival bleeding
(1984): Asikainen S+, *J Clin Periodontol* 11, 87
(1982): Ainamo J+, *J Clin Periodontol* 9, 337

Glossitis (1–10%)

Hypersensitivity
(2001): Lauerma AL, *Contact Dermatitis* 44(1), 59
(1998): Burlington B, *Ostomy Wound Manage* 44, 84
(1994): Aalto-Korte K+, *Duodecim* (Finnish) 110, 2013
(1989): Okano M+, *Arch Dermatol* 125, 50 (6 cases)
(1988): Bergqvist-Karlsson A, *Contact Dermatitis* 18, 84
(1986): Ohtoshi T+, *Clin Allergy* 16, 155
(1986): Yaacob H+, *J Oral Med* 41, 145
(1971): Wahlberg JE+, *Dermatologica* 143, 376

Oral mucosal reaction
(1982): Skoglund LA+, *Int J Oral Surg* 11, 380 (3 cases)

Stomatitis (1–10%)

Tongue irritation (1–10%)

Tongue pigmentation (>10%)

Tooth staining
(2002): Moshrefi A, *J West Soc Periodontol Periodontal Abstr* 50(1), 5

## CHLORMEZANONE

**Trade name:** Trancopal (Sanofi)
**Indications:** Anxiety
**Category:** Antianxiety agent and muscle relaxant
**Half-life:** 24 hours

### *Reactions*

#### Skin

Ankle edema

Edema

Erythema multiforme

Exanthems
(1989): Alanko K+, *Acta Derm Venereol* (Stockh) 69, 223
(1964): Welsh AL, *Med Clin North Am* 48, 459

Fixed eruption
(1998): Leal G, Fortaleza, Brazil (from Internet) (observation)
(1998): Lee Ay, *Contact Dermatitis* 38(5), 258
(1998): Mahboob A+, *Int J Dermatol* 37, 833
(1995): Rademacher D+, *Contact Dermatitis* 32, 117
(1992): el-Sayed F+, *Ann Dermatol Venereol* (French) 119, 671
(1991): Lee AY+, *Drug Intell Clin Pharm* 25, 604
(1989): Alanko K+, *Acta Derm Venereol* (Stockh) 69, 223
(1988): McFadden N, *Dermatologica* 176, 106
(1985): Kauppinen K+, *Br J Dermatol* 112, 575
(1985): Verbov J, *Dermatologica* 171, 60 (with acetaminophen)
(1983): Mohamed KN+, *Int J Dermatol* 22, 548
(1974): Kuokkanen K, *Int J Dermatol* 13, 4
(1964): Welsh AL, *Med Clin North Am* 48, 459

Flushing

Pruritus
(1964): Welsh AL, *Med Clin North Am* 48, 459

Rash (sic)
(1991): Lee AY+, *Drug Intell Clin Pharm* 25, 604 (passim)

Stevens–Johnson syndrome
(1995): Roujeau JC+, *N Engl J Med* 333, 1600
(1995): Wolkenstein P+, *Drug Saf* 13, 56

Toxic epidermal necrolysis
(1998): von Boxberg C+, *Dtsch Med Wochenschr* (German) 123, 866 (fatal)
(1996): Blum L+, *J Am Acad Dermatol* 34, 1088
(1995): Roujeau JC+, *N Engl J Med* 333, 1600
(1993): Correia O+, *Dermatology* 186, 32
(1992): Saiag P+, *J Am Acad Dermatol* 26, 567
(1991): Rosenthal E+, *Presse Med* (French) 20, 1459
(1987): Guillaume JC+, *Arch Dermatol* 123, 1166
(1983): Tagami H+, *Arch Dermatol* 119, 910

Urticaria

#### Other

Acute intermittent porphyria

Death

Dysgeusia
(1976): Rollin H, *Laryngol Rhinol Otol* (Stuttgart) (German) 55, 873

Xerostomia
(1964): Welsh AL, *Med Clin North Am* 48, 459

## CHLOROQUINE

**Trade name:** Aralen (Sanofi)
**Other common trade names:** *Avloclor; Chlorquin; Emquin; Heliopar; Lagaquin; Malarivon*
**Indications:** Malaria, rheumatoid arthritis, lupus erythematosus
**Category:** Antiprotozoal; antimalarial and antirheumatic drug; lupus erythematosus suppressant; polymorphous light eruption; and porphyria cutanea tarda
**Half-life:** 3–5 days
**Clinically important, potentially hazardous interactions with:** acitretin, antacids, cholestyramine, dapsone, furazolidone, hydroxychloroquine, methotrexate, methoxsalen, penicillamine, sulfonamides

### *Reactions*

#### Skin

Acute generalized exanthematous pustulosis (AGEP)
(1998): Janier M+, *Dermatology* 196, 271

Angioedema (<1%)
(1993): *Lakartidningen* (Swedish) 90, 54

Bullous pemphigoid
(1999): Millard TP+, *Clin Exp Dermatol* 24, 263

Contact dermatitis
(1984): Kellett JK+, *Contact Dermatitis* 11, 47
(1975): Skog E, *Contact Dermatitis* 1, 187

Ephelides
(1985): Dupre A+, *Arch Dermatol* 121, 1164

Erythema annulare centrifugum
(1982): Koralewski F, *Dermatosen* (German) 30, 125
(1967): Ashurst PJ, *Arch Dermatol* 95, 37
Erythema multiforme (<1%)
Erythroderma
(1990): Simoneaux PW, *Curr Concept Skin Dis* Winter, 15
(1986): Langtry JA+, *Br Med J Clin Res Ed* 292, 1107
(1985): Slagel GA+, *J Am Acad Dermatol* 12, 857
Exanthems (1–5%)
(1991): Ochsendorf FR+, *Hautarzt* (German) 42, 140
(1990): Simoneaux PW, *Curr Concept Skin Dis* Winter, 15
(1973): Rees RB+, *Arch Dermatol* 88, 280 (passim)
Exfoliative dermatitis
(1986): Lavrijsen APM+, *Acta Derm Venereol* (Stockh) 66, 536
(1985): Slagel GA+, *J Am Acad Dermatol* 12, 857
(1980): Koranda FC, *J Am Acad Dermatol* 4, 650 (passim)
(1973): Rees RB+, *Arch Dermatol* 88, 280 (passim)
Fixed eruption (<1%)
Lichenoid eruption
(1990): Simoneaux PW, *Curr Concept Skin Dis* Winter, 15
(1981): Koranda FC, *J Am Acad Dermatol* 4, 650 (passim)
(1979): Krebs A, *Hautarzt* (German) 30, 281
(1973): Rees RB+, *Arch Dermatol* 88, 280 (passim)
(1958): Savage J, *Br J Dermatol* 70, 181
(1948): Alving AS+, *J Clin Invest* 27, 56
Photosensitivity
(1993): *Lakartidningen* (Swedish) 90, 54
(1992): Seideman P+, *Scand J Rheumatol* 21, 101
(1991): Ochsendorf FR+, *Hautarzt* (German) 42, 140
(1989): Ortel B+, *Dermatologica* 178, 39
(1982): van Weelden H, *Arch Dermatol* 118, 290
(1973): Rees RB+, *Arch Dermatol* 88, 280 (passim)
Pigmentation
(1998): Guedira N+, *Rev Rhum Engl Ed* 65, 58
(1991): Ochsendorf FR+, *Hautarzt* (German) 42, 140
(1987): Krebs A, *Schweiz Rundsch Med Prax* (German) 76, 1069
(1982): Levy H, *S Afr Med J* 62, 735
(1981): Koranda FC, *J Am Acad Dermatol* 4, 650 (passim)
(1980): Bentsi-Enchill KO, *Trop Geogr Med* 32, 216
(1975): Marriott P+, *Proc R Soc Med* 68, 535
(1968): Stewart TW+, *Acta Derm Venereol* 48, 47
(1963): Tuffanelli D+, *Arch Dermatol* 88, 419
(1959): Dall JLC+, *BMJ* 1, 1387
Polymorphous light eruption
(1968): Reed WB+, *Arch Dermatol* 98, 327
Pruritus
(2000): Ademowo OG+, *Clin Pharm Ther* 67, 237
(1999): Millard TP+, *Clin Exp Dermatol* 24, 263
(1997): Adebayo RA+, *Br J Clin Pharmacol* 44, 157
(1997): Sowunmi A+, *Trans R Trop Med Hyg* 91, 63
(1996): George AO, *Int J Dermatol* 35, 323
(1995): Osifo NG, *Afr J Med Sci* 24, 67
(1992): Ogunranti JO+, *Eur J Clin Pharmacol* 43, 323
(1991): Ajayi AA+, *Eur J Clin Pharmacol* 41, 383
(1991): Ezeamuzie IC+, *J Trop Med Hyg* 94, 184
(1991): Mnyika KS, *East Afr Med J* 68, 139
(1991): Mnyika KS+, *J Trop Med Hyg* 94, 27 (47%)
(1991): Okor RS, *J Clin Pharm Ther* 16, 463
(1990): Abdulkadir SA+, *Trans Roy Soc Trop Med Hyg* 84, 898
(1990): Okor RS, *J Clin Pharm Ther* 15, 147
(1990): Simoneaux PW, *Curr Concept Skin Dis* Winter, 15
(1989): Abila B+, *J Trop Med Hyg* 92, 356
(1989): Burnham G+, *Trans R Soc Trop Med Hyg* 83, 527
(1989): Hallwood PM+, *Lancet* 2, 397
(1989): Osifo NG, *Afr J Med Sci* 18, 121
(1989): Soro B+, *Bull Soc Pathol Exot Filiales* (French) 82, 88
(1989): Sowunmi A+, *Lancet* 2, 213
(1987): Spencer HC+, *Ann Trop Med Parasitol* 81, 124
(1986): Harries AD+, *Ann Trop Med Parasitol* 80, 479
(1984): Bhasin V+, *J Indian Med Assoc* 82, 447
(1984): Caussade P, *Arch Fr Pediatr* (French) 41, 727
(1984): Osifo NG, *Arch Dermatol* 120, 80
(1982): Spencer HC+, *BMJ* 285, 1703
(1977): Olatunde A, *Afr J Med Sci* 6, 27
(1969): Olatunde IA, *J Nigerian Med Assoc* 6, 23
(1964): Ekpechi OL+, *Arch Dermatol* 120, 80
Psoriasis
(1993): Schopt RE+, *Dermatology* 187, 100
(1992): Vestey JP+, *J Infect* 24, 211
(1991): Damstra RJ+, *Ned Tijdschr Geneeskd* (Dutch) 135, 671
(1990): Abdulkadir SA+, *Trans R Soc Trop Med Hyg* 84, 898
(1990): Katugampola G+, *Int J Dermatol* 29, 153
(1990): Okor RS, *J Clin Pharm Ther* 15, 147
(1989): Mallett R+, *BMJ* 299, 1400
(1988): Nicolas J-F+, *Ann Dermatol Venereol* (French) 115, 289
(1985): Stone OJ, *Int J Dermatol* 24, 539
(1982): Abel EA+, *J Am Acad Dermatol* 15, 2007
(1982): Luzar MJ, *J Rheumatol* 9, 462
(1981): Olsen TG, *Ann Intern Med* 94, 546
(1980): Kuflik EG, *Cutis* 26, 153
(1966): Baker H, *Br J Dermatol* 78, 161
(1957): Cornbleet T+, *Arch Dermatol* 75, 286
Pustular eruption
(1990): Lotem M+, *Acta Derm Venereol* (Stockh) 70, 250
Pustular psoriasis
(1999): Capper N, Mobile, AL (from Internet) (observation)
(1998): Wilairatana P+, *Int J Dermatol* 37, 713
(1997): Wilairatana P+, *Int J Dermatol* 36, 634
(1987): Friedman SJ, *J Am Acad Dermatol* 16, 1256
Stevens–Johnson syndrome
(2000): Madnani N, Mumbai, India (from Internet) (observation)
(1989): Ortel B+, *Dermatologica* 178, 39
(1987): Lenox-Smith I, *J Infect* 14, 90 (fatal)
(1986): Bamber MG+, *J Infect* 13, 31 (fatal)
Toxic epidermal necrolysis (<1%)
(1994): Boffa MJ+, *Br J Dermatol* 131, 444
(1988): Phillips-Howard PA+, *Br Med J Clin Res Ed* 296, 1605
(1979): Bazarnaia NS+, *Ter Arkh* (Russian) 51, 99
(1976): Kanwar AJ+, *Indian J Dermatol* 21, 73
(1972): Shul'tsev GP+, *Sov Med* (Russian) 35, 133
Urticaria
(1990): Simoneaux PW, *Curr Concept Skin Dis* Winter, 15
(1980): Koranda FC, *J Am Acad Dermatol* 4, 650 (passim)
(1973): Rees RB+, *Arch Dermatol* 88, 280 (passim)
Vasculitis
Vitiligo
(2002): Martin R+, *World Congress Dermatol* Poster, 0114
(1997): Selvaag E, *Ann Trop Pediatr* 17, 45
(1996): Selvaag E, *Acta Derm Venereol* 76, 166
(1996): Selvaag E, *Trans R Trop Med Hyg* 90, 683
(1995): Selvaag E+, American Academy of Dermatology Meeting, New Orleans (observation)
(1992): Gonggryp LA+, *Br J Rheumatol* 31, 790
(1980): Bentsi-Enchill KO, *Trop Geogr Med* 32, 216

## Hair

Hair – alopecia
Hair – pigmentation (<1%)
(1997): Asch PH+, *Ann Dermatol Venereol* (French) 124, 552
(1992): Bublin JG+, *J Clin Pharm Ther* 17, 297
(1991): Ochsendorf FR+, *Hautarzt* (German) 42, 140
(1981): Koranda FC, *J Am Acad Dermatol* 4, 650 (passim)
(1978): Dubois EL, *Semin Arthritis Rheum* 8, 33
(1976): Sams WM, *Int J Dermatol* 15, 99
(1973): Rees RB+, *Arch Dermatol* 88, 280 (passim)
(1965): Rook A, *Br J Dermatol* 77, 115
Hair – poliosis
(1985): Dupre A+, *Arch Dermatol* 121, 1164
(1968): Pasykowa K+, *Pol Tyg Lek* (Polish) 23, 2014
(1966): Fraga S+, *An Bras Dermatol* (Portuguese) 41, 57

## Nails

Nails – discoloration
(1991): Zic JA+, *Arch Dermatol* 127, 1037
Nails – pigmentation
(1981): Koranda FC, *J Am Acad Dermatol* 4, 650 (passim)
(1963): Tuffanelli D+, *Arch Dermatol* 88, 419
Nails – shoreline
(1993): Pavithran K, *Indian J Lepr* 65, 225

## Other

Acute intermittent porphyria
(1996): Puri AS+, *Indian Pediatr* 33, 241
Death
Gingival pigmentation
(1992): Veraldi S+, *Cutis* 49, 281
Myalgia
(1998): Guedira N+, *Rev Rhum Engl Ed* 65, 58
Myopathy
(1969): Chapman RS+, *Br J Dermatol* 81, 217
Oral mucosal pigmentation
(1992): Veraldi S+, *Cutis* 49, 281
(1991): Zic JA+, *Arch Dermatol* 127, 1037
(1990): Wollina U+, *Dtsch Z Mund Kiefer Gesichtschir* (German) 14, 104
(1981): Koranda FC, *J Am Acad Dermatol* 4, 650 (passim)
(1980): Bentsi-Enchill KO, *Trop Geogr Med* 32, 216
(1971): Giansanti JS+, *Oral Surg* 31, 66
(1970): Brynolf I, *Sven Tandlak Tidskr* (Swedish) 63, 585
Oral mucosal ulceration
Porphyria
(1980): Gerwel M, *Pol Tyg Lek* (Polish) 35, 1351
(1974): Kordac V+, *Br J Dermatol* 90, 95
(1973): Knutsson F+, *Lakartidningen* (Swedish) 70, 1547
(1962): Cripps DL+, *Arch Dermatol* 86, 575
(1959): Marsden CW, *Br J Dermatol* 71, 219
(1957): Davis MJ+, *Arch Dermatol* 75, 796
(1954): Linden IH+, *Calif Med* 81, 235
Porphyria cutanea tarda
(1985): Handa F+, *Indian J Dermatol* 30, 49
Stomatitis (<1%)
Stomatopyrosis
Tinnitus

# CHLOROTHIAZIDE

**Trade names:** Aldochlor (Merck); Diuril (Merck)
**Other common trade names:** *Azide; Chlothin; Chlotride; Diurazide; Diuret; Saluretil; Saluric*
**Indications:** Hypertension, edema
**Category:** Thiazide* diuretic; antihypertensive
**Half-life:** 1–2 hours
**Clinically important, potentially hazardous interactions with:** digoxin, lithium

### *Reactions*

## Skin

Bullous eruption
Erythema multiforme
Exanthems
(1972): Kuokannen K, *Acta Allergol* 27, 407
(1966): Sherlock S+, *Lancet* 1, 1049 (10%)
(1966): Smith JW+, *Ann Intern Med* 65, 629 (1.3%)
(1960): Smirk H+, *BMJ* 1, 515
(1959): Kirkendall WM, *Circulation* 19, 933 (1.1%)
(1958): Rogin JR, *Arch Dermatol* 78, 504
Exfoliative dermatitis
Fixed eruption
(1984): Chan HL, *Int J Dermatol* 23, 607
Lichenoid eruption
(1986): Gonzalez JG+, *J Am Acad Dermatol* 15, 87
(1971): Almeyda J+, *Br J Dermatol* 85, 604
(1959): Harber LC+, *J Invest Dermatol* 33, 83
(1959): Harber LC+, *N Engl J Med* 261, 1378
Lupus erythematosus
(1966): Cohen P+, *JAMA* 197, 817
Photoreactions
Photosensitivity (<1%)
(1994): Enta T, *Can Fam Physicians* 40, 1269
(1993): Iwamoto Y, *Nippon Saikingaku Zasshi* (Japanese) 48, 523
(1984): Horio T, *Int J Dermatol* 23, 376
(1980): Stern RS+, *Arch Dermatol* 116, 1269
(1973): Stern WK, *Acta Derm Venereol* 53, 321
(1970): Zurcher K+, *Dermatologica* 141, 119
(1969): Kalivas J, *JAMA* 209, 1706
(1965): Jung EG+, *Int Arch Allergy Appl Immunol* 27, 313
(1959): Harber LC+, *J Invest Dermatol* 33, 83
(1959): Harber LC+, *N Engl J Med* 261, 1378
(1959): Norins AL, *Arch Dermatol* 79, 592
Pruritus
(1969): Kalivas J, *JAMA* 209, 1706
(1959): Norins AL, *Arch Dermatol* 79, 592
(1958): Rogin JR, *Arch Dermatol* 78, 504
Purpura
(1992): Breathnach SM+, *Adverse Drug Reactions and the Skin* Blackwell, Oxford, 46
(1980): Miescher PA+, *Clin Haematol* 9, 505
(1960): Ball P, *JAMA* 173, 663
(1959): Horowitz HI+, *N Y State J Med* 59, 1117
(1959): Nordquist P+, *Lancet* 1, 271
(1958): Jaffe MO+, *JAMA* 168, 2264
Rash (sic) (<1%)
Stevens–Johnson syndrome
Toxic epidermal necrolysis
Urticaria
(1960): Smirk H+, *BMJ* 1, 515
Vasculitis
(1965): Björnberg A+, *Lancet* 2, 982
(1960): Fitzgerald EW, *Arch Intern Med* 105, 305
(1958): Jaffe MO+, *JAMA* 168, 2264

## Hair

Hair – alopecia

## Other

Anaphylactoid reactions
Dysgeusia
Oral mucosal lesions
Paresthesias (<1%)
Xanthopsia

***Note:** Chlorothiazide is a sulfonamide and can be absorbed systemically. Sulfonamides can produce severe, possibly fatal, reactions such as toxic epidermal necrolysis and Stevens–Johnson syndrome

# CHLOROTRIANISENE

**Trade name:** Tace (Aventis)
**Other common trade names:** *Estregur; Merbentul*
**Indications:** Inoperable prostate cancer, atrophic vaginitis
**Category:** Estrogen replacement
**Half-life:** no data

### *Reactions*

## Skin

Acne pustulosa
(1964): Sneddon IB+, *Br J Dermatol* 76, 491
Candidiasis
Chloasma (<1%)
Dermatitis (sic)
Edema (>1%)
Erythema
Erythema multiforme
Erythema nodosum
Melasma (<1%)
Peripheral edema (>10%)
Photosensitivity
Rash (sic) (<1%)
Urticaria

## Hair

Hair – alopecia
Hair – hirsutism

## Other

Acute intermittent porphyria
Gynecomastia (>10%)
Mastodynia (>10%)
Porphyria cutanea tarda
(1970): Domonkos AN, *Arch Dermatol* 102, 229
(1970): Roenigk HH+, *Arch Dermatol* 102, 260
Vaginal candidiasis
Vaginitis

# CHLORPHENIRAMINE

**Trade names:** AL-R; Aller-Chlor (Rugby); Chlo-Amine; Chlor-Pro; Chlor-Trimeton (Schering); Chlorate (Major); Ornade (GSK); Phenetron (Lannett); Rynatan; Telachlor (Major); Teldrin (GSK); Triaminic (Novartis)
**Other common trade name:** *Chlor-Tripolon*
**Indications:** Allergic rhinitis, urticaria
**Category:** Antihistamine; $H_1$-blocker
**Half-life:** 20–40 hours
**Clinically important, potentially hazardous interactions with: alcohol**, anticholinergics, barbiturates, benzodiazepines, butabarbital, chloral hydrate, chlordiazepoxide, chlorpromazine, clonazepam, clorazepate, diazepam, ethchlorvynol, fluphenazine, flurazepam, hypnotics, lorazepam, MAO inhibitors, mephobarbital, mesoridazine, midazolam, narcotics, oxazepam, pentobarbital, phenobarbital, phenothiazines, primidone, prochlorperazine, promethazine, quazepam, secobarbital, sedatives, temazepam, thioridazine, tranquilizers, trifluoperazine, zolpidem

### *Reactions*

## Skin

Angioedema (1–10%)
Contact dermatitis
(2001): Hayashi K+, *Contact Dermatitis* 44(1), 38
(1990): Tosti A+, *Contact Dermatitis* 22, 55 (eye-drops)
Dermatitis (sic) (1–10%)
Diaphoresis
Photosensitivity (1–10%)

## Other

Hypersensitivity
Myalgia (<1%)
Paresthesias (<1%)
Tinnitus
Xerostomia (1–10%)

# CHLORPROMAZINE

**Trade name:** Thorazine (GSK)
**Other common trade names:** *Chloractil; Chlorazin; Chlorpromanyl; Esmino; Largactil; Novo-Chlorpromazine; Ormazine; Propaphenin; Prozin*
**Indications:** Psychosis, manic-depressive disorders
**Category:** Phenothiazine antipsychotic and antiemetic
**Half-life:** initial: 2 hours; terminal: 30 hours
**Clinically important, potentially hazardous interactions with: alcohol**, antihistamines, arsenic, chlorpheniramine, dofetilide, epinephrine, guanethidine, quinolones, sparfloxacin

**Note:** The prolonged use of chlorpromazine can produce a gray-blue or purplish pigmentation over light-exposed areas. This is a result of either dermal deposits of melanin, a chlorpromazine metabolite, or to a combination of both. Chlorpromazine melanosis is seen more often in women

### *Reactions*

## Skin

Actinic reticuloid
(1982): Amblard P+, *Ann Dermatol Venereol* (French) 109, 225
Angioedema (<1%)

(1958): Hine FR, *Am J Psychiatry* 114, 942
Bullous eruption (<1%)
(1979): Matsuo I+, *Dermatologica* 159, 46
Contact dermatitis
(1955): Lewis GM+, *JAMA* 157, 909
Dermatitis (sic)
Erythema multiforme (<1%)
(1961): Baer RL+, *Year Book of Dermatology* Chicago, 9–37
Exanthems (>5%)
(1969): Török H, *Dermatol Int* 8, 57
(1968): Raskin A, *J Nerv Ment Dis* 147, 184 (5%)
(1967): Lockey SD, *Med Sci* 18, 43
(1966): Zelickson AS, *JAMA* 198, 341
(1961): Stevanovic DV, *Br J Dermatol* 73, 233
(1957): Bernstein C+, *JAMA* 163, 930 (7–14%)
(1956): Mullins JF+, *JAMA* 162, 946
(1955): Margolis LH+, *Arch Dermatol* 72, 72 (13%)
Exfoliative dermatitis
(1961): Baer RL+, *Year Book of Dermatology* Chicago, 9–37
Fixed eruption (<1%)
Hypohidrosis (>10%)
Lichenoid eruption
(1979): Matsuo I+, *Dermatologica* 159, 46
Lupus erythematosus
(1996): Matsukawa Y+, *J Int Med Res* 24, 147
(1994): Yung RL+, *Rheum Dis Clin North Am* 20, 61
(1990): Roche-Bayard P, *Chest* 98, 1545
(1985): Pavlidakey GP+, *J Am Acad Dermatol* 13, 109
(1980): Goldman LS+, *Am J Psychiatry* 137, 1613
(1973): Ananth JV+, *Can Med Assoc J* 108, 680
(1972): Dubois EL+, *JAMA* 221, 595
(1963): Shulman LE+, *Arthritis Rheum* 6, 558
Miliaria
(1956): Mullins JF+, *JAMA* 162, 946
Peripheral edema
Photocontact dermatitis
(1962): Calnan CD+, *Trans St. Johns Hosp Derm Soc* 48, 49
Photosensitivity (1–10%)
(1995): Kim TH+, *Photodermatol Photoimmunol Photomed* 11, 170
(1993): Jeanmougin M+, *Ann Dermatol Venereol* (French) 120, 840
(1993): Wolf ME+, *Int J Clin Pharmacol* 31, 365
(1989): Hoshino T+, *Arch Dermatol Res* 281, 60
(1989): Rosen C, *Semin Dermatol* 8, 149
(1986): Lovell CR+, *Contact Dermatitis* 14, 290
(1982): Amblard P+, *Ann Dermatol Venereol* (French) 109, 225
(1979): Matsuo I+, *Dermatologica* 159, 46
(1975): Horio T, *Arch Dermatol* 111, 1469
(1974): Johnson BE, *Proc R Soc Med* 67, 871
(1973): Johnson BE, *Br J Dermatol* 89, 16
(1971): Hägermark O+, *Br J Dermatol* 84, 605
(1969): Kalivas J, *JAMA* 209, 1706 (3%)
(1968): Prien RF+, *Arch Gen Psychiatry* 18, 482 (1–22%)
(1967): Lockey SD, *Med Sci* 18, 43
(1967): Satanove A+, *JAMA* 200, 121
(1961): Stevanovic DV, *Br J Dermatol* 73, 233
(1958): Calnan CD+, *Trans St. Johns Hosp Derm Soc* 44, 26
(1957): Epstein JH+, *J Invest Dermatol* 28, 329
(1957): Winkelmann NR, *Am J Psychiatry* 113, 961 (3%)
(1956): Mullins JF+, *JAMA* 162, 946
(1955): Margolis LH+, *Arch Dermatol* 72, 72
Phototoxicity
(1997): Eberlein-Konig B+, *Dermatology* 194, 131
(1979): Matsuo I+, *Dermatologica* 159, 46
(1977): Ljunggren B, *J Invest Dermatol* 69, 383
(1975): Raffle EJ+, *Arch Dermatol* 111, 1364
(1967): Satanove A+, *JAMA* 200, 121
(1964): Greiner AC+, *Can Med Assoc J* 90, 663
Pigmentation (<1%)
(2001): Kass J+, *Cutis* 68(4), 260
(2000): Lal+, *J Psychiatry Neurosci* 25, 281
(1993): Bloom D+, *Acta Psychiatr Scand* 87, 223
(1993): Lal S+, *J Psychiatry Neurosci* 18, 173
(1993): Wolf ME+, *Int J Clin Pharmacol* 31, 365 (blue-gray)
(1988): Benning TL+, *Arch Dermatol* 124, 1541
(1988): Thompson TR+, *Acta Psychiatr Scand* 78, 763
(1975): Robins AH, *S Afr Med J* 49, 1521
(1967): Satanove A+, *JAMA* 200, 209
(1966): Hashimoto K+, *J Invest Dermatol* 47, 296
(1966): Zelickson AS, *JAMA* 198, 341
(1964): Greiner AC+, *Can Med Assoc J* 90, 663
(1964): Hays GB+, *Arch Dermatol* 90, 471
(1964): Zelickson AS+, *JAMA* 188, 394
Pruritus (1–10%)
(1968): Prien RF+, *Arch Gen Psychiatry* 18, 482 (1–22%)
(1957): Bernstein C+, *JAMA* 163, 930 (4%)
Purpura
(1987): Aram H, *J Am Acad Dermatol* 17, 139
(1967): Lockey SD, *Med Sci* 18, 43
(1965): Horowitz HI+, *Semin Hematol* 2, 287
(1957): Shannon J+, *Dermatologica* 114, 101
(1956): Mullins JF+, *JAMA* 162, 946
(1956): Wintrobe MM+, *Arch Intern Med* 98, 559
Pustular eruption
(1994): Burrows NP+, *BMJ* 309, 97
Rash (sic) (1–10%)
Seborrheic dermatitis
(1983): Binder RL+, *Arch Dermatol* 119, 473 (1–5%)
(1981): Kanwar AJ+, *Arch Dermatol* 117, 65 (passim)
(1965): Fellner MJ+, *Int J Dermatol* 19, 392
(1956): Mullins JF+, *JAMA* 162, 946
Toxic epidermal necrolysis (<1%)
(1996): Purcell P+, *Postgrad Med J* 72, 186
(1990): Ward DJ+, *Burns* 16, 97
Urticaria
(1992): Loesche C+, *Contact Dermatitis* 26, 278
(1986): Lovell CR+, *Contact Dermatitis* 14, 290
(1967): Lockey SD, *Med Sci* 18, 43
(1961): Baer RL+, *Year Book of Dermatology*, Chicago, 9–37
(1956): Mullins JF+, *JAMA* 162, 946
Vasculitis
(1987): Aram H, *J Am Acad Dermatol* 17, 139
(1969): Peterkin GAG+, *Practitioner* 202, 117
(1957): Shannon J+, *Dermatologica* 114, 101
Xerosis

## Nails

Nails – photo-onycholysis
(1985): Kechijian P, *J Am Acad Dermatol* 12, 552
Nails – pigmentation
(1971): Hägermark O+, *Br J Dermatol* 84, 605
(1966): Zelickson AS, *JAMA* 198, 341
(1965): Satanove A+, *JAMA* 200, 209
(1964): Greiner AC+, *Can Med Assoc J* 90, 663

## Other

Anaphylactoid reactions (<1%)
(2001): Nikolic S+, *Srp Arh Celok Lek* 129(7), 203
Death
(2001): Nikolic S+, *Srp Arh Celok Lek* 129(7), 203
Galactorrhea (1–10%)
Gynecomastia (1–10%)
Injection-site aseptic necrosis
Mastodynia (1–10%)
Oral mucosal eruption
Oral mucosal pigmentation
Oral ulceration

Polyarteritis nodosa
(1960): Meyler L+, *Acta Med Scand* 167, 95
Priapism (<1%)
(2001): Compton MT+, *J Clin Psychiatry* 62(5), 362 (passim)
(1999): Mutlu N+, *Int J Clin Pract* 53, 152
Pseudolymphoma
(1995): Magro CM+, *J Am Acad Dermatol* 32, 419
Tremors
(2001): Chetty M+, *Ther Drug Monit* 23(5), 556 (with oral contraceptives)
Xerostomia (1–10%)

# CHLORPROPAMIDE

**Trade name:** Diabinese (Pfizer)
**Other common trade names:** *Apo-Chlorpropamide; Arodoc C; Chlormide; Diabemide; Diabenese; Insogen; Melormin; Tesmel*
**Indications:** Diabetes
**Category:** First generation sulfonylurea* hypoglycemic and antidiuretic
**Half-life:** 30–42 hours
**Clinically important, potentially hazardous interactions with: alcohol**, phenylbutazone

## *Reactions*

### Skin

Angioedema
(1991): Chinchmanian RM+, *Therapie* (French) 46, 163
Bullous eruption (<1%)
Contact dermatitis
(1982): Fisher AA, *Cutis* 29, 551
Cutaneous side effects (sic)
(1967): McKiddie MT+, *Scott Med J* 12, 6 (1.65%)
(1965): Cervantes-Amezcua A+, *JAMA* 193, 759 (1.4%)
(1960): Duncan LJP+, *Pharmacol Rev* 12, 91 (5%)
Edema (<1%)
Erythema multiforme (<1%)
(1980): Kanefsky TM+, *Arch Intern Med* 140, 1543
(1971): Harris EL, *BMJ* 3, 29
(1966): Tullett GL, *BMJ* 1, 148 (fatal)
(1960): Rothfeld EL+, *JAMA* 172, 54 (passim)
(1960): Yaffee HS, *Arch Dermatol* 82, 636
(1959): Greenhouse B, *Ann N Y Acad Sci* 74, 643
(1959): Stewart RC+, *N Engl J Med* 261, 427
Erythema nodosum (<1%)
(1971): Harris EL, *BMJ* 3, 29
(1966): Tullett GL, *BMJ* 1, 148
Exanthems (1–5%)
(1970): Almeyda J+, *Br J Dermatol* 82, 634 (1–5%)
(1960): Rothfeld EL+, *JAMA* 172, 54 (passim)
(1959): Hamff LH+, *Ann N Y Acad Sci* 74, 820
Exfoliative dermatitis
(1971): Harris EL, *BMJ* 3, 29
(1967): Coleman WP, *Med Clin North Am* 51, 1073
(1966): Tullett GL, *BMJ* 1, 148
(1962): Hitselberger JF+, *JAMA* 180, 62
(1960): Rothfeld EL+, *JAMA* 172, 54 (passim)
(1959): Reyes JAG+, *Ann N Y Acad Sci* 74, 1012
(1959): Stewart RC+, *N Engl J Med* 261, 427
Fixed eruption
(1979): Rupp T, *Int J Dermatol* 18, 590
Flushing
(1992): Shelley WB+, *Advanced Dermatologic Diagnosis* WB Saunders, 582 (passim)
(1983): Fui SNT+, *N Engl J Med* 309, 93 (alcohol flush)
(1983): Jerntorp P+, *Eur J Clin Pharmacol* 24, 237
(1982): Ohlin H+, *Br Med J Clin Res Ed* 285, 838
(1981): Barnett AH+, *Br Med J Clin Res Ed* 283, 939
(1981): Capretti L+, *Br Med J Clin Res Ed* 283, 1361
(1981): Jentorp P+, *Acta Med Scand* Suppl 656, 33
(1981): Medback S+, *BMJ* 283, 937 (alcohol flush)
(1981): Wilkin JK, *Ann Intern Med* 95, 468
(1980): Strakosch CR+, *Lancet* 1, 394
(1979): Leslie RDG+, *Lancet* 1, 997
(1978): Leslie RDG+, *BMJ* 2, 1519 (35%)
(1978): Pyke DA+, *BMJ* 2, 1521
(1971): Fairman MJ+, *BMJ* 4, 297 (40%)
(1971): Harris EL, *BMJ* 3, 29
(1966): Muller SA, *Proc Staff Meet Mayo Clin* 41, 689 (10–30%)
(1962): FitzGerald MG+, *Diabetes* 11, 40
(1962): Larsen JA+, *Proc Soc Exp Biol Med* 109, 120
(1959): Signorelli S, *Ann NY Acad Sci* 74, 900
Granulomas
(1976): Rigberg LA+, *JAMA* 235, 409
Lichenoid eruption
(1990): Franz CB+, *J Am Acad Dermatol* 22, 128
(1984): Barnett JH+, *Cutis* 34, 542
(1971): Almeyda J+, *Br J Dermatol* 85, 604
(1968): Dinsdale RCW+, *BMJ* 1, 100
Lupus erythematosus
(1979): Rupp T, *Int J Dermatol* 18, 590
Photosensitivity (1–10%)
(1973): Feuerman E+, *Dermatologica* 146, 25
(1971): Harris EL, *BMJ* 3, 29
(1962): Hitselberger JF+, *JAMA* 180, 62
Pruritus (<3%)
(1971): Harris EL, *BMJ* 3, 29
(1962): Hitselberger JF+, *JAMA* 180, 62
Purpura
(1977): Cunliffe DJ, *Postgrad Med* 53, 87
(1971): Harris EL, *BMJ* 3, 29
(1965): Horowitz HI+, *Semin Hematol* 2, 287
(1963): FitzPatrick WJ, *Diabetes* 12, 457
(1960): Rothfeld EL+, *JAMA* 172, 54 (passim)
(1959): Grace WJ, *N Engl J Med* 260, 711
(1959): Haynes WS, *BMJ* 2, 1403
(1959): Yuen H, *Ann N Y Acad Sci* 74, 918
Rash (sic) (1–10%)
(1985): Baciewicz AM+, *Diabetes Care* 8, 200
Stevens–Johnson syndrome
(1980): Kanefsky TM+, *Arch Intern Med* 140, 1543
(1966): Coursin DB, *JAMA* 198, 113
(1960): Rothfeld EL+, *JAMA* 172, 54 (passim)
(1960): Yaffee HS, *Arch Dermatol* 82, 636
(1959): Stewart RC+, *N Engl J Med* 261, 427
Toxic epidermal necrolysis
(1989): Stern RS+, *J Am Acad Dermatol* 21, 317
(1966): Tullett GL, *BMJ* 1, 148 (fatal)
Urticaria (1–10%)
(1991): Chinchmanian RM+, *Therapie* (French) 46, 163
(1973): Feuerman E+, *Dermatologica* 146, 25
(1960): Rothfeld EL+, *JAMA* 172, 54 (passim)
Vasculitis
(1983): Batko B, *Wiad Lek* (Polish) 36, 761
(1973): Feuerman E+, *Dermatologica* 146, 25

### Hair

Hair – alopecia
(1971): Harris EL, *BMJ* 3, 29

### Other

Acute intermittent porphyria
Death
Oral lichenoid eruption
(1988): Zain RB+, *Dent J Malays* 10, 15

(1984): Barnett J+, *Cutis* 34, 542
(1968): Dinsdale RCW+, *BMJ* 1, 100
Paresthesias
Porphyria
(1965): Zarowitz H+, *N Y State J Med* 65, 2385
Porphyria cutanea tarda
(1965): Zarowitz H+, *N Y State J Med* 65, 2385
Tongue ulceration
(1984): Barnett J+, *Cutis* 34, 542

***Note:** Chlorpropamide is a sulfonamide and can be absorbed systemically. Sulfonamides can produce severe, possibly fatal, reactions such as toxic epidermal necrolysis and Stevens–Johnson syndrome

# CHLORTETRACYCLINE

**Trade name:** Aureomycin (Proter Spa)
**Other common trade name:** *Aureomicina*
**Indications:** Various infections due to susceptible organisms
**Category:** Topical and ophthalmic tetracycline antibiotic
**Half-life:** no data

### *Reactions*

## Skin
Burning (topical) (ophthalmic)
Edema (topical)
Erythema (topical)
Irritation (topical)
Photosensitivity
(1965): Verhagen AR, *Dermatologica* 130, 439
Pruritus (topical)
Rash (sic) (topical)
Stinging (topical) (ophthalmic)
Xerosis (topical)

## Other
Xerostomia (ophthalmic)

# CHLORTHALIDONE

**Trade names:** Combipres (Boehringer Ingelheim); Hygroton (Aventis); Tenoretic (AstraZeneca); Thalitone (Monarch)
**Other common trade names:** *Higroton; Hydro-Long; Hypertol; Igroton; Thalidone; Uridon*
**Indications:** Hypertension
**Category:** Thiazide* diuretic; antihypertensive
**Half-life:** 35–50 hours
**Clinically important, potentially hazardous interactions with:** digoxin, lithium

Combipres is chlorthalidone and clonidine

### *Reactions*

## Skin
Erythema multiforme
Exanthems
Exfoliative dermatitis
Lupus erythematosus
Necrotizing angiitis
Photosensitivity (1–10%)
(1989): Baker EJ+, *J Am Acad Dermatol* 21, 1026
(1988): Lehmann P+, *Hautarzt* (German) 39, 38
Psoriasis
(1987): Wolf R+, *Cutis* 40, 162
Purpura (<1%)
Rash (sic) (<1%)
Stevens–Johnson syndrome
Toxic epidermal necrolysis
(1999): Egan CA+, *J Am Acad Dermatol* 40(3), 458
Urticaria (<1%)
(1993): Neaton JD+, *JAMA 279, 713 (passim)*
Vasculitis (<1%)
(1965): Björnberg A+, *Lancet* 2, 982

## Hair
Hair – alopecia

## Other
Paresthesias (<1%)
Pseudoporphyria
(1989): Baker EJ+, *J Am Acad Dermatol* 21, 1026
Xanthopsia

***Note:** Chlorthalidone is a sulfonamide and can be absorbed systemically. Sulfonamides can produce severe, possibly fatal, reactions such as toxic epidermal necrolysis and Stevens–Johnson syndrome

# CHLORZOXAZONE

**Trade names:** Paraflex (Ortho-McNeil); Parafon Forte DSC (Ortho-McNeil)
**Other common trade names:** *Escoflex; Flexaphen; Klorzoxazon; Muscol; Prolax; Remular-S; Solaxin*
**Indications:** Painful musculoskeletal conditions
**Category:** Skeletal muscle relaxant
**Half-life:** 1–2 hours

### *Reactions*

## Skin
Angioedema (1–10%)
Ecchymoses
Erythema multiforme (<1%)
(1979): Lindholm L, *Lakartidningen* (Swedish) 76, 2795
Exanthems
Flushing (1–10%)
Petechiae
Pruritus
Rash (sic) (<1%)
Urticaria (<1%)

## Other
Anaphylactoid reactions
Hypersensitivity
Trembling (sic) (1–10%)

## CHOLESTYRAMINE

**Trade names:** Lo-Cholest; Questran (Bristol-Myers Squibb)
**Other common trade names:** *Chol-Less; Colestrol; Lismol; PMS-Cholestyramine; Prevalite; Quantalan; Questran Lite*
**Indications:** Pruritus associated with biliary obstruction, primary hypercholesterolemia
**Category:** Antihyperlipidemic; antipruritic (cholestasis); anti-diarrheal
**Half-life:** no data
**Clinically important, potentially hazardous interactions with:** acetaminophen, acitretin, aspirin, chloroquine, cyclosporine, digoxin, doxepin, fat-soluble vitamins A D E and K, hydroxychloroquine, isotretinoin, lovastatin, mycophenolate, raloxifene, sulfasalazine, sulfonylureas, tetracycline, tricyclic antidepressants, valproic acid

### *Reactions*

#### Skin
Ecchymoses
Edema
Exanthems
Rash (sic) (<1%)
Urticaria

#### Other
Dysgeusia
Paresthesias
Tinnitus
Tongue irritation (sic) (<1%)

## CHONDROITIN

**Scientific names:** *Chondroitin 4-sulfate; chondroitin 4- and 6-sulfate*
**Other common names:** CDS; Chondroitin Sulfate A; Chondroitin Sulfate C; CSA; CSC; GAG
**Family:** None
**Purported indications:** Osteoarthritis (often in combination with glucosamine), ischemic heart disease, osteoporosis, hyperlipidemia
**Other uses:** Keratoconjunctivitis, an agent in cataract surgery

### *Reactions*

#### Skin
Allergic reactions (sic)
Eyelid edema
(2000): Leeb BF+, *J Rheumatology* 27, 205
Peripheral edema

#### Hair
Hair – alopecia

## CIDOFOVIR

**Trade names:** Forvade; Vistide (Gilead)
**Indications:** Cytomegalovirus (CMV) retinitis in patients with AIDS
**Category:** Antiviral (nucleotide analog)
**Half-life:** ~2.6 hours
**Clinically important, potentially hazardous interactions with:** amphotericin B, tenofovir

### *Reactions*

#### Skin
Acne (>10%)
Allergic reactions (sic) (1–10%)
Chills (24%)
Diaphoresis (1–10%)
Edema
Facial edema
Herpes simplex
Local irritation (sic)
(1998): Zabawski EJ+, *J Am Acad Dermatol* 39, 741
Pallor (1–10%)
Pigmentation (>10%)
Pruritus (1–10%)
Rash (sic) (27%)
Urticaria (1–10%)
Xerosis

#### Hair
Hair – alopecia (22%)

#### Other
Aphthous stomatitis
Application-site reactions (sic) (39%)
(1998): Zabawski EJ+, *J Am Acad Dermatol* 39, 741
Dysgeusia (1–10%)
Myalgia
Oral candidiasis
Oral ulceration
Paresthesias (>10%)
Stomatitis (1–10%)
Tongue discoloration
Xerostomia

## CILOSTAZOL

**Synonym:** OPC13013
**Trade name:** Pletal (Otsuka)
**Indications:** Peripheral vascular disease, intermittent claudication
**Category:** Platelet aggregation inhibitor
**Half-life:** 11–13 hours
**Clinically important, potentially hazardous interactions with:** fondaparinux

### *Reactions*

#### Skin
Chills (<2%)
Ecchymoses (<2%)
Edema (<2%)
Facial edema (<2%)
Furunculosis (<2%)

Generalized edema
Hypertrophy (sic)
Infections (sic)
Peripheral edema (7–9%)
Pruritus
Purpura (<2%)
Rash (sic) (2%)
Urticaria (<2%)
Xerosis (<2%)

### Other

Hyperesthesia (2%)
Myalgia (2–3%)
Paresthesias (2%)
Tongue edema (<2%)
Vaginitis (<2%)

## CIMETIDINE

**Trade name:** Tagamet (GSK)
**Other common trade names:** *Apo-Cimetidine; Azucimet; Blocan; Cimedine; Cimehexal; Ciuk; Dyspamet; Novocimetine; Nu-Cimet; Peptol; Stomedine; Ulcedine; Zymerol*
**Indications:** Duodenal ulcer
**Category:** Histamine $H_2$-receptor antagonist
**Half-life:** 2 hours
**Clinically important, potentially hazardous interactions with:** aminophylline, anisindione, anticoagulants, buprenorphine, butorphanol, carmustine, dicumarol, dofetilide, epirubicin, fentanyl, fluorouracil, galantamine, hydromorphone, itraconazole, ketoconazole, lidocaine, midazolam, morphine, narcotic analgesics, oxycodone, pentazocine, phenytoin, propranolol, sufentanil, theophylline, warfarin, xanthines

### *Reactions*

### Skin

Acne
Angioedema (<1%)
(1985): Whelan JP, *J Clin Pharmacol* 25, 610
(1982): Sandhu BS+, *Ann Intern Med* 97, 138
(1979): Delaunois L, *N Engl J Med* 300, 1216
Baboon syndrome
(1998): Helmbold P+, *Dermatology* 197, 402
Cutaneous side effects (sic) (0.4%)
(1982): Freston JW, *Ann Intern Med* 97, 728
Erythema annulare centrifugum
(1982): Merrett AC+, *N Z J Med* 12, 107
(1981): Merrett AC+, *BMJ* 283, 698
Erythema multiforme (<1%)
(1987): Talvard O+, *Presse Med* (French) 16, 825
(1983): Guan R+, *Aust N Z J Med* 13, 182
(1982): Wallach D+, *Dermatologica* 165, 197
(1981): Bjaeldager PA, *Ugeskr Laeger* (Danish) 143, 1406
(1978): Ahmed AH+, *Lancet* 2, 433
Erythroderma
Erythrosis-like lesions (sic)
(1979): Angelini G+, *BMJ* 1, 1147
Exanthems
(1986): Peters K, *Contact Dermatitis* 15, 190
(1982): Freston JW, *Ann Intern Med* 97, 728
(1979): Hadfield WA, *Ann Intern Med* 91, 128
Exfoliative dermatitis
(1983): Mitchell GG, *Am J Med* 75, 875
(1980): Yantis PL+, *Dig Dis Sci* 25, 73
Fixed eruption
(1998): Helmbold P+, *Dermatology* 197, 402 (baboon syndrome)
(1995): Inoue A+, *Acta Derm Venereol* 75, 250
Ichthyosis
(1984): Aram H, *Int J Dermatol* 23, 458
Id reaction
(1987): Sander-Jensen K+, *Dermatologica* 174, 103
Lupus erythematosus
(1982): Davidson BL+, *Arch Intern Med* 142, 166 (exacerbation)
(1979): Littlejohn GO+, *Ann Intern Med* 91, 317
Pruritus (<1%)
(1994): Warner DMc+, *J Am Acad Dermatol* 31, 677 (passim)
(1982): Freston JW, *Ann Intern Med* 97, 728
(1982): Sandhu BS+, *Ann Intern Med* 97, 138
(1982): Wallach D+, *Dermatologica* 165, 197
(1981): Taillandier J+, *Nouv Presse Med* (French) 10, 258
(1979): Matthews CNA+, *Br J Dermatol* 101, 57
Psoriasis
(1991): Andersen M, *Ugeskr Laeger* (Danish) 153, 132
(1986): Peters K, *Contact Dermatitis* 15, 190
(1983): Mitchell GG, *Am J Med* 75, 875
(1982): Wallach D+, *Dermatologica* 165, 197
(1980): Yates VM+, *BMJ* 280, 1453
(1979): Rai GS+, *Lancet* 1, 50
Purpura
Pustular psoriasis
(1979): Rai GS+, *Lancet* 1, 50
Rash (sic) (<2%)
(1991): Marshall J+, *Chest* 99, 1016
Seborrheic dermatitis
(1981): Kanwar AJ, *Arch Dermatol* 117, 65
Stevens–Johnson syndrome
(1987): Talvard O+, *Presse Med* (French) 16, 825
(1983): Guan R+, *Aust N Z J Med* 13, 182
(1978): Ahmed AH+, *Lancet* 2, 433
Toxic dermatitis (sic)
(1981): Pasquier P+, *Nouv Presse Med* (French) 10, 2994
Toxic epidermal necrolysis (<1%)
(1998): Tidwell BH+, *Am J Health Syst Pharm* 55, 163
(1983): Dabadie H+, *Gastroenterol Clin Biol* (French) 7, 425
Urticaria
(1985): Goolamali SK, *Postgrad Med J* 61, 925
(1983): Mitchell GG, *Am J Med* 75, 875
(1982): Freston JW, *Ann Intern Med* 97, 728
(1982): Sandhu BS+, *Ann Intern Med* 97, 138
(1981): Brandrup E, *Ugeskr Laeger* (Danish) 143, 1715
(1979): Hadfield WA, *Ann Intern Med* 91, 128
Vasculitis
(1983): Mitchell GG, *Am J Med* 75, 875
(1982): Wallach D+, *Dermatologica* 165, 197
(1981): Dernbach WK+, *JAMA* 246, 331
Xerosis
(1982): Greist MC+, *Arch Dermatol* 118, 253

### Hair

Hair – alopecia
(1985): Tullio CJ+, *Clin Pharm* 4, 145
(1983): Khalsa JH+, *Int J Dermatol* 22, 202
(1981): Vircburger MI+, *Lancet* 1, 1160
(1979): Ahmad S, *Ann Intern Med* 91, 930

### Other

Anaphylactoid reactions
(1982): Knapp AB+, *Ann Intern Med* 97, 374
Galactorrhea
(1977): Bateson MC+, *Lancet* 2, 247
Gynecomastia (<1%)
(2000): Hugues FC+, *Ann Med Interne (Paris)* (French) 151, 10 (passim)

(1994): Garcia-Rodriguez LA+, *BMJ* 308, 503
(1991): Barth JA, *Zentralbl Gynakol* (German) 113, 667
(1983): Jensen RT+, *N Engl J Med* 308, 883
(1982): Peden NR+, *Br J Clin Pharmacol* 14, 565
(1979): Spence RW+, *Gut* 20, 154
(1977): Della-Fave GF+, *Lancet* 1, 1319
(1976): Hall WH, *N Engl J Med* 841, 295 (letter)

Hypersensitivity
(2000): Evans RD+, *Clin Podiatr Med Surg* 17, 371
(1986): Peters K, *Contact Dermatitis* 15, 190
(1985): Whalen JP, *J Clin Pharmacol* 25, 610

Injection-site pain

Myalgia (<1%)

Myopathy
(1982): Kaplinsky N+, *J Rheumatol* 9, 156
(1980): Feest TG+, *BMJ* 281, 1284

Porphyria
(1985): Singh R+, *J Assoc Physicians India* 33, 187

Pseudolymphoma
(1995): Magro CM+, *J Am Acad Dermatol* 32, 419

Xerostomia

# CINOXACIN

**Trade name:** Cinobac (Oclassen)
**Other common trade names:** *Cerexin; Cinobact; Cinobactin; Gugecin; Nossacin; Noxigram; Uronorm*
**Indications:** Various urinary tract infections caused by susceptible organisms
**Category:** Quinolone antibiotic
**Half-life:** 1.5 hours

## *Reactions*

### Skin

Allergic reactions (sic)
Angioedema (<3%)
Edema (<3%)
Erythema multiforme
Photosensitivity
Pruritus (<3%)
Rash (sic)
Stevens–Johnson syndrome
Toxic epidermal necrolysis
Urticaria (<3%)

### Other

Anaphylactoid reactions
(1988): Stricker BH+, *BMJ* 297, 1434

Dysgeusia (<1%)

Hypersensitivity
(1982): Scavone JM+, *Pharmacotherapy* 2, 266

Paresthesias (<1%)

Tinnitus

# CIPROFLOXACIN

**Trade names:** Ciloxan Ophthalmic (Alcon); Cipro (Bayer)
**Other common trade names:** *Ciflox; Cimogal; Ciplox; Ciprobay Uro; Cipromycin; Ciproxin; Italnik; Kenzoflex; Uniflox*
**Indications:** Various infections caused by susceptible organisms
**Category:** Synthetic fluoroquinolone antibiotic
**Half-life:** 4 hours
**Clinically important, potentially hazardous interactions with:** amiodarone, antacids, antineoplastics, arsenic, bepridil, bismuth subsalicylate, bretylium, **caffeine**, calcium salts, didanosine, disopyramide, erythromycin, iron, magnesium salts, methylxanthines, NSAIDs, phenothiazines, procainamide, quinidine, sotalol, sucralfate, theophylline, tricyclic antidepressants, zinc

Ciprofloxacin is chemically related to nalidixic acid

## *Reactions*

### Skin

Acne
(1989): Rahm V+, *Scand J Infect Dis* 60, 120
(1988): Campoli-Richards DM+, *Drugs* 35, 373
(1988): Schacht P+, *Infection* 16, S29

Allergic reactions (sic)
(2000): Burke P+, *BMJ* 320, 679

Angioedema (<1%)
(1995): Vidal C+, *Postgrad Med J* 71, 318
(1989): Davis H+, *Ann Intern Med* 111, 1041
(1989): Rahm V+, *Scand J Infect Dis* 60, 120
(1989): Schacht P+, *Am J Med* 87, 98S
(1988): Campoli-Richards DM+, *Drugs* 35, 373
(1988): Schacht P+, *Infection* 16, S29

Bullous eruption
(1988): Kaufmann I+, *Z Hautkr* (German) 63, 679

Bullous pemphigoid
(2000): Kimyadi-Asadi A+, *J Am Acad Dermatol* 42, 847

Candidiasis (<1%)
(1997): Litt JZ, Beachwood, OH (personal case) (penile) (observation)
(1989): Yangco BG+, *Clin Ther* 11, 503
(1988): Schacht P+, *Infection* 16, S29

Diaphoresis
(1990): Karimi K, *Indiana Med* 83, 266
(1989): Rahm V+, *Scand J Infect Dis* 60, 120
(1988): Campoli-Richards DM+, *Drugs* 35, 373 (0.05%)
(1988): Schacht P+, *Infection* 16, S29

Edema (<1%)
(1995): Shelley ED, Toledo, OH (personal case) (observation)

Elastolysis
(1993): Lien YH+, *Am J Kidney Dis* 22, 598

Erythema multiforme
(1994): Win A+, *Int J Dermatol* 33, 512
(1993): Imrie K+, *Am J Hematol* 43, 159

Erythema nodosum (<1%)

Erythroderma (<1%)
(1989): Wurtz RM+, *Lancet* 1, 955

Exanthems
(2002): Litt JZ, Beachwood, OH (personal case) (observation)
(2000): Litt JZ, Beachwood, OH (personal case) (observation)
(1999): Litt JZ, Beachwood, OH (anecdote from lay person on the Internet)
(1999): Litt JZ, Beachwood, OH (personal case) (observation)
(1997): Bircher AJ+, *Allergy* 52, 1246
(1996): McCarty JR, Fort Worth, TX (from Internet) (observation)

(1989): Gaut PL+, *Am J Med* 87 (Suppl 5A), 169S
(1988): Campoli-Richards DM+, *Drugs* 35, 373 (0.7%)
Exfoliative dermatitis (<1%)
Fixed eruption
(2001): Hamamoto Y+, *Clin Exp Dermatol* 26(1), 48
(2001): Rodriguez-Morales A+, *Contact Dermatitis* 44(4), 255
(2001): Sharma R, Aligarh, India (from Internet) (observation) (recurrence after fixed eruption from sparfloxacin)
(1998): Litt JZ, Beachwood, OH (personal case) (observation)
(1998): Maquirriain Gorriz MT+, *Aten Primaria* (Spanish) 21, 585
(1996): Dhar S+, *Br J Dermatol* 134, 156
(1995): Lozano-Ayllon M+, *Allergy* 50, 598
(1994): Kawada A+, *Contact Dermatitis* 31, 182
(1993): Alonso MD+, *Allergy* 48, 296
(1992): Alonso MD+, *Allergy* 47, 194
Flushing (<1%)
(1988): Campoli-Richards DM+, *Drugs* 35, 373
Linear IgA bullous dermatosis
(2001): Wiadrowski TP+, *Austral J Dermatol* 42, 196 (with vancomycin)
Livedo reticularis
(1999): Verros CD, Tripolis, Greece (from Internet) (observation) (recurred on rechallenge)
Photosensitivity (<1%)
(2000): Ferguson J+, *J Antimicrob Chemother* 45, 503
(1998): Kimura M+, *Contact Dermatitis* 38, 180
(1997): Ferguson J+, *J Antimicrob Chemother* 40, 93
(1995): Burdge DR+, *Antimicrob Agents Chemother* 39, 793
(1993): Shelley WB+, *Cutis* 51, 154 (observation)
(1993): Shelley WB+, *Cutis* 52, 27 (observation)
(1990): Ferguson J+, *Br J Dermatol* 123, 9
(1989): Granowitz EV, *J Infect Dis* 160, 910
(1989): Nedorost ST+, *Arch Dermatol* 125, 433
(1989): Rahm V+, *Scand J Infect Dis* 60, 120
(1988): Campoli-Richards DM+, *Drugs* 35, 373
(1988): Kaufmann I+, *Z Hautkr* (German) 63, 679
(1988): Schacht P+, *Infection* 16, S29
(1987): Jensen T+, *J Antimicrob Chemother* 20, 585
(1986): Ball P, *J Antimicrob Chemother* 18 (Suppl D), 187
Phototoxicity
(2000): Traynor NJ+, *Toxicol Vitr* 14, 275
(1998): Martinez LJ+ *Photochem Photobiol* 67, 399
(1993): Ferguson J+, *Br J Dermatol* 128, 285
Pigmentation (<1%)
Pruritus (<1%)
(2002): Litt JZ, Beachwood, OH (personal case) (observation)
(1999): Litt JZ, Beachwood, OH (2 personal cases) (observation)
(1989): Davis H+, *Ann Intern Med* 111, 1041
(1989): Gaut PL+, *Am J Med* 87 (Suppl 5A), 169S
(1989): Rahm V+, *Scand J Infect Dis* 60, 120
(1989): Schacht P+, *Am J Med* 87, 98S
(1989): Yangco BG+, *Clin Ther* 11, 503
(1988): Campoli-Richards DM+, *Drugs* 35, 373 (0.3%)
(1988): Sanders WE, *Rev Infect Dis* 10, 528
(1988): Schacht P+, *Infection* 16, S29
(1988): Thorsteinsson SB+, *Chemotherapy* 34, 256
Purpura
(1999): Goldberg EI+, *J Clin Dermatol* 2, 25
(1997): Sapadin A+, New York, American Academy of Dermatology Meeting (SF), Poster #110
(1994): Gamboa F+, *Ann Pharmacol* 29, 84
Radiation recall
(2001): Krishnan RS+, *J Am Acad Dermatol* 44, 1045 (with piperacillin & tobramycin)
Rash (sic) (1–10%)
(2000): Johansson A+, *Pediatr Infect Dis J* 19, 449
(2000): Talan DA+, *JAMA* 283, 1583 (4%)
(1995): Chaisson RE, *Infections in Medicine* 12, 48
(1989): Fass RJ+, *Am J Med* 87, 164S
(1989): Modai J, *Am J Med* 87, 243S
(1989): Rahm V+, *Scand J Infect Dis* 60, 120
(1989): Schacht P+, *Am J Med* 87, 98S
(1988): Sanders WE, *Rev Infect Dis* 10, 528
(1988): Schacht P+, *Infection* 16, S29
Stevens–Johnson syndrome (<1%)
(1994): Bhatia RS, *J Assoc Physicians India* 42, 344
(1994): Gohel DR+, *J Assoc Physicians India* 42, 665
(1994): Kamili MA+, *J Assoc Physicians India* 42, 755
(1994): Win A+, *Int J Dermatol* 33, 512
Toxic epidermal necrolysis (<1%)
(1997): Livasy CA+, *Dermatology* 195, 173 (fatal)
(1997): Yerasi AB+, *Ann Pharmacother* 30, 297
(1993): Moshfeghi M+, *Ann Pharmacother* 27, 1467
(1991): Sakellariou G+, *Int J Artif Organs* 14, 634
(1991): Tham TC+, *Lancet* 338, 522
Urticaria (<1%)
(1999): Litt JZ, Beachwood, OH (personal case) (observation)
(1994): Guharoy SR, *Vet Hum Toxicol* 36, 540
(1993): Litt JZ, Beachwood, OH (personal case) (observation)
(1989): Davis H+, *Ann Intern Med* 111, 1041
(1989): Rahm V+, *Scand J Infect Dis* 60, 120
(1989): Schacht P+, *Am J Med* 87, 98S
(1988): Campoli-Richards DM+, *Drugs* 35, 373 (0.05%)
(1988): Schacht P+, *Infection* 16, S29
(1986): Ball P, *J Antimicrob Chemother* 18 (Suppl D), 187
Vasculitis (<1%)
(2000): Perez Vazquez A+, *An Med Interna* (Spanish) 17, 225
(1999): Goldberg EI+, *J Clin Dermatol* 2, 25
(1997): Lieu PK+, *Allergy* 52, 593
(1997): Reano M+, *Allergy* 52, 599
(1994): Beuselinck B+, *Acta Clin Belg* 49, 173
(1993): Wagh SS+, *Indian J Pediatr* 60, 610
(1992): Stubbings J+, *BMJ* 305, 29
(1991): Kanuga J+, *Ann Allergy* 66, 76
(1989): Choe U+, *N Engl J Med* 320, 257

## Other

Anaphylactoid reactions (<1%)
(1999): Corcoy M+, *Rev Esp Anestesiol Reanim* (Spanish) 46, 419
(1999): Erdem G+, *Pediatr Infect Dis J* 18, 563
(1997): Clutterbuck DJ+, *Int J STD AIDS* 8, 707
(1997): Salon EJ+, *Ann Pharmacother* 31, 119
(1995): Assouad M+, *Ann Intern Med* 122, 396
(1994): Beuselinck B+, *Acta Clin Belg* (Dutch; French) 49, 173
(1993): Soetikno RM+, *Ann Pharmacother* 27, 1404 (in AIDS)
(1992): Berger TG+, *J Am Acad Dermatol* 26, 256
(1992): Deamer RL+, *Ann Pharmacother* 26, 1081
(1989): Davis H+, *Ann Intern Med* 111, 1041
(1989): Wurtz RM+, *Lancet* 1, 955
Anosmia
Arthralgia
(1991): Chysky V+, *Infection* 19, 289
Death
Dysesthesia (<1%)
(1995): Zehnder D+, *BMJ* 311, 1204
Dysgeusia (<1%)
(1988): Schacht P+, *Infection* 16, S29
Gynecomastia (<1%)
(1991): MacGowan AP+, *J Infect* 22, 100
Hypersensitivity
(2001): Scala E+, *Int J Dermatol* 40(9), 603
(1992): Deamer RL+, *Ann Pharmacother* 26, 1081
(1991): Bhatia RS, *J Assoc Physicians India* 39, 972
Injection-site pain
(1988): Thorsteinsson SB+, *Chemotherapy* 34, 256
(1987): Thorsteinsson SB+, *Chemotherapy* 33, 448 (with itching and burning)

Lobular panniculitis (erythematous tender nodules of extremities)
(1990): Rodriguez E+, *BMJ* 300, 1468
Oral candidiasis
(1988): Esposito S+, *Infection* 16, S57
Oral mucosal lesions
(1988): Campoli-Richards DM+, *Drugs* 35, 373
Paresthesias
(1989): Rahm V+, *Scand J Infect Dis* 60, 120
Seizures
(2001): Kushner JM+, *Ann Pharmacother* 35(10), 1194
Serum sickness
(1994): Guharoy SR, *Vet Hum Toxicol* 36, 540
(1990): Slama TG, *Antimicrob Agents Chemother* 34, 904
Stomatitis
(1989): Rahm V+, *Scand J Infect Dis* 60, 120
(1989): Schacht P+, *Am J Med* 87, 98S
(1988): Schacht P+, *Infection* 16, S29
Tendinitis
(1999): Harrell RM, *South Med J* 92, 622 (passim)
(1998): Blanco Andres C+, *Aten Primaria* (Spanish) 21, 184 (bilateral)
(1998): West MB+, *N Z Med J* 111, 18 (bilateral)
(1997): Carrasco JM+, *Ann Pharmacother* 31, 120
Tendon rupture
(2001): Malaguti M+, *J Nephrol* 14(5), 431
(2000): Casparian JM+, *South Med J* 93, 488 (2 cases)
(1998): Petersen W+, *Umfallchirurg* (German) 101, 731 (bilateral)
(1998): West MB+, *N Z Med J* 111, 18
(1997): Movin T+, *Foot Ankle Int* 18, 297 (2 cases)
(1997): Peyrade F+, *Presse Med* (French) 26, 1489
(1997): Poon CC+, *Med J Aust* 166, 665
(1997): Shinohara YT+, *J Rheumatol* 24, 238
(1996): Hugo-Persson M, *Lakartidningen* (Swedish) 93, 1520
(1996): Jagose JT+, *N Z Med J* 109, 471
(1996): McGarvey WC+, *Foot Ankle Int* 17, 496
(1993): Boulay I+, *Ann Med Interne (Paris)* (French) 144, 493
(1992): Lee TW+, *Aust N Z J Med,* 22, 500
Tinnitus
Tremors
Vaginitis (<1%)
(1990): Karimi K, *Indiana Med* 83, 266
(1987): Arcieri G+, *Am J Med* 82, 381
Xerostomia
(1989): Rahm V+, *Scand J Infect Dis* 60, 120
(1988): Campoli-Richards DM+, *Drugs* 35, 373
(1988): Schacht P+, *Infection* 16, S29

# CISATRACURIUM

**Trade name:** Nimbex (Abbott)
**Indications:** Adjunct to general anesthesia, relaxes skeletal muscle
**Category:** Non-depolarizing neuromuscular blocker (skeletal muscle relaxant)
**Half-life:** 22 minutes
**Clinically important, potentially hazardous interactions with:** aminoglycosides, clindamycin, cyclopropane, enflurane, halothane, isoflurane, methoxyflurane, piperacillin

### *Reactions*

## Skin
Flushing (0.2%)
Rash (sic) (0.1%)

## Other
Anaphylactoid reactions
(2001): Krombach J+, *Anesth Analg* 93(5), 1257
(2001): Legros CB+, *Anesth Analg* 92(3), 648
(2000): Briassoulis G+, *Paediatr Anaesth* 10(4), 429
(1999): Toh KW+, *Anesth Analg* 88(2), 462
(1997): Clendenen SR+, *Anesthesiology* 87(3), 690
Hypersensitivity
Myopathy
(1998): Davis NA+, *Crit Care Med* 26(7), 1290

# CISPLATIN

**Synonym:** CDDP
**Trade name:** Platinol (Bristol-Myers Squibb)
**Other common trade names:** *Cisplatyl; Plasticin; Platiblastin; Platinex; Platinol-AQ; Platistil*
**Indications:** Carcinomas, lymphomas
**Category:** Antineoplastic
**Half-life:** $\alpha$ phase: 25–49 minutes; $\beta$ phase: 58–73 hours
**Clinically important, potentially hazardous interactions with:** aldesleukin, methotrexate

### *Reactions*

## Skin
Acral erythema
(1998): Vakalis D+, *Br J Dermatol* 139, 750
Actinic keratosis inflammation
(1987): Johnson TM+, *J Am Acad Dermatol* 17(2 Pt 1), 192
Angioedema
(1984): Loehrer PJ+, *Ann Intern Med* 100, 704
(1983): Bronner AK+, *J Am Acad Dermatol* 9, 645 (1–5%)
(1981): Weiss RB+, *Ann Intern Med* 94, 66 (1–5%)
(1977): Rozencweig M+, *Ann Intern Med* 86, 803
Contact dermatitis
(1996): Schena D+, *Contact Dermatitis* 34, 220
Diaphoresis
(1983): Bronner AK+, *J Am Acad Dermatol* 9, 645
Erythema
(2001): Robinson JB+, *Gynecol Oncol* 82(3), 550
(1983): Bronner AK+, *J Am Acad Dermatol* 9, 645
(1980): Vogl SE+, *Cancer* 45, 11
Exanthems
(1984): Loehrer PJ+, *Ann Intern Med* 100, 704
(1981): Weiss RB+, *Ann Intern Med* 94, 66 (1–5%)
(1980): Vogl SE+, *Cancer* 45, 11
Exfoliative dermatitis
(1994): Lee TC+, *Mayo Clin Proc* 69, 80
Facial edema
(1994): Lee TC+, *Mayo Clin Proc* 69, 80
Flushing
(2001): Robinson JB+, *Gynecol Oncol* 82(3), 550
(1998): Kempf W+, *Arch Dermatol* 134, 1343
(1984): Loehrer PJ+, *Ann Intern Med* 100, 704
(1983): Bronner AK+, *J Am Acad Dermatol* 9, 645
(1980): Vogl SE+, *Cancer* 45, 11
Necrosis
(1983): Leyden M+, *Cancer Treat Rep* 67, 199
Pigmentation
(2002): Kim KJ+, *Clin Exp Dermatol* 27(2), 118
(1996): Al-Lamki Z+, *Cancer* 77, 1578
Pruritus
(2001): Robinson JB+, *Gynecol Oncol* 82(3), 550
(1994): Lee TC+, *Mayo Clin Proc* 69, 80 (passim)
(1983): Bronner AK+, *J Am Acad Dermatol* 9, 645 (1–5%)

(1981): Weiss RB+, *Ann Intern Med* 94, 66 (1–5%)
Pyoderma (verrucous)
(1982): Person JR+, *Arch Dermatol* 118, 336
Rash (sic)
Raynaud's phenomenon
(1992): Doll DC+, *Semin Oncol* 19(5), 580
(1984): Loehrer PJ+, *Ann Intern Med* 100, 704
(1981): Vogelzang NJ+, *Ann Intern Med* 95, 288
Stevens–Johnson syndrome
(1989): Brodsky A+, *J Clin Pharmacol* 29, 821
Urticaria
(1996): Schena D+, *Contact Dermatitis* 34, 220
(1994): Lee TC+, *Mayo Clin Proc* 69, 80 (passim)
(1983): Bronner AK+, *J Am Acad Dermatol* 9, 645 (1–5%)
(1981): Weiss RB+, *Ann Intern Med* 94, 66 (1–5%)
(1980): Vogl SE+, *Cancer* 45, 11

### Hair

Hair – alopecia (>10%)
(2001): Sakai H+, *Cancer Chemother Pharmacol* 48(6), 499 (with paclitaxel)
(1996): Planting AS+, *Eur J Cancer* 32A, 2026
(1992): Zaun H+, *Hautarzt* (German) 43, 215
(1989): Umeki S+, *Chemotherapy* 35, 54

### Nails

Nails – Beau's lines (transverse nail bands)
(1994): Ben-Dyan D+, *Acta Haematol* 91, 89
Nails – hypomelanosis
(1983): James WD+, *Arch Dermatol* 119, 334

### Other

Ageusia
Anaphylactoid reactions (<1%)
(1999): Ozguroglu M+, *Am J Clin Oncol* 22, 172 (intraperitoneal infusion)
(1997): Ciesielski-Carlucci C+, *Am J Clin Oncol* 20(4), 373 (with paclitaxel)
(1994): Lee TC+, *Mayo Clin Proc* 69, 80 (passim)
(1983): Bronner AK+, *J Am Acad Dermatol* 9, 645
(1982): Dunagin WG, *Semin Oncol* 9, 14
(1980): Vogl SE+, *Cancer* 45, 11
(1977): Rozencweig M+, *Ann Intern Med* 86, 803
Digital necrosis
(2000): Marie I+, *Br J Dermatol* 142, 833
Extravasation
Gingival pigmentation
(1982): Dunagin WG, *Semin Oncol* 9, 14
Hypersensitivity
(2001): Robinson JB+, *Gynecol Oncol* 82(3), 550
Injection-site cellulitis
(1994): Lee TC+, *Mayo Clin Proc* 69, 80 (passim)
(1990): Fields S+, *J Natl Cancer Inst* 82, 1649
(1989): Kerker BJ+, *Semin Dermatol* 8, 173
(1980): Lewis KP+, *Cancer Treat Rep* 64, 1162
Injection-site pain
(1998): Kempf W+, *Arch Dermatol* 134, 1343
Injection-site thrombophlebitis
Oral mucosal lesions (<1%)
(1997): Herlofson BB+, *Eur J Oral Sci* 105, 523
(1990): Al-Sarraf M+, *J Clin Oncol* 8, 1342 (>5%)
Oral ulceration (<1%)
Phlebitis
Porphyria
(1986): Aramburo-Gonzalez P+, *Med Clin (Barc)* (Spanish) 87, 738
Rhabdomyolysis
(1995): Anderlini P+, *Cancer* 76(4), 678
Tinnitus

# CITALOPRAM

**Synonym:** nitalapram
**Trade name:** Celexa (Forest)
**Indications:** Depression, obsessive-compulsive disorder, panic disorder
**Category:** Antidepressant (SSRI)
**Half-life:** 33 hours
**Clinically important, potentially hazardous interactions with:** isocarboxazid, MAO inhibitors, phenelzine, selegiline, sumatriptan, tramadol, tranylcypromine, trazodone

## *Reactions*

### Skin

Cellulitis
Dermatitis (sic)
Diaphoresis (11%)
(2001): Bostic JQ+, *J Child Adole Pyschopharmacolsc* 11(2), 159
Eczema (sic)
Exanthems
(2001): Richard MA+, *Ann Dermatol Venereol* 128(6), 759
Facial edema
Hot flashes
Hypohidrosis
Photopigmentation
(2001): Inaloz HS+, *J Dermatol* 28(12), 742
Photosensitivity
Pigmentation
(2001): Inaloz HS+, *J Dermatol* 28(12), 742
Pruritus (<10%)
(2001): Richard MA+, *Ann Dermatol Venereol* 128(6), 759
Pruritus ani
Psoriasis
(2000): Elliott P, Logan Central, Australia (from Internet) (observation)
Purpura
(2001): Robinson MJ, *Can Psychiatry* 46, 286
Rash (sic) (<10%)
Urticaria
Vasculitis
(2001): Richard MA+, *Ann Dermatol Venereol* 128(6), 759
Xerosis

### Hair

Hair – alopecia
Hair – hypertrichosis

### Other

Bruxism
(2001): Wise M, *Br J Psychiatry* 178, 182
Death
(2002): Jonasson B+, *Forensic Sci Int* 126(1), 1 (5 cases)
(2001): Dams R+, *J Anal Toxicol* 25(2), 147 (with moclobemide)
(2001): Isbister GK+, *J Anal Toxicol* 25(8), 716 (with moclobemide)
Dysgeusia
Galactorrhea
(2001): Gonzalez Pablos E+, *Actas Esp Psiquiatr* 29(6), 414
Gingival bleeding
Gingivitis
Gynecomastia
Hyperesthesia
Hypesthesia
Mastodynia
Myalgia (>2%)

Paresthesias
Priapism (clitoral)
(2002): Baptista T, *J Clin Psychiatry* 63(3), 245 (with risperidone)
(2002): Freudenreich O, *J Clin Psychiatry* 63(3), 249 (with risperidone)
(1997): Berk M+, *Int Clin Psychopharmacol* 12, 121 (3 cases)
Serotonin syndrome
(2002): Chechani V, *Crit Care Med* 30(2), 473
(2001): Dams R+, *J Anal Toxicol* 25(2), 147 (with moclobemide)
Sialorrhea
Stomatitis
Tremors (<10%)
Twitching
(2001): Rojas VM+, *J Child Adolesc Psychopharmacol* 11(3), 295
Xerostomia (20%)

## CLADRIBINE

**Synonyms:** 2-CdA; 2-chlorodeoxyadenosine
**Trade name:** Leustatin (Ortho)
**Indications:** Leukemias
**Category:** Antineoplastic; antimetabolite
**Half-life:** $\alpha$ phase: 25 minutes; $\beta$ phase: 6.7 hours

### *Reactions*

#### Skin

Allergic reactions (sic)
(1997): Robak T+, *J Med* 28, 199
Diaphoresis (1–10%)
Edema (6%)
Erythema (6%)
Exanthems (27–50%)
(1996): Meunier P+, *Acta Derm Venereol* 76, 385 (21%)
Halogenoderma (sic)
(1996): Zevin S+, *Am J Hematol* 53, 209
Petechiae (8%)
Pruritus (6%)
Purpura (10%)
Rash (sic) (27%)
(2000): Grey MR+, *Clin Lab Haematol* 22, 111
Toxic epidermal necrolysis
(1996): Meunier P+, *Acta Derm Venereol* 76, 385
Transient acantholytic dermatosis (sic)
(1997): Cohen PR+, *Acta Derm Venereol* 77, 412

#### Other

Gynecomastia
(2001): Abhyankar D+, *Leuk Lymphoma* 42(1), 243
Injection-site edema (9%)
Injection-site erythema (9%)
Injection-site pain (9%)
Injection-site phlebitis (2%)
Injection-site thrombosis (2%)
Myalgia (7%)

## CLARITHROMYCIN

**Synonym:** Cla
**Trade name:** Biaxin (Abbott)
**Other common trade names:** *Biaxin HP; Clacine; Clarith; Klacid; Klaricid; Macladin; Veclam*
**Indications:** Various infections caused by susceptible organisms
**Category:** Macrolide antibiotic
**Half-life:** 5–7 hours
**Clinically important, potentially hazardous interactions with:** alprazolam, atorvastatin, benzodiazepines, carbamazepine, chlordiazepoxide, clonazepam, clorazepate, cyclosporine, diazepam, digoxin, dihydroergotamine, disopyramide, ergot alkaloids, fluoxetine, flurazepam, fluvastatin, imatinib, lorazepam, lovastatin, methysergide, midazolam, oxazepam, paroxetine, pimozide, pravastatin, quazepam, sertraline, simvastatin, temazepam, triazolam, warfarin, zidovudine

### *Reactions*

#### Skin

Exanthems
Fixed eruption
(2001): Hamamoto Y+, *Clin Exp Dermatol* 26(1), 48
(1988): Rosina P+, *Contact Dermatitis* 38, 105
Pruritus
(1991): Poirier R, *J Antimicrob Chemother* 27 (Suppl A), 109
Psoriasis
(1994): Ellerin P, *The Schoch Letter* 44, 47 (#185) (observation)
Pustular eruption
Rash (sic) (3%)
Stevens–Johnson syndrome (<1%)
Toxic epidermal necrolysis
(2002): Masia M+, *Arch Intern Med* 162(4), 474 (with disulfiram)
Urticaria
Vasculitis
(1998): Gavura SR+, *Ann Pharmacol* 32, 543
(1993): de Vega T+, *Eur J Clin Microbiol Infect Dis* 12, 563

#### Other

Anaphylactoid reactions (<1%)
Black tongue
(1997): Greco S+, *Ann Pharmacother* 31, 1548
Death
(2002): Masia M+, *Arch Intern Med* 162(4), 474
Dysgeusia (3%)
(2001): Litt JZ, Beachwood, OH (personal case)
(2001): McCarty JM+, *Ann Allergy Asthma Immunol* 87(4), 327
(1997): Saluja A+, *Derm Surg* 23, 539
Ergotism
(2001): Ausband SC+, *J Emerg Med* 21(4), 411
Glossitis
(1997): Greco S+, *Ann Pharmacother* 31, 1548
Hypersensitivity
(1998): Igea JM+, *Allergy* 53, 107
(1998): Kruppa A+, *Dermatology* 196(3), 335
Infusion-site inflammation
(2001): Zimmerman T+, *Clin Drug Invest* 21, 527 (8%)
Infusion-site pain
(2001): Zimmerman T+, *Clin Drug Invest* 21, 527 (100%)
Injection-site pain
(1996): Peck KD+, *Pharm Res* 13, PT6028 (9 Suppl)
Oral candidiasis
Parosmia
Phlebitis

(2001): De Dios Garcia-Diaz J+, *Med Clin* (Barc) 116(4), 133 (from intravenous administration)

Pseudolymphoma
(1995): Magro CM+, *J Am Acad Dermatol* 32, 419

Rhabdomyolysis
(2001): Lee AJ, *Ann Pharmacother* 35(1), 26 (with simvastatin)
(1999): Shimada N+, *Nippon Jinzo Gakkai Shi* 41(4), 460 (with theophylline)

Stomatitis
(1997): Greco S+, *Ann Pharmacother* 31, 1548

Tremors (<1%)

Xerostomia
(2001): McCarty JM+, *Ann Allergy Asthma Immunol* 87(4), 327

# CLEMASTINE

**Trade name:** Tavist (Novartis)
**Other common trade names:** *Aller-Eze; Antihist-1; Clema; Darvine; Tavegil; Tavegyl*
**Indications:** Allergic rhinitis, urticaria
**Category:** $H_1$-receptor antihistamine
**Half-life:** 4–6 hours
**Clinically important, potentially hazardous interactions with:** barbiturates, chloral hydrate, ethylchlovynol, phenothiazines, zolpidem

### *Reactions*

## Skin

Angioedema (<1%)

Diaphoresis

Edema (<1%)

Exanthems
(1975): Todd G+, *Curr Med Res Opin* 3, 126

Flushing
(1975): Todd G+, *Curr Med Res Opin* 3, 126

Photosensitivity (<1%)
(1962): Schreiber M+, *Arch Dermatol* 86, 58

Purpura

Rash (sic) (<1%)

Toxic pustuloderma
(1996): Feind-Koopmans A+, *Clin Exp Dermatol* 21, 293

Urticaria
(1984): Savchak VI, *Vestn Dermatol Venerol* (Russian) 1, 47

## Other

Anaphylactoid reactions

Hypersensitivity

Myalgia (<1%)

Paresthesias (<1%)

Tinnitus

Xerostomia (1–10%)
(1990): Frolund L+, *Allergy* 45, 254

# CLIDINIUM

**Trade names:** Librax (ICN); Quarzan (Roche)
**Other common trade names:** *Bralix; Diporax; Epirax; Libraxin; Librocol; Nirvaxal; Spasmoten*
**Indications:** Duodenal and gastric ulcers
**Category:** Anticholinergic
**Half-life:** no data
**Clinically important, potentially hazardous interactions with:** anticholinergics, arbutamine

Librax is clidinium and chlordiazepoxide (see chlordiazepoxide)

### *Reactions*

## Skin

Flushing

Hypohidrosis

Purpura
(2001): Alexopoulou A=, *Arch Intern Med* 161(14), 1778 (with chlordiazepoxide)

Urticaria

## Other

Ageusia

Anaphylactoid reactions

Dysgeusia

Xerostomia

# CLINDAMYCIN

**Trade names:** Benzaclin (cream) (Dermik); Cleocin (Pharmacia & Upjohn); Cleocin-T (Pharmacia & Upjohn); Clindets (Stiefel)
**Other common trade names:** *Aclinda; BB; Clindacin; Dalacin; Dalacin C; Dalacine; Galecin; Sobelin*
**Indications:** Various serious infections caused by susceptible organisms
**Category:** Lincosamide antibiotic and antiprotozoal
**Half-life:** 2–3 hours
**Clinically important, potentially hazardous interactions with:** cisatracurium, erythromycin, kaolin, saquinavir

### *Reactions*

## Skin

Acute generalized exanthematous pustulosis (AGEP)
(2000): Schwab RA+, *Cutis* 65, 391

Allergic reactions (sic)
(1996): Garcia R+, *Contact Dermatitis* 35, 116

Contact dermatitis (from topical preparations)
(1995): Vejlstrup E+, *Contact Dermatitis* 32, 110
(1994): Rietschel RL, *Infect Dis Clin North Am* 8, 607
(1992): de Groot AC, *Contact Dermatitis* 8, 428
(1991): Yokayama R+, *Contact Dermatitis* 25, 125
(1983): Conde-Salazar L, *Contact Dermatitis* 9, 225
(1978): Coskey RJ, *Arch Dermatol* 114, 446
(1978): Herstoff JK, *Arch Dermatol* 114, 1402

Eczematous eruption (sic)
(1991): Yokoyama R+, *Contact Dermatitis* 25, 125

Erythema multiforme (<1%)
(1996): Munoz D+, *Contact Dermatitis* 34, 227
(1973): Fulghum DD+, *JAMA* 223, 318

Erythroderma
(2002): Horiuchi Y+, *J Dermatol* 29(2), 115

Exanthems

(2002): Lammintausta K+, *Br J Dermatol* 146, 643 (6 cases)
(1999): Mazur N+, *Ann Allergy Asthma Immunol* 82, 443
(1984): Brenner S+, *Harefuah* (Hebrew) 106, 570
(1970): Geddes AM+, *BMJ* 2, 703 (>5%)

Facial edema
(1999): Mazur N+, *Ann Allergy Asthma Immunol* 82, 443

Fixed eruption
(1998): Mahboob A+, *Int J Dermatol* 37, 833

Leukocytoclastic angiitis
(1982): Lamber WC+, *Cutis* 30, 615

Pruritus (<1%)
(1973): Fass RJ+, *Ann Intern Med* 78, 853 (10%)

Pruritus ani

Purpura

Rash (sic) (1–10%)
(2002): Maraqa NF+, *Clin Infect Dis* 34(1), 50 (1.4%)

Rosacea
(1989): de Kort WJ+, *Contact Dermatitis* 20, 72

Stevens–Johnson syndrome (<1%)
(1974): Maulide T+, *Pneumologica* (Lisbon) 5, 79
(1973): Fulghum DD+, *JAMA* 223, 318
(1973): Pickering LK, *JAMA* 223, 1392

Toxic epidermal necrolysis
(1995): Paquet P+, *Br J Dermatol* 132, 665
(1993): Correia O+, *Dermatology* 186, 32
(1992): Saiag P+, *J Am Acad Dermatol* 26, 567

Urticaria (<1%)
(1973): Fulghum DD+, *JAMA* 223, 31
(1972): Meyler L+, *Side Effects of Drugs*, Vol 7, Excerpta Medica, 389
(1970): Newell AC, *Med J Aust* 2, 321
(1969): Lattanzi WE+, *Int Med Dig* 4, 29

Vasculitis
(1982): Lambert WC+, *Cutis* 30, 615

Xerosis (from topical preparations)

### Other

Anaphylactoid reactions
(1977): Lochmann O+, *J Hyg Epiderm Microbiol Immunol* 21, 441

Dysgeusia

Edema of the lip
(1993): Segars LW+, *Ann Pharmacother* 27, 885

Hypersensitivity
(2002): Kim P+, *Clin Experiment Ophthalmol* 30(2), 147
(2002): Lammintausta K+, *Br J Dermatol* 146(4), 643

Injection-site phlebitis (<1%)

Lymphadenitis
(1997): Southern PM, *Am J Med* 103, 164

Thrombophlebitis

# CLOFAZIMINE

**Trade name:** Lamprene (Novartis)
**Other common trade names:** *Clofozine; Hansepran; Lampren; Lapren*
**Indications:** Leprosy
**Category:** Antileprotic
**Half-life:** 10 days after a single dose

## *Reactions*

### Skin

Acne (<1%)
(1992): Breathnach SM+, *Adverse Drug Reactions and the Skin* Blackwell, Oxford, 161 (passim)

Acute febrile neutrophilic dermatosis (Sweet's syndrome)
(1994): Tacke J+, *Hautarzt* (German) 45, 184

Ankle edema (<1%)
(1990): Oommen T, *Leprosy Review* 61, 289

Cheilitis (candidal) (<1%)

Discoloration (sic)
(1979): Thomsen K+, *Arch Dermatol* 115, 851

Erythroderma (<1%)

Exanthems

Exfoliative dermatitis
(1985): Pavithran K, *Int J Lepr* 53, 645

Ichthyosis (8–28%)
(1989): Patki AH+, *Indian J Lepr* 61, 92
(1987): Kumar B+, *Indian J Lepr* 59, 63
(1984): Aram H, *Int J Dermatol* 23, 458
(1982): Caver CV, *Cutis* 29, 341
(1979): Thomsen K+, *Arch Dermatol* 115, 851

Pedal edema
(1993): Tyagi PY+, *Int J Lepr Other Mycobact Dis* 61, 636

Photosensitivity (<1%)
(1992): Breathnach SM+, *Adverse Drug Reactions and the Skin* Blackwell, Oxford, 161 (passim)

Pigmentation (pink to brownish-black) (75–100%)
(1993): Krop LC+, *N Engl J Med* 329, 1582
(1992): Fitzpatrick JE, *Derm Clinics* 10, 19
(1992): Gallais V+, *Ann Dermatol Venereol* (French) 119, 471
(1991): Garrelts JC, *Ann Pharmacother* 25, 525 (orange-pink)
(1990): Job CK+, *J Am Acad Dermatol* 23, 236
(1989): Langford A+, *Oral Surg Oral Med Oral Pathol* 67, 301 (oral)
(1989): Patki AH+, *Indian J Lepr* 61, 92 (oral)
(1989): Zhang X+, *J Oral Pathol Med* 18, 471
(1988): Mensing H, *Dermatologica* 177, 232
(1987): Kossard S+, *J Am Acad Dermatol* 17, 867 (reddish-blue)
(1987): Kumar B+, *Indian J Lepr* 59, 63
(1983): Burte NP+, *Lepr India* 55, 265
(1983): Moore VJ, *Lepr Rev* 54, 327
(1981): Granstein RD+, *J Am Acad Dermatol* 5, 1 (red)
(1978): Chuaprapaisilp T+, *Br J Dermatol* 99, 303 (deep-red)
(1978): Pettit JH, *Int J Lepr Other Mycobact Dis* 46, 227
(1971): Karat ABA+, *BMJ* 4, 514
(1969): Levy L+, *Int J Lepr* 38, 404

Pruritus (1–5%)
(1992): Breathnach SM+, *Adverse Drug Reactions and the Skin* Blackwell, Oxford, 161 (passim)

Rash (sic) (1–5%)
(1995): Chaisson RE, *Infections in Medicine* 12, 48
(1992): Breathnach SM+, *Adverse Drug Reactions and the Skin* Blackwell, Oxford, 161 (passim)

Urticaria

Vitiligo
(1996): Brown-Harrell V+, *Clin Infect Dis* 22, 581

Xerosis (8–28%)
(1992): Breathnach SM+, *Adverse Drug Reactions and the Skin* Blackwell, Oxford, 161 (passim)

### Nails

Nails – discoloration
(1989): Dixit VB+, *Indian J Lepr* 61, 476
(1982): Caver CV, *Cutis* 29, 341

Nails – onycholysis
(1989): Dixit VB+, *Indian J Lepr* 61, 476

Nails – subungual hyperkeratosis
(1989): Dixit VB+, *Indian J Lepr* 61, 476

### Other

Chromhidrosis (red sweat) (1–10%)
(1987): Kumar B+, *Indian J Lepr* 59, 63
(1979): Thomsen K+, *Arch Dermatol* 115, 851
(1979): Yawalkar SJ+, *Lepr Rev* 50, 135

Dysgeusia (<1%)

## CLOFIBRATE

**Trade name:** Atromid-S (Wyeth-Ayerst)
**Other common trade names:** *Abitrate; Claripex; Col; Lipavlon; Novo-Fibrate; Regelan N; Skleromexe*
**Indications:** Type III hyperlipidemia
**Category:** Antihyperlipidemic
**Half-life:** 6–25 hours after a single dose
**Clinically important, potentially hazardous interactions with:** anisindione, anticoagulants, dicumarol, warfarin

### *Reactions*

#### Skin

Dermatitis (sic)
(1988): Murata Y+, *J Am Acad Dermatol* 18, 381
(1972): Inman WHW+, *BMJ* 3, 746
(1972): Krasno LR+, *JAMA* 219, 845
Diaphoresis
Erythema multiforme
(1988): Murata Y+, *J Am Acad Dermatol* 18, 381
Exanthems
(1988): Murata Y+, *J Am Acad Dermatol* 18, 381
(1980): Cumming A, *BMJ* 281, 1529
(1977): Heid E+, *Ann Dermatol Venereol* (French) 104, 494
(1975): Arif MA+, *Lancet* 2, 1202 (7%)
(1971): Five Year Study, *BMJ* 4, 767 (0.8%)
(1965): Hollander W, *Cardiovascular Drug Therapy* 339
Exfoliative dermatitis
(1972): Inman WHW+, *BMJ* 3, 746
Facial dermatitis
(1967): Orgain ES+, *Arch Intern Med* 119, 80
Lupus erythematosus
(1973): Howard EJ+, *JAMA* 226, 1358
Photosensitivity
(1990): Leroy D+, *Photodermatology* 7, 136
(1988): Murata Y+, *J Am Acad Dermatol* 18, 381
(1977): Heid E+, *Ann Dermatol Venereol* (French) 104, 494
(1967): Orgain ES+, *Arch Intern Med* 119, 80
Pruritus (<1%)
Purpura
(1975): Arif MA+, *Lancet* 2, 1202
Rash (sic) (<1%)
Sarcoidosis
(1986): Yamada S+, *J Dermatol* (Tokio) 13, 217
Stevens–Johnson syndrome
(1994): Wong SS, *Acta Derm Venereol* 74, 475
Toxic epidermal necrolysis
Urticaria (<1%)
Vesiculobullous eruption
(1977): Heid E+, *Ann Dermatol Venereol* (French) 104, 494
Xerosis

#### Hair

Hair – alopecia (<1%)
(1971): Five Year Study, *BMJ* 4, 767 (0.8%)
Hair – dry (<1%)

#### Other

Dysgeusia
Gynecomastia
Hypogeusia
Myalgia
Myopathy (<1%)
(1976): Rumpf KW+, *Lancet* 1, 249
(1975): Pierides AM+, *Lancet* 2, 1279
(1968): Langer T+, *N Engl J Med* 279, 856
Oral ulceration
(1973): Howard EJ+, *JAMA* 226, 1358
Rhabdomyolysis
(1977): Smals AG+, *N Engl J Med* 296(16), 942
Stomatitis

## CLOMIPHENE

**Trade names:** Clomid (Aventis); Serophene (Serono)
**Other common trade names:** *Clom 50; Clomifen; Dyneric; Milophene; Omifin; Pergotime; Phenate; Serophene*
**Indications:** Ovulatory failure
**Category:** Infertility therapy adjunct; ovulation stimulator
**Half-life:** 5–7 days

### *Reactions*

#### Skin

Acne
(2001): Guzick ND, Houston, TX (from Internet) (several observations)
Allergic reactions (sic)
Dermatitis (sic) (<1%)
Diaphoresis
Edema
Erythema
Erythema multiforme
Erythema nodosum
(1980): Salvatore MA+, *Arch Dermatol* 116, 557
Exanthems
(1996): Coots NV+, *Cutis* 57, 91
(1966): Johnson JE+, *Pacif Med Surg* 74, 153 (0.8%)
Flushing (10%)
(1966): Johnson JE+, *Pacif Med Surg* 74, 153 (14%)
Hot flashes (>10%)
Melanoma
(1999): Fuller PN, *Am J Obstet Gynecol* 180, 1499
(1995): Rossing MA+, *Melanoma Res* 5, 123
(1992): Kuppens E+, *Melanoma Res* 2, 71
Pruritus
Purpura (palpable)
(1996): Coots NV+, *Cutis* 57, 91
Rash (sic) (<1%)
Urticaria
(1969): *Drug and Therapeutic Bulletin* (London), 7, 34

#### Hair

Hair – alopecia (<1%)
(1969): *Drug and Therapeutic Bulletin* (London), 7, 34 (0.4%)
(1966): Johnson JE+, *Pacif Med Surg* 74, 153 (0.3%)
Hair – hypertrichosis
(2001): Smith KC, Niagara Falls, ON, Canada (from Internet) (several observations)

#### Other

Gynecomastia (1–10%)
(1978): Check JH+, *Fertility and Sterility* 30, 713
Mastodynia (1–10%)
Myalgia

# CLOMIPRAMINE

**Trade name:** Anafranil (Novartis)
**Other common trade names:** *Anafranil Retard; Apo-Clomipramine; Clofranil; Clopress; Placil*
**Indications:** Obsessive-compulsive disorder
**Category:** Tricyclic antidepressant
**Half-life:** 21–31 hours
**Clinically important, potentially hazardous interactions with:** amprenavir, arbutamine, clonidine, epinephrine, formoterol, guanethidine, isocarboxazid, linezolid, MAO inhibitors, phenelzine, quinolones, sparfloxacin, tranylcypromine

### *Reactions*

#### Skin

Acne (2%)
Allergic reactions (sic) (<3%)
Cellulitis (2%)
Cheilitis
Chloasma
Contact dermatitis
(1991): Ljunggren B+, *Contact Dermatitis* 24, 259
Dermatitis (sic) (2%)
Diaphoresis (29%)
(1992): Guelfi JD+, *Br J Psychiatry* 160, 519
(1990): McTavish D+, *Drugs* 38, 19 (43%)
Edema (2%)
Erythema
Exanthems
Flushing (8%)
Folliculitis
Photosensitivity (<1%)
(1991): Ljunggren B+, *Contact Dermatitis* 24, 259
(1989): Tunca Z+, *Am J Psychiatry* 146, 552
(1979): Parkes JD+, *Lancet* 2, 1085
Pigmentation (pseudocyanotic)
(1989): Tunca Z+, *Am J Psychiatry* 146, 552
Pruritus (6%)
Psoriasis
Purpura (3%)
Pustular eruption
Rash (sic) (8%)
Seborrhea
Urticaria (1%)
Vasculitis
Xerosis (2%)

#### Hair

Hair – alopecia (<1%)
Hair – alopecia areata
(1993): Kubota T+, *Acta Neurol Napoli* (Italian) 15, 200
Hair – hypertrichosis

#### Other

Ageusia
Black tongue
Dysgeusia (8%)
Galactorrhea (<1%)
Gingival bleeding
Gingivitis
Glossitis
Gynecomastia (2%)
Mastodynia (1%)
Myalgia (13%)
Paresthesias
Sialorrhea
Stomatitis
Tongue ulceration
Vaginitis (2%)
Xerostomia (84%)
(1992): Cohen DJ+, *Psychiatr Clin North Am* 15, 109
(1992): DeVeaugh-Geiss J+, *J Am Acad Child Adolesc Psychiatry* 31, 45
(1992): Guelfi JD+, *Br J Psychiatry* 160, 519
(1990): McTavish D+, *Drugs* 38, 19

# CLONAZEPAM

**Trade name:** Klonopin (Roche)
**Other common trade names:** *Clonex; Iktorivil; Landsen; Lonazep; Rivotril*
**Indications:** Petit mal and myoclonic seizures
**Category:** Benzodiazepine anticonvulsant and antipanic
**Half-life:** 18–50 hours
**Clinically important, potentially hazardous interactions with:** amprenavir, chlorpheniramine, clarithromycin, efavirenz, esomeprazole, imatinib, indinavir, nelfinavir

### *Reactions*

#### Skin

Allergic reactions (sic) (1–10%)
Angioedema
(1976): Pinder RM+, *Drugs* 12, 321
Ankle edema
Dermatitis (sic) (1–10%)
Diaphoresis (>10%)
Erythema multiforme
(1998): Amichai B+, *Clin Exp Dermatology* 23, 206
Exanthems
(1976): Pinder RM+, *Drugs* 12, 321
Facial edema
Hypermelanosis
(1976): Pinder RM+, *Drugs* 12, 321
Pruritus
Pseudo-mycosis fungoides
(1996): Gordon KB+, *J Am Acad Dermatol* 34, 304
Purpura
(1976): Pinder RM+, *Drugs* 12, 321
Rash (sic) (>10%)
Urticaria

#### Hair

Hair – alopecia
(2000): Mercke Y+, *Ann Clin Psychiatry* 12, 35
Hair – hirsutism

#### Other

Black tongue
(2000): Heymann WR, *Cutis* 66, 25
Burning mouth syndrome
(2001): Culhane NS+, *Ann Pharmacother* 35(7), 874
Dysgeusia
(2000): Heymann WR, *Cutis* 66, 25
Gingivitis
Injection-site phlebitis
Injection-site thrombosis
Oral mucosal eruption
(1986): Bernard K, *Lijec Vjesn* (Serbo-Croatian-Roman) 108, 235

Oral ulceration
Paresthesias
Pseudolymphoma
(1995): Magro CM+, *J Am Acad Dermatol* 32, 419
Sialopenia (>10%)
Sialorrhea (1–10%)
Xerostomia (>10%)
(2000): Heymann WR, *Cutis* 66, 25

# CLONIDINE

**Trade names:** Catapres (Boehringer Ingelheim); Combipres (Boehringer Ingelheim)
**Other common trade names:** *Barclyd; Catapresan; Daipres; Dixarit; Duraclon; Haemiton; Nu-Clonidine; Sulmidine*
**Indications:** Hypertension
**Category:** Alpha$_2$-adrenergic agonist; antihypertensive
**Half-life:** 6–24 hours
**Clinically important, potentially hazardous interactions with:** acebutolol, amitriptyline, amoxapine, atenolol, betaxolol, carteolol, clomipramine, desipramine, doxepin, esmolol, imipramine, metoprolol, nadolol, nortriptyline, penbutolol, pindolol, propranolol, protriptyline, timolol, tricyclic antidepressants, trimipramine, verapamil

Combipres is clonidine and chlorthalidone

### *Reactions*

## Skin

Angioedema (<1%)
(1995): Waldfahrer F+, *HNO* (German) 43, 35
Contact dermatitis (from patch) (20%)
(2002): Prisant LM, *J Clin Hypertens* (Greenwich) 4(2), 136
(1999): Polster AM+, *Cutis* 63, 154
(1997): Shelley ED+, *J Geriatr Dermatol* 4, 192
(1995): Corazza M+, *Contact Dermatitis* 32, 246
(1994): Tom GR+, *Ann Pharmacother* 28, 889
(1992): Breathnach SM+, *Adverse Drug Reactions and the Skin* Blackwell, Oxford, 226 (passim)
(1991): Ito MK+, *Am J Med* 91, 42S
(1991): McChesney JA, *West J Med* 154, 736
(1990): Hogan DJ+, *J Am Acad Dermatol* 22, 811
(1990): Scheper RJ+, *Contact Dermatitis* 23, 81
(1989): Fillingim JM+, *Clin Ther* 11, 398
(1989): Holdiness MR, *Contact Dermatitis* 20, 3
(1988): Horning JR+, *Chest* 93, 941
(1987): Bigby M+, *JAMA* 258, 1819 (letter)
(1987): Maibach HI, *Contact Dermatitis* 16, 1
(1986): Hollifield J, *Am Heart J* 112, 900
(1986): Weber MA, *Am Heart J* 112, 906
(1986): White TM+, *West J Med* 145, 104
(1985): Grattan CEH+, *Contact Dermatitis* 2, 225
(1985): Maibach H, *Contact Dermatitis* 12, 192
(1984): van Ketel WG, *Ned Tijdschr Geneeskd* (Dutch) 128, 34
(1983): Boekhorst JC, *Lancet* 2, 1031
(1983): Groth H+, *Lancet* 2, 850
Depigmentation
(2002): Prisant LM, *J Clin Hypertens* (Greenwich) 4(2), 136
(1995): Doe N+, *Arch Intern Med* 155, 2129 (from patch)
Diaphoresis
(1990): Leeman CP, *J Clin Psychiatry* 51, 258
Eczematous eruption (sic)
(1987): Dick JBC+, *Lancet* 1, 516
(1985): Grattan CEH+, *Contact Dermatitis* 12, 225
Edema
Erythema
(2002): Prisant LM, *J Clin Hypertens* (Greenwich) 4(2), 136
(1987): Dick JBC+, *Lancet* 1, 516
Exanthems
Excoriations
(2002): Prisant LM, *J Clin Hypertens* (Greenwich) 4(2), 136
Herpes simplex
(1987): Wiser TH+, *J Am Acad Dermatol* 17, 143
Induration
(2002): Prisant LM, *J Clin Hypertens* (Greenwich) 4(2), 136
Irritation (from patch)
(1999): Dias VC+, *Am J Ther* 6, 19
Lupus erythematosus
(1994): Heilmann G+, *Dtsch Med Wochenschr* (German) 119, 858
(1992): Breathnach SM+, *Adverse Drug Reactions and the Skin* Blackwell, Oxford, 226 (passim)
(1981): Witman G+, *R I Med J* 64, 147
Pemphigoid (anogenital and cicatricial)
(1980): van Joost T+, *Br J Dermatol* 102, 715
Peripheral edema
Pigmentation
(2002): Prisant LM, *J Clin Hypertens* (Greenwich) 4(2), 136
(1987): Wiser TH+, *J Am Acad Dermatol* 17, 143 (from patch)
Pityriasis rosea
(1998): Reed BR, Denver, CO (2 cases – in siblings) (from Internet) (observation)
(1992): Breathnach SM+, *Adverse Drug Reactions and the Skin* Blackwell, Oxford, 226 (passim)
Pruritus (>5%)
(1999): Dias VC+, *Am J Ther* 6, 19
(1987): Dick JBC+, *Lancet* 1, 516
(1984): Weber MA+, *Arch Intern Med* 144, 1211
(1984): Weber MA+, *Lancet* 1, 9
(1983): Boekhorst JC, *Lancet* 2, 1031
Psoriasis
(1981): Wilkin J, *Arch Dermatol* 117, 4
Rash (sic) (1–10%)
(1988): Glassman AH, *JAMA* 259, 2863
Raynaud's phenomenon (<1%)
Scaling
(2002): Prisant LM, *J Clin Hypertens* (Greenwich) 4(2), 136
Ulcer (1–10%)
Urticaria (<1%)
Vesiculation
(2002): Prisant LM, *J Clin Hypertens* (Greenwich) 4(2), 136

## Hair

Hair – alopecia (<1%)

## Other

Acute intermittent porphyria
Application-site vesiculation
(1987): Dick JBC+, *Lancet* 1, 516
Dysgeusia (from patch)
Gynecomastia (<1%)
Hyperesthesia (1–10%)
Immune complex disease
(1989): Petersen HH+, *Acta Derm Venereol* (Stockh) 69, 519
Pseudolymphoma
(1997): Shelley WB+, *Lancet* 350, 1223 (at site of patch)
Xerostomia (40%)
(2000): Geyer O+, *Graefes Arch Clin Exp Ophthalmol* 238, 149
(2000): Litt JZ, Beachwood, OH (personal case) (observation)
(1999): Dias VC+, *Am J Ther* 6, 19
(1988): Glassman AH, *JAMA* 259, 2863
(1984): Weber MA+, *Arch Intern Med* 144, 1211
(1984): Weber MA+, *Lancet* 1, 9
(1983): Boekhorst JC, *Lancet* 2, 1031

# CLOPIDOGREL

**Trade name:** Plavix (Bristol-Myers Squibb)
**Indications:** Atherosclerotic events
**Category:** Oral antiplatelet (thienopyridine derivative)
**Half-life:** ~8 hours
**Clinically important, potentially hazardous interactions with:** anisindione, anticoagulants, dicumarol, fondaparinux, warfarin

### *Reactions*

## Skin

Allergic reactions (sic) (1–2.5%)
Bullous eruption (1–2.5%)
Eczema (sic) (1–2.5%)
Edema (3–5%)
Exanthems (1–2.5%)
(2001): Blumenthal HL, Beachwood, OH (personal communication)
(1999): Smith JG, Mobile, AL (from Internet) (observation) (generalized)
Flu-like syndrome (sic) (7.5%)
Pruritus (3.3%)
(1999): Smith JG, Mobile, AL (from Internet) (observation)
Purpura (5.3%)
(2001): Nara W+, *Am J Med Sci* 322(3), 170
(2000): Brooker JZ, *N Engl J Med* 343(16), 1192
(2000): Cheung RT, *N Engl J Med* 343(16), 1192
(2000): Goldstein MR, *N Engl J Med* 343(16), 1192
(2000): Salliere D+, *N Engl J Med* 343(16), 1191
(2000): Trontell AE+, *N Engl J Med* 343(16), 1191
Rash (sic) (4.2%)
Thrombocytopenic purpura
(2001): Briguori C+, *Ital Heart J* 2(12), 935
(2001): Medina PJ+, *Curr Opin Hematol* 8(5), 286
(2001): Nara W+, *Am J Med Sci* 322(3), 170
(2000): Bennett CL+, *N Engl J Med* 342, 1773 (11 patients)
(2000): Chinnakotla S+, *Transplantation* 70, 550
(2000): SoRelle R, *Circulation* 101, E9036
(1999): Carwile JM+, *Blood* 94, 1:78
(1999): Connors JM+, *Transfusion* 39, 56S
Toxic skin reaction (sic)
(2001): El-Majjaoui S+, *J Mal Vasc* 26(3), 207
Ulceration (1–2.5%)
Urticaria (1–2.5%)
(1997): Coukell AJ+, *Drugs* 54, 745

## Other

Ageusia
(2000): Golka K+, *Lancet* 355, 465
Hypersensitivity
(2001): Sarrot-Reynauld F+, *Ann Intern Med* 135(4), 305
Hypesthesia (1–2.5%)
Paresthesias (1–2.5%)

# CLORAZEPATE

**Trade name:** Tranxene (Abbott)
**Other common trade names:** *Gen-XENE; Novoclopate; Transene; Tranxal; Tranxen; Tranxilen; Tranxilium*
**Indications:** Anxiety and panic disorders
**Category:** Benzodiazepine anxiolytic and sedative-hypnotic; anticonvulsant
**Half-life:** 48–96 hours
**Clinically important, potentially hazardous interactions with:** amprenavir, antacids, carbamazepine, carmustine, chlorpheniramine, clarithromycin, efavirenz, esomeprazole, imatinib, indinavir, itraconazole, ketoconazole, MAO inhibitors, midazolam, moclobemide, nelfinavir, phenytoin, sucralfate, theophylline, warfarin

### *Reactions*

## Skin

Blistering (sic)
(1979): Herschthal D+, *Arch Dermatol* 115, 499
Dermatitis (sic) (1–10%)
Diaphoresis (>10%)
Exanthems
(2001): Sachs B+, *Br J Dermatol* 144(2), 316 (generalized)
Photosensitivity
(1989): Torras H+, *J Am Acad Dermatol* 21, 1304
Pruritus
Purpura
Rash (sic) (>10%)
Urticaria
(1981): Bonnetblanc JM+, *Ann Dermatol Venereol* (French) 108, 177
Vasculitis
(1985): Sanchez NP+, *Arch Dermatol* 121, 220

## Nails

Nails – photo-onycholysis
(1989): Torras H+, *J Am Acad Dermatol* 21, 1304

## Other

Oral ulceration
Paresthesias
Porphyria
(2001): Rassiat E+, *Gastroenterol Clin Biol* 25(8), 832
Sialopenia (>10%)
Sialorrhea (1–10%)
Tremors
Xerostomia (>10%)

# CLOTRIMAZOLE

**Trade names:** Gyne-Lotrimin (Schering); Lotrimin (Lotrimin ); Mycelex (Bayer)
**Other common trade names:** *Agisten; Candid; Canestene; Imazol; Taon*
**Indications:** Candidiasis, dermatophyte infections of the skin
**Category:** Imidazole antifungal
**Half-life:** No data

### *Reactions*

## Skin

Burning

(1994): Binet O+, *Mycoses* 37, 455
(1983): Higashide K+, *J Int Med Res* 11, 21 (from vaginal tablets)
Contact dermatitis
(1999): Cooper SM+, *Contact Dermatitis* 41, 168
(1999): Erdmann S+, *Contact Dermatitis* 40, 47
(1997): Dharmagunawardena B+, *Contact Dermatitis* 32, 187
(1995): Baes H, *Contact Dermatitis* 32, 187
(1994): Valsecchi R+, *Contact Dermatitis* 30, 248
(1987): Raulin C+, *Derm Beruf Umwelt* (German) 35, 64
(1985): Balato N+, *Contact Dermatitis* 12, 110
(1985): Kalb RE+, *Cutis* 36, 240
(1978): Roller JA, *Br Med J* 2, 737
Edema
Erythema
Exfoliation
Irritation (sic)
(1994): Binet O+, *Mycoses* 37, 455
Pruritus
Stinging
Urticaria
Vesiculation

### Other
Dysgeusia

## CLOXACILLIN

**Trade names:** Cloxapen (GSK); Tegopen (Mead Johnson)
**Other common trade names:** *Alclox; Apo-Cloxi; Ekvacillin; Loxavit; Nu-Cloxi; Orbenin; Orbenine*
**Indications:** Various infections caused by susceptible organisms
**Category:** Penicillinase-resistant penicillin antibiotic
**Half-life:** 0.5–1.1 hours
**Clinically important, potentially hazardous interactions with:** anticoagulants, cyclosporine, demeclocycline, doxycycline, methotrexate, minocycline, oxytetracycline, tetracycline

#### *Reactions*

### Skin
Angioedema
Contact dermatitis
(1996): Gamboa P+, *Contact Dermatitis* 34, 75
Ecchymoses
Erythema multiforme
Exanthems
Exfoliative dermatitis
Hematomas
Jarisch–Herxheimer reaction
Pruritus
Rash (sic) (<1%)
(1979): Puri V+, *Indian Pediatr* 16, 1153
Stevens–Johnson syndrome
Urticaria

### Nails
Nails – onycholysis
Nails – shedding
(1984): Daniel CR, *J Am Acad Dermatol* 10, 250
(1969): Eastwood JB+, *Br J Dermatol* 81, 750

### Other
Anaphylactoid reactions
Black tongue
Glossitis
Glossodynia
Hypersensitivity
Injection-site pain
Oral candidiasis
Serum sickness (<1%)
Stomatitis
Vaginitis

## CLOZAPINE

**Trade name:** Clozaril (Novartis)
**Other common trade names:** *Entumin; Entumine; Leponex; Lozapin; Sizopin*
**Indications:** Schizophrenia
**Category:** Tricyclic antipsychotic
**Half-life:** 8–12 hours
**Clinically important, potentially hazardous interactions with:** carbamazepine, fluoxetine, risperidone, ritonavir

#### *Reactions*

### Skin
Acute generalized exanthematous pustulosis (AGEP)
(1997): Bosonnet S+, *Ann Dermatol Venereol* (French) 124, 547
Dermatitis (sic) (<1%)
Diaphoresis (6%)
(2001): Kane JM+, *Arch Gen Psychiatry* 58(10), 965
(2001): Richardson C+, *Am J Psychiatry* 158(8), 1329
(1991): Safferman A+, *Schizophr Bull* 17, 247 (31%)
(1990): Fitton A+, *Drugs* 40, 722
Eczematous eruption (sic) (<1%)
(1994): Shelley WB+, *Cutis* 53, 33 (observation)
Edema (<1%)
Erythema (<1%)
Erythema multiforme (<1%)
Exanthems
Facial erosions
(1994): Shelley WB+, *Cutis* 53, 33 (observation)
Lupus erythematosus
(1994): Wickert WA+, *Postgrad Med J* 70, 940
Pedal edema
(2000): Durst R+, *Isr Med Assoc* 2, 485
Periorbital edema (<1%)
Petechiae (<1%)
(1994): Shelley WB+, *Cutis* 53, 33 (observation)
Photosensitivity
(1995): Howanitz E+, *J Clin Psychiatry* 56, 589
Pruritus (<1%)
Purpura (<1%)
Rash (sic) (2%)
Stevens–Johnson syndrome (<1%)
Urticaria (<1%)
Vasculitis (<1%)

### Other
Death
(2002): Levin TT+, *Psychosomatics* 43(1), 71
(2001): Gillespie JA, *Ann Pharmacother* 35(12), 1671
(2001): Hoehns JD+, *Ann Pharmacother* 35(7), 862 (with sertaline)
(2001): Tie H+, *J Clin Psychopharmacol* 21(6), 630
Dysgeusia (<1%)
Glossodynia (1%)
Mastodynia (<1%)

Priapism
(2001): Bongale RN+, *Am J Psychiatry* 158(12), 2087
(2001): Compton MT+, *J Clin Psychiatry* 62(5), 363 (passim)
(2000): Compton MT+, *Am J Psychiatry* 157, 659
(1994): Barbieri NB+, *Can J Psychiatry* 39, 128
Rhabdomyolysis
(1996): Meltzer HY+, *Neuropsychopharmacology* 15(4), 395
Seizures
(2002): Duggal HS+, *Am J Psychiatry* 159(2), 315
(2001): Landry P, *Am J Psychiatry* 158(11), 1930
(2001): Navarro V+, *Am J Psychiatry* 158(6), 968
Sialorrhea (31%)
(2001): Bai YM+, *J Clin Psychopharmacol* 21(6), 608
(2001): Kane JM+, *Arch Gen Psychiatry* 58(10), 965
(2000): Miller DD, *J Clin Psychiatry* 61, 14
(2000): Wahlbeck K+, *Cochran Database Syst Rev* (2):CD000059
(1999): Antonello C+, *J Psychiatry Neurosci* 24, 250
(1999): Campbell M+, *Br J Clin Pharmacol* 47, 13
(1998): Young CR+, *Schizophr Bull* 24, 381
(1997): Spivak B+, *Int Clin Psychopharmacol* 12, 213
(1995): Fritze J+, *Lancet* 346, 1034
(1991): Bourgeois JA+, *Hosp Community Psychiatry* 42, 1174
(1991): Calabrese JR+, *J Clin Psychopharmacol* 11, 396
(1991): Copp PJ+, *Br J Psychiatry* 159, 166
(1991): Goumeniouk AD+, *Can J Psychiatry* 36, 234
(1991): Kahn N+, *Neurology* 41, 1699
(1991): Ogle MR+, *Indiana Med* 84, 606
(1991): Safferman A+, *Schizophr Bull* 17, 247
(1990): Fitton A+, *Drugs* 40, 722
Tremors (1–10%)
Xerostomia (6%)
(2001): Kane JM+, *Arch Gen Psychiatry* 58(10), 965
(1991): Safferman A+, *Schizophr Bull* 17, 247 (6%)
(1990): Fitton A+, *Drugs* 40, 722

# CO-TRIMOXAZOLE

**Synonyms:** sulfamethoxazole-trimethoprim; SMX-TMP; SMZ-TMP; TMP-SMX; TMP-SMZ
**Trade names:** Bactrim (Roche); Cotrim (Teva); Septrin (GSK)
**Other common trade names:** *Anitrim; Apo-Sulfatrim; Bactelan; Batrizol; Ectaprim; Esteprim; Isobac; Pro-Trin; Roubac; Sulfatrim; Trimzol; Trisulfa*
**Indications:** Various infections caused by susceptible organisms
**Category:** Antibacterial and antiprotozoal
**Half-life:** 6–10 hours
**Clinically important, potentially hazardous interactions with:** anticoagulants, cyclosporine, dofetilide, isotretinoin, methotrexate, warfarin

Co-trimoxazole is sulfamethoxazole* and trimethoprim

## *Reactions*

### Skin

Acute febrile neutrophilic dermatosis (Sweet's syndrome)
(1996): Walker DC+, *J Am Acad Dermatol* 34, 918
(1989): Cobb MW, *J Am Acad Dermatol* 21, 339 (passim)
(1986): Su WPD+, *Cutis* 37, 167
Acute generalized exanthematous pustulosis (AGEP)
(1995): Moreau A+, *Int J Dermatol* 34, 263 (passim)
Allergic reactions (sic)
(1999): ter Hofstede HJ+, *Br Clin Pharmacol* 47, 571
Angioedema
(1988): Fihn SD+, *Ann Intern Med* 108, 350 (1–5%)
Bullous eruption
(1989): Caumes E+, *Presse Med* (French) 18, 1708
Cutaneous side effects (sic)
(1994): Roudier C+, *Arch Dermatol* 130, 1383 (48% in AIDS patients)
(1971): Koch-Weser J+, *Arch Intern Med* 128, 399. (2.1%)
Dermatitis (sic)
(1989): Atahan IL+, *Br J Radiol* 62, 1107 (at previously irradiated area)
(1987): Vukelja SJ+, *Cancer Treat Rep* 71, 668 (at previously irradiated area)
(1984): Shelley WB+, *J Am Acad Dermatol* 11, 53 (at site of previous sunburn)
(1971): Cotterill JA+, *Br J Dermatol* 84, 366
Erythema multiforme
(1999): Lehman DF+, *J Clin Pharmacol* 39, 533
(1998): Siegfried EC+, *J Am Acad Dermatol* 39, 797 (passim)
(1997): Rieder MJ+, *Pediatr Infect Dis J* 16, 1028 (70% in children with HIV)
(1995): Jick H+, *Pharmacotherapy* 15, 428
(1991): Tilden ME+, *Arch Ophthalmol* 109, 67
(1990): Chan HL+, *Arch Dermatol* 126, 43
(1989): Alanko K+, *Acta Derm Venereol* (Stockh) 69, 223
(1988): Hira SK+, *J Am Acad Dermatol* 19, 451
(1988): Platt R+, *J Infect Dis* 158, 474
(1987): Penmetcha M, *BMJ* 295, 556
(1987): Schöpf E, *Infection* 15 (Suppl 5P), S254
(1985): Heer M+, *Gastroenterology* 88, 1954
(1982): Brettle RP+, *J Infect* 4, 149
(1979): Beck MH+, *Clin Exp Dermatol* 4, 201
(1978): Assaad D+, *Can Med Assoc J* 118, 154
(1978): Azinge NO+, *J Allergy Clin Immunol* 62, 125
(1975): Bernstein LS, *Can Med Assoc J* 112 (Suppl), 96
(1971): Koch-Weser J+, *Arch Intern Med* 128, 399 (0.15%)
Erythema nodosum
(1974): Delaney TJ+, *Br J Dermatol* 90, 205
(1971): Koch-Weser J+, *Arch Intern Med* 128, 399
Erythroderma
(1979): Kennedy C+, *BMJ* 1, 1356
Exanthems
(1999): Iborra C+, *Arch Dermatol* 135, 350
(1998): Blumenthal HL, Beachwood, OH (personal case) (observation)
(1998): Hattori N+, *J Dermatol* 25, 269
(1998): Litt JZ, Beachwood, OH (personal case) (observation)
(1997): Blumenthal HL, Beachwood, OH (personal case) (observation)
(1997): Palau LA+, *Infect Med* 14, 846
(1996): Caumes E, *Rev Mal Respir* (French) 13, 101 (passim)
(1995): Hertl M+, *Br J Dermatol* 132, 215
(1995): Wolkenstein P+, *Arch Dermatol* 131, 544
(1994): Litt JZ, Beachwood, OH (personal case) (observation)
(1993): Agarwal BR+, *Indian Pediatr* 30, 1026
(1993): Litt JZ, Beachwood, OH (personal case) (observation)
(1993): Malnick SDH+, *Ann Pharmacotherapy* 27, 1139
(1990): Medina I+, *N Engl J Med* 323, 776 (47% in AIDS)
(1988): DeRaeve L+, *Br J Dermatol* 119, 521
(1988): Fihn SD+, *Ann Intern Med* 108, 350 (1–5%)
(1988): Sattler FR+, *Ann Intern Med* 109, 280 (44% in AIDS)
(1988): Weinke T+, *Dtsch Med Wochenschr* (German) 113, 1129 (25% in AIDS)
(1987): Goa KL+, *Drugs* 33, 242 (65% in AIDS)
(1987): Schöpf E, *Infection* 15 (Suppl 5P), S254
(1986): Sonntag MR+, *Schweiz Med Wochenschr* (German) 116, 142
(1985): DeHovitz JA+, *Ann Intern Med* 103, 479
(1985): Maayan S+, *Arch Intern Med* 145, 1607
(1984): Gordon FM+, *Ann Intern Med* 100, 495 (51% in AIDS)
(1984): Kovacs JA+, *Ann Intern Med* 100, 663 (29% in AIDS)
(1983): Mitsuyasu R+, *N Engl J Med* 308, 1535 (69% in AIDS)
(1982): Goetz MB+, *JAMA* 247, 3118

(1980): Fennell RS+, *Clin Pediatr* 19, 124
(1979): Abengowe CU, *Curr Med Res Opin* 5, 749 (3.2%)
(1977): Taylor B+, *BMJ* 2, 552 (12%)
(1976): Arndt KA+, *JAMA* 235, 918 (5.9%)
(1976): Gower PE+, *BMJ* 1, 684 (>5%)
(1975): Bernstein LS, *Can Med Assoc J* 112 (Suppl), 96 (1.9%)
(1975): Gleckman RA, *JAMA* 233, 427 (0.84%)
(1975): Sallam MA+, *Curr Med Res Opin* 3, 229 (3.4%)
(1972): Halpern GM, *BMJ* 1, 691
(1971): Koch-Weser J+, *Arch Intern Med* 128, 399 (1%)

Exfoliative dermatitis
(1990): Ponte CD+, *Drug Intell Clin Pharm* 24, 140 (feet)
(1975): Bernstein LS, *Can Med Assoc J* 112 (Suppl), 96
(1971): Koch-Weser J+, *Arch Intern Med* 128, 399

Fixed eruption
(2002): Litt JZ, Beachwood, OH (personal case) (glans penis) (recurrent)
(2001): Bayazit-Ozkaya E+, *J Am Acad Dermatol* 45(5), 712
(2000): Ozkaya-Bayazit E+, *Eur J Dermatol* 10, 288
(1999): Mohamed KB, *J Pediatr* 135, 396
(1999): Morelli JG+, *J Pediatr* 134, 365
(1998): Lee AY, *Contact Dermatitis* 38(5), 258
(1998): Mahboob A+, *Int J Dermatol* 37, 833
(1998): Ozkaya-Bayazit E+, *Contact Dermatitis* 39, 87 (trimethoprim)
(1997): Gruber F+, *Clin Exp Dermatol* 22, 144
(1997): Ozkaya-Bayazit E+, *Br J Dermatol* 137, 1028 (linear) (trimethoprim)
(1996): Sharma VK+, *J Dermatol* 23, 530
(1995): Wolkenstein P+, *Arch Dermatol* 131, 544
(1993): Oleaga JM+, *Contact Dermatitis* 29, 155
(1993): Ramam M+, *Indian Pediatr* 30, 110 (in an infant)
(1992): Lim JT+, *Ann Acad Med Singapore* 21, 408
(1991): Jain VK+, *Ann Dent* 50, 9 (oral mucous membrane)
(1991): Smoller BR+, *J Cutan Pathol* 18, 13
(1991): Thankappen TP+, *Int J Dermatol* 30, 867 (36.3%)
(1990): Gaffoor PMA+, *Cutis* 45, 242 (genitalia)
(1989): Basomba A+, *J Allergy Clin Immunol* 84, 409
(1989): Bharija SC+, *Australas J Dermatol* 30, 43
(1989): Gupta R, *Indian J Dermatol* 55, 181 (in an infant)
(1989): Varsano I+, *Dermatologica* 178, 232
(1988): Baird BJ+, *Int J Dermatol* 27, 170 (bullous and generalized)
(1988): Bharija SC+, *Dermatologica* 176, 108 (in an infant)
(1987): Amir J+, *Drug Intell Clin Pharm* 21, 41
(1987): Hughes BR+, *Br J Dermatol* 116, 241
(1987): Van Voorhees A+, *Am J Dermatopathol* 9, 528
(1986): Kanwar AJ+, *Dermatologica* 172, 230
(1985): Gomez B+, *Allergol Immunopathol Madr* (Spanish) 13, 87
(1984): Pandhi RK+, *Sex Transm Dis* 11, 164
(1982): Gibson JR, *BMJ* 284, 1529
(1980): Talbot MD, *Practitioner* 224, 823
(1978): Verbov J, *Arch Dermatol* 114, 963
(1972): Aoyama H+, *Jpn J Dermatol* B 82, 16

Flushing
(1984): Jick SS+, *Lancet* 2, 631

Genital ulceration
(2001): Cherian G, *Int J Clin Pract* 55(2), 151

Jarisch-Herxheimer reaction
(2001): Peschard S+, *Presse Med* 30(31), 1549

Lichenoid eruption
(1994): Berger TG+, *Arch Dermatol* 130, 609

Linear IgA bullous dermatosis
(2002): Cohen LM+, *J Am Acad Dermatol* 46, S32 (passim)
(1997): Paul C+, *Br J Dermatol* 136, 406
(1994): Kuechle MK+, *J Am Acad Dermatol* 30, 187

Lupus erythematosus
(1985): Stratton MA, *Clin Pharm* 4, 657
(1975): Grennan DM+, *BMJ* 4, 385

Mucocutaneous syndrome
(1982): Brettle RP+, *J Infect* 4, 149

Photosensitivity
(1994): Berger TG+, *Arch Dermatol* 130, 609 (in HIV-infected) (4 cases)
(1994): Shelley WB+, *Cutis* 53, 162 (observation)
(1987): Schöpf E, *Infection* 15 (Suppl 5P), S254
(1986): Chandler MJ, *J Infect Dis* 153, 1001

Pruritus
(1997): Caumes E+, *Arch Dermatol* 133, 465
(1997): Thaler D, Monona, WI (from internet) (observation)
(1996): Litt JZ, Beachwood, OH (from Internet) (observation)
(1990): Medina I+, *N Engl J Med* 323, 776 (1–5%)
(1987): Colebunders R+, *Ann Intern Med* 107, 599 (4% in AIDS)
(1986): Sher MR, *J Allergy Clin Immunol* 77, 133
(1984): Kramer BS+, *Cancer* 53, 329
(1975): Gleckman RA, *JAMA* 233, 427 (0.84%)
(1971): Koch-Weser J+, *Arch Intern Med* 128, 399 (0.15%)

Pruritus vulvae
(1981): *Modern Medicine* 49, 111

Psoriasis
(1979): Kennedy C+, *BMJ* 1, 1356

Purpura
(1993): Kaufman DW+, *Blood* 82, 2714
(1989): Saxena SK, *J Assoc Physicians India* 37, 479
(1971): Koch-Weser J+, *Arch Intern Med* 128, 399

Purpuric "gloves and socks syndrome"
(1999): van Rooijen MM+, *Hautarzt* (German) 50, 280

Pustular eruption
(1994): Spencer JM+, *Br J Dermatol* 130, 514
(1990): Guy C+, *Nouv Dermatol* (French) 9, 540
(1989): Grattan CEH, *Dermatologica* 179, 57 (passim)
(1986): Macdonald KJS+, *BMJ* 293, 1279
(1978): Braun-Falco O+, *Hautarzt* (German) 29, 371
(1977): Knudsen L+, *Ugeskr Laeger* (Danish) 139, 1007

Radiation recall
(1990): Leslie MD+, *Br J Radiol* 63, 661
(1987): Vukelja SJ+, *Cancer Treat Rep* 71, 668 (at previously irradiated area)
(1984): Shelley WB+, *J Am Acad Dermatol* 11, 53 (at site of previous sunburn)

Rash (sic) (>10%)
(2001): Meyers B+, *Liver Transpl* 7(8), 750
(2000): Talan DA+, *JAMA* 283, 1583 (14%)
(1995): Williams JW+, *JAMA* 273, 1015
(1993): Malnick SD+, *Ann Pharmacother* 27, 1139
(1984): Gordin FM+, *Ann Intern Med* 100, 495
(1978): Lawson DH+, *Am J Med Sci* 275, 53

Stevens–Johnson syndrome (1–10%)
(2001): Brett AS+, *South Med J* 94, 342
(1998): Arola O+, *Lancet* 351, 1102 (trimethoprim)
(1998): Siegfried EC+, *J Am Acad Dermatol* 39, 797 (passim)
(1997): Douglas R+, *Clin Infect Dis* 25, 1480 (2 cases)
(1997): Rieder MJ+, *Pediatr Infect Dis J* 16, 1028 (10% in children with HIV)
(1996): Caumes E, *Rev Mal Respir* (French) 13, 101
(1996): Eastham JH+, *Ann Pharmacother* 30, 606
(1996): McCarty J, Fort Worth, TX (from Internet) (observation)
(1995): Kuper K+, *Ophthalmologe* (German) 92, 823
(1995): Lewis RJ, *Br J Rheumatol* 34, 84
(1995): Sharma VK+, *Pediatr Dermatol* 12, 178
(1995): Wolkenstein P+, *Arch Dermatol* 131, 544
(1994): Shelley WB+, *Cutis* 53, 159 (observation)
(1993): Litt JZ, Beachwood, OH (personal case) (observation)
(1990): Chan HL+, *Arch Dermatol* 126, 43
(1988): Platt R+, *J Infect Dis* 158, 474
(1985): Heer M+, *Gastroenterology* 88, 1954
(1982): Brettle RP+, *J Infect* 4, 149
(1979): Beck MH+, *Clin Exp Dermatol* 4, 201
(1978): Assaad D+, *Can Med Assoc* 118, 154

(1978): Azinge NO+, *J Allergy Clin Immunol* 62, 125
(1978): Kikuchi S+, *Lancet* 2, 580
(1978): Thorpe JA+, *Lancet* 1, 276 (fatal)
(1975): Bernstein LS, *Can Med Assoc J* 112 (Suppl), 96
(1970): Shaw DJ+, *Johns Hopkins Med J* 126, 130

Toxic epidermal necrolysis (1–10%)
(2002): Correia O+, *Arch Dermatol* 138, 29 (three cases)
(2002): John T+, *Ophthalmology* 109(2), 351
(2002): Nassif A+, *J Invest Dermatol* 118(4), 728
(2001): Paquet P+, *Burns* 27(6), 652
(2001): See S+, *Ann Pharmacother* 35(6), 694
(2001): Spies M+, *Pediatrics* 108, 1162
(2000): Moussala M+, *J Fr Ophtalmol* (French) 23, 229
(2000): Yang CH+, *Int J Dermatol* 39, 621 (with methotrexate)
(1999): Egan CA+, *J Am Acad Dermatol* 40, 458 (6 cases)
(1998): Arora VK+, *Indian J Chest Dis Allied Sci* 40, 125
(1998): Rademaker M+, *New Zealand Adverse Drug Reactions Committee*, April, 1998 (from Internet)
(1998): Siegfried EC+, *J Am Acad Dermatol* 39, 797 (passim)
(1996): Caumes E, *Rev Mal Respir* (French) 13, 101
(1996): Rehbein H, Jacksonville, FL (from Internet) (observation)
(1996): Wagner FF+, *N Engl J Med* 334, 922
(1995): Jick H+, *Pharmacotherapy* 15, 428
(1995): Sharma VK+, *Pediatr Dermatol* 12, 178
(1995): Wolkenstein P+, *Arch Dermatol* 131, 544 (7 cases)
(1993): Correia O+, *Dermatology* 186, 32
(1990): Chan HL+, *Arch Dermatol* 126, 43
(1990): Kobza Black A+, *Br J Dermatol* 123, 277
(1990): Roujeau JC+, *Arch Dermatol* 126, 37
(1990): Ward DJ+, *Burns* 16, 97
(1989): Carmichael AJ+, *Lancet* 2, 808
(1989): Whittington RM, *Lancet* 2, 574
(1988): De Raeve L+, *Br J Dermatol* 119, 521 (passim)
(1987): Guillaume JC+, *Arch Dermatol* 123, 1166
(1987): Schöpf E, *Infection* 15 (Suppl 5P), S254
(1986): Miller KD+, *Am J Trop Med Hyg* 33, 451
(1986): Revuz J, *J Dermatol Paris* 153 (abstract)
(1986): Roman O+, *Rev Pediatr Obstet Ginecol Pediatr* (Romanian) 35, 261
(1984): Fong PH+, *Singapore Med J* 25, 184
(1984): Westly ED+, *Arch Dermatol* 120, 721
(1983): Petersen P+, *Ugeskr Laeger* (Danish) 145, 3345
(1982): Ortiz JE+, *Ann Plast Surg* 9, 249
(1978): Anhalt G+, *Plastic Reconstr Surg* 61, 905
(1978): Assaad D+, *Can Med Assoc J* 118, 154
(1978): Petricevic I+, *Lijec Vjesn* (Serbo-Croatian-Roman) 100, 596
(1975): Bernstein LS, *Can Med Assoc J* 112 (Suppl), 96
(1973): Beyvin AJ+, *Anesth Analg Paris* (French) 30, 767
(1972): Chanial G+, *J Med Lyon* (French) 53, 859
(1971): Chanial G+, *Bull Soc Fr Dermatol Syphiligr* (French) 78, 565

Urticaria
(1994): Blumenthal HL, Beachwood, OH (personal case) (observation)
(1993): Litt JZ, Beachwood, OH (personal case) (observation)
(1991): Greenberger PA, *JAMA* 265, 458
(1987): Schöpf E, *Infection* 15 (Suppl 5P), S254
(1985): Goolamali SK, *Postgrad Med J* 61, 925
(1985): Maayan S+, *Arch Intern Med* 145, 1607
(1984): Kramer BS+, *Cancer* 53, 329
(1981): Abi-Mansur P+, *Am J Gastroenterol* 76, 356
(1971): Koch-Weser J+, *Arch Intern Med* 128, 399

Vasculitis
(1998): Tonev S+, *J Eur Acad Dermatol Venereol* 11, 165
(1995): Lewis RJ, *Br J Rheumatol* 34, 84
(1989): Verne-Pignatelli J+, *Postgrad Med J* 65, 51
(1987): Schöpf E, *Infection* 15 (Suppl 5P), S254
(1978): Braun-Falco O+, *Hautarzt* (German) 29, 371
(1978): Coquin Y+, *Nouv Presse Med* (French) 7, 3145
(1976): Wåhlin A+, *Lancet* 2, 1415
(1971): Koch-Weser J+, *Arch Intern Med* 128, 399

Vulvovaginitis
(1985): Wong ES+, *Ann Intern Med* 102, 302

## Hair

Hair – straight
(1999): Oakley A, Hamilton, New Zealand (from Internet) (observation)

## Nails

Nails – loss
(2000): Canning DA, *J Urol* 163, 1386

## Other

Anaphylactoid reactions
(1998): Bijl AM+, *Clin Exp Allergy* 28, 510 (trimethoprim)
(1998): Siegfried EC+, *J Am Acad Dermatol* 39, 797 (passim)
(1988): Arnold PA+, *Drug Intell Clin Pharm* 22, 43
(1985): Gossius G+, *Scand J Infect Dis* 16, 373

Aphthous stomatitis
(1981): *J Antimicrob Chemother* 7, 179

Black tongue
(1993): Blumenthal HL, Beachwood, OH (personal case) (observation)

Dysgeusia
(1988): Fischl MA+, *JAMA* 259, 1185

Gingival hyperplasia
(1997): Caron F+, *Therapie* (French) 52, 73

Glossitis

Hypersensitivity
(2001): Moran KA+, *South Med J* 94(3), 350 ('sepsis-like')
(2000): Pirmohamed M+, *Pharmacogenetics* 10(8), 705
(1999): Lehman DF+, *J Clin Pharmacol* 39, 533
(1999): Pakianathan MR+, *AIDS* 13, 1787
(1998): Mohanasundaram J+, *J Indian Med Assoc* 96, 21
(1998): Ryan C+, *WMJ* 97, 23
(1997): Hicks ME+, *Ann Pharmacother* 31, 1259
(1994): Carr A+, *AIDS* 8, 333
(1993): Marinac JS+, *Clin Infect Dis* 16, 178
(1993): Martin GJ+, *Clin Infect Dis* 16, 175
(1993): Mathelier-Fusade P+, *Presse Med* (French) 22, 1363
(1993): Mehta J+, *J Assoc Physicians India* 41, 235

Myalgia

Oral mucosal eruption
(1991): Tilden ME+, *Arch Ophthalmol* 109, 67
(1988): Fihn SD+, *Ann Intern Med* 108, 350 (1–5%)

Oral ulceration
(1987): Hughes WT+, *N Engl J Med* 316, 1627
(1981): Orenstein WA+, *Am J Med Sci* 282, 27

Pseudolymphoma
(1978): Laugier P+, *Z Hautkr* (German) 53, 353

Rhabdomyolysis
(1988): Arnold PA+, *Drug Intell Clin Pharm* 22, 43

Serum sickness (<1%)
(1988): Platt R+, *J Infect Dis* 158, 474

Stomatitis (<1%)
(1999): Iborra C+, *Arch Dermatol* 135, 350

Tinnitus

Tongue ulceration
(1981): *J Antimicrob Chemother* 7, 179

Tremors
(1999): Patterson RG+, *Pharmacotherapy* 19, 1456

***Note:** Co-trimoxazole is a sulfonamide and can be absorbed systemically. Sulfonamides can produce severe, possibly fatal, reactions such as toxic epidermal necrolysis and Stevens–Johnson syndrome

## COCAINE

**Trade name:** Cocaine
**Indications:** Topical anesthesia
**Category:** Topical anesthetic; substance abuse drug
**Half-life:** 75 minutes
**Clinically important, potentially hazardous interactions with:** epinephrine

**Note:** Cocaine is a benzoylmethylecogonine alkaloid derived from the leaves of the *Erythroxylon coca* tree. Street names for cocaine include: coke; flake; snow; toot, etc. Crack cocaine is a highly potent smokable form of cocaine

### *Reactions*

#### Skin

Angioedema
(1999): Castro-Villamor MA+, *Ann Emerg Med* 34, 296
Bullous eruption
(1985): Tomecki KJ+, *J Am Acad Dermatol* 12, 585
Cutaneous nodules (sic)
(1989): Heng MCY+, *J Am Acad Dermatol* 21, 570
Diaphoresis
Formication
Granulomas (foreign body)
(1985): Posner DI+, *J Am Acad Dermatol* 13, 869
Hyperkeratosis (fingers and palms)
(1992): Feeney CM+, *Cutis* 50, 193 (from crack cocaine)
Necrosis
(2000): Carter EL+, *Cutis* 65, 73 (mid-facial)
(1988): Zamora-Quezada JC+, *Ann Intern Med* 108, 564
Scleroderma (reversible)
(1992): Lam M+, *N Engl J Med* 326, 1435
(1991): Bourgeois P+, *Baillieres Clin Rheumatol* 5, 13
(1989): Kerr HD, *South Med J* 82, 1275
Urticaria
(1999): Castro-Villamor MA+, *Ann Emerg Med* 34, 296
Vasculitis
(1999): Hofbauer GF+, *Br J Dermatol* 141, 600
Warts (snorters' warts)
(1987): Schuster DS, *Arch Dermatol* 123, 571

#### Other

Ageusia (>10%)
Anosmia (>10%)
Black tongue
(1999): Burnett LB+, *Online Textbook of Emergency Medicine* (from crack cocaine)
Bruxism
(1999): Fazzi M+, *Minerva Stomatol* (Italian) 48, 485
Gingival ulceration
(1999): Fazzi M+, *Minerva Stomatol* (Italian) 48, 485
Injection-site scarring
(1968): Yaffee HS, *Cutis* 4, 286
Nasal septal perforation
(2001): Millard DR+, *Plast Reconstr Surg* 107(2), 419
(2000): Patel R+, *J Natl Med Assoc* 92, 39
(1986): Schwartz RH+, *Am Fam Physician* 43, 187
Necrosis of palate
(1999): Fazzi M+, *Minerva Stomatol* (Italian) 48, 485
Porphyria
(1987): Dick AD+, *Lancet* 2, 1150
Priapism
(1999): Altman AL+, *J Urol* 161, 1817
(1998): Myrick H+, *Ann Clin Psychiatry* 10, 8 (with trazodone)
Rhabdomyolysis
(2000): Richards JR, *J Emerg Med* 19(1), 51
(1999): Hedetoft C+, *Ugeskr Laeger* 161(50), 6907
(1996): Bakir AA+, *Curr Opin Nephrol Hypertens* 5(2), 122
(1996): Lampley EC+, *Obstet Gynecol* 87(5), 804
(1994): Villalba Garcia MV+, *An Med Interna* 11(3), 119
(1992): Garcia Castano J+, *An Med Interna* 9(7), 340 (13 cases)
(1992): Zele I+, *Minerva Med* 83(12), 847 (24%)
(1991): Horst E+, *South Med J* 84(2), 269
(1989): Loper KA, *Med Toxicol Adverse Drug Exp* 4(3), 174
(1989): VanDette JM+, *Clin Pharm* 8(6), 401
Thrombophlebitis
(1987): Heng MC+, *J Am Acad Dermatol* 16, 462
Tremors (1–10%)

## CODEINE

**Synonym:** methylmorphine
**Trade names:** Calcidrine; Cheracol; Guaituss AC; Halotussin; Novahistine DH; Nucofed; Robitussin AC; Tussar-2; Tussi-Organidin
**Other common trade names:** *Actacode; Codicept; Codiforton; Paveral; Solcodein; Tricodein*
**Indications:** Pain, cough suppressant
**Category:** Opioid (narcotic) analgesic; antitussive
**Half-life:** 2.5–4 hours
**Clinically important, potentially hazardous interactions with: alcohol**, CNS depressants, MAO inhibitors

### *Reactions*

#### Skin

Acute generalized exanthematous pustulosis (AGEP)
(1995): Lee S+, *Australas J Dermatol* 36, 25
Angioedema
(1992): Breathnach SM+, *Adverse Drug Reactions and the Skin* Blackwell, Oxford, 211 (passim)
(1960): Schoenfeld MR, *N Y State J Med* 60, 2591
Bullous eruption
(1992): Breathnach SM+, *Adverse Drug Reactions and the Skin* Blackwell, Oxford, 211 (passim)
Contact dermatitis
(1995): Waclawski ER+, *Contact Dermatitis* 33, 51
(1983): Romaguera C+, *Contact Dermatitis* 9, 170
Diaphoresis
Edema
(2001): Estrada JL+, *Contact Dermatitis* 44(3), 185 (generalized)
Erythema multiforme (<1%)
(1992): Breathnach SM+, *Adverse Drug Reactions and the Skin* Blackwell, Oxford, 211 (passim)
(1983): Ponte CD, *Drug Intell Clin Pharm* 17, 128
(1975): Vanderveen TW+, *Am J Hosp Pharm* 32, 1149
(1968): Bianchine JR+, *Am J Med* 7, 390
Erythema nodosum (<1%)
(1992): Breathnach SM+, *Adverse Drug Reactions and the Skin* Blackwell, Oxford, 211 (passim)
Exanthems
(1985): Hunskaar S+, *Ann Allergy* 54, 240
(1980): Voorhorst R+, *Ann Allergy* 44, 116
(1976): Nishioka K+, *Nippon Rinsho* (Japanese) 34, 3123
(1969): Török H, *Int J Dermatol* 8, 57
(1960): Heijer A, *Acta Derm Venereol* (Stockh) 40, 35
(1934): Scheer M+, *JAMA* 102, 908
Exfoliative dermatitis
(1995): Rodriguez F+, *Contact Dermatitis* 32, 120
Facial edema
Fixed eruption (<1%)

(1996): Gonzalo-Garijo MA+, *Br J Dermatol* 135, 498
(1992): Breathnach SM+, *Adverse Drug Reactions and the Skin* Blackwell, Oxford, 211 (passim)
(1990): Gaffoor PMA+, *Cutis* 45, 242 (passim)
(1974): Kuokkanen K, *Int J Dermatol* 13, 4
(1969): Török H, *Int J Dermatol* 8, 57
(1960): Heijer A, *Acta Derm Venereol* (Stockh) 40, 35

Flushing
(1983): Shanahan EC+, *Anaesthesia* 38, 40

Pityriasis rosea
(1993): Yosipovitch G+, *Harefuah* (Hebrew) 124, 198; 247

Pruritus (<1%)
(1986): de Groot AC+, *Contact Dermatitis* 14, 209
(1976): von Muhlendahl KE+, *Lancet* 2, 303
(1934): Scheer M+, *JAMA* 102, 908

Radiation recall (sunlight and electronic beam)
(1984): Shelley WB+, *J Am Acad Dermatol* 11, 53

Rash (sic) (1–10%)
(1976): von Muhlendahl KE+, *Lancet* 2, 303

Toxic epidermal necrolysis (<1%)
(1973): Steigleder GK, *Hautarzt* (German) 24, 261
(1972): Monnat A, *Schweiz Med Wochenschr* (French) 102, 1876

Urticaria (1–10%)
(2000): Vidal C+, *Allergy* 55, 416
(1986): de Groot AC+, *Contact Dermatitis* 4, 209
(1986): Rosenstreich DL, *J Allergy Clin Immunol* 78, 1099
(1985): Hunskaar S+, *Ann Allergy* 54, 240
(1976): von Muhlendahl KE+, *Lancet* 2, 303
(1960): Heijer A, *Acta Derm Venereol* (Stockh) 40, 35
(1960): Schoenfeld MR, *N Y State J Med* 60, 2591

### Nails

Nails – shoreline
(1985): Shelley WB+, *Cutis* 35, 220

### Other

Anaphylactoid reactions
Dysgeusia
Injection-site pain (1–10%)
Oral ulceration
Paresthesias
Seizures
(2001): Zolezzi M+, *Ann Pharmacother* 35(10), 1211
Trembling (sic) (<1%)
Xerostomia (1–10%)

## COENZYME Q-10

**Scientific names:** *Mitoquinone; Ubidecarenone; Ubiquinone*
**Other common names:** Co Q10; Co-Enzyme Q10; Co-Q10; coenzyme Q10; CoQ; CoQ-10;CcoQ10; Q10
**Family:** none
**Purported indications:** Congestive heart failure, angina, diabetes, hypertension, breast cancer, increasing exercise tolerance
**Other uses:** Muscular dystrophy, chronic fatigue, life extension, male infertility, preventing 'statin-indiced' myopathy, muscular dystrophy

#### *Reactions*

### Skin

None

**Note:** CoQ-10 was first identified in 1957. It is widely used in Japan where millions of Japanese patients receive CoQ-10 as part of their treatment for congestive heart failure. CoQ-10 is manufactured from fermenting beets and sugar cane with special strains of yeast

## COLCHICINE

**Trade name:** ColBenemid* (Merck)
**Other common trade names:** *Cochiquim; Colchineos; Colgout; Goutnil; Kolkicin; Konicine*
**Indications:** Gouty arthritis
**Category:** Uricosuric; antigout anti-inflammatory
**Half-life:** 20 minutes
**Clinically important, potentially hazardous interactions with:** erythromycin, troleandomycin

ColBenemid is colchicine and probenecid

#### *Reactions*

### Skin

Angioedema
Bullous eruption (<1%)
(1957): Ott H+, *Dtsch Med Wochenschr* (German) 82, 1163

Cutaneous side effects (sic) (14%)
(1957): Ott H+, *Dtsch Med Wochenschr* (German) 82, 1163

Erythema nodosum
(2002): Guven AG+, *Pediatrics* 109(5), 971

Erythroderma
(1971): Durkalec J+, *Pol Tyg Lek* (Polish) 26, 1048

Exanthems
Fixed eruption
(1996): Mochida K+, *Dermatology* 192, 61

Flushing
Lichenoid eruption
(1974): Sayag J+, *Bull Soc Fr Dermatol Syphiligr* (French) 81, 94

Necrosis
Photocontact dermatitis
(1992): Foti C+, *Contact Dermatitis* 27, 201

Pruritus (<1%)
(1957): Hollander L, *Arch Dermatol* 75, 872
(1957): Ott H+, *Dtsch Med Wochenschr* (German) 82, 1163

Purpura
Pyoderma
(1957): Ott H+, *Dtsch Med Wochenschr* (German) 82, 1163

Rash (sic) (<1%)
Staphylococcal scalded skin syndrome
(1993): Khuong MA+, *Dermatology* 186, 153
(1967): Halprin KM, *JAMA* 202, 137

Toxic epidermal necrolysis
(1994): Alfandari S+, *Infection* 22, 365
(1990): Roujeau JC+, *Arch Dermatol* 126, 37

Urticaria
(1991): Anderson MH+, *Ann Allergy* 66, 207

Vasculitis
(1993): Barash J+, *Isr J Med Sci* 29, 310
(1964): Sinaly NP, *Ann Intern Med* 60, 470

Vesicular eruptions (palms)
(1957): Hollander L, *Arch Dermatol* 75, 872

### Hair

Hair – alopecia (1–10%)
(2002): Guven AG+, *Pediatrics* 109(5), 971
(1980): Harms M, *Hautarzt* (German) 31, 161 (20–50%)
(1977): Naidus RM+, *Arch Intern Med* 137, 394
(1970): Wallace S+, *Am J Med* 48, 443
(1967): Spanopoulos GJ, *Practitioner* 198, 426

### Other

Anaphylactoid reactions
Death
(2002): Maxwell MJ+, *Emerg Med J* 19(3), 265 (overdose)

Hypersensitivity
Injection-site thrombophlebitis
Muscle pain
(2002): Guven AG+, *Pediatrics* 109(5), 971
Myalgia
(2002): Fernandez C+, *Acta Neuropathol* (Berlin) 103(2), 100
Myopathy (<1%)
(1999): Gruberg L+, *Transplant Proc* 31, 2157
(1998): Duarte J+, *Muscle Nerve* 21, 550
(1997): Ducloux D+, *Nephrol Dial Transplant* 12, 2389
(1997): Sinsawaiwong S+, *J Med Assoc Thai* 80, 667
(1992): Himmelmann F+, *Acta Neuropathologica* 83, 440
Porphyria cutanea tarda
(1971): Kuokkanen K, *Acta Derm Venereol* (Stockh) 51, 318
Rhabdomyolysis
(2001): Chattopadhyay I+, *Postgrad Med J* 77(905), 191
(1997): Dawson TM+, *J Rheumatol* 24(10), 2045

***Note:** Colchicine, by itself, is generic

# COLESEVELAM

**Trade name:** Welchol (Sankyo Parke Davis)
**Indications:** Hypercholesterolemia
**Category:** Antilipemic; bile acid sequestrant
**Half-life:** no data

### *Reactions*

## Skin
Flu-like syndrome (sic)

## Other
Myalgia (2%)
Oral ulceration

# COLESTIPOL

**Trade name:** Colestid (Pharmacia & Upjohn)
**Other common trade names:** *Cholestabyl; Lestid*
**Indications:** Primary hypercholesterolemia
**Category:** Antilipidemic
**Half-life:** no data

### *Reactions*

## Skin
Dermatitis (sic) (<1%)
Edema
Exanthems (<1%)
Urticaria (<1%)

# CORTICOSTEROIDS

**Generic names:**
**Alclometasone [Al]**
Trade name: Aclovate (GSK)
Topical
**Amcinonide [A]**
Trade name: Cyclocort (Fujisawa)
Topical
**Beclomethasone [Be]**
Trade names: Beclovent (GSK), Vanceril (Schering), Beconase (GSK), Vancenase (Schering)
Systemic
**Betamethasone [B]**
Trade names: Celestone (Schering), Betaderm (Stiefel), Diprosone (Schering), Luxig (Connetics)
Systemic/Topical
**Budesonide [Bu]**
Trade name: Rhinocort (AstraZeneca)
Systemic
**Clobetasol**
Trade names: Temovate (Elan), Embeline (HealthPoint), Olux (Connetics)
Topical/Systemic
**Cortisone [C]**
Trade name: Cortone (Merck)
Systemic
**Desonide**
Trade name: DesOwen (Galderma)
Topical
**Desoximetasone**
Trade name: Topiccort (Medicis)
Topical
**Dexamethasone [D]**
Trade name: Decadron [Merck]
Systemic/Topical
**Fludrocortisone**
Trade name: Florinef (Apothecon)
Systemic
**Flumetasone**
Trade names: Locacorten (Bioglan), Locasalen (Bioglan)
Topical
**Flunisolide**
Trade names: Aerobid (Forest), Nasalide (Dura)
Systemic
**Fluocinolone**
Trade names: Capex (Galderma), Synalar (Bioglan), Synemol (Medicis)
Topical
**Fluocinonide**
Topical
**Flurandrenolide**
Trade name: Cordran (Oclassen)
Topical
**Fluticasone [Ft]**
Trade names: Cutivate (Elan); Flonase (GSK)
Topical/Systemic
**Halcinonide**
Trade name: Halog (BMS)
Topical
**Halobetasol**
Trade name: Ultravate (BMS)
Topical
**Halomethasone**
Trade name: Sicorten (Bioglan)
Topical
**Hydrocortisone [H]**
Trade names: Hytone (Dermik); Cortef; Solu-Cortef
Systemic/Topical
**Methylprednisolone [M]**
Trade names: Medrol; Depo-Medrol (Pharmacia); Solu-Medrol (Pharmacia)
Systemic
**Mometasone**
Trade names: Elocon (Schering); Elocom (Schering)
Topical
**Prednicarbate**
Trade name: Dermatop (Ortho)
Topical

**Prednisolone [Prl]**
Trade names: Delta-Cortef (Pharmacia); Hydeltra (Merck); Hydeltrasol (Merck)
**Prednisone [Pr]**
Trade names: Deltasone (Pharmacia); Meticorten (Schering); Orasone
Systemic
**Triamcinolone [T]**
Trade names: Aristocort (Fujisawa); Azmacort (Aventis); Kenalog, Nasocort (Fujisawa)
Topical/Systemic
**Tixocortol [Tx}**
Trade name: (not available in USA)
Topical

**Category:** Anti-inflammatory

**Clinically important, potentially hazardous interactions with:** acitretin, aldesleukin, anticholinesterases, cyclosporine, didanosine, doxycycline, **echinacea**, edrophonium, imatinib, isotretinoin, **mistletoe**, mycophenolate, rifabutin, rifampin, rifapentine, **smallpox vaccine**, tetracycline, **varicella vaccine**

## *Reactions*

### Skin

Acanthosis nigricans
(1982): Bailin PL+, *Clin Rheum Dis* 8, 493 (passim)
(1980): Gottlieb NL+, *JAMA* 243, 1260 ([Pr])
(1968): Brown J+, *Medicine* 47, 33

Acne
(2001): Werth V, *Dermatology Times* 18
(2000): Fung MA+, *Dermatology* 200, 43
(2000): Stein RB+, *Drug Saf* 23, 429
(1993): Monk B+, *Clin Exp Dermatol* 18, 148
(1982): Bailin PL+, *Clin Rheum Dis* 8, 493 (passim)
(1953): Smith RC+, *Arch Dermatol* 67, 630

Acute generalized exanthematous pustulosis (AGEP)
(1996): Demitsu T+, *Dermatology* 193, 56 ([D])

Allergic reactions (sic)
(1999): Alexiou C+, *Laryngorhinootologie* (German) 78, 573 ([Pr])

Angioedema
(1980): Ashord RFU+, *Postgrad Med J* 56, 437 ([H])

Atrophy
(1990): Ford MD+, *Ophthalmic Surg* 21, 215 ([T])
(1978): Gottlieb NL+, *JAMA* 240, 559 ([Pr])
(1975): Kikuchi I+, *Arch Dermatol* 111, 795
(1974): Kikuchi I+, *Arch Dermatol* 109, 558
(1974): Rimbaud P+, *Presse Med* (French) 3, 665
(1972): Di Stefano V+, *Clin Orthop* 87, 254
(1966): Cassidy JT+, *Ann Intern Med* 65, 1008
(1964): Ayres S, *Arch Dermatol* 90, 242

Bacterial infection

Bullous eruption
(1999): Lew DB+, *Pediatr Dermatology* 16, 146 ([P])

Calcification
(1979): Leigh IM+, *Br J Dermatol* 101, 71

Contact dermatitis
(2001): Weber F+, *Contact Dermatitis* 44(2), 105
(2000): Chew AL+, *Cutis* 65, 307 ([T, Pr, D, P])
(1997): Murata Y+, *Arch Dermatol* 133, 1053
(1997): Vestergaard L+, *Ugeskr Laeger* (Danish) 159, 5662 ([Bu, H, Tx])
(1995): Bircher AJ+, *Acta Derm Venereol* 75, 490 ([P, B])
(1995): Lepoittevin J-P+, *Arch Dermatol* 131, 31
(1993): Elsner P, *Curr Prob Dermatol* 21, 170
(1993): Fedler R+, *Hautarzt* (German) 44, 91 ([A])
(1993): Hisa T+, *Contact Dermatitis* 28, 174 ([B, Bu, F, A, H])
(1985): Hayakawa R+, *Contact Dermatitis* 12, 213 ([A])
(1985): Yoshikawa K+, *Contact Dermatitis* 12, 55 ([H])

Depigmentation
(1974): Rimbaud P+, *Presse Med* (French) 3, 665
(1972): Bloomfield E, *BMJ* 3, 766
(1972): Glick EN, *BMJ* 4, 300

Dermal thinning
(1992): Breathnach SM+, *Adverse Drug Reactions and the Skin* Blackwell, Oxford, 267 (passim)
(1990): Capewell S+, *BMJ* 300, 1548 ([Pr])

Dermatitis (sic)
(2000): Harris A+, *Australas J Dermatol* 41, 124 ([Pr])
(1994): Whitmore SE, *Br J Dermatol* 131, 296 ([D]) (generalized)

Dermatofibromas
(1991): Cohen PR, *Int J Dermatol* 30, 266
(1991): Margolis DJ, *Int J Dermatol* 30, 750

Diaphoresis
(1999): Alexiou C+, *Laryngorhinootologie* (German) 78, 573 ([Pr])

Ecchymoses
(1992): Breathnach SM+, *Adverse Drug Reactions and the Skin* Blackwell, Oxford, 267 (passim)
(1991): Anderson B+, *Intern Med* 151, [M, T] ([M, T])

Eczematous eruption (sic)
(1993): Belsito DV, *Cutis* 52, 291
(1993): Torres V+, *Contact Dermatitis* 29, 106 ([H])
(1992): Lauerma AI+, *Arch Dermatol* 128, 275 ([H])
(1988): Lindehof B, *Contact Dermatitis* 18, 309

Erythema (diffuse and widespread)
(1999): Alexiou C+, *Laryngorhinootologie* (German) 78, 573 ([Pr])
(1995): Saff DM+, *Arch Dermatol* 131, 742 ([T]) (localized) (intralesional triamcinolone)
(1993): Fedler R+, *Hautarzt* 44, 91 ([A])
(1993): Räsänen L+, *Br J Dermatol* 128, 407

Erythema multiforme
(1999): Lew DB+, *Pediatr Dermatol* 16, 146 ([P])

Exanthems
(1995): Ijsselmuiden O+, *Acta Derm Venereol* (Stockh) 75, 57 ([T]) (intraarticular triamcinolone)
(1995): Whitmore SE, *Contact Dermatitis* 32, 193
(1987): Maucher OM+, *Hautarzt* (German) 38, 577 ([B,D])

Facial edema
(2001): Werth V, *Dermatology Times* 18
(1995): Whitmore SE, *Contact Dermatitis* 32, 193

Fixed eruption
(2001): Sener O+, *Ann Allergy Asthma* 86(3), 335 (solitary, non-pigmenting) ([T])

Flushing
(1999): Alexiou C+, *Laryngorhinootologie* (German) 78, 573 ([P])
(1980): Gottlieb NL+, *JAMA* 243, 1547

Fungal infection

Herpes simplex

Herpes zoster

Infections (sic)
(2002): Beeh KM+, *Pneumologie* 56(2), 91 (2.7%)

Kaposi's sarcoma
(1993): Trattner A+, *J Am Acad Dermatol* 29, 890
(1991): Soria C+, *J Am Acad Dermatol* 24, 1027
(1981): Ilie B+, *Dermatologica* 163, 455
(1981): Leung F+, *Am J Med* 71, 320

Leucoderma acquisitum
(1972): Cahn BJ+, *Cutis* 9, 509

Linear atrophy
(1988): Friedman SJ+, *J Am Acad Dermatol* 19, 537
(1988): Jemec GBE, *J Dermatol Surg Oncol* 14, 88
(1987): Gupta A+, *Pediatr Dermatol* 4, 259
(1985): Litt JZ, *Arch Dermatol* 121, 26

Linear hypopigmentation
(1999): George WM+, *Cutis* 64, 61 (also perilinear)
(1988): Friedman SJ+, *J Am Acad Dermatol* 19, 537
(1985): Litt JZ, *Arch Dermatol* 121, 26

(1984): McCormack PC+, *Arch Dermatol* 120, 708
(1980): Gottlieb L+, *Arch Dermatol* 140, 1507 ([Pr])
(1962): Goldman L, *JAMA* 182, 614

Lupus erythematosus
(1973): Hardin JG, *Ann Intern Med* 78, 558

Mycotic infection

Necrosis
(1974): Rimbaud P+, *Presse Med* (French) 3, 665

Perianal ulcerations
(2002): Adams BB+, *Cutis* 69, 67 (Be for 3 months)

Perioral dermatitis
(1992): Breathnach SM+, *Adverse Drug Reactions and the Skin* Blackwell, Oxford, 267 (passim)

Photocontact dermatitis
(1978): Rietchel RL, *Contact Dermatitis* 4, 334

Pigmentation (sic)
(1992): Breathnach SM+, *Adverse Drug Reactions and the Skin* Blackwell, Oxford, 267 (passim)
(1982): Bailin PL+, *Clin Rheum Dis* 8, 493 (passim)

Pityriasis rosea
(1981): Leonforte JF, *Dermatologica* 163, 480

Porokeratosis
(1980): Feuerman EJ+, *Acta Derm Venereol* (Stockh) 85, 59

Pruritus
(1999): Alexiou C+, *Laryngorhinootologie* (German) 78, 573 ([Pr])
(1999): Lew DB+, *Pediatr Dermatology* 16, 146 ([P])
(1998): Klein-Gitelman MS+, *J Rheumatol* 25, 1995
(1995): Saff DM+, *Arch Dermatol* 131, 742 ([T]) (localized) (intralesional T)

Pseudoxanthoma elasticum
(1982): Miki Aso+, *J Dermatol* (Tokio) 9, 207

Purpura
(2000): Rosen R, Sydney, Australia (from Internet) (observation) (from inhaled steroid)
(1990): Capewell S+, *BMJ* 300, 1548 ([Pr])
(1982): Bailin PL+, *Clin Rheum Dis* 8, 493 (passim)
(1980): Gottlieb NL+, *JAMA* 243, 1260

Pustular psoriasis
(1982): Bailin PL+, *Clin Rheum Dis* 8, 493 (passim)

Redness of face (sic)

Staphylococcal scalded skin syndrome
(1998): Shirin S+, *Cutis* 62, 223 ([Pr]) (in an adult)

Striae
(2001): Werth V, *Dermatology Times* 18
(1982): Bailin PL+, *Clin Rheum Dis* 8, 493 (passim)
(1975): Nikolowski W, *Akt Dermatol* (German) 1, 9

Telangiectases
(1989): Hogan DJ+, *J Am Acad Dermatol* 20, 1129
(1982): Bailin PL+, *Clin Rheum Dis* 8, 493 (passim)
(1972): DiStefano V+, *Clin Orthop* 87, 254

Urticaria
(2001): Borja JM+, *Allergy* 56(8), 802 ([H])
(2001): Nettis E+, *Allergy* 56(8), 791 ([H])
(2001): Pollack B+, *Br J Dermatol* 144, 1228 ([M])
(2001): Rasanen L+, *Allergy* 56, 352 ([H])
(2001): Werth V, *Dermatology Times* 18
(1995): Ijsselmuiden OE+, *Acta Derm Venereol* 75, 57 ([T])
(1995): Whitmore SE, *Contact Dermatitis* 32, 193
(1993): Fedler R+, *Hautarzt* 44, 91 ([A])
(1980): Ashford RF+, *Postgrad Med J* 56, 437 ([Pr])

Vasculitis
(1995): Wolkenstein P+, *Drug Saf* 13, 56
(1982): Bailin PL+, *Clin Rheum Dis* 8, 493 (passim)
(1969): Rosenberg AL+, *Arthritis Rheum* 12, 317
(1967): Main RA, *Br J Dermatol* 79, 68

Viral infection

## Hair

Hair - alopecia
(2001): Werth V, *Dermatology Times* 18

Hair – hirsutism

Hair – hypertrichosis
(1988): Holman GA+, *Pediatrics* 81, 452
(1982): Bailin PL+, *Clin Rheum Dis* 8, 493 (passim)

## Other

Anaphylactoid reactions
(2001): Werth V, *Dermatology Times* 18
(2000): Alexander J, Tulsa, OK [T] (from Internet) (observation) (triamcinolone)
(2000): Heeringa M+, *BMJ* 321(7266), 927 ([Bu])
(2000): Vedamurthy M, Chennai, India, [T] (from Internet) (observation) (triamcinolone)
(1999): Kamm GL+, *Ann Pharmacother* 33, 451
(1998): Klein-Gitelman MS+, *J Rheumatol* 25, 1995
(1995): Jacqz-Aigrain E+, *Arch Pediatr* (French) 2, 353 ([P, Pr, B])
(1992): Coronminas N+, *Pharm Weekbl Sci* 14, 93 ([H])
(1985): Peller JS+, *Ann Allergy* 54, 302 ([H])
(1981): Dajani BM+, *J Allergy Clin* 68, 201 ([H])
(1974): Mendelson LM+, *J Allergy Clin Immunol* 54, 125
(1960): King RA, *Lancet* 2, 1093

Black tongue

Buffalo hump
(1982): Bailin PL+, *Clin Rheum Dis* 8, 493 (passim)

Hypersensitivity
(2000): Brancaccio RR+, *Cutis* 65, 31 ([T]) (at injection site)
(1993): Chan AT, *BMJ* 306, 109 ([D])

Impaired wound healing
(1992): Breathnach SM+, *Adverse Drug Reactions and the Skin* Blackwell, Oxford, 267 (passim)

Injection-site aseptic necrosis

Injection-site lipoatrophy
(2000): Anderson B+, *Arch Intern Med* 151, 153 ([M, T])
(1975): Nikolowski W, *Akt Dermatol* (German) 1, 9
(1974): Kikuchi I+, *Arch Dermatol* 109, 558
(1974): Rimbaud P+, *Presse Med* (French) 3, 665
(1963): Schetman D+, *Arch Dermatol* 88, 820

Moon face
(1982): Bailin PL+, *Clin Rheum Dis* 8, 493 (passim)

Myopathy
(1992): Decramer M+, *Am Rev Resp Dis* 146, 800
(1990): Shee CD, *Respiratory Medicine* 84, 229 ([H])
(1986): Knox AJ+, *Thorax* 41, 411 ([H])
(1985): Bowyer SL+, *J Allerg Clin Immunol* 2, 234
(1982): Mastaglia FL, *Drugs* 24, 304
(1980): Van Marle W+, *BMJ* 281, 271 ([H])

Oral candidiasis
(2002): Beeh KM+, *Pneumologie* 56(2), 91
(1998): Reed CE+, *J Allergy Clin Immunol* 101, 14 ([Be])
(1984): Clissold SP+, *Drugs* 28, 485 ([Bu])

Panniculitis
(1988): Saxena AK+, *Cutis* 43, 241

Stomatitis
(1990): Yamaguchi M+, *Kyobu Shikkan Gakkai Zasshi* (Japanese) 28, 1410 ([Be])

# CREATINE

**Scientific names:** *N-(aminoiminomethyl)-N methyl glycine; N-amidinosarcosine*
**Other common names:** Cr; Creatine monohydrate
**Family:** none
**Purported indications:** To improve exercise performance & increase muscle mass in athletes & older adults
**Other uses:** Heart failure, neuromuscular disease, cholesterol-lowering, amyotrophic lateral sclerosis (ALS), rheumatoid arthritis, cardiac surgery (IV)

### *Reactions*

#### Skin

Acne
(1998): Gregg LJ, Tulsa, OK (from Internet) (2 observations)
Facial rash (sic)
(1998): US Food & Drug Administration
Periorbital edema
(1998): US Food & Drug Administration

#### Other

Anaphylactoid reactions
(1998): US Food & Drug Administration
Myalgia
(1998): US Food & Drug Administration
Polymyositis
(1998): US Food & Drug Administration
Rhabdomyolysis
(2001): Ray TR+, *South Med J* 94(6), 608
(2000): Robinson SJ, *J Am Board Fam Pract* 13(2), 134
(1998): US Food & Drug Administration

***Note:** Creatine is found primarily in skeletal muscle (95%), also in heart, brain, testes & other tissues. The body synthesizes 1 to 2 grams of creatine a day

****Note:** Creatine use is widespread among amateur and professional athletes including, Mark McGuire, Sammy Sosa, John Elway and others. The annual consumption of creatine in the US exceeds 10 million pounds

# CROMOLYN

**Synonyms:** cromolyn sodium; disodium cromoglycate
**Trade names:** Gastrocrom (Medeva); Intal (Aventis)
**Other common trade names:** *Colimune; Cromlom; Cromoptic; Fivent; Nalcrom; Opticrom; Rynacrom*
**Indications:** Allergic rhinitis, asthma, mastocytosis
**Category:** Mast cell stabilizer
**Half-life:** 80 minutes

### *Reactions*

#### Skin

Angioedema (1–10%)
(1992): Breathnach SM+, *Adverse Drug Reactions and the Skin* Blackwell, Oxford, 235 (passim)
(1979): Settipane GA+, *JAMA* 241, 811
(1975): Sheffer AL+, *N Engl J Med* 293, 1220
(1974): Crisp J+, *JAMA* 229, 787
Contact dermatitis
(1997): Camarasa JG+, *Contact Dermatitis* 36, 160 (from eye drops)
(1993): Lewis FM+, *Contact Dermatitis* 28, 246
(1988): Kudo H+, *Contact Dermatitis* 19, 312
Dermatitis (sic) (generalized)
(1979): Settipane GA+, *JAMA* 241, 811
Eczematous eruption (sic)
Edema
Erythema
Exanthems
Exfoliative dermatitis
Facial dermatitis (sic)
(1979): Settipane GA+, *JAMA* 241, 811
(1974): Brogden RN+, *Drugs* 7, 164
Flushing
Photosensitivity
Pruritus
(1975): Sheffer AL+, *N Engl J Med* 293, 1220
Rash (sic) (<1%)
Rosacea
(1979): Mayberry JF+, *BMJ* 2, 1366
Urticaria (<1%)
(1992): Breathnach SM+, *Adverse Drug Reactions and the Skin,* Blackwell, Oxford, 235 (passim)
(1977): Menon MP+, *Scand J Respir Dis* 58, 145
(1975): Sheffer AL+, *N Engl J Med* 293, 1220
Vasculitis
(1978): Rosenberg JL+, *Arch Intern Med* 138, 989

#### Other

Anaphylactoid reactions (<1%)
(1996): Ibanez MD+, *Ann Allergy Asthma Immunol* 77, 185
(1996): Shearer WT, *Ann Allergy Asthma Immunol* 77, 165
(1992): Breathnach SM+, *Adverse Drug Reactions and the Skin* Blackwell, Oxford, 235 (passim)
(1983): Ahmad S, *Ann Intern Med* 99, 882
(1975): Sheffer AL+, *N Engl J Med* 293, 1220
Anosmia
(1998): Graedon J+, Newspaper anecdote from *People's Pharmacy* column
Dysgeusia (>10%)
Hypersensitivity (immediate type)
(1987): Skarpass IJK, *Allergy* 42, 318
Myalgia
Myopathy
(1979): Settipane GA+, *JAMA* 241, 811
Paresthesias
Serum sickness
Xerostomia (1–10%)

# CYANOCOBALAMIN

**Synonym:** vitamin $B_{12}$
**Trade names:** Berubigen; Crysti-12; Cyanoject (Mayrand); Cyomin (Forest); Ener-B; Nascobal (Schwarz); Rubramin (Bristol-Myers Squibb); Vitamin $B_{12}$
**Other common trade names:** *Anacobin; Betolvex; Cobex; Crystamine; Cytamen; Dobetin; Lifaton $B_{12}$; Redisol; Rubesol-1000; Sytobex; Vicapan N*
**Indications:** Vitamin $B_{12}$ deficiency, pernicious anemia
**Category:** Water-soluble nutritional supplement and antianemic
**Half-life:** 6 days

### *Reactions*

#### Skin

Acne
(1991): Sherertz EF, *Cutis* 48, 119

(1979): Dupre A+, *Cutis* 24, 210
(1976): Braun-Falco O+, *Münch Med Wochenschr* (German) 118, 155
(1969): Dugois P+, *Bull Soc Fr Dermatol Syphiligr* (French) 76, 382
(1969): Dugois P+, *Lyon Med* (French) 221, 1165
(1967): Puissant A+, *Bull Soc Fr Derm Syphiligr* (French) 74, 813
(1966): Goldblatt S, *Hautarzt* (German) 17, 106

Allergic reactions (sic)
(1986): Bigby M+, *JAMA* 256, 3358 (1.79%)

Angioedema
(1952): Bedford PD, *BMJ* 1, 690

Bullous eruption (<1%)
(1977): Pevny I+, *Hautarzt* (German) 28, 600

Cheilitis
(1981): Price ML+, *Contact Dermatitis* 7, 352

Contact dermatitis
(1994): Rodriguez A+, *Contact Dermatitis* 31, 271
(1975): Malten KE, *Contact Dermatitis* 1, 325

Eczematous eruption (sic)
(1977): Pevny I+, *Hautarzt* (German) 28, 600

Exanthems
(1986): Woodliff HJ, *Med J Aust* 144, 223
(1977): Pevny I+, *Hautarzt* (German) 28, 600
(1976): Arndt KA+, *JAMA* 235, 918

Folliculitis
(1989): Gallastegui C+, *Drug Intell Clin Pharm* 23, 1033

Pruritus (1–10%)
(1974): Nalivko F+, *Vestn Dermatol Venerol* (Russian) 8, 66

Rosacea fulminans
(2001): Jansen T+, *J Eur Acad Dermatol Venereol* 15(5), 484

Systemic eczematous contact dermatitis

Urticaria (<1%)
(1996): Denis R+, *Clin Lab Haematol* 18, 129
(1986): Woodliff HJ, *Med J Aust* 144, 223
(1977): Pevny I+, *Hautarzt* (German) 28, 600
(1974): Nalivko F+, *Vestn Dermatol Venerol* (Russian) 8, 66
(1971): James J+, *BMJ* 2, 262
(1969): Meyer de Schmid JJ+, *Bull Soc Fr Dermatol Syphiligr* (French) 76, 670
(1952): Bedford PD, *BMJ* 1, 690

### Other

Anaphylactoid reactions (<1%)
(1998): Tordjman R+, *Eur J Haematol* 60, 269
(1984): Sobolevskii AI+, *Vestn Dermatol Venerol* (Russian) April, 66
(1977): Pevny I+, *Hautarzt* (German) 28, 600
(1971): James J+, *BMJ* 2, 262
(1968): Hovding G, *BMJ* 3, 102

Embolia cutis medicamentosa (Nicolau syndrome)
(2002): Poletti E+, *World Congress Dermatol* Poster, 0124
(1995): Kunzi T+, *Schweiz Rundsch Med Prax* (German) 84, 640

Hypersensitivity
(1974): Nalivko SN+, *Vestn Dermatol Venerol* (Russian) August, 66

Injection-site aseptic necrosis
(1995): Kunzi T+, *Schweiz Rundsch Med Prax* (German) 84, 640

Injection-site pain

Paresthesias

Porphyria cutanea tarda
(1965): DeFeo CP, *Arch Dermatol* 92, 330

## CYCLAMATE

**Trade name:** Sucaryl (Abbott)
**Indications:** Sweetening
**Category:** Sulfonamide* sweetener
**Half-life:** no data

#### *Reactions*

### Skin

Angioedema
(1968): Feingold BF, *Ann Allergy* 26, 309

Bullous eruption
(1968): Feingold BF, *Ann Allergy* 26, 309

Exanthems
(1965): Boros E, *JAMA* 194, 571

Photosensitivity
(1981): Fujita M+, *Arch Dermatol* 117, 246 (passim)
(1972): Jung EG, *Z Haut Geschlechtskr* (German) 47, 329
(1970): *Nutr Rev* 28, 122
(1969): Yong JM+, *Lancet* 2, 1273
(1968): Feingold BF, *Ann Allergy* 26, 309
(1968): Turk JL+, *Br J Dermatol* 80, 200
(1966): Kobori T+, *J Asthma Res* 3, 213

Pruritus
(1968): Feingold BF, *Ann Allergy* 26, 309
(1967): Lamberg SI, *JAMA* 201, 747
(1965): Boros E, *JAMA* 194, 571

Urticaria
(1981): Fujita M+, *Arch Dermatol* 117, 246
(1968): Feingold BF, *Ann Allergy* 26, 309

### Other

Hypersensitivity (nonallergic)
(1998): Ehlers I+, *Allergy* 53, 1074

Paresthesias
(1992): Shelley WB+, *Advanced Dermatologic Diagnosis* WB Saunders, 1039

***Note:** Cyclamate is a sulfonamide and can be absorbed systemically. Sulfonamides can produce severe, possibly fatal, reactions such as toxic epidermal necrolysis and Stevens–Johnson syndrome

## CYCLOBENZAPRINE

**Trade name:** Flexeril (Merck)
**Other common trade names:** *Benzamin; Cloben; Cyben; Flexiban; Novo-Cycloprine; Yurelax*
**Indications:** Muscle spasms
**Category:** Skeletal muscle relaxant
**Half-life:** 1–3 days

#### *Reactions*

### Skin

Allergic reactions (sic)
Angioedema (<1%)
Dermatitis (sic) (<1%)
Diaphoresis
(1984): Heckerling PS+, *Ann Intern Med* 101, 881
Facial edema (<1%)
Flushing
Photosensitivity
Pruritus (<1%)
Purpura
Rash (sic) (<1%)

Urticaria (<1%)

### Hair

Hair – alopecia

### Other

Ageusia (<1%)
Anaphylactoid reactions (<1%)
Dysgeusia (3%)
Galactorrhea
Gynecomastia
Paresthesias (<1%)
Stomatitis
Tinnitus
Tongue edema (<1%)
Tongue pigmentation
Xerostomia (27%)
(1988): Bennett RM+, *Arthritis Rheum* 31, 1535
(1988): Katz WA+, *Clin Ther* 10, 216

# CYCLOPHOSPHAMIDE

**Synonyms:** CPM; CTX; CYT
**Trade names:** Cytoxan (Bristol-Myers Squibb); Neosar (Pharmacia & Upjohn)
**Other common trade names:** *Cycloblastin; Cyclostin; Endoxan; Endoxana; Genoxal; Ledoxina; Procytox; Sendoxan*
**Indications:** Lymphomas
**Category:** Antineoplastic and immunosuppressant
**Half-life:** 4–7 hours
**Clinically important, potentially hazardous interactions with:** aldesleukin, azathioprine, cyclosporine, mycophenolate, **vaccines**

## *Reactions*

### Skin

Acral erythema
(1995): Komamura H+, *J Dermatol* 22(2), 116 (with vincristine, doxorubicin and G-CSF)
(1993): Vukelja SJ+, *Cutis* 52, 89
(1986): Crider MK+, *Arch Dermatol* 122, 1023
Allergic reactions (sic)
(2001): Stratton J+, *Nephrol Dial Transplant* 16(8), 1724
Angioedema
(1977): Ross WE+, *Cancer Treat Rep* 61, 495
Condylomata acuminata
(1996): D'Hondt L+, *Acta Gastroenterol Belg* (French) 59, 254
Contact dermatitis
(1967): Maguire HC, *J Invest Dermatol* 48, 39
Dermatitis herpetiformis
(1986): Gottlieb D+, *Med J Aust* 145, 241
Dermatofibromas
(1986): Bargman HB+, *J Am Acad Dermatol* 14, 351
Diaphoresis
Eccrine squamous syringometaplasia
(1997): Valks R+, *Arch Dermatol* 133, 873
Erythema multiforme (<1%)
Erythrodysesthesia syndrome
(1989): Matsuyama JR+, *Drug Intell Clin Pharm* 23, 776
Exanthems
(1992): Breathnach SM+, *Adverse Drug Reactions and the Skin* Blackwell, Oxford, 289 (passim)
(1992): Hann SK+, *J Dermatol* 20, 94
(1982): Bailin PL+, *Clin Rheum Dis* 8, 493 (passim)
Facial burning
(1994): Kosirog-Glowacki JL+, *Ann Pharmacother* 28, 197
Flushing (1–10%)
(1994): Dhar S+, *Dermatology* 188, 332
Graft-versus-host reaction
(2001): Valks R+, *Arch Dermatol* 137, 61 (3 cases)
Keratoacanthoma
(1972): Lowney ED, *Arch Dermatol* 105, 924
Lupus erythematosus
(2001): McClain S, New York, NY (from Internet) (observation)
Lymphoma
(1992): Pandya AG+, *Arch Dermatol* 128, 1626 (passim)
(1983): Goslen JB+, *Arch Dermatol* 119, 326
Myxedema
(1971): Coffey VJ, *BMJ* 4, 682
Palmar–plantar erythema
(1990): Pagliuca A+, *Postgrad Med J* 66, 242
Pigmentation (<1%)
(2001): Viana G, *Belo Horizonte* (Brazil) (from Internet) (observation)
(1993): Pai BH, *J Assoc Physicians India* 41, 124
(1992): Babu KG, *J Assoc Physicians India* 40, 211
(1992): Pandya AG+, *Arch Dermatol* 128, 1626 (passim)
(1991): Dutta TK+, *J Assoc Physicians India* 39, 230
(1991): Singal R+, *Pediatr Dermatol* 8, 231
(1981): Nixon DW+, *Cutis* 27, 181
(1975): No Author, *Lancet* 2, 128
(1975): Shah PC+, *Lancet* 2, 548 (palmar)
(1974): Romankiewicz JA, *Am J Hosp Pharm* 31, 1074
(1973): Levantine A+, *Br J Dermatol* 89, 105
(1973): Mani MK+, *J Assoc Physicians India* 21, 799
(1972): Amar Inalsingh CH, *Arch Dermatol* 106, 765 (palmar)
(1972): Harrison BM+, *BMJ* 2, 352
(1966): Solidoro A+, *Cancer Chemotherapy* 50, 265
Polyarteritis nodosa
(1983): Goslen JB+, *Arch Dermatol* 119, 326
Pruritus
(1978): Krutchik AN+, *Arch Intern Med* 138, 1725
Purpura
Rash (sic) (1–10%)
Squamous cell carcinoma
(1992): Pandya AG+, *Arch Dermatol* 128, 1626 (passim)
(1972): Lowney ED, *Arch Dermatol* 105, 924
Stevens–Johnson syndrome
(1996): Assier-Bonnet H+, *Br J Dermatol* 135, 864
(1985): Leititis JU+, *Klin Padiatr* (German) 197, 441
Toxic epidermal necrolysis (<1%)
Ultraviolet light recall
(1993): Williams BJ+, *Clin Exp Dermatol* 18, 452
(1984): Andersen KE+, *Photodermatol* 1, 129
Urticaria
(1992): Breathnach SM+, *Adverse Drug Reactions and the Skin* Blackwell, Oxford, 289 (passim)
(1987): Grosbois B+, *Rev Med Interne* (French) 8, 208
(1982): Anku V, *Cancer Treat Rep* 66, 2106
(1980): Diaz-Rubio E+, *Rev Clin Esp* (Spanish) 156, 461
(1978): Krutchik AN+, *Arch Intern Med* 138, 1725
(1978): Legha SS+, *Cancer Treat Rep* 62, 180
(1977): Ross WE+, *Cancer Treat Rep* 61, 495
(1976): Lakin JD+, *J Allergy Clin Immunol* 58, 160
Vasculitis
(1989): Green RM+, *Aust N Z J Med* 19, 55

### Hair

Hair – alopecia (universal and severe in one-third)
(2001): Viana G, *Belo Horizonte* (Brazil) (from Internet) (observation)
(2000): Tran D+, *Australas J Dermatology* 41, 106
(1996): Infanti L+, *Haematologica* 81, 521
(1992): Pandya AG+, *Arch Dermatol* 128, 1626 (passim)
(1987): David J+, *Nurs Times* 83, 36

(1987): Parker R, *Oncol Nurs Forum* 14, 49
(1985): Middleton J+, *Cancer Treat Rep* 69, 373
(1984): Ahmed AR+, *J Am Acad Dermatol* 11, 1115
(1984): Cline BW, *Cancer Nurs* 7, 221
(1982): Bailin PL+, *Clin Rheum Dis* 8, 493 (passim)
(1980): Maxwell MB, *Am J Nursing* 80, 900
(1979): Holmes W, *ANA Publ* (NP-59), 223
(1972): Harrison BM+, *BMJ* 2, 352
(1966): Herzberg JJ, *Arch Klin Exp Dermatol* (German) 227, 452
(1966): Simister JM, *BMJ* 2, 1138

### Nails

Nails – Beau's lines (transverse nail bands)
(1994): Ben-Dyan D+, *Acta Haematol* 91, 89
Nails – dystrophy
(1992): Breathnach SM+, *Adverse Drug Reactions and the Skin* Blackwell, Oxford, 289 (passim)
Nails – onychodermal band
(1993): Kowal-Vern A+, *Cutis* 52, 43
Nails – pigmentation (<1%)
(2002): Srikant M+, *Br J Haematol* 117(1), 2
(2001): Viana G, *Belo Horizonte* (Brazil) (from Internet) (observation)
(1992): Bianchi L+, *Dermatology* 185, 216 (longitudinal)
(1983): Manigand G+, *Sem Hop* (French) 59, 1840
(1982): Bailin PL+, *Clin Rheum Dis* 8, 493 (passim)
(1981): Adam BA, *Singapore Med J* 22, 35
(1980): Daniel CR+, *Cutis* 25, 595
(1980): Sulis E+, *Eur J Cancer* 16, 1517
(1978): Shah PC+, *Br J Dermatol* 98, 675
(1975): Markenson AL+, *Lancet* 2, 128 (pigmented banding)
(1975): Shah PC+, *Lancet* 2, 548
(1973): Mani MK+, *J Assoc Physicians of India* 21, 799
(1972): Amar Inalsingh CH, *Arch Dermatol* 106, 765
(1966): Solidoro A+, *Cancer Chemother* 50, 265
Nails – transverse leukonychia (Meuhrcke's lines)
(1992): Bianchi L+, *Dermatology* 185, 216 (longitudinal)
(1990): Bader-Meunier B+, *Ann Pediatr Paris* (French) 37, 337
(1983): James WD+, *Arch Dermatol* 119, 334

### Other

Acute intermittent porphyria
Anaphylactoid reactions (<1%)
(1992): Breathnach SM+, *Adverse Drug Reactions and the Skin* Blackwell, Oxford, 289 (passim)
(1979): Murti L+, *J Pediatr* 94, 844
(1977): Karchmer RK+, *JAMA* 237, 475
Gingival pigmentation
(1979): Krutchik AN+, *South Med J* 72, 1615
(1972): Harrison BM+, *BMJ* 2, 352
Hypersensitivity
(1996): Popescu NA+, *J Allergy Clin Immunol* 97, 26
(1992): Weiss RB, *Semin Oncol* 19, 458
(1978): Legha SS+, *Cancer Treat Rep* 62, 180
Injection-site pain
Oral mucosal ulceration
(1992): Pandya AG+, *Arch Dermatol* 128, 1626 (passim)
(1982): Bailin PL+, *Clin Rheum Dis* 8, 493 (passim)
Oral mucositis
(2000): Wardley AM+, *Br J Haematol* 110, 292
Porphyria cutanea tarda
(1988): Manzione NC+, *Gastroenterology* 95, 1119
Rhabdomyolysis
Scalp burning
(1994): Kosirog-Glowacki JL+, *Ann Pharmacother* 28, 197
Stomatitis (10%)
(1982): Bailin PL+, *Clin Rheum Dis* 8, 493 (passim)
(1975): Carter SK, *Cancer Treat Rev* 2, 295
Tooth discoloration
(1972): Harrison BM+, *BMJ* 2, 352

## CYCLOSERINE

**Trade name:** Seromycin (Dura)
**Other common trade names:** *Closerin; Closerina; Cyclomycin; Cyclorine; Cycosin; Orientomycin*
**Indications:** Tuberculosis
**Category:** Tuberculostatic
**Half-life:** 10 hours

#### *Reactions*

### Skin

Allergic reactions (sic)
Dermatitis (sic)
(1972): Levantine A+, *Br J Dermatol* 86, 651
(1971): Nava C, *Med Lav* (Italian) 62, 351
Exanthems
(1985): Holdiness R, *Int J Dermatol* 24, 280
(1973): Mühlberger F, *Schweiz Med Wochenschr* (German) 103, 126
(1969): Agrawal R, *BMJ* 4, 540
(1959): Bereston ES, *J Invest Dermatol* 33, 427
Lichenoid eruption
(1995): Shim JH+, *Dermatology* 191, 142
Pruritus
Rash (sic) (<1%)
Stevens–Johnson syndrome
(1997): Akula SK+, *Int J Tuberc Lung Dis* 1, 187 (in AIDS)
Urticaria
(1959): Bereston ES, *J Invest Dermatol* 33, 427

### Other

Oral mucosal lesions
Paresthesias

## CYCLOSPORINE

**Synonyms:** CsA; CyA; cyclosporin A
**Trade names:** Neoral (Novartis); Sandimmune (Novartis)
**Other common trade names:** *Ciclosporin; Consupren; Implanta; Sandimmun*
**Indications:** Prophylaxis of organ rejection in transplants
**Category:** Immunosuppressant
**Half-life:** 10–27 hours (adults)
**Clinically important, potentially hazardous interactions with:** amiloride, aminoglycosides, amphotericin B, ampicillin, anisindione, anticoagulants, atorvastatin, azithromycin, azothioprine, bacampicillin, basiliximab, bosentan, carbenicillin, caspofungin, cholestyramine, clarithromycin, cloxacillin, co-trimoxazole, corticosteroids, cyclophosphamide, danazol, dicloxacillin, dicumarol, digoxin, diltiazem, disulfiram, **echinacea**, erythromycin, ethotoin, etoposide, fluoxymesterone, fluvastatin, foscarnet, fosphenytoin, gemfibrozil, imatinib, imipenem cilastatin, ketoconazole, lovastatin, mephenytoin, methicillin, methoxsalen, methyltestosterone, mezlocillin, mycophenolate, nafcillin, NSAIDs, orlistat, oxacillin, penicillins, phenytoin, pravastatin, rifabutin, rifampin, rifapentine, ritonavir, simvastatin, spironolactone, **St John's wort**, sulfacetamide, sulfadiazine, sulfamethoxazole, sulfisoxazole, sulfonamides, tacrolimus, testosterone, ticarcillin, triamterene, troleandomycin, **vaccines**

**Note:** A good discussion of cyclosporine in dermatology can be found in (1989): Gupta AK+, *J Am Acad Dermatol* 21, 1245

#### *Reactions*

### Skin

Acne

(2001): Reitamo S+, *Br J Dermatol* 145(3), 438 (13%) (with sirolimus)
(2001): Werth V, *Dermatology Times* 15

Acne keloid
(2001): Carnero L+, *Br J Dermatol* 144(2), 429 (nuchal scalp)

Angioedema
(1980): Isenberg DA+, *N Engl J Med* 303, 754

Angiomas
(1998): De Felipe I+, *Arch Dermatol* 134, 1487

Ankle edema
(1997): Berthe-Jones J+, *Br J Dermatol* 136, 76

Basal cell carcinoma
(2001): Otley CC+, *Arch Dermatol* 137, 459
(1992): Pakula A+, *J Am Acad Dermatol* 26, 139
(1987): Penn I, *Transplantation* 43, 32

Bullous eruption (1%)
(1990): Petit D+, *J Am Acad Dermatol* 22, 851

Buschke–Lowenstein penile carcinoma
(1993): Piepkorn M+, *J Am Acad Dermatol* 29, 321

Cutaneous neoplasms (sic)
(1995): Kohler LD+, *Hautarzt* (German) 46, 638

Eccrine squamous syringometaplasia
(1997): Valks R+, *Arch Dermatol* 133, 873

Edema
(1997): Shapiro J+, *J Am Acad Dermatol* 36, 114

Epidermal cysts
(1993): Richter A+, *Hautarzt* (German) 44, 521
(1993): Valicenti JMK+, *Arch Dermatol* 129, 794 (passim)
(1992): Schoendorff C+, *Cutis* 50, 36 (epidermoid)
(1986): Bencini PL+, *Dermatologica* 172, 24

Erythema
(2001): Takamatsu Y+, *Bone Marrow Transplant* 28(4), 421

Exanthems
(1985): Chapius B+, *N Engl J Med* 312, 1259

Facial edema
(1986): Schmitz-Schumann M, *Prog Allergy* 38, 436

Fixed eruption
(2002): Verma SB (Baroda) (India) (from Internet) (observation)

Flushing (>3%)
(2000): Ramsay HM+, *Br J Dermatol* 142, 832
(1992): Goodman MM+, *J Am Acad Dermatol* 27, 594
(1992): Shelley WB+, *Advanced Dermatologic Diagnosis* WB Saunders, 583 (passim)
(1990): Gupta AK+, *J Am Acad Dermatol* 22, 242
(1986): Kahan BD+, *World J Surg* 10, 348

Folliculitis
(2001): Werth V, *Dermatology Times* 15
(1995): Ojeda-Vargas M+, *Enferm Infecc Microbiol Clin* (Spanish) 13, 637
(1993): Richter A+, *Hautarzt* (German) 44, 521
(1993): Sepp N+, *Br J Dermatol* 128, 213
(1993): Valicenti JMK+, *Arch Dermatol* 129, 794 (passim)
(1986): Bencini PL+, *Dermatologica* 172, 24

Herpes simplex
(1993): Sepp N+, *Br J Dermatol* 128, 213
(1993): Valicenti JMK+, *Arch Dermatol* 129, 794 (passim)
(1986): Bencini PL+, *Dermatologica* 172, 24

Herpes zoster
(1986): Bencini PL+, *Dermatologica* 172, 24

Hidradenitis
(1984): Palestine AG+, *Am J Med* 4:77, 652

Hot flashes
(2001): Reitamo S+, *Br J Dermatol* 145(3), 438 (12%) (with sirolimus)

Hyperkeratosis (follicular spiny)
(1995): Izakovic J+, *Hautarzt* (German) 46, 841

Hypohidrosis
(1990): Gupta AK+, *Arch Dermatol* 126, 339

Ichthyosis
(1986): Bencini PL+, *Dermatologica* 172, 24

Kaposi's sarcoma
(1997): Vella JP+, *N Engl J Med* 336, 1761
(1996): Ozen S+, *Nephrol Dial Transplant* 11, 1162
(1988): Bencini PL+, *Br J Dermatol* 118, 709
(1987): Penn I, *Transplantation* 43, 32

Keratoses
(1995): Yamamoto T+, *J Dermatol* 22, 298
(1993): Piepkorn M+, *J Am Acad Dermatol* 29, 321
(1992): Ross M+, *J Am Acad Dermatol* 26, 128

Keratosis pilaris
(1993): Valicenti JMK+, *Arch Dermatol* 129, 794 (passim)
(1986): Bencini PL+, *Dermatologica* 172, 24

Lichenoid eruption
(1995): Shim JH+, *Dermatology* 191, 142

Linear IgA bullous dermatosis
(1990): Petit D+, *J Am Acad Dermatol* 22, 851

Lupus erythematosus
(1990): Cooper KD, *Dermatology* 1(2), 3

Lymphocytic infiltration
(1992): Bagot M+, *J Am Acad Dermatol* 26, 283
(1991): Sabourin JC, *Ann Pathol* 11, 208
(1990): Gupta AK+, *J Am Acad Dermatol* 22, 242
(1990): Gupta AK+, *J Am Acad Dermatol* 23, 1137
(1988): Brown MD+, *Arch Dermatol* 124, 1097

Lymphoma
(1993): Masouye I+, *Arch Dermatol* 129, 914
(1992): Koo JY+, *J Am Acad Dermatol* 26, 836
(1992): Zijlmans JM+, *N Engl J Med* 326, 1363
(1991): Tomson CR+, *Nephrol Dial Transplant* 6, 896
(1989): Walker RJ+, *Aust N Z J Med* 19, 154
(1987): Penn I, *Transplantation* 43, 32
(1984): Beveridge T+, *Lancet* 1, 788
(1983): Inglehart JK, *N Engl J Med* 309, 123

Melanoma
(1990): Merot Y+, *Br J Dermatol* 123, 237

Mycosis fungoides
(1990): Fradin MS+, *J Am Acad Dermatol* 23, 1265

Nodular cutaneous T-lymphocyte infiltrate
(1988): Brown MD+, *Arch Dermatol* 124, 1097

Papillomas (facial)
(1993): Valicenti JMK+, *Arch Dermatol* 129, 794

Papulo-vesicular lesions (sic)
(1988): Frosch PJ+, *Hautarzt* (German) 39, 611

Pigmentation
(1997): Oakley A, Hamilton, New Zealand (from Internet) (observation)

Poikiloderma
(1986): Bencini PL+, *Dermatologica* 172, 24

Porokeratosis (superficial actinic)
(1997): Matsushita S+, *J Dermatol* 24, 110

Pruritus (<2%)
(1992): Goodman MM+, *J Am Acad Dermatol* 27, 594

Psoriasis
(1986): Bencini PL+, *Dermatologica* 172, 24

Purpura (3%)
(1998): Roberts P+, *Transplant Proc* 30, 1512
(1986): Bencini PL+, *Dermatologica* 172, 24

Pustular psoriasis
(1998): Mahendran R+, *Br J Dermatol* 139, 934
(1997): Drugge R, Stamford, CT (from Internet) (observation)

Pyogenic granuloma
(2001): al-Zayer M+, *Spec Care Dentist* 21(5), 187

Rash (sic) (10%)
(1992): Goodman MM+, *J Am Acad Dermatol* 27, 594

Raynaud's phenomenon
(1986): Deray G+, *Lancet* 2, 1092

Sebaceous hyperplasia
(1998): Walther T+, *Dtsch Med Wochenschr* 123, 798
(1993): Valicenti JMK+, *Arch Dermatol* 129, 794 (passim)
(1992): Pakula A+, *J Am Acad Dermatol* 26, 139
(1986): Bencini PL+, *Dermatologica* 172, 24
Squamous cell carcinoma
(2001): Marcil I+, *Lancet* 358(9287), 1042
(2001): Otley CC+, *Arch Dermatol* 137, 459
(1997): van de Kerkhof PC+, *Br J Dermatol* 136, 275
(1996): Cox NH, *Clin Exp Dermatol* 21, 323
(1993): Piepkorn M+, *J Am Acad Dermatol* 29, 321 (penis)
(1990): Fradin MS+, *J Am Acad Dermatol* 23, 1265 (passim)
(1989): Bos JD+, *J Am Acad Dermatol* 21, 1305
(1985): Bencini PL+, *Br J Dermatol* 113, 373
(1985): Price ML+, *N Engl J Med* 313, 1420
(1985): Thompson JF+, *Lancet* 1, 158
(1983): Mortimer PS+, *J R Soc Med* 76, 786
Striae
(1986): Bencini PL+, *Dermatologica* 172, 24
Thrombocytopenic purpura
(2001): Medina PJ+, *Curr Opin Hematol* 8(5), 286
Toxic epidermal necrolysis
(1997): Jarrett P+, *Clin Exp Dermatol* 22, 254
Ulceration (1%)
Urticaria
(2001): Takamatsu Y+, *Bone Marrow Transplant* 28(4), 421 (with tacrolimus)
(1985): Ptachcinski RJ+, *Lancet* 1, 636
Vasculitis
(2000): Gupta MN+, *Ann Rheum Dis* 59, 319
(1994): Henckes M+, *Transpl Int* 7, 292
Verruca vulgaris
(1998): Irimajiri J+, *J Dermatol* 25, 688
Vitiligo
(1986): Bencini PL+, *Dermatologica* 172, 24

## Hair

Hair – alopecia (3%)
(1998): Hunt M, *Cosmetic Dermatology* 23
(1987): Keown PA+, *Hospital Practice* 22, 207
Hair – alopecia areata
(1999): Cerottini JP+, *Dermatology* 198, 415
(1996): Misciali C+, *Arch Dermatol* 132, 843 (universalis)
(1996): Parodi A+, *Br J Dermatol* 135, 657 (universalis)
(1995): Davies MG+, *Br J Dermatol* 132, 835
(1994): Roger D+, *Acta Derm Venereol* 74, 154
Hair – breakage
Hair – growth
(1995): Mannes GP+, *Transpl Int* 8, 247 ("delightful")
(1994): Yamamoto S+, *J Dermatol Sci* 7 Suppl: s47
Hair – hypertrichosis (19%)
(2001): Werth V, *Dermatology Times* 15
(2000): Ionnides D+, *Arch Dermatol* 136, 868
(1997): Avci O+, *J Am Acad Dermatol* 36, 796
(1997): Brehler R+, *J Am Acad Dermatol* 36, 983 (passim)
(1997): Ellis CN, *Int J Dermatol* 36 (Supplement), 7 (passim)
(1997): Shapiro J+, *J Am Acad Dermatol* 36, 114
(1997): Shupack J+, *J Am Acad Dermatol* 36, 423
(1996): el Shahawy MA+, *Nephron* 72, 679
(1996): Jayamanne DG+, *Nephrol Dial Transplant* 11, 1159 (eyelashes)
(1995): Honeyman JF+, *Int J Dermatol* 34, 583
(1993): Sepp N+, *Br J Dermatol* 128, 213
(1993): Valicenti JMK+, *Arch Dermatol* 129, 794 (passim)
(1992): Humphreys TR+, *J Am Acad Dermatol* 29, 490 (passim)
(1990): Fradin MS+, *J Am Acad Dermatol* 23, 1265
(1988): Frosch PJ+, *Hautarzt* (German) 39, 611
(1988): Penmetcha M+, *Int J Dermatol* 27, 53
(1987): Keown PA+, *Hospital Practice* 22, 207
(1987): Wysocki GP+, *Clin Exp Dermatol* 12, 191
(1986): Bencini PL+, *Br J Dermatol* 114, 396
(1986): Kahan BD+, *World J Surg* 10, 348
(1984): Harper JL+, *Br J Dermatol* 110, 469
Hair – perifolliculitis barbae
(2002): Moderer M+, *World Congress Dermatol* Poster, 0117
Hair – pseudofolliculitis barbae
(1997): Lear J+, *Br J Dermatol* 136, 132

## Nails

Nails – abnormal growth
(1986): Gratwohl A+, *Prog Allergy* 38, 404
Nails – brittle (<2%)
Nails – disorder (sic)
(1994): Wakelin SH+, *Br J Dermatol* 131, 147
Nails – ingrown
(1993): Olujohungbe A+, *Lancet* 342, 1111
Nails – leukonychia
(1986): Bencini PL+, *Dermatologica* 172, 24
Nails – periungual granulation tissue
(1995): Higgins EM+, *Br J Dermatol* 132, 829

## Other

Acromegaloid features
(1987): Reznik VM, *Lancet* 1, 1405
Anaphylactoid reactions (<1%)
(2001): Ebo DG+, *Ann Allergy Asthma Immunol* 87(3), 243
(2001): Riegert-Johnson DL+, *Bone Marrow Transplant* 28(12), 1176
(2001): Takamatsu Y+, *Bone Marrow Transplant* 28(4), 421
(1989): Gupta AK+, *J Am Acad Dermatol* 21, 1245
(1985): Chapuis B+, *N Engl J Med* 312, 1259
(1985): Leunissen KML+, *Lancet* 1, 636
(1985): Ptachcinski RJ+, *Lancet* 1, 636
Angiosarcoma (fatal)
(2001): Schulze R+, *Internist* 42, 119
Aphthous stomatitis
(2001): Reitamo S+, *Br J Dermatol* 145(3), 438 (9%) (with sirolimus)
(1986): Bencini PL+, *Dermatologica* 172, 24
Breast lumps (sic)
(1980): Rolles K+, *Lancet* 2, 795
Dysesthesia
(2000): Capper N, Mobile, AL (from Internet) (observation)
(1990): Gupta AK+, *J Am Acad Dermatol* 22, 242
Fibroadenoma
(2001): Muttarak M+, *Australas Radiol* 45(4), 517
(2001): Weinstein SP+, *Radiology* 220(2), 465
Gingival bleeding
Gingival hyperplasia (>10%)
(2002): Keglevich T+, *Fogorv Sz* 95(1), 15
(2001): Brennan MT+, *Oral Surg Oral Med Oral Pathol Oral Radiol Endod* 92(5), 503
(2001): Buduneli N+, *Acta Odontol Scand* 59(6), 367
(2001): Bustos DA+, *J Periodontol* 72(6), 741
(2001): Irshied J+, *J Clin Pediatr Dent* 26(1), 93
(2001): Oettinger-Barak O+, *J Periodontol* 72(9), 1236
(2001): Thomas DW+, *J Clin Periodontol* 28(7), 706
(2001): Uzel MI+, *J Periodontol* 72(7), 921
(2001): Vallejo C+, *Haematologica* 86(1), 110
(2001): Werth V, *Dermatology Times* 15
(2001): Wondimu B+, *Int J Paediatr Dent* 11(6), 424
(2000): Czech W+, *J Am Acad Dermatol* 42, 653
(2000): Hernandez G+, *J Periodontol* 71(10), 1630
(2000): Kirby B+, *Clin Exp Dermatol* 25, 97
(2000): Oettinger-Barak O+, *J Periodontol* 71, 650
(2000): Thomas DW+, *Transplantation* 69, 522
(1999): Spratt H+, *Oral Dis* 5, 27
(1999): Wirnsberger GH+, *Transplantation* 67, 1289

(1998): Cebeci I+, *J Periodontol* 69, 1435
(1998): Desai P+, *J Can Dent Assoc* 64, 263
(1998): Jucgla A+, *Br J Dermatol* 138, 198
(1998): Kohnle M+, *Transplant Proc* 30, 2122
(1998): Mattson JS+, *J Am Dent Assoc* 129, 78
(1998): Nash MM+, *Transplantation* 65, 1611
(1998): Nohl F+, *Ther Umsch* (German) 55, 573
(1998): Nowicki M+, *Ann Transplant* 3, 25
(1998): Pilloni A+, *J Periodontol* 69, 791
(1998): Varga E+, *J Clin Periodontol* 25, 225
(1998): Wirnsberger GH+, *Transplant Proc* 30, 2117
(1997): Avci O+, *J Am Acad Dermatol* 36, 796
(1997): Brehler R+, *J Am Acad Dermatol* 36, 983 (passim)
(1997): Cecchin E+, *Ann Intern Med* 126, 409
(1997): Dodd DA, *J Heart Lung Transplant* 16, 579
(1997): Ellis CN, *Int J Dermatol* 36 (Supplement), 7 (passim)
(1997): Gómez E+, *Nephrol Dial Transplant* 12, 2694
(1997): Hall EE, *Curr Opin Peridontology* 4, 59 (passim)
(1997): Iacopino AM+, *J Periodontol* 68, 73
(1997): Jackson C+, *N Y State Dent J* 63, 46
(1997): Puig JM+, *Transplant Proc* 29, 2379
(1997): Silverstein LH+, *Gen Dent* 45, 371
(1996): Ashrafi SH+, *Scanning Microsc* 10, 219
(1996): Boran M+, *Transplant Proc* 28, 2316
(1996): Cebeci I+, *J Periodontol* 67, 1201
(1996): Darbar UR+, *J Clin Periodontol* 23, 941
(1996): Montebugnoli L+, *J Clin Periodontol* 23, 868
(1996): Somacarrera ML+, *Spec Care Dent* 16, 18
(1995): Moghadam BKH+, *Cutis* 56, 46 (passim)
(1995): Wahlstrom E+, *N Engl J Med* 332, 753
(1994): Wong W+, *Lancet* 343, 986
(1993): King GN+, *J Clin Periodontol* 20, 286
(1993): Seymour RA, *Adverse Drug React Toxicol Rev* 12, 215
(1993): Seymour RA+, *J R Coll Surg Edinb* 38, 328
(1993): Thomason JM+, *J Clin Periodontol* 20, 37
(1993): Valicenti JMK+, *Arch Dermatol* 129, 794 (passim)
(1992): Humphreys TR+, *J Am Acad Dermatol* 29, 490 (passim)
(1992): Mastrolonardo M+, *Dermatol Clin* (Italian) 4, 246
(1992): Seymour RA+, *J Clin Periodontol* 19, 1
(1991): Puelacher W+, *Z Stomatol* (German) 88, 7
(1990): Cooper KD, *Dermatology* 1(2), 3
(1989): Ross PJ+, *J Dent Child* 56, 56
(1988): Frosch PJ+, *Hautarzt* (German) 39, 611
(1988): Veraldi S+, *Int J Dermatol* 27, 730
(1987): Keown PA+, *Hospital Practice* 22, 207
(1987): Reznik VM, *Lancet* 1, 1405
(1986): Kahan BD+, *World J Surg* 10, 348

Gingivitis (4%)

Glossitis (atrophic)
(1986): Bencini PL+, *Dermatologica* 172, 24

Gynecomastia (>3%)
(1998): Kollias J+, *Aust N Z J Surg* 68, 679
(1994): Jacobs U+, *Transplant Proc* 26, 3122
(1987): Beris P+, *Schweiz Med Wochenschr* (German) 117, 1751

Hyperesthesia
(1987): Keown PA+, *Hospital Practice* 22, 207

Hypersensitivity
(2001): Sumpton JE+, *Transplant Proc* 33(6), 3015

Lingual fungiform papillae hypertrophy (sic)
(1996): Silverberg NB+, *Lancet* 348, 967

Lymphoproliferative disease
(1989): Walker RJ+, *Aust N Z J Med* 19, 154
(1988): Brown MD+, *Arch Dermatol* 124, 1097

Myalgia
(2001): Kappers-Klunne MC+, *Br J Haematol* 114(1), 121
(1988): Brown MD+, *Arch Dermatol* 124, 1097 (passim)

Myopathy
(1990): Fernandez-Sola J+, *Lancet* 335, 362
(1989): Chassagne P+, *Lancet* 2, 1104

Oral ulceration
(1986): Bencini PL+, *Dermatologica* 172, 24

Paresthesias (>8%)
(2001): Capper RN, Mobile, AL (from Internet) (observation) (tingling lips & fingers)
(2001): Laws RA, Providence, RI (from Internet) (observation) (hands & feet)
(2001): Thaler D, Monona, WI (from Internet) (observation) (numb lips)
(2000): Baumgaertnet J, LaCrosse, WI (from Internet) (3 observations)
(2000): Lepine EM, Rock Hill, SC (from Internet) (observation)
(2000): Thaler D, Monona, WI (from internet) (observation)
(1997): Berthe-Jones J+, *Br J Dermatol* 136, 76
(1997): Ellis CN, *Int J Dermatol* 36 (Supplement), 7 (passim)
(1997): Shupack J+, *J Am Acad Dermatol* 36, 423
(1992): Goodman MM+, *J Am Acad Dermatol* 27, 594
(1990): Cooper KD, *Dermatology* 1(2), 3
(1988): Bennett WM+, *Ann Rev Med* 37, 215 (passim)
(1987): Dougados M+, *Arthritis Rheum* 30, 83

Parkinsonism
(2002): Kim HC+, *Nephrol Dial Transplant* 17(2), 319

Pseudolymphoma
(1988): Thestrup-Pedersen K+, *Dermatologica* 177, 376

Rhabdomyolysis
(1999): Maltz HC+, *Ann Pharmacother* 33(11), 1176 (with atorvastatin)
(1995): Meier C+, *Schweiz Med Wochenschr* 125(27), 1342 (with simvastatin)
(1992): Blaison G+, *Rev Med Interne* 13(1), 61 (with simvastatin)
(1988): Tobert JA, *Am J Cardiol* 62, 28J (with lovastatin)

Shivering (sic)
(2000): Lepine EM, Rock Hill, SC (from Internet) (observation)

Stomatitis (7%)

Tinnitus

Tremors (>10%)

Tumors
(2001): Werth V, *Dermatology Times* 15

# CYCLOTHIAZIDE

**Trade name:** Anhydron (Lilly)
**Other common trade names:** *Doburil; Valmiran*
**Indications:** Edema, hypertension
**Category:** Thiazide* diuretic
**Half-life:** no data
**Clinically important, potentially hazardous interactions with:** digoxin

### *Reactions*

---

## Skin

Exanthems (<1%)
Photosensitivity
Purpura
Rash (sic)
Urticaria
Vasculitis

## Other

Paresthesias

***Note:** Cyclothiazide is a sulfonamide and can be absorbed systemically. Sulfonamides can produce severe, possibly fatal, reactions such as toxic epidermal necrolysis and Stevens–Johnson syndrome

## CYPROHEPTADINE

**Trade name:** Periactin (Merck)
**Other common trade names:** *Ciplactin; Ciproral; Nuran; Periactine; Periactinol; Peritol; Sigloton*
**Indications:** Allergic rhinitis, urticaria
**Category:** $H_1$-receptor antihistamine and appetite stimulant
**Half-life:** 1–4 hours
**Clinically important, potentially hazardous interactions with:** anticholenergic, MAO inhibitors, phenelzine, tranylcypromine

### *Reactions*

#### Skin
Allergic reactions (sic) (<1%)
Angioedema (<1%)
Contact dermatitis
(1995): Li LF+, *Contact Dermatitis* 33, 50
Dermatitis (sic)
Diaphoresis
Edema (<1%)
Erythema
Exanthems
(1964): Gould AH+, *Med Clin North Am* 48, 411
Flushing
Lichenoid eruption
(1971): Baer RL+, in Fitzpatrick, *Dermatology in General Medicine*, McGraw-Hill 1281
Lupus erythematosus
Peripheral edema
Photosensitivity
(1971): Kalivas J, *JAMA* 216, 526
Purpura
Rash (sic) (<1%)
Urticaria
Vasculitis
(1984): Ekenstam E+, *Arch Dermatol* 120, 484

#### Other
Anaphylactoid reactions
Dysgeusia
(1997): Neufeld-Kaiser W+, *Arch Dermatol* 133, 251
Myalgia (<1%)
Paresthesias (<1%)
Tinnitus
Xerostomia (1–10%)
(1990): Kardinal CG+, *Cancer* 65, 2657
(1990): Pontius EB, *J Clin Psychopharmacol* 8, 230

## CYTARABINE

**Synonyms:** arabinosylcytosine; ara-C
**Trade names:** Cytosar-U (Pharmacia & Upjohn); Tarabine (Pharmacia & Upjohn)
**Other common trade names:** *Alexan; Arabitin; Arace; Aracytine; Cytarbel; Cytosar; Uducil*
**Indications:** Leukemias
**Category:** Antineoplastic; antimetabolite
**Half-life:** initial: 10–15 minutes
**Clinically important, potentially hazardous interactions with:** aldesleukin

### *Reactions*

#### Skin
Acral erythema
(2001): Takeuchi M+, *Rinsho Ketsueki* 42(3), 216
(1999): Azurdia RM+, *Clin Exp Dermatol* 24, 64
(1998): Calista D+, *J Eur Acad Dermatol Venereol* 10, 274
(1997): Arranz FR+, *Arch Dermatol* 133, 499
(1997): Demircay Z+, *Int J Dermatol* 36, 593
(1995): Dechaufour F+, *Ann Dermatol Venereol* (French) 120, 219
(1992): Doll DC+, *Semin Oncol* 19(5), 580
(1992): Rongioletti F+, *J Am Acad Dermatol* 26, 284
(1991): Brown J+, *J Am Acad Dermatol* 24, 1023
(1991): Rongioletti F+, *J Cutan Pathol* 18, 453
(1989): Alexander J, *Oncol Nurs Forum* 16, 829
(1989): Kroll SS+, *Ann Plast Surg* 23, 263
(1989): Oksenhendler E+, *Eur J Cancer Clin Oncol* 25, 1181
Acral erythrodysesthesia syndrome (hand–foot syndrome)
(1993): Waltzer JF+, *Arch Dermatol* 129, 43 (bullous variety)
(1991): Baack BR+, *J Am Acad Dermatol* 24, 457
(1989): Kampmann KK+, *Cancer* 63, 2482 (bullous variety)
(1988): Shall L+, *Br J Dermatol* 119, 249
(1986): Crider MK+, *Arch Dermatol* 122, 1023 (>5%)
(1985): Baer MR+, *Ann Intern Med* 102, 556 (bullous variety)
(1985): Cardonnier C+, *Ann Intern Med* 97, 783
(1985): Levine LE+, *Arch Dermatol* 121, 102
(1985): Peters WG+, *Ann Intern Med* 103, 805 (bullous variety)
(1985): Walker IR+, *Arch Dermatol* 121(10), 1240 (10–67%) (dose-related)
(1983): Herzig RH+, *Blood* 62, 361 (1–5%)
(1982): Burgdorf WHC+, *Ann Intern Med* 97, 61
Actinic keratoses (with pruritus and erythema)
(1989): Kerker BJ+, *Semin Dermatol* 8, 173
Acute febrile neutrophilic dermatosis (Sweet's syndrome)
(1993): Torri O+, *Ann Dermatol Venereol* (French) 120, 884
Allergic edema (sic)
Bullous eruption
(1992): Richards C+, *Oncol Nurs Forum* 19, 1191
Desquamation
(1992): Richards C+, *Oncol Nurs Forum* 19, 1191
Erythema
(1998): Taverna C+, *Schweiz Med Wochenschr* (German) 128, 1117
(1992): Richards C+, *Oncol Nurs Forum* 19, 1191
Erythema and swelling of ears
(1990): Krulder JWM+, *Eur J Cancer* 26, 649
Erythroderma (generalized)
(1988): Benson PM+, *J Assoc Military Derm* XIV, 28 (passim)
Exanthems
(1988): Benson PM+, *J Assoc Military Derm* XIV, 28
(1986): Morant R+, *Schweiz Med Wochenschr* (German) 116, 1415 (60%)
(1983): Herzig RH+, *Blood* 62, 361 (1–5%)

(1983): Shah SS+, *Cancer Treat Rep* 67, 405*
Exfoliative dermatitis
(1989): Williams SF+, *Br J Haematol* 73, 274
Freckles (1–10%)
Herpes zoster
(1973): Stevens DA+, *N Engl J Med* 289, 873
Neutrophilic eccrine hidradenitis
(1997): Jegasothy SM+, Pittsburgh, American Academy of Dermatology Meeting (SF) (gross and microscopic)
(1995): Kanzaki H+, *J Dermatol* 22, 137
(1993): Thorisdottir K+, *J Am Acad Dermatol* 28, 775
(1992): Bernstein EF+, *Br J Dermatol* 127, 529 (recurrent)
(1991): Vion B+, *Dermatologica* 183, 70
(1990): Hurt MA+, *Arch Dermatol* 126, 73
(1989): Bailey DL+, *Pediatr Dermatol* 6, 33
(1989): Kerker BJ+, *Semin Dermatol* 8, 173
(1987): Katsanis E+, *Am J Pediatr Hematol Oncol* 9, 204
(1984): Flynn TC+, *J Am Acad Dermatol* 11, 584
Petechiae
(1998): Taverna C+, *Schweiz Med Wochenschr* (German) 128, 1117
Pruritus (1–10%)
Rash (sic) (>10%)
Seborrheic keratoses (inflammation of) (Leser–Trélat syndrome)
(1999): Williams JV+, *J Am Acad Dermatol* 40, 643
(1979): Kechijian P+, *Ann Intern Med* 91, 868
Syringosquamous metaplasia (sic)
(1990): Bhawan J+, *Am J Dermatopathol* 12, 1
Toxic epidermal necrolysis
(2001): Özkan A+, *Pediatr Dermatol* 18(1), 38
(1998): Figueiredo MS+, *Rev Assoc Med Bras* (Portuguese) 44, 53
Ulceration
(1969): Bodey GP+, *Cancer Chemother Rep* 53, 59
Urticaria
Vasculitis*
(1998): Ahmed I+, *Mayo Clin Proc* 73, 239
(1989): Kerker BJ+, *Semin Dermatol* 8, 173
(1989): Williams SF+, *Br J Haematol* 73, 274

## Hair

Hair – alopecia (1–10%)
(1988): Benson PM+, *J Assoc Military Derm* XIV, 28 (passim)
(1986): Morant R+, *Schweiz Med Wochenschr* (German) 116, 1415 (100%)
(1970): Upjohn Company, *Clin Pharmacol Ther* 11, 155
(1969): Bodey GP+, *Cancer Chemother Rep* 53, 59

## Nails

Nails – Mees' lines
(1982): Jeanmougin M+, *Ann Dermatol Venereol* (French) 109, 169
Nails – transverse leukonychia
(1990): Bader-Meunier B+, *Ann Pediatr Paris* (French) 37, 337

## Other

Anal ulceration (>10%)
Anaphylactoid reactions
(1997): Blanca M+, *Allergy* 52, 1009
(1989): Williams SF+, *Br J Haematol* 73, 274
(1980): Rassiga AL+, *Arch Intern Med* 104, 425
Hypersensitivity
(1992): Weiss RB, *Semin Oncol* 19, 458
Injection-site cellulitis (1–10%)
Myalgia (1–10%)
Oral mucosal lesions
(1986): Morant R+, *Schweiz Med Wochenschr* (German) 116, 1415 (1–5%)
(1978): Levine N+, *Cancer Treat Rev* 5, 67
(1974): Levantine A+, *Br J Dermatol* 90, 239 (66%)
(1971): Lang HN+, *Med J Aust* 2, 187
(1968): Howard JP+, *Cancer* 21, 341
Oral ulceration (>10%)
Pseudotumor cerebri
(1999): Fort JA+, *Ann Pharmacother* 33, 576
Stomatitis
(1988): Benson PM+, *J Assoc Military Derm* XIV, 28 (passim)
Thrombophlebitis (>10%)

***Note:** Vasculitis, a part of the cytarabine syndrome, consists of fever, malaise, myalgia, conjunctivitis, arthralgia and a diffuse erythematous maculopapular eruption that occurs from 6 to 12 hours following the administration of the drug

## DACARBAZINE

**Synonym:** DIC
**Trade name:** DTIC-Dome (Bayer)
**Other common trade names:** *D.T.I.C; Dacatic; Deticene; Detimedac*
**Indications:** Malignant melanoma, carcinomas
**Category:** Antineoplastic
**Half-life:** initial: 20–40 minutes
**Clinically important, potentially hazardous interactions with:** aldesleukin

### *Reactions*

#### Skin

Actinic keratosis inflammation
(1987): Johnson TM+, *J Am Acad Dermatol* 17(2 Pt 1), 192
Angioedema
(1981): Wassilew SW+, *Hautarzt* (German) 32 (Suppl 5), 453
Erythema
Exanthems
(1981): Wassilew SW+, *Hautarzt* (German) 32 (Suppl 5), 453
Fixed eruption
(1982): Koehn GG+, *Arch Dermatol* 118, 1018
Flushing (1–10%)
(1982): Dunagin WG, *Semin Oncol* 9, 14
(1978): Levine N+, *Cancer Treat Rev* 5, 67 (100%)
Photosensitivity (<1%)
(1989): Serrano G+, *Photodermatol* 6, 140
(1982): Koehn GG+, *Arch Dermatol* 118, 1018
(1981): Bonifazi E+, *Contact Dermatitis* 7, 161
(1981): Wassilew SW+, *Hautarzt* (German) 32 (Suppl 5), 453
(1981): Yung CW+, *J Am Acad Dermatol* 4, 541
(1980): Beck TM+, *Cancer Treat Rep* 64, 725
(1980): Bolling R+, *Hautarzt* (German) 31, 602
(1980): Ippen H, *Dtsch Med Wochenschr* (German) 105, 531
(1980): Kunze J+, *Z Hautkr* (German) 55, 100
Rash (sic) (1–10%)
Urticaria
(1995): Bourry C+, *Therapie* (French) 50, 588
(1981): Wassilew SW+, *Hautarzt* (German) 32 (Suppl 5), 453
Vasculitis

#### Hair

Hair – alopecia (1–10%)
(1978): Levine N+, *Cancer Treat Rev* 5, 67

#### Nails

Nails – pigmentation
(1984): Daniel CR+, *J Am Acad Dermatol* 10, 250

#### Other

Anaphylactoid reactions (1–10%)
Death
(2001): Ramanathan RK+, *Ann Oncol* 12(8), 1139
Depression
(2001): Ramanathan RK+, *Ann Oncol* 12(8), 1139
Dysgeusia (1–10%) (metallic taste)
Hypersensitivity
(1992): Weiss RB, *Semin Oncol* 19, 458
Injection-site burning (>10%)
Injection-site cellulitis
(1989): Kerker BJ+, *Semin Dermatol* 8, 173
Injection-site dermatitis
(1987): Dufresne RG, *Cutis* 39, 197
Injection-site necrosis (>10%)
(1987): Dufresne RG, *Cutis* 39, 197
Injection-site pain (>10%)
Injection-site phlebitis
(1989): Kerker BJ+, *Semin Dermatol* 8, 173
Myalgia (1–10%)
Paresthesias (facial)
Rhabdomyolysis
(1995): Anderlini P+, *Cancer* 76(4), 678
Stomatitis (<1%)

## DACTINOMYCIN

**Synonyms:** ACT; actinomycin D
**Trade name:** Cosmegen (Merck)
**Other common trade names:** *Ac-De; Cosmegen Lyovac; Lyovac*
**Indications:** Melanonas, sarcomas
**Category:** Antineoplastic antibiotic
**Half-life:** 36 hours
**Clinically important, potentially hazardous interactions with:** aldesleukin

### *Reactions*

#### Skin

Acne (>10%)
(1993): Blatt J+, *Med Pediatr Oncol* 21, 373
(1983): Bronner AK+, *J Am Acad Dermatol* 9, 645
(1982): Dunagin WG, *Semin Oncol* 9, 14
(1974): Levantine A+, *Br J Dermatol* 90, 239 (>5%)
(1969): Epstein EH+, *N Engl J Med* 281, 1094
Actinic keratosis inflammation
(1987): Johnson TM+, *J Am Acad Dermatol* 17(2 Pt 1), 192
Bullous pemphigoid
(1982): Amer MH+, *Int J Dermatol* 21, 32
Cellulitis
(1989): Kerker BJ+, *Semin Dermatol* 8, 173
Cheilitis
Dermatitis (sic)
(1975): Cassady JR+, *Radiology* 115, 171
Erythema
Erythema, brawny localized
(1997): Coppes MJ+, *Med Pediatr Oncol* 29, 226
Erythema multiforme
Exanthems
Folliculitis
(1981): Henkes J+, *Actas Dermosifiliogr* (Spanish) 72, 469
(1969): Epstein EH+, *N Engl J Med* 281, 1094
Keratoses (reactivation of)
(1989): Kerker BJ+, *Semin Dermatol* 8, 173
Pigmentation
(1995): Kanwar VS+, *Med Pediatr Oncol* 24, 329
(1978): Levine N+, *Cancer Treat Rev* 5, 67 (100%)
(1971): Ma HK+, *J Obstet Gynaecol Br Commonw* 78, 166
Pruritus
(1989): Kerker BJ+, *Semin Dermatol* 8, 173
Pustular eruption
(1983): Bronner AK+, *J Am Acad Dermatol* 9, 645
(1969): Epstein EH+, *N Engl J Med* 281, 1094
Radiation recall (>10%)
(1997): Coppes MJ+, *Med Pediatr Oncol* 29, 226
(1978): Levine N+, *Cancer Treat Rev* 5, 67 (50%)
(1975): Dreizen S+, *Postgrad Med* 58, 150
(1974): Levantine A+, *Br J Dermatol* 90, 239 (>5%)
Serpentine supravenous hyperpigmentation (sic)
(2000): Marcoux D+, *J Am Acad Dermatol* 43, 540 (with vincristine)

Toxic epidermal necrolysis
Urticaria

### Hair

Hair – alopecia (>10%)
(1964): Falkson G+, *Br J Dermatol* 76, 309

### Other

Anaphylactoid reactions (<1%)
Injection-site extravasation (>10%)
(1997): Coppes MJ+, *Med Pediatr Oncol* 29, 226
Injection-site necrosis (>10%)
(1987): Dufresne RG, *Cutis* 39, 197
Injection-site phlebitis (>10%)
Myalgia
Oral mucosal lesions
(1983): Bronner AK+, *J Am Acad Dermatol* 9, 645 (>5%)
(1975): Dreizen S+, *Postgrad Med* 58, 150
(1972): Cridland MD, *Drugs* 3, 352
Phlebitis
(1989): Kerker BJ+, *Semin Dermatol* 8, 173
Stomatitis (ulcerative) (>5%)

## DALTEPARIN

**Trade name:** Fragmin (Pharmacia & Upjohn)
**Other common trade name:** *Fragmine*
**Indications:** Prophylaxis of deep vein thrombosis
**Category:** Anticoagulant; low molecular weight heparin
**Half-life:** 4–8 hours
**Clinically important, potentially hazardous interactions with:** butabarbital, danaparoid

#### *Reactions*

### Skin

Allergic reactions (sic) (1–10%)
Bullous eruption (1–10%)
(1999): Tong, M, Kota Kinabalu, Malaysia (from Internet) (observation)
Exanthems (<1%)
Pruritus (1–10%)
Rash (sic) (1–10%)

### Hair

Hair – alopecia
(2001): Apsner R+, *Blood* 97(9), 2914–5
(2000): Barnes C, *Blood* 96, 1618

### Other

Anaphylactoid reactions (1–10%)
Injection-site edema
(2000): Szolar-Platzer C+, *J Am Acad Dermatol* 43, 920
Injection-site hematoma (1–10%)
Injection-site pain (1–10%)
Injection-site pruritus
(2000): Szolar-Platzer C+, *J Am Acad Dermatol* 43, 920
Necrosis

## DAN-SHEN

**Scientific names:** *Gansu danshen; Salvia miltiorrhiza (red sage); Southern danshen*
**Other common names:** Chinese Red Sage; Huang Ken; Red Rooted Sage; Red Sage; Salvia Root; Tzu Tan-Ken
**Family:** Labiatae; Lamiaceae
**Purported indications:** Circulation problems, ischemic stroke, angina pectoris, cardiovascular disease
**Other uses:** menstrual problems, chronic hepatitis, abdominal masses, insomnia, acne, psoriasis, eczema, bruising

#### *Reactions*

### Skin

Pruritus

## DANAPAROID

**Trade name:** Orgaran (Organon)
**Indications:** Prevention of postoperative deep thrombosis
**Category:** Anticoagulant
**Half-life:** ~24 hours
**Clinically important, potentially hazardous interactions with:** butabarbital, dalteparin, enoxaparin, heparin

#### *Reactions*

### Skin

Allergic reactions (sic) (<1%)
(2000): de Saint-Blanquat L+, *Ann Fr Anesth Reanim* 19, 751
Edema (2.6%)
Infections (sic) (2.1%)
Peripheral edema (3.3%)
Pruritus (3.9%)
Purpura
Rash (sic) (2.1–4.8%)
(1999): Wutschert R+, *Drug Saf* 20, 515

### Other

Injection-site hematoma (5%)
Injection-site infiltrated plaques
(2000): Koch P+, *J Am Acad Dermatol* 42, 612
(2000): Martin L+, *Contact Dermatitis* 42, 295
(2000): Szolar-Platzer C+, *J Am Acad Dermatol* 43, 920
Injection-site pain (7.6–13.7%)
Injection-site reactions
(2001): Figarella I+, *Ann Dermatol Venereol* 128, 35
Paresthesias

# DANAZOL

**Trade name:** Danocrine (Sanofi)
**Other common trade names:** *Azol; Bonzol; Cyclomen; D-Zol; Danol; Ladogal; Winobanin; Zoldan-A*
**Indications:** Endometriosis, fibrocystic breast disease
**Category:** Synthetic pituitary gonadotropin inhibitor
**Half-life:** ~4.5 hours
**Clinically important, potentially hazardous interactions with:** acitretin, cyclosporine, oral contraceptives, tacrolimus, warfarin

### *Reactions*

## Skin

Acne (>10%)
(1982): Madanes AE+, *Ann Intern Med* 96, 625 (20%)
(1980): Hosea SW+, *Ann Intern Med* 93, 809 (8%)
(1979): Greenberg RD, *Cutis* 24, 431
(1977): Spooner JB+, *J Int Med Res* 5 (Suppl 3), 15
Angioedema
(1993): Litt JZ, Beachwood, OH (personal case) (observation)
(1988): Guillet G+, *Dermatologica* 177, 370
Diaphoresis (3%)
(1977): Spooner JB+, *J Int Med Res* 5 (Suppl 3), 15
Edema (>10%)
(1977): Spooner JB+, *J Int Med Res* 5 (Suppl 3), 15
Erythema multiforme
(1992): Reynolds NJ+, *Clin Exp Dermatol* 17, 140
(1988): Gately LE+, *Ann Intern Med* 109, 85
Exanthems
(1993): Litt JZ, Beachwood, OH (personal case) (observation)
(1989): Ahn YS+, *Ann Intern Med* 111, 723 (6%)
(1982): Madanes AE+, *Ann Intern Med* 96, 625
(1975): 13, 94
Flushing
(1988): Henzl MR+, *N Engl J Med* 318, 485 (68%)
(1980): Hosea SW+, *Ann Intern Med* 93, 809 (12%)
(1977): Spooner JB+, *J Int Med Res* 5 (Suppl 3), 15
(1975): 13, 94
Guillain–Barré syndrome
(1985): Hory B+, *Am J Med* 79, 111
Lupus erythematosus
(1991): Sassolas B+, *Br J Dermatol* 125, 190
(1988): Guillet G+, *Dermatologica* 177, 370
(1982): Fretwell MD, *Allergy Clin Immunol* 69, 306
Lymphomatoid papulosis
(1985): Wise C+, *Fertil Steril* 44, 702
Petechiae
Photosensitivity (<1%)
Pruritus
(1989): Ahn YS+, *Ann Intern Med* 111, 723 (3.5%)
Purpura
(1990): Taillan B+, *Presse Med* (French) 19, 721
Rash (sic) (3%)
(1977): Spooner JB+, *J Int Med Res* 5 (Suppl 3), 15
Seborrhea
(1989): Ahn YS+, *Ann Intern Med* 111, 723
(1982): Madanes AE+, *Ann Intern Med* 96, 625 (30%)
(1981): Duff P+, *Am J Obstet Gynecol* 141, 349 (passim)
(1977): Spooner JB+, *J Int Med Res* 5 (Suppl 3), 15
Stevens–Johnson syndrome
Urticaria

## Hair

Hair – alopecia
(1989): Ahn YS+, *Ann Intern Med* 111, 723 (3.5%)
(1981): Duff P+, *Am J Obstet Gynecol* 141, 349
(1980): Hosea SW+, *Ann Intern Med* 93, 809 (17%)
Hair – hirsutism (<10%)
(1991): Bates GW+, *Clin Obstet Gynecol* 34, 848
(1989): Ahn YS+, *Ann Intern Med* 111, 723 (3.5%)
(1982): Madanes AE+, *Ann Intern Med* 96, 625 (7%)
(1980): Hosea SW+, *Ann Intern Med* 93, 809 (8%)

## Other

Acute intermittent porphyria
Bleeding gums
Breast changes (sic)
(1977): Spooner JB+, *J Int Med Res* 5 (Suppl 3), 15
Candidal vaginitis (<1%)
(1977): Spooner JB+, *J Int Med Res* 5 (Suppl 3), 15
Death
(2001): Hayashi T+, *J Gastroenterol* 36(11), 783
Gingivitis
Paresthesias
Rhabdomyolysis
(1994): Dallaire M+, *CMAJ* 150(12), 1991 (with lovastatin)
Vaginal dryness (sic)

# DANTROLENE

**Trade name:** Dantrium (Procter & Gamble)
**Other common trade names:** *Dantamacrin; Dantrolen*
**Indications:** Spasticity, malignant hyperthermia
**Category:** Skeletal muscle relaxant
**Half-life:** 8.7 hours
**Clinically important, potentially hazardous interactions with:** verapamil

### *Reactions*

## Skin

Acne
(1981): Pembroke AC+, *Br J Dermatol* 104, 465
(1980): Dykes MHM, *JAMA* 231, 862
Chills (1–10%)
Dermatitis (sic)
Diaphoresis
Erythema
Exanthems
(1980): Dykes MHM, *JAMA* 231, 862
Photosensitivity
Pruritus
Rash (sic) (>10%)
Urticaria

## Hair

Hair – abnormal growth

## Other

Anaphylactoid reactions
Dysgeusia
Malignant lymphoma
(1980): Wan HH+, *Postgrad Med J* 56, 261
Myalgia
Thrombophlebitis
Tremors

# DAPSONE

**Trade name:** Dapsone (Jacobus)
**Other common trade names:** *Avlosulfon; Dapson; Dapson-Fatol; Protogen; Sulfona*
**Indications:** Leprosy, dermatitis herpetiformis
**Category:** Antileprotic; dermatitis herpetiformis suppressant
**Half-life:** 10–50 hours
**Clinically important, potentially hazardous interactions with:** chloroquine, didanosine, furazolidone, ganiciclovir, hydroxychloroquine, methotrexate, pyrimethamine, rifabutin, rifampin, sulfonamides

## *Reactions*

### Skin

Bullous eruption (<1%)
(1984): Alarcon GS+, *Arthritis Rheum* 27, 1071
Cyanosis
(1981): Editorial, *Lancet* 2, 184
Dapsone syndrome*
(1998): Kumar RH+, *Indian J Lepr* 70, 271 (17 cases)
(1997): McKenna KE+, *Br J Dermatol* 137, 657
(1994): Barnard GF+, *Am J Gastroenterol* 89, 2057
(1994): Hiran S+, *J Assoc Physicians India* 42, 497
(1994): Risse L+, *Ann Dermatol Venereol* (French) 121, 242
(1994): Saito S+, *Clin Exp Dermatol* 19, 152
(1994): Stephen G+, *J Assoc Physicians India* 42, 72
(1992): Kraus A+, *J Rheumatol* 19, 178
(1991): Ramanan C+, *Indian J Lepr* 63, 226
(1988): Grayson ML+, *Lancet* 1, 531
(1987): Khare AK+, *Indian J Lepr* 59, 106
(1985): Sharma VK+, *Indian J Lepr* 57, 807
(1982): Kromann NP+, *Arch Dermatol* 118, 531
(1981): Tomecki KJ+, *Arch Dermatol* 117, 38
Epidermolysis bullosa
(1992): Kong LN, *Chung Hua Li Tsa Chih* (Chinese) 27, 495
Erythema multiforme (<1%)
(2001): Werth V, *Dermatology Times* 15
(1994): Pertel P+, *Clin Infect Dis* 18, 630
(1993): Stern RS, *Arch Dermatol* 129, 301 (passim)
(1981): Frey HM+, *Ann Intern Med* 94, 777
(1980): Dutta RK, *Lepr India* 52, 306
(1970): Millikan LE+, *Arch Dermatol* 102, 220
(1961): Browne SG+, *BMJ* 1, 550 (passim)
Erythema nodosum
(1993): Stern RS, *Arch Dermatol* 129, 301 (passim)
(1981): Editorial, *Lancet* 2, 184
(1970): Millikan LE+, *Arch Dermatol* 102, 220
Erythroderma
(1989): Patki AH+, *Lepr Rev* 60, 274
Exanthems (1–5%)
(2002): Thong BY+, *Ann Allergy Asthma Immunol* 88(5), 527 (with pyrimethamine)
(2001): Werth V, *Dermatology Times* 15
(1993): Stern RS, *Arch Dermatol* 129, 301 (passim)
(1986): Lindskov R+, *Dermatologica* 172, 214 (6%)
(1981): Frey HM+, *Ann Intern Med* 94, 777
(1981): Tomecki KJ+, *Arch Dermatol* 117, 38
(1970): Millikan LE+, *Arch Dermatol* 102, 220
(1968): Ramanujam K+, *Lepr India* 40, 6
(1965): Rosenthal AL+, *Arch Intern Med* 115, 73 (1–5%)
(1964): Browne SG, *BMJ* 2, 1041
(1963): Browne SG, *BMJ* 2, 664 (2%)
Exfoliative dermatitis (<1%)
(1993): Stern RS, *Arch Dermatol* 129, 301 (passim)
(1981): Frey HM+, *Ann Intern Med* 94, 777
(1981): Tomecki KJ+, *Arch Dermatol* 117, 38
(1980): Lal S+, *Lepr India* 52, 302
(1971): Browne SG, *BMJ* 2, 558 (passim)
(1970): Millikan LE+, *Arch Dermatol* 102, 220
(1963): Browne SG, *BMJ* 2, 664
(1961): Browne SG+, *BMJ* 1, 550 (passim)
Fixed eruption
(1988): Tham SN+, *Singapore Med J* 29, 300
(1982): Sinha MR, *Lepr India* 54, 152
(1964): Browne SG, *BMJ* 2, 1041 (1–5%)
Flu-like syndrome
(2001): Werth V, *Dermatology Times* 15
Lichenoid eruption
Lupus erythematosus (<1%)
(1992): Kraus A+, *J Rheumatol* 19, 178
(1984): Alarcon GS+, *Arthritis Rheum* 27, 1071 (bullous)
(1979): Fine RM, *Int J Dermatol* 18, 811
(1979): Lang PG, *J Am Acad Dermatol* 1, 479
(1974): Vandersteen PR+, *Arch Dermatol* 110, 95
Photosensitivity (<1%)
(2001): Stockel S+, *Eur J Dermatol* 11(1), 50
(1994): Berger TG+, *Arch Dermatol* 130, 609 (in HIV-infected) (4 cases)
(1989): Dhanapaul S, *Lepr Rev* 60, 147
(1988): Fumey SM+, *Z Hautkr* (German) 63, 53
(1987): Joseph MS, *Lepr Rev* 58, 425
(1979): Lang PG, *J Am Acad Dermatol* 1, 479
Pigmentation
(1997): David KP+, *Trans R Soc Trop Med Hyg* 91, 204 ("hyperpigmented dermal macules")
(1977): Sakurai I+, *Int J Lepr Other Mycobact Dis* 45, 343
(1976): Shelley WB+, *Br J Dermatol* 95, 79 (bluish-gray)
(1964): Browne SG, *BMJ* 2, 1041
(1963): Browne SG, *BMJ* 2, 664
(1961): Browne SG+, *BMJ* 1, 550
Pruritus
(1964): Browne SG, *BMJ* 2, 1041
Purpura
(1968): Ramanujam K+, *Lepr India* 40, 6
Rash (sic)
(2000): Chogle A+, *Indian J Gastroenterol* 19, 85
(1996): Beumont MG+, *Am J Med* 100, 611
Scleroderma
(1990): May DG+, *Clin Pharm Ther* 48, 286
Stevens–Johnson syndrome
(1994): Pertel P+, *Clin Infect Dis* 18, 630
(1961): Browne SG+, *BMJ* 1, 550 (passim)
Subcorneal pustular dermatosis
(1983): Halevy S+, *Acta Derm Venereol* (Stockh) 63, 441
Toxic epidermal necrolysis (<1%)
(1993): Fitzpatrick TB+, *Dermatologic Capsule and Comment* 15, 10 (observation)
(1993): Stern RS, *Arch Dermatol* 129, 301 (passim)
(1988): Phillips-Howard PA+, *Br Med J Clin Res Ed* 296, 1605
(1983): Katoch K+, *Lepr India* 55, 133
(1981): Editorial, *Lancet* 2, 184
(1961): Browne SG+, *BMJ* 1, 550
Toxic erythema (sic)
(1993): Stern RS, *Arch Dermatol* 129, 301 (passim)
Urticaria
(1970): Millikan LE+, *Arch Dermatol* 102, 220

### Nails

Nails – Beau's lines (transverse nail bands)
(1989): Patki AH+, *Lepr Rev* 60, 274
(1988): Grayson ML+, *Lancet* 1, 531
(1984): Daniel CR+, *J Am Acad Dermatol* 10, 250

### Other

Acute intermittent porphyria
Hypersensitivity*
(2002): Thong BY+, *Ann Allergy Asthma Immunol* 88(5), 527 (with pyrimethamine)
(2001): Rao PN+, *Lepr Rev* (72(1) (57)
(2001): Werth V, *Dermatology Times* 15
(2000): Chogle A+, *Indian J Gastroenterol* 19, 85
(1998): Pei-Lin Ng P+, *J Am Acad Dermatol* 39, 646
(1998): Schlienger RG+, *Epilepsia* 39, S3 (passim)
(1998): Siegfried EC+, *J Am Acad Dermatol* 39, 797 (passim)
(1996): Prussick R+, *J Am Acad Dermatol* 35, 346
(1995): Bocquet H+, *Ann Dermatol Venereol* (French) 122, 514
(1984): Mohamed KN, *Lepr Rev* 55, 385
Nodular panniculitis
(1986): Uplekar MW+, *Indian J Lepr* 58, 286
Oral mucosal eruption
(1981): Frey HM+, *Ann Intern Med* 94, 777
Oral mucosal fixed eruption
Oral mucosal pigmentation
(1964): Browne SG, *BMJ* 2, 1041
Porphyria cutanea tarda
(1992): Shelley WB+, *Advanced Dermatologic Diagnosis* WB Saunders, 414 (passim)
Tinnitus

***Note:** A hypersensitivity reaction – termed the "sulfone syndrome" or "dapsone syndrome" – may infrequently develop during the first six weeks of treatment. This syndrome consists of exfoliative dermatitis, fever, malaise, nausea, anorexia, hepatitis, jaundice, lymphadenopathy and hemolytic anemia. See (1982): Kromann NP+, *Arch Dermatol* 118, 531

## DAUNORUBICIN

**Synonyms:** daunomycin; DNR; rubidomycin
**Trade names:** Cerubidine (Bedford); DaunoXome (Nexstar)
**Other common trade name:** *Daunoxome*
**Indications:** Acute leukemias
**Category:** Antineoplastic
**Half-life:** 14–20 hours
**Clinically important, potentially hazardous interactions with:** aldesleukin

#### *Reactions*

### Skin

Angioedema
(1983): Bronner AK+, *J Am Acad Dermatol* 9, 645
(1981): Weiss RB+, *Ann Intern Med* 94, 66 (1–5%)
(1978): Levine N+, *Cancer Treat Rev* 5, 67
(1970): Freeman AI, *Cancer Chemother Rep* 54, 475
Chills (<1%)
Contact dermatitis
(1986): Eddy JL+, *Oncol Nurs Forum* 13, 9
(1975): Reich SD+, *Cancer Chemother Rep* 59, 677
Erythema
Exanthems
(1978): Levine N+, *Cancer Treat Rev* 5, 67 (2%)
(1970): Zanoni G+, *Blut* (German) 25, 20
Flushing
Folliculitis
(1997): Fournier S+, *Arch Dermatol* 133, 918 (disseminated)
Hypopigmentation
(1975): Dreizen S+, *Postgrad Med* 58, 150
Neutrophilic eccrine hidradenitis
(1993): Thorisdottir K+, *J Am Acad Dermatol* 28, 775
Pigmentation
(2002): Kroumpouzos G+, *J Am Acad Dermatol* 46(2), S1 (generalized)
(1992): Anderson LL+, *J Am Acad Dermatol* 26, 255
(1984): Kelly TM+, *Arch Dermatol* 120, 262
Pruritus
Rash (sic) (<1%)
Urticaria (<1%)
(1983): Bronner AK+, *J Am Acad Dermatol* 9, 645
(1981): Weiss RB+, *Ann Intern Med* 94, 66 (1–5%)
(1970): Freeman AI, *Cancer Chemother Rep* 54, 475

### Hair

Hair – alopecia (>10%)
(1997): Fournier S+, *Arch Dermatol* 133, 918
(1972): Cridland MD, *Drugs* 3, 352
(1972): Jacquillat C+, *BMJ* 4, 468
(1969): Bonadonna G+, *BMJ* 3, 503

### Nails

Nails – pigmentation (<1%)
(1983): James WD+, *Arch Dermatol* 119, 334
(1982): Daniel CR+, *Cutis* 30, 348
(1979): Hanada T+, *Nippon Naika Gakkai Zasshi* (Japanese) 68, 1319 (bands)
(1978): de Marinis M+, *Ann Intern Med* 89, 516

### Other

Anaphylactoid reactions
Death
(2002): Fassas A+, *Br J Haematol* 116(2), 308
Infusion-site extravasation
(2000): Kassner E, *J Pediatr Oncon Nurs* 17, 135
Injection-site cellulitis
(1989): Kerker BJ+, *Semin Dermatol* 8, 173
Injection-site necrosis (1–10%)
(1987): Dufresne RG, *Cutis* 39, 197
(1979): Dragon LH+, *Ann Intern Med* 91, 58
Injection-site phlebitis
(1989): Kerker BJ+, *Semin Dermatol* 8, 173
Injection-site ulceration (1–10%)
(1984): Cox RF, *Am J Hosp Pharm* 41, 2410
Mucositis
(2002): Fassas A+, *Br J Haematol* 116(2), 308
Oral mucosal lesions
(1983): Bronner AK+, *J Am Acad Dermatol* 9, 645 (>5%)
(1975): Dreizen S+, *Postgrad Med* 58, 75
Stomatitis (>10%)
(1969): Bonadonna G+, *BMJ* 3, 503

## DEFEROXAMINE

**Trade name:** Desferal (Novartis)
**Other common trade name:** *Desferin*
**Indications:** Hemochromatosis, acute iron overload
**Category:** Chelating agent; antidote
**Half-life:** 6.1 hours
**Clinically important, potentially hazardous interactions with:** ascorbic acid

#### *Reactions*

### Skin

Acne
Angioedema
(1984): Romeo MA+, *J Inherited Metab Dis* 7, 121

Depigmentation
(2001): Lopez L+, *Dermatol Surg* 27(9), 795
Dermatitis (sic)
(1988): Venencie PY+, *Ann Dermatol Venereol* (French) 115, 1174
Edema (<1%)
Erythema (<1%)
Erythema multiforme
Exanthems
Flushing (<1%)
Pigmentation
Pruritus (<1%)
(1984): Romeo MA+, *J Inherited Metab Dis* 7, 121
Purpura
Rash (sic) (<1%)
Toxic epidermal necrolysis
Urticaria (<1%)

### Other

Anaphylactoid reactions (<1%)
Arthralgia
(2001): Taher A+, *Eur J Haematol* 67(1), 30
Injection-site erythema
Injection-site inflammation (1–10%)
Injection-site pain (1–10%)
Oral mucosal lesions
Tinnitus

## DELAVIRDINE

**Synonym:** U-90152S
**Trade name:** Rescriptor (Pharmacia & Upjohn)
**Indications:** HIV-1 infection
**Category:** Antiretroviral; non-nucleoside reverse transcriptase inhibitor
**Half-life:** 5.8 hours
**Clinically important, potentially hazardous interactions with:** alprazolam, anisindione, anticoagulants, dicumarol, dihydroergotamine, ergot, indinavir, methysergide, midazolam, phenytoin, quinidine, rifampin, triazolam, warfarin

***Reactions***

### Skin

Allergic reactions (sic) (<2%)
Angioedema (<2%)
Dermatitis (sic) (<2%)
Desquamation (<2%)
Diaphoresis (<2%)
Ecchymoses (<2%)
Edema of the lip (<2%)
Epidermal cyst (<2%)
Erythema (<2%)
Erythema multiforme (<2%)
Exanthems (6.6%)
Folliculitis (<2%)
Fungal dermatitis (sic) (<2%)
Nodule (sic) (<2%)
Peripheral edema (<2%)
Petechiae (<2%)
Pruritus (<2%)
Purpura (<2%)
Rash (sic) (9.8%)
Seborrhea (<2%)
Stevens–Johnson syndrome (<2%)
Urticaria (<2%)
Vasculitis (<2%)
Vesiculobullous eruption (<2%)
Xerosis (<2%)

### Hair

Hair – alopecia (<2%)

### Nails

Nails – disorder (sic) (<2%)

### Other

Aphthous stomatitis (<2%)
Dysgeusia (<2%)
Gingivitis (<2%)
Gynecomastia (<2%)
Hyperesthesia (<2%)
Hypesthesia (<2%)
Myalgia (<2%)
Oral ulceration (<2%)
Paresthesias (<2%)
Rhabdomyolysis
(2002): Castro JG+, *Am J Med* 112(6), 505 (with atorvastatin)
Sialorrhea (<2%)
Stomatitis (<2%)
Tingling (<2%)
Tongue edema (<2%)
Vaginal candidiasis (<2%)
Xerostomia (<2%)

## DEMECLOCYCLINE

**Trade name:** Declomycin (Lederle)
**Other common trade names:** *Ledermicina; Ledermycin; Rynabron*
**Indications:** Various infections caused by susceptible organisms
**Category:** Tetracycline antibiotic and antiprotozoal
**Half-life:** 10–17 hours
**Clinically important, potentially hazardous interactions with:** amoxicillin, ampicillin, antacids, bacampicillin, calcium carbonate, carbenicillin, cloxacillin, digoxin, methotrexate, methoxyflurane, mezlocillin, nafcillin, oxacillin, penicillins, piperacillin, ticarcillin

***Reactions***

### Skin

Acne
(1969): Weary PE+, *Arch Dermatol* 100, 179
Angioedema
Bullous eruption
Candidiasis
Exanthems
Exfoliative dermatitis (<1%)
Fixed eruption
(1978): Jolly HW+, *Arch Dermatol* 114, 1484
(1970): Delaney TJ, *Br J Dermatol* 83, 357
(1970): Savin JA, *Br J Dermatol* 83, 546
(1968): Sarkany I, *Proc R Soc Med* 61, 891
Lichenoid eruption
(1972): Jones HE+, *Arch Dermatol* 106, 58
Lupus erythematosus
Perianal rash

Photosensitivity (1–10%)
(1984): Kromann N+, *Ugeskr Laeger* (Danish) 146, 515
(1980): Stern RS+, *Arch Dermatol* 116, 1269
(1974): Maibach HI+, *Arch Dermatol* 109, 97 (1.5%) (lichenoid)
(1972): Jones HE+, *Arch Dermatol* 106, 58 (lichenoid)
(1971): Frost P+, *JAMA* 216, 326 (90%)
(1971): Ippen H, *Hautarzt* (German) 22, 549
(1971): Kahn G+, *Arch Dermatol* 103, 94
(1968): Stratigos JD+, *Br J Dermatol* 80, 391
(1967): Kotani Y, *Acta Dermatol Kyoto Engl Ed* (Japanese) 62, 188
(1965): Clendenning WE, *Arch Dermatol* 91, 628 (20%)
(1962): de Veber LL, *Can Med Assoc J* 86, 168
(1962): Hicks JH, *South Med J* 55, 357
(1961): Orentreich N+, *Arch Dermatol* 83, 68
(1961): Shapiro JL+, *JAMA* 176, 596
(1960): Carey BW, *JAMA* 172, 1196 (1.5%)
(1960): Falk MS, *JAMA* 172, 1156
(1960): Fuhrman DL+, *Arch Dermatol* 82, 244
(1960): Morris WE, *JAMA* 172, 1155
Phototoxicity
(1968): Blank H+, *Arch Dermatol* 97, 1 (90%)
(1961): Cahn MM+, *Arch Dermatol* 84, 485
(1961): Saslaw S, *N Engl J Med* 264, 1301
Pigmentation
Pruritus (<1%)
Pruritus ani
Purpura
Stevens–Johnson syndrome
Toxic epidermal necrolysis
(1988): Massullo RE+, *J Am Acad Dermatol* 19, 358
Urticaria

### Nails
Nails – onycholysis
Nails – photo-onycholysis
(1977): Bethell HJN, *BMJ* 2, 96
(1974): Bettley FR+, *Proc R Soc Med* 67, 600
(1973): Verma KC+, *Indian J Dermatol* 18, 23
(1972): Cabre J+, *Actas Dermosifiliogr* (Spanish) 63, 211
(1962): de Veber LL, *Can Med Assoc J* 86, 168
(1961): Orentreich N+, *Arch Dermatol* 83, 68
Nails – pigmentation (<1%)

### Other
Anaphylactoid reactions (<1%)
Glossitis
Mucous membrane pigmentation
Oral mucosal eruption
(1964): Martin WJ, *Med Clin North Am* 48, 255
Paresthesias (<1%)
Porphyria
(1979): Boissonnas A+, *Nouv Presse Med* (French) 8, 210
Pseudotumor cerebri
Tongue pigmentation
Tooth discoloration

## DENILEUKIN

**Trade name:** Ontak (Ligand)
**Indications:** Cutaneous T-cell lymphoma
**Category:** Antineoplastic
**Half-life:** distribution: 2–5 minutes; terminal: 70–80 minutes

#### *Reactions*

### Skin
Allergic reactions (sic) (1%)
Bullous eruption
Chills (81%)
Diaphoresis (10%)
Ecchymoses
Edema (47%)
Exanthems
Flushing
Infections (sic) (48%)
Petechiae
Pruritus (20%)
Purpura
Rash (sic) (34%)
Urticaria
Vesicular eruptions

### Other
Anaphylactoid reactions (1%)
Hypersensitivity (69%)
Infusion-site reactions (sic) (8%)
Myalgia (18%)
Paresthesias (13%)
Phlebitis
Thrombophlebitis

## DESIPRAMINE

**Trade name:** Norpramin (Aventis)
**Other common trade names:** *Deprexan; Nebril; Nortimil; Pertofran; Pertofrane; Petylyl; PMS-Desipramine*
**Indications:** Depression
**Category:** Tricyclic antidepressant and antipanic
**Half-life:** 7–60 hours
**Clinically important, potentially hazardous interactions with:** amprenavir, arbutamine, clonidine, epinephrine, fluoxetine, formoterol, guanethidine, isocarboxazid, linezolid, MAO inhibitors, phenelzine, quinolones, sparfloxacin, tranylcypromine

#### *Reactions*

### Skin
Acne
Allergic reactions (sic) (<1%)
(1987): Joffe RT+, *Can J Psychiatry* 32, 695
(1987): Richter MA+, *Am J Psychiatry* 144, 526
Angioedema
(1963): Mann AM+, *Can Med Assoc J* 88, 1102
Diaphoresis (1–10%)
(1965): Editorial, *JAMA* 194, 82
Ecchymoses
(1968): Rachmilewitz EA+, *Blood* 32, 524
Edema
Erythema

Exanthems
(1988): Biederman J+, *J Clin Psychiatry* 49, 178 (5.8%)
(1988): McLean JD, *Can J Psychiatry* 33, 331
(1987): Ellsworth A+, *Drug Intell Clin Pharm* 21, 510
(1987): Joffe RT+, *Can J Psychiatry* 32, 695 (6.2%)
(1968): Powell WJ+, *JAMA* 206, 642
Exfoliative dermatitis
(1968): Powell WJ+, *JAMA* 206, 642
Flushing
(1965): Editorial, *JAMA* 194, 82
Petechiae
(1968): Rachmilewitz EA+, *Blood* 32, 524
Photosensitivity (1.4%)
(1965): Editorial, *JAMA* 194, 82
Pigmentation (blue-gray) (photosensitive)
(1993): Narurkar V+, *Arch Dermatol* 129, 474
(1993): Steele TE+, *J Clin Psychopharmacol* 13, 76
Pruritus
(1988): Biederman J+, *J Clin Psychiatry* 49, 178
(1987): Ellsworth A+, *Drug Intell Clin Pharm* 21, 510
(1987): Pohl R+, *Am J Psychiatry* 144, 237
(1968): Powell WJ+, *JAMA* 206, 642
Purpura
(1980): Miescher PA+, *Clin Haematol* 9, 505
(1968): Rachmilewitz EA+, *Blood* 32, 524
Rash (sic)
(1965): Editorial, *JAMA* 194, 82
Urticaria
(1991): Bajwa WK+, *J Nerv Ment Dis* 179, 108
(1988): Biederman J+, *J Clin Psychiatry* 49, 178
(1987): Pohl R+, *Am J Psychiatry* 144, 237
Vasculitis
Xerosis

### Hair
Hair – alopecia (<1%)
(1991): Warnock JK+, *J Nerv Ment Dis* 179, 441

### Other
Black tongue
Bromhidrosis
Dysgeusia (>10%)
Galactorrhea (<1%)
Gynecomastia (<1%)
Hypersensitivity
Mucous membrane desquamation
(1968): Powell WJ+, *JAMA* 206, 642
Paresthesias
Pseudolymphoma
(1995): Magro CM+, *J Am Acad Dermatol* 32, 419
Stomatitis
Tinnitus
Xerostomia (>10%)
(1993): Pataki CS+, *J Am Acad Child Adolesc Psychiatry* 32, 1065
(1965): Editorial, *JAMA* 194, 82

## DESLORATADINE

**Trade name:** Clarinex (Schering)
**Indications:** Allergic rhinitis, urticaria
**Category:** Antihistamine
**Half-life:** 27 hours

#### *Reactions*

### Skin
None

### Other
Anaphylactoid reactions
Hypersensitivity
Myalgia
Xerostomia

## DESMOPRESSIN

**Trade names:** DDAVP (Aventis); Stimate (Centeon)
**Other common trade names:** *Defirin; Desmospray; Minirin; Minurin; Octostim*
**Indications:** Primary nocturnal enuresis
**Category:** Antidiuretic; antihemophilic; antihemorrhagic; posterior pituitary hormone
**Half-life:** 75 minutes

#### *Reactions*

### Skin
Allergic reactions (sic)
(1982): Yokota M+, *Endocrinol Jpn* 29, 475
Diaphoresis
(1985): Richardson DW+, *Ann Intern Med* 103, 228
Edema
Flushing (1–10%)
(1985): Richardson DW+, *Ann Intern Med* 103, 228 (1–5%)
Rash (sic)

### Other
Injection-site edema
Injection-site erythema
Injection-site pain (1–10%)

## DEXCHLORPHENIRAMINE

**Trade names:** Dexchlor; Poladex; Polaramine (Schering)
**Other common trade names:** *Delamin; Polaramin; Polaronil; Polazit; Trenolone*
**Indications:** Allergic rhinitis, urticaria
**Category:** Antihistamine; $H_1$-blocker
**Half-life:** 20–24 hours
**Clinically important, potentially hazardous interactions with:** barbiturates, chloral hydrate, ethchlorvynol, glutethimide, phenothiazines, zolpidem

#### *Reactions*

### Skin
Angioedema (<1%)
Chills

Contact dermatitis
(1989): Cusano F+, *Contact Dermatitis* 21, 340
Diaphoresis
Edema (<1%)
Photosensitivity (<1%)
Rash (sic) (<1%)
Urticaria

### Other

Anaphylactoid reactions
Myalgia (<1%)
Paresthesias (<1%)
Xerostomia (1–10%)

## DEXMEDETOMIDINE

**Trade name:** Precedex (Abbott)
**Indications:** Sedation for intensive care unit intubation
**Category:** Alpha-adrenergic agonist; sedative
**Half-life:** 2 hours

### *Reactions*

### Skin

Diaphoresis (<1%)
Infections (sic) (2%)
Pain (3%)
Photopsia (<1%)
Xerosis

### Other

Sialopenia
(1990): Aantaa RE+, *Anesth Analg* 70, 407

## DEXTROAMPHETAMINE

**Trade names:** Adderall (Shire Richwood); Dexedrine (GSK)
**Other common trade names:** *Dexamphetamine; Dexamphetamini; Dextrostat; Ferndex; Oxydess*
**Indications:** Narcolepsy, attention deficit disorder (ADD)
**Category:** Central nervous system stimulant; amphetamine
**Half-life:** 10–12 hours
**Clinically important, potentially hazardous interactions with:** fluoxetine, fluvoxamine, MAO inhibitors, paroxetine, phenelzine, sertraline, tranylcypromine

### *Reactions*

### Skin

Chills
Diaphoresis (1–10%)
Rash (sic) (<1%)
Toxic epidermal necrolysis
(1975): Giallorenzi AF+, *Oral Surg Oral Med Oral Pathol* 40, 611
Urticaria (<1%)

### Other

Dysgeusia
Rhabdomyolysis
(2000): Richards JR, *J Emerg Med* 19(1), 51
(1999): Hedetoft C+, *Ugeskr Laeger* 161(50), 6907
(1998): Robertsen A+, *Tidsskr Nor Laegeforen* 118(28), 4340
(1996): Hofland E+, *Ned Tijdschr Geneeskd* 140(12), 681
(1996): Roebroek RM+, *Ned Tijdschr Geneeskd* 140(29), 1519
(1996): Roebroek RM+, *Ned Tijdschr Geneeskd* 140(4), 205
(1996): Sultana SR+, *J R Coll Surg Edinb* 41(6), 419
(1992): Kao CH+, *Clin Nucl Med* 17(2), 101
(1990): Yamazaki F+, *Nippon Naika Gakkai* 79(1), 100
(1977): Kendrick WC+, *Ann Intern Med* 86(4), 381 (5 cases)
Xerostomia (1–10%)

## DEXTROMETHORPHAN

**Trade names:** Benylin; Cheracol-D; Drixoral; Pertussin; Robitussin; Sucrets; Suppress; Trocal; Vicks Formula 44
**Other common trade names:** *Balminil; Delsym; Koffex; Triaminic DM*
**Indications:** Nonproductive cough
**Category:** Antitussive (nonnarcotic)
**Half-life:** no data
**Clinically important, potentially hazardous interactions with:** linezolid, phenelzine, sibutramine, tranylcypromine, valdecoxib

### *Reactions*

### Skin

Bullous eruption
(1999): Sahn EE, *Dermatology Times* April, 5 (infant with urticaria pigmentosa)
(1996): Cook J+, *Pediatr Dermatol* 13, 410 (infant with urticaria pigmentosa)
Fixed eruption
(1991): Smoller BR+, *J Cutan Pathol* 18, 13
(1990): Stubb S+, *Arch Dermatol* 126, 970

### Other

Anaphylactoid reactions
(1998): Knowles SR+, *J Allergy Clin Immunol* 102, 316

## DIACETYLMORPHINE

(See HEROIN)

## DIAZEPAM

**Trade names:** Diastat (Elan); Dizac; Valium (Roche)
**Other common trade names:** *Assival; Dialar; Diapax; Diazemuls; Ducene; E-Pam; Meval; Novazam; Solis; Vivol*
**Indications:** Anxiety
**Category:** Benzodiazepine anxiolytic and sedative-hypnotic; anticonvulsant
**Half-life:** 20–70 hours
**Clinically important, potentially hazardous interactions with: alcohol**, amprenavir, barbiturates, chlorpheniramine, clarithromycin, CNS depressants, efavirenz, esomeprazole, fluroquinolone antibiotics, imatinib, indinavir, ivermectin, macrolide antibiotics, MAO inhibitors, methadone, narcotics, nelfinavir, phenothiazines, ritonavir, SSRIs

### *Reactions*

### Skin

Acne
(1962): Grayson LD, *Gen Pract* 25, 9

Allergic reactions (sic)
(1982): Allin DM, *Curr Med Res Opin* 8, 33
(1977): Padfield A+, *BMJ* 1, 575
Angioedema
(1974): Felix RH+, *Lancet* 1, 1017
Bullous eruption
(1977): Varma AJ+, *Arch Intern Med* 137, 1207
Contact dermatitis
(1995): Fisher AA, *Cutis* 55, 327 (systemic)
(1995): Kampgen E+, *Contact Dermatitis* 33, 356
(1994): Garcia-Bravo B+, *Contact Dermatitis* 30, 40
Dermatitis (sic) (1–10%)
Diaphoresis (>10%)
Eczematous eruption (sic)
(1974): Felix RH+, *Lancet* 1, 1017
Exanthems
(1986): Bigby M+, *JAMA* 256, 3358 (0.04%)
(1981): Adverse Drug Reaction List, *Jpn Med Gaz* (Japanese) 18:6–7, 16
(1976): Arndt KA+, *JAMA* 235, 918 (0.38%)
(1967): Jenner FA+, *Dis Nerv Syst* 28, 245
(1964): Holt KS, *Ann Physiol Med* (Suppl) 16
(1963): Love J, *Dis Nerv Syst* 24, 674
Exfoliative dermatitis
(1967): Satyadas JS+, *J Indian Med Assoc* 3, 49
(1963): Love J, *Dis Nerv Syst* 24, 674
Fixed eruption (<1%)
(1979): Olumide F, *Int J Dermatol* 18, 818
(1966): Jadassohn W+, *Dermatologica* 133, 91
Flushing
(1964): Holt KS, *Ann Physiol Med* (Suppl) 16
Granuloma disciformis (Miescher)
(1969): Clarke DM, *Australas J Dermatol* 10, 194
Melanoma
(1981): Adam S+, *Lancet* 2, 1344
Pellagra
(1982): Stadler R+, *Hautarzt* (German) 33, 276
Pigmentation
(1980): Ferreira JA, *Aesthetic Plast Surg* 4, 343
Pruritus
(1995): Kampgen E+, *Contact Dermatitis* 33, 356
Purpura
(1985): Ambriz-Fernandez R+, *Rev Invest Clin* (Spanish) 37, 347
(1980): Miescher PA+, *Clin Haematol* 9, 505
(1977): Cimo PL+, *Am J Hematol* 2, 65
(1977): Ghosh JS, *BMJ* 1, 902
Rash (sic) (>10%)
(1983): O'Brien JE+, *Curr Ther Res* 34, 825
Urticaria
(1987): Deardon DJ+, *Br J Anaesth* 59, 391
Vasculitis
(1999): Olcina GM+, *Am J Psychiatry* 156, 972

### Nails

Nails – parrot-beak nails
(1971): Kandil E, *J Med Liban* 24, 433

### Other

Anaphylactoid reactions
(1987): Deardon DJ+, *Br J Anaesth* 59, 391
Gynecomastia
(2000): Hugues FC+, *Ann Med Interne (Paris)* (French) 151, 10 (passim)
(1994): Llop R+, *Ann Pharmacother* 28, 671
(1979): Moerck HJ+, *Lancet* 1, 1344 (letter)
Injection-site phlebitis (>10%)
(1981): Clarke RSJ, *Drugs* 22, 26 (39%)
(1980): Schou-Olesen A+, *Br J Anaesth* 52, 609
Paresthesias
Porphyria
(1979): Stone DR+, *Br J Anaesth* 51, 809
(1978): Mees DE+, *South Med J* 68, 29
Porphyria variegata
Rhabdomyolysis
(1982): Bogaerts Y+, *Clin Nephrol* 17(4), 206
Sialorrhea
Tongue, coated
Xerostomia (>10%)

# DIAZOXIDE

**Trade name:** Hyperstat (Schering)
**Other common trade names:** *Eudimine; Proglicem; Proglycem; Sefulken*
**Indications:** Hypoglycemia, hypertension
**Category:** Antihypoglycemic; antihypertensive
**Half-life:** 20–36 hours
**Clinically important, potentially hazardous interactions with:** phenytoin

## *Reactions*

### Skin

Candidiasis
Cellulitis (<1%)
Diaphoresis
Edema
Exanthems
Flushing (<1%)
Herpes (sic)
Leukomelanoderma (sic)
(1967): Saito T+, *Acta Dermatol* (Kyoto) 61, 207
Lichenoid eruption
(1975): Burton JL+, *Br J Dermatol* 93, 707
(1973): Menter MA, *Proc R Soc Med* 66, 326
Photosensitivity
(1967): Saito T+, *Acta Dermatol* (Kyoto) 61, 207
Pruritus
Purpura
Rash (sic) (<1%)
Urticaria
Xerosis
(1975): Burton JL+, *Br J Dermatol* 93, 707

### Hair

Hair – alopecia
(1975): Burton JL+, *Br J Dermatol* 93, 707
(1972): Milner RD+, *Arch Dis Child* 47, 537
Hair – hypertrichosis (<1%)
(1989): Rousseau C+, *Dermatologica* 179, 221
(1988): Prigent F+, *Ann Dermatol Venereol* (French) 115, 191
(1987): Turpin G+, *Presse Med* (French) 16, 398
(1983): Schiazza L+, *G Ital Dermatol Venereol* (Italian) 118, 113
(1981): Perez-Mijares R+, *Rev Clin Esp* (Spanish) 162, 225
(1975): Burton JL+, *Br J Dermatol* 93, 707 (>5%)
(1973): Menter MA, *Proc R Soc Med* 66, 326
(1972): Leng JJ+, *Pediatr Clin North Am* 19, 681
(1972): Milner RD+, *Arch Dis Child* 47, 537
(1968): Koblenzer PJ+, *Ann N Y Acad Sci* 150, 373

### Other

Ageusia
Dysgeusia
Hypersensitivity

Injection-site pain (<1%)
Injection-site phlebitis (<1%)
Paresthesias
Sialorrhea
Tinnitus
Xerostomia

# DICLOFENAC

**Trade names:** Arthrotec (Pharmacia); Solaraze Gel (Bioglan); Voltaren (Novartis)
**Other common trade names:** *Allvoran; Apo-Diclo; Fenac; Galedol; Liroken; Monoflam; Nu-Diclo; Remethan; Taks; Voltarene; Voltarol*
**Indications:** Rheumatoid and osteoarthritis
**Category:** Nonsteroidal anti-inflammatory (NSAID)
**Half-life:** 1–2 hours
**Clinically important, potentially hazardous interactions with:** methotrexate

Arthrotec is diclofenac and misoprostol

### *Reactions*

## Skin

Allergic reactions (sic)
(1992): Schiavino D+, *Contact Dermatitis* 26, 357
(1979): Ciucci AG, *Rheum Rehab* 18 (Suppl 2), 116
Angioedema (1–3%)
(2000): Hadar A+, *Harefuah* (Hebrew) 138, 211 (from suppository)
Bullous eruption (1–3%)
(1982): Valsecchi R+, *G Ital Derm Venereol* (Italian) 117, 221
(1981): Gabrielsen TO+, *Acta Derm Venereol* (Stockh) 61, 439
Contact dermatitis
(1998): Ueda K+, *Contact Dermatitis* 39, 323
(1996): Gonzalo MA+, *Dermatology* 193, 59
(1996): Valsecchi R+, *Contact Dermatitis* 34, 150
(1994): Gebhardt M+, *Contact Dermatitis* 30, 183
(1994): Romano A+, *Allergy* 49, 57
Dermatitis (sic) (1–3%)
Dermatitis herpetiformis
(1989): Grob JJ+, *Dermatologica* 178, 58
(1981): Gabrielsen TO+, *Acta Derm Venereol* (Stockh) 61, 439
Dermatomyositis
(1989): Grob JJ+, *Dermatologica* 178, 58
Diaphoresis (<1%)
Eczema (sic) (1–3%)
Edema
Erythema (sic)
(1998): Schaad HJ+, *Ther Umsch* (German) 55, 586 (generalized)
(1992): Barrett PJ+, *Anaesthesia* 47, 83
(1979): Ciucci AG, *Rheum Rehab* 18 (Suppl 2), 116
Erythema multiforme (<1%)
(1999): Emmett SD, Solana Beach, CA (from internet) (observation)
(1996): Delrio FG+, *Am J Med Sci* 312(2), 95
(1995): Dhar S+, *Dermatology* 191, 76
(1993): Khalil H+, *Arch Intern Med* 153, 1649
(1988): Todd PA+, *Drugs* 35, 244
(1985): Morris BAP+, *Can Med Assoc J* 133, 665
(1982): Seigneuric C+, *Ann Dermatol Venereol* (French) 109, 287
Erythema nodosum (<1%)
Exanthems (1–5%)
(1994): Romano A+, *Allergy* 49, 57
(1992): Breathnach SM+, *Adverse Drug Reactions and the Skin* Blackwell, Oxford, 188 (passim)
(1988): Todd PA+, *Drugs* 35, 244
(1986): Halevy S+, *Harefuah* (Hebrew) 110, 30
(1985): Morris BAP+, *Can Med Assoc J* 133, 665
(1979): Ciucci AG, *Rheum Rehab* 18 (Suppl 2), 116
Exfoliative dermatitis (<1%)
Fixed eruption
(1998): Mahboob A+, *Int J Dermatol* 37, 833
Flushing (<1%)
Lichenoid eruption
(1999): Fetterman M, Miami, FL (from Internet) (observation)
Linear IgA bullous dermatosis
(2002): Cohen LM+, *J Am Acad Dermatol* 46, S32 (passim)
(1997): Paul C+, *Br J Dermatol* 136, 406
(1982): Valsecchi R+, *G Ital Derm Venereol* (Italian) 117, 221
(1981): Gabrielsen TO+, *Acta Derm Venereol* (Stockh) 61, 439
Lupus erythematosus
Pemphigus
(1997): Matz H+, *Dermatology* 195, 48
Peripheral edema
Photosensitivity (1–3%)
(1998): Encinas S+, *Chem Res Toxicol* 11, 946
(1997): O'Reilly FM+, American Academy of Dermatology Meeting, Poster #14
(1996): Becker L+, *Acta Derm Venereol* (Stockh) 76, 337
(1992): Le Corre Y+, *Ann Dermatol Venereol* (French) 119, 923 (granuloma annulare type)
(1988): Todd PA+, *Drugs* 35, 244
Pruritus (1–10%)
(1995): Litt JZ, Beachwood, OH (personal case) (observation)
(1994): Litt JZ, Beachwood, OH (personal case) (observation)
(1992): Breathnach SM+, *Adverse Drug Reactions and the Skin* Blackwell, Oxford, 188 (passim)
(1988): Todd PA+, *Drugs* 35, 244
(1981): Gabrielsen TO+, *Acta Derm Venereol* (Stockh) 61, 439
(1979): Ciucci AG, *Rheum Rehab* 18 (Suppl 2), 116
Pseudoreactions (sic)
(1991): VanArsdel PP, *JAMA* 266, 3343
Psoriasis
(1999): Dintiman B, Fairfax, VA (from Internet) (observation)
(1999): Fetterman M, Miami, FL (from Internet) (observation)
(1987): Sendagorta E+, *Dermatologica* 175, 300 (pustular)
Purpura (1–3%)
(1988): Todd PA+, *Drugs* 35, 244
(1979): Ciucci AG, *Rheum Rehab* 18 (Suppl 2), 116
Pustular psoriasis
(1999): Dintiman B, Fairfax, VA (from Internet) (observation)
(1999): Fetterman M, Miami, FL (from Internet) (observation)
(1987): Sendagorta E+, *Dermatologica* 175, 300
Rash (sic) (>10%)
(1978): Abrams GJ+, *S Afr Med J* 53, 442
Skin reactions (sic)
(1986): Catalano MA, *Am J Med* 80, 81
Stevens–Johnson syndrome (1–3%) (1 fatal case)
(1988): Todd PA+, *Drugs* 35, 244
(1979): Ciucci AG, *Rheum Rehab* 18 (Suppl 2), 116
Still's disease
(1985): Wouters JM+, *J Rheumatol* 12, 791
Toxic epidermal necrolysis
(1998): Choi KL, Toronto, Canada (from Internet) (observation)
(1993): Correia O+, *Dermatology* 186, 32
(1985): Kamanabroo D+, *Arch Dermatol* 121, 1548
Toxic shock
(1998): Schaad HJ+, *Ther Umsch* (German) 55, 586
Urticaria (1–3%)
(1998): Gala G+, *Allergy* 53, 623
(1995): Litt JZ, Beachwood, OH (personal case) (observation)

(1995): Rademaker M, *N Z Med J* 108, 165
(1992): Breathnach SM+, *Adverse Drug Reactions and the Skin* Blackwell, Oxford, 188 (passim)
(1988): Todd PA+, *Drugs* 35, 244
(1979): Ciucci AG, *Rheum Rehab* 18 (Suppl 2), 116

Vasculitis
(1999): Emmet S, Solana Beach, CA (from Internet) (from ophthalmic solution) (observation)
(1997): Morros R+, *Br J Rheumatol* 36, 503
(1992): Breathnach SM+, *Adverse Drug Reactions and the Skin* Blackwell, Oxford, 188 (passim)
(1982): Bonafe JL+, *Ann Dermatol Venereol* (French) 109, 283

## Hair

Hair – alopecia (1–3%)

## Other

Acute intermittent porphyria
Anaphylactoid reactions (1–3%)
(2000): Hadar A+, *Harefuah* (Hebrew) 138, 211 (from suppository)
(2000): Ray M+, *Indian Pediatr* 36, 1067 (fatal)
(1999): Enrique E+, *Allergy* 54, 529
(1996): Levy JH+, *N Engl J Med* 335, 1925
(1993): Alkhawajah AM+, *Forensic Sci Int* 60, 107
(1993): van der Klauw MM+, *Br J Clin Pharmacol* 35, 400
(1992): *Australian Adverse Drug Reactions Bulletin* 11, 7
Aphthous stomatitis
(1988): Todd PA+, *Drugs* 35, 244
Death
Dysgeusia (1–3%)
Embolia cutis medicamentosa (Nicolau syndrome)
(2002): Poletti E+, *World Congress Dermatol* Poster, 0124
(1999): Forsbach Sanchez G+, *Rev Invest Clin* (Spanish) 51, 71
Hypersensitivity
(2000): del Pozo MD+, *Allergy* 55, 412
(1998): Romano A+, *Ann Allergy Asthma Immunol* 81, 373
Injection-site necrosis
(1989): Tweedie DG, *Anaesthesia* 44, 932
Injection-site pain
(1998): Schaad HJ+, *Ther Umsch* (German) 55, 586
Oral ulceration
(2000): Madinier I+, *Ann Med Interne (Paris)* (French) 151, 248
Paresthesias (<1%)
Pseudolymphoma
(2001): Werth V, *Dermatology Times* 18
Rhabdomyolysis
(1996): Delrio FG+, *Am J Med Sci* 312(2), 95
Serum sickness
Stomatitis (<1%)
Tinnitus
Tongue edema (1–3%)
Xerostomia (1–3%)
(1988): Todd PA+, *Drugs* 35, 244

# DICLOXACILLIN

**Trade names:** Dycill (GSK); Dynapen (Mead Johnson)
**Other common trade names:** *Brispen; Dichlor-Stapenor; Diclo; Diclocil; Diclocillin; Diclox; Novapen; Pathocil; Posipen*
**Indications:** Infections due to penicillinase-producing staphylococci
**Category:** Penicillinase-resistant penicillin antibiotic
**Half-life:** 0.5–1.0 hours
**Clinically important, potentially hazardous interactions with:** anticoagulants, cyclosporine, methotrexate, tetracyclines

### *Reactions*

## Skin

Angioedema
Bullous eruption
Dermatitis (sic)
Ecchymoses
Erythema multiforme
(1991): Porteous DM+, *Arch Dermatol* 127, 740
Erythema nodosum
Erythroderma
(1985): Shelley WB+, *Cutis* 220, 224
Exanthems (<1%)
Exfoliative dermatitis (<1%)
Hematomas
Jarisch–Herxheimer reaction
Pruritus
(1998): Siegfried EC+, *J Am Acad Dermatol* 39, 797 (passim)
Purpura
Rash (sic) (<1%)
Stevens–Johnson syndrome
(1991): Porteous DM+, *Arch Dermatol* 127, 740
Toxic epidermal necrolysis
Urticaria
(1998): Siegfried EC+, *J Am Acad Dermatol* 39, 797 (passim)
(1985): Green RL+, *JAMA* 254, 531 (postcoital)
Vasculitis
Vesicular eruptions

## Nails

Nails – shoreline
(1985): Shelley WB+, *Cutis* 220, 224

## Other

Anaphylactoid reactions
(1998): Siegfried EC+, *J Am Acad Dermatol* 39, 797 (passim)
Black tongue
Dysgeusia
Glossitis
Glossodynia
Hypersensitivity (<1%)
Injection-site pain
Myalgia
Oral candidiasis
Serum sickness (<1%)
Stomatitis
Stomatodynia
Vaginitis (<1%)
Xerostomia

## DICUMAROL

**Synonym:** bishydroxycoumarin
**Trade name:** Dicumarol (Abbott)
**Other common trade names:** *Apekumarol; Dicumol; Embolin*
**Indications:** Atrial fibrillation, pulmonary embolism, venous thrombosis
**Category:** Oral anticoagulant
**Half-life:** 1–4 days
**Clinically important, potentially hazardous interactions with:** allopurinol, amiodarone, amobarbital, anabolic steroids, anti-thyroid agents, aprobarbital, aspirin, barbiturates, bivalirubin, butabarbital, butalbital, cimetidine, clofibrate, clopidogrel, cyclosporine, delavirdine, disulfiram, fenofibrate, fluconazole, gemfibrozil, glutethimide, imatinib, itraconazole, ketoconazole, levothyroxine, liothyronine, mephobarbital, methimazole, metronidazole, miconazole, penicillins, pentobarbital, phenobarbital, phenylbutazones, piperacillin, primidone, propylthiouracil, quinidine, quinine, rifabutin, rifampin, rifapentine, rofecoxib, salicylates, secobarbital, sulfinpyrazone, sulfonamides, testosterone, thyroids, zileuton

***Reactions***

### Skin

Acral purpura
(1986): Stone MS+, *J Am Acad Dermatol* 14, 796
Angioedema (<1%)
Bullous eruption
(1986): Stone MS+, *J Am Acad Dermatol* 14, 796 (passim)
Dermatitis (sic)
(1992): Breathnach SM+, *Adverse Drug Reactions and the Skin* Blackwell, Oxford, 248 (passim)
(1991): Quintavalla R+, *Int Angiol* 10, 103
Ecchymoses
(1988): Cole MS+, *Surgery* 103, 271 (passim)
Exanthems
(1989): Kruis-de Vries MH+, *Dermatologica* 178, 109
(1988): Cole MS+, *Surgery* 103, 271 (passim)
(1978): Kwong P+, *JAMA* 239, 1884
(1968): Schiff BL+, *Arch Dermatol* 98, 136
(1960): Adams CW+, *Circulation* 22, 947
Hemorrhagic skin infarcts
(1989): Geoghegan+, *BMJ* 298, 902
(1988): Cole MS, *Surgery* 103, 271
(1980): Schleicher SM+, *Arch Dermatol* 116, 444
Necrosis
(2002): Cirafici P+, *Dermatology* 204(2), 157
(1992): Sharafuddin MA+, *Arch Dermatol* 128, 105
(1989): Grimaudo V+, *BMJ* 289, 233
(1988): Cole MS+, *Surgery* 103, 271
(1987): Gladson CL+, *Arch Dermatol* 123, 1701a
(1984): Slutzki S+, *Int J Dermatol* 23, 117
(1982): Faraci PA, *Int J Dermatol* 21, 329
(1981): Horn JR+, *Am J Hosp Pharm* 38, 1763
(1976): Kirby JD+, *Br J Dermatol* 94, 97
(1971): Danilov B+, *Rev Med Chir Soc Med Nat Iasi* (Romanian) 75, 479
Pigmentation
(1978): Rebhun J, *Ann Allergy* 40, 44
Pruritus (<1%)
Purplish erythema (sic) (feet and toes)
(1978): Kwong P+, *JAMA* 239, 1884
(1961): Feder W+, *Ann Intern Med* 55, 911
Purpura
(1988): Cole MS+, *Surgery* 103, 271 (passim)
(1965): Selye H+, *Arch Klin Exp Dermatol* (German) 223, 527
Rash (sic)
Urticaria
(1988): Cole MS+, *Surgery* 103, 271 (passim)
(1986): Stone MS+, *J Am Acad Dermatol* 14, 796 (passim)
(1959): Sheps ES+, *Am J Cardiol* 3, 118
Vesicular eruptions
(1986): Stone MS+, *J Am Acad Dermatol* 14, 796 (passim)

### Hair

Hair – alopecia (1–10%)
(1989): Kruis-de Vries MH+, *Dermatologica* 178, 109 (passim)
(1988): Umlas J+, *Cutis* 42, 63
(1986): Stone MS+, *J Am Acad Dermatol* 14, 796 (passim)
(1969): Baker H+, *Br J Dermatol* 81, 236
(1957): Cornbleet T+, *Arch Dermatol* 75, 440

### Other

Hypersensitivity
Oral ulceration
Priapism

## DICYCLOMINE

**Trade names:** Antispaz; Bemote; Bentyl (Aventis); Byclomine; Di-Spaz; Dibent; Neoquess; OrTyl; Spasmoject
**Other common trade names:** *Bentylol; Formulex; Lomine; Merbentyl; Notensyl; Panakiron; Spasmoban; Swityl*
**Indications:** Irritable bowel syndrome
**Category:** Anticholinergic; antispasmodic
**Half-life:** initial: 1.8 hours; terminal: 9–10 hours
**Clinically important, potentially hazardous interactions with:** anticholinergics, arbutamine

***Reactions***

### Skin

Exanthems
(1987): Castleden CM+, *J Clin Exp Gerontol* 9, 265
(1952): Pakula SF, *Postgrad Med* 11, 123
Flushing
Hypohidrosis (>10%)
Pruritus
(1951): Ausman DC+, *Wisconsin Med J* 50, 1089
Rash (sic) (<1%)
(1975): Hennessy WB, *Med J Aust* 2, 421
(1951): Chamberlain DT, *Gastroenterology* 17, 224
Urticaria
Xerosis (>10%)

### Other

Ageusia
Anaphylactoid reactions
Dysgeusia
Injection-site reactions (sic) (>10%)
Tremors
Xerostomia (>10%)
(1975): Hennessy WB, *Med J Aust* 2, 421

# DIDANOSINE

**Trade name:** Videx (Bristol-Myers Squibb)
**Indications:** Advanced HIV infection
**Category:** Antiretroviral; nucleoside reverse transcriptase inhibitor (NRTI)
**Half-life:** 1.5 hours
**Clinically important, potentially hazardous interactions with:** ciprofloxacin, corticosteroids, dapsone, itraconazole, ketoconazole, lomefloxacin, sulfones, tenofovir, tetracycline

### *Reactions*

## Skin

Acral erythema
(1993): Pedailles S+, *Ann Dermatol Venereol* (French) 120, 837
Chills
Diaphoresis
Erythema multiforme
(2001): Scully C+, *Oral Dis* 7(4), 205 (passim)
(1992): Parneix-Spake A+, *Lancet* 340, 847
Exanthems
Pruritus (9%)
Purpura
Rash (sic) (9%)
Stevens–Johnson syndrome
(1992): Parneix-Spake A+, *Lancet* 340, 847
Urticaria
Vasculitis
(1994): Herranz P+, *Lancet* 344, 680

## Hair

Hair – alopecia (<1%)

## Other

Anaphylactoid reactions (<1%)
Death
(2001): Hwang SW+, *Singapore Med J* 42(6), 247 (2 cases) (with stavudine)
Gynecomastia
(2001): Aquilina C+, *Int J STD AIDS* 12(7), 481 (with stavudine)
(2001): Manfredi R+, *Ann Pharmacother* 35(4), 438 (with stavudine)
Hypersensitivity (<1%)
Lipodystrophy
(2001): Aquilina C+, *Int J STD AIDS* 12(7), 481 (with didanosine)
Myalgia
Myopathy
Paresthesias
Xerostomia
(2001): Scully C+, *Oral Dis* 7(4), 205 (up to 33%) (passim)

# DIDEOXYCYTIDINE (ddC)

(See ZALCITABINE)

# DIETHYLPROPION

**Synonym:** amfepramone
**Trade name:** Tenuate (Aventis)
**Other common trade names:** *Anorex; Linea; Nobesine; Prefamone; Regenon; Tenuate Retard; Tepanil*
**Indications:** Weight reduction
**Category:** Anorexiant; CNS stimulant
**Half-life:** 4–6 hours
**Clinically important, potentially hazardous interactions with:** fluoxetine, fluvoxamine, MAO inhibitors, paroxetine, phenelzine, sertraline, tranylcypromine

### *Reactions*

## Skin

Diaphoresis (<1%)
Ecchymoses
Erythema (<1%)
Erythema multiforme
(1997): Thaler D, Monona, WI (from internet) (observation)
Exanthems (<1%)
Flushing (<1%)
Pruritus (<1%)
Purpura (<1%)
Rash (sic)
Scleroderma
(1991): Bourgeois P+, *Baillieres Clin Rheumatol* 5, 13
(1990): Aeschlimann A+, *Scand J Rheumatol* 19, 87
Systemic sclerosis
(1984): Tomlinson, JW+, *J Rheumatol* 11, 254
Urticaria

## Hair

Hair – alopecia (<1%)

## Other

Dysgeusia
Gynecomastia
Myalgia (<1%)
Tremors
Xerostomia

# DIETHYLSTILBESTROL

**Synonyms:** DES; stilbestrol
**Trade names:** Diethylstilbestrol (Lilly); Stilphostrol
**Other common trade names:** *Diethyl Stilbestrol; Distilbene; Honvol; Stilboestrol*
**Indications:** Metastatic prostate carcinoma, progressive breast cancer
**Category:** Estrogen; antineoplastic; osteoporosis prophylactic
**Half-life:** 2–3 days

### *Reactions*

## Skin

Acanthosis nigricans
(1974): Banuchi SR+, *Arch Dermatol* 109, 544
(1971): Curth HO, *Birth Defects* 7, 31
Acneform eruption
Angioedema
(1942): Saphir WS+, *JAMA* 119, 557

Bullous eruption
(1971): Kuchera LK, *JAMA* 218, 562
Chloasma (<1%)
Edema
Erythema multiforme
Erythema nodosum
Exanthems
(1984): Lee M+, *J Urol* 131, 767
Exfoliative dermatitis
(1942): Kasselberg LA, *JAMA* 120, 117
Flushing
(1981): Ingle JN+, *N Engl J Med* 304, 16 (3%)
Hyperkeratosis of nipples
(1980): Mold DE+, *Cutis* 26, 95
Lupus erythematosus
(1989): Collins D, *J Rheumatol* 16, 408
Melasma (<1%)
Peripheral edema (>10%)
Pruritus
(1971): Kuchera LK, *JAMA* 218, 562
Purpura
(1984): Lee M+, *J Urol* 131, 767
Rash (sic) (<1%)
Urticaria
(1989): Collins D, *J Rheumatol* 16, 408
(1984): Lee M+, *J Urol* 131, 767

### Hair

Hair – alopecia
Hair – hirsutism
(1982): Peress MR+, *Am J Obstet Gynecol* 144, 135

### Other

Gynecomastia (>10%)
Mastodynia (>10%)
Periarteritis nodosa
(1967): Keyloun V+, *Vasc Dis* 4, 21
Porphyria cutanea tarda
(1989): Coulson IH+, *Br J Urol* 63, 648
(1978): Weimar VM+, *J Urol* 120, 643
(1972): Reginster JP, *Arch Belg Dermatol Syphiligr* (French) 28, 179
(1970): Domonkos AN, *Arch Dermatol* 102, 229
(1970): Roenigk HH+, *Arch Dermatol* 102, 260
(1969): Degos R+, *Ann Dermatol Syphiligr Paris* (French) 96, 5
(1967): Thivolet J+, *Dermatologica* (French) 135, 455
(1967): Vail JT, *JAMA* 201, 671
(1966): Copeman PW+, *BMJ* 5485, 461
(1966): Levere RD, *Blood* 28, 569
(1965): Becker FT, *Arch Dermatol* 92, 252
(1964): Theologides H+, *Metabolism* 13, 391
(1963): Hurley HJ, *Arch Dermatol* 88, 233
(1963): Walshe M, *Br J Dermatol* 75, 298
Vaginal candidiasis

# DIFLUNISAL

**Trade name:** Dolobid (Merck)
**Other common trade names:** *Ansal; Apo-Diflunisal; Diflonid; Diflusal; Dolobis; Donobid; Fluniget; Flustar; Nu-Diflunisal*
**Indications:** Rheumatoid and osteoarthritis
**Category:** Nonsteroidal anti-inflammatory (NSAID); analgesic
**Half-life:** 8–12 hours
**Clinically important, potentially hazardous interactions with:** indomethacin

## *Reactions*

### Skin

Angioedema (<1%)
Bullous eruption
(1989): Street ML+, *J Am Acad Dermatol* 20, 850
Diaphoresis (<1%)
(1986): Muncie HL+, *J Fam Pract* 23, 125
(1979): Papatheodossiou N, *Curr Med Res Opinion* 6, 154
Edema (<1%)
Erythema multiforme (<1%)
(1986): Grom JA+, *Hosp Formul Manage* 21, 353
(1985): Bigby M+, *J Am Acad Dermatol* 12, 866 (5%)
(1985): O'Brien WM+, *J Rheumatol* 12, 13
(1982): Dubois A+, *Presse Med* (French) 11, 606
(1978): Hunter JA+, *BMJ* 2, 1088
Erythroderma
(1989): Street ML+, *J Am Acad Dermatol* 20, 850
(1980): Chan LK+, *BMJ* 280, 84
Exanthems
(1992): Breathnach SM+, *Adverse Drug Reactions and the Skin* Blackwell, Oxford, 180 (passim)
(1988): Cook DJ+, *Can Med Assoc J* 138, 1029
(1985): Bigby M+, *J Am Acad Dermatol* 12, 866 (5%)
(1985): Bocanegra TS+, *Curr Res Med Opin* 9, 568 (1.7%)
Exfoliative dermatitis (<1%)
(1985): Bigby M+, *J Am Acad Dermatol* 12, 866
Fixed eruption
(1998): Mahboob A+, *Int J Dermatol* 37, 833
(1991): Roetzheim RG+, *J Am Acad Dermatol* 24, 1021 (non-pigmenting)
Flushing (<1%)
Lichenoid eruption
(1989): Street ML+, *J Am Acad Dermatol* 20, 850
Peripheral edema
Photosensitivity (<1%)
(1989): Street ML+, *J Am Acad Dermatol* 20, 850
Pruritus (1–10%)
(1992): Breathnach SM+, *Adverse Drug Reactions and the Skin* Blackwell, Oxford, 180 (passim)
(1986): Hurme M+, *Int J Clin Pharmacol Res* 6, 53
(1985): Bigby M+, *J Am Acad Dermatol* 12, 866 (5%)
Purpura
Rash (sic) (3–9%)
(1987): Masden JJ+, *Curr Ther Res* 42, 319
(1986): Bennett RM, *Clin Ther* 9, 27
(1986): Turner RA+, *Clin Ther* 9, 37
Skin reactions (sic)
(1985): Lee P+, *J Rheumatol* 12, 544
(1983): McQueen EG, *N Z Med J* 96, 95
Stevens–Johnson syndrome (<1%)
(1992): Breathnach SM+, *Adverse Drug Reactions and the Skin* Blackwell, Oxford, 180 (passim)
(1986): Grom JA+, *Hosp Formul Manage* 21, 353
(1986): Szczeklik A, *Drugs* 32 (Suppl 4), 148

(1985): Bigby M+, *J Am Acad Dermatol* 12, 866
(1982): Dubois A+, *Presse Med* (French) 11, 606
(1979): *Curr Probl* 4, 2
(1978): Hunter JA+, *BMJ* 2, 1088
Toxic epidermal necrolysis (<1%)
(1990): Roujeau JC+, *Arch Dermatol* 126, 37
Urticaria (>1%)
(1995): Arias J+, *Ann Allergy Asthma Immunol* 74, 160
(1992): Breathnach SM+, *Adverse Drug Reactions and the Skin* Blackwell, Oxford, 180 (passim)
(1987): Morse DR+, *Clin Ther* 9, 500
(1985): Bigby M+, *J Am Acad Dermatol* 12, 866 (5%)
(1983): Griffin JP, *Practitioner* 227, 1283 (passim)
(1980): Chan LK+, *BMJ* 280, 84
Vasculitis (<1%)

### Hair
Hair – alopecia
(1978): Bresnihan B+, *Curr Med Res Opinion* 5, 556

### Nails
Nails – onycholysis

### Other
Anaphylactoid reactions (<1%)
Aphthous stomatitis
Hypersensitivity (<1%)
Oral lichen planus
(1983): Hamburger J+, *BMJ* 287, 1258
Oral ulceration
Paresthesias (<1%)
Pseudolymphoma
(2001): Werth V, *Dermatology Times* 18
Pseudoporphyria
(1987): Taylor BJ+, *N Z Med J* 100, 322
Stomatitis (<1%)
Tinnitus
Trembling (<1%)
Xerostomia
(1982): Ankri J+, *Clin Ther* 5, 85

## DIGOXIN

**Trade names:** Lanoxicaps (GSK); Lanoxin (GSK)
**Other common trade names:** *Cardigox; Digacin; Digoxine; Eudigox; Lanicor; Lenoxin; Novo-Digoxin*
**Indications:** Congestive heart failure, atrial fibrillation
**Category:** Cardiac glycoside; inotropic; antiarrhythmic
**Half-life:** 36–48 hours
**Clinically important, potentially hazardous interactions with:** alprazolam, amiodarone, amphotericin B, arbutamine, bendroflumethiazide, benzthiazide, bumetanide, chlorothiazide, chlorthalidone, cholestyramine, clarithromycin, cyclosporine, cyclothiazide, demeclocycline, doxycycline, erythromycin, esomeprazole, ethacrynic acid, furosemide, hydrochlorothiazide, hydroflumethiazide, indapamide, methyclothiazide, metolazone, minocycline, **mistletoe**, oxytetracycline, polythiazide, propafenone, propantheline, quinethazone, quinidine, rifampin, **siberian ginseng**, tetracycline, thiazide diuretics, trichlormethiazide, verapamil

***Reactions***

### Skin
Angioedema
Bullous eruption
(1992): Breathnach SM+, *Adverse Drug Reactions and the Skin* Blackwell, Oxford, 216 (passim)
Diaphoresis
(1980): Lofgren RP, *N Engl J Med* 302, 919
Exanthems (1.6%)
(1994): Martin SJ+, *JAMA* 271, 1905 (generalized)
(1994): Shelley WB+, *Cutis* 54, 76 (observation)
(1992): Breathnach SM+, *Adverse Drug Reactions and the Skin* Blackwell, Oxford, 216 (passim)
Pruritus
(1994): Martin SJ+, *JAMA* 271, 1905 (generalized)
Psoriasis
(1981): David M+, *J Am Acad Dermatol* 5, 702
Purpura
(1992): Breathnach SM+, *Adverse Drug Reactions and the Skin* Blackwell, Oxford, 216 (passim)
Rash (sic)
Urticaria
(1994): Shelley WB+, *Cutis* 54, 76 (observation)
(1992): Breathnach SM+, *Adverse Drug Reactions and the Skin* Blackwell, Oxford, 216 (passim)
Vasculitis
(1972): Brauner GJ+, *Cutis* 10, 441

### Hair
Hair – alopecia

### Nails
Nails – shedding (finger- and toenails)

### Other
Dyschromatopsia (green vision)
Gynecomastia
(2000): Hugues FC+, *Ann Med Interne (Paris)* (French) 151, 10 (passim)
Xanthopsia

## DIHYDROERGOTAMINE

**Trade names:** D.H.E. 45 (Novartis); Migranal Nasal Spray (Novartis)
**Other common trade names:** *Dergiflux; Dihydergot; Ergont; Ergovasan; Ikaran; Orstanorm; Seglor; Verladyn; Verteblan*
**Indications:** Prevention of vascular headaches
**Category:** Ergot alkaloid
**Half-life:** 1.3–3.9 hours
**Clinically important, potentially hazardous interactions with:** almotriptan, amprenavir, clarithromycin, delavirdine, efavirenz, erythromycin, indinavir, naratriptan, nelfinavir, ritonavir, rizatriptan, saquinavir, sibutramine, sumatriptan, troleandomycin, zolmitriptan

***Reactions***

### Skin
Edema (>10%)
Pruritus

### Other
Dysgeusia
Injection-site reactions (sic)
Myalgia
Paresthesias (>10%)
Xerostomia (>10%)

# DIHYDROTACHYSTEROL

**Trade names:** DHT (Roxane); Hytakerol (Sanofi-Winthrop)
**Other common trade names:** *AT 10; Dihydral; Dygratyl; Vitamin D*
**Indications:** Hypocalcemia associated with hypoparathyroidism
**Category:** Fat soluble vitamin
**Half-life:** no data

### *Reactions*

## Skin

Exanthems
Livedo reticularis
(1985): Michel B+, *Schweiz Med Wochenschr* (German) 115, 418
Pruritus (1–10%)

## Other

Calcification
(1985): Michel B+, *Schweiz Med Wochenschr* (German) 115, 418
Dysgeusia (metallic taste)
Myalgia
Ulcerative necrosis
(1985): Michel B+, *Schweiz Med Wochenschr* (German) 115, 418
Xerostomia

# DILTIAZEM

**Trade names:** Cardizem (Aventis); Cartia-XT; Dilacor XR (Watson); Diltia-XT; Teczem (Aventis); Tiazac (Forest)
**Other common trade names:** *Alti-Diltiazem; Britiazem; Calcicard; Deltazen; Dilrene; Diltahexal; Nu-Diltiaz; Presoken; Tiamate; Tilazem; Tildiem*
**Indications:** Angina, essential hypertension
**Category:** Calcium channel blocker; antianginal; antiarrhythmic and antihypertensive
**Half-life:** 5–8 hours (for extended-release capsules)
**Clinically important, potentially hazardous interactions with:** amiodarone, carbamazepine, cyclosporine, epirubicin, **mistletoe**, simvastatin

Teczem is diltiazem and enalapril

### *Reactions*

## Skin

Acne
(1989): Stern R+, *Arch Intern Med* 149, 829
Acute generalized exanthematous pustulosis (AGEP)
(1998): Jan V+, *Dermatology* 197, 274
(1998): Knowles S+, *J Am Acad Dermatol* 38, 201 (passim)
(1997): Blodgett TP+, *Cutis* 60, 45
(1997): Vincente-Calleja JM+, *Br J Dermatol* 137, 837
(1996): Wolkenstein P+, *Contact Dermatitis* 35, 234
(1995): Krasovec M+, *Schweiz Rundsch Med Prax* (German) 84, 814
(1995): Moreau A+, *Int J Dermatol* 34, 263 (passim)
(1995): Wakelin SH+, *Clin Exp Dermatol* 20, 341
(1993): Janier M+, *Br J Dermatol* 129, 354
(1992): Wittal RA+, *Australas J Dermatol* 33, 11
(1988): Lambert DG+, *Br J Dermatol* 118, 308
Angioedema
(1998): Knowles S+, *J Am Acad Dermatol* 38, 201 (passim)
(1989): Sadick NS+, *J Am Acad Dermatol* 21, 132
Ankle edema
(1994): Litt JZ, Beachwood, OH (personal case) (observation)
Capillaritis (Schamberg's)
(1999): Eastern JS, Belleville, NJ (from Internet) (observation)
Cutaneous side effects (sic)
(1993): Kitamura K+, *J Dermatol* 20, 279 (psoriasiform) (31%)
(1993): Sousa-Basto A+, *Contact Dermatitis* 29, 44
Dermatitis (sic)
Diaphoresis
(1988): Lambert DG+, *Br J Dermatol* 118, 308 (passim)
(1985): Scolnick B+, *Ann Intern Med* 102, 558
Ecchymoses (<1%)
Edema (1–10%)
(2001): Chugh SK+, *J Cardiovasc Pharmacol* 38(3), 356
(1998): Knowles S+, *J Am Acad Dermatol* 38, 201 (passim)
(1982): Hossack KF, *Am J Cardiol* 49, 567
(1982): McGraw BF, *Drug Intell Clin Pharm* 16, 366
Erythema
(1998): Knowles S+, *J Am Acad Dermatol* 38, 201 (passim)
(1982): McGraw BF, *Drug Intell Clin Pharm* 16, 366
Erythema multiforme (<1%)
(1998): Knowles S+, *J Am Acad Dermatol* 38, 201 (passim)
(1995): Avila JR+, *Ann Pharmacother* 29, 317
(1993): Kitamura K+, *J Dermatol* 20, 279 (psoriasiform) (31%)
(1993): Sanders CJ+, *Lancet* 341, 967
(1993): Sousa-Basto A+, *Contact Dermatitis* 29, 44
(1992): Wittal RA+, *Australas J Dermatol* 33, 11
(1989): Berbis P+, *Dermatologica* 179, 90
(1989): Brown FH+, *Ann Dent* 48, 39
(1989): Stern R+, *Arch Intern Med* 149, 829
Exanthems
(2000): Heymann WR, *Cutis* 66, 129
(1998): Knowles S+, *J Am Acad Dermatol* 38, 201 (passim)
(1994): Baker BA+, *Ann Pharmacother* 28, 118
(1993): Kitamura K+, *J Dermatol* 20, 279 (psoriasiform) (31%)
(1993): Sousa-Basto A+, *Contact Dermatitis* 29, 44
(1992): Romano A+, *Ann Allergy* 69, 31
(1992): Wittal RA+, *Australas J Dermatol* 33, 11 (erythroderma)
(1990): Wirebaugh SR+, *Drug Intell Clin Pharm* 24, 1046
(1989): Jones SK+, *Clin Exp Dermatol* 14, 457
(1989): Stern R+, *Arch Intern Med* 149, 829
(1988): Hammentgen R+, *Dtsch Med Wochenschr* (German) 113, 1283
(1988): Lambert DG+, *Br J Dermatol* 118, 308 (passim)
(1988): Wakeel RA+, *BMJ* 296, 1071 (passim)
(1986): Gibson RS+, *N Engl J Med* 315, 423 (0.7%)
(1985): Chaffman M+, *Drugs* 29, 387 (1.3%)
(1985): Scolnick B+, *Ann Intern Med* 102, 558
Exfoliative dermatitis (<1%)
(1998): Knowles S+, *J Am Acad Dermatol* 38, 201 (passim)
(1997): Odeh M, *J Toxicol Clin Toxicol* 35, 101
(1993): Sousa-Basto A+, *Contact Dermatitis* 29, 44
(1989): Stern R+, *Arch Intern Med* 149, 829
(1988): Wakeel RA+, *BMJ* 296, 1071 (passim)
(1986): Lavrijsen APM+, *Acta Derm Venereol* 66, 536 (in a patient with psoriasis)
Flushing (1–10%)
(1992): Shelley WB+, *Advanced Dermatologic Diagnosis* WB Saunders, 583 (passim)
(1988): Lambert DG+, *Br J Dermatol* 118, 308 (passim)
(1985): Chaffman M+, *Drugs* 29, 387 (0.1–1%)
(1983): Lewis JG, *Drugs* 25, 196
(1982): McGraw BF, *Drug Intell Clin Pharm* 16, 366
Hyperkeratosis (feet)
(1992): Ilia R+, *Int J Cardiol* 35, 115
Lichenoid eruption (photosensitive)
(2001): Gladstone GC, *Dermatology Times* Worcester, MA (personal communication)
(1988): Lambert DG+, *Br J Dermatol* 118, 308
Lupus erythematosus
(1998): Callen JP, Academy '98 Meeting (4 patients)

(1998): Knowles S+, *J Am Acad Dermatol* 38, 201 (passim)
(1995): Crowson AN+, *N Engl J Med* 333, 1429
(1989): Stern R+, *Arch Intern Med* 149, 829

Palmar–plantar desquamation
(1985): Scolnick B+, *Ann Intern Med* 102, 558

Periorbital edema
(1993): Friedland S+, *Arch Ophthalmol* 111, 1027

Peripheral edema (5–8%)
(2002): No Author, *Medscape Primary Care* 4

Petechiae (<1%)

Photosensitivity (<1%)
(1998): Knowles S+, *J Am Acad Dermatol* 38, 201 (passim)
(1997): O'Reilly FM+, American Academy of Dermatology Meeting, Poster #14
(1996): Seggev JS+, *J Allergy Clin Immunol* 97, 852
(1994): Shelley WB+, *Cutis* 53, 161 (observation)
(1992): Wittal RA+, *Australas J Dermatol* 33, 11 (erythroderma)
(1990): Young L+, *Clin Exp Dermatol* 15, 467
(1989): Berbis P+, *Dermatologica* 179, 90
(1988): Lambert DG+, *Br J Dermatol* 118, 308
(1986): Lavrijsen APM+, *Acta Derm Venereol* 66, 536
(1979): Hashimoto M+, *Acta Dermatol* (Kyoto) 74, 181
(1976): Fujiwara N+, *Nippon Rinsho* (Japanese) 34, 3121

Pigmentation
(2002): Chwala A+, *Arch Dermatol* 46, 468

Pruritus (<1%)
(2001): Gladstone GC, *Dermatology Times* (personal communication)
(2000): Heymann WR, *Cutis* 66, 129
(1998): Knowles S+, *J Am Acad Dermatol* 38, 201 (passim)
(1994): Baker BA+, *Ann Pharmacother* 28, 118
(1989): Stern R+, *Arch Intern Med* 149, 829
(1986): Gibson RS+, *N Engl J Med* 315, 423 (0.7%)
(1982): McGraw BF, *Drug Intell Clin Pharm* 16, 366

Psoriasis
(2001): Smith KC, Niagara Falls, Ontario (from Internet) (observation)
(1998): Knowles S+, *J Am Acad Dermatol* 38, 201 (passim)
(1993): Kitamura K+, *J Dermatol* 20, 279 (psoriasiform) (31%)

Purpura (<1%)
(2001): Inui S+, *J Dermatol* 28(2), 100 (lichenoid)
(1998): Knowles S+, *J Am Acad Dermatol* 38, 201 (passim)
(1992): Kuo M+, *Ann Pharmacother* 26, 1089

Pustular eruption
(1993): Janier M+, *Br J Dermatol* 129, 354
(1988): Lambert DG+, *Br J Dermatol* 118, 308

Pustular psoriasis
(1989): Stern R+, *Arch Intern Med* 149, 829

Rash (sic) (1.3%)
(1998): Knowles S+, *J Am Acad Dermatol* 38, 201 (passim)
(1989): Stern R+, *Arch Intern Med* 149, 829
(1982): McGraw BF, *Drug Intell Clin Pharm* 16, 366

Skin thickening (sic)
(1998): Knowles S+, *J Am Acad Dermatol* 38, 201 (passim)
(1992): Ilia R+, *Int J Cardiol* 35, 115

Stevens–Johnson syndrome
(1998): Knowles S+, *J Am Acad Dermatol* 38, 201 (passim)
(1993): Sanders CJ+, *Lancet* 341, 967
(1990): Taylor J+, *Clin Pharmacy* 9, 948
(1989): Stern R+, *Arch Intern Med* 149, 829

Subcorneal pustular dermatosis
(2001): Reed B, Denver, CO (from Internet) (observation)
(1992): Wittal RA+, *Australas J Dermatol* 33, 11

Toxic dermatitis (sic)
(1988): Wakeel RA+, *BMJ* 296, 1071

Toxic epidermal necrolysis
(1998): Knowles S+, *J Am Acad Dermatol* 38, 201 (passim)
(1991): No Author, *Lakartidningen* (Swedish) 88, 3489
(1989): Stern R+, *Arch Intern Med* 149, 829
(1988): Wakeel RA+, *BMJ* 296, 1071 (passim)

Toxic erythema
(1998): Knowles S+, *J Am Acad Dermatol* 38, 201 (passim)
(1988): Wakeel RA+, *BMJ* 296, 1071

Toxic skin eruptions (sic)
(1993): Barbaud A+, *Therapie* (French) 48, 499

Ulcerations of legs
(1989): Jones SK+, *Clin Exp Dermatol* 14, 457
(1988): Carmichael AJ+, *BMJ* 297, 562 (vasculitic)

Urticaria (<1%)
(1998): Knowles S+, *J Am Acad Dermatol* 38, 201 (passim)
(1989): Jones SK+, *Clin Exp Dermatol* 14, 457
(1989): Sadick NS+, *J Am Acad Dermatol* 21, 132
(1989): Stern R+, *Arch Intern Med* 149, 829

Vasculitis (<1%)
(1998): Knowles S+, *J Am Acad Dermatol* 38, 201 (passim)
(1992): Kuo M+, *Ann Pharmacother* 26, 1089
(1992): Wittal RA+, *Australas J Dermatol* 33, 11
(1989): Stern R+, *Arch Intern Med* 149, 829
(1988): Sheehan-Dare RA+, *Br J Dermatol* 119, 134
(1988): Sheehan-Dare RA+, *Postgrad Med J* 64, 467

## Hair

Hair – alopecia (<1%)
(1998): Knowles S+, *J Am Acad Dermatol* 38, 201 (passim)
(1989): Stern R+, *Arch Intern Med* 149, 829

Hair – hirsutism
(1989): Stern R+, *Arch Intern Med* 149, 829

## Nails

Nails – dystrophy
(1989): Stern R+, *Arch Intern Med* 149, 829

## Other

Dysgeusia (<1%)
(2000): Zervakis J+, *Physiol Behav* 68, 405

Erythromyalgia
(1989): Stern R+, *Arch Intern Med* 149, 829

Gingival hyperplasia (21%)
(1999): Ellis JS+, *J Periodontol* 70, 63 (74%)
(1998): Knowles S+, *J Am Acad Dermatol* 38, 201 (passim)
(1995): Moghadam BKH+, *Cutis* 56, 46 (passim)
(1993): King GN+, *J Clin Periodontol* 20, 286
(1990): Brown RS+, *Oral Surg* 70, 593
(1987): Giustiniani S+, *Int J Cardiol* 15, 247

Gynecomastia
(1994): Otto C+, *Arch Intern Med* 154, 351

Hypersensitivity
(1998): Knowles S+, *J Am Acad Dermatol* 38, 201 (passim)

Lymphadenopathy
(1985): Scolnick B+, *Ann Intern Med* 102, 558

Parageusia (<1%)

Paresthesias (<1%)
(1982): McGraw BF, *Drug Intell Clin Pharm* 16, 366

Parkinsonism
(2001): Remblier C+, *Therapie* 56(1), 57

Pseudolymphoma
(1995): Magro CM+, *J Am Acad Dermatol* 32, 419

Rhabdomyolysis
(2001): Kanathur N+, *Tenn Med* 94(9), 339 (with simvastatin)
(2001): Peces R+, *Nephron* 89(1), 117 (with simvastatin)

Tinnitus

Tremors (<1%)

Xerostomia (<1%)
(1983): Lewis JG, *Drugs* 25, 196
(1981): Pepine CJ+, *Am Heart J* 101, 719

# DIMENHYDRINATE

**Trade names:** Calm-X; Dimetabs; Dramamine; Marmine; Nico-Vert; Tega-Cert; Tega-Vert; Triptone; Vertab; Wehamine
**Other common trade names:** *Andrumin; Lomarin; Nauseatol; Nausicalm; Travel Tabs; Vomacur; Vomex A; Vomisen*
**Indications:** Motion sickness, dizziness, nausea, vomiting
**Category:** $H_1$-receptor antihistamine and antinauseant
**Half-life:** no data

### *Reactions*

## Skin

Angioedema (<1%)
Diaphoresis
Eczematous eruption (sic)
Edema (<1%)
Exanthems
Fixed eruption (<1%)
(2000): Ozkaya-Bayazit E+, *Eur J Dermatol* 10, 288
(2000): Saenz de San Pedro B+, *Allergy* 55, 297
(2000): Smith KC, Niagara Falls, Ontario (from Internet) (observation) (recurrent)
(1999): Gallagher W, *The Schoch Letter,* 49, #1, 2
(1998): Smola H+, *Br J Dermatol* 138, 920
(1997): Gonzalo-Garijo MA+, *Br J Dermatol* 135, 661
(1992): Hatzis J+, *Cutis* 50, 50
(1989): Hogan DJ+, *J Am Acad Dermatol* 20, 503
(1982): Schnyder UW+, *Dermatologica* 165, 292
(1960): Kirshbaum BA+, *Am J Med Sci* 240, 512
(1960): Stritzler C+, *J Invest Dermatol* 34, 319
Flushing
Photosensitivity (<1%)
(1976): Horio T, *Arch Dermatol* 112, 1125
Rash (sic) (<1%)
Systemic eczematous contact dermatitis
Urticaria

## Other

Acute intermittent porphyria
Anaphylactoid reactions
Injection-site pain (<1%)
Myalgia (<1%)
Paresthesias (<1%)
Xerostomia (1–10%)

# DIPHENHYDRAMINE

**Trade names:** Allermax; Benadryl (Parke-Davis); Benylin (Warner-Lambert); Compoz; Sominex 2 (GSK); Valdrene
**Other common trade names:** *Allerdryl; Allermin; Banophen; Benahist; Dibrondrin; Dolestan; Genahist; Insomnal; Nytol; Resmin; Sediat*
**Indications:** Allergic rhinitis, urticaria
**Category:** Antihistamine; antidyskinetic; antiemetic; sedative-hypnotic
**Half-life:** 2–8 hours
**Clinically important, potentially hazardous interactions with: alcohol**, anticholinergics, chloral hydrate, CNS depressants, glutethimide, MAO inhibitors

### *Reactions*

## Skin

Allergic reactions (sic)
(1970): Fidel VG, *Klin Med Mosk* (Russian) 48, 109
Angioedema (<1%)
(1988): Self F+, *J R Soc Med* 81, 544
Contact dermatitis
(1998): Yamada S+, *Contact Dermatitis* 38, 282
(1983): Coskey RJ, *J Am Acad Dermatol* 8, 204
(1976): Horio T, *Arch Dermatol* 112, 1124
(1972): Shelley WB+, *Acta Derm Venereol* (Stockh) 52, 376
Diaphoresis
Eczema (sic)
(1981): Lawrence CM+, *Contact Dermatitis* 7, 276
(1972): Shelley WB+, *Acta Derm Venereol* (Stockh) 52, 376
Edema (<1%)
Exanthems
(1965): Davenport PM+, *Arch Dermatol* 92, 577
Fixed eruption
(1993): Dwyer CM+, *J Am Acad Dermatol* 29, 496
(1973): Csonka GW, *Br J Vener Dis* 49, 316
(1970): Savin JA, *Br J Dermatol* 83, 546
(1961): Welsh AM, *Arch Dermatol* 84, 1004
Livedo reticularis
(1996): Morell A+, *Dermatology* 193, 50
Photosensitivity (<1%)
(2000): Danby FW, Manchester, NH (from Internet) (observation)
(1976): Horio T, *Arch Dermatol* 112, 1124
(1974): Emmett EA, *Arch Dermatol* 110, 249
(1962): Schreiber M+, *Arch Dermatol* 86, 58
Pruritus
(1998): Litt JZ, Beachwood, OH (personal case) (observation) (following varicella)
(1972): Shelley WB+, *Acta Derm Venereol* (Stockh) 52, 376
(1965): Davenport PM+, *Arch Dermatol* 92, 577
Purpura
(1996): Morell A+, *Dermatology* 193, 50
Rash (sic) (<1%)
Toxic epidermal necrolysis
(1991): Epishin AV+, *Klin Med Mosk* (Russian) 69, 92
(1978): Soskin IaM+, *Akush Ginekol Kruglikova* (Russian) January, 67
(1972): Timperman J+, *Z Rechtsmed* (German) 71, 139
Urticaria
Vasculitis
(1965): Davenport PM+, *Arch Dermatol* 92, 577

## Other

Anaphylactoid reactions
(1998): Barranco P+, *Allergy* 53, 814

(1995): Manhart AR+, J *Toxicol Clin Toxicol* 33, 189
(1994): Watanabe T+, *J Toxicol Clin Toxicol* 32, 593
(1980): Sandler BB, *Sov Med* (Russian) (9) 119

Hypersensitivity

Injection-site gangrene
(1989): Ramsdell WM, *J Am Acad Dermatol* 21, 1318

Injection-site necrosis
(1989): Ramsdell WM, *J Am Acad Dermatol* 21, 1318

Myalgia (<1%)

Paresthesias (<1%)

Rhabdomyolysis
(1996): Emadian SM+, *Am J Emerg Med* 14(6), 574

Tinnitus

Tremors

Xerostomia (1–10%)

# DIPHENOXYLATE

**Trade names:** Logen; Lomanate; Lomotil (Searle); Lonox (Geneva)
**Other common trade names:** *Lamocot; Lofene; Low-Quel*
**Indications:** Diarrhea
**Category:** Antidiarrheal
**Half-life:** 2.5 hours

***Note:** Diphenoxylate is almost always prescribed with atropine sulfate

### *Reactions*

## Skin

Angioedema
Diaphoresis (<1%)
Flushing
Pruritus (<1%)
Urticaria (<1%)

## Other

Anaphylactoid reactions
Gingivitis
Paresthesias
Xerostomia (3%)

# DIPHENYLHYDANTOIN

(See PHENYTOIN)

# DIPYRIDAMOLE

**Trade names:** Aggrenox (Boehringer Ingelheim); Persantine (Boehringer Dupont)
**Other common trade names:** *Cardoxin; Cleridium; Coronarine; Coroxin; Curantyl N; Dipridacot; Lodimol; Novo-Dipiradol; Persantin*
**Indications:** Thromboembolic complications following cardiac valve replacement
**Category:** Platelet aggregation inhibitor and coronary vasodilator
**Half-life:** 10–12 hours
**Clinically important, potentially hazardous interactions with:** fondaparinux, reteplase

Aggrenox is dipyridamole and aspirin

### *Reactions*

## Skin

Allergic reactions (sic) (<1%)

Angioedema
(1971): Sullivan JM+, *N Engl J Med* 284, 1391

Diaphoresis (0.4%)

Edema (0.3%)

Erythema multiforme

Exanthems
(1971): Sullivan JM+, *N Engl J Med* 284, 1391

Flushing (3.4%)

Pruritus
(1971): Sullivan JM+, *N Engl J Med* 284, 1391

Psoriasis
(1971): Sullivan JM+, *N Engl J Med* 284, 1391

Purpura (1.4%)
(1993): Kaufman DW+, *Blood* 82, 2714

Rash (sic) (2.3%)
(1971): Sullivan JM+, *N Engl J Med* 284, 1391

Stevens–Johnson syndrome
(1971): Sullivan JM+, *N Engl J Med* 284, 1391

Toxic epidermal necrolysis
(1993): Seoane-Leston JM+, *Rev Stomatol Chir Maxillofac* (French) 94, 281

Ulceration (<1%)

Urticaria
(1971): Sullivan JM+, *N Engl J Med* 284, 1391

## Other

Anaphylactoid reactions
(1994): Weinmann P+, *Am J Med* 97, 488

Dysgeusia (0.1%)

Gingival bleeding (<1%)

Hypesthesia (0.5%)

Injection-site pain (0.1%)

Injection-site reactions (sic) (0.4%)

Mastodynia (0.03%)

Myalgia (0.9%)

Paresthesias (1.3%)

Pseudopolymyalgia rheumatica
(1990): Chassagne P+, *BMJ* 301, 875

Tremors (<1%)

## DIRITHROMYCIN

**Trade name:** Dynabac (Sanofi)
**Indications:** Various infections caused by susceptible organisms
**Category:** Macrolide antibiotic
**Half-life:** 8 hours
**Clinically important, potentially hazardous interactions with:** pimozide, warfarin

### *Reactions*

#### Skin
Allergic reactions (sic) (<1%)
Bullous eruption
Diaphoresis (<1%)
Edema (<1%)
Flu-like syndrome (sic) (<1%)
Peripheral edema (<1%)
Pruritus (1.2%)
Rash (sic) (1.4%)
Urticaria (1.2%)

#### Other
Anaphylactoid reactions
Dysgeusia (<1%)
Myalgia (<1%)
Oral ulceration (<1%)
Paresthesias (<1%)
Tremors (<1%)
Vaginal candidiasis (<1%)
Vaginitis (<1%)
Xerostomia (<1%)

## DISOPYRAMIDE

**Trade name:** Norpace (Searle)
**Other common trade names:** *Dimodan; Dirythmin SA; Disonorm; Durbis; Isorythm*
**Indications:** Ventricular arrhythmias
**Category:** Antiarrhythmic
**Half-life:** 4–10 hours
**Clinically important, potentially hazardous interactions with:** arsenic, ciprofloxacin, clarithromycin, enoxacin, erythromycin, gatifloxacin, lomefloxacin, moxifloxacin, norfloxacin, ofloxacin, quinolones, sparfloxacin

### *Reactions*

#### Skin
Angioedema
Dermatitis (sic)
Edema (1–3%)
Erythema nodosum
(1985): Niv Y+, *Harefuah* (Hebrew) 108, 490
Exanthems (1–5%)
(1987): Brogden RN+, *Drugs* 34, 151 (1–2%)
(1973): 11, 3
Lupus erythematosus (<1%)
(1985): Epstein A+, *Arthritis Rheum* 28, 158
(1981): Wanner WR+, *Am Heart J* 101, 687
Photosensitivity
(1987): Brogden RN+, *Drugs* 34, 151
Pruritus (1–3%)
Purpura
(1987): Brogden RN+, *Drugs* 34, 151
Rash (sic) (generalized) (1–3%)
Urticaria
Xerosis

#### Hair
Hair – alopecia

#### Other
Gynecomastia (<1%)
Oral mucosal lesions (40%)
(1987): Brogden RN+, *Drugs* 34, 151
Paresthesias (<1%)
Xerostomia (32%)
(1987): Brogden RN+, *Drugs* 34, 151 (40%)

## DISULFIRAM

**Trade name:** Antabuse (Wyeth-Ayerst)
**Other common trade names:** *Antabus; Busetal; Esperal; Nocbin; Refusal; Tetradin*
**Indications:** Alcoholism
**Category:** Deterrent to alcohol consumption
**Half-life:** no data
**Clinically important, potentially hazardous interactions with: alcohol**, anisindione, anticoagulants, cyclosporine, dicumarol, ethanolamine, ethotoin, fosphenytoin, mephenytoin, metronidazole, phenytoin, warfarin

### *Reactions*

#### Skin
Acne
(1967): Hitch JM, *JAMA* 200, 879
(1964): Fegeler F, *Arch Klin Exp Dermatol* (German) 219, 335
(1953): Barefoot SW, *JAMA* 147, 1653
Allergic reactions (sic)
Bullous eruption
(1990): Larbre B+, *Ann Dermatol Venereol* (French) 117, 721
(1979): Webb PK+, *JAMA* 241, 2061
Contact dermatitis (on exposure to rubber)
(1996): Rebandel P+, *Contact Dermatitis* 35, 48
(1995): Fisher AA, *Cutis* 56, 131
(1994): Mathelier-Fusade P+, *Contact Dermatitis* 31, 121
(1992): Baptista A+, *Contact Dermatitis* 26, 140
(1989): Minet A+, *Ann Dermatol Venereol* (French) 116, 543
(1988): Olfson M, *Am J Psychiatry* 145, 651
(1984): van Hecke E+, *Contact Dermatitis* 10, 254
(1982): Fisher AA, *Cutis* 30, 461 (passim)
(1979): *Contact Dermatitis* 5, 199
(1979): Webb PK+, *JAMA* 241, 2061
(1976): Lachapelle JM+, *Nouv Presse Med* (French) 5, 1536
(1975): Lachapelle JM, *Contact Dermatitis* 1, 218
(1974): Kobayasi T+, *Arch Dermatol Forsch* (German) 249, 125
(1970): Gunther WW, *Med J Aust* 1, 1177
(1968): van Ketel WG, *Ned Tijdschr Geneeskd* (Dutch) 112, 406
Dermatitis recall (nickel)
(1993): Gamboa P+, *Contact Dermatitis* 28, 255
(1992): Klein LR+, *J Am Acad Dermatol* 26, 645
(1987): Grondahl-Hansen V+, *Ugeskr Laeger* (Danish) 149, 2401
(1987): Kaaber K+, *Derm Beruf Umwelt* (German) 35, 209
Diaphoresis (<1%) (with alcohol)
Eczematous eruption (sic)
(1994): Mathelier-Fusade P+, *Contact Dermatitis* 31, 121
(1981): Goitre M+, *Contact Dermatitis* 7, 272

Exanthems
(1992): Breathnach SM+, *Adverse Drug Reactions and the Skin* Blackwell, Oxford, 204 (passim)
(1989): Minet A+, *Ann Dermatol Venereol* (French) 116, 543
Fixed eruption (<1%)
(2000): Sorkin M, Denver, CO (from Internet) (observation)
(1961): Welsh AL+, *Arch Dermatol* 84, 1004
(1950): Lewis HM+, *JAMA* 142, 1141
Flushing (<1%) (with alcohol)
(1992): Breathnach SM+, *Adverse Drug Reactions and the Skin* Blackwell, Oxford, 204 (passim)
(1992): Shelley WB+, *Advanced Dermatologic Diagnosis* WB Saunders, 582 (passim)
(1982): Fisher AA, *Cutis* 30, 461 (passim)
(1981): Wilkins JK, *Ann Intern Med* 95, 468
Periarteritis nodosa
(1975): Telerman-Toppet N+, *Acta Clin Belg* (French) 30, 101
Purpura
(1982): Thompson CC+, *J Am Dent Assoc* 105, 465
Pustular eruption
(1990): Larbre R+, *Ann Dermatol Venereol* (French) 117, 721
Rash (sic) (1–10%)
Skin reaction (sic) (from beer-containing shampoo)
(1980): Stoll D+, *JAMA* 244, 2045
Systemic eczematous contact dermatitis (sic)
(1966): Fisher AA, *Ann Allergy* 24, 406
Toxic epidermal necrolysis
(1989): Stern RS+, *J Am Acad Dermatol* 21, 317
Urticaria
(1992): Breathnach SM+, *Adverse Drug Reactions and the Skin* Blackwell, Oxford, 204 (passim)
(1989): Minet A+, *Ann Dermatol Venereol* (French) 116, 543
(1982): Fisher AA, *Cutis* 30, 461 (passim)
Vasculitis
(1985): Sanchez NP+, *Arch Dermatol* 121, 220
Yellow palms
(1997): Santonastaso M+, *Lancet* 350, 266

### Other

Dysgeusia (metallic or garlic aftertaste) (1–10%)
Hypogeusia
Paresthesias
Periarteritis nodosa
(1970): Zanini S+, *Fracastoro* (Italian) 63, 117

## DIVALPROEX

(See VALPROIC ACID)

## DOBUTAMINE

**Trade name:** Dobutrex (Lilly)
**Other common trade names:** *Cardiject; Dobril; Dobuject; Dobutamin; Inotrex; Oxiken; Tobrex*
**Indications:** Cardiac surgery, heart failure
**Category:** Vasopressor; adrenergic agonist; sympathomimetic
**Half-life:** 2 minutes
**Clinically important, potentially hazardous interactions with:** furazolidone

#### *Reactions*

### Skin

Cellulitis
(1994): Cernek PK, *Ann Pharmacother* 28, 964
Dermal hypersensitivity (sic)
(1991): Wu CC+, *Chest* 99, 1547
Erythema
(1991): Wu CC+, *Chest* 99, 1547
Necrosis
(1979): Hoff JV+, *N Engl J Med* 300, 1280
Pruritus
(1991): Wu CC+, *Chest* 99, 1547
(1986): McCauley CS+, *Ann Intern Med* 105, 966 (scalp)

### Other

Injection-site pain
Injection-site phlebitis
Paresthesias (1–10%)
Phlebitis

## DOCETAXEL

**Trade name:** Taxotere (Aventis)
**Indications:** Metastatic breast cancer
**Category:** Antineoplastic
**Half-life:** 11–18 hours
**Clinically important, potentially hazardous interactions with:** aldesleukin

#### *Reactions*

### Skin

Allergic reactions (sic)
(2001): Talla M+, *Therapie* 56(5), 632
Angioedema
Ankle edema
(1995): Zimmerman GC+, *Arch Dermatol* 131, 202
Edema (1–20%)
(1996): Edmonson JH+, *Am J Clin Oncon* 19, 574
(1993): Schrijvers D+, *Ann Oncol* 4, 610 (20%)
Erythema (0.9%)
(1995): Cortes JE+, *J Clin Oncol* 13, 2643
Erythrodysesthesia syndrome
(1995): Zimmerman GC+, *Arch Dermatol* 131, 202
(1994): Zimmerman GC+, *J Natl Cancer Inst* 86, 557
(1993): Vukelja SJ+, *J Natl Cancer Inst* 85, 1432
Exanthems
(1995): Cortes JE+, *J Clin Oncol* 13, 2643
(1995): Zimmerman GC+, *Arch Dermatol* 131, 202
Fibrosis
(2000): Cleveland MG+, *Cancer* 88, 1078 (generalized)
Fixed eruption (erythematous plaque)
(2000): Chu CY+, *Br J Dermatol* 142, 808
Flushing
Peripheral edema (1–10%)
Photo-recall phenomenon
(1995): Zimmerman GC+, *Arch Dermatol* 131, 202
Photosensitivity
(1995): Zimmerman GC+, *Arch Dermatol* 131, 202
Pruritus
(1995): Cortes JE+, *J Clin Oncol* 13, 2643
Radiation recall
(2002): Morkas M+, *J Clin Oncol* 20(3), 867
Rash (sic) (0.9%)
(1996): Edmonson JH+, *Am J Clin Oncon* 19, 574
Recall dermatitis
(2001): Giesel BU+, *Strahlenther Onkol* 177(9), 487
Scleroderma

(2001): Hassett G+, *Clin Exp Rheumatol* 19(2), 197
(1995): Battafarano DF+, *Cancer* 76,110
Seborrheic keratoses
(2001): Chu CY+, *Acta Derm Venereol* 81(4), 316
Squamous syringometaplasia
(2002): Karam A+, *Br J Dermatol* 146(3), 524
Toxic epidermal necrolysis
(2002): Dourakis SP+, *J Clin Oncol* 20(13), 3030
Urticaria
Xerosis
(1995): Cortes JE+, *J Clin Oncol* 13, 2643

### Hair

Hair – alopecia (80%)
(1995): Lemenager M+, *Lancet* 346, 371

### Nails

Nails – Beau's lines (transverse nail bands)
(1999): Correia O+, *Dermatology* 198, 288
Nails – changes (sic)
(2002): Pavithran K+, *Br J Dermatol* 146(4), 709
(2001): Kuroi K+, *Gan To Kagaku Ryoho* (Japanese) 28(6), 797
(2001): Wasner G+, *Lancet* 357(9260), 910
Nails – onycholysis
(1999): Correia O+, *Dermatology* 198, 288
(1998): Obermair A+, *Ann Oncol* 9, 230
(1996): Dreyfuss AL+, *J Clin Oncol* 14, 1672
(1996): Trudeau ME, *Semin Oncol* 22, 17
(1995): Zimmerman GC+, *Arch Dermatol* 131, 202
Nails – paronychia
(1999): Correia O+, *Dermatology* 198, 288 (painful)
Nails – pigmentation
(1999): Correia O+, *Dermatology* 198, 288 (orange discoloration)
(1998): Jacob CI+, *Arch Dermatol* 134, 1167 ("nail bed dyschromia")
Nails – subungual abscess
(2000): Vanhooteghem O+, *Br J Dermatol* 143, 462
Nails – subungual hemorrhage
(1999): Correia O+, *Dermatology* 198, 288
Nails – subungual hyperkeratosis
(1999): Correia O+, *Dermatology* 198, 288
Nails – transverse superficial loss of nail plate
(1999): Correia O+, *Dermatology* 198, 288
(1997): Llombart-Cussac A+, *Arch Dermatol* 133, 1466

### Other

Dysesthesia (3.9%)
Hypersensitivity (0.9%)
(2002): Denman JP+, *J Clin Oncol* 20(11), 2760 (previous hypersensitivity to paclitaxel)
(1996): Hudis CA+, *J Clin Oncol* 14, 58
(1995): Bedikian AY+, *J Clin Oncol* 13, 2895
(1993): Schrijvers D+, *Ann Oncol* 4, 610 (28%)
Infusion-site erythema
(1995): Zimmerman GC+, *Arch Dermatol* 131, 202
Infusion-site exanthems
(2002): Hirai K+, *Gynecol Obstet Invest* 53(2), 118
Infusion-site extravasation
(2000): Raley J+, *Gynecol Oncol* 78, 259
Infusion-site fixed eruption
(1995): Zimmerman GC+, *Arch Dermatol* 131, 202
Infusion-site hyperpigmentation
(2000): Schrijvers D+, *Br J Dermatol* 142, 1069
(1995): Zimmerman GC+, *Arch Dermatol* 131, 202
Infusion-site inflammation
(1995): Zimmerman GC+, *Arch Dermatol* 131, 202
Injection-site dermatitis
(2002): Hirai K+, *Gynecol Obstet Invest* 53(2), 118
Injection-site erythema
(2002): Hirai K+, *Gynecol Obstet Invest* 53(2), 118
Myalgia (>10%)
Paresthesias (3.9%)
Stomatitis (42.3%)
(1996): Edmonson JH+, *Am J Clin Oncon* 19, 574

## DOCUSATE

**Trade names:** Colase; Dialose; Diocto; Disonate; DOK; Doxinate; Modane; Regutol; Sulfalax; Surfak
**Other common trade names:** *Coloxyl; Doxate-S; Hisof; Jamylene; Lambanol; Mollax; Regulex; Selax; SoFlax; Softon*
**Indications:** Constipation
**Category:** Laxative; stool softener
**Onset of action:** 12–72 hours

#### *Reactions*

### Skin

Contact dermatitis
(1998): Lee AY+, *Contact Dermatitis* 38, 355
Diaphoresis
Exanthems (1%)
Rash (sic)

### Other

Dysgeusia

## DOFETILIDE

**Trade name:** Tikosyn (Pfizer)
**Indications:** Conversion of atrial fibrillation and atrial flutter to normal sinus rhythm
**Category:** Class III antiarrhythmic
**Half-life:** 10 hours
**Clinically important, potentially hazardous interactions with:** chlorpromazine, cimetidine, co-trimoxazole, fluphenazine, ketoconazole, medroxyprogesterone, megestrol, mesoridazine, phenothiazines, prochlorperazine, progestins, promethazine, thioridazine, trifluoperazine, trimethoprim, verapamil

#### *Reactions*

### Skin

Angioedema (<2%)
Diaphoresis (>2%)
Edema
Flu-like syndrome (sic) (4%)
Peripheral edema (>2%)
Rash (sic) (3%)

### Other

Paresthesias (<2%)

# DOLASETRON

**Trade name:** Anzemet (Aventis)
**Indications:** Prevention of nausea and vomiting
**Category:** Antiemetic and antinauseant
**Half-life:** 7.3 hours

### *Reactions*

#### Skin
Chills (>2%)
Diaphoresis
Edema
Facial edema
Flushing
Peripheral edema
Pruritus
Purpura
Rash (sic)
Urticaria

#### Other
Anaphylactoid reactions
Dysgeusia
Myalgia
Paresthesias
Photophobia
Thrombophlebitis
Twitching (sic)

# DOMPERIDONE

**Trade names:** Evoxin; Motilium (Janssen)
**Indications:** Inverigational antiemetic, gastroesophageal reflux disease (GERD), nausea and vomiting
**Category:** Peripherally acting dopamine2-receptor antagonist
**Half-life:** 7-8 hours

**Note:** Domperamol is domperidone & acetaminophen

### *Reactions*

#### Skin
Diaphoresis
Edema
Edema of the lip
Facial edema
Facial erythema
Lupus erythematosus
(1986): Yasue T+, *J Dermatol* 13(4), 292
Pruritus
Rash (sic)
(1981): Nagler J+, *Am J Gastroenterol* 76(6), 495
Redness of face
Urticaria

#### Other
Anaphylactoid reactions
Breast changes (sic)
Death
(1984): Giaccone G+, *Lancet* 2(8415):1336 (2 cases)
(1982): Joss RA+, *Lancet* 1(8279):1019
Depression
(1999): Patterson D+, *Am J Gastroenterol* 95(5), 1230
Dry mucous membranes
Galactorrhea
(1992): Bozzolo M+, *Schweiz Rundsch Med Prax* 81:1511
(1991): Nijhawan S+, *Indian J Gastroenterol* 10(3), 113
(1986): Maddern GJ+, *J Clin Gastroenterol* 8(2), 135
(1983): Cann PA+, *BMJ (Clin Res Ed)* 286(6375), 1395
(1983): Maddern GJ, *Med J Aust* 2(11), 539
Gynecomastia
(1991): Keating JP+, *Postgrad Med J* 67(786), 401
(1982): van der Steen M+, *Lancet* 2(8303), 884 (in a male infant)
Hypersensitivity
Neruoleptic malignant syndrome (<0.1%)
(1992): Spirt MJ+, *Dig Dis Sci* 37(6), 946
Parkinsonism
(1994): Llau ME+, *Rev Neurol* (Paris) (French) 150:757
Tremors

# DONEPEZIL

**Synonym:** E2020
**Trade name:** Aricept (Eisai)
**Indications:** Mild dementia of the Alzheimer's type
**Category:** Reversible acetylcholinesterase inhibitor for Alzheimer's disease; cholinergic agent
**Half-life:** 50–70 hours
**Clinically important, potentially hazardous interactions with:** galantamine

### *Reactions*

#### Skin
Dermatitis (sic) (<1%)
Diaphoresis (>1%)
Ecchymoses (4%)
Erythema (<1%)
Facial edema (<1%)
Flushing
(1996): Rogers SL+, *Dementia* 7, 293 (3%)
Hyperkeratosis (sic) (<1%)
Neurodermatitis (sic) (<1%)
Neuroleptic malignant syndrome
(2001): Ueki A+, *Nippon Ronen Igakkai Zasshi* 38(6), 822 (with bromperidol)
Periorbital edema (<1%)
Pigmentation (<1%)
Pruritus (>1%)
Purpura (1–10%)
(1998): Bryant CA+, *BMJ* 317, 787
Striae (<1%)
Ulceration (<1%)
Urticaria (>1%)

#### Hair
Hair – alopecia (<1%)
Hair – hirsutism (<1%)

#### Other
Dysgeusia (<1%)
Gingivitis (<1%)
Paresthesias (<1%)
Tongue edema (<1%)
Vaginitis (<1%)
Xerostomia (<1%)

## DOPAMINE

**Trade names:** Dopastat; Intropin
**Other common trade names:** *Cardiosteril; Dopamin; Dopamin AWD; Dynatra; Revimine*
**Indications:** Hemodynamic imbalances present in shock
**Category:** Adrenergic agonist; sympathomimetic; vasopressor
**Half-life:** 2 minutes
**Clinically important, potentially hazardous interactions with:** ethotoin, fosphenytoin, furazolidone, MAO inhibitors, mephenytoin, phenelzine, phenytoin, tranylcypromine

### *Reactions*

#### Skin
Dermal necrosis
(2001): Subhani M+, *J Perinatol* 21(5), 324
Exanthems
Piloerection (goose bumps)
Pruritus
Raynaud's phenomenon (<1%)
Urticaria

#### Hair
Hair – alopecia

#### Other
Injection-site extravasation
(1998): Chen JL+, *Ann Pharmacother* 32, 545
(1989): Denkler KA+, *Plast Reconstr Surg* 84, 811
Injection-site gangrene
(1977): Boltax RS+, *N Engl J Med* 296, 823
Injection-site necrosis (<1%)
(1992): Breathnach SM+, *Adverse Drug Reactions and the Skin* Blackwell, Oxford, 233 (passim)
(1982): Pillgram-Larsen J+, *Tidsskr Nor Laegeforen* (Norwegian) 102, 1583
(1976): Green SI+, *N Engl J Med* 294, 114
Injection-site piloerection and vasoconstriction (sic)
(1991): Ross M, *Arch Dermatol* 127, 586
Peripheral ischemia
(1983): Coakley J, *Lancet* 2, 633
Symmetric peripheral gangrene (sic)
(1997): Weinberg JM+, *Arch Dermatol* 133, 249

## DORZOLAMIDE

**Trade names:** Cosopt (Merck); Trusopt (Merck)
**Indications:** Glaucoma, ocular hypertension
**Category:** Carbonic anhydrase inhibitor (a sulfonamide)*
**Half-life:** about 4 months

Cosopt is dorzolamide and timolol

### *Reactions*

#### Skin
Contact blepharoconjunctivitis
(2001): Mancuso G+, *Contact Dermatitis* 45(4), 243
Contact dermatitis
(2001): Shimada M+, *Contact Dermatitis* 45(1), 52
(1998): Aalto-Korte K, *Contact Dermatitis* 39, 206
Eyelid edema
(1998): Adamsons IA+, *J Glaucoma* 7, 395
Periorbital dermatitis
(2002): Delaney YM+, *Br J Ophthalmol* 86(4), 378
Rash (sic) (<1%)
Stinging (ocular) (33%)
(2000): Stewart WC+, *Am J Ophthalmol* 129, 723
(1998): Adamsons IA+, *J Glaucoma* 7, 395

#### Other
Dysgeusia (25%)
Ocular burning (33%)

***Note:** Dorzolamide is a sulfonamide and can be absorbed systemically. Sulfonamides can produce severe, possibly fatal, reactions such as toxic epidermal necrolysis and Stevens–Johnson syndrome

## DOXACURIUM

**Trade name:** Nuromax (GSK)
**Indications:** Neuromuscular blockade
**Category:** Skeletal muscle relaxant; neuromuscular blocker
**Half-life:** 100–200 minutes
**Clinically important, potentially hazardous interactions with:** amikacin, aminoglycosides, carbamazepine, cyclopropane, enflurane, gentamicin, halothane, isoflurane, kanamycin, methoxyflurane, neomycin, piperacillin, streptomycin, tobramycin

### *Reactions*

#### Skin
Rash (sic)
Urticaria (<1%)

## DOXAPRAM

**Trade name:** Dopram (Robins)
**Indications:** Chronic obstructive pulmonary disease, drug-induced CNS depression
**Category:** Respiratory stimulant; CNS stimulant
**Duration of action:** 3.4 hours

### *Reactions*

#### Skin
Diaphoresis (<1%)
Flushing
(1972): 10, 43
Pruritus
(1972): 10, 43

#### Other
Injection-site erythema
Injection-site pain
Injection-site phlebitis (<1%)
Oral mucosal lesions
Paresthesias

## DOXAZOSIN

**Trade name:** Cardura (Pfizer)
**Other common trade names:** *Alfadil; Cardoxan; Cardular; Dedralen; Diblocin; Supressin*
**Indications:** Hypertension
**Category:** Alpha-adrenergic blocking agent; antihypertensive
**Half-life:** 19–22 hours

### *Reactions*

#### Skin

Bruising
(1991): Anon, *Arch Intern Med* 151, 1413
Diaphoresis (1.4%)
(1988): Young JL+, *Drugs* 35, 525
Eczema (sic) (<0.5%)
Edema (4%)
Exanthems (1.7%)
(1988): Young JL+, *Drugs* 35, 525
Facial edema (1%)
Flu-like syndrome (sic) (1.1%)
Flushing (1%)
(1991): Anon, *Arch Intern Med* 151, 1413
Hot flashes (<1%)
Lichen planus
(2001): Madnani N, Mumbai, India (from Internet) (observation)
Lichenoid eruption
(2002): Mittal A, *Udaipur* (India) (from Internet) (observation)
Lupus erythematosus
(1992): Feurle GE, *Dtsch Med Wochenschr* (German) 117, 157
Pallor (<1%)
Peripheral edema
Pruritus (1%)
Purpura (<0.5%)
Rash (sic) (1%)
(1991): Anon, *Arch Intern Med* 151, 1413
Urticaria
(1991): Anon, *Arch Intern Med* 151, 1413
Xerosis (<0.5%)

#### Hair

Hair – alopecia (<0.5%)
(1991): Anon, *Arch Intern Med* 151, 1413
Hair – growth (sic)
(1991): Anon, *Arch Intern Med* 151, 1413

#### Other

Dysgeusia (<0.5%)
(1991): Anon, *Arch Intern Med* 151, 1413
Hypesthesia (<1%)
Mastodynia (<1%)
Myalgia (1%)
Paresthesias
Parosmia (<0.05%)
Tinnitus
Xerostomia (2%)
(1991): Anon, *Arch Intern Med* 151, 1413

## DOXEPIN

**Trade names:** Sinequan (Pfizer); Zonalon (topical) (Bioglan)
**Other common trade names:** *Adapin; Alti-Doxepin; Anten; Aponal; Doneurin; Gilex; Mareen; Novo-Doxepin; Sinquan; Triadapin*
**Indications:** Mental depression, anxiety
**Category:** Tricyclic antidepressant; antipanic and antipruritic
**Half-life:** 6–8 hours
**Clinically important, potentially hazardous interactions with: alcohol**, amprenavir, arbutamine, cholestyramine, clonidine, CNS depressants, epinephrine, formoterol, guanethidine, isocarboxazid, linezolid, MAO inhibitors, phenelzine, QT interval prolonging agents, quinolones, selegiline, sparfloxacin, sympathomimetics, tranylcypromine

### *Reactions*

#### Skin

Allergic reactions (sic)
Ankle edema
(1991): Dalack GW+, *Am J Psychiatry* 148, 1601
Contact dermatitis (from topical)
(1999): Wakelin SH+, *Contact Dermatitis* 40, 214
(1997): Koehn G, *The Schoch Letter* 47, 20 (observation)
(1996): Bilbao I+, *Contact Dermatitis* 35, 254
(1996): Rapaport MJ, *Arch Dermatol* 132, 1516
(1996): Shama S, *The Schoch Letter* 46, 36 (observation)
(1996): Shelley WB+, *J Am Acad Dermatol* 34, 143
(1996): Smith KC, Niagara Falls, Ontario (from Internet) (observation)
(1996): Taylor JS+, *Arch Dermatol* 132, 515
(1995): Goldblum O, *The Schoch Letter* 45, 26 (observation)
(1995): Greenberg JH, *Contact Dermatitis* 33, 281
(1995): Porres J, *The Schoch Letter* 45, 39 (observation)
Diaphoresis (1–10%)
Edema
Erythema
Exanthems
(1970): Pöldinger P+, *Praxis* 59, 1006 (0.4%)
Flushing
(1998): Foster M+, *J Clin Dermatol* Winter, 7
Photosensitivity (<1%)
(1985): Walter-Ryan WG+, *JAMA* 254, 357
(1982): *Patient Care* June 15, 208 (list)
Pruritus
(1970): Pöldinger P+, *Praxis* 59, 1006
Purpura
(1972): Nixon DD, *JAMA* 220, 418
Rash (sic)
(1991): Roose SP+, *J Clin Psychiatry* 52, 338
Red, dry skin (sic)
(1991): Kastrup O+, *Dtsch Med Wochenschr* (German) 116, 1748
Toxic dermatitis (sic)
(1995): Vo MY, *Arch Dermatol* 131, 1468
Urticaria
Vasculitis

#### Hair

Hair – alopecia (<1%)

#### Other

Aphthous stomatitis
(1980): Ives TJ+, *Am J Hosp Pharm* 37, 1551 (passim)
Application-site burning
Application-site edema

Dysgeusia (>10%)
Galactorrhea (<1%)
Glossalgia
(1980): Ives TJ+, *Am J Hosp Pharm* 37, 1551 (passim)
Glossitis
(1980): Ives TJ+, *Am J Hosp Pharm* 37, 1551
Gynecomastia (<1%)
Paresthesias
Parkinsonism
Pseudolymphoma
(1995): Magro CM+, *J Am Acad Dermatol* 32, 419
Rhabdomyolysis
(1988): Hojgaard AD+, *Acta Med Scand* 223, 79 (with nitrazepam)
Stomatitis
(1981): Salem RB+, *Drug Intell Clin Pharm* 15, 992
Tinnitus
Tremors
Xerostomia (>10%)
(1998): Foster M+, *J Clin Dermatol* Winter, 7 (5%)
(1989): Assalian P+, *Drugs* 38(Suppl 1), 32
(1989): Lose G+, *J Urol* 142, 1024

# DOXERCALCIFEROL

**Trade name:** Hectorol (Bone Care)
**Indications:** Secondary hyperparathyroidism
**Category:** Vitamin D analog (prohormone)
**Half-life:** 32–37 hours

## *Reactions*

### Skin

Edema (34.4%)
Pruritus (8.2%)

# DOXORUBICIN

**Trade names:** Adriamycin (Pharmacia & Upjohn); Doxil (Alza); Rubex (Bristol-Myers Squibb)
**Other common trade names:** *Adiblastine; Adriablastine; Adriacin; Adriblatina; Farmablastina*
**Indications:** Carcinomas, leukemias, sarcomas
**Category:** Anthracycline and antibiotic; antineoplastic
**Half-life:** $\alpha$ phase: 0.6 hours; $\beta$ phase: 16.7 hours
**Clinically important, potentially hazardous interactions with:** aldesleukin

## *Reactions*

### Skin

Acral erythema
(1995): Komamura H+, *J Dermatol* 22(2), 116 (with vincristine, cyclophosphamide and G-CSF)
Acral erythrodysesthesia syndrome (hand–foot syndrome)
(2002): Numico G+, *Lung Cancer* 35(1), 59
(2001): Goram AL+, *Pharmacotherapy* 21(6), 751
(2001): Verschraegen CF+, *Cancer* 92(9), 2327
(1995): Gordon KB+, *Cancer* 75, 2169
(1991): Baack BR+, *J Am Acad Dermatol* 24, 457
(1989): Jones AP+, *Br J Cancer* 59, 814
(1985): Levine LE+, *Arch Dermatol* 121, 102
(1985): Vogelzang NJ+, *Ann Intern Med* 103, 303
(1985): Walker IR+, *Arch Dermatol* 121, 1240
(1984): Lokich JJ+, *Ann Intern Med* 101, 798
(1982): Cordonnier C+, *Ann Intern Med* 97, 783
Actinic keratosis inflammation
(2001): Eisner J, Mt. Vernon, WA (from Internet) (observation)
(1987): Johnson TM+, *J Am Acad Dermatol* 17(2 pT 1), 192
Allergic reactions (sic) (<1%)
(1979): Fallah-Sohy E+, *JAMA* 241, 1108
Angioedema
(1984): Collins JA, *Drug Intell Clin Pharm* 18, 402
(1983): Bronner AK+, *J Am Acad Dermatol* 9, 645
(1981): von Eyben FE+, *Cancer* 48, 1535 (passim)
(1981): Weiss RB+, *Ann Intern Med* 94, 66
(1979): Maldonado JE, *N Engl J Med* 301, 386
Cellulitis
Contact dermatitis
(1975): Reich SD+, *Cancer Chemother Rep* 59, 677
Dermatitis herpetiformis
(1986): Gottlieb D+, *Med J Aust* 145, 241
Exanthems
(1987): Lee M+, *J Urol* 138, 143
(1984): Collins JA, *Drug Intell Clin Pharm* 18, 402
Exfoliative dermatitis
(1975): Manalo FB+, *JAMA* 233, 56
Flushing (1–10%)
(1992): Curran CF, *Arch Dermatol* 128, 1408
(1987): Lee M+, *J Urol* 138, 143
Intertrigo
(2000): Lotem M+, *Arch Dermatol* 136, 1475
Keratoderma
(1975): Manalo FB+, *JAMA* 233, 56
Melanotic macules
(2000): Lotem M+, *Arch Dermatol* 136, 1475
Necrosis (local)
(1998): Bekerecioglu M+, *J Surg Res* 75, 61
(1982): Riegels-Nielsen P+, *Ugeskr-Laeger* (Danish) 144, 1313
(1981): von Eyben FE+, *Cancer* 48, 1535 (passim)
(1976): Rudolph R+, *Cancer* 38, 1087
Palmar–plantar erythema (painful)
(1990): Pagliuca A+, *Postgrad Med J* 66, 242
(1989): Jones AP+, *Br J Cancer* 59, 814
(1989): Oksenhendler E+, *Eur J Cancer Clin Oncol* 25, 1181
(1988): Shall L+, *Br J Dermatol* 119, 249
Palmar–plantar erythrodysesthesia syndrome
(2000): Lotem M+, *Arch Dermatol* 136, 1475
Pigmentation
(1996): Schulte-Huermann P+, *Dermatology* 191, 65
(1992): Konohana A, *J Dermatol* 19, 250
(1990): Curran CF, *N Z Med J* 103, 517
(1990): Kumar L+, *N Z Med J* 103, 165
(1987): Loureiro C+, *J Clin Oncol* 5, 1705
(1983): Bronner AK+, *J Am Acad Dermatol* 9, 645 (palms and soles)
(1982): Alagaratnam TT+, *Aust N Z J Surg* 52, 531
(1981): Granstein RD+, *J Am Acad Dermatol* 5, 1 (brown-black)
(1980): Orr LE+, *Arch Dermatol* 116, 273
(1977): Kew MC+, *Lancet* 1, 811
(1976): Rubegni M+, *Nouv Presse Med* (French) 5, 798
(1974): Pratt CB+, *JAMA* 228, 460 (dermal creases)
(1974): Rothberg H+, *Cancer Chemother Rep* 58, 749
Postirradiation erythema
Pruritus
(1987): Lee M+, *J Urol* 138, 143
(1984): Solimando DA+, *Drug Intell Clin Pharm* 18, 808
Purpura
(1987): Lee M+, *J Urol* 138, 143
(1971): Wang JJ+, *Cancer* 28, 837
Pustular psoriasis

(2001): Kreuter A+, *Acta Derm Venereol* 81(3), 224
Radiation recall (<1%)
(1976): Greco FA+, *Ann Intern Med* 85, 294
(1975): Dreizen S+, *Postgrad Med* 58, 150
(1974): Etcubanas E+, *Cancer Chemother Rep* 58, 757
Radiation recall (sunlight)
(2000): Lotem M+, *Arch Dermatol* 136, 1475
Rash (sic)
(2000): Israel VP+, *Gynecol Oncol* 78, 143
(1981): Karlin DA+, *Lancet* 2, 534
Raynaud's phenomenon
(1993): von Gunten CF+, *Cancer* 72, 2004
Scrotal skin toxicity (sic)
(2000): Toma S+, *Anticancer Res* 20, 485
Skin reactions (sic)
(2001): Verschraegen CF+, *Cancer* 92(9), 2327
Toxic epidermal injury (sic)
(1981): von Eyben FE+, *Cancer* 48, 1535
Urticaria (<1%)
(1986): Wandt H, *Dtsch Med Wochenschr* (German) 111, 356
(1984): Collins JA, *Drug Intell Clin Pharm* 18, 402
(1984): Solimando DA+, *Drug Intell Clin Pharm* 18, 808
(1983): Bronner AK+, *J Am Acad Dermatol* 9, 645
(1981): Hatfield AK+, *Cancer Treat Rep* 65, 353
(1981): von Eyben FE+, *Cancer* 48, 1535 (passim)
(1981): Weiss RB+, *Ann Intern Med* 94, 66
(1978): Souhami J+, *JAMA* 240, 1624
(1974): Pratt CB+, *Am J Dis Child* 127, 534
(1974): Pratt CB+, *JAMA* 228, 460 (passim)

## Hair

Hair – alopecia (>10%)
(2000): Lotem M+, *Arch Dermatol* 136, 1475 (passim)
(1995): Bonadonna G+, *JAMA* 273, 542 (96%)
(1994): Bogner JR+, *J Acquir Immune Defic Syndr* 7, 463
(1994): Rodrigeuz R+, *Ann Oncol* 5, 769
(1989): Henderson IC+, *J Clin Oncol* 7, 560 (>5%)
(1988): Giaccone G+, *Cancer Nurs* 11, 170
(1986): Martin-Jiminez M+, *N Engl J Med* 315, 894
(1986): Perez JE+, *Cancer Treat Rep* 70, 1213
(1984): Satterwhite B+, *Cancer* 54, 34
(1984): Wheelock JB+, *Cancer Treat Rep* 68, 1387
(1983): Howard N+, *Br J Radiol* 56, 963
(1983): Tigges FJ, *MMW Munch Med Wochenschr* (German) 125, 19
(1982): Gregory RP+, *Br Med J Clin Res Ed* 284, 1674
(1982): Hunt JM+, *Cancer Nurs* 5, 25
(1981): Anderson JE+, *Br Med J Clin Res* 282, 423
(1981): Cooke T+, *Br Med J Clin Res Ed* 282, 734
(1981): Hallett N, *Nurs Mirror* 152, 32
(1981): Tigges FJ, *MMW Munch Med Wochenschr* (German) 123, 737
(1980): Presser SE, *N Engl J Med* 302, 921
(1980): Timothy AR+, *Lancet* 1, 663
(1979): Dean JC+, *N Engl J Med* 301, 1427
(1979): Lovejoy NC, *Cancer Nurs* 2, 117
(1978): Soukop M+, *Cancer Treat Rep* 62, 489
(1977): Edelstyn GA+, *Lancet* 2, 253
(1975): Manalo FB+, *JAMA* 233, 56
(1974): Blum RH+, *Ann Intern Med* 80, 249 (85–100%)
(1974): Cortes EP+, *JAMA* 221, 1132 (100%)
(1974): Pratt CB+, *Am J Dis Child* 127, 534 (80%)
(1974): Pratt CB+, *JAMA* 228, 460 (passim)
(1971): Middleman E, *Cancer* 25, 844
(1971): Wang JJ+, *Cancer* 28, 837
(1969): Bonadonna G+, *BMJ* 3, 503 (60–100%)

## Nails

Nails – Beau's lines (transverse nail bands)
(1994): Ben-Dayan D+, *Acta Haematol* 91, 89
Nails – onycholysis
(1990): Curran CF, *Arch Dermatol* 126, 1244
(1989): Jones AP+, *Br J Cancer* 59, 814
(1985): Kechijian P, *J Am Acad Dermatol* 12, 552
(1980): Runne U+, *Z Haut* (German) 55, 1590
(1975): Manalo FB+, *JAMA* 233, 56
Nails – pigmentation (1–10%)
(1983): Manigand G+, *Sem Hop* (French) 59, 1840
(1982): Sans-Ortiz J+, *Med Clin (Barc)* (Spanish) 79, 49
(1981): Giacobetti R+, *Am J Dis Child* 135, 317
(1980): Runne U+, *Z Haut* (German) 55, 1590
(1980): Sulis E+, *Eur J Cancer* 16, 1517
(1977): Kew MC+, *Lancet* 1, 811
(1974): Pratt CB+, *JAMA* 228, 460 (21%)
Nails – pigmentation ('alternate brown black and white lines')
(1999): Ghoshal UC+, *J Diarrhoeal Dis Res* 17, 43
Nails – pigmented bands
(1983): Bronner AK+, *J Am Acad Dermatol* 9, 645
(1983): James WD+, *Arch Dermatol* 119, 334 (white lines)
(1981): Giacobetti R+, *Am J Dis Child* 135, 317
(1977): Morris D+, *Cancer Chemother Rep* 61, 499
(1976): Nixon DW, *Arch Intern Med* 113, 1117
(1975): Priestman TJ+, *Lancet* 1, 3337

## Other

Anaphylactoid reactions (<1%)
(1984): Collins JA, *Drug Intell Clin Pharm* 18, 402
(1982): Dunagin WG, *Semin Oncol* 9, 14
Infusion-site reactions
(2001): Verschraegen CF+, *Cancer* 92(9), 2327
Injection-site erythema
(1984): Collins JA, *Drug Intell Clin Pharm* 18, 402
(1983): Bronner AK+, *J Am Acad Dermatol* 9, 645
(1982): Dunagin WG, *Semin Oncol* 9, 14
(1981): von Eyben FE+, *Cancer* 48, 1535 (passim)
(1981): Weiss RB+, *Ann Intern Med* 94, 66 (>5%)
(1978): Souhami J+, *JAMA* 240, 1624
(1974): Etcubanas E+, *Cancer Chemother Rep* 58, 757 (>5%)
Injection-site extravasation (>10%)
(2000): Kassner E, *J Pediatr Oncon Nurs* 17, 135
(2000): Lotem M+, *Arch Dermatol* 136, 1475
(1999): Fleming A+, *J Hand Surg [Br]* 24, 390
(1998): Emiroglu M+, *Ann Plast Surg* 41, 103
(1989): Harwood KV+, *Oncol Nurs Forum* 16, 10
(1984): Hankin FM+, *J Pediatr Orthop* 4, 96
(1984): Sonneveld P+, *Cancer Treat Rep* 68, 895
(1983): Cohen FJ+, *J Hand Surg Am* 8, 43
(1983): Olver IN+, *Cancer Treat Rep* 67, 407
(1983): Pitkanen J+, *J Surg Oncol* 23, 259
(1980): Barden GA, *South Med J* 73, 1543
(1978): Bowers DG+, *Plast Reconstr Surg* 61, 86
Injection-site necrosis (>10%)
(1998): Bekerecioglu M+, *J Surg Res* 75, 61
(1987): Dufresne RG, *Cutis* 39, 197
(1983): Bronner AK+, *J Am Acad Dermatol* 9, 645
(1978): Souhami J+, *JAMA* 240, 1624
(1976): Rudolph R+, *Cancer* 38, 1087
Injection-site ulceration (>10%)
(1979): Petro JA+, *Surg Forum* 30, 535
(1979): Zweig JI+, *Cancer Treat Rep* 63, 2101
(1978): Mehta P+, *Clin Pediatr Phila* 17, 663
(1977): Reilly JJ+, *Cancer* 40, 2053
Mucositis
(2001): Verschraegen CF+, *Cancer* 92(9), 2327
(2000): Lotem M+, *Arch Dermatol* 136, 1475
Oral mucosal lesions
(1975): Dreizen S+, *Postgrad Med* 58, 75 (71%)
(1974): Blum RH+, *Ann Intern Med* 80, 249 (79%)

(1974): Cortes EP+, *JAMA* 221, 1132 (61%)
(1974): Pratt CB+, *Am J Dis Child* 127, 534 (37%)
(1971): Middleman E, *Cancer* 25, 844
(1971): Wang JJ+, *Cancer* 28, 837
(1969): Bonadonna G+, *BMJ* 3, 503 (100%)

Oral mucosal pigmentation
(1989): Kerker BJ+, *Semin Dermatol* 8, 173

Oral ulceration
(1974): Pratt CB+, *JAMA* 228, 460 (passim)

Stomatitis (>10%)
(2002): Numico G+, *Lung Cancer* 35(1), 59
(2001): Goram AL+, *Pharmacotherapy* 21(6), 751
(2001): Verschraegen CF+, *Cancer* 92(9), 2327
(2000): Israel VP+, *Gynecol Oncol* 78, 143
(2000): Lotem M+, *Arch Dermatol* 136, 1475
(1994): Bogner JR+, *J Acquir Immune Defic Syndr* 7, 463
(1989): Henderson IC+, *J Clin Oncol* 7, 560 (8.4%)
(1981): von Eyben FE+, *Cancer* 48, 1535 (passim)
(1975): Dreizen S+, *Postgrad Med* 58, 75 (>5%)
(1975): Manalo FB+, *JAMA* 233, 56
(1969): Bonadonna G+, *BMJ* 3, 503 (60–100%)

Tongue pigmentation
(1989): Kerker BJ+, *Semin Dermatol* 8, 173
(1976): Rao SP+, *Cancer Treat Rep* 60, 1402

# DOXYCYCLINE

**Trade names:** Adoxa; Doryx (Warner-Chilcott); Monodox (Oclassen); Vibra-Tabs (Pfizer); Vibramycin (Pfizer)
**Other common trade names:** *Apo-Dox; Apo-Doxy; Atridox; Azudoxat; Bactidox; Doximed; Doxy-100; Doxylin; Doxytec; Vibramycine; Vibravenos*
**Indications:** Various infections caused by susceptible organisms
**Category:** Tetracycline antibiotic
**Half-life:** 12–22 hours
**Clinically important, potentially hazardous interactions with:** amoxicillin, ampicillin, antacids, bacampicillin, bismuth, calcium, carbenicillin, cloxacillin, corticosteroids, digoxin, iron, methoxyflurane, mezlocillin, nafcillin, oxacillin, penicillins, piperacillin, retinoids, ticarcillin, zinc

### *Reactions*

## Skin

Acute generalized exanthematous pustulosis (AGEP)
(1993): Trueb RM+, *Dermatology* 186, 75

Allergic reactions (sic) (0.47%)
(1986): Bigby M+, *JAMA* 256, 3358

Angioedema
(1997): Shapiro LE+, *Arch Dermatol* 133, 1224

Erythema multiforme
(1988): Lewis-Jones MS+, *Clin Exp Dermatol* 13, 245
(1987): Curley RK+, *Clin Exp Dermatol* 12, 124
(1985): Albengres E+, *Therapie* (French) 38, 577

Exanthems
(1987): Bryant SG+, *Pharmacotherapy* 7, 125 (4.4%)

Exfoliative dermatitis

Fixed eruption (<1%)
(2002): Walfish AE+, *Cutis* 69, 207 (Metronidazole, in the same patient, also produced a Fixed Eruption)
(1999): Correia O+, *Clin Exp Dermatol* 24, 137 (genital) (with minocycline)
(1996): Marmelzat J, Los Angeles, CA (from Internet) (observation)
(1989): Alanko K+, *Acta Derm Venereol* (Stockh) 69, 223
(1988): Budde J+, *Aktuel Dermatol* (German) 14, 304
(1987): Jolly HW+, *Arch Dermatol* 114, 1484
(1984): Bargman H, *J Am Acad Dermatol* 11, 900

Lupus erythematosus

Painful eruption of hands (sic)
(1995): Levine N, *Geriatrics* 50, 23

Photosensitivity (<1%)
(2002): Litt JZ, Beachwood, OH (personal observation)
(1997): O'Reilly FM+, American Academy of Dermatology Meeting, Poster #14
(1997): Shapiro LE+, *Arch Dermatol* 133, 1224
(1997): Tanaka N+, *Contact Dermatitis* 37, 93
(1995): Nowakowski J+, *J Am Acad Dermatol* 32, 223
(1992): Bennett MJ, *J R Army Med Corps* 138, 56
(1987): Edwards R, *N Z Med J* 100, 640
(1980): Möller H+, *Acta Derm Venereol* (Stockh) 60, 495
(1977): Rey M+, *Nouv Presse Med* (French) 6, 3755
(1973): Zuehlke RL, *Arch Dermatol* 108, 837
(1968): Blank H+, *Arch Dermatol* 97, 1 (20%)

Phototoxicity
(2002): Bohannon JS, Midlothian, VA (from Internet) (observation)
(2002): Fishman CB, San Luis Obispo, CA (from Internet) (observation)
(2002): Litt JZ, Beachwood, OH (personal case) (observation)
(2002): Sorkin M, Denver, CO (from Internet) (observation)
(2002): Thaler D, Monona, WI (from Internet) (observation)
(1999): Litt JZ, Beachwood, OH (personal case) (observation)
(1996): McCarty JR, Fort Worth, TX (from Internet) (observation)
(1995): Smith EL+, *Br J Dermatol* 132, 316
(1994): Bjellerup AM+, *Br J Dermatol* 130, 356
(1993): Layton A+, *Clin Exp Dermatol* 18, 425
(1993): Shea CR+, *J Invest Dermatol* 101, 329
(1982): Rosen K+, *Acta Derm Venereol* 62, 246
(1972): Frost P+, *Arch Dermatol* 105, 681

Pigmentation
(1999): Westermann GW+, *J Intern Med* 246, 591
(1980): Möller H+, *Acta Derm Venereol* (Stockh) 60, 495

Pruritus ani

Psoriasis
(1988): Tsankov NK+, *Australas J Dermatol* 29, 111

Purpura

Rash (sic) (<1%)
(1997): Shapiro LE+, *Arch Dermatol* 133, 1224

Seborrhea (sic)
(1997): Rademaker M, New Zealand (from Internet) (observation)

Stevens–Johnson syndrome
(1987): Curley RK+, *Clin Exp Dermatol* 12, 124

Toxic epidermal necrolysis
(1999): Egan CA+, *J Am Acad Dermatol* 40, 458
(1974): Aksnes K, *Tidsskr Nor Laegeforen* (Norwegian) 94, 1254

Urticaria
(1997): Shapiro LE+, *Arch Dermatol* 133, 1224
(1992): Deluze C+, *Allergol Immunopathol Madr* (Spanish) 20, 215
(1989): Alanko K+, *Acta Derm Venereol* (Stockh) 69, 223

Vasculitis
(1981): Rockl H, *Hautarzt* (German) 32, 467

## Nails

Nails – discoloration (painful)
(1993): Coffin SE+, *Pediatr Infect Dis J* 12, 702

Nails – onycholysis

Nails – photo-onycholysis
(2000): Yong CK+, *Pediatrics* 106, E13
(1995): Shapero H, *The Schoch Letter* 45 #6, 21 (observation)
(1988): Quirce-Gancedo S+, *Med Clin (Barc)* (Spanish) 90, 636
(1987): Baran R+, *J Am Acad Dermatol* 17, 1012

(1985): Gventer M+, *J Am Podiatr Med Assoc* 75, 658
(1982): Jeanmougin M+, *Ann Dermatol Venereol* (French) 109, 165
(1981): Cavens TR, *Cutis* 27, 53
(1972): Ramelli G+, *Cutis* 10, 155
(1971): Frank SB+, *Arch Dermatol* 103, 520

### Other

Anaphylactoid reactions
Anosmia
(1990): Bleasel AF+, *Med J Aust* 152, 440
Dysgeusia
(2001): Bunker C, United Kingdom (personal communication)
Glossitis
Hypersensitivity
Hypesthesia
(2002): Sorkin M, Denver, CO (from Internet) (two observations)
Injection-site phlebitis (<1%)
Paresthesias
(1995): Shapero H, *The Schoch Letter* 45, 21 (observation)
(1994): Blanchard L, *The Schoch Letter* 44, #6 (observation)
(1994): Liss W, *The Schoch Letter* 44, 16 (observation)
(1993): Held J, *The Schoch Letter* 43, 27 (observation)
Phlebitis (<1%)
Pseudotumor cerebri
Serum sickness
(1997): Shapiro LE+, *Arch Dermatol* 133, 1224
Tongue pigmentation
Tooth discoloration (>10%) (in children)
(1998): Lochary ME+, *Pediatr Infect Dis J* 17, 429 (staining of permanent teeth)
Vaginitis
(1995): Nowakowski J+, *J Am Acad Dermatol* 32, 223

## DRONABINOL

**Synonyms:** tetrahydrocannabinol; THC
**Trade name:** Marinol (Roxane)
**Indications:** Chemotherapy-induced nausea
**Category:** Antiemetic; appetite stimulant
**Half-life:** 19–24 hours

### *Reactions*

### Skin

Diaphoresis (<1%)
Flushing (<1%)

### Other

Myalgia (<1%)
Paresthesias
Tinnitus
Xerostomia (1–10%)

## DROPERIDOL

**Trade names:** Droperidol (AstraZeneca); Inapsine (Akorn)
**Other common trade names:** *Dehydrobenzperidol; Droleptan; Inapsin; Sintodian*
**Indications:** Tranquilizer and antiemetic in surgical procedures
**Category:** Antiemetic; antipsychotic
**Half-life:** 2.3 hours

### *Reactions*

### Skin

Chills
Diaphoresis
Shivering (sic)

### Other

Death
(2001): Glassman AH+, *Am J Psychiatry* 158(11), 1774

# ECHINACEA

**Scientific names:** *Echinacea angustifola; Echinacea pallida; Echinacea purpurea*
**Other common names:** American Cone Flower; Black Sampson; Black Susans; Comb Flower; Indian Head; Purple-Cone Flower; Snakeroot
**Family:** Asteraceae; Compositae
**Purported indications:** Colds and upper respiratory infections, antiseptic, antiviral, immune stimulant, peripheral vasodilator, urinary tract infections, yeast infections
**Other uses:** skin wounds, skin ulcers, psoriasis, herpes simplex, septicemia, tonsillitis, boils, abscesses, rheumatism, migraines, dyspepsia, pain, eczema, rattlesnake bites, syphilis, typhoid, malaria, diphtheria, bee stings and hemorrhoids
**Clinically important, potentially hazardous interactions with:** corticosteroids, cyclosporine

### *Reactions*

#### Skin
Allergic reactions (sic)
Angioedema
(2000): www.aaaai.org/media/pressreleases/2000/03/000307.html
Erythema nodosum
(2001): Crawford R, *J Am Acad Dermatol* 44, 298 (recurrent)
Urticaria
(2000): www.aaaai.org/media/pressreleases/2000/03/000307.html

#### Other
Anaphylactoid reactions
(2000): www.aaaai.org/media/pressreleases/2000/03/000307.html
(1998): Mullins RJ, *Med J Aust* 168, 170
Hypersensitivity
(2000): www.aaaai.org/media/pressreleases/2000/03/000307.html (23 cases)
Paresthesias
Sialorrhea

**Note:** Individuals with atopy may be more likely to experience an allergic reaction when taking Echinacea

# EDROPHONIUM

**Trade names:** Enlon (Baxter); Reversol (Organon); Tensilon (ICN)
**Indications:** Myasthenia gravis diagnosis
**Category:** Neuromuscular blocking agent; cholinesterase inhibitor; antidote
**Half-life:** 1.8 hours
**Clinically important, potentially hazardous interactions with:** corticosteroids, galantamine

### *Reactions*

#### Skin
Diaphoresis (>10%)
Flushing
Rash (sic)
Urticaria

#### Other
Anaphylactoid reactions
Hypersensitivity (<1%)
Sialorrhea (>10%)
Thrombophlebitis (<1%)

# EFAVIRENZ

**Trade name:** Sustiva (DuPont)
**Indications:** HIV infection
**Category:** Antiretroviral non-nucleoside reverse transcriptase inhibitor (NNRTI)
**Half-life:** 52–76 hours
**Clinically important, potentially hazardous interactions with:** alprazolam, benzodiazepines, chlordiazepoxide, clonazepam, clorazepate, diazepam, dihydroergotamine, ergot, flurazepam, lorazepam, methysergide, midazolam, oral contraceptives, oxazepam, quazepam, temazepam, triazolam

### *Reactions*

#### Skin
Eczema (sic) (<2%)
Exanthems (27%)
(2001): Hartmann M+, *HIV Clin Trials* 2(5), 421
(1998): Adkins JC+, *Drugs* 56, 1055
Exfoliation (sic) (<2%)
Flushing (<2%)
Folliculitis (<2%)
Hot flashes (<2%)
Peripheral edema (<2%)
Photosensitivity
(2000): Newell A+, *Sex Transm Infect* 76, 221
Pruritus (<2%)
Rash (sic) (5–20%)
Urticaria (<2%)
Vasculitis
(2002): Domingo P+, *Arch Intern Med* 162(3), 355

#### Hair
Hair – alopecia (<2%)

#### Other
Dysgeusia (<2%)
Gynecomastia
(2002): Qazi NA+, *AIDS* 16(3), 506
(2001): Arranz Caso JA+, *AIDS* 15(11), 1447
(2001): Caso JA+, *AIDS* 15(11), 1447
(2001): Mercie P+, *AIDS* 15(1), 126
Hypersensitivity
(2000): Bossi P+, *Clin Infect Dis* 30, 227
Hypesthesia (1–2%)
Myalgia (<2%)
Paresthesias (<2%)
Parosmia (<2%)
Thrombophlebitis (<2%)
Tremors (<2%)
Xerostomia (<2%)

## EFLORNITHINE

**Synonym:** DFMO
**Trade names:** Ornidyl; Vaniqa (Bristol-Myers Squibb)
**Indications:** Sleeping sickness, hypertrichosis
**Category:** Ornithine decarboxylase inhibitor
**Half-life:** IV: 3–3.5 hours; topical: 8 hours

### *Reactions*

#### Skin

Acne (24.3%)
(2001): Thaler D, Monona, WS (perioral) (from Internet) (observation) )
Burning skin (4.3%)
Cheilitis (<1%)
Contact dermatitis (<1%)
Edema of the lip (<1%)
Erythema (1.3%)
(2001): Hickman JG+, *Curr Med Res Opin* 16, 235
Facial edema (0.3–3%)
Folliculitis (0.5%)
Herpes simplex (<1%)
Irritation (1%)
Pruritus (3.8%)
(2001): Hickman JG+, *Curr Med Res Opin* 16, 235
Rash (sic) (2.8%)
Rosacea (<1%)
Stinging (7.9%)
Xerosis (1.8%)
(2001): Hickman JG+, *Curr Med Res Opin* 16, 235

#### Hair

Hair – alopecia (1.5%)
Hair – ingrown (0.3–2%)
Hair – pseudofollicultis barbae (5–15%)

#### Other

Paresthesias (3.6%)

## ELETRIPTAN

**Trade name:** Relpax (Pfizer)
**Indications:** Migraine headaches
**Category:** Serotonin agonist
**Half-life:** 4-5 hours

### *Reactions*

#### Skin

Abscess (<1%)
Allergic reactions (sic) (<1%)
Candidiasis (<1%)
Chills (<1%)
Diaphoresis (<1%)
Edema (<1%)
Exanthems (<1%)
Exfoliative dermatitis (<1%)
Facial edema (<1%)
Peripheral edema (<1%)
Pigmentation (<1%)
Pruritus (<1%)
Psoriasis (<1%)
Rash (sic) (<1%)
Urticaria (<1%)
Xerosis (<1%)

#### Hair

Hair – alopecia

#### Other

Arthralgia (<1%)
Depression (<1%)
Dysgeusia (<1%)
Foetor ex ore (halitosis) (<1%)
Gingivitis (<1%)
Hyperesthesia (<1%)
Hypesthesia (<1%)
Mastodynia (<1%)
Myalgia (<1%)
Myopathy (<1%)
Paresthesias (<1%)
Parosmia (<1%)
Sialorrhea (<1%)
Stomatitis (<1%)
Tinnitus (<1%)
Tongue disorder (<1%)
Tooth disorder (sic) (<1%)
Tremors (<1%)
Twitching (<1%)
Vaginitis (<1%)

## ENALAPRIL

**Trade names:** Lexxel (AstraZeneca); Teczem (Aventis); Vasotec (Merck)
**Other common trade names:** *Amprace; Apo-Enalapril; Enaladil; Enapren; Glioten; Innovace; Pres; Renitec; Reniten; Xanef*
**Indications:** Hypertension
**Category:** Angiotensin-converting enzyme (ACE) inhibitor; antihypertensive and vasodilator
**Half-life:** 11 hours
**Clinically important, potentially hazardous interactions with:** amiloride, spironolactone, triamterene

Lexxel is enalapril and felodipine; Teczem is enalapril and diltiazem; Vaseretic is enalapril and hydrochlorothiazide

### *Reactions*

#### Skin

Acantholysis (sic)
(1999): Lo Schiavo A+, *Dermatology* 198, 391
Angioedema (<1%)
(2002): Kaur S+, *J Dermatol* 29(6), 336
(2001): Cohen EG+, *Ann Otol Rhinol Laryngol* 110(8), 701 (64 cases)
(2000): Babadzhan VD+, *Lik Sprava* (Russian) Apr-Jun, (3–4), 54
(1998): *Prescrire Int* 7, 92
(1998): Leuwer A+, *HNO* (German) 46, 56 (9 cases)
(1997): Brown NJ+, *JAMA* 278, 232
(1996): Kind B+, *Schweiz Rundsch Med Prax* (German) 85, 567
(1996): Langauer-Messmer S+, *Postgrad Med J* 72, 383
(1996): Mullins RJ+, *Med J Aust* 165, 319 (visceral)
(1996): Pillans PI+, *Eur J Clin Pharmacol* 51, 123
(1995): Forslund T+, *J Intern Med* 238, 179
(1995): Juarez-Giminez JC+, *Ann Pharmacother* 29, 317
(1995): Kozel MM+, *Clin Exp Dermatol* 20, 60
(1995): Waldfahrer F+, *HNO* (German) 43, 35

(1994): Dupasquier E, *Arch Mal Coeur Vaiss* (French) 87, 1371
(1994): Dyer PD, *J Allergy Clin Immunol* 93, 947
(1994): Farraye FA+, *Am J Gastroenterol* 89, 1117
(1994): Lehmke J, *Med Klin* (German) 89, 508
(1994): Nielsen EW+, *Tidsskr Nor Laegeforen* (Norwegian) 114, 804
(1994): Varma JR+, *J Am Board Fam Pract* 7, 433
(1993): Oike Y+, *Intern Med* 32, 308 (fatal)
(1993): Thompson T+, *Laryngoscope* 103, 10
(1992): Bielory L+, *Allergy Proc* 13, 85
(1992): Diehl KL+, *Dtsch Med Wochenschr* (German) 117, 727
(1992): Dobroschke R+, *Anasthesiol Intensivmed Notfallmed Schmerzther* (German) 27, 510
(1992): Finley CJ+, *Am J Emerg Med* 10, 550
(1992): Hedner T+, *BMJ* 304, 941
(1992): Jain M+, *Chest* 102, 871
(1992): Venable RJ, *J Fam Pract* 34, 201
(1991): Abidin MR+, *Arch Otolaryngol Head Neck Surg* 117, 1059
(1991): Candelaria LM+, *J Oral Maxillofac Surg* 49, 1237
(1991): Lanting PJ+, *Ned Tijdschr Geneeskd* (Dutch) 135, 335
(1991): Roberts JR+, *Ann Emerg Med* 20, 555
(1990): Chin HL+, *Ann Intern Med* 112, 312
(1990): DiNardo LJ+, *Trans Pa Acad Ophthalmol Otolaryngol* 42, 998
(1990): Gannon TH+, *Laryngoscope* 100, 1156
(1990): Gianos ME+, *Am J Emerg Med* 8, 124
(1990): Gonnering RS+, *Am J Ophthalmol* 110, 566
(1990): McAreavey D+, *Drugs* 40, 326 (0.2%)
(1990): Orfan N+, *JAMA* 264, 1287
(1990): Seidman MD+, *Otolaryngol Head Neck Surg* 102, 727
(1990): Zech J+, *HNO* (German) 38, 143
(1989): Barna JS+, *Va Med* 116, 147
(1989): Giannoccaro PJ+, *Can J. Cardiol* 5, 335 (fatal)
(1989): Huwyler T+, *Schweiz Med Wochenschr* (German) 119, 1253
(1989): Smith ME+, *Otolaryngol Head Neck Surg* 101, 93
(1989): Todd PA+, *Drugs* 37, 141 (<0.1%)
(1989): Werber JL+, *Otolaryngol Head Neck Surg* 101, 96
(1988): Inman WH+, *BMJ* 297, 826
(1988): Schilling H+, *Z Kardiol* 77 (German) (Suppl 3), 47
(1988): Slater EE+, *JAMA* 260, 967 (0.1%)
(1988): Wernze H, *Z Kardiol* (German) 77, 61
(1987): Ferner RE+, *BMJ* 294, 1119
(1987): Inman WHW, *BMJ* 294, 578
(1987): Vaillant L+, *Therapie* (French) 42, 411
(1987): Wood SM+, *BMJ* 294, 91
(1986): Marichal JF+, *Therapie* (French) 41, 517

Bullous pemphigoid
(1994): Mullins PD+, *BMJ* 309, 1411
(1993): Smith EP+, *J Am Acad Dermatol* 29, 879

Diaphoresis (<1%)
(1994): Nachbar F+, *Dtsch Med Wochenschr* (German) 119, 321

Erythema
(1993): Carrington PR+, *Cutis* 51, 121

Erythema multiforme (<1%)

Exanthems
(1993): Carrington PR+, *Cutis* 51, 121
(1990): McAreavey D+, *Drugs* 40, 326 (1.4%)
(1990): Ruiz AM+, *Drugs* 39 (Suppl 2) 77 (0.9%)
(1989): Todd PA+, *Drugs* 37, 141
(1988): Warner NJ+, *Drugs* 35 (Suppl 5), 89 (1.4%)
(1986): Gavras H, *Clin Ther* 9, 24
(1986): Todd PA+, *Drugs* 31, 198 (0.5%)
(1984): Kubo SH+, *Ann Intern Med* 100, 616
(1983): Barnes JN+, *Lancet* 2, 41

Exfoliative dermatitis (<1%)

Flushing (<1%)
(1989): Healey LA+, *N Engl J Med* 321, 763
(1987): Ferner RE+, *BMJ* (Clin Res) 294, 1119

Herpes zoster (<1%)

Lichenoid eruption
(1995): Roten SV+, *J Am Acad Dermatol* 32, 293
(1993): Kanwar AJ+, *Dermatology* 187, 80 (photosensitive)

Lupus erythematosus
(1990): Schwarz D+, *Lancet* 336, 187

Mycosis fungoides
(1986): Furness PN+, *J Clin Pathol* 39, 902

Pemphigus
(2001): Thami GP+, *Dermatology* 202(4), 341
(1997): Brenner S+, *J Am Acad Dermatol* 36, 919
(1996): Mitchell DF, Charleston, SC (from Internet) (observation)
(1995): Frangogiannis NG+, *Ann Intern Med* 122, 803 (larynx and esophagus)
(1994): Kuechle MK+, *Mayo Clin Proc* 69, 1166
(1994): Wolf R+, *Dermatology* 189, 1
(1993): Brenner S+, *Clin Dermatol* 11, 501
(1992): Ruocco V+, *Int J Dermatol* 31, 33

Pemphigus foliaceus
(2000): Ong CS+, *Australas J Dermatol* 41(4), 242
(1991): Shelton RM, *J Am Acad Dermatol* 24, 503

Pemphigus vegetans
(1994): Bastiaens MT+, *Int J Dermatol* 33, 168 (3 cases)

Photodermatitis
(1993): Shelley WB+, *Cutis* 52, 81 (observation)

Photosensitivity (<1%)
(1997): O'Reilly FM+, American Academy of Dermatology Meeting, Poster #14
(1993): Kanwar AJ+, *Dermatology* 187, 80

Pruritus (<1%)
(1993): Litt JZ, Beachwood, OH (personal case) (observation)
(1990): Heckerling PS, *Ann Intern Med* 112, 879 (vulvovaginal)
(1987): Nugent LW+, *J Clin Pharmacol* 27, 461
(1986): Gavras H, *Clin Ther* 9, 24 (0.75%)

Psoriasis
(1993): Coulter DM+, *N Z Med J* 106, 392
(1990): Wolf R+, *Dermatologica* 181, 51

Purpura
(1989): Grosbois B+, *BMJ* 298, 189 (with quinidine)

Rash (sic) (1.4%)
(2000): Babadzhan VD+, *Lik Sprava* (Russian) Apr–Jun, (3–4), 54
(1986): DiBianco R, *Med Toxicol* 1, 122 (passim)
(1986): Irvin JD+, *Am J Med* 81, 46
(1984): Davies RO+, *Am J Med* 77, 23
(1984): McFate Smith W+, *J Hypertens* Suppl 2, S113

Stevens–Johnson syndrome (<1%)

Toxic epidermal necrolysis (<1%)

Toxic pustuloderma
(1996): Ferguson JE+, *Clin Exp Dermatol* 21, 54

Urticaria (<1%)
(1996): Pillans PI+, *Eur J Clin Pharmacol* 51, 123
(1993): Carrington PR+, *Cutis* 51, 121
(1988): Inman WH+, *BMJ* 297, 826
(1988): Slater EE+, *JAMA* 260, 967
(1987): Wood SM+, *BMJ* 294, 91

Vasculitis (<1%)
(1993): Carrington PR+, *Cutis* 51, 121
(1991): Ayani I+, *Med Clin* (Barc) (Spanish) 95, 596

## Hair

Hair – alopecia (<1%)
(1991): Ahmad S, *Arch Intern Med* 151, 404

## Nails

Nails – dystrophy
(1986): Gupta S+, *BMJ* 293, 140

## Other

Ageusia
(1988): Rumboldt Z+, *Int J Clin Pharmacol Res* 8(3), 181

(1984): Davies RO+, *Am J Med* 77, 23
(1984): McFate Smith W+, *J Hypertens* Suppl 2, S113
Anaphylactoid reactions (<1%)
(1989): Todd PA+, *Drugs* 37, 141
Anosmia (<1%)
Cough
(2002): Coca A+, *Clin Ther* 24(1), 126
(2001): Adigun AQ+, *West Afr J Med* 20(1), 46
(2001): Lee SC+, *Hypertension* 38(2), 166
(2001): Rake EC+, *J Hum Hypertens* 15(12), 863 (23%)
(2000): Babadzhan VD+, *Lik Sprava* (Russian) Apr–Jun, (3–4), 54
(1988): Rumboldt Z+, *Int J Clin Pharmacol Res* 8(3), 181
Death
(2001): Gonzalez de la Puente MA+, *Ann Pharmacother* 35(11), 1492
Dysesthesia (<1%)
Dysgeusia (1–10%)
(2000): Zervakis J+, *Physiol Behav* 68, 405
(1988): Schilling H+, *Z Kardiol* (German) 77 (Suppl 3), 47
(1986): DiBianco R, *Med Toxicol* 1, 122
(1986): Irvin JD+, *Am J Med* 81, 46
(1984): Davies RO+, *Am J Med* 77, 23
Glossitis (<1%)
Glossopyrosis
(1989): Drucker CR+, *Arch Dermatol* 125, 1437
Gynecomastia
(1994): Llop R+, *Ann Pharmacother* 28, 671
Myalgia (<1%)
Oral bleeding (sic)
(1984): Kubo SH+, *Ann Intern Med* 100, 616
Oral mucosal lesions
(1986): Gavras H, *Clin Ther* 9, 24 (0.37%)
(1986): Todd PA+, *Drugs* 31, 198 (0.5%)
(1985): Gomez HJ+, *Drugs* 30 (Suppl 1), 13
(1984): Kubo SH+, *Ann Intern Med* 100, 616
Oral mucosal lichenoid eruption
(1989): Firth NA+, *Oral Surg Oral Med Oral Pathol* 67, 41
Oral ulceration
(2000): Madinier I+, *Ann Med Interne (Paris)* 151, 248
(1982): Viraben R+, *Arch Dermatol* 118, 959
Paresthesias (<1%)
Pseudopolymyalgia
(1989): Leloët X+, *BMJ* 298, 325
Scalded mouth (sic)
(1982): Vlasses PH+, *BMJ* 284, 1672
Stomatitis (<1%)
Tinnitus
Tongue edema
(1996): Litt JZ, Beachwood, OH (personal case) (observation)
(1990): Zech J+, *HNO* (German) 38, 143
(1986): Marichal JF+, *Therapie* (French) 41, 517
Xerostomia (<1%)

# ENFLURANE

**Trade name:** Ethrane (Ohmeda)
**Other common trade names:** *Alyrane; Efrane; Etrane*
**Indications:** Maintenance of general anesthesia
**Category:** General anesthetic
**Half-life:** N/A
**Clinically important, potentially hazardous interactions with:** cisatracurium, doxacurium, pancuronium, rapacuronium

### *Reactions*

## Skin
None
Shivering

## Other
Rhabdomyolysis
(1987): Lee SC+, *J Oral Maxillofac Surg* 45(9), 789 (with succinylcholine)

# ENOXACIN

**Trade name:** Penetrex (Aventis)
**Other common trade names:** *Bactidan; Comprecin; Enoxacine; Enoxen; Enoxor; Gyramid*
**Indications:** Urinary tract infections
**Category:** Fluoroquinolone antibiotic
**Half-life:** 3–6 hours
**Clinically important, potentially hazardous interactions with:** amiodarone, arsenic, bepridil, bretylium, disopyramide, erythromycin, phenothiazines, procainamide, quinidine, sotalol, tricyclic antidepressants

### *Reactions*

## Skin
Chills (<1%)
Diaphoresis (<1%)
Edema (<1%)
Erythema multiforme (<1%)
Erythema nodosum
Exanthems
(1988): Henwood JM+, *Drugs* 32, 32 (0.57%)
Exfoliative dermatitis (<1%)
Photoreactions
(1990): Schauder S, *Z Hautkr* (German) 65, 253
Photosensitivity (<1%)
(1993): Kang JS+, *Photodermatol Photoimmunol Photomed* 9, 159
(1992): Izu R+, *Photodermatol Photoimmunol Photomed* 9, 86
(1990): Schauder S, *Z Hautkr* (German) 65, 253
(1989): Kawabe Y+, *Photodermatology* 6, 57
(1988): Henwood JM+, *Drugs* 32, 32 (0.57%)
Phototoxicity
(1998): Martinez LJ+ *Photochem Photobiol* 67, 399
(1994): Fujita H+, *Photodermatol Photoimmunol Photomed* 10, 202
(1990): Przybilla B+, *Dermatologica* 181, 98
(1990): Schauder S, *Z Hautkr* (German) 65, 253
Pigmentation
Pruritus (<1%)
Purpura (<1%)
Rash (sic) (<1%)
Stevens–Johnson syndrome (<1%)

Toxic epidermal necrolysis (<1%)
Urticaria (<1%)
(1988): Henwood JM+, *Drugs* 32, 32 (0.57%)

### Other
Dysgeusia
Hypersensitivity
Injection-site phlebitis
Myalgia (<1%)
Paresthesias (<1%)
Stomatitis (<1%)
Tendon rupture (<1%)
Tinnitus
Tremors (<1%)
Vaginal candidiasis (<1%)
Vaginitis (<1%)
Xerostomia (<1%)

## ENOXAPARIN

**Trade name:** Lovenox (Aventis)
**Other common trade names:** *Clexan; Clexane 40; Klexane*
**Indications:** Prevention of deep vein thrombosis
**Category:** Anticoagulant (heparin; low weight)
**Half-life:** 4.5 hours
**Clinically important, potentially hazardous interactions with:** butabarbital, danaparoid

#### *Reactions*

### Skin
Cutaneous side effects (sic) (0.2%)
(2000): Enrique E+, *Contact Dermatitis* 42, 43
Ecchymoses (2%)
Edema (3%)
Erythema (1–10%)
(1993): Phillips JK+, *Br J Haematol* 85, 837
Exanthems
(2001): Kim K & Lynfield Y, New York, NY (personal communication)
Peripheral edema (3%)
Pruritus
(2001): Kim K & Lynfield Y, New York, NY (personal communication)
Purpura (1–10%)
Urticaria
(1997): Downham TF, Taylor, MI (from Internet) (observation)
Vesicular eruptions (<1%)

### Other
Anaphylactoid reactions (<1%)
Fat necrosis
(2001): Davies J+, *Postgrad Med* 77(903), 43112
Hypersensitivity
(2000): Romero Ortega MR+, *Aten Primaria* (Spanish) 25, 521
(1998): Cabanas R+, *J Investig Allergol Clin Immunol* 8, 383
(1998): Mendez J+, *Allergy* 53, 999
(1996): Koch P+, *Contact Dermatitis* 34, 156
(1996): Mendez J+, *Allergy* 51, 853
Injection-site erythema
(2001): Kim K & Lynfield Y, New York, NY (personal communication)
Injection-site exanthems
(2000): Szolar-Platzer C+, *J Am Acad Dermatol* 43, 920
Injection-site infiltrated plaques
(1998): Mendez J+, *Allergy* 53, 999
(1998): Valdes F+, *Allergy* 53, 625
Injection-site necrosis
(1997): Lefebvre I+, *Ann Dermatol Venereol* (French) 124, 397
(1997): Tonn ME+, *Ann Pharmacother* 31, 323
(1996): Fried M+, *Ann Intern Med* 125, 521
Injection-site pain
Injection-site pruritus
(2000): Szolar-Platzer C+, *J Am Acad Dermatol* 43, 920
Necrosis (<1%)
(2002): Toll A+, *World Congress Dermatol* Poster, 0130

## ENTACAPONE

**Trade name:** Comtan (Novartis)
**Other common trade name:** *Comtess*
**Indications:** Parkinsonism
**Category:** Antiparkinsonian; reverse COMT inhibitor
**Half-life:** 2.4 hours
**Clinically important, potentially hazardous interactions with:** MAO inhibitors, phenelzine, tranylcypromine

#### *Reactions*

### Skin
Bacterial infection (sic) (1%)
Diaphoresis (2%)
Purpura (2%)

### Other
Dysgeusia (1%)
Xerostomia (3%)

## EPHEDRA

**Scientific names:** *Ephedra distachya; Ephedra equisetina; Ephedra gerardiana; Ephedra intermedia; Ephedra sinica*
**Other common names:** Desert Herb; Joint Fir; Ma Huang; Mahuang; Popotillo; Sea Grape; Teamster's Tea; Yellow Astringent; Yellow Horse
**Family:** Ephedraceae
**Purported indications:** Bronchospasm, asthma, bronchitis, allergic disorders, central nervous stimulant, cardiovascular stimulant, appetite suppressant
**Other uses:** Colds, flu, fever, chills, edema, headache, anhidrosis, diuretic, joint and bone pain
**Clinically important, potentially hazardous interactions with:** olmesartan

#### *Reactions*

### Skin
Flushing

### Other
Eosinophilia–myalgia syndrome
(1999): Zaacks SM+, *J Toxicol Clin Toxicol* 37, 485
Hypersensitivity
Myalgia
Myopathy
Tremors

## EPHEDRINE

**Trade names:** Ectasule; Efedron; Ephedsol; Marax; Pretz-D; Rynatuss; Vicks Vatronol
**Indications:** Nasal congestion, acute hypotensive states, asthma
**Category:** Adrenergic agonist; sympathomimetic bronchodilator
**Half-life:** 3–6 hours
**Clinically important, potentially hazardous interactions with:** antihypertensives, furazolidone, guanethidine, MAO inhibitors, methyldopa, phenelzine, phenylpropanolamine, selegiline, tranylcypromine, tricyclic antidepressants

### *Reactions*

#### Skin

Bullous eruption
(1944): Lewis G, *Arch Dermatol* 49, 379
Contact dermatitis (following topical application)
(1945): Spencer GA, *Arch Dermatol* 51, 48
(1944): Lewis G, *Arch Dermatol* 49, 379
(1936): Hollander L, *JAMA* February 29, 706
Dermatitis (sic)
(1993): Villas-Martinez F+, *Contact Dermatitis* 29, 215
(1991): Audicana M+, *Contact Dermatitis* 24, 223
Diaphoresis (1–10%)
Edema
Exanthems
(1933): Abramovitz EW+, *Br J Dermatol* XLV, 236
Exfoliative dermatitis
(1981): Serup J, *Ugeskr Laeger* (Danish) 143, 1660
Fixed eruption
(2000): Tanimoto K+, *Masui* 49(12), 1374
(1997): Garcia Ortiz JC+, *Allergy* 52, 229
(1994): Krivda SJ+, *J Am Acad Dermatol* 31, 291 (non-pigmenting)
(1968): Brownstein MH, *Arch Dermatol* 97, 115
(1960): Englehardt AW, *Hautarzt* (German) 11, 49
Pallor (1–10%)
Purpura
(1933): Abramovitz EW+, *Br J Dermatol* XLV, 236
Urticaria
(1978): Speer F+, *Ann Allergy* 40, 32
(1933): Abramovitz EW+, *Br J Dermatol* XLV, 236
Vasculitis
(1978): Speer F+, *Ann Allergy* 40, 32

#### Other

Trembling (1–10%)
Tremors (1–10%)
Xerostomia (1–10%)

## EPINEPHRINE

**Synonym:** adrenaline
**Trade names:** Adrenalin (Parke-Davis); AsthmaHaler; Bronitin; Bronkaid; Epifrin (Allergan); Epipen (CTR Labs); MedihalerEpi; Primatene; Sus-Phrine (Forest)
**Other common trade names:** *Adrenaline; Ana-Guard; Epi E-Z Pen; Eppy; Eppystabil; Isopto-Epinal; Primatene Mist; S-2; Simplene*
**Indications:** Cardiac arrest, hay fever, asthma, anaphylaxis
**Category:** Adrenergic agonist; sympathomimetic bronchodilator
**Duration of action:** 1–4 hours
**Clinically important, potentially hazardous interactions with:** albuterol, alpha-blockers, amitriptyline, amoxapine, atenolol, beta-blockers, carteolol, chlorpromazine, clomipramine, cocaine, desipramine, doxepin, ergotamine, furazolidone, halothane, imipramine, MAO inhibitors, metoprolol, nadolol, nortriptyline, penbutolol, phenelzine, phenoxybenzamine, phenylephrine, pindolol, prazosin, propranolol, protriptyline, sympathomimetics, terbutaline, thioridazine, timolol, tranylcypromine, tricyclic antidepressants, trimipramine, vasopressors

### *Reactions*

#### Skin

Contact dermatitis
(1993): Gaspari AA, *Contact Dermatitis* 28, 35
(1980): Romaguera C+, *Contact Dermatitis* 6, 364
(1976): Alani SD+, *Contact Dermatitis* 2, 147
(1970): Gibbs RC, *Arch Dermatol* 101, 92
Diaphoresis (1–10%)
Exanthems
Fixed eruption
Flushing (1–10%)
Necrosis
(1984): Antrum RM+, *Br J Clin Pract* 38, 191
Pallor (<1%)
Pemphigoid (cicatricial)
(1981): Vadot E+, *Bull Soc Ophtalmol Fr* (French) 81, 693
(1977): Norn MS, *Am J Ophthalmol* 83, 138
Urticaria

#### Hair

Hair – alopecia
(1972): Kass MA+, *Arch Ophthalmol* 88, 429 (eyelashes)

#### Other

Injection-site necrosis
Injection-site pain
Injection-site urticaria
Trembling (1–10%)
Xerostomia (<1%)

# EPIRUBICIN

**Trade name:** Ellence (Pharmacia & Upjohn)
**Indications:** Adjuvant therapy in primary breast cancer
**Category:** Antineoplastic
**Half-life:** 33 hours
**Clinically important, potentially hazardous interactions with:** amlodipine, bepridil, cimetidine, diltiazem, felodipine, isradipine, nicardipine, nifedipine, nimodipine, nisoldipine, verapamil

### *Reactions*

## Skin

Cutaneous reactions (sic)
(1999): Ormrod D+, *Drugs Aging* 15, 389
Erythema
Exfoliative dermatitis
Facial flushing
Hot flashes (5–39%)
Photosensitivity
Pigmentation
Pruritus (9%)
Radiation recall
Rash (sic) (1–9%)
Recall phenomenon
(1999): Wilson J+, *Clin Oncol (R Coll Radiol)* 11, 424
Skin changes (sic) (0.7–5%)
Ulceration
Urticaria

## Hair

Hair – alopecia (69–95%) (reversible)
(1999): Ormrod D+, *Drugs Aging* 15, 389
(1991): Carmo-Pereira J+, *Cancer Chemother Pharmacol* 27, 394 (95%)
(1991): Fountzilas G+, *Tumori* 77, 232 (81%)
(1986): Kimura K+, *Gan To Kagaku Ryoho* (Japanese) 13, 2440 (71.4%)
(1986): Sakata Y+, *Gan To Kagaku Ryoho* (Japanese) 13, 1887
(1986): Tominaga T+, *Gan To Kagaku Ryoho* (Japanese) 13, 2187 (66.7%)
(1985): Holdener EE+, *Invest New Drugs* 3, 63 (54%)
(1984): Lopez M+, *Invest New Drugs* 2, 315
(1984): Schutte J+, *J Cancer Res Clin Oncol* 107, 38 (88%)
(1980): Bonfante V+, *Recent Results Cancer Res* 74, 192

## Nails

Nails – pigmentation

## Other

Anaphylactoid reactions
Hypersensitivity
Injection-site extravasation
(1999): Fleming A+, *J Hand Surg [Br]* 24, 390
Injection-site inflammation
Injection-site necrosis
Injection-site reactions (sic) (3–20%)
Injection-site ulceration
Mucositis
(1999): Ormrod D+, *Drugs Aging* 15, 389
Myalgia
(1995): Fountzilas G+, *Med Pediatr Oncol* 24, 23 (55%)
Oral ulceration
Phlebitis
Stomatitis
(1995): Fountzilas G+, *Med Pediatr Oncol* 24, 23
(1991): Carmo-Pereira J+, *Cancer Chemother Pharmacol* 27, 394 (35%)
(1991): Fountzilas G+, *Tumori* 77, 232 (24%)
(1986): Kimura K+, *Gan To Kagaku Ruoho* (Japanese) 13, 2440 (12.5%)
(1986): Sakata Y+, *Gan To Kagaku Ryoho* (Japanese) 13, 1887
(1980): Bonfante V+, *Recent Results Cancer Res* 74, 192

# EPOETIN ALFA

**Synonyms:** erythropoietin; EPO
**Trade names:** Epogen (Amgen); Procrit (Ortho)
**Other common trade names:** *Epoxitin; Eprex; Erypo*
**Indications:** Anemia
**Category:** Colony stimulating factor; growth factor
**Half-life:** 4–13 hours (in patients with chronic renal failure)

### *Reactions*

## Skin

Acne
(1989): Faulds D+, *Drugs* 38, 863
Angioedema (1–5%)
Contact dermatitis
(1993): Hardwick N+, *Contact Dermatitis* 28, 123
Edema (17%)
Exanthems
(1990): Schröder-Kolb B, *Derm Beruf Umwelt* (German) 38, 12 (papular)
Lichenoid eruption
(1997): Puritz E, Smithtown, NY (from Internet) (observation)
Photosensitivity
(1992): Harvey E+, *J Pediatr* 121, 749
Pruritus
(1990): Schröder-Kolb B, *Derm Beruf Umwelt* (German) 38, 12 (papular)
(1989): Faulds D+, *Drugs* 38, 863
Rash (sic) (1–10%)
Urticaria

## Hair

Hair – alopecia
(2001): Reddy V+, *Nephrol Dial Transplant* 16(7), 1525
Hair – alopecia totalis
(2001): Reddy V+, *Nephrol Dial Transplant* 16(7), 1525
Hair – hypertrichosis
(1991): Kleiner MJ+, *Am J Kidney Dis* 18, 689

## Other

Anaphylactoid reactions
Hypersensitivity (<1%)
Injection-site pain
(1998): Veys N+, *Clin Nephrol* 49, 41
Injection-site reactions (sic) (7%)
Injection-site thrombophlebitis
Injection-site ulceration
(1997): Siegel DM, New York, NY (from Internet) (observation)
Myalgia
Paresthesias (11%)
Porphyria cutanea tarda
(1992): Harvey E+, *J Pediatr* 121, 749

## EPROSARTAN

**Trade name:** Teveten (Solvay)
**Indications:** Hypertension
**Category:** Angiotensin II receptor antagonist; antihypertensive
**Half-life:** 5–9 hours

### *Reactions*

#### Skin

Angioedema
Diaphoresis (<1%)
Eczema (sic) (<1%)
Exanthems (<1%)
Facial edema (<1%)
Furunculosis (<1%)
Herpes simplex (<1%)
Hot flashes (<1%)
Peripheral edema (<1%)
Pruritus (<1%)
Purpura (<1%)
Rash (sic) (<1%)

#### Other

Cough
(2001): Rake EC+, *J Hum Hypertens* 15(12), 863 (5%)
Gingivitis (<1%)
Myalgia
Paresthesias (<1%)
Tendinitis (<1%)
Tremors (<1%)
Xerostomia (<1%)

## EPTIFIBATIDE

**Trade name:** Integrilin (COR)
**Indications:** Acute coronary syndrome, unstable angina
**Category:** Antiplatelet; platelet aggregation inhibitor
**Half-life:** 2.5 hours
**Clinically important, potentially hazardous interactions with:** fondaparinux

### *Reactions*

#### Skin

None

#### Other

Anaphylactoid reactions (<1%)
Injection-site reactions (sic)

## ERGOCALCIFEROL

**Synonyms:** viosterol; vitamin $D_2$
**Trade names:** Calciferol (Schwarz); Deltalin (Lilly); Drisdol (Sanofi); Vitamin D
**Other common trade names:** *Kalciferol; Ostoforte; Radiostol Forte; Sterogyl-15; Vigantol; Vitaminol*
**Indications:** Rickets, hypoparathyroidism
**Category:** Fat-soluble nutritional supplement; antihypocalcemic and antihypoparathyroid
**Half-life:** 19–48 hours

### *Reactions*

#### Skin

Granulomas (perforating)
(1982): Aliaga A+, *Dermatologica* 164, 62
Pruritus (1–10%)

#### Other

Dysgeusia (1–10%) (metallic taste)
Myalgia
Xerostomia

## ERTAPENEM

**Synonyms:** L-749,345; MK-0826
**Trade name:** Invanz (Merck)
**Indications:** Severe resistant bacterial infections caused by susceptible organisms
**Category:** Carbapenem antibiotic
**Half-life:** 4 hours
**Clinically important, potentially hazardous interactions with:** probenecid

### *Reactions*

#### Skin

Candidiasis (>1%)
Chills (>1%)
Dermatitis (sic) (>1%)
Desquamation (>1%)
Diaphoresis (>1%)
Edema (3%)
Erythema (1–2%)
Facial edema (>1%)
Flushing (>1%)
Hematomas (<1%)
Necrosis (<1%)
Pruritus (1–2%)
Rash (sic) (2–3%)
Urticaria (>1%)
Vaginal pruritus (>1%)
Vulvovaginitis (>1%)

#### Other

Anaphylactoid reactions (some fatal)
Cough (1–2%)
Death (2.5%)
Depression (>1%)
Dysgeusia (>1%)
Hiccups (<1%)
Hypersensitivity

Hypesthesia (>1%)
Infusion-site extravasation (0.7–2%)
Injection-site induration (>1%)
Injection-site pain (>1%)
Leg pain (0.4–1%)
Oral candidiasis (0.1%)
Oral ulceration (>1%)
Pain (>1%)
Paresthesias (>1%)
Phlebitis (1.5–2%)
Seizures (0.5%)
Stomatitis (>1%)
Thrombophlebitis (1.5–2%)
Tremors (>1%)
Vaginal candidiasis (>1%)
Vaginitis (1–3%)

# ERYTHROMYCIN

**Trade names:** E.E.S; E-Mycin; Eramycin; Ery-Ped; Ery-Tab; Eryc; Erypar; Erythrocin; Eryzole*; Ilosone; Ilotycin; PCE; Pediazole*; Robimycin; Wintrocin; Wyamicin S
**Other common trade name:** *Too numerous to list*
**Indications:** Various infections caused by susceptible organisms
**Category:** Bacteriostatic macrolide antibiotic
**Half-life:** 1.4–2 hours
**Clinically important, potentially hazardous interactions with:** alfentanil, aminophylline, amoxicillin, ampicillin, anticonvulsants, astemizole, atorvastatin, benzodiazepines, bromocriptine, carbamazepine, ciprofloxacin, cisapride, clindamycin, colchicine, cyclosporine, digoxin, dihydroergotamine, disopyramide, enoxacin, ergotamine, fluoxetine, fluvastatin, gatifloxacin, imatinib, lomefloxacin, lorazepam, lovastatin, methadone, methysergide, midazolam, moxifloxacin, norfloxacin, ofloxacin, paroxetine, pimozide, pravastatin, quinolones, sertraline, sildenafil, simvastatin, sparfloxacin, tacrolimus, terfenadine, theophylline, triazolam, vinblastine, warfarin

***Note:** Eryzole and Pediazole are combinations of erythromycin and sulfisoxazole

### *Reactions*

## Skin

Acne
(1969): Weary PE+, *Arch Dermatol* 100, 179
Acute generalized exanthematous pustulosis (AGEP)
(1995): Moreau A+, *Int J Dermatol* 34, 263 (passim)
(1991): Roujeau J-C+, *Arch Dermatol* 127, 1333
Allergic reactions (sic) (<1%)
(1986): Bigby M+, *JAMA* 256, 3358 (2.04%)
(1976): Arndt KA+, *JAMA* 235, 918 (2.3%)
(1967): Nichols JT+, *Oral Surg Oral Med Oral Pathol* 24, 323
Baboon syndrome
(1997): Goossens C+, *Dermatology* 194, 421
Contact dermatitis (systemic)
(1996): Valsecchi R+, *Contact Dermatitis* 34, 428
(1995): Martins C+, *Contact Dermatitis* 33, 360
(1994): Fernandez Redondo V+, *Contact Dermatitis* 30, 311
(1994): Fernandez Redondo V+, *Contact Dermatitis* 30, 43
Eczema (sic)
Erythema multiforme
(1985): Ting HC+, *Int J Dermatol* 24, 587
Exanthems (1–5%)
(1995): Litt JZ, Beachwood, OH (personal case) (observation)
(1991): Igea JM+, *Ann Allergy* 66, 216
(1989): Pendleton N+, *Br J Clin Prac* 43, 464
(1979): Hartigan DA+, *Lancet* 2, 411
(1973): Shapera RM+, *JAMA* 226, 531 (3.5%)
Fixed eruption
(1998): Mahboob A+, *Int J Dermatol* 37, 833
(1991): Florido-Lopez JF+, *Allergy* 46, 77
(1991): Mutalik S, *Int J Dermatol* 30, 751
(1986): Kanwar AJ+, *Dermatologica* 172, 315
(1984): Pigatto PD, *Acta Derm Venereol* (Stockh) 64, 272
(1976): Naik RPC+, *Dermatologica* 152, 177 (bullous)
Pruritus
Pustular eruption
(1993): Manu Shah R+, *Eur J Dermatol* 3, 576
Rash (sic) (<1%)
(1992): Shirin H+, *Ann Pharmacother* 26, 1522
(1989): Pendleton N+, *Br J Clin Pract* 43, 464
(1983): Furniss LD, *Drug Intell Clin Pharm* 17, 631
Red neck syndrome
(1992): Estrada V+, *Rev Clin Esp* (Spanish) 190, 100
Stevens–Johnson syndrome
(1998): N Z Medicines Adverse Reactions Committee (from Internet) (observation)
(1995): Lestico MR+, *Am J Health Syst Pharm* 52, 1805
(1995): Pandha HS+, *N Z Med J* 108, 13
(1993): Leenutaphong V+, *Int J Dermatol* 32, 428
(1983): Fischer PR+, *Am J Dis Child* 137, 914
Toxic epidermal necrolysis
(1995): Kuper K+, *Ophthalmologe* (German) 92, 823
(1995): Raymond F+, *Arch Pediatr* (French) 2, 494
(1993): Leenutaphong V+, *Int J Dermatol* 32, 428
(1991): Porteous DM+, *Arch Dermatol* 127, 740 (in AIDS)
(1987): Guillaume JC+, *Arch Dermatol* 123, 1166
(1985): Lund-Kofoed ML+, *Contact Dermatitis* 13, 273
(1974): Czaplinska W+, *Pol Tyg Lek* (Polish) 29, 1263
Urticaria
(1998): Siegfried EC+, *J Am Acad Dermatol* 39, 797 (passim)
(1993): Lopez-Serrano C+, *Allergol Immunopathol Madr* (Spanish) 21, 225
(1976): van Ketel WG, *Contact Dermatitis* 2, 363
(1960): Prasard AS, *N Engl J Med* 262, 139
Vasculitis
(1985): Sanchez NP+, *Arch Dermatol* 121 220

## Other

Anaphylactoid reactions
(1998): Siegfried EC+, *J Am Acad Dermatol* 39, 797 (passim)
(1996): Jorro G+, *Ann Allergy Asthma Immunol* 77, 456
Enamel hypoplasia (teeth)
(1965): Adno J+, *SA Tydskrif vir Geneeskunde* (English), 1124
Gingival hyperplasia
(1992): Valsecchi R+, *Acta Derm Venereol* (Stockh) 72, 157
Glossodynia
Hypersensitivity (1–10%)
(1999): Gallardo MA+, *Cutis* 64, 129
(1998): Kruppa A+, *Dermatology* 196(3), 335
(1982): Lombardi P+, *Contact Dermatitis* 8, 416
Infusion-site inflammation
(2001): Zimmerman T+, *Clin Drug Invest* 21, 527 (58%)
Infusion-site pain
(2001): Zimmerman T+, *Clin Drug Invest* 21, 527 (25%)
Infusion-site phlebitis (1–10%)
(1987): David LM, *Am J Hosp Pharm* 44, 732
(1986): Holt RJ+, *Clin Pharm* 5, 787
Injection-site irritation
(1983): Marlin GE+, *Hum Toxicol* 3, 593
Oral candidiasis (1–10%)

Oral ulceration
(1980): Evens RP+, *Drug Intell Clin Pharm* 14, 217
Phlebitis
(2001): de Dios Garcia-Diaz J+, *Med CLin* (Barc) 116(4), 133 (from intravenous administration)
Rhabdomyolysis
(1988): Tobert JA, *Am J Cardiol* 62, 28J (with Cyclosporine)
Stomatodynia
Thrombophlebitis
Tinnitus
Tooth discoloration
(1965): Adno J+, *SA Tydskrif vir Geneeskunde* (English), 1124

# ESMOLOL

**Trade name:** Brevibloc (Baxter)
**Indications:** Tachyarrhythmias, tachycardia
**Category:** Beta-adrenergic blocker; antiarrhythmic class II; antihypertensive
**Half-life:** 9 minutes
**Clinically important, potentially hazardous interactions with:** clonidine, verapamil

### *Reactions*

## Skin
Acne (<1%)
Cold extremities (sic)
Diaphoresis (>10%)
Eczema (<1%)
Edema (<1%)
Erythema (<1%)
Exfoliative dermatitis (<1%)
Facial edema
Flushing (<1%)
Necrosis (<1%)
Pallor (<1%)
Pigmentation (<1%)
Psoriasis (<1%)
Purpura
Rash (sic)
Urticaria

## Hair
Hair – alopecia

## Other
Dysgeusia
Infusion-site reactions (sic) (1–10%)
Injection-site inflammation
(1987): Benfield P+, *Drugs* 33, 392
Injection-site pain (8%)
Paresthesias (<1%)
Thrombophlebitis (<1%)
Xerostomia (<1%)

# ESOMEPRAZOLE

**Synonyms:** Perprazole; H 19918
**Trade name:** Nexium (AstraZeneca)
**Indications:** Gastroesophageal Reflux Disease (GERD)
**Category:** Proton pump inhibitor
**Half-life:** 1.5 hours
**Clinically important, potentially hazardous interactions with:** benzodiazepines, chlordiazepoxide, clonazepam, clorazepate, diazepam, digoxin, flurazepam, lorazepam, midazolam, oxazepam, quazepam, temazepam

### *Reactions*

## Skin
Acne (<1%)
Allergic reactions (sic) (<1%)
Angioedema (<1%)
Candidiasis (<1%)
Dermatitis (sic) (<1%)
Diaphoresis (<1%)
Edema, generalized (<1%)
Exanthems (<1%)
Facial flushing (<1%)
Flushing (<1%)
Fungal infection (sic) (<1%)
Peripheral edema (<1%)
Pruritus (<1%)
Pruritus ani (<1%)
Urticaria (<1%)

## Other
Arthralgia (<1%)
Depression (<1%)
Dysgeusia (<1%)
Fibromyalgia (<1%)
Hypesthesia (<1%)
Paresthesias (<1%)
Parosmia (<1%)
Polymyalgia (<1%)
Tinnitus (<1%)
Tongue edema (<1%)
Ulcerative stomatitis (<1%)
Vaginitis (<1%)
Xerostomia

# ESTAZOLAM

**Trade name:** ProSom (Abbott)
**Other common trade names:** *Domnamid; Esilgan; Eurodin; Kainever; Nuctalon; Tasedan*
**Indications:** Insomnia
**Category:** Benzodiazepine sedative-hypnotic
**Half-life:** 10–24 hours
**Clinically important, potentially hazardous interactions with:** indinavir, ritonavir

### *Reactions*

## Skin
Acne (<1%)
Allergic reactions (sic) (<1%)
Chills (<1%)

Dermatitis (sic) (<1%)
Diaphoresis (1–10%)
Edema (<1%)
Eyelid edema (<1%)
Flushing (1–10%)
Photosensitivity
Pruritus (1–10%)
Purpura (<1%)
Rash (sic) (>10%)
Urticaria (1–10%)
Vaginal pruritus (1–10%)
Xerosis (<1%)

### Other

Dysgeusia (1–10%)
Glossitis
Gynecomastia (<1%)
Myalgia (1–10%)
Oral ulceration (<1%)
Paresthesias (1–10%)
Sialopenia (>10%)
Sialorrhea (<1%)
Xerostomia (>10%)

## ESTRAMUSTINE

**Trade name:** Emcyt (Pharmacia & Upjohn)
**Other common trade name:** *Cellmusin*
**Indications:** Prostate carcinoma
**Category:** Antineoplastic; nitrogen mustard
**Half-life:** 20 hours
**Clinically important, potentially hazardous interactions with:** aldesleukin

#### *Reactions*

### Skin

Allergic reactions (sic)
(2001): Zelek L+, *Ann Oncol* 12(9), 1265
Edema (>10%)
Exanthems
(1971): Anderes A+, *Praxis* (German) 60, 1276
Flushing (1%)
Hot flashes (<1%)
Night sweats (<1%)
Pigmentary changes (sic) (<1%)
Pruritus (2%)
(1976): Nagel R+, *Med Klin* (German) 71, 1724
Purpura (3%)
Rash (sic) (1%)
Urticaria
Xerosis (2%)

### Hair

Hair – alopecia (<1%)

### Other

Death
(2001): Zelek L+, *Ann Oncol* 12(9), 1265
Gynecomastia (>10%)
Injection-site thrombophlebitis (1–10%)
(1976): Nagel R+, *Med Klin* (German) 71, 1724
Mastodynia (66%)
Thrombophlebitis (3%)
Tinnitus

## ESTROGENS

**Generic:**
**Chlorotrianisene**
Trade name: Tace
**Diethylstilbestrol**
Trade names: Cyren A; Destrol; Stilphostrol
**Estradiol**
Trade names: Estrace; Estraderm
**Estrogens, conjugated**
Trade name: Premarin
**Estrogens, esterified**
Trade names: Estratab; Menest
**Estrone**
Trade names: Estroject; Estronol; Gynogen; Theelin, etc.
**Estropipate**
Trade name: Ogen
**Ethinyl estradiol**
Trade name: Estinyl
**Quinestrol**
Trade name: Estrovis

#### *Reactions*

### Skin

Acanthosis nigricans
(1974): Banuchi SR+, *Arch Dermatol* 109, 544
Acne
Angioedema
(2000): McGlinchey PG+, *Am J Med Sci* 320, 212
(1942): Saphir WS+, *JAMA* 119, 557
Ankle edema
Bullous eruption
(1971): Kuchera LK, *JAMA* 218, 562
Chloasma (<1%)
Contact dermatitis
(1981): Ljunggren B, *Contact Dermatitis* 7, 141,
Dermatitis (sic)
(1995): Shelley WB+, *J Am Acad Dermatol* 32, 25
Eczema (sic)
(1995): Shelley WB+, *J Am Acad Dermatol* 32, 25
Edema (<1%)
Erythema multiforme
(1998): Moghadam BK+, *Oral Surg Oral Med Oral Pathol Oral Radiol Endod* 85, 537
Erythema nodosum
(1990): Bartelsmeyer JA+, *Clin Obstet Gynecol* 33, 777
(1980): Salvatore MA+, *Arch Dermatol* 116, 557
Exanthems
(1999): Coustou D+, *Ann Dermatol Venereol* 125, 484
(1999): Kumar A+, *Australas J Dermatol* 40, 96
(1997): Litt JZ, Beachwood, OH (personal case) (observation)
(1984): Lee M+, *J Urol* 131, 767
Exfoliative dermatitis
(1942): Kasselberg LA, *JAMA* 120, 117
Fixed eruption (<1%)
Flushing
(1981): Ingle JN+, *N Engl J Med* 304, 16 (3%)
(1973): Delius L, *Dtsch Med Wochenschr* (German) 98, 1512
Hot flashes
(2001): Spetz AC+, *J Urol* 166(2), 517
Hyperkeratosis of nipples
(1980): Mold DE+, *Cutis* 26, 95
Irritation (sic) (from transdermal system)
Livedo reticularis
Lupus erythematosus
(1989): Colins D, *J Rheumatol* 16, 408

(1986): Barrett C+, *Br J Rheumatol* 25, 300
(1973): Elias PM, *Arch Dermatol* 108, 716
(1971): Kay DR+, *Arthritis Rheum* 14, 239 (5%) (ANA only)
(1971): Laugier P+, *Bull Soc Fr Syphiligr* (French) 78, 623 (SLE-induced)
(1969): Bole CG+, *Lancet* 1, 323
(1968): Hadida E+, *Bull Soc Fr Syphiligr* (French) 75, 616
(1968): Schleicher EM, *Lancet* 1, 821
(1966): Pimstone BL, *S Afr J Obstet Gynecol* 3, 62

Melasma (<1%)
(1992): Breathnach SM+, *Adverse Drug Reactions and the Skin* Blackwell, Oxford, 274 (passim)
(1967): Resnic S, *JAMA* 199, 601

Mucha–Habermann disease
(1973): Hollander A+, *Arch Dermatol* 107, 465

Papulovesicular eruption
(1999): Coustou D+, *Ann Dermatol* 125, 484
(1998): Coustou D+, *Ann Dermatol Venereol* (French) 125, 505

Peripheral edema

Photoreactions

Photosensitivity
(1970): Mathison IW+, *Obstet Gynecol Surv* 25, 389
(1968): Erickson LR+, *JAMA* 203, 980
(1965): Daniels F, *Med Clin North Am* 49, 565

Pigmentation
(1999): Oakley A, Auckland, New Zealand (from Internet) (observation) (from topical, over vulva)
(1972): Ippen H+, *Hautarzt* (German) 23, 21 (chloasma)
(1967): Resnic S, *JAMA* 199, 601

Pruritus
(2000): Siepmann M+, *Dtsch Med Wochenschr* (German) 125, 557
(1999): Coustou D+, *Ann Dermatol Venereol* 125, 484
(1999): Kumar A+, *Australas J Dermatol* 40, 96
(1998): Coustou D+, *Ann Dermatol Venereol* (French) 125, 505
(1995): Shelley WB+, *J Am Acad Dermatol* 32, 25
(1971): Kuchera LK, *JAMA* 218, 562

Purpura
(1984): Lee M+, *J Urol* 131, 767

Rash (sic) (<1%)

Raynaud's phenomenon
(1998): Fraenkel L+, *Ann Intern Med* 129, 208

Scleroderma
(2000): D'Cruz D, *Toxicol Lett* 112 and 421

Spider nevi
(1992): Breathnach SM+, *Adverse Drug Reactions and the Skin* Blackwell, Oxford, 274 (passim)

Striae

Telangiectases
(1970): Aram H+, *Acta Derm Venereol* 50, 302

Urticaria
(1998): Moghadam BK+, *Oral Surg Oral Med Oral Pathol Oral Radiol Endod* 85, 537
(1995): Shelley WB+, *J Am Acad Dermatol* 32, 25
(1984): Lee M+, *J Urol* 131, 767
(1964): Beall GN, *Medicine* (Baltimore) 43, 131

Vasculitis (cutaneous polyarteritis nodosa)
(1998): Cvancara JL+, *J Am Acad Dermatol* 39, 643

Vesicular eruptions
(1999): Kumar A+, *Australas J Dermatol* 40, 96

## Hair

Hair – alopecia
(1992): Breathnach SM+, *Adverse Drug Reactions and the Skin* Blackwell, Oxford, 233 (passim)

Hair – hirsutism
(1971): Fusi S+, *Folia Endocrinol* (Italian) 24, 412

Hair – straight
(1994): Litt JZ, Beachwood, OH (personal case) (observation)

## Nails

Nails – onycholysis
(1976): Byrne JP+, *Post Grad Med J* 52, 535

## Other

Acute intermittent porphyria

Dry eye syndrome
(2001): Schaumberg DA+, *JAMA* 286(17), 2114

Galactorrhea

Gingival hyperplasia

Gynecomastia (>10%)
(2000): Felner EI+, *Pediatrics* 105, E55 (3 prepubertal boys from an estrogen cream)
(1987): Schmidt KU+, *Dtsch Med Wochenschr* (German) 112, 926
(1984): Gottswinter JM+, *Haarwasser Med Klin* (German) 79, 181
(1978): Gabilove JL+, *Arch Dermatol* 114, 1672
(1969): Degos R+, *Ann Dermatol Syphiligr Paris* (French) 96, 5
(1969): Goebel M, *Hautarzt* (German) 20, 521
(1968): Stewart WM+, *Bull Soc Fr Dermatol Syphiligr* (French) 75, 294

Injection-site pain (1–10%)

Mastodynia (>10%)
(2002): Arrenbrecht S+, *Osteoporos Int* 13(2), 176 (17%)

Oral mucosal eruption
(1998): Moghadam BK+, *Oral Surg Oral Med Oral Pathol Oral Radiol Endod* 85, 537

Oral mucosal pigmentation
(1991): Perusse R+, *Cutis* 48, 61

Osteoma cutis
(2002): Stockel S+, *Hautarzt* 53(1), 37

Porphyria
(1994): Siersema PD+, *Eur J Gastroenterol Hepatol* 6, 371
(1989): CoulsonDH+, *Br J Urol* 63, 648

Porphyria cutanea tarda
(1995): Nonaka S+, *Nippon Rinsho* (Japanese) 53, 1427
(1990): Roger D+, *Ann Dermatol Venereol* (French) 117, 127
(1982): Enriquez de Salamanca R+, *Arch Dermatol Res* 274, 179
(1979): Grossman ME+, *Am J Med* 67, 277
(1979): Sweeney GD+, *Can Med Assoc J* 120, 803
(1978): Benedetto AV+, *Cutis* 21, 483
(1976): Byrne JP+, *Post Grad Med J* 52, 535
(1975): Haberman HF+, *Can Med Assoc J* 113, 653
(1975): Malina L+, *Br J Dermatol* 92, 707
(1975): Wanscher B, *Ugeskr Laeger* (Danish) 137, 623
(1973): Gajdos A+, *Nouv Presse Med* (French) 2, 1131
(1973): Palma-Carlos AG+, *Nouv Presse Med* (French) 2, 1996
(1971): Barth J+, *Dermatol Monatsschr* (German) 157, 160
(1971): Stein KM+, *Obstet Gynecol* 38, 755
(1970): Roenigk HH+, *Arch Dermatol* 102, 260
(1969): Duverne+, *Lyon Med* (French) 221, 1097
(1966): Levere RD, *Blood* 28, 569
(1965): Becker FT, *Arch Dermatol* 92, 252
(1964): Theologides H+, *Metabolism* 13, 391
(1963): Hurley HJ, *Arch Dermatol* 88, 233
(1963): Walshe M, *Br J Dermatol* 75, 298

Vaginal candidiasis

# ETANERCEPT

**Trade name:** Enbrel (Immunex)
**Indications:** Rheumatoid arthritis
**Category:** Antirheumatic; biologic response modifying; anti-arthritic
**Half-life:** 98–300 hours

### *Reactions*

## Skin

Allergic reactions (sic) (<3%)
Cellulitis
(2002): Gorman JD+, *N Engl J Med* 346, 1349
Erythema
Exanthems
(2002): Conaghan P+, *Skin & Allergy News* June, 40
Herpes zoster
(2001): Hogarty T, (from Internet) (observation) (generalized)
Infections (sic) (<3%)
(2002): Gorman JD+, *N Engl J Med* 346, 1349
(2002): Phillips K+, *Arthritis Rheum* 47(1), 17
(2002): Steensma DP+, *Blood* 99(6), 2252
(2001): Baghai M+, *Mayo Clin Proc* 76(6), 653
Lupus erythematosus
(2002): Shakoor N+, *Lancet* 359 (4 cases)
(2001): Bleumink GS+, *Rheumatology* (Oxford) 40, 1317
(2001): Werth V, *Dermatology Times* 18
(1999): Brion PH+, *Ann Intern Med* 131, 634 (discoid)
Malignancies (sic) (<3%)
Pruritus
Rash (sic) (5%)
(2000): *Nurses' Drug Alert*, 24, 4
(1999): Brion PH+, *Ann Int Med* 131, 634
Skin disorders (sic)
(2001): Sandborn WJ+, *Gastroenterology* 121(5), 1088
Squamous cell carcinoma
(2001): Smith KJ+, *J Am Acad Dermatol* 45(6), 953 (7 cases)
(2000): Smith KJ+, Academy of Dermatology Meeting San Francisco Poster Exhibit
Ulceration
Upper respiratory tract infection
(2001): Alldred A, *Expert Opin Pharmacother* 2(7), 1137
Urticaria
(2000): Skytta E+, *Clin Exp Rheumatol* 18, 533
Vasculitis
(2002): Conaghan P+, *Skin & Allergy News* June, 40
(2001): Werth V, *Dermatology Times* 18
(2000): Galaria NA+, *J Rheumatol* 27, 2041 (leukocytoclastic)
(1999): Brion PH+, *Ann Intern Med* 131, 634 (necrotizing)

## Other

Death
(2002): Phillips K+, *Arthritis Rheum* 47(1), 17
(2001): Baghai M+, *Mayo Clin Proc* 76(6), 653
Injection-site reactions (20–40%)
(2002): Gorman JD+, *N Engl J Med* 346, 1349
(2002): Steensma DP+, *Blood* 99(6), 2252
(2001): Alldred A, *Expert Opin Pharmacother* 2(7), 1137
(2001): Girolomoni G+, *Arch Dermatol* 137, 784
(2001): Sandborn WJ+, *Gastroenterology* 121(5), 1088
(2001): Werth V, *Dermatology Times* 18
(2001): Werth VP+, *Arch Dermatol* 137(7), 953
(2001): Zeltser R+, *Arch Dermatol* 137(7), 893
(2001): Zeltser R+, *Arch Dermatol* 137, 893 (20%)
(2000): Bathon JM+, *N Engl J Med* 343, 1586
(2000): Lovell DJ+, *N Engl J Med* 342, 763
(2000): Mease PJ, *Lancet* 356, 385
(2000): Murphy FT+, *Arch Dermatol* 136, 556
(1999): Jarvis B+, *Drugs* 57, 945
(1999): Moreland LW+, *Ann Intern Med* 130, 478
(1999): Moreland LW+, *Arthritis Rheum* 41, S364 (Suppl)
(1999): Weinblatt ME+, *N Engl J Med* 340, 253
Multiple sclerosis
(2001): Sicotte NL+, *Neurology* 57(10), 1885
Rheumatoid nodules (sic)
(2002): Kekow J+, *Arthritis Rheum* 46(3), 843
Tinnitus
(2002): Gorman JD+, *N Engl J Med* 346, 1349

# ETHACRYNIC ACID

**Trade name:** Edecrin (Merck)
**Other common trade names:** *Edecril; Edecrina; Hydromedin; Reomax*
**Indications:** Edema
**Category:** Loop diuretic
**Half-life:** 2–4 hours
**Clinically important, potentially hazardous interactions with:** amikacin, aminoglycosides, digoxin, gentamicin, kanamycin, neomycin, streptomycin, tobramycin

### *Reactions*

## Skin

Allergic reactions (sic)
Chills (<1%)
Exanthems
(1966): Sherlock S+, *Lancet* 1, 1049
Photosensitivity
Purpura (<1%)
Rash (sic) (<1%)
Urticaria
Vasculitis
(1992): Breathnach SM+, *Adverse Drug Reactions and the Skin* Blackwell, Oxford, 229 (passim)
(1967): Bar-on H+, *Isr J Med Sci* 3, 113

## Other

Injection-site pain
Thrombophlebitis (<1%)
Tinnitus
Xerostomia

# ETHAMBUTOL

**Trade name:** Myambutol (Dura)
**Other common trade names:** *Apo-Ethambutol; Dexambutol; EMB; Etapiam; Etibi; Stambutol*
**Indications:** Tuberculosis
**Category:** Antimycobacterial
**Half-life:** 3–4 hours

### *Reactions*

## Skin

Acne
Angioedema
(1985): Holdiness MR, *Int J Dermatol* 24, 280
Bullous eruption

(1985): Holdiness MR, *Int J Dermatol* 24, 280
(1981): Frentz G+, *Acta Derm Venereol* (Stockh) 61, 89
Chills
Contact dermatitis
(1986): Holdiness MR, *Contact Dermatitis* 15, 282
(1986): Holdiness MR, *Contact Dermatitis* 15, 96
Dermatitis (sic)
Diaphoresis
(1985): Holdiness MR, *Int J Dermatol* 24, 280
Erythema multiforme
(1985): Holdiness MR, *Int J Dermatol* 24, 280
(1981): Frentz G+, *Acta Derm Venereol* (Stockh) 61, 89
Exanthems
(1985): Holdiness MR, *Int J Dermatol* 24, 280
(1981): Frentz G+, *Acta Derm Venereol* (Stockh) 61, 89 (1–5%)
(1977): Pasricha JS+, *Arch Dermatol* 113, 1122
Exfoliative dermatitis
(1985): Holdiness MR, *Int J Dermatol* 24, 280
Lichenoid eruption
(1995): Grossman ME+, *J Am Acad Dermatol* 33, 675
(1981): Frentz G+, *Acta Derm Venereol* (Stockh) 61, 89
Lupus erythematosus
(1986): Layer P+, *Dtsch Med Wochenschr* (German) 111,1603
(1977): Djawari D, *Z Hautkr* (German) 53, 180
Photosensitivity
(1994): Berger TG+, *Arch Dermatol* 130, 609 (in HIV-infected)
Pruritus (<1%)
(1985): Holdiness MR, *Int J Dermatol* 24, 280
(1981): Frentz G+, *Acta Derm Venereol* (Stockh) 61, 89
(1969): Council on Drugs, *JAMA* 208, 2463
Purpura
(1972): Levantine A+, *Br J Dermatol* 86, 651
Rash (sic) (<1%)
(1995): Chaisson RE, *Infections in Medicine* 12, 48
(1995): Wong PC+, *Eur Respir J* 8, 866
Stevens–Johnson syndrome
(1979): Surjapranata FJ+, *Paediatr Indones* 19, 195
Toxic epidermal necrolysis
(1985): Heng MCY, *Br J Dermatol* 106, 107
(1981): Pegram PS+, *Arch Intern Med* 141, 1677
Urticaria
(1985): Holdiness MR, *Int J Dermatol* 24, 280
(1981): Frentz G+, *Acta Derm Venereol* (Stockh) 61, 89

### Hair

Hair – alopecia
(1985): Holdiness MR, *Int J Dermatol* 24, 280

### Other

Anaphylactoid reactions (<1%)
Dyschromatopsia
Hypersensitivity
(1995): Dhamgaye T+, *Tuber Lung Dis* 76,181
Paresthesias

## ETHANOLAMINE

**Trade name:** Ethamolin (Cypros)
**Other common trade name:** *Ethanolamine oleate*
**Indications:** Bleeding esophageal varices
**Category:** Sclerosing agent
**Half-life:** no data
**Clinically important, potentially hazardous interactions with:** acitretin, amobarbital, aprobarbital, butabarbital, disulfiram, insulin, mephobarbital, pentobarbital, phenobarbital, primidone, secobarbital, thiopental

### *Reactions*

### Skin

Contact dermatitis
(1995): Kock P, *Contact Dermatitis* 33, 273
(1994): Aranzabal A+, *Contact Dermatitis* 31, 121
(1994): Ortiz-Frutos FJ+, *Contact Dermatitis* 31, 193
(1994): Schnuch A, *Contact Dermatitis* 30, 243

### Other

Anaphylactoid reactions (<1%)
Injection-site necrosis

## ETHCHLORVYNOL

**Trade name:** Placidyl (Abbott)
**Other common trade names:** *Arvynol; Nostel*
**Indications:** Insomnia
**Category:** Sedative-hypnotic
**Half-life:** 10–20 hours
**Clinically important, potentially hazardous interactions with:** antihistamines, brompheniramine, buclizine, chlorpheniramine, dexchlorpheniramine, meclizine, tripelennamine

### *Reactions*

### Skin

Allergic reactions (sic)
Bullous eruption (from overdose)
(1990): Yell RP, *Am J Emerg Med* 8, 246
(1980): Brodin MD+, *J Cutan Pathol* 7, 326
Diaphoresis
Facial numbness (sic)
Fixed eruption
(1965): Auerbach R, *Arch Dermatol* 92, 184
Pruritus
Purpura
(1972): Jakobson ES, *Ann Intern Med* 77, 73 (fatal)
Rash (sic) (1–10%)
Urticaria

### Other

Acute intermittent porphyria
Death
Dysgeusia (>10%)
Hypersensitivity
Paresthesias
Pressure necrosis
(1990): Chamberlain JM+, *Am J Emerg Med* 8, 467

## ETHIONAMIDE

**Trade name:** Trecator-SC (Wyeth-Ayerst)
**Other common trade names:** *Ethatyl; Etiocidan; Myobid-250; Tubermin*
**Indications:** Tuberculosis
**Category:** Tuberculostatic
**Half-life:** 2–3 hours

### *Reactions*

#### Skin

Acne
(1992): Breathnach SM+, *Adverse Drug Reactions and the Skin* Blackwell, Oxford (passim)
(1965): 3, 61
(1963): Lees AW, *Am Rev Respir Dis* 88, 347
Allergic reactions (sic)
(1971): *Med Lett* 13, 55 (1%)
Butterfly eruptions on the face (sic)
(1992): Breathnach SM+, *Adverse Drug Reactions and the Skin* Blackwell, Oxford (passim)
Eczema (sic) (chiefly involving the forehead)
(1992): Breathnach SM+, *Adverse Drug Reactions and the Skin* Blackwell, Oxford, 159 (passim)
Exanthems
(1969): Agrawal R, *BMJ* 4, 540
(1965): Carey VCI, *Tubercle* 46, 287
Ichthyosis
(1972): Levantine A+, *Br J Dermatol* 86, 651
Lupus erythematosus
(1973): Desmons MF, *Bull Soc Fr Dermatol Syphiligr* (French) 80, 168
Pellagra
(1987): Schmutz JL+, *Ann Dermatol Venereol* (French) 114, 569
Photosensitivity
(1966): Baran R, *Hôpital* (French) 54, 445
(1966): Friedmann ME, *Bull Soc Franc Dermatol Syphiligr* (French) 73, 510
Purpura
(1992): Breathnach SM+, *Adverse Drug Reactions and the Skin* Blackwell, Oxford (passim)
Rash (sic) (<1%)
Seborrheic dermatitis
(1972): Levantine A+, *Br J Dermatol* 86, 651
Urticaria (1–5%)

#### Hair

Hair – alopecia (<1%)
(1992): Breathnach SM+, *Adverse Drug Reactions and the Skin* Blackwell, Oxford, 159 (passim)
(1966): Baran R, *Hôpital* (French) 54, 445

#### Other

Dysgeusia (1–10%) (metallic taste)
Gynecomastia (<1%)
Oral ulceration
Sialorrhea
Stomatitis (<1%)
(1992): Breathnach SM+, *Adverse Drug Reactions and the Skin* Blackwell, Oxford (passim)
Stomatodynia
Xerostomia

## ETHOSUXIMIDE

**Trade name:** Zarontin (Parke-Davis)
**Other common trade names:** *Emeside; Ethymal; Petnidan; Pyknolepsinum; Simatin; Zarondan*
**Indications:** Absence (petit mal) seizures
**Category:** Succinimide anticonvulsant
**Half-life:** 50–60 hours

### *Reactions*

#### Skin

Cutaneous side effects (sic) (3.4%)
(1966): Weinstein AW+, *Am J Dis Child* 111, 63
Erythema multiforme (<1%)
(1966): Coursin DB, *JAMA* 198, 113
Exanthems (1–5%)
(1991): Pelekanos J+, *Epilepsia* 32, 554
(1966): Weinstein AW+, *Am J Dis Child* 111, 63 (2.2%)
Exfoliative dermatitis (<1%)
Lupus erythematosus (>10%)
(1996): Miyasaka N, *Intern Med 35, 527*
(1996): Takeda S+, *Intern Med* 35, 587
(1996): Wallace SJ, *Drug Saf* 15, 378
(1994): Riviello JJ+, *J Epilepsy* 7, 23
(1993): Ansell BM, *Lupus* 2, 193
(1993): Drory VE+, *Clin Neuropharmacol* 16, 19 (passim)
(1985): Lovisetto P+, *Recenti Prog Med* (Italian) 76, 84
(1984): Koike K+, *Rinsho Ketsueki* 25, 1635
(1979): Tor J+, *Med Clin (Barc)* (Spanish) 73, 443
(1976): Singsen BH+, *Pediatrics* 57, 529
(1975): Teoh PC+, *Arch Dis Child* 50, 658 (morphea-like)
(1973): Beernink DH+, *J Pediatr* 82, 113
(1970): Alter BP, *J Pediatr* 77, 1093
(1970): Dabbous IA+, *J Pediatr* 76, 617
(1968): Livingston S+, *JAMA* 203, 731
(1968): Monnet P+, *Lyon Med* (French) 220, 467
Periorbital edema
Pruritus
Purpura
(1967): Kontsouliers E, *Lancet* 2, 310
Rash (sic) (<1%)
Raynaud's phenomenon
(1990): Rose CD+, *Arthritis Rheum* 33 (Suppl) R23
(1975): Taaffe A+, *Br Dent J* 138, 172
(1966): Coursin DB, *JAMA* 198, 113
Stevens–Johnson syndrome (>10%)
(1975): Taaffe A+, *Br Dent J* 138, 172
Urticaria (1–5%)
(1966): Weinstein AW+, *Am J Dis Child* 111, 63 (1%)

#### Hair

Hair – alopecia
Hair – hirsutism

#### Other

Acute intermittent porphyria
Gingival hyperplasia
Oral ulceration
Tongue edema

## ETHOTOIN

**Trade name:** Peganone (Abbott)
**Other common trade name:** *Accenon*
**Indications:** Tonic–clonic (grand mal) seizures
**Category:** Hydantoin anticonvulsant
**Half-life:** 3–9 hours
**Clinically important, potentially hazardous interactions with:** chloramphenicol, cyclosporine, disulfiram, dopamine, imatinib, itraconazole

### *Reactions*

#### Skin
Bullous eruption
Fixed eruption
Lupus erythematosus
Purpura
(1967): Coleman WP, *Med Clin North Am* 51, 1073
Rash (sic)

#### Other
Gingival hyperplasia

## ETIDRONATE

**Trade name:** Didronel (MGI)
**Other common trade names:** *Didronate; Difosfen; Dinol; Diphos; Osteum*
**Indications:** Paget's disease, osteoporosis
**Category:** Bone resorption inhibitor; antihypercalcemic
**Half-life:** 6 hours

### *Reactions*

#### Skin
Angioedema (<1%)
Exanthems
Pruritus
(1985): Holzmann H+, *Hautarzt* (German) 36, 326
Rash (sic) (<1%)
Stevens–Johnson syndrome
Toxic epidermal necrolysis
(1995): Coakley G+, *Br J Rheumatol* 34, 798
Urticaria

#### Hair
Hair – alopecia

#### Other
Ageusia
Dysgeusia (<1%)
Glossitis
Hypersensitivity (<1%)
Paresthesias
Stomatitis

## ETODOLAC

**Trade name:** Lodine (Wyeth-Ayerst)
**Other common trade names:** *Antilak; Ecridoxan; Edolan; Elderin; Lonine; Tedolan; Utradol; Zedolac*
**Indications:** Pain
**Category:** Nonsteroidal anti-inflammatory (NSAID)
**Half-life:** 7 hours
**Clinically important, potentially hazardous interactions with:** aspirin, methotrexate

### *Reactions*

#### Skin
Angioedema (<1%)
(1991): Astorga-Paulsen G+, *Curr Med Res Opin* 12, 401
Bullous eruption
Dermatitis (sic)
Diaphoresis
Ecchymoses
Edema
Erythema multiforme (<1%)
Exanthems
(1998): Litt JZ, Beachwood, OH (personal case) (observation)
(1997): Litt JZ, Beachwood, OH (personal case) (observation)
(1990): Schattenkirchner M, *Eur J Rheumatol Inflamm* 10, 56
(1986): Lynch S+, *Drugs* 31, 288 (3%)
Exfoliation (sic)
Exfoliative dermatitis
Facial edema
(1991): Astorga-Paulsen G+, *Curr Res Med Opin* 12, 401
(1990): Freitas GG, *Curr Med Res Opin* 12, 255
Fixed eruption
(1997): Blumenthal HL, Beachwood, OH (personal case) (observation)
Flushing
(1991): Astorga-Paulsen G+, *Curr Med Res Opin* 12, 401
Furunculosis
(1987): Waltham-Weeks CD, *Curr Med Res Opin* 10, 540
Peripheral edema
(1990): Freitas GG, *Curr Med Res Opin* 12, 255
Photosensitivity
(1987): Waltham-Weeks CD, *Curr Med Res Opin* 10, 540
Pigmentation
Pruritus (1–10%)
(1998): Litt JZ, Beachwood, OH (personal case) (observation)
(1991): Astorga-Paulsen G+, *Curr Res Med Opin* 12, 401
(1991): Balfour JA+, *Drugs* 42, 274
(1991): Bianchi-Porro G+, *J Intern Med* 229, 5
(1991): *Med Lett Drug Ther* 33, 79
(1991): Karbowski A, *Curr Med Res Opin* 12, 309
(1990): Schattenkirchner M, *Eur J Rheumatol Inflamm* 10, 56
(1989): Ciocci A, *Curr Med Res Opin* 11, 471
Purpura
Rash (sic) (>10%)
(1991): Anon, *Med Lett Drug Ther* 33, 79
(1991): Astorga-Paulsen G+, *Curr Med Res Opin* 12, 401
(1991): Balfour JA+, *Drugs* 42, 274
(1989): Ciocci A, *Curr Med Res Opin* 11, 471
(1989): Williams PI+, *Curr Med Res Opin*
Stevens–Johnson syndrome (<1%)
Toxic epidermal necrolysis (<1%)
Urticaria (<1%)
(2000): Mitchell D, Thomasville, GA (from Internet) (observation)

(1996): Thaler D, Monona, WI (personal case) (pressure) (observation)
Vasculitis
(1996): Lie JT+, *J Rheumatol* 23, 183 (hypersensitivity)
(1989): Willemin B+, *Ann Méd Int* (French) 140, 529
Vesiculobullous eruption

### Hair

Hair – alopecia

### Other

Gingival ulceration
Glossitis
Gynecomastia
Parageusia
Paresthesias
Sialorrhea
Stomatitis
Tinnitus
Ulcerative stomatitis
Xerostomia

## ETOPOSIDE

**Synonyms:** epipodophyllotoxin; VP-16; VP-16–213
**Trade name:** VePesid (Bristol-Myers Squibb)
**Other common trade names:** *Aside; Etopos; Etosid; Lastet; Serozide; Vepeside; VP-TEC*
**Indications:** Lymphomas, carcinomas
**Category:** Antineoplastic
**Half-life:** terminal: 4–15 hours
**Clinically important, potentially hazardous interactions with:** aldesleukin, cyclosporine

#### *Reactions*

### Skin

Allergic reactions (sic) (1–2%)
Diaphoresis
Ecchymoses
Eccrine squamous syringometaplasia
(1997): Valks R+, *Arch Dermatol* 133, 873
Erythema
(1994): Portal I+, *Cancer Chemother Pharmacol* 34, 181 (acral)
(1993): Dechaufour F+, *Ann Dermatol Venereol* (French) 120, 219 (acral)
(1993): Vukelja SJ+, *Cutis* 52, 89 (acral)
Erythema multiforme
(1987): Yokel BK+, *J Cutan Pathol* 14, 326
Exanthems
(1992): Beyer J+, *Bone Marrow Transplant* 10, 491
(1992): Breathnach SM+, *Adverse Drug Reactions and the Skin* Blackwell, Oxford, 301 (passim)
(1987): Yokel BK+, *J Cutan Pathol* 14, 326
(1981): Weiss RB+, *Ann Intern Med* 94, 66
Facial edema
Flushing (<1%)
(1990): Henwood JM+, *Drugs* 39, 438
(1988): Ogle KM+, *Am J Clin Oncol* 11, 663
(1985): Tucci E+, *Chemioterapia* 4, 460
Pigmentation
(2001): Mutafoglu-Uysal K+, *Turk J Pediatr* 43(2), 172
(1991): Singal R+, *Pediatr Dermatol 8, 231*
Pruritus
Purpura
Radiation recall
(1993): Williams BJ+, *Clin Exp Dermatol* 18, 452 (ultraviolet)
(1992): Breathnach SM+, *Adverse Drug Reactions and the Skin* Blackwell, Oxford, 301 (passim)
(1987): Yokel BK+, *J Cutan Pathol* 14, 326
Rash (sic)
Stevens–Johnson syndrome
(1992): Breathnach SM+, *Adverse Drug Reactions and the Skin* Blackwell, Oxford, 301 (passim)
(1987): Yokel BK+, *J Cutan Pathol* 14, 326
(1983): Jameson CH+, *Cancer Treat Rep* 67, 1050
Urticaria

### Hair

Hair – alopecia (8–66%)
(1990): Henwood JM+, *Drugs* 39, 438 (100%, dose-dependent)
(1989): Smit EF+, *Thorax* 44, 631
(1989): Wander HE+, *Cancer Chemother Pharmacol* 24, 261
(1989): Yoshino M+, *Jpn J Clin Oncol* 19, 120 (57%)

### Nails

Nails – Beau's lines (transverse nail bands)
(1994): Ben-Dayan D+, *Acta Haematol* 91, 89
Nails – onycholysis
(1995): Obermair A+, *Gynecol Oncol* 57, 436

### Other

Anaphylactoid reactions (<2%)
(1989): Siddall SJ+, *Lancet* 1, 394
(1989): Wander HE+, *Cancer Chemother Pharmacol* 24, 261
Dysgeusia
Hypersensitivity (<1%)
(2002): Siderov J+, *Br J Cancer* 86(1), 12
(2001): Mutafoglu-Uysal K+, *Turk J Pediatr* 43(2), 172
(1993): Hudson MM+, *J Clin Oncol* 11, 1080
(1992): Weiss RB, *Semin Oncol* 19, 458
(1991): Kellie SJ+, *Cancer* 67, 1070
(1988): Ogle KM+, *Am J Clin Oncol* 11, 663
(1985): Tucci E+, *Chemioterapia* 4, 460
(1984): O'Dwyer PJ+, *Cancer Treat Rep* 68, 959
Injection-site pain
Mucositis (>10%)
Oral mucosal lesions
(1990): Henwood JM+, *Drugs* 39, 438 (1–5%)
Paresthesias
Stomatitis (1–10%)
Thrombophlebitis (<1%)
Tongue edema

## EXEMESTANE

**Trade name:** Aromasin (Pharmacia & Upjohn)
**Indications:** advanced breast cancer
**Category:** antineoplastic (steroidal aromatase inactivator)
**Half-life:** 24 hours

#### *Reactions*

### Skin

Diaphoresis (6%)
(2000): Clemett D+, *Drugs* 59, 1279
(1997): Thurlimann B+, *Eur J Cancer* 33, 1767 (12%)
Edema (7%)
Flu-like syndrome
Hot flashes (13%)
(2000): Clemett D+, *Drugs* 59, 1279
(1999): Jones S+, *J Clin Oncol* 17, 3418

(1998): Paridaens R+, *Anticancer Drugs* 9, 675 (30%)
(1997): Thurlimann B+, *Eur J Cancer* 33, 1767 (21%)
Infections (sic)
Lymphedema (2–5%)
Peripheral edema
(1997): Thurlimann B+, *Eur J Cancer* 33, 1767 (9%)
Pruritus (2–5%)
Rash (sic) (2–5%)

## Hair

Hair – alopecia (2–5%)

## Other

Hypesthesia
Paresthesias (2–5%)
Tumor-site pain
(1998): Paridaens R+, *Anticancer Drugs* 9, 675 (30%)

## FAMCICLOVIR

**Trade name:** Famvir (Novartis)
**Indications:** Acute herpes zoster, recurrent genital herpes
**Category:** Antiviral
**Half-life:** 2–3 hours

### *Reactions*

#### Skin
Dermatitis (sic)
(1996): Sacks SL+, *JAMA* 276, 44
Pruritus (3.7%)

#### Other
Hypersensitivity
(2001): Kawsar M+, *Sex Transm Infect* 77(3), 204
Paresthesias (2.6%)

## FAMOTIDINE

**Trade name:** Pepcid (Merck)
**Other common trade names:** *Amfamox; Apo-Famotidine; Durater; Famodil; Famoxal; Ganor; Gastro; Motiax; Mylanta AR; Nu-Famotidine; Pepcidine; Pepdul; Sigafam*
**Indications:** Duodenal ulcer, Gastroesophageal Reflux Disease (GERD)
**Category:** Histamine $H_2$-receptor antagonist and anti-ulcer
**Half-life:** 2.5–3.5 hours
**Clinically important, potentially hazardous interactions with:** cefditoren

### *Reactions*

#### Skin
Acne (<1%)
Allergic reactions (sic) (<1%)
Angioedema
(1986): Campoli-Richards DM+, *Drugs* 32, 197 (0.05%)
Contact dermatitis
(1994): Guimaraens D+, *Contact Dermatitis* 31, 259
(1990): Monteseirin J+, *Contact Dermatitis* 22, 290
Cutaneous side effects (sic)
(1986): Campoli-Richards DM+, *Drugs* 32, 197 (0.4%)
Dermographism
(1994): Warner DMc+, *J Am Acad Dermatol* 31, 677
Erythema multiforme
(1999): Horiuchi Y+, *Ann Intern Med* 131, 795
Exanthems
Facial edema
Flushing
(1986): Campoli-Richards DM+, *Drugs* 32, 197 (0.2%)
Periorbital edema
Pruritus (<1%)
(1994): Warner DMc+, *J Am Acad Dermatol* 31, 677
(1990): Edge DP, *N Z Med J* 103, 150
Purpura
(1996): Kallal SM+, *West J Med* 164, 446
Rash (sic)
(1989): McCullough AJ+, *Gastroenterology* 97, 860
(1989): Schunack W, *J Int Med Res* 17 (Suppl 1), 9A
Toxic epidermal necrolysis
(1995): Brunner M+, *Br J Dermatol* 133, 814
Urticaria (<1%)
(1994): Warner DMc+, *J Am Acad Dermatol* 31, 677
(1986): Campoli-Richards DM+, *Drugs* 32, 197 (0.1%)
Vasculitis
(1993): Torralba M+, *An Med Interna* (Spanish) 10, 621
(1990): Andreo JA+, *Med Clin<D (Barc) (Spanish) 95, 234*
Xerosis (<1%)

#### Hair
Hair – alopecia

#### Other
Dysgeusia
Gynecomastia
Injection-site pain
Myalgia
Oral mucosal lesions
(1986): Campoli-Richards DM+, *Drugs* 32, 197 (0.15%)
Paresthesias (<1%)
(1997): Litt JZ, Beachwood, OH (personal case) (observation)
(1997): Litt JZ, Beachwood, OH (personal case) (observation) (prickly sensation)
Tinnitus
Xerostomia
(1986): Campoli-Richards DM+, *Drugs* 32, 197 (0.15%)

## FELBAMATE

**Trade name:** Felbatol (Wallace)
**Other common trade names:** *Felbamyl; Taloxa*
**Indications:** Partial seizures
**Category:** Antiepileptic
**Half-life:** 13–23 hours

### *Reactions*

#### Skin
Acne (3.4%)
Bullous eruption (<1%)
Diaphoresis
Edema
Facial edema (3.4%)
Flushing
Lichen planus
Livedo reticularis
Lupus erythematosus
Photosensitivity (<0.01%)
Pruritus (>1%)
Purpura
Pustular eruption
(1994): Shelley WB+, *Cutis* 53, 282 (observation)
Rash (sic) (3.5%)
Stevens–Johnson syndrome
(1994): Jackel RA, *Epilepsia* 35, 98
Toxic epidermal necrolysis
(1995): Travaglini MT+, *Pharmacotherapy* 15, 260
Urticaria (<1%)

#### Hair
Hair – alopecia

#### Other
Anaphylactoid reactions (<0.01%)
Dysgeusia (6.1%)
Foetor ex ore (halitosis)
Gingival bleeding
Glossitis

Myalgia (2.6%)
Oral mucosal edema (>1%)
Paresthesias (3.5%)
Thrombophlebitis
Xerostomia (2.6%)

# FELODIPINE

**Trade names:** Lexxel (AstraZeneca); Plendil (Zeneca Merck)
**Other common trade names:** *AGON SR; Hydac; Modip; Munobal; Penedil; Renedil; Splendil*
**Indications:** Hypertension
**Category:** Calcium channel blocker; antihypertensive
**Half-life:** 11–16 hours
**Clinically important, potentially hazardous interactions with:** carbamazepine, epirubicin, imatinib

Lexxel is enalapril and felodipine

### *Reactions*

## Skin

Ankle edema
(1992): Morgan TO+, *Am J Hypertens* 5, 238
(1992): Morgan TO+, *Kidney Int* Suppl 36, S78
(1991): Dimenas E+, *Eur J Clin Pharmacol* 40, 141
(1991): Liedholm H+, *Drug Intell Clin Pharm* 25, 1007
Diaphoresis
(1988): Saltiel E+, *Drugs* 36, 387
Edema
(1991): *Med Lett Drugs Ther* 33, 115
Erythema (1.5%)
Exanthems
(1993): Litt JZ, Beachwood, OH (personal case) (observation)
(1985): Lorimer AR+, *Drugs* 29 (Suppl 2), 154
Facial edema (1.5%)
Flu-like syndrome (sic) (<1%)
Flushing
(1992): Morgan TO+, *Am J Hypertens* 5, 238
(1991): Dimenas E+, *Eur J Clin Pharmacol* 40, 141
(1991): Frewin DB+, *Eur J Clin Pharmacol* 41, 393
(1991): *Med Lett Drugs Ther* 33, 115
(1991): Liedholm H+, *Drug Intell Clin Pharm* 25, 1007
(1991): Yedinak KC+, *Drug Intell Clin Pharm* 25, 1193
(1988): Saltiel E+, *Drugs* 36, 387 (5–30%; dose-related)
(1987): Elmfeldt D+, *Drugs* 34 (Suppl 3), 132
(1985): Aberg H+, *Drugs* 29 (Suppl 2), 117 (44%)
(1985): Lorimer AR+, *Drugs* 29 (Suppl 2), 154 (25%)
Peripheral edema (22%)
(1991): Frewin DB+, *Eur J Clin Pharmacol* 41, 393
Pruritus (<1%)
Purpura
(1991): Capewell S+, *Eur J Clin Pharmacol* 41, 95
Rash (sic) (1.5%)
Telangiectases
(2001): Silvestre JF+, *J Am Acad Dermatol* 45, 323 (facial; photodistributed)
(1998): Karonen T+, *Dermatology* 196, 272 (truncal)
Urticaria (1.5%)

## Nails

Nails – brittle
(1985): Aberg H+, *Drugs* 29 (Suppl 2), 117 (44%)

## Other

Gingival hyperplasia (2–10%)
(1998): Young PC+, *Cutis* 62, 41
Gynecomastia (<1%)
Myalgia (1.5%)
Paresthesias (2.5%)
Tinnitus
Xerostomia (<1%)
(1991): Dimenas E+, *Eur J Clin Pharmacol* 40, 141

# FENOFIBRATE

**Synonyms:** procetofene; proctofene
**Trade name:** Tricor (Abbott)
**Other common trade name:** *Apo-Fenofibrate*
**Indications:** Hyperlipidemia
**Category:** Fibric acid cholesterol-lowering agent
**Half-life:** 20 hours
**Clinically important, potentially hazardous interactions with:** dicumarol, lovastatin, nicotinic acid, warfarin

### *Reactions*

## Skin

Exanthems
(1990): Balfour JA+, *Drugs* 40, 260
Photoreactions
(1996): Jeanmougin M+, *Ann Dermatol Venereol* (French) 123, 251
Photosensitivity
(1997): Leroy D+, *Photodermatol Photoimmunol Photomed* 13, 93
(1997): Machet L+, *J Am Acad Dermatol* 37, 808
(1996): Diemer S+, *J Dermatol Sci* 13, 172
(1996): Leenutaphong V+, *J Am Acad Dermatol* 35, 775
(1994): Miranda MA+, *Photochem Photobiol* 59, 171
(1993): Gardeazabal J+, *Photodermatol Photoimmunol Photomed* 9, 156
(1993): Jeanmougin M+, *Ann Dermatol Venereol* (French) 120, 549
(1992): Serrano G+, *J Am Acad Dermatol* 27, 204
(1990): Leroy D+, *Photodermatol Photoimmunol Photomed* 7, 136
(1989): Merino MV+, *Actas Dermo-Sif* (Spanish) 80, 703
Phototoxicity
(1993): Vargas F+, *Photochem Photobiol* 58, 471
(1990): Merino V+, *Contact Dermatitis* 23, 284
Pruritus (4%)
Rash (sic) (4–8%)
(1989): Blane GF, *Cardiology* 76, 1
(1989): *Am J Med* 83, 26 (2%)
Skin reactions (sic) (1–10%)
(1989): Goldberg AC+, *Clin Ther* 11, 69
Toxic epidermal necrolysis
(2002): Correia O+, *Arch Dermatol* 138, 29 (two cases)
Urticaria

## Hair

Hair – alopecia
(1990): Gollnick H+, *Z Hautkr* (German) 65, 1128

## Other

Muscle tenderness
(1989): *Am J Med* 83, 26 (1%)
Muscle toxicity (sic)
(1989): Muller JP+, *Presse Med* (French) 18, 1033
(1982): Giraud P+, *Rev Rhum Mal Osteartic* (French) 49, 162
Myalgia (<1%)
(2001): Rabasa-Lhoret R+, *Diabetes Metab* 27(1), 66
Myopathy

(1991): Solsona L+, *Med Clin (Barc)* (Spanish) 97, 677
Paresthesias
Polymyositis
(1991): Sauvaget F+, *Rev Med Interne* (French) 12, 52
Rhabdomyolysis
(2000): Duda-Krol W+, *Wiad Lek* 53(7), 454
(1992): Raimondeau J+, *Presse Med* 21(14), 663 (with pravastatin)
Septic–Toxic shock (sic)
(2000): Duda-Krol W+, *Wiad Lek* 53(7), 454
Vaginitis

# FENOPROFEN

**Trade name:** Nalfon (Dista)
**Other common trade names:** *Fenoprex; Fenopron; Fepron; Feprona; Nalgesic; Progesic*
**Indications:** Arthritis
**Category:** Nonsteroidal anti-inflammatory (NSAID)
**Half-life:** 2.5–3 hours
**Clinically important, potentially hazardous interactions with:** methotrexate

### *Reactions*

## Skin

Acne
(1974): Wojtulewski JA+, *BMJ* 2, 475
Angioedema (<1%)
Bruising (<1%)
Bullous eruption
Diaphoresis (<0.5%)
Erythema multiforme (<1%)
(1988): Stotts JS+, *J Am Acad Dermatol* 18, 755
Exanthems
(1985): Bigby M+, *J Am Acad Dermatol* 12, 866
(1977): Davis JD+, *Clin Pharmacol Ther* 21, 52
Exfoliative dermatitis (<1%)
Hot flashes (<1%)
Peripheral edema (<1%)
Pruritus (3–9%)
(1992): Breathnach SM+, *Adverse Drug Reactions and the Skin* Blackwell, Oxford, 186 (passim)
(1985): Bigby M+, *J Am Acad Dermatol* 12, 866
(1977): Davis JD+, *Clin Pharmacol Ther* 21, 52
Purpura (<1%)
(1992): Breathnach SM+, *Adverse Drug Reactions and the Skin* Blackwell, Oxford, 186 (passim)
(1978): Simpson RE+, *N Engl J Med* 298, 629
Rash (sic) (>10%)
Stevens–Johnson syndrome (<1%)
Toxic epidermal necrolysis (<1%)
(1988): Stotts JS+, *J Am Acad Dermatol* 18, 755
Urticaria (1–3%)
(1992): Breathnach SM+, *Adverse Drug Reactions and the Skin* Blackwell, Oxford, 186 (passim)
(1985): Bigby M+, *J Am Acad Dermatol* 12, 866
Vesiculobullous eruption
(1992): Breathnach SM+, *Adverse Drug Reactions and the Skin* Blackwell, Oxford, 186 (passim)

## Hair

Hair – alopecia (<1%)

## Other

Anaphylactoid reactions
Aphthous stomatitis (<1%)
Dysgeusia (<1%) (metallic taste)
Glossopyrosis (<1%)
Mastodynia (<1%)
Oral ulceration
Stomatitis
Tinnitus
Xerostomia (>1%)

# FENTANYL

**Trade names:** Actiq (Abbott); Duragesic (Janssen)
**Other common trade names:** *Beatryl; Durogesic; Fentanest; Leptanal; Sublimaze*
**Indications:** Chronic pain
**Category:** Narcotic agonist analgesic
**Half-life:** 1.5–6 hours
**Clinically important, potentially hazardous interactions with:** amiodarone, amprenavir, cimetidine, indinavir, nelfinavir, ranitidine, ritonavir, saquinavir

### *Reactions*

## Skin

Cold, clammy skin (<1%)
Diaphoresis (>10%)
(2001): Litt JZ, Beachwood, OH (personal case) (observation)
(1992): Calis KA+, *Clin Pharm* 11, 22
(1992): Friesen RH+, *Anesthesiology* 76, 46
Edema
(1990): Ducker P+, *Z Hautkr* (German) 65, 734
Erythema (at application site) (<1%)
(1992): Mosser KH, *Am Fam Physician* 45, 2289
(1990): Ducker P+, *Z Hautkr* (German) 65, 734
Exanthems
Exfoliative dermatitis
Fixed eruption
(2001): Vaughan K, Lakewood, WA (from Internet) (observation) (from patch)
Flushing (3–10%)
Papular eruption (sic) (>1%)
Pruritus (3–44%)
(2002): Nelson KE+, *Anesthesiology* 96(5), 1070
(1999): Herman NL+, *Anesth Analg* 89, 378
(1996): Larijani GE+, *Pharmacotherapy* 16, 958
(1994): Gerwels JW+, *J Dermatol Surg Oncol* 20, 823
(1992): Badner NH+, *Can J Anaesth* 39, 330
(1992): Belzarena SD, *Anesth Analg* 74, 653
(1992): Calis KA+, *Clin Pharm* 11, 22
(1992): Friesen RH+, *Anesthesiology* 76, 46 (facial)
(1992): Mosser KH, *Am Fam Physician* 45, 2289
(1992): Mourisse J+, *Acta Anaesthesiol Scand* 36, 70
(1992): Paech MJ, *Anaesth Intensive Care* 20, 15
(1992): Sandler ES+, *Pediatrics* 89, 631
(1992): Varrassi G+, *Anaesthesia* 47, 558
(1992): White MJ+, *Can J Anaesth* 39, 594
(1989): Ackerman WE+, *Can J Anaesth* 36, 388
(1989): Jorrot JC+, *Ann Fr Anesth Réanim* (French) 8, 321 (22%)
(1988): Davies GG+, *Anesthesiology* 69, 763
(1988): Monk JP+, *Drugs* 36, 286 (40%)
(1986): Shipton EA+, *S Afr Med J* 70, 325 (13%)
Purpura
(2001): Tweed WA+, *Anesth Analg* 92, 1442
Pustules (sic) (<1%)
Rash (sic) (>1%)

(1992): Sandler ES+, *Pediatrics* 89, 631
(1992): Stoukides CA+, *Clin Pharm* 11, 222
Urticaria (<1%)

### Other

Anaphylactoid reactions
(2001): Girgis Y, *Anaesthesia* 56(10), 1016
(2001): Konarzewski W+, *Anaesthesia* 56(5), 497 (with propofol) (fatal)
(2001): Lewis S+, *Anaesthesia* 56(11), 1128
(1990): Ducker P+, *Z Hautkr* (German) 65, 734
Cough
(2001): Tweed WA+, *Anesth Analg* 92(6), 1442
Death
(2001): Girgis Y, *Anaesthesia* 56(10), 1016
Dysesthesia (<1%)
Dysgeusia (<1%)
Paresthesias (<1%)
Xerostomia (>10%)
(2001): Litt JZ, Beachwood, OH (personal case) (observation)
(1992): Calis KA+, *Clin Pharm* 11, 22

## FEVERFEW

**Scientific names:** *Chrysanthemum parthenium; Pyrethrum parthenium; Tanacetum parthenium*
**Other common names:** Atamisa; Bachelor's Button; Featerfoiul; Featherfew; Featherfoil; Santa Maria
**Family:** Asteraceae; Compositae
**Purported indications:** fever, headache, migraine, menstrual irregularites, arthritis, psoriasis, allergies, asthma, tinnitus, vertigo, nausea, vomiting
**Other uses:** Infertility, cancer, common cold, earache, liver disease, prevention of miscarriage, orthopedic disorders, swollen feet, diarrhea, dyspepsia. General stimulant and tonic

#### *Reactions*

### Skin

Angioedema (lips)
(1998): Awang DVC, *Int Med* 1, 11
(1985): Johnson ES+, *BMJ* (*Clin Res Ed*) 291, 569
Contact dermatitis
(1996): Lamminpaa A+, *Contact Dermatitis* 34, 330
Prurigo nodularis
(2000): Sharma VK+, *Contact Dermatitis* 42(4), 235

### Other

Ageusia
(1998): Awang DVC, *Int Med* 1, 11
(1985): Johnson ES+, *BMJ* (*Clin Res Ed*) 291, 569
Oral ulceration
(1998): Awang DVC, *Int Med* 1, 11
(1985): Johnson ES+, *BMJ* (*Clin Res Ed*) 291, 569

## FEXOFENADINE

**Trade name:** Allegra (Aventis)
**Indications:** Allergic rhinitis, pruritus, urticaria
**Category:** $H_1$-receptor antagonist; antihistamine (nonsedating)
**Half-life:** 14.4 hours

#### *Reactions*

### Skin

Acne
(1998): Litt JZ, Beachwood, OH (personal case) (observation)
Viral infection (sic) (2.5%)

## FILGRASTIM

(See GRANULOCYTE COLONY-STIMULATING FACTOR (GCSF))

## FINASTERIDE

**Trade names:** Propecia (Merck); Proscar (Merck)
**Other common trade names:** *Pro-Cure; Proscar 5*
**Indications:** Benign prostatic hypertrophy, male-pattern baldness
**Category:** Androgen hormone inhibitor; antineoplastic; hair growth stimulant
**Half-life:** 4.8–6 hours

#### *Reactions*

### Skin

Folliculitis
(2000): Price VH+, *J Am Acad Dermatol* 43, 768
Rash (sic)
(1999): Cather JC+, *Cutis* 64, 167
Urticaria

### Hair

Hair – hypotrichosis (sic)
(1998): Panagotacos PJ (from Internet) (observation) ("reversal of graying hair")
Hair – patchy hair, loss of beard (sic)
(1999): Mitchell D, Thomasville, GA (from Internet) (observation)
(1998): Drayton GE, Los Angeles, CA (from Internet) (observation)

### Nails

Nails – onychomycosis
(1999): Mitchell D, Thomasville, GA (from Internet) (observation)

### Other

Gynecomastia
(2002): Ferrando J+, *Arch Dermatol* 138, 543
(2000): Wade MS+, *Australas J Dermatol* 41, 55 (painful and reversible)
(2000): Zimmerman RL+, *Arch Pathol Lab Med* 124, 625
(1999): Cather JC+, *Cutis* 64, 167 (passim)
(1999): Miller JA+, *South Med J* 92, 615
(1997): Carlin BI+, *J Urol* 158, 547
(1997): Staiman VR+, *Urology* 50, 929
(1996): Green L+, *New Engl J Med* 335, 823

(1996): Wilton L+, *Br J Urol* 78, 379
(1995): Volpi R+, *Am J Med Sci* 309, 322
Lip swelling
Mastodynia (<1%)
Myopathy (severe)
(1999): Cather JC+, *Cutis* 64, 167

# FLAVOXATE

**Trade name:** Urispas (Alza)
**Other common trade names:** *Bladderon; Genurin; Harnin; Patricin; Spasuret; Urispadol; Uronid*
**Indications:** Dysuria, urgency, nocturia
**Category:** Urinary antispasmodic agent
**Half-life:** no data*
**Clinically important, potentially hazardous interactions with:** anticholinergics, arbutamine

### *Reactions*

## Skin

Exanthems
Rash (sic) (<1%)
(1999): Enomoto U+, *Contact Dermatitis* 40, 337
Urticaria

## Other

Hypersensitivity
(1986): Hirohata S+, *Arch Intern Med* 146, 2409
Oral ulceration
(1972): Strouthidis TM+, *Lancet* 1, 72
Xerostomia (>10%)

***Note:** Onset of action: 55–60 minutes

# FLECAINIDE

**Trade name:** Tambocor (3M)
**Other common trade names:** *Almarytm; Apocard; Corflene; Flecaine; Tabco*
**Indications:** Atrial fibrillation
**Category:** Antiarrhythmic
**Half-life:** 7–22 hours
**Clinically important, potentially hazardous interactions with:** ritonavir

### *Reactions*

## Skin

Diaphoresis (<3%)
Edema (3.5%)
Exanthems
(1985): Holmes B+, *Drugs* 27, 301 (1.4%)
Exfoliative dermatitis (<1%)
Flushing (<3%)
Pruritus (<1%)
Psoriasis
(1988): Mancuso G+, *G Ital Dermatol Venerol* (Italian) 123, 171
(1985): Holmes B+, *Drugs* 27, 301
Rash (sic) (<3%)
Urticaria (<1%)

## Hair

Hair – alopecia (<1%)

## Other

Dysgeusia (<1%) (metallic taste)
Hypesthesia (1–10%)
Myalgia (<1%)
Oral edema
Paresthesias (<1%)
Tinnitus
Tongue edema (<1%)
Tremors (5%)
Xerostomia (<1%)

# FLUCONAZOLE

**Trade name:** Diflucan (Pfizer)
**Other common trade names:** *Biozolene; Flucazol; Flukezol; Fluzone; Fungata; Triflucan*
**Indications:** Candidiasis
**Category:** Broad-spectrum bis-triazole antifungal
**Half-life:** 25–30 hours
**Clinically important, potentially hazardous interactions with:** alprazolam, amphotericin B, anisindione, anticoagulants, dicumarol, methadone, midazolam, phenobarbital, phenytoin, sulfonylureas, vinblastine, vincristine, warfarin

### *Reactions*

## Skin

Acne
(1998): Drake L, *J Am Acad Dermatol* 38, S87
Acute generalized exanthematous pustulosis (AGEP)
(2002): Alsadhan A+, *J Cutan Med Surg* 6(2), 122
(2002): Di Lernia V (Italy) (personal communication) (from Internet) (observation)
Angioedema
(1999): Errico MR, Buenos Aires, Argentina (from Internet) (observation)
(1991): Abbott M+, *Lancet* 2, 633
Bullous eruption
(1994): Gupta AK+, *J Am Acad Dermatol* 30, 911
Erythema multiforme
(1994): Gupta AK+, *J Am Acad Dermatol* 30, 911
(1991): Gussenhoven MJE+, *Lancet* 338, 120
Exanthems
(2001): Altman EM, West Orange, NJ (from Internet) (observation)
(1990): Grant SM+, *Drugs* 39, 877 (1.8%) (in AIDS patients)
Exfoliative dermatitis
(1994): Gupta AK+, *J Am Acad Dermatol* 30, 911 (passim)
(1990): Grant SM+, *Drugs* 39, 877
Fixed eruption
(2002): Ghislain P-D, *J Am Acad Dermatol* 46, 47 (recurrence)
(2001): Hudson TF, Conway AR (from Internet) (observation)
(2000): Heikkilä H+, *J Am Acad Dermatol* 42, 883
(1997): Danby B, Kingston, Ontario (from Internet) (observation)
(1997): Jaffe P, Columbia, SC (from Internet) (observation)
(1994): Morgan JM+, *BMJ* 308, 454
Pallor (<1%)
Petechiae
(1995): Mercurio MG+, *J Am Acad Dermatol* 32, 525
Pruritus

(1999): Errico MR, Buenos Aires, Argentina (from Internet) (observation)
(1991): Neuhaus G+, *BMJ* 302, 1341
Purpura
(1990): Agarwal A+, *Ann Intern Med* 113, 899
Rash (sic) (1.8%)
(1998): Scher RK+, *J Am Acad Dermatol* 38, S77
(1995): Powderly WG, *Infections in Medicine*, 257 (passim)
(1994): Gupta AK+, *J Am Acad Dermatol* 30, 911 (1.8%)
Skin hypertrophy (sic)
(1998): Drake L+, *J Am Acad Dermatol* 38, S87
Stevens–Johnson syndrome
(1995): Powderly WG, *Infections in Medicine*, 257 (passim)
(1991): Gussenhoven MJE+, *Lancet* 1, 120
(1990): Sugar AM+, *Rev Infect Dis* 12, S338
Toxic epidermal necrolysis
(1993): Azon-Masoliver A+, *Dermatology* 187, 268
(1990): Grant SM+, *Drugs* 39, 877
Urticaria

### Hair
Hair – alopecia
(2001): Ondo A, *Las Cruces, NM* (from Internet) (observation)
(1996): Goldsmith LA, *Ann Intern Med* 125, 153
(1995): Pappas PG+, *Ann Intern Med* 123, 354
(1993): Weinroth SE+, *Ann Intern Med* 119, 637

### Nails
Nail – disorder (sic)
(1998): Drake L+, *J Am Acad Dermatol* 38, S87
(1998): Ling MR+, *J Am Acad Dermatol* 38, S95
Nail – melanonychia (longitudinal)
(1998): Kar HK, *Int J Dermatol* 37, 719

### Other
Anaphylactoid reactions (in AIDS patients)
Dysgeusia
(1998): Quart AM+, *Infect Med* 15, 379
(1991): Neuhaus G+, *BMJ* 302, 1341
Hypersensitivity (1–4%)
(1997): Craig TJ, *J Am Osteopath Assoc* 97, 584
Oral ulceration
(1998): Ling MR+, *J Am Acad Dermatol* 38, S95
(1991): Abbott M+, *Lancet* 2, 633
Paresthesias
(1991): Neuhaus G+, *BMJ* 302, 1341
Xerostomia
(1998): Quart AM+, *Infect Med* 15, 379

## FLUCYTOSINE

**Trade name:** Ancobon (ICN)
**Other common trade names:** *5-FC; Alcobon; Ancotil*
**Indications:** Candidal and cryptococcal infections
**Category:** Antifungal
**Half-life:** 3–8 hours

#### *Reactions*

### Skin
Exanthems
(1987): Thyss A+, *Ann Dermatol Venereol* (French) 114, 1131
(1972): Editorial, *N Engl J Med* 286, 777
Photosensitivity (<1%)
(1987): Thyss A+, *Ann Dermatol Venereol* (French) 114, 1131
(1983): Shelley WB+, *J Am Acad Dermatol* 8, 229
Pruritus
Purpura
Rash (sic) (1–10%)
Urticaria

### Other
Anaphylactoid reactions (<1%)
Paresthesias (<1%)
Parkinsonism (<1%)
Xerostomia

## FLUDARABINE

**Trade name:** Fludara (Berlex)
**Indications:** Chronic lymphocytic leukemia (B-cell)
**Category:** Purine nucleoside antineoplastic
**Half-life:** 9 hours
**Clinically important, potentially hazardous interactions with:** aldesleukin

#### *Reactions*

### Skin
Chills (>10%)
Edema (>10%)
Exanthems
Paraneoplastic pemphigus
(2001): Gooptu C+, *Br J Dermatol* 144(6), 1255 (3 cases)
(1995): Bazarbachi A+, *Ann Oncol* 6, 730
Petechiae
(2001): Churn M+, *Clin Oncol* 13, 273
Rash (sic) (>10%)
Squamous cell carcinoma
(1997): Davidovitz Y+, *Acta Haematol* 98, 44 (flare-up)

### Hair
Hair – alopecia (1–10%)

### Other
Dysgeusia (<1%) (metallic taste)
Myalgia (>10%)
Paresthesias (>10%)
Stomatitis (>10%)

## FLUMAZENIL

**Trade name:** Romazicon (Roche)
**Other common trade names:** *Anexate; Lanexat*
**Indications:** Benzodiazepine overdose
**Category:** Benzodiazepine antidote
**Half-life:** terminal: 41–79 minutes
**Clinically important, potentially hazardous interactions with: alcohol**, neuromuscular blockers

#### *Reactions*

### Skin
Diaphoresis (3–9%)
Flushing (1–3%)
Hot flashes (1–10%)
Rash (sic)
Urticaria (<1%)

### Other

Hypesthesia
Injection-site pain (3–9%)
Injection-site reactions (sic)
Paresthesias (1–10%)
Thick tongue (sic) (<1%)
Thrombophlebitis
Tinnitus
Tremors (1–10%)
Xerostomia (1–10%)

# FLUOROURACIL

**Trade names:** Adrucil (Pharmacia & Upjohn); Efudex (ICN); Fluoroplex (Allergan)
**Other common trade names:** *Efudix; Efurix*
**Category:** Antineoplastic antimetabolite
**Half-life:** 8–20 minutes
**Clinically important, potentially hazardous interactions with:** aldesleukin, cimetidine, metronidazole

## *Reactions*

### Skin

Acral erythema
(1995): Esteve E+, *Ann Med Interne Paris* (French) 146, 192
(1992): Doll DC+, *Semin Oncol* 19(5), 580
(1989): Vukelja SJ+, *Ann Intern Med* 111, 688
Acral erythrodysesthesia syndrome (hand–foot syndrome)
(2002): Cure H+, *J Clin Oncol* 20(5), 1175 (38%)
Actinic keratosis inflammation (sic)
(1999): Nabai H+, *Cutis* 64, 43
(1987): Johnson TM+, *J Am Acad Dermatol* 17(2 Pt 1), 192
(1969): Omura EF+, *JAMA* 208, 150
(1962): Falkson G+, *Br J Dermatol* 74, 229
Angioedema
Bullous eruption
(1970): Bart BJ+, *Arch Dermatol* 102, 457
Contact dermatitis
(1999): Sanchez-Perez J+, *Contact Dermatitis* 41, 106
(1997): Anderson LL+, *J Am Acad Dermatol* 36, 478
(1996): Nadal C+, *Contact Dermatitis* 35, 124 (systemic)
(1977): Goette DK+, *Arch Dermatol* 113, 1058
Dermatitis (sic) (>10%)
Eczematous eruption (sic)
(1977): Bernstein T, *New Engl J Med* 297, 337
Erythema
(1980): Hrushesky WJ, *Cutis* 26, 181
(1962): Falkson G+, *Br J Dermatol* 74, 229
Erythema multiforme
(1980): Ueki H+, *Hautarzt* (German) 31, 207
Erythematous eruption, linear serpentine (sic)
(1998): Pujol RM+, *J Am Acad Dermatol* 39, 839
Exanthems (1–10%)
(1994): Leo S+, *J Chemother* 6, 423
(1994): Sollitto RB+, *Arch Dermatol* 130, 1194 (sun-exposed areas)
Fissuring
Folliculitis (forehead)
(2001): Schmid-Wendtner M-H+, *Lancet* 358, 1575 (passim)
Keratoderma (palms)
(2001): Schmid-Wendtner M-H+, *Lancet* 358, 1575 (passim)
Keratoses
(2001): Kurzman MA, Staten Island, NY (from Internet) (observation)
(2001): Lamberts RJ, Grand Rapids, MI (from Internet) (observation) (inflammation)
Necrosis
(1980): Yaffee HS+, *Cutis* 25, 649 ("ecdysis")
Palmar–plantar erythrodysesthesia syndrome (hand–foot syndrome)
(2001): Elasmar SA+, *Jpn J Clin Oncol* 31(4), 172 (passim)
(1997): Chiara S+, *Eur J Cancer* 33, 967
(1997): Iurio A+, *Acta Oncol* 36, 653
(1997): Thaler D, Monona, WI (from internet) (observation)
(1995): Banfield GK+, *J R Soc Med* 88, 356
(1994): Leo S+, *J Chemother* 6, 423
(1993): Beard JS+, *J Am Acad Dermatol* 29, 325
(1991): Jorda E+, *Int J Dermatol* 30, 653
(1989): Curran CF+, *Ann Intern Med* 111, 858
(1989): Vukelja SJ+, *Ann Intern Med* 111, 688
(1988): Guillaume J-C+, *Ann Dermatol Venereol* (French) 115, 1167
(1987): Molina R+, *Proc Am Soc Clin Oncol* 4, 92
(1985): Atkins JN, *Ann Intern Med* 102, 419
(1985): Feldman LD+, *JAMA* 254, 3479
(1984): Lokich JJ+, *Ann Intern Med* 101, 798
Palmar–plantar pigmentation
(2001): Schmid-Wendtner M-H+, *Lancet* 358, 1575 (passim)
Pellagra
(1992): Breathnach SM+, *Adverse Drug Reactions and the Skin* Blackwell, Oxford, 193 (passim)
Photosensitivity (<1%)
(1999): von Moos R+, *Schweiz Med Wochenschr* (German) 129, 52
(1992): Breathnach SM+, *Adverse Drug Reactions and the Skin* Blackwell, Oxford, 193 (passim)
(1962): Falkson G+, *Br J Dermatol* 74, 229
Phototoxicity
Pigmentation (<1%)
(1997): Miller BH+, *J Am Acad Dermatol* 36, 72
(1995): Allen BJ+, *Int J Dermatol* 34, 219 (reticulate)
(1994): Leo S+, *J Chemother* 6, 423
(1991): Vukelja SJ+, *J Am Acad Dermatol* 25, 905 (serpentine)
(1980): Hrushesky WJ, *Cutis* 26, 181 (sun-exposed areas)
(1977): Goette DK+, *Arch Dermatol* 113, 1058
(1962): Falkson G+, *Br J Dermatol* 74, 229
Pruritus
Radiation recall
(1992): Breathnach SM+, *Adverse Drug Reactions and the Skin* Blackwell, Oxford, 193 (passim)
Reactivation phenomenon (sic)
(1997): Anderson LL+, *J Am Acad Dermatol* 36, 478
(1993): Prussick R+, *Arch Dermatol* 129, 644
Seborrheic dermatitis
(1962): Falkson G+, *Br J Dermatol* 74, 229
Urticaria
Xerosis (1–10%)

### Hair

Hair – alopecia (>10%)
(2002): Sloan JA+, *J Clin Oncol* 20(6), 1491
(2001): Madnani N, Mumbai, India (from Internet) (observation)
(1992): Breathnach SM+, *Adverse Drug Reactions and the Skin* Blackwell, Oxford, 193 (passim)
(1962): Falkson G+, *Br J Dermatol* 74, 229

### Nails

Nails – onycholysis
Nails – pigmentation (<1%)
(2001): Schmid-Wendtner M-H+, *Lancet* 358, 1575 (passim)
(1962): Falkson G+, *Br J Dermatol* 74, 229

### Other

Anaphylactoid reactions

(1992): Breathnach SM+, *Adverse Drug Reactions and the Skin* Blackwell, Oxford, 193 (passim)
Dysgeusia
Ectropion
(1997): Lewis JE, *Int J Dermatol* 36, 79
(1994): Hecker D+, *Cutis* 53, 137
Infusion-site pigmentation
(2001): Schmid-Wendtner M-H+, *Lancet* 358, 1575 (passim)
Injection-site burning
(1998): Kraus S+, *J Am Acad Dermatol* 38, 438
(1997): Miller BH+, *J Am Acad Dermatol* 36, 72
Injection-site desquamation
(1998): Kraus S+, *J Am Acad Dermatol* 38, 438
(1997): Miller BH+, *J Am Acad Dermatol* 36, 72
(1997): Swinehart JM+, *Arch Dermatol* 133, 67
(1992): Breathnach SM+, *Adverse Drug Reactions and the Skin* Blackwell, Oxford, 193 (passim)
Injection-site edema
(1997): Miller BH+, *J Am Acad Dermatol* 36, 72
(1997): Swinehart JM+, *Arch Dermatol* 133, 67
(1992): Breathnach SM+, *Adverse Drug Reactions and the Skin* Blackwell, Oxford, 193 (passim)
Injection-site erythema
(1998): Kraus S+, *J Am Acad Dermatol* 38, 438
(1997): Miller BH+, *J Am Acad Dermatol* 36, 72
(1997): Swinehart JM+, *Arch Dermatol* 133, 67
(1992): Breathnach SM+, *Adverse Drug Reactions and the Skin* Blackwell, Oxford, 193 (passim)
Injection-site necrosis
(1998): Kraus S+, *J Am Acad Dermatol* 38, 438
(1997): Swinehart JM+, *Arch Dermatol* 133, 67
Injection-site pain
(1998): Kraus S+, *J Am Acad Dermatol* 38, 438
(1997): Swinehart JM+, *Arch Dermatol* 133, 67
Injection-site ulceration
(1997): Miller BH+, *J Am Acad Dermatol* 36, 72
(1997): Swinehart JM+, *Arch Dermatol* 133, 67
Mucositis (1–10%)
(2002): Cure H+, *J Clin Oncol* 20(5), 1175 (26%)
(2001): Hejna M+, *Eur J Cancer* 37(16), 1994
Paresthesias (<1%)
Stomatitis (>10%)
(2002): Ito A+, *Gan To Kagaku Ryoho* 29(4), 563
(2002): Sloan JA+, *J Clin Oncol* 20(6), 1491
(2002): Ueno H+, *Cancer Chemother Pharmacol* 49(2), 155
Tongue pigmentation
(2001): Schmid-Wendtner M-H+, *Lancet* 358, 1575 (passim)

# FLUOXETINE

**Trade name:** Prozac (Dista)
**Other common trade names:** *Adofen; Apo-Fluoxetine; Dom-Fluoxetine; Fluctin; Fluctine; Fludac; Fluoxac; Fluoxeren; Fluxil; Fontex*
**Indications:** Depression, obsessive-compulsive disorder
**Category:** Selective serotonin reuptake inhibitor (SSRI); antidepressant and antiobsessional
**Half-life:** 2–3 days
**Clinically important, potentially hazardous interactions with:** alprazolam, amphetamines, clarithromycin, clozapine, desipramine, dextroamphetamine, diethylpropion, erythromycin, haloperidol, imipramine, isocarboxazid, linezolid, lithium, MAO inhibitors, mazindol, meperidine, methamphetamine, midazolam, moclobemide, nortriptyline, phendimetrazine, phenelzine, phentermine, phenylpropanolamine, phenytoin, pimozide, pseudoephedrine, selegiline, serotonin agonists, sibutramine, **St John's wort**, sumatriptan, sympathomimetics, tramadol, tranylcypromine, trazodone, tricyclic antidepressants, troleandomycin, **tryptophan**

## *Reactions*

### Skin

Acne (<1%)
Angioedema
(1991): Olfson M+, *J Nerv Mental Dis* 179, 504
Bruising
(1996): Pai VB+, *Ann Pharmacother* 30, 786
Bullous eruption (<1%)
Candidiasis
Cellulitis
Contact dermatitis (<1%)
Cutaneous reactions (sic)
(1998): Beauquier B+, *Encephale* (French) 24, 62
Diaphoresis (8.4%)
(1985): Wernicke JF, *J Clin Psychiatry* 46, 59
Eczema (sic) (<1%)
Erythema multiforme
(1985): Wernicke JF, *J Clin Psychiatry* 46, 59
Erythema nodosum (<1%)
Exanthems (4%)
(1993): Gupta MA+, *Cutis* 51, 386 (3%) (passim)
(1993): Gupta RK+, *Med J Aust* 158, 722
(1993): Litt JZ, Beachwood, OH (personal case) (observation)
(1991): Olfson M+, *J Nerv Mental Dis* 159, 504
(1989): Miller LG+, *Am J Psychiatry* 146, 1616
(1988): Cooper GL, *Br J Psychiatry* 153, 77
(1985): Wernicke JF, *J Clin Psychiatry* 46, 59
Exfoliative dermatitis
Facial edema (<1%)
Flushing (<2%)
Furunculosis (<1%)
Herpes simplex (reactivation)
(1991): Reed SM+, *Am J Psychiatry* 148, 949
Herpes zoster
Hot flashes
Lichenoid eruption
Lupus erythematosus (discoid)
Mycosis fungoides (exacerbation)
(1996): Vermeer MH+, *J Am Acad Dermatol* 35, 635
Peripheral edema (<1%)
Petechiae (<1%)

Photosensitivity
(1998): Pazzagli L+, *Pharm World Sci* 20, 136 (with alprazolam)
Phototoxicity (<1%)
(1995): Gaufberg E+, *J Clin Psychiatry* 56, 486
(1995): O'Brien T, *Australas J Dermatology* 36, 103
Pigmentation (<1%)
Pruritus (2.4%)
(1993): Gupta RK+, *Med J Aust* 158, 722
(1991): Olfson M+, *J Nerv Mental Dis* 159, 504
(1985): Wernicke JF, *J Clin Psychiatry* 46, 59
Pseudo-mycosis fungoides (sic)
(1996): Gordon KB+, *J Am Acad Dermatol* 34, 304
Psoriasis (<1%)
(1992): Hemlock C+, *Ann Pharmacother* 26, 211
Purpura (<1%)
Pustular eruption (<1%)
Rash (sic) (6%)
(1989): Miller LG+, *Am J Psychiatry* 146, 1616
(1987): Zerbe RL, *Int J Obes* 11 (Suppl 3), 191
(1985): Wernicke JF, *J Clin Psychiatry* 46, 59
Raynaud's phenomenon
(2000): De Broucker+, *Ann Med Interne* (Paris) 151(5), 424
Seborrhea (<1%)
Stevens–Johnson syndrome
(1998): N Z Medicines Adverse Reactions Committee (from Internet) (observation)
(1992): Bodokh I+, *Therapie* (French) 47, 441
Subcutaneous nodule (sic)
Toxic epidermal necrolysis
(1992): Bodokh I+, *Therapie* (French) 47, 441
(1991): Rosenthal E+, *Presse Med* (French) 20, 1459
Ulcers (<1%)
Urticaria (4%)
(1994): Blumenthal HL, Beachwood, OH (personal case) (observation)
(1993): Gupta RK+, *Med J Aust* 158, 722
(1992): Leznoff A+, *J Clin Psychopharmacol* 12, 355
(1991): Olfson M+, *J Nerv Mental Dis* 159, 504
(1989): Miller LG+, *Am J Psychiatry* 146, 1616
Vasculitis
(1999): Fisher A+, *Aust N Z J Med* 29, 375 (focal necrotizing)
(1995): Roger D+, *Dermatology* 191, 164
Xerosis

### Hair

Hair – alopecia (<1%)
(2000): Murlidhar MD, Madras, India (from Internet) (observation)
(1996): Bhatara VS+, *J Clin Psychiatry* 57, 227
(1995): Seifritz E+, *Can J Psychiatry* 40, 362
(1995): Shelley WB+, *Cutis* 55, 144 (observation)
(1994): Mareth TR, *J Clin Psychiatry* 55, 163
(1994): Shelley WB+, *Cutis* 53, 282 (observation)
(1993): Ogilvie AD, *Lancet* 342, 1423
(1991): Ananth J+, *J Psychiatry* 36, 621
(1991): Gupta S+, *Br J Psychiatry* 159, 737
(1991): Jenike MA, *Am J Psychiatry* 148, 392
Hair – hirsutism (<1%)

### Other

Ageusia (<1%)
Anaphylactoid reactions (<1%)
Aphthous stomatitis (<1%)
Black tongue
(2000): Heymann WR, *Cutis* 66, 25
Dysgeusia (1.8%)
(2000): Heymann WR, *Cutis* 66, 25
Galactorrhea
(2001): Peterson MC, *Mayo Clin Proc* 76, 215
Gingivitis (<1%)
Glossitis (<1%)
Glossodynia
(1994): Shelley WB+, *Cutis* 53, 242 (observation)
Gynecomastia (<1%)
Hyperesthesia (<1%)
Hypersensitivity
(1994): Beer K+, *Arch Dermatol* 130, 803
Hypesthesia (<1%)
Mastodynia (<1%)
Myalgia
Myopathy (<1%)
Oral ulceration (<1%)
(2000): Madinier I+, *Ann Med Interne (Paris)* (French) 151, 248
Paresthesias
(2001): Ribeiro L+, *Braz J Med Biol Res* 34(10), 1303
(1996): Bhatara VS+, *J Clin Psychiatry* 57, 227
Parosmia (<1%)
Priapism (<1%)
Pseudolymphoma
(1995): Crowson AN+, *Arch Dermatol* 131, 925
(1995): Magro CM+, *J Am Acad Dermatol* 32, 419
Rhabdomyolysis
(1990): Lazarus A, *J Clin Psychopharacol* 10 (overdose)
Serotonin syndrome
(2002): Chechani V, *Crit Care Med* 30(2), 473
(2000): Manos GH, *Ann Pharmacother* 34(7–8), 871 (with buspirone)
Serum sickness
(1991): Vincent A+, *Am J Psychiatry* 148, 1602
(1989): Miller LG+, *Am J Psychiatry* 146, 1616
Sialorrhea (<1%)
Stomatitis (<1%)
Thrombophlebitis (<1%)
Tinnitus
Tongue edema (<1%)
Tongue pigmentation (<1%)
Tremors (2–10%)
Vaginal anesthesia
(1993): King VL+, *Am J Psychiatry* 150, 984
Xerostomia (12%)
(2000): Heymann WR, *Cutis* 66, 25
(1993): Beasley CM+, *Ann Clin Psychiatry* 5, 199
(1985): Wernicke JF, *J Clin Psychiatry* 46, 59

## FLUOXYMESTERONE

**Trade names:** Android-F; Halotensin (Pharmacia & Upjohn)
**Other common trade names:** *Stenox; Vewon*
**Indications:** Breast carcinoma, hypogonadism, anemia
**Category:** Androgen; antineoplastic; antianemic
**Half-life:** 9.2 hours
**Clinically important, potentially hazardous interactions with:** anticoagulants, cyclosporine, warfarin

#### *Reactions*

### Skin

Acne (>10%)
(1992): Fryand O+, *Acta Derm Venereol* 72, 148
(1990): Fuchs E+, *J Am Acad Dermatol* 23, 125
(1989): Fryand O+, *Tidsskr Nor Laegeforen* (Norwegian) 109, 239

(1989): Hartmann AA+, *Monatsschr Kinderheilkd* (German) 137, 466
(1989): Heydenreich G, *Arch Dermatol* 125, 571 (fulminans)
(1989): Scott MJ+, *Cutis* 44, 30
(1989): von Muhlendahl KE+, *Dtsch Med Wochenschr* (German) 114, 712
(1988): Traupe H+, *Arch Dermatol* 124, 414 (fulminans)
(1987): Kiraly CL+, *Am J Dermatopathol* 9, 515
(1984): Lamb DR, *Am J Sports Med* 12, 31
(1965): Kennedy BJ, *J Am Geriatr Soc* 13, 230
(1965): Rook A, *Br J Dermatol* 77, 115

Contact dermatitis
(1989): Holdiness MR, *Contact Dermatitis* 20, 3 (from patch)

Edema (>10%)

Exanthems

Flushing (1–5%)
(1965): Kennedy BJ, *J Am Geriatr Soc* 13, 230

Furunculosis
(1989): Scott MJ+, *Cutis* 44, 30

Lichenoid eruption
(1989): Aihara M+, *J Dermatol* (Tokio) 16, 330

Lupus erythematosus
(1978): Robinson HM, *Z Haut* (German) 53, 349

Pruritus

Psoriasis
(1990): O'Driscoll JB+, *Clin Exp Dermatol* 15, 68

Purpura

Seborrhea (sic)

Seborrheic dermatitis
(1989): Scott MJ+, *Cutis* 44, 30

Striae
(1989): Scott MJ+, *Cutis* 44, 30

Urticaria

### Hair

Hair – alopecia
(1989): Scott MJ+, *Cutis* 44, 30
(1965): Kennedy BJ, *J Am Geriatr Soc* 13, 230

Hair – hirsutism (1–10%)
(1994): Castillo-Ceballos A+, *Med Clin (Barc)* (Spanish) 102, 78
(1991): Bates GW+, *Clin Obstet Gynecol* 34, 848
(1991): No Author, *Obstet Gynecol* 78, 474
(1991): Parker LU+, *Cleve Clin J Med* 58, 43
(1991): Urman B+, *Obstet Gynecol* 77, 595
(1989): Scott MJ+, *Cutis* 44, 30
(1974): Baron J, *Zentralbl Gynakol* (German) 96, 129
(1971): Fusi S+, *Folia Endocrinol* (Italian) 24, 412
(1965): Kennedy BJ, *J Am Geriatr Soc* 13, 230

### Other

Anaphylactoid reactions
Gynecomastia (<1%)
Hypersensitivity (<1%)
Injection-site pain
Mastodynia (>10%)
Paresthesias
Priapism (>10%)
Stomatitis

# FLUPHENAZINE

**Trade names:** Permitil (Schering); Prolixin (Bristol-Myers Squibb)
**Other common trade names:** *Anatensol; Apo-Fluphenazine; Dapatum D25; Dapotum D; Fludecate; Modecate; Moditen*
**Indications:** Psychoses
**Category:** Phenothiazine antipsychotic
**Half-life:** 84–96 hours
**Clinically important, potentially hazardous interactions with:** antihistamines, arsenic, chlorpheniramine, dofetilide, quinolones, sparfloxacin

## *Reactions*

### Skin

Angioedema (<1%)
Contact dermatitis
Dermatitis (sic)
Diaphoresis
Eczema (sic)
Edema
Erythema
Exanthems
Exfoliative dermatitis
Hypohidrosis (>10%)

Lupus erythematosus
(1975): Gallien M+, *Ann Med Psychol* (Paris) (French) 1, 237

Peripheral edema
Photosensitivity

Pigmentation (<1%) (blue-gray)
(1987): Krebs A, *Schweiz Rundsch Med Prax* (German) 76, 1069

Pruritus (<1%)
Purpura
Rash (sic) (1–10%)
Seborrhea

Toxic epidermal necrolysis
(1972): Carli-Basset C+, *Sem Hôp* (French) 48, 497

Urticaria

Vitiligo
(1987): Krebs A, *Schweiz Rundsch Med Prax* (German) 76, 1069
(1985): Rampertaap MP, *Mo Med* 82, 24

Xerosis

### Other

Anaphylactoid reactions
Galactorrhea (1–10%)
Gynecomastia (1–10%)
Injection-site reactions
Mastodynia (1–10%)
Parkinsonism

Priapism (<1%)
(1986): Fishbain DA, *Psychosomatics* 27, 538
(1985): Fishbain DA, *Ann Emerg Med* 14, 600

Rhabdomyolysis
(1978): Mann SC+, *Am J Psychiatry* 135, 1097

Sialorrhea
(1973): Johnson DAW, *Br J Psychiatry* 123, 519

Trembling (sic) (fingers)
Xerostomia (<1%)

# FLURAZEPAM

**Trade name:** Flurazepam
**Other common trade names:** *Apo-Flurazepam; Benozil; Dalmadorm; Flunox; Nergart; Novoflupam; Som Pam; Somnol; Valdorm*
**Indications:** Insomnia
**Category:** Benzodiazepine hypnotic-sedative
**Half-life:** 40–114 hours
**Clinically important, potentially hazardous interactions with:** amprenavir, chlorpheniramine, clarithromycin, efavirenz, esomeprazole, imatinib, indinavir, nelfinavir, ritonavir

### *Reactions*

#### Skin

Dermatitis (sic) (1–10%)
Diaphoresis (>10%)
Exanthems
(1976): Arndt KA+, *JAMA* 235, 918 (0.05%)
Flushing
Pruritus
Purpura
Rash (sic) (>10%)
Urticaria

#### Other

Acute intermittent porphyria
Dysgeusia (3.4%) (metallic taste)
(1984): Greenblatt DJ+, *J Clin Psychiatry* 45, 192 (3%)
Oral mucosal lesions
(1984): Greenblatt DJ+, *J Clin Psychiatry* 45, 192 (3%)
Paresthesias
Sialopenia (>10%)
Sialorrhea (1–10%)
Xerostomia (>10%)

# FLURBIPROFEN

**Trade name:** Ansaid (Pharmacia & Upjohn)
**Other common trade names:** *Apo-Flurbiprofen; Cebutid; Flurofen; Flurozin; Froben; Lapole; Nu-Flurprofen*
**Indications:** Arthritis
**Category:** Nonsteroidal anti-inflammatory (NSAID)
**Half-life:** 3–4 hours
**Clinically important, potentially hazardous interactions with:** methotrexate

### *Reactions*

#### Skin

Angioedema (<1%)
(1997): Romano A+, *J Intern Med* 241, 81
Burning (ophthalmic)
Contact dermatitis
(2000): Kawada A+, *Contact Dermatitis* 42, 167
Cutaneous side effects (sic) (6%)
(1986): Buson M, *J Int Med Res* 14, 1
(1977): Sheldrake FE+, *Curr Med Res Opin* 5, 106
Dermatitis herpetiformis
(1994): Tousignant J+, *Int J Dermatol* 33, 199
Diaphoresis
Discoloration (sic)
Eczema (sic) (3–9%)
Edema (3–9%)
Erythema multiforme (<1%)
Exanthems
(1997): Romano A+, *J Intern Med* 241, 81
(1977): Cardoe N, *Curr Med Res Opin* 5, 99
(1974): Calin A+, *BMJ* 4, 496 (3%)
Exfoliative dermatitis (<1%)
Fixed eruption
(1993): *Dermatology* 186, 164
Flushing
Furunculosis
Herpes simplex
Herpes zoster
Hot flashes (<1%)
Peripheral edema
Photosensitivity (<1%)
Pruritus (1–5%)
(1977): Cardoe N, *Curr Med Res Opin* 5, 99
Pseudoreactions (sic)
(1991): VanArsdel PP, *JAMA* 266, 3343
Purpura
Rash (sic) (1–3%)
Seborrhea
Stevens–Johnson syndrome (<1%)
Stinging (ophthalmic)
Toxic epidermal necrolysis (<1%)
(1987): Gillaume JC+, *Arch Dermatol* 123, 1166
Ulceration
Urticaria (<1%)
Vasculitis
(1990): Wei M, *Ann Intern Med* 112, 550
Vulvovaginitis
Xerosis

#### Hair

Hair – alopecia (<1%)

#### Nails

Nails – disorder (sic) (<1%)
Nails – pigmentation

#### Other

Anaphylactoid reactions (<1%)
Aphthous stomatitis
Dysgeusia (<1%)
Hypersensitivity
(1997): Romano A+, *J Intern Med* 241, 81
Oral lichenoid eruption
(2000): Madinier I+, *Ann Med Interne (Paris)* (French) 151, 248
(1983): Hamburger J+, *BMJ* 287, 1258
Paresthesias (<1%)
Parosmia (<1%)
Stomatitis
Tinnitus
Xerostomia (<1%)

# FLUTAMIDE

**Trade name:** Eulexin (Schering)
**Other common trade names:** *Drogenil; Euflex; Eulexine; Flucinom; Fluken; Flulem; Fugerel; Novo-Flutamide*
**Indications:** Metastatic prostate carcinoma
**Category:** Antineoplastic (prostate carcinoma); antiandrogen
**Half-life:** 6 hours

### *Reactions*

## Skin

Bullous eruption
Diaphoresis
(1992): Schmeller N, *Internist Berl* (German) 33, 284
Edema (4%)
Erythema
Exanthems
(1999): Fisher BJ, Toronto, Ontario (from Internet) (observation) (generalized)
(1989): Brogden RN+, *Drugs* 38, 185
Flu-like syndrome (sic) (<1%)
Hot flashes (61%)
Lupus erythematosus
(1998): Reid MB+, *J Urol* 159, 2098
Photosensitivity
(1999): Tsien C+, *J Urol* 162, 494
(1998): Vilaplana J+, *Contact Dermatitis* 38, 68
(1998): Yokote R+, *Eur J Dermatol* 8, 427
(1996): Fujimoto M+, *Br J Dermatol* 135, 496
(1991): Moraillon I+, *Photodermatol Photoimmunol Photomed* 8, 264
Rash (sic) (3%)
Toxic epidermal necrolysis
Urticaria

## Other

Gynecomastia (9%)
(1997): Staiman VR+, *Urology* 50, 929
(1993): Aso Y+, *Hinyokika Kiyo* (Japanese) 39, 391
Injection-site irritation (3%)
Paresthesias (1–10%)
Pseudoporphyria
(1999): Mantoux F+, *Ann Dermatol Venereol* (French) 126, 150
(1999): Schmutz JL+, *Ann Dermatol Venereol* (French) 126, 374
(1998): Borroni G+, *Br J Dermatol* 138, 711

# FLUVASTATIN

**Trade name:** Lescol (Novartis)
**Other common trade names:** *Cranoc; Locol*
**Indications:** Hypercholesterolemia
**Category:** Antihyperlipidemic; HMG-CoA reductase inhibitor
**Half-life:** 1.2 hours
**Clinically important, potentially hazardous interactions with:** azithromycin, bosentan, clarithromycin, cyclosporine, erythromycin, gemfibrozil, imatinib

### *Reactions*

## Skin

Allergic reactions (sic) (2.6%)
Angioedema
Discoloration (sic)
Erythema multiforme
Flu-like syndrome (sic)
Flushing
Lupus erythematosus
(1998): Sridhar MK+, *Lancet* 352, 114 (fatal)
Photosensitivity
Pruritus
Purpura
Rash (sic) (2.7%)
(1998): N Z Medicines Adverse Reactions Committee (from Internet) (observation) (2 patients)
Stevens–Johnson syndrome
Toxic epidermal necrolysis
Upper respiratory infection (16%)
Urticaria
Vasculitis
Xerosis

## Hair

Hair – alopecia
(2002): Litt JZ, Beachwood, OH (personal case) (observation)
Hair – changes (sic)

## Nails

Nails – changes (sic)

## Other

Anaphylactoid reactions
Death
Dysgeusia
Gynecomastia
Myalgia (5–6%)
(1997): Australian Adverse Drug Reactions Bulletin 16(1), February
Myopathy
(1997): Australian Adverse Drug Reactions Bulletin 61(1), February
(1995): Garnett WR, *Am J Health Syst Pharm* 52(15), 1639
Myositis
(1997): Australian Adverse Drug Reactions Bulletin 16(1), February
Paresthesias
Rhabdomyolysis
(2002): Sica DA+, *Am J Geriatr Cardiol* 11(1), 48
(2002): Sica DA+, *Curr Opin Nephrol Hypertens* 11(2), 123
(1999): Bottorff M, *Atherosclerosis* 147(Suppl 1), S23
(1995): Farmer JA+, *Baillieres Clin Endocrinol Metab* 9(4), 825
(1995): Garnett WR, *Am J Health Syst Pharm* 52(15), 1639

# FLUVOXAMINE

**Trade name:** Luvox (Solvay)
**Other common trade names:** *Apo-Fluvoxamine; Dumirox; Dumyrox; Faverin; Favoxil; Fevarin; Maveral*
**Indications:** Obsessive-compulsive disorder, depression
**Category:** Selective serotonin reuptake inhibitor (SSRI); antidepressant
**Half-life:** 15 hours
**Clinically important, potentially hazardous interactions with:** alprazolam, amphetamines, dextroamphetamine, diethylpropion, isocarboxazid, linezolid, MAO inhibitors, mazindol, methamphetamine, phendimetrazine, phenelzine, phentermine, phenylpropanolamine, pseudoephedrine, selegiline, sibutramine, sumatriptan, sympathomimetics, tacrine, tramadol, tranylcypromine, trazodone, troleandomycin

### *Reactions*

#### Skin

Acne (<1%)
Allergic reactions (sic) (<1%)
Angioedema
(1993): No Author, *Lakartidningen* (Swedish) 90, 54
Bullous eruption
Cutaneous reactions (sic)
(1998): Beauquier B+, *Encephale* (French) 24, 62
Dermatitis (sic) (<1%)
Diaphoresis (7%)
(1986): Benfield P+, *Drugs* 32, 313 (5%)
Ecchymoses (<1%)
Edema (<1%)
Exanthems
Exfoliative dermatitis (<1%)
Furunculosis (<1%)
Photosensitivity (<1%)
(1996): Gillet-Terver MN+, *Australas J Dermatol* 37, 62
(1993): *Lakartidningen* (Swedish) 90, 54
Pigmentation (<1%)
Pruritus
Purpura (<1%)
Rash (sic)
Seborrhea (<1%)
Stevens–Johnson syndrome
Toxic epidermal necrolysis (<1%)
(1993): Wolkenstein P+, *Lancet* 342, 304
Urticaria (<1%)
Xerosis (<1%)

#### Hair

Hair – alopecia (<1%)
Hair – alopecia areata
(1996): Parameshwar E, *Am J Psychiatry* 153, 581

#### Other

Ageusia (<1%)
Anaphylactoid reactions
Dysgeusia (3%)
Gingivitis (<1%)
Glossitis (<1%)
Mastodynia (<1%)
Myalgia
Myopathy (<1%)
Oral mucosal lesions
(1986): Benfield P+, *Drugs* 32, 313 (10%)
Paresthesias
Parosmia (<1%)
Priapism
Serotonin syndrome
(2001): Demers JC+, *Ann Pharmacother* 35(10), 1217 (with mirtazapine)
(2001): Isbister GK+, *Ann Pharmacother* 35(12), 1674 (with mirtazapine)
(2001): Kaneda Y+, *Int J Neurosci* 109(3), 165
Sialorrhea
Stomatitis (<1%)
Vaginitis (<1%)
Xerostomia (14%)
(1986): Benfield P+, *Drugs* 32, 313 (10%)

# FOLIC ACID

**Synonyms:** folacin; folate; vitamin $B_9$
**Trade name:** Folvite (Lederle)
**Other common trade names:** *Acfol; Apo-Folic; Dalisol; Flodine; Folacin; Folina; Folinsyre; Folitab; Folsan; Lexpec*
**Indications:** Anemias
**Category:** Nutritional supplement; water-soluble vitamin
**Half-life:** no data

### *Reactions*

#### Skin

Acne
(1964): Fegeler F, *Arch Klin Exp Dermatol* (German) 219, 335
Allergic reactions (sic) (<1%)
Dermatitis (sic)
(1966): Pedersen JT, *Ugeskr Laeger* (Danish) 128, 708
Erythema
(1966): Pedersen JT, *Ugeskr Laeger* (Danish) 128, 708
Exanthems
(1985): Sparling R+, *Clin Lab Haematol* 7, 184
(1964): Fegeler F, *Arch Klin Exp Dermatol* (German) 219, 335
Flushing (<1%)
Pruritus (<1%)
(1966): Mathur BP, *Indian J Med Sci* 20, 133
(1966): Pedersen JT, *Ugeskr Laeger* (Danish) 128, 708
Rash (sic) (<1%)
Urticaria
(1985): Sparling R+, *Clin Lab Haematol* 7, 184

#### Other

Anaphylactoid reactions
(2000): Dykewicz MS+, *J Allergy Clin Immunol* 106, 386
(1966): Woodliff HJ, *Med J Aust* 53, 351

# FONDAPARINUX

**Trade name:** Arixtra (Sanofi)
**Indications:** Prophylaxis of deep vein thrombosis
**Category:** Faxtor Xa Inhibitor
**Half-life:** 17–21 hours
**Clinically important, potentially hazardous interactions with:** abciximab, anagrelide, anticoagulants, cilostazol, clopidogrel, dipyridamole, eptifibatide, many **herbals** that possess anticoagulant or antiplatelet activity, salicylates, ticlopidine, tirofiban

### *Reactions*

#### Skin
Bullous eruption (3%)
Edema (9%)
Pain (2%)
Purpura (4%)
Rash (sic) (8%)

#### Other
Injection-site bleeding (1–10%)
Injection-site pruritus (1–10%)
Injection-site rash (sic) (1–10%)

# FORMOTEROL

**Synonym:** Formoterol fumarate
**Other common trade name:** *Oxeze*
**Indications:** Asthma, bronchospasm
**Category:** Beta2-adrenergic agonist
**Half-life:** 10–14 hours
**Clinically important, potentially hazardous interactions with:** clomipramine, desipramine, doxepin, imipramine, nortriptyline, protriptyline, trimipramine

### *Reactions*

#### Skin
Angioedema
Erythema
Infections (sic) (3%)
Pruritus
Rash (sic) (1.1%)
Urticaria
Viral infection (17.2%)

#### Other
Anaphylactoid reactions (1%)
Cough
(1990): Schultze-Werninghaus G, *Lung* 168 (Suppl 83-9)
Hypesthesia
(1995): van den Berg BT+, *Fundam Clin Pharmacol* 9(6), 593
Myalgia
Tremors (1.9%)
(1998): Bartow RA+, *Drugs* 55(2), 303
(1995): van den Berg BT+, *Fundam Clin Pharmacol* 9(6), 593
(1992): Lipworth BJ, *Drug Saf* 7(1), 54
(1991): Faulds D+, *Drugs* 42(1), 115
(1990): Schultze-Werninghaus G, *Lung* 168 (Suppl 83–9) (6%)
Xerostomia
(1990): Schultze-Werninghaus G, *Lung* 168 (Suppl 83–9) (1%)

# FOSCARNET

**Trade name:** Foscavir (AstraZeneca)
**Other common trade name:** *Foscovir*
**Indications:** Cytomegalovirus retinitis in patients with AIDS
**Category:** Antiviral; inhibits various viral DNA and RNA polymerases
**Half-life:** ~3 hours
**Clinically important, potentially hazardous interactions with:** cyclosporine

### *Reactions*

#### Skin
Acne
Dermatitis (sic) (<1%)
Diaphoresis (>5%)
Edema (<1%)
Eosinophilic pustular folliculitis
(2001): Roos TC+, *J Am Acad Dermatol* 44, 546
Exanthems (>5%)
(2001): Roos TC+, *J Am Acad Dermatol* 44, 546
(1990): Green ST, *J Infection* 21, 227
Facial edema (>5%)
Fixed eruption
(1990): Connolly GM+, *Genitourin Med* 66, 97
Flushing (1–5%)
Herpes simplex (<1%)
Leg edema (<1%)
Penile ulcers
(1997): English JC+, *J Am Acad Dermatol* 37, 1
(1996): Agcaoili DJ+, *Infect Med* 13, 35
(1996): Papini M+, *Ann Dermatol Venereol* (French) 123, 679
(1995): Fitzgerald E+, *Arch Dermatol* 131, 1447
(1993): Bodian AB, *Int J Dermatol* 32, 526
(1993): Brockmeyer NH+, *Int J Clin Pharmacol Ther Toxicol* 31, 204
(1993): Gross AS+, *Clin Infect Dis* 17, 1076
(1993): Moyle G+, *AIDS* 7, 140
(1993): Schiff TA+, *Int J Dermatol* 32, 526
(1992): Evans LM+, *J Am Acad Dermatol* 27, 124
(1992): Katlama C+, *J Acquir Immune Defic Syndr* 5 (Suppl 1), S18
(1991): Chrisp P+, *Drugs* 41, 104
(1990): Fégueux S+, *Lancet* 335, 547
(1990): Gilquin J+, *Lancet* 335, 287
(1990): Lernestedt J-O+, *Lancet* 335, 548
(1990): Moyle G+, *Lancet* 335, 547 (4.7%)
(1990): Van Der Pijl JW+, *Lancet* 335, 286 (30%)
Periorbital edema
Peripheral edema (<1%)
Pigmentation (>5%)
Pruritus (>5%)
(2001): Roos TC+, *J Am Acad Dermatol* 44, 546
Pruritus ani (<1%)
Psoriasis (<1%)
Rash (sic) (generalized) (>5%)
(1991): Blanshard C, *J Infect* 23, 336
(1990): Green ST+, *J Infect* 21, 227
Seborrhea (>5%)
Toxic epidermal necrolysis
(1999): Wharton JR+, *Cutis* 63, 333
(1997): Lauglin CL, Little Rock, Arkansas, American Academy of Dermatology Meeting, (SF) (gross and microscopic)
Ulceration (>5%)
Urticaria (<1%)
(2001): Roos TC+, *J Am Acad Dermatol* 44, 546

Vulvar ulceration
(1993): Caumes E+, *J Am Acad Dermatol* 28, 799 (erosion)
(1992): Lacey HB+, *Genitourin Med* 68, 182
Warts (<1%)
Xerosis (<1%)

### Hair

Hair – alopecia (<1%)

### Other

Dysgeusia (>5%)
Gynecomastia (<1%)
Hyperesthesia (<1%)
Hypesthesia
Injection-site pain (1–10%)
Injection-site thrombophlebitis
(1991): Chrisp P+, *Drugs* 41, 104
Myalgia (>5%)
Oral leukoplakia
Oral ulceration
(2000): Madinier I+, *Ann Med Interne (Paris)* (French) 151, 248
(1990): Fégueux S+, *Lancet* 335, 547
(1990): Gilquin J+, *Lancet* 335, 287
(1990): Moyle G+, *Lancet* 335, 547
Paresthesias (1–10%)
(1990): Safrin S+, *J Infect Dis* 161, 1078
Stomatitis (<1%)
Thrombophlebitis (<1%)
Tinnitus
Tongue ulceration (<1%)
Ulcerative stomatitis (>5%)
Xerostomia

# FOSFOMYCIN

**Trade name:** Monurol (Forest)
**Indications:** Urinary tract infections
**Category:** Antibiotic (acute cystitis)
**Half-life:** 3–9 hours

## *Reactions*

### Skin

Angioedema
Exanthems (<1%)
Pruritus (<1%)
Rash (sic) (1.4%)

### Other

Anaphylactoid reactions
(1998): Rosales MJ+, *Allergy* 53, 905
Myalgia (<1%)
Paresthesias (<1%)
Vaginitis (7.6%)
Xerostomia (<1%)

# FOSINOPRIL

**Trade name:** Monopril (Bristol-Myers Squibb)
**Other common trade names:** *Acenor-M; Dynacil; Fosinorm; Fozitec; Staril; Vasopril*
**Indications:** Hypertension
**Category:** Angiotensin-converting enzyme (ACE) inhibitor; antihypertensive
**Half-life:** 11.5 hours
**Clinically important, potentially hazardous interactions with:** amiloride, spironolactone, triamterene

## *Reactions*

### Skin

Angioedema (<1%)
(2001): Cohen EG+, *Ann Otol Rhinol Laryngol* 110(8), 701 (64 cases)
(1997): Graumuller S+, *HNO* (German) 45, 1016
Bullous pemphigoid
Diaphoresis (<1%)
Edema (<1%)
Eosinophilic vasculitis
Exfoliative dermatitis
Flu-like syndrome (sic) (<1%)
Flushing
Pemphigus
(2002): Parodi A+, *Dermatology* 204, 139
Pemphigus foliaceus
(2000): Ong CS+, *Australas J Dermatol* 41(4), 242
Photosensitivity (<1%)
Pruritus (<1%)
(2001): Nunes AC+, *Eur J Gastroenterol Hepatol* 13, 279
Rash (sic) (<1%)
(1990): Pool JL, *Clin Ther* 12, 520 (0.9%)
Scleroderma
Urticaria (<1%)
Vasculitis

### Other

Ageusia (<1%)
Anaphylactoid reactions
Cough
(2001): Adigun AQ+, *West Afr J Med* 20(1), 46–7
(2001): Lee SC+, *Hypertension* 38(2), 166
Dysgeusia (<1%)
(1992): Murdoch D+, *Drugs* 43, 123
Gynecomastia
Myalgia (<1%)
Paresthesias (<1%)
Tinnitus
Tremors (<1%)
Xerostomia (<1%)

# FOSPHENYTOIN

**Trade name:** Cerebyx (Pfizer)
**Indications:** Seizure prophylaxis, status epilepticus
**Category:** Anticonvulsant
**Half-life:** 15 minutes
**Clinically important, potentially hazardous interactions with:** chloramphenicol, cyclosporine, disulfiram, dopamine, imatinib, itraconazole

Fosphenytoin is a prodrug of phenytoin

## *Reactions*

### Skin

Acne (<1%)
Bullous eruption
(2001): Hebert AA+, *J Clin Psychiatry* 62(suppl 14), 22
Chills (sic)
Ecchymoses
Erythema multiforme (<1%)
(2001): Hebert AA+, *J Clin Psychiatry* 62(suppl 14), 22
Exanthems
Exfoliative dermatitis (<1%)
(2001): Hebert AA+, *J Clin Psychiatry* 62(suppl 14), 22
Facial edema
Lupus erythematosus
(2001): Hebert AA+, *J Clin Psychiatry* 62(suppl 14), 22
Pruritus (48.9%)
(2001): Hebert AA+, *J Clin Psychiatry* 62(suppl 14), 22
(1998): Knapp LE+, *J Child Neurol* 13, S15
(1998): Luer MS, *Neurol Res* 20, 178
Rash (sic) (<1%)
Stevens–Johnson syndrome
Toxic epidermal necrolysis

### Other

Dysgeusia (3.3%)
Gingival hyperplasia
(2001): Hebert AA+, *J Clin Psychiatry* 62(suppl 14), 22
Hyperesthesia (2.2%)
Hypesthesia
Injection-site pain
Paresthesias (4.4%)
(1998): Luer MS, *Neurol Res* 20, 178
Tongue disorder (sic)
Xerostomia (4.4%)

# FROVATRIPTAN

**Trade name:** Frova
**Indications:** Migraine headaches
**Category:** 5-HT1 (serotonin) receptor agonist; antimigraine
**Half-life:** 26 hours

## *Reactions*

### Skin

Bullous eruption (<1%)
Cheilitis (<1%)
Conjunctivitis (<1%)
Diaphoresis (1%)
Flushing (4%)
Hot flashes (<1%)
Pain (1%)
Pruritus (<1%)
Purpura (<1%)
Rash (sic)

### Other

Arthralgia (<1%)
Depression (<1%)
Dysesthesia (1%)
Dysgeusia (<1%)
Hyperesthesia (<1%)
Hypesthesia (1%)
Myalgia (<1%)
Paresthesias (4%)
(2001): Easthope SE+, *CNS Drugs* 15(12), 969
Sialopenia (3%)
Sialorrhea (<1%)
Skeletal pain (3%)
Stomatitis (<1%)
Tinnitus (1%)
Toothache (1%)
Tremors (<1%)
Xerostomia

# FULVESTRANT

**Synonyms:** ICI 182; 780
**Trade name:** Faslodex (AstraZeneca)
**Indications:** Metastatic breast cancer
**Category:** Antineoplastic; estrogen receptor antagonist
**Half-life:** ~40 days

## *Reactions*

### Skin

Diaphoresis (5%)
Edema (9%)
Flu-like syndrome (7.1%)
Hot flashes
(2002): Lynn J, *Cancer Nurs* 25, 12S
Peripheral edema
Rash (sic) (7%)

### Other

Arthritis (3%)
Back pain (14%)
Bone pain (16%)
Cough (10%)
Depression (6%)
Injection-site reactions (11%)
(2002): Lynn J, *Cancer Nurs* 25, 12S
Myalgia (<1%)
Pain (19%)
Paresthesias (6%)

# FURAZOLIDONE

**Trade name:** Furoxone (Roberts)
**Other common trade names:** *Furion; Furoxona; Fuxol*
**Indications:** Various infections caused by susceptible organisms
**Category:** Nitrofuran antibiotic; antidiarrheal; antiprotozoal
**Half-life:** no data
**Clinically important, potentially hazardous interactions with:** amphetamines, chloroquine, dapsone, dobutamine, dopamine, ephedrine, epinephrine, meperidine, morphine, phenylephrine, phenylpropanolamine, pseudoephedrine, sympathomimetics

### *Reactions*

## Skin

Contact dermatitis
(1990): de Groot AC+, *Contact Dermatitis* 22, 202
(1980): Goette DK+, *Cutis* 26, 406
(1978): Novak M, *Cesk Dermatol* (Czech) 53, 128
(1974): Bleumink E+, *Hautarzt* (German) 25, 403
Disulfiram-like reaction (with alcohol) (<1%)*
Erythema multiforme
(1986): Fisher AA, *Cutis* 37, 158
(1980): Goette DK+, *Cutis* 26, 406
Exanthems (<1%)
Flushing (with alcohol) (<1%)
Photosensitivity
(1980): Goette DK+, *Cutis* 26, 406
Pruritus
Pruritus ani
Rash (sic) (<1%)
Urticaria (<1%)
(1969): Aaronson CM, *JAMA* 210, 557

## Other

Serum sickness
(1978): Wolfe MS+, *Am J Trop Med Hyg* 27, 762

***Note:** The disulfiram-like reaction consists of facial flushing, diaphoresis, tachycardia, and pounding headache

# FUROSEMIDE

**Trade name:** Lasix (Aventis)
**Other common trade names:** *Apo-Furosemide; Discoid; Dryptal; Edenol; Frusid; Furorese; Furoside; Fusid; Henexal; Lasilix; Novo-Semide; Urex; Uritol*
**Indications:** Edema
**Category:** Sulfonamide* loop diuretic; antihypertensive
**Half-life:** 0.5–1 hour
**Clinically important, potentially hazardous interactions with:** amikacin, aminoglycoside amphotericin, digoxin, gentamicin, kanamycin, neomycin, streptomycin, tobramycin

### *Reactions*

## Skin

Acute febrile neutrophilic dermatosis (Sweet's syndrome)
(1989): Cobb MW, *J Amer Acad Dermatol* 21, 339
Acute generalized exanthematous pustulosis (AGEP)
(1995): Moreau A+, *Int J Dermatol* 34, 263 (passim)
Bullous eruption (<1%)
(1995): Tamimi NA+, *Nephrol Dial Transplant* 10, 1943
(1993): Landor M+, *Ann Allergy* 70, 196
(1992): Van Olden RW+, *Am J Nephrol* 12, 351 (photosensitive)
(1989): Sfar Z+, *Tunis Med* (French) 67, 805
(1985): Anderson CD+, *Photodermatol* 2, 111
(1982): Hallan H+, *Tidsskr Nor Laegeforen* (Norwegian) 102, 630
(1980): Guin JD, *Cutis* 25, 534
(1980): Rees RB+, *J Am Acad Dermatol* 2, 244
(1977): Hertzenberg S, *Tidsskr Nor Laegeforen* (Norwegian) 97, 792
(1977): Heydenreich G+, *Acta Med Scand* 202, 61
(1977): Heydenreich G+, *Ugeskr Laeger* (Danish) 139, 1847
(1976): Burry JN+, *Ann Intern Med* 84, 493
(1976): Coles GA+, *BMJ* 2, 525
(1976): Gilchrist B+, *Ann Intern Med* 84, 494
(1976): Keczkes K+, *BMJ* 2, 236
(1975): Gilchrist B+, *Ann Intern Med* 83, 480
(1969): Ebringer A+, *Med J Aust* 1, 768
Bullous pemphigoid
(2002): Thaler D, Monona, WI (from Internet) (observation)
(1997): Panayiotou BN+, *Br J Clin Pract* 51, 49 (2 patients)
(1996): Koch CA+, *Cutis* 58, 340
(1995): Siddiqui MA+, *J Am Geriatr Soc* 43, 1183
(1991): Shelley WB+, *Cutis* 48, 367 (passim)
(1986): Ingber A+, *Z Hautarzt* (German)
(1984): Halevy S+, *Harefuah* (Hebrew) 106, 125
(1981): Castel T, *Clin Exp Dermatol* 6, 635
(1980): Neufeld R+, *Cutis* 26, 290
(1976): Fellner J+, *Arch Dermatol* 112, 75
Cutaneous side effects (sic)
(1986): Bigby M+, *JAMA* 256, 3358 (0.05%)
(1976): Arndt KA+, *JAMA* 235, 918 (0.26%)
Diaphoresis
Epidermolysis bullosa
(1976): Kennedy AC+, *BMJ* 1, 1509
(1976): Kennedy AC, *Br J Dermatol* 94, 495
Erythema multiforme (<1%)
(1980): Zugerman C, *Arch Dermatol* 116, 518
(1970): Gibson TP+, *JAMA* 212, 1709
(1969): Ebringer A+, *Med J Aust* 1, 768
Erythema nodosum
(1975): Dargie HJ+, *Meyler's Side Effects of Drugs*, Vol 8, Amsterdam, Excerpta Medica, 483
Exanthems
(1999): Litt JZ, Beachwood, OH (personal case) (observation)
(1988): Lin RY, *N Y State J Med* 88, 439
(1979): Lowe J+, *BMJ* 2, 360 (0.2%)
(1979): Naranjo CA+, *Clin Pharmacol Ther* 25, 154 (0.6%)
(1978): Bjoerndal N+, *Ugeskr Laeger* (Danish) 140, 1084
(1977): Greenblatt DJ+, *Am Heart J* 94, 6 (0.2%)
(1970): Gibson TP+, *JAMA* 212, 1709
(1966): Sherlock S+, *Lancet* 1, 1049 (12%)
Exfoliative dermatitis
(1992): Breathnach SM+, *Adverse Drug Reactions and the Skin* Blackwell, Oxford, 230 (passim)
(1978): Bjoerndal N+, *Ugeskr Laeger* (Danish) 140, 1084
(1975): Dargie HJ+, *Meyler's Side Effects of Drugs*, Vol 8, Amsterdam, Excerpta Medica, 483
Flushing
(1977): Greenblatt DJ+, *Am Heart J* 94, 6
Grinspan's syndrome**
(1990): Lamey PJ+, *Oral Surg Oral Med Oral Path* 70, 184
Lichenoid eruption
(1990): West AJ+, *J Am Acad Dermatol* 23, 689
(1981): Ota J+, *Skin Res* (Japanese) 23, 639
Linear IgA bullous dermatosis
(1999): Cerottini J-P+, *J Am Acad Dermatol* 41, 103
Lupus erythematosus
(1988): Lin RY, *N Y State J Med* 88, 439
Periorbital edema

(1987): Hansbrough JR+, *J Allergy Clin Immunol* 80, 538
Photosensitivity (1–10%)
(1989): Cobb MW, *J Amer Acad Dermatol* 21, 339
(1977): Heydenreich G+, *Acta Med Scand* 202, 61
Phototoxicity
(1998): Vargas F+, *J Photochem Photobiol B* 42, 219
(1976): Burry JN+, *Ann Intern Med* 84, 493
(1976): Burry JN, *Br J Dermatol* 94, 495
Porokeratosis (disseminated superficial)
(2000): Kroiss MM+, *Acta Derm Venereol* 80, 52
Pruritus (<1%)
(1993): Litt JZ, Beachwood, OH (personal case) (observation)
(1987): Hansbrough JR+, *J Allergy Clin Immunol* 80, 538
(1978): Sibbald RG+, *Can Med Assoc J* 118, 142
Purpura
(1989): Nishioka K+, *J Dermatol* 16, 220 (pigmented)
(1983): Michel M+, *Rev Geriat* (French) 8/10, 505
(1969): Ebringer A+, *Med J Aust* 1, 768
Pustular eruption
(1990): Mothiron C+, *Presse Med* (French) 19, 1504
(1989): Cobb MW, *J Am Acad Dermatol* 21, 339
(1973): Macmillan AL, *Dermatologica* 146, 285
Rash (sic) (<1%)
Stevens–Johnson syndrome
(1991): Chan JC+, *Drug Saf* 6, 230
(1978): Ward B+, *Am J Ophthalmol* 86, 133
Toxic epidermal necrolysis
(1999): Egan CA+, *J Am Acad Dermatol* 40, 458
Urticaria
(1987): Hansbrough JR+, *J Allergy Clin Immunol* 80, 538
(1967): Milla Santos J, *Summa Med* (Spanish) 10, 3
(1966): Atkins LL, *Geriatrics* 21, 143
Vasculitis
(1990): Bourgain C+, *Presse Med* (French) 19, 1504
(1989): Cobb MW, *J Amer Acad Dermatol* 21, 339
(1988): Lin RY, *N Y State J Med* 88, 439
(1982): de la Chapelle C+, *LARC Med* (French) 2, 760
(1978): Sibbald RG+, *Can Med Assoc J* 118, 142
(1977): Hendricks WM+, *Arch Dermatol* 113, 375 (necrotizing)
(1971): Pathy MS, *Gerontol Clin* 13, 261

## Other

Acute intermittent porphyria
Anaphylactoid reactions
(1987): Hansbrough JR+, *J Allergy Clin Immunol* 80, 538
Injection-site erythema (<1%)
Injection-site pain
Paresthesias
Porphyria
(1984): Harber LC+, *J Invest Dermatol* 82, 207
Porphyria cutanea tarda
(1992): Shelley WB+, *Advanced Dermatologic Diagnosis* WB Saunders, 414 (passim)
(1983): Goldsman CI+, *Cleve Clin Q* 50, 151
(1977): Rufli T+, *Schweiz Med Wochenschr* (German) 107, 1093
Pseudolymphoma
(1995): Magro CM+, *J Am Acad Dermatol* 32, 419
Pseudoporphyria cutanea tarda
(1998): Breier F+, *Dermatology* 197, 271
Thrombophlebitis
Tinnitus
Ulcerative stomatitis
(1988): Lin RY, *N Y State J Med* 88, 439
Xanthopsia
Xerostomia
(1967): Milla Santos J, *Summa Med* (Spanish) 10, 3

***Note:** Furosemide is a sulfonamide and can be absorbed systemically. Sulfonamides can produce severe, possibly fatal, reactions such as toxic epidermal necrolysis and Stevens–Johnson syndrome

****Note:** Grinspan's syndrome is the triad of oral lichen planus, diabetes mellitus, and hypertension

# GABAPENTIN

**Trade name:** Neurontin (Pfizer)
**Indications:** Seizures
**Category:** Anticonvulsant
**Half-life:** 5–6 hours

### *Reactions*

#### Skin

Acne (>1%)
Acute febrile neutrophilic dermatosis (Sweet's syndrome)
(2001): Popescu C, Bucharest, Romania (from Internet) (observation)
(1999): Smith W (from Internet) (observation)
Exanthems
Facial edema (<1%)
Peripheral edema (1.7%)
(1998): Rowbotham M+, *JAMA* 280, 1837
Pruritus (1.3%)
Purpura (<1%)
Rash (sic) (>1%)
Stevens–Johnson syndrome
(1998): Gonzalez-Sicilia L+, *Am J Med* 105, 455
Urticaria

#### Hair

Hair – alopecia
(1997): Picard C+, *Ann Pharmacother* 31, 1260

#### Other

Foetor ex ore (halitosis)
(1998): Backonja M+, *JAMA* 280, 1831
Gingivitis (<1%)
Glossitis
Gynecomastia
(2000): Zylicz Z, *J Pain Symptom Manage* 20, 2
Myalgia (2%)
Paresthesias (<1%)
Priapism
(2001): Matthews SC+, *Psychosomatics* 42(3), 280
Sialorrhea
Stomatitis
Tinnitus
Tooth discoloration
Tremors (1–10%)
Xerostomia (1.7%)

# GALANTAMINE

**Trade name:** Reminyl (Janssen)
**Indications:** Alzheimer's Disease
**Category:** Acetylcholinesterase Inhibitor
**Half-life:** 6–8 hours
**Clinically important, potentially hazardous interactions with:** bethanechol, cimetidine, donepezil, edrophonium, pilocarpine, rivastigmine, succinylcholine, tacrine

**Note:** Derived from snowdrop (*Galanthus* sp) bulbs

### *Reactions*

#### Skin

Acute generalized exanthematous pustulosis (AGEP)
(2002): Gantcheva M+, *World Congress Dermatol* Poster, 1588
Edema
Peripheral edema (>2%)
Purpura (>2%)
Upper respiratory infection (>2%)

#### Other

Depression (5%)
Paresthesias
Sialorrhea
Tremors (1–10%)
Xerostomia

# GANCICLOVIR

**Trade name:** Cytovene (Roche)
**Other common trade names:** *Cymevan; Cymeven; Cymevene; Vitrasert*
**Indications:** Cytomegalovirus retinitis in immunocompromised patients
**Category:** Antiviral
**Half-life:** 2.5–3.6 hours
**Clinically important, potentially hazardous interactions with:** amphotericin B, imipenem cilastatin, zidovudine

### *Reactions*

#### Skin

Acne (<1%)
Bullous eruption (<1%)
Chills (<1%)
Diaphoresis
Edema (<1%)
Exanthems (<1%)
(1987): Chachoua A+, *Ann Intern Med* 107, 133 (4.9%)
(1979): Eyanson S+, *Arch Dermatol* 115, 54 (2%)
Exfoliative dermatitis
Facial edema (<1%)
Fixed eruption (<1%)
Photosensitivity (<1%)
Pigmentation (<1%)
Pruritus (5%)
Psoriasis
Purpura
Rash (sic) (>10%)
Stevens–Johnson syndrome
Urticaria (<1%)

#### Hair

Hair – alopecia (<1%)
(1990): Faulds D+, *Drugs* 39, 597

#### Other

Anaphylactoid reactions
Anosmia
Dysgeusia (<1%)
Gingival hypertrophy
Hypesthesia (<1%)
Injection-site edema (<1%)
Injection-site inflammation (2%)
Injection-site pain
(1990): Faulds D+, *Drugs* 39, 597 (4%)
Mastodynia (<1%)
Myalgia (<1%)

Oral ulceration (<1%)
Paresthesias (6–10%)
Phlebitis (2%)
Tongue disorder (sic) (<1%)
Tremors (<1%)
Xerostomia (<1%)

# GANIRELIX

**Trade name:** Antagon (Organon)
**Indications:** Infertility
**Category:** Antigonadotropic hormone
**Half-life:** 16.2 hours

### *Reactions*

## Skin

Hot flashes (4–5%)
Pruritus

## Other

Injection-site reactions
(2001): Fluker M+, *Fertil Steril* 75(1), 38 (11.9%)
(2000): Gillies PS+, *Drugs* 59, 107
(2000): Oberye J+, *Hum Reprod* 15, 245

# GARLIC

**Scientific name:** *Allium sativum*
**Other common names:** Ail; Ajo; Allium; Camphor of the Poor; Clove Garlic; Nectar of the Gods; Poor Man's Treacle; Rust Treacle; Stinking Rose
**Family:** Liliaceae
**Purported indications:** Hypertension, hypercholesterolemia, preventing atherosclerosis, earaches, menstrual disorders, cancer prevention, immune system stimulation
**Other uses:** Diabetes, allergies, 'flu, arthritis, traveler's diarrhea, bacterial and fungal infections, tinea corporis, tinea pedis and onychomycosis, vaginitis. Flavor component
**Clinically important, potentially hazardous interactions with:** olmesartan, saquinavir

### *Reactions*

## Skin

Bullous eruption
(1993): Garty BZ, *Pediatrics* 91, 658
Burns
(2000): Hviid K+, *Ugeskr Laeger* 162(50), 6853
(2000): Rafaat M+, *Peditar Dermatol* 17(6), 475
(1997): Roberge RJ+, *Am J Emerg Med* 15(5), 548
(1987): Parish RA+, *Pediatr Emerg Care* 3(4), 258
Contact dermatitis
(2001): McGovern TW+, *Cutis* 67, 193
(1999): Eming SA+, *Br J Dermatol* 141(2), 391 (toxic)
(1999): Jappe U+, *Am J Contact Dermat* 10, 37
(1997): Bruynzeel DP, *Contact Dermatitis* 37, 70
(1996): Delaney TA+, *Australas J Dermatol* 37, 109
(1996): Kanerva L+, *Contact Dermatitis* 35(3), 157
(1993): Acciai MC+, *Contact Dermatitis* 29, 48
(1992): McFadden JP+, *Contact Dermatitis* 27(5), 333
(1991): Lee TY+, *Contact Dermatits* 24(3), 193
(1991): Lembo G+, *Contact Dermatitis* 25(5), 330
(1987): Cronin E, *Contact Dermatitis* 17, 265
(1985): Fernandez de Corres L+, *Allergol Immunopathol* (Madr) 13(4), 291
(1983): Papegeorgiou C+, *Arch Dermatol Res* 275(4), 229
(1981): Martinescu E, *Rev Med Chir Soc Med Nat Iasi* 85(3), 541
(1980): Mitchell JC, *Contact Dermatitis* 6(5), 356
(1978): van Ketel WF+, *Contact Dermatitis* 4(1), 53
(1977): Sinha SM+, *Arch Dermatol* 113(6), 776
Pemphigus
(1996): Ruocco V+, *Dermatology* 192(4), 373
Urticaria
(2001): McGovern TW+, *Cutis* 67, 193 (passim)

## Other

Anaphylactoid reactions
(1999): Perez-Pimiento AJ+ 54(6), 626
Foetor ex ore (halitosis)
Hypersensitivity
(2001): McGovern TW+, *Cutis* 67, 193 (passim)
(1982): Campolmi P+, *Contact Dermatitis* 8(5), 352
Stomatodynia

# GATIFLOXACIN

**Trade name:** Tequin (Bristol-Myers Squibb)
**Indications:** Various infections caused by susceptible organisms
**Category:** Fluoroquinolone antibiotic
**Half-life:** 7–14 hours
**Clinically important, potentially hazardous interactions with:** amiodarone, arsenic, bepridil, bretylium, disopyramide, erythromycin, phenothiazines, procainamide, quinidine, sotalol, tricyclic antidepressants

### *Reactions*

## Skin

Allergic reactions (sic) (0.1–3%)
Angioedema
Burning (sic)
Candidiasis
Cheilitis (<0.1%)
Chills (0.1–3%)
Diaphoresis (0.1–3%)
Ecchymoses (<0.1%)
Edema (<0.1%)
Erythema
Exanthems (<0.1%)
Facial edema (<0.1%)
Fixed eruption
(2000): Zabawski E, Longwood, TX (from Internet) (observation)
Peripheral edema (0.1–3%)
Photosensitivity
(2000): Stein GE+, *Inf Med* 17, 564
Pruritus (<0.1%)
Rash (sic) (0.1–3%)
Stevens–Johnson syndrome
Toxic epidermal necrolysis
Urticaria
Vasculitis
Vesiculobullous eruption (<0.1%)

## Other

Anaphylactoid reactions
Dysgeusia (0.1–3%)

(2000): Stein GE+, *Inf Med* 17, 564
Foetor ex ore (halitosis) (<1%)
Gingivitis (<0.1%)
Glossitis (0.1–3%)
Hyperesthesia (<0.1%)
Hypersensitivity
Injection-site reactions (sic) (5%)
(2002): Perry CM+, *Drugs* 62(1), 169
(2000): Gajjar DA+, *Pharmacotherapy* 20, 49S
Mastodynia (<0.1%)
Myalgia (<0.1%)
Oral candidiasis (0.1–3%)
Oral ulceration (0.1–3%)
Paresthesias (0.1–3%)
Parosmia (<0.1%)
Serum sickness
Stomatitis (0.1–3%)
Tendinitis
Tendon rupture
Tongue edema (<0.1%)
Tremors (0.1–3%)
Vaginitis (6%)
(2000): Stein GE+, *Inf Med* 17, 564

## GEMCITABINE

**Trade name:** Gemzar (Lilly)
**Indications:** Pancreatic carcinoma
**Category:** Antineoplastic nucleoside analogue
**Half-life:** 42–94 minutes
**Clinically important, potentially hazardous interactions with:** aldesleukin

### *Reactions*

#### Skin

Allergic reactions (sic) (4%)
Dermatitis (sic)
(2001): Fogarty G+, *Lung Cancer* 33(2), 299
Diaphoresis
Edema (13%)
(2000): Geffen DB+, *Isr Med Assoc J* 2, 552
(1995): Tonato M+, *Anticancer Drugs* 6, 27
Erysipeloid rash (sic)
(2000): Brandes A+, *Anticancer Drugs* 11, 15 (confined to areas of lymphedema)
Exanthems
(2001): Chu CY+, *Acta Derm Venereol* 81(6), 426
(1996): Chen YM+, *J Clin Oncol* 14, 1743
Flu-like syndrome (sic) (>10%)
(2002): Eckel F+, *Cancer Invest* 20(2), 180
Infections (sic) (16%)
Lipodermatosclerosis
(2001): Chia-Yu C+, *Acta Dermato-Venereol* 81(6), 426
Lymphedema
(2000): Brandes A+, *Anticancer Drugs* 11, 15 (confined to areas of erysipeloid rash)
Peripheral edema (20%)
(2002): Voorburg AM+, *Lung Cancer* 36(2), 203 (with cisplatin)
(1995): Tonato M+, *Anticancer Drugs* 6, 27
(1994): Abratt RP+, *J Clin Oncol* 12, 1535
Petechiae (16%)
Pruritus (13%)
Pruritus ani
(1999): Hejna M+, *N Engl J Med* 340, 655
Radiation recall
(2002): Jeter MD+, *Int J Radiat Oncol Biol Phys* 53(2), 394
(2001): Bar-Sela G+, *Tumori* 87(6), 428
(2001): Fogarty G+, *Lung Cancer* 33(2–3), 299
(2000): Burstein HJ, *J Clin Oncol* 18, 693
Radiation recall (myositis)
(2001): Fogarty G+, *Lung Cancer* 33(2–3), 299
Rash (sic) (30%)
Vasculitis
(2002): Voorburg AM+, *Lung Cancer* 36(2), 203
(2000): Banach MJ+, *Arch Ophthalmol* 118, 726 (necrotizing)

#### Hair

Hair – alopecia (15%)
(2002): Brugnatelli S+, *Oncology* 62(1), 33
(2001): Chu CY+, *Acta Derm Venereol* 81(6), 426 (passim)
(1999): Akrivakis K+, *Anticancer Drugs 1999* 10, 525
(1995): Tonato M+, *Anticancer Drugs* 6, 27
(1994): Abratt RP+, *J Clin Oncol* 12, 1535

#### Other

Anaphylactoid reactions
Dysgeusia
(2001): Johnson FM, *Cancer Nurs* 24(2), 149
Injection-site reactions (4%)
Mucositis
(2002): Eckel F+, *Cancer Invest* 20(2), 180
Myalgia (>10%)
(2002): Voorburg AM+, *Lung Cancer* 36(2), 203 (with cisplatin)
Myositis
(2001): Fogarty G+, *Lung Cancer* 33(2), 299
Paresthesias (10%)
Pseudolymphoma
(2001): Marucci G+, *Br J Dermatol* 145(4), 650
Stomatitis (11%)
(2002): Bass AJ+, *J Clin Oncol* 20(13), 2995
(2002): Brugnatelli S+, *Oncology* 62(1), 33

## GEMFIBROZIL

**Trade name:** Lopid (Parke-Davis)
**Other common trade names:** *Bolutol; Decrelip; Fibrocit; Gemlipid; Gen-Fibro; Gevilon Uno; Jezil; Lipur; Nu-Gemfibrozil*
**Indications:** Hyperlipidemia
**Category:** Antihyperlipidemic
**Half-life:** 1.5 hours
**Clinically important, potentially hazardous interactions with:** atorvastatin, bexarotene, cyclosporine, dicumarol, fluvastatin, lovastatin, nicotinic acid, pravastatin, simvastatin, warfarin

### *Reactions*

#### Skin

Abscess
Acanthosis nigricans
Angioedema
Basal cell carcinoma
Dermatitis (sic) (0.4%)
(1988): Todd PA+, *Drugs* 36, 314
Dermatomyositis (<1%)
Eczema (sic) (1.9%)
Erythema multiforme
Exanthems
(1990): Fusella J+, *J Rheumatol* 17, 572

(1988): Todd PA+, *Drugs* 36, 314 (2.1%)
Exfoliative dermatitis (<1%)
Ichthyosis
Lichen planus
Lupus erythematosus
Melanoma
Petechiae
Pruritus (0.8%)
(1988): Todd PA+, *Drugs* 36, 314
Psoriasis
(1989): Frick MH, *Arch Dermatol* 125, 132
(1988): Fisher DA+, *Arch Dermatol* 124, 854
Rash (sic) (1.7%)
Raynaud's phenomenon (<1%)
(1993): Smith GW+, *Br J Rheumatol* 32, 84
Seborrhea
Skin thickening (sic)
Urticaria (0.1%)
(1988): Todd PA+, *Drugs* 36, 314
Vasculitis (<1%)
(1993): Smith GW+, *Br J Rheumatol* 32, 84
Xerosis

### Hair
Hair – alopecia
Hair – hirsutism

### Nails
Nails – discoloration
(1990): Klein ME, *The Schoch Letter* 40 (#7), 29 (#120) (observation)
Nails – increased growth (sic)

### Other
Anaphylactoid reactions
Death
(2001): Federman DG+, *South Med J* 94(10), 1023
(2000): Ozdemir O+, *Angiology* 51(8), 695 (with cerivastatin)
Dysgeusia (<1%)
Hyperesthesia (<1%)
Hypesthesia (<1%)
Myalgia (<1%)
(2001): Litt JZ (personal case) (observation)
Myopathy
Myositis
Paresthesias (<1%)
Polymyositis
(1990): Fusella J+, *J Rheumatol* 17, 572
Pseudolymphoma
(1995): Magro CM+, *J Am Acad Dermatol* 32, 419
Rhabdomyolysis
(2002): Carretero MM+, *Br J Gen Pract* 52(476), 235 (with cerivastatin)
(2001): Bosch Rovira T+, *Rev Clin Esp* 201(12), 731 (with cerivastatin)
(2001): Bruno-Joyce J+, *Ann Pharmacother* 35(9), 1016 (with cerivastatin)
(2001): de Arriba Mendez JJ+, *Med Clin* (Barc) 117(7), 278 (with cerivastatin)
(2001): Federman DG+, *South Med J* 94(10), 1023 (with simvastatin)
(2001): Hendriks F+, *Nephrol Dial Transplant* 16(12), 2418 (with cerivastatin)
(2001): Tomlinson B+, *Am J Med* 110(8), 669 (with cerivastatin)
(2000): Oldemeyer JB+, *Cardiology* 94(2), 127 (with simvastatin)
(2000): Ozdemir O+, *Angiology* 51(8), 695 (with cerivastatin)
(1998): Torbet JA, *Am J Cardiol* 62, 28J (with cyclosporine)
(1990): Pierce LR+, *JAMA* 264(1), 71 (with lovastatin)

## GEMTUZUMAB

**Trade name:** Mylotarg (Wyeth-Ayerst)
**Indications:** Acute myeloid leukemia
**Category:** Antineoplastic monoclonal antibody
**Half-life:** 45 hours (initial dose)

#### *Reactions*

### Skin
Chills (66%)
(2001): Larson RA, *Semin Hematol* 38(Suppl 6), 24
Ecchymoses (15%)
Herpes simplex (22%)
Infections (sic) (28%)
(2001): Larson RA, *Semin Hematol* 38(Suppl 6), 24 (23%)
(2001): Sievers EL+, *Curr Opin Oncol* 13(6), 522
(2001): Sievers EL+, *J Clin Oncol* 19(13), 3244 (28%)
Peripheral edema (21%)
Petechiae (21%)
Rash (sic) (23%)

### Other
Arthralgia (10%)
Infusion-related syndrome
(2001): Larson RA, *Semin Hematol* 38(Suppl 6), 24
Local reaction (sic) (25%)
Mucositis (25%)
(2001): Larson RA, *Semin Hematol* 38(Suppl 6), 24 (4%)
(2001): Sievers EL+, *Curr Opin Oncol* 13(6), 522
(2001): Sievers EL+, *J Clin Oncol* 19(13), 3244 (4%)
Pain
(2001): Larson RA, *Semin Hematol* 38(SUppl 6), 24
Stomatitis (32%)

## GENTAMICIN

**Trade names:** Garamycin (Schering); Genoptic; Gentacidin; Jenamicin; Ocumycin
**Other common trade names:** *Alcomicin; Cidomycin; Diogent; Garatec; Gentalline; Gentalol; I-Gent; Refobacin; Sedanazin*
**Indications:** Various infections caused by susceptible organisms
**Category:** Aminoglycoside antibiotic
**Half-life:** 2–4 hours
**Clinically important, potentially hazardous interactions with:** aldesleukin, aminoglycosides, atracurium, bumetanide, carbenicillin, cephalexin, cephalothin, doxacurium, ethacrynic acid, furosemide, methoxyflurane, non-polarizing muscle relaxants, pancuronium, pipecuronium, polypeptide antibiotics, rocuronium, succinylcholine, torsemide, tubocurarine, vecuronium

#### *Reactions*

### Skin
Contact dermatitis
(2001): Sanchez-Perez J+, *Contact Dermatitis* 44(1), 54 (with kanamycin)
(1996): Merlob P+, *Cutis* 57, 429 (neonatal orbital)
(1996): Munoz-Bellido FJ+, *Allergy* 51, 758
(1989): van Ketel WG+, *Contact Dermatitis* 20, 303
(1988): Robinson PM, *J Laryngol Otol* 102, 577
(1970): Lynfield YL, *N Y State J Med* 70, 2235
(1969): Braun W+, *Hautarzt* (German) 20, 108

Eczematous eruption (sic)
(1988): Ghadially R+, *J Am Acad Dermatol* 19, 428
Edema (1–10%)
Erythema (1–10%)
Exanthems
(2002): Spigarelli MG+, *Pediatr Pulmonol* 33(4), 311
(1990): Flax SH+, *Cutis* 46, 59
(1974): Hewitt WL, *Postgrad Med* 50 (Suppl 7), 55 (0.3%)
(1971): Tümmers H+, *Med Welt* (German) 22, 1404 (1%)
(1969): Braun W+, *Hautarzt* (German) 20, 108
Exfoliative dermatitis
(1989): Guin JD+, *Cutis* 43, 564
Photosensitivity (<1%)
(1990): Flax SH+, *Cutis* 46, 59 (photo recall)
(1966): Hough CE+, *Clin Med Surg* 73, 55
Pruritus (1–10%)
Purpura
(1974): Hewitt WL, *Postgrad Med* 50 (Suppl 7), 55 (0.3%)
Rash (sic)
(2002): Spigarelli MG+, *Pediatr Pulmonol* 33(4), 311
Toxic epidermal necrolysis
(1984): Sluchenkova LD+, *Pediatriia* (Russian) July, 57
Urticaria
(1974): Hewitt WL, *Postgrad Med* 50 (Suppl 7), 55 (0.14%)
Vasculitis
(1980): Bonnetblanc JM+, *Ann Dermatol Vénéréol* (French) 107, 1089

### Hair

Hair – alopecia
(1973): Levantine A+, *Br J Dermatol* 89, 549
(1970): Yoshioka H+, *JAMA* 211, 123

### Other

Anaphylactoid reactions
(1983): Fisher AA, *Cutis* 32, 510
Hypersensitivity
(2002): Spigarelli MG+, *Pediatr Pulmonol* 33(4), 311
Injection-site erythema
(1990): Shen K, *Lancet* 336, 689
Injection-site induration
Injection-site necrosis
(1990): Grob JJ+, *Dermatologica* 180, 258
(1985): Doutre MS+, *Therapie* (French) 40, 266
(1985): Duterque M+, *Ann Dermatol Venereol* (French) 112, 707
(1984): Penso D+, *Presse Méd* (French) 13, 1575
(1984): Taillandier J+, *Presse Méd* (French) 13, 1574
Injection-site pain (<1%)
Paresthesias
Phlebitis
Pseudotumor cerebri (<1%)
Sialorrhea (<1%)
Stomatitis
Thrombophlebitis
Tinnitus
Tremors (<1%)

# GINGER

**Scientific name:** *Zingiber officinale*
**Other common names:** African Ginger; Black Ginger; Cochin Ginger; Gingembre; Ginger Root; Jamaica Ginger; Race Ginger; Zingiberis rhizoma
**Family:** Zingiberaceae
**Purported indications:** Motion sickness, colic, dyspepsia, flatulence, rheumatoid arthritis, loss of appetite, post-surgical nausea and vomiting, discontinuing SSRI drug therapy
**Other uses:** Anorexia, upper respiratory infections, cough, bronchitis. thermal burns, flavoring agent, fragrance component in soaps and cosmetics

## *Reactions*

### Skin

Contact dermatitis
(1996): Kanerva L+, *Contact Dermatitis* 35(3), 157
Dermatitis (sic)

# GINKGO BILOBA

**Scientific name:** *Ginkgo biloba*
**Other common names:** Fossil Tree; Ginkgo; Ginkgo Folium; Ginkyo; Japanese Silver Apricot; Kew Tree; Maidenhair Tree; Salisburia
**Family:** Ginkgoaceae
**Purported indications:** Dementia, Alzheimer's disease, memory loss, headache, tinnitus, vertigo, dizziness, mood disturbances, hearing disorders, intermittent claudication, attention deficit hyperactivity disorder
**Other uses:** Premenstrual syndrome, thrombosis, heart disease, hypercholesterolemia, dysentery, filariasis, diabetic retinopathy. Wound dressings, psychiatric conditions in the elderly
**Clinically important, potentially hazardous interactions with:** aspirin, diuretics, phenytoin, thiazide diuretics, warfarin

## *Reactions*

### Skin

Allergic reactions (sic)
Contact dermatitis
(1989): Lepoittevin JP+, *Arch Dermatol* 281, 227
(1988): Tomb RR+, *Contact Dermatitis* 19, 281
Erythema
Exanthems
(2002): Chiu AE+, *J Am Acad Dermatol* 46(1), 145
Pruritus
Rash (sic)
Vasculitis
Vesicular eruptions

### Other

Phlebitis
Rectal burning (sic)
Spontaneous bleeding
(1998): Matthews MK, *Neurology* 50, 1933
(1997): Gilbert GJ, *Neurology* 48, 1137
(1997): Rosenblatt M+, *N Engl J Med* 336, 1108
(1996): Rowen J+, *Neurology* 46, 1775
Stomatitis

**Note:** *Ginkgo biloba* is the oldest living tree species in the world. Ginkgo is the most frequently prescribed herbal medicine in Germany

## GINSENG

**Scientific name:** *Panax ginseng*
**Other common names:** Asian Ginseng; Asiatic Ginseng; Chinese Ginseng; Ginseng Radix; Ginseng Root; Japanese Ginseng; Jintsam; Korean Ginseng; Korean Red; Ninjin; Oriental Ginseng; Panax Ginseng; Red Ginseng; Ren She; Sang; Seng
**Family:** Araliaceae
**Purported indications:** General tonic, stimulating the immune system. improving physical stamina, athletic stamina and cognitive function, concentration and work efficiency, diuretic, antidepressant
**Other uses:** Premature ejaculation, anemia, diabetes, gastritis, neurasthenia, impotence, fever and hangover. Used in soaps, cosmetics and flavorings
**Clinically important, potentially hazardous interactions with: alcohol**, aspirin, olmesartan, phenelzine

### *Reactions*

#### Skin

Allergic reactions (sic)
Edema
Pruritus
Stevens–Johnson syndrome
(1996): Dega H+, *Lancet* 313, 756

#### Other

Mastodynia
(1978): Palmer BV+, *BMJ* 1, 1284
Penile pain

**Note:** Ginseng has been used for medicinal purposes for more than 2000 years. Approximately 6,000,000 Americans use it regularly

## GLIMEPIRIDE*

**Trade name:** Amaryl (Aventis)
**Indications:** Non-insulin dependent diabetes type II
**Category:** Second generation sulfonylurea* antidiabetic
**Half-life:** 5–9 hours

### *Reactions*

#### Skin

Allergic reactions (sic) (<1%)
Diaphoresis
Edema (<1%)
Erythema (<1%)
Exanthems (<1%)
Exfoliation (sic)
Photosensitivity (<1%)
Pruritus (<1%)
Psoriasis
(1997): Leal G, Fortaleza, Brazil (from Internet) (observation)
Rash (sic) (<1%)
(2001): Deerochanawong C+, *J Med Assoc Thai* 84(9), 1221
Urticaria (<1%)

#### Other

Porphyria cutanea tarda

***Note:** Glimepiride is a sulfonamide and can be absorbed systemically. Sulfonamides can produce severe, possibly fatal, reactions such as toxic epidermal necrolysis and Stevens–Johnson syndrome

## GLIPIZIDE*

**Trade name:** Glucotrol (Pfizer)
**Other common trade names:** *Glibenese; Glipid; Glyde; Melizide; Mindiab; Minidiab; Minodiab*
**Indications:** Non-insulin dependent diabetes type II
**Category:** Second generation sulfonylurea* antidiabetic
**Half-life:** 2–4 hours

### *Reactions*

#### Skin

Eczema (sic)
Edema (<1%)
Erythema (<1%)
Exanthems (<1%)
Exfoliation (sic)
Flushing (<1%)
Grinspan's syndrome**
(1990): Lamey PJ+, *Oral Surg Oral Med Oral Path* 70, 184
Lichenoid eruption
Photosensitivity (1–10%)
Phototoxicity
(2000): Vargas F+, *In Vitr Mol Toxicol* 13, 17
Pigmented purpuric dermatosis
(1999): Adams BB+, *J Am Acad Dermatol* 41, 827
Pruritus (<3%)
Psoriasis (induced)
(1994): Litt JZ, Beachwood, OH (2 personal cases) (observation)
Purpura
Rash (sic) (1–10%)
Urticaria (1–10%)

#### Other

Hypesthesia (<3%)
Myalgia (<3%)
Oral lichen planus
(1990): Lamey PJ+, *Oral Surg Oral Med Oral Path* 70, 184
Paresthesias (<3%)
Porphyria (coproporphyria-like)
(1991): Moder KG+, *Mayo Clin Proc* 66, 312
Porphyria cutanea tarda

***Note:** Glipizide is a sulfonamide and can be absorbed systemically. Sulfonamides can produce severe, possibly fatal, reactions such as toxic epidermal necrolysis and Stevens–Johnson syndrome

****Note:** Grinspan's syndrome: the triad of oral lichen planus, diabetes mellitus, and hypertension

## GLUCAGON

**Trade name:** Glucagon Emergency Kit (Lilly)
**Indications:** Hypoglycemic reactions
**Category:** Antihypoglycemic; antispasmodic; antidote
**Half-life:** 3–10 minutes
**Clinically important, potentially hazardous interactions with:** warfarin

### *Reactions*

#### Skin

Acute febrile neutrophilic dermatosis (Sweet's syndrome)
(1996): Glass LF+, *J Am Acad Dermatol* 34, 455 (passim)
(1994): Fukutoku M+, *Br J Haematol* 86, 645

(1994): Johnson ML+, *Arch Dermatol* 130, 77
(1993): Paydas S+, *Br J Haematol* 85, 191
(1992): Karp DL, *Ann Intern Med* 117, 875
(1992): Park JW+, *Ann Intern Med* 116, 996
(1991): Cohen PR+, *J Am Acad Dermatol* 25, 734

Angioedema
(1985): Gelfand DW+, *Am J Roentgenol* 144, 405

Epidermolysis bullosa acquisita
(1992): Ward JC+, *Br J Haematol* 81, 27

Erythema multiforme
(1980): Edell SL, *Am J Roentgenol* 134, 385

Erythema nodosum
(1994): Nomiyama J+, *Am J Hematol* 47, 333

Exanthems
(1996): Glass LF+, *J Am Acad Dermatol* 34, 455
(1995): Scott GA, *Am J Dermatopathol* 17, 107
(1994): Sasaki O+, *Intern Med* 33, 641
(1993): Peters MS+, *J Cutan Pathol* 20, 465
(1993): Yamashita N+, *J Dermatol* 20, 473
(1992): Mehregan DR+, *Arch Dermatol* 128, 1055
(1976): Barber SG+, *Lancet* 20, 1138

Folliculitis
(1996): Glass LF+, *J Am Acad Dermatol* 34, 455 (passim)
(1992): Ostlere LS+, *Br J Dermatol* 127, 193

Glucagonoma syndrome (necrolytic migratory erythema)
(1988): Benhamou PY+, *Ann Dermatol Venereol* (French) 115, 717

Pyoderma gangrenosum
(1996): Glass LF+, *J Am Acad Dermatol* 34, 455 (passim)
(1994): Johnson ML+, *Arch Dermatol* 130, 77
(1991): Ross HJ+, *Cancer* 68, 441 (bullous)

Rash (sic)
(1979): Barber SG+, *Ann Intern Med* 91, 213
(1976): Barber SG+, *Lancet* 2, 1138

Urticaria (1–10%)
(1985): Gelfand DW+, *Am J Roentgenol* 144, 405
(1975): Kitabchi AE+, *J Clin Endocrinol Metab* 41, 863

Vasculitis
(1996): Glass LF+, *J Am Acad Dermatol* 34, 455 (passim)
(1995): Couderc LJ+, *Respir Med* 89, 237
(1995): Vidarsson B+, *Am J Med* 98, 589
(1994): Jain KK, *J Am Acad Dermatol* 31, 213
(1994): Johnson ML+, *Arch Dermatol* 130, 77
(1994): van Kamp H+, *Br J Haematol* 86, 415
(1991): Wodzinski MA+, *Br J Haematol* 77, 249
(1990): Welte Z+, *Blood* 75, 1056
(1989): Dreicer R+, *Ann Intern Med* 111, 91

### Other

Injection-site reactions (sic)
(1996): Glass LF+, *J Am Acad Dermatol* 34, 455 (passim)
(1993): Samlaska CP+, *Arch Dermatol* 129, 645
(1992): Mehregan DR+, *Arch Dermatol* 128, 1055

# GLYBURIDE

**Synonyms:** glibenclamide; glybenclamide
**Trade names:** Diabeta (Aventis); Glucovance (Bristol-Myers Squibb); Glynase (Pharmacia & Upjohn); Micronase (Pharmacia & Upjohn)
**Other common trade names:** *Albert Glyburide; Daonil; Euglucan; Euglucon; Glimel; Glucal; Hemi-Daonil; Med-Glibe; Miglucan; Norboral*
**Indications:** Non-insulin dependent diabetes type II
**Category:** Second generation sulfonylurea* antidiabetic
**Half-life:** 5–16 hours
**Clinically important, potentially hazardous interactions with:** bosentan

Glucovance is glyburide and metformin

## *Reactions*

### Skin

Allergic reactions (sic) (0.21%)
(1986): Bigby M+, *JAMA* 256, 3358

Angioedema

Bullous eruption
(1981): Wongpaitoon V+, *Postgrad Med J* 57, 244

Eczema (sic)

Erythema (1–5%)
(1988): Chee Ching S, *Photodermatol* 5, 42

Exanthems (1–5%)
(1971): Editorial, *BMJ* 2, 644
(1970): O'Sullivan DJ+, *BMJ* 2, 572 (0.5–1%)
(1969): Müller R+, *Horm Metab Res* 1, 88

Exfoliation (sic)

Eyelid edema
(1985): Yitalo P+, *Arzneimittelforsch* (German) 35, 1596

Flushing
(1971): Fairman MJ+, *BMJ* 4, 297
(1971): Wardle EN+, *BMJ* 3, 309

Lichenoid eruption

Linear IgA bullous dermatosis
(1983): Väätäinen N+, *Acta Derm Venereol* (Stockh) 63, 169

Pellagra
(1988): Berova N+, *Dermatol Monatsschr* (German) 174, 50

Pemphigus
(1993): Paterson AJ+, *J Oral Pathol Med* 22, 92

Photosensitivity (1–10%)
(1995): Fujii S+, *Am J Hematol* 50, 223
(1994): Shelley WB+, *Cutis* 53, 287 (observation)
(1994): Shelley WB+, *Cutis* 53, 77 (observation)
(1988): Chee-Ching S, *Photodermatology* 5, 42
(1988): Sun CC, *Photodermatol* 5, 42
(1987): Henrietta G, *Nursing* 17, 56
(1969): Müller R+, *Horm Metab Res* 1, 88

Pruritus (1–10%)
(1988): Chee Ching S, *Photodermatol* 5, 42
(1987): *Physicians Drug Alert* 7, 71
(1970): O'Sullivan DJ+, *BMJ* 2, 572

Psoriasis
(1988): Milner JE, *The Schoch Letter* 38(5), Item 64 (observation)
(1987): Goh CL, *Australas J Dermatol* 28, 30

Purpura
(1986): Dickey W+, *BMJ* 293, 823
(1983): Väätäinen N+, *Acta Derm Venereol* (Stockh) 63, 169

Rash (sic) (1–10%)

Urticaria (1–5%)
(1994): Shelley WB+, *Cutis* 53, 77 (observation)

(1991): Chichmanian RM+, *Therapie* (French) 46, 163
(1986): Jordan NS+, *Hosp Pharm* 21, 462
(1986): Kure J, *NC Med J* 47, 149
(1969): Müller R+, *Horm Metab Res* 1, 88
Vasculitis
(1986): Dickey W+, *BMJ* 293, 823
(1980): Ingelmo M+, *Med Clin (Barc)* (Spanish) 75, 306
(1974): Clarke BF+, *Diabetes* 23, 739
(1970): O'Sullivan DJ+, *BMJ* 2, 572
Vesiculobullous eruption
(1993): Landor M+, *Ann Allergy* 70, 196

## Other

Dysgeusia
Hypersensitivity (generalized)
(1974): Clarke BF+, *Diabetes* 23, 739
Myalgia
Paresthesias (<1%)
Porphyria cutanea tarda

***Note:** Glyburide is a sulfonamide and can be absorbed systemically. Sulfonamides can produce severe, possibly fatal, reactions such as toxic epidermal necrolysis and Stevens–Johnson syndrome

# GLYCOPYRROLATE

**Trade name:** Robinul (Robins)
**Other common trade names:** *Gastrodyn; Sroton; Strodin*
**Indications:** Duodenal ulcer, irritable bowel syndrome
**Category:** Anticholinergic; antispasmodic
**Half-life:** no data
**Clinically important, potentially hazardous interactions with:** anticholinergics, arbutamine

### *Reactions*

## Skin

Allergic reactions (sic)
Flushing
Hypohidrosis (>10%)
Photosensitivity (1–10%)
Rash (sic) (<1%)
Urticaria
Xerosis (>10%)

## Other

Anhidrosis
Dysgeusia
Injection-site irritation (>10%)
Xerostomia (>10%)
(2001): Patel PS+, *Spec Care Dentist* 21(5), 176

# GOLD and GOLD COMPOUNDS

**Generic names:**
**Auranofin**
Trade name: Ridaura (GSK)
**Aurothioglucose**
Trade name: Solganal (Schering)
**Gold sodium thiomalate (sodium aurothiomalate)**
Trade name: Myochrysine (Merck)
**Other common trade names:** *Aureotan; Aurolate; Aurothio; Miocrin; Myocrisine; Shiosol; Tauredon*
**Indications:** Rheumatoid arthritis
**Category:** Antiarthritic
**Half-life:** 5 days

### *Reactions*

## Skin

Acne
(1982): Bailin PL+, *Clin Rheum Dis* 8, 493 (passim)
(1977): Hjortshoj A, *Acta Derm Venereol* (Stockh) 57, 165
Angioedema (<1%)
(1989): Herbst WM+, *Hautarzt* (German) 40, 568
Angiofibromatosis
(1989): Herbst WM+, *Hautarzt* (German) 40, 568
Bullous eruption
(1970): Almeyda J+, *Br J Dermatol* 83, 707
(1951): Jaeger H, *Dermatologica* 103, 280
(1940): Wile UJ+, *Arch Dermatol* 42, 1005 (passim)
Bullous pemphigoid
(1983): Wozel G+, *Dermatol Monatsschr* (German) 169, 125
Cheilitis
(1982): Bailin PL+, *Clin Rheum Dis* 8, 493 (passim)
(1974): Penneys NS+, *Arch Dermatol* 109, 372
Chrysiasis (blue-green pigmentation)
(2001): Werth V, *Dermatology Times* 18
Contact dermatitis
(2002): Ahlgren C+, *Acta Derm Venereol* 82(1), 41 (dental gold alloy)
(2001): Lee AY+, *Contact Dermatitis* 45(4), 214
(2000): Trattner A+, *Contact Dermatitis* 42, 301
(2000): Vamnes JS+, *Contact Dermatitis* 42, 128
(1999): Bruze M+, *Contact Dermatitis* 40, 295
(1999): Fowler JF, *Skin and Allergy News* September, 34 (9.5%)
(1999): Räsänen L+, *Br J Dermatol* 141, 683
(1998): Estlander T+, *Contact Dermatitis* 38, 40
(1998): Moller H+, *Am J Contact Dermat* 9, 15
(1998): Wiesner M+, *Contact Dermatitis* 38, 52
(1997): Armstrong DK+, *Br J Dermatol* 136, 776
(1997): Fleming C+, *Contact Dermatitis* 37, 298 (lymphomatoid)
(1997): Hostynek JJ, *Food Chem Toxicol* 35, 839
(1997): Kilpikari I, *Contact Dermatitis* 37, 130
(1997): Moller H+, *Acta Derm Venereol* 77, 370
(1997): Silva R+, *Contact Dermatitis* 37, 78
(1996): Sabroe RA+, *Contact Dermatitis* 34, 345
(1996): Tan E+, *Australas J Dermatol* 37, 218
(1994): Björkner B+, *Contact Dermatitis* 30, 144
(1994): Bruze M+, *J Am Acad Dermatol* 31, 579
(1994): Collet E+, *Ann Dermatol Venereol* (French) 121, 21
(1994): Osawa J+, *Contact Dermatitis* 31, 89
(1994): Webster CG+, *Cutis* 54, 25
(1993): Aro T+, *Contact Dermatitis* 28, 276
(1993): Hisa T+, *Contact Dermatitis* 28, 174
(1993): Koga T+, *Br J Dermatol* 128, 227
(1993): Koga T+, *Contact Dermatitis* 28, 303
(1990): Miller RA+, *J Am Acad Dermatol* 23, 360
(1990): Wijnands MJ+, *Lancet* 335, 867

(1989): Camarasa JG+, *Med Cutan Ibero Lat Am* (Spanish) 17, 187
(1988): Fowler JF, *Arch Dermatol* 124, 181
(1988): Goh CL, *Contact Dermatitis* 18, 122
(1988): Wicks IP+, *Ann Rheum Dis* 47, 421
(1987): Fisher AA, *Cutis* 39, 473
(1987): Fisher AA, *J Am Acad Dermatol* 17, 853
(1985): Kalamkarian AA+, *Vestn Dermatol Venerol* (Russian) August, 4
(1985): Rapson WS, *Contact Dermatitis* 13, 56
(1985): Silvennoinen-Kassinen S+, *Contact Dermatitis* 11, 156
(1985): Tosi S+, *Int J Clin Pharmacol Res* 5, 265
(1983): Monti M+, *Contact Dermatitis* 9, 150
(1982): Iwatsuki K+, *Arch Dermatol* 118, 608
(1980): Raith L+, *Dermatol Monatsschr* (German) 166, 382
(1978): Budden MG+, *Contact Dermatitis* 4, 172
(1977): Dick D, *BMJ* 1, 51
(1977): Fisher AA, *Cutis* 19, 156
(1977): Rennie N, *BMJ* 1, 446
(1975): Klaschka F, *Contact Dermatitis* 1, 264
(1975): Roeleveld CG+, *Contact Dermatitis* 1, 333
(1973): Petros H+, *Br J Dermatol* 88, 505
(1971): Nava C+, *Med Lav* (Italian) 62, 572
(1971): Rytter M+, *Dermatologica* (German) 142, 209
(1971): Walzer R+, *Arch Dermatol* 104, 107

Cutaneous eruption (sic)
(1998): Pandya AG+, *Arch Dermatol* 134, 1104

Dermatitis (sic)
(2000): ter Borg EJ+, *Arthritis Rheum* 43, 1420
(1999): Räsänen L+, *Br J Dermatol* 141, 683
(1997): Choy EH+, *Br J Rheumatol* 36, 1054
(1996): Bonnetblanc JM, *Presse Med* (French) 25, 1555
(1986): Minghetti G+, *G Ital Dermatol Venereol* (Italian) 121, 425
(1985): Kalamkarian AA+, *Vestn Dermatol Venerol* (Russian) Aug, 4
(1983): Sigler JW, *Am J Med* 75, 59
(1958): Smith RT+, *JAMA* 167, 1197
(1940): Wile UJ+, *Arch Dermatol* 42, 1005 (passim)

Eczematous eruption (sic)
(1994): Lizeaux-Parneix V+, *Ann Dermatol Venereol* (French) 121, 793
(1986): Hofmann C+, *Z Rheumatol* (German) 45, 100
(1976): Rennie JAN, *BMJ* 2, 1294

Erythema annulare centrifugum
(1992): Tsuji T+, *J Am Acad Dermatol* 27, 284

Erythema multiforme
(1982): Bailin PL+, *Clin Rheum Dis* 8, 493 (passim)
(1966): Cameron AJ+, *BMJ* 2, 1125

Erythema nodosum
(1998): Pandya AG+, *Arch Dermatol* 134, 1104 (passim)
(1982): Bailin PL+, *Clin Rheum Dis* 8, 493 (passim)
(1974): Penneys NS+, *Arch Dermatol* 109, 372
(1973): Stone RL+, *Arch Dermatol* 107, 602

Exanthems (>5%)
(1999): Räsänen L+, *Br J Dermatol* 141, 683
(1998): Pandya AG+, *Arch Dermatol* 134, 1104 (passim)
(1996): Bonnetblanc JM, *Presse Med* (French) 25, 1555
(1994): Shelley WB+, *Cutis* 52, 87 (observation)
(1977): Voigt K+, *Hautarzt* (German) 28, 421
(1974): Penneys NS+, *Arch Dermatol* 109, 372
(1972): Walzer RA+, *Arch Dermatol* 106, 231
(1940): Wile UJ+, *Arch Dermatol* 42, 1005 (passim)

Exfoliative dermatitis
(2000): Lancucki J+, *Wiad Lek* (Polish) 21, 1347 (erythroderma)
(1998): Pandya AG+, *Arch Dermatol* 134, 1104 (passim)
(1996): Sigurdsson V+, *J Am Acad Dermatol* 35, 53
(1991): Wilson CL+, *Int J Dermatol* 30, 148
(1989): Ranki A+, *Am J Dermatopathol* 11, 22
(1984): Adachi JD+, *J Rheumatol* 11, 355
(1982): Bailin PL+, *Clin Rheum Dis* 8, 493 (passim)
(1974): Penneys NS+, *Arch Dermatol* 109, 372
(1940): Wile UJ+, *Arch Dermatol* 42, 1005 (passim)

Fixed eruption

Graft-versus-host reaction
(1998): Jappe U+, *Hautarzt* (German) 49, 126 (passim)

Granuloma annulare
(1990): Martin N+, *Arch Dermatol* 126, 1370
(1980): Rothwell RS+, *Arch Dermatol* 116, 863

Herpes zoster
(1981): Fam AG+, *Ann Intern Med* 94, 712

Lichen planus
(1996): Russell MA+, *N Engl J Med* 334, 603
(1990): Torrelo A+, *Actas Dermo-Sif* (Spanish) 81, 743
(1986): Hofmann C+, *Z Rheumatol* (German) 45, 100
(1986): Ingber A+, *Z Hautkr* (German) 61, 315
(1982): Bailin PL+, *Clin Rheum Dis* 8, 493 (passim)
(1979): Krebs A, *Hautarzt* (German) 30, 281
(1977): Hjorthsoj A, *Acta Derm Venereol* (Stockh) 57, 165
(1974): Delaby MC, *Arch Belg Dermatol* 30, 111
(1974): Penneys NS+, *Arch Dermatol* 109, 372 (32%)
(1937): Hartfall SJ+, *Lancet* 2, 838

Lichen spinulosus
(1932): Throne B+, *Arch Dermatol* 25, 494

Lichenoid eruption
(2001): Werth V, *Dermatology Times* 18
(1999): Räsänen L+, *Br J Dermatol* 141, 683
(1998): Pandya AG+, *Arch Dermatol* 134, 1104 (passim)
(1997): Choy EH+, *Br J Rheumatol* 36, 1054
(1996): Bonnetblanc JM, *Presse Med* (French) 25, 1555
(1994): Alzieu PH+, *Ann Dermatol Venereol* (French) 121, 798
(1994): Lizeaux-Parneix V+, *Ann Dermatol Venereol* (French) 121, 793
(1971): Almeyda J+, *Br J Dermatol* 85, 604

Lupus erythematosus
(1988): Balsa A+, *Rev Clin Esp* (Spanish) 182, 505
(1969): Goerz G, *Dtsch Med Wochenschr* (German) 94, 2040
(1967): Kapp W+, *Praxis* (German) 56, 1594

Lymphocytoma cutis
(1992): Kobayashi Y+, *J Am Acad Dermatol* 27, 457

Lymphomatoid eosinophilic reaction (sic)
(1999): Park YM+, *Contact Dermatitis* 40, 216

Pemphigus
(1978): Miyamoto Y+, *Arch Dermatol* 114, 1855

Photosensitivity
(1973): Machtey I, *Harefuah* (Hebrew) 85, 517
(1970): Almeyda J+, *Br J Dermatol* 83, 707

Pigmentation (chrysiasis)
(1998): Pandya AG+, *Arch Dermatol* 134, 1104 (passim)
(1997): Miller ML+, *Cutis* 59, 256
(1996): Fleming CJ+, *J Am Acad Dermatol* 34, 349
(1992): Cremer B+, *Dtsch Med Wochenschr* (German) 117, 558
(1990): Bonet M+, *Clin Rheumatol* 9, 254
(1984): Fam AG+, *Arthritis Rheum* 27, 119
(1984): Larsen FS+, *Clin Exp Dermatol* 9, 174
(1984): Pelachyk IM+, *J Cutan Pathol* 11, 491
(1982): Bailin PL+, *Clin Rheum Dis* 8, 493 (passim)
(1982): Beckett VL+, *Mayo Clin Proc* 57, 773
(1981): Granstein RD+, *J Am Acad Dermatol* 5, 1 (blue-gray)
(1975): Altmeyer P+, *Hautarzt* (German) 26, 330
(1974): Gottlieb NL+, *Arthritis Rheum* 17, 56
(1973): Cox AJ+, *Arch Dermatol* 108, 655
(1973): Levantine A+, *Br J Dermatol* 89, 105
(1971): Franken E, *Dtsch Gesundheitsw* (German) 26, 653
(1965): Bianchi O+, *Arch Argent Dermatol* (Spanish) 15, 464
(1941): Schmidt OEL, *Arch Dermatol* 44, 446
(1928): Hansborg H, *Acta Tuberc Scand* 4, 124

Pityriasis rosea
(1999): Räsänen L+, *Br J Dermatol* 141, 683
(1998): Pandya AG+, *Arch Dermatol* 134, 1104 (passim)

(1994): Lizeaux-Parneix V+, *Ann Dermatol Venereol* (French) 121, 793
(1992): Tsuji T+, *J Am Acad Dermatol* 27, 284
(1986): Hofmann C+, *Z Rheumatol* (German) 45, 100
(1982): Bailin PL+, *Clin Rheum Dis* 8, 493 (passim)
(1977): Maize JC+, *Arch Dermatol* 113, 1457
(1974): Penneys NS+, *Arch Dermatol* 109, 372
(1940): Wile UJ+, *Arch Dermatol* 42, 1005

Pruritus
(1998): Pandya AG+, *Arch Dermatol* 134, 1104
(1996): Bonnetblanc JM, *Presse Med* (French) 25, 1555
(1982): Bailin PL+, *Clin Rheum Dis* 8, 493 (passim)
(1975): Gordon MH+, *Ann Intern Med* 82, 47
(1974): Pennys NS+, *Arch Dermatol* 109, 372 (84%)
(1958): Smith RT+, *JAMA* 167, 1197
(1940): Wile UJ+, *Arch Dermatol* 42, 1005 (passim)

Psoriasis
(1991): Smith DL+, *Arch Dermatol* 127, 268

Purpura
(1984): Adachi JD+, *J Rheumatol* 11, 355
(1982): Bailin PL+, *Clin Rheum Dis* 8, 493 (passim)
(1966): Saphir JR+, *JAMA* 195, 782

Pyoderma gangrenosum

Radiation keratosis
(1996): Helm KF+, *Cutis* 57, 435

Rash (sic) (>10%)
(1990): Fremont-Smith P+, *Ann Rheum Dis* 49, 271
(1989): Caspi D+, *Ann Rheum Dis* 48, 730
(1984): Grindulis KA+, *Ann Rheum Dis* 43, 398
(1982): Smith PJ+, *Br Med J (Clin Res Ed)* 285, 595
(1979): Kean WF+, *Arthritis Rheum* 22, 495
(1961): Bayles TB, *Med Clin North Am* 5, 1229
(1956): Bayles TB+, *Ann Rheum Dis* 15, 394

Seborrheic dermatitis
(1982): Bailin PL+, *Clin Rheum Dis* 8, 493 (passim)
(1981): Kanwar AJ+, *Arch Dermatol* 117, 65 (passim)
(1951): Merliss RR+, *Ann Intern Med* 35, 352

Squamous cell carcinoma
(1990): Miller RA+, *J Am Acad Dermatol* 23, 360 (from radioactive gold)
(1973): Holubar K+, *Hautarzt* (German) 24, 489 (from radioactive gold)

Toxic dermatitis (sic)
(1958): Smith RT+, *JAMA* 167, 1197

Toxic epidermal necrolysis
(1998): Pandya AG+, *Arch Dermatol* 134, 1104 (passim)
(1982): Braun-Falco O+, *MMM Munch Med Wochenschr* (German) 124, 757 (with benoxaprofen)
(1982): Feldman C+, *Rheumatol Rehabil* 21, 222 (with benoxaprofen)
(1951): Jaeger H, *Dermatologica* 103, 280

Urticaria (1–10%)
(1998): Pandya AG+, *Arch Dermatol* 134, 1104 (passim)
(1994): Lizeaux-Parneix V+, *Ann Dermatol Venereol* (French) 121, 793
(1982): Bailin PL+, *Clin Rheum Dis* 8, 493 (passim)
(1974): Penneys NS+, *Arch Dermatol* 109, 372
(1970): Almeyda J+, *Br J Dermatol* 83, 707
(1940): Wile UJ+, *Arch Dermatol* 42, 1005 (passim)
(1936): Roche H, *BMJ* 1, 31

Vasculitis
(1984): Hauteville D+, *Rev Rhum Mal Osteoartic* (French) 51, 56
(1982): Bailin PL+, *Clin Rheum Dis* 8, 493 (passim)
(1974): Roenigk HR+, *Arch Dermatol* 109, 253
(1974): Steele DR, *Arch Dermatol* 110, 297

Vitiligo
(1933): Pillsbury DM+, *Arch Dermatol* 27, 36

Xerosis
(1984): Grindulis KA+, *Ann Rheum Dis* 43, 398

## Hair

Hair – alopecia (1–10%)
(1998): Pandya AG+, *Arch Dermatol* 134, 1104 (passim)
(1984): Grindulis KA+, *Ann Rheum Dis* 43, 398
(1982): Bailin PL+, *Clin Rheum Dis* 8, 493 (passim)
(1975): Gordon MH+, *Ann Intern Med* 82, 47
(1972): Walzer RA+, *Arch Dermatol* 106, 231

Hair – pigmentation
(1974): Gottlieb NL+, *Arthritis Rheum* 17, 56

## Nails

Nails – dystrophy
(1977): Voigt K+, *Hautarzt* (German) 28, 421

Nails – exfoliation
(1938): Boon TH, *BMJ* 1, 780

Nails – lichen planus
(1990): Torrelo A+, *Actas Dermo-Sif* (Spanish) 81, 743

Nails – onycholysis
(1977): Voigt K+, *Hautarzt* (German) 28, 421

Nails – pigmentation
(1984): Fam AG+, *Arthritis Rheum* 27, 119 (gold nails)
(1974): Gottlieb NL+, *Arthritis Rheum* 17, 56

Nails – shedding
(2000): ter Borg EJ+, *Arthritis Rheum* 43, 1420

Nails – yellow
(2001): Roest MA+, *Br J Dermatol* 145, 186

## Other

Acute intermittent porphyria

Anaphylactoid reactions

Aphthous stomatitis
(1989): Caspi D+, *Ann Rheum Dis* 48, 730
(1979): Kean WF+, *Arthritis Rheum* 22, 495
(1976): Kuffer R+, *Rev Stomatol Chir Maxillofac* (French) 77, 747

Burning mouth syndrome
(1994): Laeijendecker R+, *J Am Acad Dermatol* 30, 205

Dysgeusia
(1996): Bonnetblanc JM, *Presse Med* (French) 25, 1555
(1974): Pennys NS+, *Arch Dermatol* 109, 372 (metallic taste)
(1970): Almeyda J+, *Br J Dermatol* 83, 707
(1940): Wile UJ+, *Arch Dermatol* 42, 1005 (passim)

Gingivitis (>10%)
(1976): Adams D+, *J Rheumatol Rehabilitation* 15, 245
(1970): Almeyda J+, *Br J Dermatol* 83, 707

Gingivostomatitis
(1982): Izumi AK, *Arch Dermatol Res* 272, 387 (allergic contact)

Glossitis (>10%)
(1976): Adams D+, *J Rheumatol Rehabilitation* 15, 245
(1975): Gordon MH+, *Ann Intern Med* 82, 47

Hypersensitivity
(1972): Walzer RA+, *Arch Dermatol* 106, 231

Injection-site pain
(1984): Grindulis KA+, *Ann Rheum Dis* 43, 398

Mucocutaneous reaction
(1996): Cheatum DE, *J Rheumatol* 23, 944
(1995): Klinkhoff AV+, *J Rheumatol* 22, 1657

Oral lichen planus
(1994): Laeijendecker R+, *J Am Acad Dermatol* 30, 205
(1994): Lizeaux-Parneix V+, *Ann Dermatol Venereol* (French) 121, 793
(1993): Brown RS+, *Cutis* 51, 183

Oral lichenoid eruption
(1990): Vallejo-Irastorza G+, *Av Odontoestomatol* (Spanish) 6, 131

Oral mucosal eruption
(1968): Bardadin T+, *Reumatologia* (Polish) 6, 287

Oral mucosal pigmentation
(1990): Torrelo A+, *Actas Dermo-Sif* (Spanish) 81, 743

(1984): Sutak J+, *Prakt Zubn Lek* (Czech) 32, 166
Oral ulceration
(2000): Madinier I+, *Ann Med Interne (Paris)* (French) 151, 248
(1999): Räsänen L+, *Br J Dermatol* 141, 683
(1984): Glenert U, *Oral Surg* 58, 52
(1982): Bailin PL+, *Clin Rheum Dis* 8, 493 (passim)
(1979): Kean WF+, *Arthritis Rheum* 22, 495
(1976): Adams D+, *J Rheumatol Rehabilitation* 15, 245
Pseudolymphoma
(2002): Kim KJ+, *Br J Dermatol* 146, 882 (gold acupuncture)
(1996): Kalimo K+, *J Cutan Pathol* 23, 328
Stomatitis (>10%)
(2001): Werth V, *Dermatology Times* 18
(1997): Tosti A+, *Semin Cutan Med Surg* 16, 314
(1996): Bonnetblanc JM, *Presse Med* (French) 25, 1555
(1994): Laeijendecker R+, *J Am Acad Dermatol* 30, 205
(1992): Svensson A+, *Ann Rheum Dis* 51, 326
(1989): Caspi D+, *Ann Rheum Dis* 48, 730
(1987): Tumiati B+, *J Rheumatol* 14, 177
(1984): Glenert U, *Oral Surg* 58, 52
(1983): Sigler JW, *Am J Med* 75, 59
(1982): Bailin PL+, *Clin Rheum Dis* 8, 493 (passim)
(1979): Belkahaia C+, *Tunis Med* (French) 57, 234
(1979): Fregert S+, *Contact Dermatitis* 5, 63
(1975): Gordon MH+, *Ann Intern Med* 82, 47
(1971): Myers AR, *Mod Treat* 8, 761
(1970): Almeyda J+, *Br J Dermatol* 83, 707
(1970): Schopf E+, *Hautarzt* (German) 21, 422
(1958): Smith RT+, *JAMA* 167, 1197
Vaginitis
(1978): Webster JC+, *Am J Obstet Gynecol* 131, 700

**Note:** Adverse reactions can occur months after therapy has been discontinued

## GOSERELIN

**Trade name:** Zoladex (AstraZeneca)
**Other common trade name:** *Prozoladex*
**Indications:** Breast and prostate carcinoma, endometriosis
**Category:** Gonadotropin-releasing analog hormone
**Half-life:** 5 hours

### *Reactions*

#### Skin

Chills
Diaphoresis (1–10%)
Edema (1–10%)
Hot flashes (>10%)
(1993): Bressler LR+, *Ann Pharmacother* 27, 182
Rash (sic) (1–10%)
Urticaria

#### Other

Anaphylactoid reactions
(1996): Raj SG+, *Am J Med Sci* 312, 187
Gynecomastia (>10%)
Hypersensitivity
(1996): Raj SG+, *Am J Med Sci* 312, 187
Injection-site pain (1–10%)
Injection-site papules & nodules (sic)
(2002): Cunha AP+, *World Congress Dermatol* Poster, 0095
Mastodynia (1–10%)
Relapsing polychondritis
(1997): Labarthe MP+, *Dermatology* 195, 391

## GRANISETRON

**Trade name:** Kytril (Roche)
**Other common trade name:** *Kevatril*
**Indications:** Chemotherapy-related emesis
**Category:** Antiemetic and antinauseant; serotonin antagonist
**Half-life:** 3–4 hours; cancer patients: 10–12 hours

### *Reactions*

#### Skin

Allergic reactions (sic)
(2001): Kanny G+, *J Allergy Clin Immunol* 108(6), 1059
Exanthems
Hot flashes (<1%)
Rash (sic)
Urticaria

#### Hair

Hair – alopecia (3%)

#### Other

Anaphylactoid reactions
Dysgeusia (2%)
Hypersensitivity

## GRANULOCYTE COLONY-STIMULATING FACTOR (GCSF)

**Generic name:**
**Filgrastim (rG-CSF)**
Trade name: Neupogen (Amgen)
**Sargramostin (rGM-CSF)**
Trade names: Leukine (Immunex); Prokine
**Other common trade names:** *Grasin; Leucogen; Neupogen 30*
**Indications:** Bone marrow allograft and autograft
**Category:** Hematopoietic growth factor; neutrophil stimulator
**Half-life:** filgrastim: 3.5 hours; sargramostin: 2–3 hours

### *Reactions*

#### Skin

Acne
(1996): Lee PK+, *J Am Acad Dermatol* 34, 855
Acral erythema
(1995): Komamura H+, *J Dermatol* 22(2), 116
Acute febrile neutrophilic dermatosis (Sweet's syndrome)
(2002): Brazzelli V+, *World Congress Dermatol* Poster, 0089
(2001): Matsumura T+, *Br J Haematol* 113(1), 1
(2001): Prendiville J+, *Pediatr Dermatol* 18(5), 417 (2 cases)
(2000): Malone JC+, *Arch Dermatol* 345 (passim)
(1999): Arbetter KR+, *Am J Hematol* 61, 126
(1999): Veres K+, *Orv Hetil* (Hungarian) 140, 1059
(1998): Chao SC+, *J Formos Med Assoc* 96, 276
(1998): Hasegawa M+, *Eur J Dermatol* 8, 503 (2 patients)
(1998): Merkel PA, *Curr Opin Rheumatol* 10, 45
(1996): Garty BZ+, *Pediatrics* 97, 401
(1996): Jain KK, *Cutis* 57, 107
(1996): Petit T+, *Lancet* 347, 690
(1996): Prevost-Blank PL+, *J Am Acad Dermatol* 35, 995
(1996): Richard MA+, *J Am Acad Dermatol* 35, 629
(1996): Shimizu T+, *J Pediatr Hematol Oncol* 18, 282
(1995): Shiga Y+, *Rinsho Ketsueki* (Japanese) 36, 353
(1995): Suzuki Y+, *Br J Dermatol* 133, 483
(1994): Fukutoku M+, *Br J Haematol* 86, 645

(1994): Johnson ML+, *Arch Dermatol* 130, 77
(1994): Reuss-Borst MA+, *Leuk Lymphoma* 15, 261
(1994): van Kamp H+, *Br J Haematol* 86, 415
(1993): Paydas S+, *Br J Haematol* 85, 191
(1992): Karp DL, *Ann Intern Med* 117, 875
(1992): Park JW+, *Ann Intern Med* 116, 996
(1991): Ross HJ+, *Cancer* 68, 441
(1990): Morioka N+, *J Am Acad Dermatol* 23, 247
(1989): Groopman JE+, *N Engl J Med* 321, 1449
(1989): Kluin-Nelemans JC+, *Br J Haematol* 73, 419

Diaphoresis
(2000): Khoury H+, *Bone Marrow Transplant* 25, 1197

Erythema
(1990): Farmer KL+, *Arch Dermatol* 126, 1243
(1989): Groopman JE+, *N Engl J Med* 321, 1449

Erythema nodosum
(1994): Nomiyama J+, *Am J Hematol* 47, 333

Exanthems
(1996): Glass LF+, *J Am Acad Dermatol* 34, 455
(1995): McMullin MF+, *Clin Rheumatol* 14, 204
(1995): Scott GA, *Am J Dermatopathol* 17, 107
(1994): Sasaki O+, *Intern Med* 33, 641
(1993): Samlaska CP+, *Arch Dermatol* 129, 645
(1993): Yamashita N+, *J Dermatol* 20, 473
(1991): Cohen PR+, *J Am Acad Dermatol* 25, 734
(1991): Horn TD+, *Arch Dermatol* 127, 49 (>5%)
(1990): Farmer KL+, *Arch Dermatol* 126, 1243
(1990): Lazarus H+, *Proc Am Soc Clin Oncol* 9, 15
(1988): Brandt SJ+, *N Engl J Med* 318, 869 (63%)

Exfoliative dermatitis
(1988): Brandt SJ+, *N Engl J Med* 318, 869 (10%)

Flushing (>10%)
(2000): Khoury H+, *Bone Marrow Transplant* 25, 1197

Folliculitis
(1992): Ostlere LS+, *Br J Dermatol* 127, 193

Lichenoid reaction
(2002): Brazzelli V+, *World Congress Dermatol* Poster, 0089

Linear IgA bullous dermatosis
(1999): Kano Y+, *Eur J Dermatol* 9, 122

Neutrophilic eccrine hidradenitis
(1998): Bachmeyer C+, *Br J Dermatol* 139, 354

Panniculitis, necrotizing
(2000): Dereure O+, *Br J Dermatol* 142, 834

Peripheral edema (1–10%)

Pruritus
(1990): Farmer KL+, *Arch Dermatol* 126, 1243
(1990): Steward WP+, *Int J Cell Cloning* 8, 335
(1989): Steward WP+, *Br J Cancer* 59, 142 (1–5%)

Psoriasis
(2001): Yonei T+, *Nihon Kokyuki Gakkai Zasshi* 39(6), 438
(1998): Cho SG+, *J Korean Med Sci* 13, 685
(1996): Kavanaugh A, *Am J Med* 101, 567

Pyoderma gangrenosum
(1998): Merkel PA, *Curr Opin Rheumatol* 10, 45
(1991): Ross HJ+, *Cancer* 68, 441

Rash (sic)

Urticaria

Vasculitis
(1999): Andavolu MV+, *Ann Hematol* 78, 79
(1998): Merkel PA, *Curr Opin Rheumatol* 10, 45
(1995): Couderc LJ+, *Respir Med* 89, 237
(1995): Farhey YD+, *J Rheumatol* 22, 1179
(1995): Vidarsson B+, *Am J Med* 98, 589
(1994): Jain KK, *J Am Acad Dermatol* 31, 213
(1994): Johnson ML+, *Arch Dermatol* 130, 77
(1990): Farmer KL+, *Arch Dermatol* 126, 1243
(1989): Kluin-Nelemans JC+, *Br J Haematol* 73, 419

## Hair

Hair – alopecia (>10%)
(1990): Lazarus H+, *Proc Am Soc Clin Oncol* 9, 15

## Other

Anaphylactoid reactions (<1%)
(2000): Khoury H+, *Bone Marrow Transplant* 25, 1197
(1999): Dupre D+, *Ann Dermatol Venereol* (French) 126, 161
(1999): Keung YK+, *Bone Marrow Transplant* 23, 200

Injection-site bullous eruption
(1990): Farmer KL+, *Arch Dermatol* 126, 1243

Injection-site erythema
(1995): Scott GA, *Am J Dermatopathol* 17, 107

Injection-site lichenoid reaction
(1999): Viallard AM+, *Dermatology* 198, 301

Injection-site nodules (sic)
(1990): Farmer KL+, *Arch Dermatol* 126, 1243

Injection-site pain (1–10%)

Injection-site pruritus
(1990): Farmer KL+, *Arch Dermatol* 126, 1243

Injection-site urticaria
(1995): Scott GA, *Am J Dermatopathol* 17, 107

Lymphoproliferative disease
(1994): De la Rubia J+, *Bone Marrow Transplantation* 14, 475
(1994): Kawach Y+, *Leukemia and Lymphoma* 13, 509

Mucositis
(1999): Crawford J+, *Cytokines Cell Mol Ther* 5, 187

Myalgia (>10%)

Oral mucosal lesions
(1990): Lazarus H+, *Proc Am Soc Clin Oncol* 9, 15

Stomatitis (>10%)

# GREEN TEA

**Scientific names:** *Camellia sinensis; Camellia thea; Camellia theifera; Thea bohea; Thea sinensis; Thea viridis*
**Other common names:** Chinese tea; tea
**Family:** Theaceae
**Purported indications:** Improving cognitive performance, stomach disorders, nausea, vomiting, diarrhea, headaches
**Other uses:** Crohn's disease, reduces risk of prostate and colon cancer, protects against heart disease, dental caries, kidney stones. Prevents skin cancer related to UV radiation. Topically, green tea bags are used as a wash to soothe sunburn, a compress for headaches, a poultice for bags under eyes, to stop bleeding of gum sockets, to stop increased sweating.

### *Reactions*

## Skin

None

**Note:** Tea is consumed as a beverage

## GREPAFLOXACIN*

**Indications:** Various infections caused by susceptible organisms
**Category:** Fluoroquinolone antibiotic
**Half-life:** 5–12 hours

### *Reactions*

#### Skin

Acne (<1%)
Balanitis (<1%)
Cheilitis (<1%)
Diaphoresis (<1%)
Edema (<1%)
Exanthems (<1%)
Exfoliative dermatitis (<1%)
Facial edema (<1%)
Fungal dermatitis (sic) (<1%)
Herpes simplex (<1%)
Peripheral edema (<1%)
Photosensitivity
(1997): Ferguson J+, *J Antimicrob Chemother* 40, 93
(1997): Stahlmann R+, *J Antimicrob Chemother* 40, 83
Phototoxicity (2%)
(2000): Traynor NJ+, *Toxicol Vitr* 14, 275
(1998): Lode H, *Infect Med* 15 (Suppl 1), 28
Pruritus (<1%)
Rash (sic) (1.9%)
(1998): Lode H, *Infect Med* 15 (Suppl 1), 28
(1997): Stahlmann R+, *J Antimicrob Chemother* 40, 83
Toxic epidermal necrolysis (<1%)
Urticaria (<1%)
Vesiculobullous eruption (<1%)
Xerosis (<1%)

#### Hair

Hair – alopecia (<1%)

#### Other

Ageusia (<1%)
Bromhidrosis (<1%)
Dysgeusia (17%) (metallic taste)
(1998): Chodosh S+, *Antimicrob Agents Chemother* 42, 114
(1998): Lode H, *Infect Med* 15 (Suppl 1), 28
(1997): Stahlmann R+, *J Antimicrob Chemother* 40, 83
Gingivitis (<1%)
Glossitis (<1%)
Hypersensitivity
Hypesthesia (<1%)
Myalgia (<1%)
Oral candidiasis (<1%)
Oral ulceration (<1%)
Paresthesias (<1%)
Parosmia (<1%)
Stomatitis (<1%)
Tendinitis
Tendon rupture
Tongue disorder (sic) (<1%)
Tongue edema (<1%)
Tongue pigmentation (<1%)
Vaginitis (3.3%)
Xerostomia (1.1%)

***Note:** Grepafloxacin has been withdrawn in the USA

## GRISEOFULVIN

**Trade names:** Fulvicin (Schering); Grifulvin V (Ortho); Gris-PEG (Allergan); Grisactin (Wyeth-Ayerst)
**Other common trade names:** *Fulcin; Fulvina P/G; Grisefuline; Griseostatin; Grisovin; Likudin M; Polygris*
**Indications:** Fungal infections of the skin, hair and nails
**Category:** Antifungal
**Half-life:** 9–24 hours
**Clinically important, potentially hazardous interactions with: alcohol**, midazolam

### *Reactions*

#### Skin

Allergic reactions (sic) (1–5%)
(1971): *Med Lett* 13, 55
Angioedema (<1%)
(1994): Gupta AK+, *J Am Acad Dermatol* 30, 677 (passim)
(1989): Rustin MHA+, *Br J Dermatol* 120, 455
(1961): Goldblatt S, *Arch Dermatol* 83, 936
Angular stomatitis
(1994): Gupta AK+, *J Am Acad Dermatol* 30, 677 (passim)
Bullous eruption (<1%)
(1995): Meffert JJ+, *Cutis* 56, 279
(1960): O'Farrell NM, *Arch Dermatol* 82, 424
Candidiasis
(1972): Bessiere L, *Bull Soc Fr Dermatol Syphiligr* (French) 79, 560
Cold urticaria
(1989): Rustin MHA+, *Br J Dermatol* 120, 455
(1965): Chang T, *JAMA* 193, 848
Erythema multiforme (<1%)
(1994): Gupta AK+, *J Am Acad Dermatol* 30, 677 (passim)
(1990): Almeida L+, *J Am Acad Dermatol* 23, 855
(1989): Rustin MHA+, *Br J Dermatol* 120, 455
(1981): Walinga H+, *Ned Tijdschr Geneeskd* (Dutch) 125, 729
(1961): Sternberg TH+, *Med Clin North Am* 45, 781
Exanthems
(1997): Litt JZ, Beachwood, OH (personal case) (observation in a 10-year-old boy)
(1994): Gupta AK+, *J Am Acad Dermatol* 30, 677 (passim)
(1993): Gaudin JL+, *Gastroenterol Clin Biol* 17, 145
(1992): Breathnach SM+, *Adverse Drug Reactions and the Skin* Blackwell, Oxford, 169 (passim)
(1989): Miyagawa S+, *Am J Med* 87, 100
(1972): Von Pohler M+, *Dermatol Monatsschr* (German) 158, 383
Exfoliative dermatitis
(1989): Rustin MHA+, *Br J Dermatol* 120, 455
(1964): Reaves LE, *J Am Geriatr Soc* 12, 889
Fixed eruption (<1%)
(1998): Mahboob A+, *Int J Dermatol* 37, 833
(1994): Gupta AK+, *J Am Acad Dermatol* 30, 677 (passim)
(1989): Boudghene-Stambouli O+, *Dermatologica* 179, 92
(1989): Rustin MHA+, *Br J Dermatol* 120, 455
(1984): Feinstein A+, *J Am Acad Dermatol* 10, 915
(1981): Thyagarajan K+, *Mykosen* (German) 24, 482
(1977): Savage J, *Br J Dermatol* 97, 107
Flushing
(1992): Shelley WB+, *Advanced Dermatologic Diagnosis* WB Saunders, 582 (passim)
Hemorrhagic eruption (sic)
(1992): Breathnach SM+, *Adverse Drug Reactions and the Skin* Blackwell, Oxford, 169 (passim)
Herpes zoster
(1969): Chistiakov AM, *Vestn Dermatol Venerol* (Russian) 43, 76
Hypohidrosis

(1986): Duvanel T, *Ann Dermatol Venereol* (French) 113, 471
Jarisch–Herxheimer reaction
(1993): Amita DB+, *Clin Exp Dermatol* 18, 389
Leprosy (exacerbation)
(1982): Shulman DG+, *Arch Dermatol* 118, 909
Lichenoid eruption
(1994): Gupta AK+, *J Am Acad Dermatol* 30, 677 (passim)
(1961): Sternberg TH+, *Med Clin North Am* 45, 781
Lupus erythematosus
(1995): Bonilla-Felix M+, *Pediatr Nephrol* 9, 478
(1994): Gupta AK+, *J Am Acad Dermatol* 30, 677 (passim)
(1990): Okazaki H+, *Ryumachi* (Japanese) 30, 418
(1989): Miyagawa S+, *Am J Med* 87, 100
(1989): Miyagawa S+, *J Am Acad Dermatol* 21, 343
(1985): Madhok R+, *BMJ* 291, 249 (fatal)
(1976): Watsky MS+, *Cutis* 17, 361
(1968): Shinskii GE+, *Sov Med* (Russian) 31, 92
(1966): Anderson W+, *J Med Soc N J* 63, 161
(1966): Lee SL+, *Arch Intern Med* 117, 620
(1963): Steagall RW, *Arch Dermatol* 88, 218
(1962): Alexander S, *Br J Dermatol* 74, 72
Mucocutaneous lymph node syndrome (Kawasaki syndrome)
Petechiae
(1994): Gupta AK+, *J Am Acad Dermatol* 30, 677 (passim)
(1960): Smith NG, *Arch Dermatol* 81, 981
Photosensitivity (1–10%)
(1994): Gupta AK+, *J Am Acad Dermatol* 30, 677 (passim)
(1989): Kojima K+, *J Dermatol* (Tokio) 15, 76
(1989): Miyagawa S+, *Am J Med* 87, 100
(1989): Rustin MHA+, *Br J Dermatol* 120, 455
(1988): Kawabe Y+, *Photodermatol* 5, 272
(1988): Kojima T+, *J Dermatol* 15, 76
(1986): Ljunggren B+, *Photodermatol* 3, 26
(1983): Hawk JLM, *Clin Exp Dermatol* 9, 300
(1977): Martins JE+, *Rev Hosp Clin Fac Med Sao Paulo* (Portuguese) 32, 1
(1976): Jarratt M, *Int J Dermatol* 15, 317
(1972): Gotz H, *Arch Dermatol Forsch* (German) 244, 391
(1969): Kalivas J, *JAMA* 209, 1706
(1967): Tarsitani F+, *Policlinico Prat* (Italian) 74, 329
(1966): Kobori T+, *J Asthma Res* 3, 213
(1965): Chang T, *JAMA* 193, 848
(1961): Lamb JH+, *Arch Dermatol* 83, 568
(1961): Sternberg TH+, *Med Clin North Am* 45, 781
(1960): Quero R, *J Invest Dermatol* 34, 283
Pigmentation
(1968): Vollum DI, *Trans St Johns Hosp Dermatol Soc* 54, 204
(1964): Durand P+, *Minerva Med* (Italian) 55, 2422
Pityriasis rosea
Pruritus (<1%)
(1994): Gupta AK+, *J Am Acad Dermatol* 30, 677 (passim)
(1989): Rustin MHA+, *Br J Dermatol* 120, 455
(1960): Quero R, *J Invest Dermatol* 34, 283
(1960): Smith NG, *Arch Dermatol* 81, 981
Purpura
(1967): Lockey SD, *Med Sci* 18, 43
Rash (sic) (>10%)
Seborrheic dermatitis
(1962): Brodthagen H, *Acta Derm Venereol* (Stockh) 42, 345
Stevens–Johnson syndrome
(1989): Rustin MHA+, *Br J Dermatol* 120, 455
(1981): Walinga H+, *Ned Tijdschr Geneeskd* (Dutch) 125, 729
(1973): Belkin BG+, *Vestn Dermatol Venerol* (Russian) 47, 61
Toxic epidermal necrolysis
(1991): Correia O+, *Ann Fr Anesth Reanim* (French) 10, 493
(1990): Mion G+, *Ann Fr Anesth Reanim* (French) 9, 305 (fatal)
(1989): Mion G+, *Lancet* 2, 1331 (fatal)
(1988): Taylor B+, *J Am Acad Dermatol* 19, 565
Urticaria (>10%)
(1989): Rustin MHA+, *Br J Dermatol* 120, 455
(1984): Feinstein A+, *J Am Acad Dermatol* 10, 915
(1963): Driscoll BJO, *BMJ* 2, 503
(1963): Fisher AA, *Arch Dermatol* 87, 660
(1961): Goldblatt S, *Arch Dermatol* 83, 936
Vasculitis
(1994): Gupta AK+, *J Am Acad Dermatol* 30, 677 (passim)
(1970): Livingood CS+, *Cutis* 6, 1346

## Nails

Nails – subungual hemorrhages
Nails – yellow
(1986): Duvanel T, *Ann Dermatol Venereol* (French) 113, 471

## Other

Acute intermittent porphyria
(1965): Berman A+, *JAMA* 192, 1005
Anaphylactoid reactions
(1977): Fel'ker Ala+, *Vestn Dermatol Venerol* (Russian) February, 78
Black tongue
(1994): Gupta AK+, *J Am Acad Dermatol* 30, 677 (passim)
Death
Dysgeusia
(1995): Hofmann H+, *Arch Dermatol* 131, 919
(1994): Gupta AK+, *J Am Acad Dermatol* 30, 677 (passim)
(1971): Fogan L, *Ann Intern Med* 74, 795
Glossodynia
(1994): Gupta AK+, *J Am Acad Dermatol* 30, 677 (passim)
Gynecomastia
(1994): Gupta AK+, *J Am Acad Dermatol* 30, 677 (passim)
(1968): Vollum DI, *Trans St Johns Hosp Dermatol Soc* 54, 204
Hypogeusia
(1971): Fogan L, *Ann Intern Med* 74, 795
Oral candidiasis (1–10%)
(1994): Gupta AK+, *J Am Acad Dermatol* 30, 677 (passim)
Paresthesias
(1994): Gupta AK+, *J Am Acad Dermatol* 30, 677 (passim)
Porphyria
(1980): Smith AG+, *Clin Haematol* 9, 399
(1969): Kalivas J, *JAMA* 209, 1706
(1968): Watson CJ+, *Arch Dermatol* 98, 451
(1967): Lochhead AC+, *Br J Dermatol* 79, 96
(1966): Ziprowski L+, *Arch Dermatol* 93, 21
(1965): Berman A+, *JAMA* 192, 1005
(1964): Redeker AG+, *JAMA* 188, 466
(1963): Editorial, *Lancet* 1, 870
(1963): Rimington C+, *Lancet* 2, 318
Porphyria cutanea tarda
(1970): Thiers H+, *Arch Belg Dermatol Syphiligr* (French) 26, 463
Protoporphyria
(1990): Gederaas OA+, *Photodermatol Photoimmunol Photomed* 7, 82
(1983): Poh-Fitzpatrick MB+, *J Clin Invest* 72, 1449
(1970): Perrot H+, *Experientia* (French) 26, 256
Serum sickness
(1994): Gupta AK+, *J Am Acad Dermatol* 30, 677 (passim)
(1989): Rustin MHA+, *Br J Dermatol* 120, 455
Stomatodynia
Xerostomia
(1994): Gupta AK+, *J Am Acad Dermatol* 30, 677 (passim)

# GUANABENZ

**Trade name:** Wytensin (Wyeth-Ayerst)
**Other common trade names:** *Rexitene; Wytens*
**Category:** $Alpha_2$ adrenergic agonist; antihypertensive
**Half-life:** 7–10 hours

### *Reactions*

#### Skin
Edema (<3%)
Hyperhidrosis
Pruritus (<3%)
Rash (sic) (<3%)

#### Other
Dysgeusia (<3%)
Gynecomastia (<3%)
Sialorrhea
Xerostomia (28%)
(1988): Bork K, *Cutaneous Side Effects of Drugs* WB Saunders, 307

# GUANADREL

**Trade name:** Hylorel (Medeva)
**Indications:** Hypertension
**Category:** Adrenergic blocking agent; antihypertensive
**Half-life:** 5–45 hours (terminal)

### *Reactions*

#### Skin
Peripheral edema (28.6%)

#### Other
Glossitis (8.4%)
Paresthesias (25.1%)
Xerostomia (1.7%)

# GUANETHIDINE

**Trade name:** Ismelin (Novartis)
**Other common trade names:** *Apo-Guanethidine; Ismeline*
**Indications:** Hypertension
**Category:** $Alpha_2$ adrenergic agonist; antihypertensive
**Half-life:** 5–10 days
**Clinically important, potentially hazardous interactions with:** amitriptyline, amoxapine, chlorpromazine, clomipramine, desipramine, doxepin, ephedrine, imipramine, insulin, minoxidil, nortriptyline, protriptyline, tricyclic antidepressants, trimipramine

### *Reactions*

#### Skin
Dermatitis (sic)
Exanthems
Fixed eruption
(1966): Rastogi SK, *J Indian Med Assoc* 47, 31
Lupus erythematosus
Peripheral edema (>10%)
Purpura
Urticaria
Vasculitis
(1964): Dewar HA+, *BMJ* 2, 609 (polyarteritis nodosa?)

#### Hair
Hair – alopecia

#### Other
Glossitis (5%)
Myalgia
Paresthesias (16%)
Priapism
Sialorrhea
Xerostomia (1–10%)

# GUANFACINE

**Trade name:** Tenex (Robins)
**Other common trade names:** *Entulic; Estulic*
**Indications:** Hypertension
**Category:** $Alpha_2$ adrenergic agonist; antihypertensive
**Half-life:** 10–30 hours

### *Reactions*

#### Skin
Dermatitis (sic) (<3%)
Diaphoresis (<3%)
(1991): Wilson MF+, *J Clin Pharmacol* 31, 318
(1990): Mosqueda-Garcia R, *Am J Med Sci* 299, 73
(1986): Sorkin EM+, *Drugs* 31, 301 (3%)
Edema
Exanthems
Exfoliative dermatitis
Peripheral edema
(1991): Oster JR+, *Arch Intern Med* 151, 1638
Pruritus (<3%)
(1991): Wilson MF+, *J Clin Pharmacol* 31, 318
Purpura (<3%)
Rash (sic)
(1990): Lewin A+, *J Clin Pharmacol* 30, 1081
Urticaria

#### Hair
Hair – alopecia

#### Other
Dysgeusia (<3%)
(1988): Cornish LA, *Clin Pharm* 7, 187
Paresthesias (<3%)
Sialorrhea
Tinnitus
Xerostomia (47%)
(1991): Wilson MF+, *J Clin Pharmacol* 31, 318
(1990): Lewin A+, *J Clin Pharmacol* 30, 1081
(1990): Mosqueda-Garcia R, *Am J Med Sci* 299, 73
(1988): Board AW+, *Clin Ther* 10, 761
(1988): Cornish LA, *Clin Pharm* 7, 187
(1988): Van Zweiten PA, *Am J Cardiol* 61, 6D

# HALOPERIDOL

**Trade name:** Haldol (Ortho-McNeil)
**Other common trade names:** *Dozic; Duraperidol; Haloper; Peridol; Seranace; Serenace*
**Indications:** Psychoses, Tourette's disorder
**Category:** Phenothiazine; antipsychotic and sedative
**Half-life:** 20 hours
**Clinically important, potentially hazardous interactions with:** fluoxetine, lithium, methotrexate, propranolol

### *Reactions*

## Skin

Acne
Cellulitis
(1982): Sacks HS, *Hosp Pract Off Ed* 17, 179
Contact dermatitis (<1%)
Diaphoresis
(2001): Kane JM+, *Arch Gen Psychiatry* 58(10), 965
Exanthems
Exfoliative dermatitis
Flushing
(1972): Meyler L+, *Side Effects of Drugs Annual* 7, Excerpta Medica, Amsterdam
Neuroleptic malignant syndrome
(2002): Neu P+, *Pharmacopsychiatry* 35(1), 26
(2001): Reeves RR+, *Ann Pharmacother* 35(6), 698 (with risperidone and mirtazapine)
(2001): Russell CS+, *Obstet Gynecol* 98(5), 906
(2001): Wang HC+, *Mov Disord* 16(4), 765
Photosensitivity (<1%)
(2002): Thami GP+, *Postgrad Med* 78(916), 116 (pellagra-like)
(1970): *Med Lett* 12, 104
(1964): Gerle B, *Acta Psychiatr Scand* 40, 65
Pigmentation (<1%)
Pruritus (<1%)
Purpura
Rash (sic) (<1%)
Seborrheic dermatitis
(1984): Binder RL+, *J Clin Psychiatry* 45, 125
(1983): Binder RL+, *Arch Dermatol* 119, 473
Urticaria

## Hair

Hair – alopecia (<1%)
(2000): Mercke Y+, *Ann Clin Psychiatry* 12, 35
Hair – alopecia areata
(1994): Kubota T+, *Jpn J Psychiatry Neurol* 48, 579
(1993): Kubota T+, *Acta Neurol Napoli* 15, 200 (3 cases)
Hair – depigmentation
(1964): Simpson GM+, *Clin Pharmacol Ther* 5, 310 (graying and fading)

## Other

Death
(2001): Glassman AH+, *Am J Psychiatry* 158(11), 1774
Galactorrhea (<1%)
Gynecomastia (<1%)
Injection-site hypersensitivity
(1992): Hay J, *J Clin Psychiatry* 53, 256
Injection-site pain and itching
(1990): Hamann GL+, *J Clin Psychiatry* 51, 502
Injection-site reactions (sic)
(1995): Maharaj K+, *J Clin Psychiatry* 56, 172
(1992): Reinke M+, *J Clin Psychiatry* 53, 415
(1990): Hamann GL+, *J Clin Psychiatry* 51, 502
Mastodynia
Parkinsonism (pseudo)
Priapism (<1%)
Rhabdomyolysis
(1996): Meltzer HY+, *Neuropsychopharmacology* 15(4), 395
(1984): Cavanaugh JJ+, *J Clin Psychiatry* 45, 356
Sialorrhea
(2001): Kane JM+, *Arch Gen Psychiatry* 58(10), 965
Tremors
(2001): Russell CS+, *Obstet Gynecol* 98(5), 906
Xerostomia (<1%)
(2001): Kane JM+, *Arch Gen Psychiatry* 58(10), 965

# HALOTHANE

**Trade name:** Fluothane (Wyeth-Ayerst)
**Other common trade names:** *Halothan; Trothane*
**Indications:** Induction and maintenance of general anesthesia
**Category:** Anesthetic
**Half-life:** no data
**Clinically important, potentially hazardous interactions with:** aminophylline, atracurium, cisatracurium, doxacurium, epinephrine, non-depolarizing muscle relaxants, pancuronium, rapacuronium, rifampin, theophylline, vecuronium, xanthines

### *Reactions*

## Skin

Acne
(1987): Guldager H, *Lancet* 1, 1211
(1973): Gomez SW, *Anesth Analg* 52, 861
(1973): Soper LE+, *Anesth Analg* 52, 125
Angioedema
(1988): Slegers-Karsmakers S+, *Anesthesia* 43, 506
Exanthems
(1988): Slegers-Karsmakers S+, *Anesthesia* 43, 506
Sensitivity (sic)
(1979): Bodman R, *Br J Anaesth* 51, 1092 (to vapors)
Urticaria
(1964): Cole WHJ, *Med J Aust* 2, 925

## Hair

Hair – alopecia
(1990): Gollnick H+, *Z Haut* (German) 65, 1128

## Other

Rhabdomyolysis
(1987): Rubiano R+, *Anesthesiology* 67(5), 856
(1985): Sodano R+, *Minerva Anestesiol* 51(3), 109
(1979): Bomholt A, *Ugeskr Laeger* 141, 925
(1976): Moore WE+, *Anesth Analg* 55(5), 680 (with succinylcholine)

## HAWTHORN (FRUIT, LEAF, FLOWER EXTRACT)

**Scientific names:** *Crataegus calpodendron; Crataegus chrysocarpa; Crataegus douglasii; Crataegus laevigata; Crataegus monogyna; Crataegus oxyacantha; Crataegus pentagyna; Crataegus phenophyrum; Crataegus pinnatifida*
**Other common names:** Aubepine; bianco spino; crataegi fructus; crataegus fruit; English hawthorn; epine blanche; epine de Mai; fructus oxyacanthae; Haagdorn; Hagedorn; harthorne; haw; hawthorne; hedgethorne; May; May blossom; May bush; Maythorn; Meelbeebaum; Meidorn; Nan Shanzha; Oneseed Hawthorn; Shanzha; Thorn Plum; Weissdorn; whitethorn
**Family:** Rosaceae
**Purported indications:** Amenorrhea, angina, arrhythmias, arteriosclerosis, atherosclerosis, congestive heart failure, coronary heart disease, diuretic, hyperlipidemia, hypertension, hypotension, sedative
**Other uses:** Appetite stimulant, arthritis, enteritis, indigestion, sore throats, stomach aches. Used topically for boils, sores and ulcers

**Note:** The American Herbal Products Association (AHPA) gives hawthorn a class I safety rating, indicating that it is very safe. However, hawthorn should be used with caution in patients with heart disease

### *Reactions*

#### Skin

Allergic reactions (sic)
Diaphoresis
Rash (sic) (hands)
- (1996): Newall CA+, *A Guide For Healthcare Professionals* (London UK, Pharmaceutical Press)

Toxiderma
- (1984): Rogov VD, *Vestn Dermatol Venerol* 7, 46

#### Other

Hypersensitivity
- (1984): Steinman HK+, *Contact Dermatitis* 11(5), 321

## HENNA*

**Scientific names:** *Lawsonia alba; Lawsonia inermis*
**Other common names:** Alcanna; Egyptian Privet; Hennae folium; Hinai; Hinna; Inai; Jamaica Kina; Lawsone (2-hydroxy-1:4naphthaquione); Mehandi; Mehndi; Smooth Lawsonia
**Family:** Lythraceae
**Purported indications:** Anti-inflammatory, analgesic, antipyretic, seborrheic dermatitis, fungal infections, gastrointestinal ulcers, sunscreen, dandruff, scabies, amebic dysentery, cancer, enlarged spleen, headache, jaundice, and for decorative henna tattoos
**Other uses:** In manufacturing, henna is used in cosmetics, as a body paint, in hair dyes and hair care products, and as dye for nails, hands and clothing

**Note:** Black Henna is Henna plus paraphenylenediamine (PPD). PPD is added to henna to make it stain black. PPD is a transdermal toxin and may be used alone as hair dye or to stain skin black. Other products called 'black henna' may have indigo or food dyes added, and are generally not harmful to the skin. The (+PPD) following the references, below, indicates that this is Black Henna

### *Reactions*

#### Skin

Allergic reactions (sic)
- (2000): US Food and Drug Administration, Office of Cosmetics and Colors Fact Sheet
- (1970): Blohm SG+, *Acta Derm Venereol* 50, 49
- (1970): Rajka G+, *Acta Derm Venereol* 50, 51

Bullous eruption
Burns
Contact dermatitis
- (2001): Di Lando A+, *Am J Contact Dermat* 12(3), 186
- (2001): Kulkarni PD+, *Cutis* 68(3):187, 229 (+PPD)
- (2001): Lauchl S+, *Swiss Med Wkly* 131, 199 (+PPD)
- (2001): Onder M+, *Int J Dermatol* 40(9), 577 (+PPD)
- (2001): Oztass MO+, *J Eur Acad Dermatol Venereol* 15(1), 91
- (2001): Thami GP+, *Allergy* 56(10), 1013
- (2000): Le Coz CJ+, *Arch Dermatol* 136(12), 1515 (+PPD)
- (2000): Lyon MJ+, *Arch Dermatol* 136(1), 124
- (2000): Nikkels AF+, *J Eur Acad Dermatol Venereol* 15(2), 140 (+PPD)
- (2000): Raison-Peyron N+, *Ann Dermatol Venereol* 127(12), 1083 (+PPD)
- (2000): Sidbury R+, *Am J Contact Dermat* 11(3), 182 (+PPD)
- (2000): Tosti A+, *Contact Dermatitis* 42(6), 356
- (1999): Gallo R+, *Contact Dermatitis* 40(1), 57
- (1999): Lestringant GG+, *Br J Dermatol* 141(3), 598
- (1999): Lewin PK, *CMAJ* 160(3), 310
- (1998): Nigam PK+, *Contact Dermatitis* 18(1), 55
- (1998): Wakelin SH+, *Contact Dermatitis* 39(2), 92 (+PPD)
- (1997): Downs AMR+, *Br Med J* 315, 1772 (+PPD)
- (1997): Etienne A+, *Contact Dermatitis* 37(4), 183
- (1997): Garcia Ortiz JC+, *Int Arch Allergy Immunol* 114(3), 298
- (1996): al-Sheik OA+, *Int J Dermatol* 35(7), 493
- (1992): Wantke F+, *Contact Dermatitis* 27(5), 346 (from Azo dyes)
- (1986): Gupta BN+, *Contact Dermatitis* 15(5), 303
- (1980): Pasricha JS+, *Contact Dermatitis* 6(4), 288

Edema
- (2001): Lauchl S+, *Swiss Med Wkly* 131, 199 (+PPD)
- (2001): Wohrl S+, *Eur Acad Dermatol Venereol* 15(5), 470 (+PPD)

Erythema
- (2002): Schultz E+, *Int J Dermatol* 41(5), 301
- (2001): Lauchl S+, *Swiss Med Wkly* 131, 199 (+PPD)

Erythema multiforme
- (2001): Jappe U+, *Contact Dermatitis* 45(4), 249 (+PPD)

Keloid
- (1999): Lewkin PK, *CMAJ* 160(3), 310

Lichenoid dermatitis
- (2002): Ferrer P+, *Cosmetic Dermatology* 15, 11

Lichenoid reaction
- (2002): Chung WH+, *Arch Dermatol* 138(1), 88 (+PPD)
- (2002): Schultz E+, *Int J Dermatol* 41(5), 301
- (2000): Rubegni P+, *Contact Dermatitis* 42(2), 117

Photosensitivity
Pigmentation
- (2001): Wohrl S+, *J Eur Acad Dermatol Venereol* 15(5), 470 (+PPD)

Pruritus
- (2001): Lauchl S+, *Swiss Med Wkly* 131, 199 (+PPD)
- (2000): Sidbury R+, *Am J Contact Dermat* 11(3), 182 (+PPD)

Psoriasis
- (1991): El-Gammal SY, *Bull Indian Inst Hist Med Hyderabad* 121(2), 125

Rash (sic)
Urticaria
(1997): Downs AMR+, *Br Med J* 315, 1722
(1996): Majoie IM+, *Am J Contact Dermat* 7(1), 38

## Other

Death
(2001): Devecioglu C+, *Turk J Pediatr* 43(1), 65
(2001): Raupp P+, *Arch Dis Child* 85(5), 411
(1992): Sir Hashim M+, *Ann Trop Paediatr* 12(1), 3 (+PDD)
Hypersensitivity
(2001): Bolhaar ST+, *Allergy* 56(3), 248
(2001): Kulkarni PD+, *Cutis* 68(3), 187 (+PPD)
(2000): Lyon MJ+, *Arch Dermatol* 136(1), 124
(2000): Nikkels AF+, *J Eur Acad Dermatol Venereol* 15(2), 140 (+PPD)
(1996): Abdulla KA+, *Lancet* 348(9028), 658 (+PPD)
(1996): Majoie IM+, *Am J Contact Dermat* 7(1), 38
(1996): Ozsoylu S, *Lancet* 348(9035), 1173
(1982): Starr JC+, *Ann Allergy* 48(2), 98
(1979): Cronin E, *Contact Dermatitis* 5(3), 198
(1976): Pepys J+, *Clin Allergy* 6(4), 399

***Note:** Adverse side effects to pure henna is rare; those reported above may be due to additives. Henna tattoos were popularized by Madonna. Her black patterns, however, were created with body paint, not henna

# HEPARIN

**Trade names:** Hep-Flush (Wyeth-Ayerst); Hep-Lock (Elkins-Sinn); Liquaemin (Organon)
**Other common trade names:** *Calcilean; Calciparin; Caprin; Hepalean; Heparin-Leo; Heparine; Liquemin; Uniparin*
**Indications:** Venous thrombosis, pulmonary embolism
**Category:** Anticoagulant
**Half-life:** 1.5 hours
**Clinically important, potentially hazardous interactions with:** aspirin, bivalirudin, butabarbital, danaparoid, salicylates, tirofiban

### *Reactions*

## Skin

Allergic reactions (sic) (1–10%)
(1997): Hermes B+, *Acta Derm Venereol* 77, 35
(1972): Lebeaupin R+, *Anesth Analg* (Paris) (French) 29, 487
Angioedema (<1%)
Baboon syndrome
(1993): Herfs H+, *Hautarzt* (German) 44, 466
Burning (sic) (soles)
(1992): Breathnach SM+, *Adverse Drug Reactions and the Skin*, Blackwell,Oxford, 249 (passim)
Chills
Contact dermatitis
(1996): Boehncke WH+, *Contact Dermatitis* 35, 73
(1996): Koch P+, *Contact Dermatitis* 34, 1256
(1995): Krasovec M+, *Contact Dermatitis* 32, 135
(1992): Valsecchi R+, *Contact Dermatitis* 26, 129
(1988): Young E, *Contact Dermatitis* 19, 152
Ecchymoses
(1985): Tuneu A+, *J Am Acad Dermatol* 12, 1072
(1979): Stavorovsky M+, *Dermatologica* 158, 451
Erythema
Erythematous plaques (sic)
Exanthems
(1996): Warkentin TE, *Br J Haematol* 92, 494
(1994): Greiner D+, *Hautarzt* (German) 45, 569
Fixed eruption
(1995): Mohammed KN, *Dermatology* 190, 91
Hemorrhage
(1992): Breathnach SM+, *Adverse Drug Reactions and the Skin* Blackwell, Oxford, 249 (passim)
(1986): Levine M+, *Semin Thromb Hemost* 12, 39
Livedo reticularis
(1993): Gross AS+, *Int J Dermatol* 32, 276
Necrosis
(2002): Wong G+, *World Congress Dermatol* Poster, 0133
(2001): Andolfatto S+, *Ann Biol Clin* (Paris) 59(5), 651 (2 cases)
(2001): Denton MD+, *Am J Nephrol* 21(4), 289
(1997): Carter RL, *N Engl J Med* 336, 589
(1997): Kumar PD, *N Engl J Med* 336, 588
(1997): Libow LF+, *Cutis* 59, 242
(1997): McCloskey RV, *N Engl J Med* 336, 588
(1997): Schechter FG, *N Engl J Med* 336, 589
(1996): Christiaens GC+, *N Engl J Med* 335, 715
(1996): Whitmore SE+, *Arch Dermatol* 132, 341
(1995): Balestra B, *Schweiz Med Wochenschr* (German) 125, 361
(1994): Griffin JP, *Adverse Drug React Toxicol Rev* 13, 157
(1994): Leblanc M+, *Nephron* 68, 133
(1994): Peluso AM+, *Eur J Dermatol* 4, 127
(1994): Yoon TY+, *Ann Dermatol* 6, 74
(1993): Humphries JE, *Acta Haematol* 90, 52
(1993): Warkentin TE+, *Am J Med* 95, 662
(1993): Yates P+, *Clin Exp Dermatol* 18, 138
(1992): Calzavara-Pinton PG+, *EJD* 2, 171
(1992): Soundararajan R+, *Am J Med* 93, 467
(1992): Thomas D+, *Chest* 102, 1578
(1991): Humphries JE+, *Am J Kidney Dis* 17, 233
(1991): Ritchie AJ+, *Ulster Med* J 60, 248
(1990): Adcock DM+, *Semin Thromb Hemost* 16, 283
(1990): Bircher AJ+, *Br J Dermatol* 123, 507 (passim)
(1990): Fowlie J+, *Postgrad Med J* 66, 573
(1989): Armengol R+, *Med Clin (Barc)* (Spanish) 93, 699
(1989): Diem E, *Hautarzt* (German) 40, 239
(1989): Rongioletti F+, *Dermatologica* 178, 47
(1989): Vinti H+, *Presse Med* (French) 18, 128
(1988): Cohen GR+, *Obstet Gynecol* 73, 498
(1988): Hartman AR+, *J Vasc Surg* 7, 781
(1987): Alegre A+, *Med Clin (Barc)* (Spanish) 88, 170
(1987): Jones BF+, *Australas J Dermatol* 28, 117
(1986): Lim KB+, *Singapore Med J* 27, 356
(1985): Barthelemy H+, *Ann Dermatol Venereol* (French) 112, 245
(1985): Tuneu A+, *J Am Acad Dermatol* 12, 1072
(1984): Hasegawa GR, *Drug Intell Clin Pharm* 18, 313
(1984): Mathieu A+, *Ann Dermatol Venereol* (French) 111, 733
(1984): Monreal M+, *Lancet* 2, 820
(1984): Nodel'son SE+, *Ter Arkh* (Russian) 56, 118
(1984): Ulrick PJ+, *Med J Aust* 140, 287
(1983): Jehn U+, *Dtsch Med Wochenschr* (German) 108, 1148
(1983): Levine LE+, *Arch Dermatol* 119, 400
(1982): Isaacs P+, *Br Med J Clin Res Ed* 284, 201
(1982): No Author, *Am J Hosp Pharm* 39, 412
(1982): Shelley WB+, *J Am Acad Dermatol* 7, 674
(1981): Berkessy S+, *Orv Hetil* (Hungarian) 122, 3075
(1981): Jackson AM+, *Br Med J Clin Res Ed* 283, 1087
(1981): Kelly RA+, *JAMA* 246, 1582
(1980): Hall JC+, *JAMA* 244, 1831
(1979): White PW+, *Ann Surg* 190, 595
Peripheral edema
(1993): Phillips JK+, *Br J Haematol* 84, 349
Petechiae
(1979): Stavorovsky M+, *Dermatologica* 158, 451
Pruritus (<1%)
Purpura (>10%)
Rash (sic)

Scleroderma
(1985): Barthelemy H+, *Ann Dermatol Venereol* (French) 112, 245
Skin lesions (sic)
(1996): Warkentin TE, *Br J Haematology* 92, 494
Toxic dermatitis (sic)
(1996): Gallais V+, *Presse Med* (French) 25, 1040
Toxic epidermal necrolysis
(1991): Lemziakov TG+, *Vrach Delo* (Ukrainian) November, 113
(1985): Leung A, *JAMA* 253, 201
Ulceration
(2001): Denton MD+, *Am J Nephrol* 21(4), 289
Urticaria (<1%)
(1992): Breathnach SM+, *Adverse Drug Reactions and the Skin* Blackwell, Oxford, 249 (passim)
(1990): Bircher AJ+, *Br J Dermatol* 123, 507 (passim)
(1975): Hancock BW+, *BMJ* 3, 746
(1964): Zinn WJ, *Am J Cardiol* 14, 36
(1962): Rajka G+, *Acta Derm Venereol* (Stockh) 42, 27
Vasculitis
(1989): Guillet G+, *J Am Acad Dermatol* 20, 1130
(1989): Korstanje MJ+, *Contact Dermatitis* 20, 283
(1982): Kearsley JH+, *Aust N Z J Med* 12, 288
(1979): Ranft K+, *Med Welt* (German) 30, 1489
(1979): Stavorovsky M+, *Dermatologica* 158, 451

### Hair
Hair – alopecia
(1980): Jaques LB, *Pharmacol Rev* 31, 99
(1969): Baker H+, *Br J Dermatol* 81, 236

### Nails
Nails – discoloration of lunulae

### Other
Anaphylactoid reactions
(1992): Breathnach SM+, *Adverse Drug Reactions and the Skin* Blackwell, Oxford, 249 (passim)
(1990): Bircher AJ+, *Br J Dermatol* 123, 507 (passim)
Gingival bleeding (>10%)
Hypersensitivity
(2002): Nicolie B+, *Allerg Immunol (Paris* (Paris) 34(2), 47
(2000): Koch P+, *J Am Acad Dermatol* 42, 612
(1995): Sanders MN+, *Int J Dermatol* 34, 443
(1994): Patriarca G+, *Allergy* 49, 292
(1993): Dupin N+, *Ann Dermatol Venereol* (French) 120, 845
(1993): O'Donnell BF+, *Br J Dermatol* 129, 634
(1992): de Kort WJ+, *Ned Tijdschr Geneeskd* (Dutch) 136, 2379
(1992): Manoharan A, *Eur J Haematol* 48, 234
(1991): Rivers JK+, *Aust N Z J Surg* 61, 865
(1989): Korstanje MJ+, *Contact Dermatitis* 20, 383
(1989): Patrizi A+, *Contact Dermatitis* 20, 309
(1973): Curry N+, *Arch Intern Med* 132, 744
Injection-site eczematous patches (<1%)
(2000): Koch P+, *J Am Acad Dermatol* 42, 612
(1995): Mathelier-Fusade P+, *Presse Med* (French) 24, 323
(1993): Phillips JK+, *Br J Haematol* 84, 349 (erythema)
(1990): Bircher AJ+, *Br J Dermatol* 123, 507
Injection-site hematoma
Injection-site induration
(1993): Phillips JK+, *Br J Haematol* 84, 349
(1989): Guillet G+, *J Am Acad Dermatol* 20, 1130
(1989): Klein GF+, *J Am Acad Dermatol* 21, 703
(1987): Mayou SC+, *Br J Dermatol* 117, 664
Injection-site necrosis (<1%)
(1995): Mar AW+, *Australas J Dermatol* 36, 201
(1988): Cohen GR+, *Obstet and Gyn* 72, 498
(1984): Hasegawa GR, *Drug Intell Clin Pharm* 18, 313
(1980): Hall JC+, *JAMA* 244, 1831
Injection-site pain
(2001): Chan H, *J Adv Nurs* 35(6), 882
Injection-site plaques
(2000): Koch P+, *J Am Acad Dermatol* 42, 612
(1990): Bircher AJ+, *Br J Dermatol* 123, 507
Injection-site purpura
(2001): Chan H, *J Adv Nurs* 35(6), 882
Injection-site urticaria
(1995): Mathelier-Fusade P+, *Presse Med* (French) 24, 323
Priapism
(2001): Bauduer F+, *Presse Med* 30(8), 376
(2001): Bschleipfer TH+, *Int J Impot rES* 13(6), 357

## HEPATITIS B VACCINE

**Trade names:** Engerix B (GSK); Recombivax HB (Merck)
**Other common trade name:** *Heptavax-B*
**Indications:** For immunization of infection caused by all known subtypes of hepatitis B virus
**Category:** Vaccine
**Half-life:** N/A

### *Reactions*

### Skin
Allergic granulomatous angiitis (Churg–Strauss syndrome)
(1998): Vanoli M+, *Ann Rheum Dis* 57(4), 256
Anetoderma
(1997): Daoud MS+, *J Am Acad Dermatol* 36 (5 Pt 1), 779
Angioedema
(1998): Barbaud A+, *Br J Dermatol* 139(5), 925
Bullous pemphigoid
(2002): Erbagci Z, *World Congress Dermatol* Poster 0315
Chills
Dermatomyositis
(1998): Fernandez-Funez A+, *Med Clin* (Barc) 111(17), 675
Diaphoresis
Eczematous reaction (sic)
(1999): Mc Kenna KE, *Contact Dermatitis* 40(3), 158
Erythema
Erythema multiforme
(2000): Loche F+, *Clin Exp Dermatol* 25(2), 167
(1994): Di Lernia+, *Pediatr Dermatol* 11(4), 363
Erythema nodosum
(1993): Castresana-Isla CJ+, *J Rheumatol* 20(8), 1417
(1990): Rogerson SJ+, *BMJ* 301, 345
(1989): Goolsby PL, *N Engl J Med* 321, 1198
Flushing
Gianotti–Crosti syndrome
(2001): Tay YK, *Pediatr Dermatol* 18(3), 262
Granuloma (necrobiotic)
(1998): Ajithkumar K+, *Clin Exp Dermatol* 23(5), 222
Granuloma annulare
(1998): Wolf F+, *Eur J Dermatol* 8(6), 435 (generalized)
Guillain–Barré syndrome
(2000): Sinsawaiwong S+, *J Med Assoc Thai* 83(9), 1124
(1997): Kakar A+, *Indian J Pediatr* 64(5), 710
Herpes zoster
Lichen planus
(2002): Calista D+, *World Congress Dermatol* Poster, 0090
(2001): Al-Khenaizan S, *J Am Acad Dermatol* 45(4), 614
(2001): Aron-Moar A+, *Lupus* 10(3), 237
(2000): Agrawal S+, *J Dermatol* 27(9), 618
(1999): Rebora A+, *Dermatology* 198(1), 1
(1999): Schupp P+, *Int J Dermatol* 38(10), 799
(1998): Ferrando MN+, *Br J Dermatol* 139(2), 350

(1998): Merigou D+, *Ann Dermatol Venereol* 125(6-7), 399
(1997): Gisserot O+, *Presse Med* 26(16), 760
(1995): Lefort A+, *Ann Dermatol Venereol* 122(10), 701
(1994): Aubin F+, *Arch Dermatol* 130(10), 1329
(1993): Trevisan G+, *Acta Derm Venereol* 73(1), 73
(1990): Ciaccio M+, *Br J Dermatol* 122, 424

Lichenoid eruption
(2001): Usman A+, *Pediatr Dermatol* 18(2), 123
(1997): Saywell CA+, *Australas J Dermatol* 38(3), 152

Lupus erythematosus
(2000): Maillefert JF+, *Arthritis Rheum* 43(2), 468
(1999): Senecal JL+, *Arthritis Rheum* 42(6), 1307
(1998): Grotto I+, *Vaccine* 16(4), 329
(1996): Grezard P+, *Ann Dermatol Venereol* 123(10), 657
(1996): Guiserix J, *Nephron* 74(2), 441
(1994): Mamoux V+, *Arch Pediatr* 1(3), 307
(1992): Tudela P+, *Nephron* 62(2), 236

Morphea
(2000): Schmutz JL+, *Presse Med* 29(19), 1046

Petechiae

Purpura
(2002): Chave TA+, *World Congress Dermatol* Poster, 0093
(2001): Conesa V+, *Haematologica* 86(3), E09
(1999): Lliminana C+, *Med Clin* (Barc) 113(1), 39
(1999): Muller A+, *Eur J Pediatr* 158 Suppl 3, S209
(1998): Ronchi F+, *Arch Dis Child* 78(3), 273 (3 cases)
(1994): Poullin P+, *Lancet* 344(8932), 1293

Rash (sic)

Raynaud's phenomenon
(1990): Cockwell P+, *BMJ* 301, 1281

Reiter's syndrome
(1994): Fraser PA+, *BMJ* 309(6967), 1513
(1994): Hassan W+, *BMJ* 309(6947), 94

Sjøgren's syndrome
(2000): Toussirot E+, *Arthritis Rheum* 43(9), 2139

Stevens–Johnson syndrome

Urticaria
(2000): Barbaud A+, *Ann Dermatol Venereol* 127(6-7), 662
(1998): Barbaud A+, *Br J Dermatol* 139(5), 925
(1998): Grotto I+, *Vaccine* 16(4), 329

Vasculitis
(2001): Saadoun D+, *Rev Med Interne* 22(2), 172
(1999): Le Hello C, *Pathol Biol* (Paris) 47(3), 252
(1999): Le Hello+, *J Rheumatol* 26(1), 191 (3 cases)
(1998): Bui-Quang D+, *Presse Med* 27(26), 1321
(1998): Grotto I+, *Vaccine* 16(4), 329
(1998): Masse I+, *Presse Med* 27(20), 965
(1997): Kerleau JM+, *Rev Interne Med* 18(6), 491 (necrotizing)
(1993): Allen MB+, *Thorax* 48(5), 580
(1990): Cockwell P+, *BMJ* 301, 1281

## Hair

Hair – alopecia
(1997): Wise RP+, *JAMA* 278(14), 1176 (46 cases)

## Other

Anaphylactoid reactions
(2000): *Prescrire Int* 9(46), 59
(1998): Grotto I+, *Vaccine* 16(4), 329
(1996): *MMWR Morb Mortal Wkly Rep* 45(RR-12), 1
(1994): Stratton KR+, *JAMA* 271(20), 1602

Aphthous stomatitis
(1996): Grezard P+, *Ann Dermatol Venereol* 123(10), 657

Arthralgia

Arthus reaction
(2001): Froelich H+, *Clin Infect Dis* 33(6), 906 (with skin necrosis)

Death
(1999): Niu MT+, *Pediatr Adolesc Med* 153(12), 1279

Erythermalgia
(1999): Rabaud C+, *J Rheumatol* 26(1), 233

Hypersensitivity

Hypesthesia

Injection-site ecchymoses

Injection-site edema

Injection-site erythema

Injection-site induration

Injection-site nodules (sic)

Injection-site pain

Injection-site pruritus

Injection-site soreness (22%)

Myalgia

Oral lichenoid eruption
(2000): Pemberton MN+, *Oral Surg Oral Med Oral Pathol Oral Radiol Endod* 89(6), 717

Paresthesias

Periarteritis nodosa
(2001): Saadoun D+, *Rev Med Interne* 22(2), 172
(1988): Le Goff P+, *Presse Med* 17, 1763

Polymyalgia rheumatica
(2001): Saadoun D+, *Rev Med Interne* 22(2), 172

Sclerotic plaques (sic)
(1998): Gout O+, *Rev Neurol* (Paris) 154(3), 205

Serum sickness

Still's disease
(1998): Grasland A+, *Rev Med Interne* 19(2), 134

Tinnitus

White dot syndrome (retinal)
(1996): Baglivo E+, *Am J Ophthalmol* 122(3), 431

# HEROIN

**Trade name:** Heroin
**Indications:** Recreational drug
**Category:** Diacetylmorphine; a semisynthetic narcotic; substance abuse drug
**Half-life:** no data

### *Reactions*

## Skin

Abscess
(1990): Rasokat H, *Z Haut* (German) 65, 351
(1987): Muller F+, *Infection* 15, 201
(1987): Podzamczer D+, *J Am Acad Dermatol* 16, 386
(1984): O'Sullivan M+, *Ir Med J* 77, 68
(1980): Espiritu MB+, *Laryngoscope* 90, 1111 (neck)
(1979): Webb D+, *West J Med* 130, 200
(1971): Young AW+, *Arch Dermatol* 104, 80

Acanthosis nigricans
(1973): Young AW+, *Am Fam Physician* 7, 79
(1971): Young AW+, *Arch Dermatol* 104, 80

Acne
(1973): Young AW+, *Am Fam Physician* 7, 79

Angioedema
(1973): Young AW, *N Y State J Med* 73, 1681

Blistering (arms)
(1995): Mielke-Ibrahim R+, *Dtsch Med Wochenschr* (German) 120, 55

Bullous impetigo
(1973): Young AW, *N Y State J Med* 73, 1681

Candidiasis
(1987): Bielsa I+, *Int J Dermatol* 26, 314 (systemic)
(1987): Puig L+, *Int J Dermatol* 26, 257

(1985): Calandra T+, *Eur J Clin Microbiol* 4, 340 (disseminated)
Cellulitis
(1988): O'Rourke MG+, *Med J Aust* 148, 54
(1984): Alguire PC, *Cutis* 34, 93 (necrotizing of the scrotum)
(1975): Lewis RJ+, *JAMA* 232, 54
Contact dermatitis
(1973): Young AW+, *Am Fam Physician* 7, 79
Cutaneous side effects (sic) (85%)
Ecthyma
(1990): Rasokat H, *Z Haut* (German) 65, 351
Ecthyma gangrenosum
(1977): Mandell IN+, *Arch Dermatol* 113, 199
Edema
(1990): Rasokat H, *Z Haut* (German) 65, 351
(1973): McCabe WP+, *Plast Reconstr Surg* 52, 538
(1973): Young AW+, *Am Fam Physician* 7, 79
(1973): Young AW, *N Y State J Med* 73, 1681 (eyelids)
(1971): Weidman AJ+, *N Y State J Med* 71, 2643 (eyelids)
(1971): Young AW+, *Arch Dermatol* 104, 80
Exanthems
(1973): Young AW, *N Y State J Med* 73, 1681
(1970): Vollum DI, *BMJ* 2, 647
Excoriations
(1990): Rasokat H, *Z Haut* (German) 65, 351
Fixed eruption
(1983): Westerhof W+, *Br J Dermatol* 109, 605 (tongue)
(1973): Young AW, *N Y State J Med* 73, 1681
Folliculitis (candidal)
(1987): Cristobal-Rodriguez P+, *Med Cutan Ibero Lat Am* (Spanish) 15, 411
(1986): Darcis JM+, *Am J Dermatopathol* 8, 501 (with septicemia)
(1986): Leclerc G+, *Int J Dermatol* 25, 100
(1985): Calandra T+, *Eur J Clin Microbiol* 4, 340
Glucagonoma syndrome (necrolytic migratory erythema)
(1994): Bencini PL+, *Dermatology* 189, 72
Kaposi's sarcoma
(1986): Schofer H+, *Hautarzt* (German) 37, 159
Necrosis
(1990): Rasokat H, *Z Haut* (German) 65, 351
(1972): Dunne JH+, *Arch Dermatol* 105, 544
Necrotizing fasciitis
(1990): Rasokat H, *Z Haut* (German) 65, 351
Pemphigus
(1989): Civatte J, *Dermatol Monatsschr* (German) 175, 1
Pemphigus erythematosus
(1978): Fellner MJ+, *Int J Dermatol* 17, 308
Pemphigus vegetans
(1998): Downie JB+, *J Am Acad Dermatol* 39, 872
Perforating collagenosis
(1989): Bank DE+, *J Am Acad Dermatol* 21, 371
Photosensitivity
(1973): Young AW, *N Y State J Med* 73, 1681
(1971): Young AW+, *Arch Dermatol* 104, 80
Pigmentation
(1990): Rasokat H, *Z Haut* (German) 65, 351
(1973): Young AW+, *Am Fam Physician* 7, 79
(1973): Young AW, *N Y State J Med* 73, 1681 (photolocalized)
(1971): Young AW+, *Arch Dermatol* 104, 80 (photolocalized)
Polyarteritis nodosa
(1982): Ojeda E+, *Rev Clin Esp* (Spanish) 167, 275
Pruritus
(1990): Rasokat H, *Z Haut* (German) 65, 351
(1973): Young AW+, *Am Fam Physician* 7, 79
(1973): Young AW, *N Y State J Med* 73, 1681
(1971): Young AW+, *Arch Dermatol* 104, 80
(1970): Vollum DI, *BMJ* 2, 647
(1967): Minkin W+, *N Engl J Med* 277, 473
Purpura
(1973): Young AW+, *Am Fam Physician* 7, 79
Pustular eruption
(1993): Badillet G+, *Ann Dermatol Venereol* (French) 110, 691 (candidal)
(1992): Gallais V+, *Presse Med* (French) 21, 677 (candidal)
(1990): Altes J+, *Enferm Infecc Microbiol Clin* (Spanish) 8, 464
(1985): Cabre L+, *Med Clin (Barc)* (Spanish) 84, 542 (candidal)
(1984): Pinilla-Moraza J+, *Med Clin (Barc)* (Spanish) 83, 557
Toxic epidermal necrolysis
(1990): Llibre LM+, *Med Clin (Barc)* (Spanish) 94, 799
(1974): Lewis RJ, *JAMA* 230, 375
Ulceration
(1990): Abidin MR+, *Ann Plast Surg* 24, 268
(1990): Rasokat H, *Z Haut* (German) 65, 351
(1973): McCabe WP+, *Plast Reconstr Surg* 52, 538
(1971): Young AW+, *Arch Dermatol* 104, 80
Urticaria
(1990): Shaikh WA, *Allergy* 45, 555
(1973): Young AW+, *Am Fam Physician* 7, 79
(1973): Young AW, *N Y State J Med* 73, 1681
Vasculitis
(1984): Rosman JB+, *Neth J Med* 27, 50
(1979): Redmond WJ, *Arch Dermatol* 115, 111

## Other

Death
(1996): Amoiridis G+, *Nervenarzt* 67(12), 1023
Dental decay
(1999): Fazzi M+, *Minerva Stomatol* (Italian) 48, 485
Hypersensitivity
(1990): Rasokat H, *Z Haut* (German) 65, 351
Injection-site scarring
(1990): Rasokat H, *Z Haut* (German) 65, 351
Injection-site ulceration
(1995): Hatton MQ+, *Clin Oncol R Coll Radiol* 7, 268
(1982): White WB+, *Cutis* 29, 63 (penis)
(1973): Bennett RG+, *Arch Dermatol* 107, 121
Myopathy
(1990): Shoji S, *Nippon Rinsho* (Japanese) 48, 1517
Necrotizing vasculitis (tongue)
(1995): Jurgensen O+, *Schweiz Monatsschr Zahnmed* (German; French) 105, 54
Oral mucosal ulceration (tongue)
(1983): Westerhof W+, *Br J Dermatol* 109, 605
Rhabdomyolysis
(2000): Richards JR, *J Emerg Med* 19(1), 51
(1996): Amoiridis G+, *Nervenarzt* 67(12), 1023 (fatal)
(1992): Zele I+, *Minerva Med* 83(12), 847 (30%)
(1991): Nolte KB+, *Am J Forensic Med Pathol* 12(3), 273
(1990): Larpin R+, *Presse Med* 19(30), 1403
(1988): Hecker E+, *Schweiz Med Wochenschr* 118(52), 1982 (5 cases)
(1988): Uzan M+, *Nephrologie* 9(5), 217 (13 cases)
(1981): Palmucci L+, *Ital J Neurol Sci* 2(3), 275
Serum sickness
(1971): Weidman AJ+, *N Y State J Med* 71, 2643
Sweat gland necrosis
(1986): Rocamora A+, *J Dermatol* 13, 49
Tongue pigmentation (fixed eruption)
(1983): Westerhof W+, *Br J Dermatol* 109, 605

## HORSE CHESTNUT – BARK

**Scientific name:** *Aesculus hippocastanum*
**Other common names:** Buckeye; Hippocastani Cortex (bark); Marron Europeen
**Family:** Hippocastanaceae
**Purported indications:** Orally, used for malaria & dysentery. Topically, used for lupus & skin ulcers
**Other uses:** In combination with other herbs, it is used to treat varicose veins, hemorrhoids & rectal problems

### *Reactions*

#### Skin

Purpura
(1998): Brinker F, *Herb Contraindications & Interactions* Eclectic Medical Publications (2nd Ed)

***Note:** Horse chestnut bark's active ingredient contains the toxic glycoside, escin, which seems to have weak diuretic activity

## HORSE CHESTNUT – FLOWER

**Scientific name:** *Aesculus hippocastanum*
**Other common names:** Buckeye; Hippocastani Flos (flower); Marron Europeen
**Family:** Hippocastanaceae
**Purported indications:** Hemorrhoids, rectal problems, strengthening veins, improving circulation
**Other uses:** Ringing in the ears, bile flow disturbances, pancreatitis

### *Reactions*

#### Skin

Contact dermatitis
(1980): Comaish JS+, *Contact Dermatitis* 6(2), 150
Purpura
(1998): Brinker F, *Herb Contraindications & Interactions* Eclectic Medical Publications (2nd Ed)

## HORSE CHESTNUT – LEAF

**Scientific name:** *Aesculus hippocastanum*
**Other common names:** Buckeye; Hippocastani folium; Marron Europeen
**Family:** Hippocastanaceae
**Purported indications:** Chronic venous insufficiency, eczema, phlebitis, hemorrhoids
**Other uses:** Cough remedy, arthritis, rheumatism

### *Reactions*

#### Skin

Purpura
(1998): Brinker F, *Herb Contraindications & Interactions* Eclectic Medical Publications (2nd Ed)

***Note:** Horse chestnut leaf's active ingredient contains the toxic glycoside, esculin, which purportedly strengthens the veins and helps to prevent vascular leakage. It is likely unsafe when taken orally

## HORSE CHESTNUT – SEED

**Scientific name:** *Aesculus hippocastanum*
**Other common names:** Chestnut; Escine; Hippocastani Semen; Marron Europeen; Venostat; Venostatin Retard
**Purported indications:** Hemorrhoids, varicose veins, phlebitis, improving circulation
**Other uses:** Phlebitis, diarrhea, fever, enlarged prostate

### *Reactions*

#### Skin

Purpura
(1998): Brinker F, Herb Contraindications & Interactions, Eclectic Medical Publications (2nd Ed)

#### Other

Anaphylactoid reactions
(1998): Gruenwald J+, PDR for Herbal Medicines. 1st ed. Montvale, NJ: Medical Economics Company, Inc
Depression
Twitching

***Note:** Horse chestnut seed's active ingredient contains the toxic glycoside, esculin, which purportedly strengthens the veins and helps to prevent vascular leakage

## HYDRALAZINE

**Trade names:** Apresazide (Novartis); Apresoline (Novartis); Ser-Ap-Es (Novartis)
**Other common trade names:** *Alphapress; Apdormin; Apresolin; Novo-Hylazin; Nu-Hydral; Solesorin; Stable*
**Indications:** Hypertension
**Category:** Vasodilator; antihypertensive
**Half-life:** 3–7 hours

Apresazide is hydralazine and hydrochlorothiazide; Ser-Ap-Es is hydralazine, reserpine and hydrochlorothiazide

### *Reactions*

#### Skin

Acute febrile neutrophilic dermatosis (Sweet's syndrome)
(1995): Gilmour E+, *Br J Dermatol* 133, 490
(1991): Juanola X+, *J Rheumatol* 18, 948
(1990): Ramsay-Goldman R+, *J Rheumatol* 17, 682
(1987): Servitje O+, *Arch Dermatol* 123, 1436
(1986): Sequeira W+, *Am J Med* 81, 558
Allergic reactions (sic)
(1986): Bigby M+, *JAMA* 236, 3358
Angioedema (<1%)
Bullous eruption
(1988): Dodd HJ+, *Br J Dermatol* 119 (Suppl 33), 27
Chills
Diaphoresis
Edema (<1%)
Erythema nodosum
(1984): Peterson LL, *J Am Acad Dermatol* 10, 379
Exanthems
(1984): Peterson LL, *J Am Acad Dermatol* 10, 379
(1984): Schapel GJ, *Med J Aust* 141, 765
(1981): Finlay AY+, *BMJ* 282, 1703
(1967): Alarcon-Segovia D+, *Medicine* (Baltimore) 46, 1
Fixed eruption (<1%)

(1986): Sehgal VN+, *Int J Dermatol* 25, 394
Flushing (>10%)
(1967): Alarcon-Segovia D+, *Medicine* (Baltimore) 46, 1
Lupus erythematosus
(1998): Hari CK+, *J Laryngol Otol* 112, 875
(1997): Yung R+, *Arthritis Rheum* 40, 1436
(1996): Miyasaka N, *Intern Med* 35, 587
(1996): Pirmohamed M, *Hum Exp Toxicol* 15, 361
(1994): Cohen MG, *J Rheumatol* 21, 578
(1994): Hofstra AH, *Drug Metab Rev* 26, 485
(1994): Nassberger L+, *Scand J Rheumatol* 23, 206
(1992): Rubin RL, *Clin Biochem* 25, 223
(1992): Skaer TL, *Clin Ther* 14, 496
(1992): Yonga GO, *East Afr Med J* 69, 649
(1991): Alarcon-Segovia D+, *Baillieres Clin Rheumatol* 5, 1
(1991): Hess EV, *Curr Opin Rheumatol* 3, 809
(1991): Juanola X+, *J Rheumatol* 18, 948
(1990): Mulder H, *Eur J Clin Pharmacol* 38, 303
(1990): Nassberger L+, *Clin Exp Immunol* 81, 380
(1990): Ramsay-Goldman R+, *J Rheumatol* 17, 682
(1990): Richards FM+, *Am J Med* 88, 56N
(1989): Fleming MG+, *Int J Dermatol* 28, 321 (bullous)
(1989): Mitchell JA+, *Clin Exp Immunol* 78, 354
(1989): Palsson L+, *Clin Pharmacol Ther* 46, 177
(1989): Sim E, *Complement Inflamm* 6, 119
(1989): Speirs C+, *Lancet* 1, 922
(1989): Yemini M+, *Eur J Obstet Gynecol Reprod Biol* 30, 193
(1988): Chong WK+, *BMJ* 297, 660
(1988): Dodd HJ+, *Br J Dermatol* 119 (Suppl 33), 27
(1988): Jiang M, *Chung Kuo I Hsueh Yuan Hsueh Pao* (Chinese) 10, 379
(1988): Sturman SG+, *Lancet* 2, 1304 (fatal)
(1988): Uetrecht JP, *Chem Res Toxicol* 1, 133
(1987): Andersson OK, *Eur J Clin Pharmacol* 31, 741
(1987): Craft JE+, *Arthritis Rheum* 30, 689
(1987): Martinez-Vea A+, *Am J Nephrol* 7, 71
(1987): Servitje O+, *Arch Dermatol* 123, 1436
(1986): Asherson RA+, *Ann Rheum Dis* 45, 771
(1986): Innes A+, *Br J Rheumatol* 25, 225
(1986): Sequeira W+, *Am J Med* 81, 558
(1985): Cush JJ+, *Am J Med Sci* 290, 36
(1985): Doherty M+, *Br Med J Clin Res Ed* 290, 675
(1985): Epstein A+, *Arthritis Rheum* 28, 158
(1985): Kale SA, *Postgrad Med* 77, 231
(1985): Lovisetto P+, *Recenti Prog Med* (Italian) 76, 110
(1985): Stratton MA, *Clin Pharm* 4, 657
(1985): Totoritis MC+, *Postgrad Med* 78, 149
(1984): Brand C+, *Lancet* 1, 462
(1984): Cameron HA+, *BMJ* 289, 410 (6.7%)
(1984): Christophidis N, *Lancet* 2, 868
(1984): French WJ, *Ala J Med Sci* 21, 427
(1984): Naparstek Y+, *Arthritis Rheum* 27, 822
(1984): No Author, *Lancet* 2, 441
(1984): Peterson LL, *J Am Acad Dermatol* 10, 379
(1984): Ramsay LE+, *Br Med J Clin Res Ed* 289, 1310
(1984): Shapiro KS+, *Am J Kidney Dis* 3, 270
(1984): Sim E+, *Lancet* 2, 422
(1984): Timbrell JA+, *Eur J Clin Pharmacol* 27, 555
(1984): Weiser GA+, *Arch Intern Med* 144, 2271
(1984): Wollina U, *Z Gesamte Inn Med* (German) 39, 69
(1983): Macleod WN, *Scott Med J* 28, 181
(1983): Shoenfeld Y+, *Br Med J Clin Res Ed* 286, 224
(1982): Aylward PE+, *Aust N Z J Med* 12, 546
(1982): Freestone S+, *Br Med J Clin Res Ed* 285, 1536
(1982): Harmon CE+, *Clin Rheum Dis* 8, 121
(1982): Hess EV, *Arthritis Rheum* 25, 857
(1982): Mansilla-Tinoco R+, *BMJ* 284, 936
(1982): Ohe A+, *Osaka City Med J* 28, 149
(1982): Ramsay LE+, *Br Med J Clin Res Ed* 284, 1711
(1981): Chisholm JC, *J Natl Med Assoc* 73, 278
(1981): Dubroff LM+, *Arthritis Rheum* 24, 1082
(1981): Neville E+, *Postgrad Med* 57, 378
(1981): Perry HM, *Arthritis Rheum* 24, 1093
(1981): Reidenberg MM, *Arthritis Rheum* 24, 1004
(1981): Sinclair AJ+, *Hum Toxicol* 1, 65
(1980): Batchelor JR+, *Lancet* 1, 1107
(1980): Harland SJ+, *BMJ* 281, 273
(1980): Weinstein A, *Prog Clin Immunol* 4, 1
(1979): Kissin MW+, *BMJ* 2, 1330
(1979): Ryan PF+, *Lancet* 2, 1248
(1978): Anderson B+, *JAMA* 239, 1392
(1978): Jones WN+, *Ariz Med* 35, 16
(1978): Weinstein J, *Am J Med* 65, 553
(1976): Berkowitz HS, *S Afr Med J* 50, 797
(1976): Demay-Wechsler P, *Rev Stomatol Chir Maxillofac* (French) 77, 727
(1976): Hess EV+, *Arthritis Rheum* 19, 122
(1975): Irias JJ, *Am J Dis Child* 129, 862
(1975): Johansson M+, *Lakartidningen* (Swedish) 72, 153
(1975): Lee SL+, *Semin Arthritis Rheum* 5, 83
(1974): Blumenkrantz N+, *Acta Med Scand* 195, 443
(1973): Almeyda J+, *Br J Dermatol* 88, 313 (13%)
(1973): Perry HM, *Am J Med* 54, 58 (12%)
(1971): Alkalay I+, *Ann Allergy* 29, 35
(1967): Alarcon-Segovia D+, *Medicine* (Baltimore) 46, 1
(1966): White AB, *J Am Geriatr Soc*, 14, 361
(1963): Shulman LE+, *Arthritis Rheum* 6, 558 (1–3%)
Photosensitivity
(1967): Alarcon-Segovia D+, *Medicine* (Baltimore) 46, 1
Pruritus
(1984): Peterson LL, *J Am Acad Dermatol* 10, 379
Purpura
(1984): Peterson LL, *J Am Acad Dermatol* 10, 379
(1980): Petty R+, *BMJ* 280, 482
(1967): Alarcon-Segovia D+, *Medicine* (Baltimore) 46, 1
Pyoderma gangrenosum
(1984): Peterson LL, *J Am Acad Dermatol* 10, 379
Rash (sic) (<1%)
Sjøgren's syndrome
(1988): Darwaza A+, *Int J Oral Maxillopfac* 17, 92
Systemic eczematous contact dermatitis
(1964): van Ketel WG, *Acta Derm Venereol* (Stockh) 44, 49
Ulceration
(1980): Brooks AP+, *BMJ* 280, 482
(1980): Petty R+, *BMJ* 280, 482
Urticaria
Vasculitis
(1998): Merkel PA, *Curr Opin Rheumatol* 10, 45
(1993): Reynolds NJ+, *Br J Dermatol* 129, 82
(1982): Kincaid-Smith P+, *Lancet* 2, 348
(1981): Finlay AY+, *Br Med J Clin Res Ed* 282, 1703
(1981): Peacock A+, *BMJ* 282, 1121
(1980): Bernstein RM+, *BMJ* 280, 156
(1980): Brooks AP+, *BMJ* 280, 482

## Other

Death
Hypersensitivity
Myalgia
Oral ulceration
(1984): Peterson LL, *J Am Acad Dermatol* 10, 379
(1980): Brooks AP+, *BMJ* 280, 482
Orogenital ulceration
(1984): Peterson LL, *J Am Acad Dermatol* 10, 379
(1981): Neville E+, *Postgrad Med* 57, 378
Paresthesias
Relapsing polychondritis
(1983): Dahlqvist A+, *Acta Otolaryngol Stockh* 96, 355
Tremors

# HYDROCHLOROTHIAZIDE

**Trade names:** Aldactazide; Aldoril; Apresazide; Avalide (Sanofi-Synthelab); Capozide; Dyazide (GSK); E-Zide; Esidrix; Hydro-Chlor; Hydro-D; Hydro-Par; HydroDIURIL; Maxzide (Bertek); Microzide; Oretic; Prinizide; Ser-Ap-Es.; Zestoretic (AstraZeneca)
**Other common trade names:** *Apo-Hydro; Clothia; Dichlotride; Diu-Melsin; Diuchlor H; Esidrex; Hydrosaluric; Urozide*
**Indications:** Edema
**Category:** Thiazide diuretic*; antihypertensive
**Half-life:** 5.6–14.8 hours
**Clinically important, potentially hazardous interactions with:** digoxin, lithium

Aldactazide is spironolactone and hydrochlorothiazide; Aldoril is methyldopa and hydrochlorothiazide; Avalide is irbesartan and hydrochlorothiazide; Capozide is captopril and hydrochlorothiazide; Dyazide is triamterene and hydrochlorothiazide; Maxzide is triamterene and hydrochlorothiazide; Moduretic is amiloride and hydrochlorothiazide; Prinizide is lisinopril and hydrochlorothiazide; Ser-Ap-Es is reserpine, hydralazine and hydrochlorothiazide

## *Reactions*

### Skin

Actinic reticuloid
(1985): Robinson HN+, *Arch Dermatol* 121, 522
Acute generalized exanthematous pustulosis (AGEP)
(2001): Petavy-Catala C+, *Acta Derm Venereol* 81(3), 209
Bullous eruption (<1%)
Dermatitis (sic)
(1984): Fisher RS+, *J Am Acad Dermatol* 11, 146
(1960): Smirk H+, *BMJ* 1, 515
Diaphoresis
(1979): Fan WJ+, *Pediatrics* 64, 698
Erythema annulare centrifugum
(1988): Goette DK+, *Int J Dermatol* 27, 129
(1973): Rekant SI+, *Arch Dermatol* 107, 424
Erythema multiforme (<1%)
(1985): Ting HC+, *Int J Dermatol* 24, 587
Exanthems
(1960): Smirk H+, *BMJ* 1, 515
Exfoliative dermatitis
Fixed eruption
(1985): Kauppinen K+, *Br J Dermatol* 112, 575
Lichenoid eruption
(1986): Halevy S+, *Ann Allergy* 56, 402
(1971): Almeyda J+, *Br J Dermatol* 85, 604
(1959): Harber LC+, *J Invest Dermatol* 33, 83
(1959): Harber LC+, *N Engl J Med* 261, 1378
Lupus erythematosus
(2002): Boye T+, *World Congress Dermatol* Poster, 0088
(1998): Callen JP, Academy '98 Meeting (5 patients)
(1996): Litt JZ, Beachwood, OH (personal case) (observation)
(1995): Brown CW+, *Clin Toxicol* 33, 729
(1995): Rich MW+, *J Rheumatol* 22, 1001
(1993): Goodrich AL+, *J Am Acad Dermatol* 28, 1001
(1991): Wollenberg A+, *Hautarzt* (German) 42, 709
(1989): Alanko K+, *Acta Derm Venereol* (Stockh) 69, 223
(1989): Fine RM, *Int J Dermatol* 28, 375 (Comment)
(1989): Parodi A+, *Photodermatology* 6, 100
(1988): Darken M+, *J Am Acad Dermatol* 18, 38
(1986): Berbis Ph, *Ann Dermatol Venereol* 113, 1245 (thiazides)
(1985): Reed BR+, *Ann Intern Med* 103, 49
(1977): Weiss RB, *W V Med J* 73, 101
Photoreactions
(1994): Bielan B, *Dermatol Nurs* 6, 30
(1985): Reed BR+, *Ann Intern Med* 103, 49
(1965): Fellner MJ+, *Med Clin North Am* 49, 709
(1959): Harber LC+, *J Invest Dermatol* 33, 83
(1959): Harber LC+, *N Engl J Med* 261, 1378
Photosensitivity (<1%)
(2000): Wagner SN+, *Contact Dermatitis* 43, 245 (with ramipril)
(1994): Shelley WB+, *Cutis* 53, 287 (observation)
(1994): Shelley WB+, *Cutis* 53, 77 (observation)
(1987): Addo HA+, *Br J Dermatol* 116, 749
(1985): Reed BR+, *Ann Intern Med* 103, 49
(1985): Robinson HN+, *Arch Dermatol* 121, 522
(1984): Ophir O+, *Harefuah* (Hebrew) 107, 14
(1983): White IR, *Contact Dermatitis* 9, 237
(1982): No Author, *Ugeskr Laeger* (Danish) 144, 1101
(1981): Journet M, *Union Med Can* 110, 356
(1980): Okrasinski H, *Lakartidningen* (Swedish) 77, 2718
(1980): Torinuki W, *J Dermatol* (Tokio) 7, 293
(1969): Kalivas J, *JAMA* 209, 1706
(1965): Jung EG+, *Int Arch Allergy Appl Immunol* 27, 313
(1959): Harber LC+, *J Invest Dermatol* 33, 83
(1959): Harber LC+, *N Engl J Med* 261, 1378
(1959): Norins AL, *Arch Dermatol* 79, 592
Phototoxicity
(1989): Diffey BL, *Arch Dermatol* 125, 1355
(1987): Addo HA+, *Br J Dermatol* 116, 749
(1982): Rosen K+, *Acta Derm Venereol* (Stockh) 62, 246
Porokeratosis (Mibelli)
(1984): Inamoto N+, *J Am Acad Dermatol* 11, 359
Pruritus (<1%)
(1992): Shelley WB+, *Cutis* 49, 391 (observation)
(1969): Kalivas J, *JAMA* 209, 1706
Purpura
(1980): Miescher PA+, *Clin Haematol* 9, 505
(1971): Eisner EW+, *JAMA* 215, 480
(1966): Smith JW+, *Ann Intern Med* 65, 629
(1963): Bettman JW, *Arch Intern Med* 112, 840
(1960): Ball P, *JAMA* 173, 663
(1960): Gesink MH+, *JAMA* 172, 556
Rash (sic)
(1976): Weisburst M+, *South Med J* 69, 126
Stevens–Johnson syndrome
(1978): Assaad D+, *Can Med Assoc* 118, 154
Systemic eczematous contact dermatitis
Toxic epidermal necrolysis
(1978): Assaad D+, *Can Med Assoc J* 118, 154
(1973): Björnberg A, *Acta Derm Venereol* (Stockh) 53, 149
Urticaria
(1960): Smirk H+, *BMJ* 1, 515
Vasculitis
(1989): Grunwald MH+, *Isr J Med Sci* 25, 572
(1965): Björnberg A+, *Lancet* 2, 982

### Other

Dysgeusia
(2000): Zervakis J+, *Physiol Behav* 68, 405
Oral lichenoid eruption (erosive)
(1990): Espana A+, *Med Clin (Barc)* (Spanish) 94, 559
Paresthesias
Pseudoporphyria
(1990): Motley RJ, *BMJ* 300, 1468
Xanthopsia
Xerostomia

***Note:** Hydrochlorothiazide is a sulfonamide and can be absorbed systemically. Sulfonamides can produce severe, possibly fatal, reactions such as toxic epidermal necrolysis and Stevens–Johnson syndrome

## HYDROCODONE*

**Trade names:** Bacomine; Ban-Tuss HC; Codamine; Duratuss; Hycodan; Hycomine; Hycophen; Hydromine; Hydrophen; Lorcet; Lortab; Morcomine; Propachem; Ru-Tuss; Tussgen; Tussionex; Tussogest; Vicodin; Vicoprofen; Zydone
**Indications:** Acute pain, coughing
**Category:** Narcotic analgesic and antitussive
**Half-life:** 3.8 hours

### *Reactions*

**Skin**

Diaphoresis
Edema
Erythema multiforme
Exanthems
(2000): Litt JZ, Beachwood, OH (personal case) (observation)
Flushing
Hot flashes
Pruritus (1–10%)
(2000): Litt JZ, Beachwood, OH (personal case) (observation)
(1999): Litt JZ, Beachwood, OH (personal case) (observation)
(1999): Sorkin MJ, Denver, CO (from Internet) (observation)
Rash (sic) (>10%)
Stevens–Johnson syndrome
Toxic epidermal necrolysis
Urticaria (>10%)

**Other**

Xerostomia

***Note:** Hydrocodone is included in many combination drugs. Other medications that can be included in these preparations include: phenylpropanolamine, phenylephrine, pyrilamine, pseudoephedrine, acetaminophen, ibuprofen, and others

## HYDROFLUMETHIAZIDE*

**Trade name:** Diucardin (Wyeth-Ayerst)
**Other common trade names:** *Diademil; Hydravern; Hydrenox; Leodrine; Rivosil; Rontyl*
**Indications:** Hypertension, edema
**Category:** Thiazide* diuretic; antihypertensive
**Duration of action:** 12–24 hours
**Clinically important, potentially hazardous interactions with:** digoxin, lithium

### *Reactions*

**Skin**

Photosensitivity (<1%)
Purpura
Rash (sic) (<1%)
Urticaria
Vasculitis

**Other**

Dysgeusia
Paresthesias (<1%)
Xanthopsia

***Note:** Hydroflumethiazide is a sulfonamide and can be absorbed systemically. Sulfonamides can produce severe, possibly fatal, reactions such as toxic epidermal necrolysis and Stevens–Johnson syndrome

## HYDROMORPHONE

**Trade name:** Dilaudid (Abbott)
**Other common trade names:** *Dilaudid HP; HydroStat IR; Palladone*
**Indications:** Pain
**Category:** Narcotic analgesic; antitussive
**Half-life:** 1–3 hours
**Clinically important, potentially hazardous interactions with:** cimetidine

### *Reactions*

**Skin**

Diaphoresis
Exanthems
(1992): de Cuyper C+, *Contact Dermatitis* 27, 220 (generalized)
Flushing (1–10%)
Pruritus (<1%)
(1992): Chaplan SR+, *Anesthesiology* 77, 1090 (11.5%)
Rash (sic) (<1%)
Urticaria (<1%)

**Hair**

Hair – alopecia

**Other**

Dysgeusia
Injection-site reactions (sic)
Paresthesias
Xerostomia (1–10%)

## HYDROXYCHLOROQUINE

**Trade name:** Plaquenil (Sanofi)
**Other common trade names:** *Ercoquin; Oxiklorin; Plaquinol; Quensyl; Toremonil; Yuma*
**Indications:** Malaria, lupus erythematosus, rheumatoid arthritis
**Category:** Antimalarial; anti-lupus and antirheumatic
**Half-life:** elimination in blood: 50 days
**Clinically important, potentially hazardous interactions with:** chloroquine, cholestyramine, dapsone, penicillamine

### *Reactions*

**Skin**

Acute generalized exanthematous pustulosis (AGEP)
(1996): Assier-Bonnet H+, *Dermatology* 193, 70
(1995): Bonnetblanc JM+, *Ann Dermatol Venereol* (French) 122, 604
(1995): Moreau A+, *Int J Dermatol* 34, 263 (passim)
(1993): Assier H+, *Ann Dermatol Venereol* (French) 120, 848
Angioedema (<1%)
Bullous eruption
(2001): Klein AD, Statesboro, GA (from Internet) (observation)
(1995): Kutz DC+, *Arthritis Rheum* 38, 440 Statesboro, GA (from Internet) (observation)
Contact dermatitis
(1999): Meier H+, *Hautarzt* (German) 50, 665
Cutaneous atrophy
(2001): Vassallo C+, *Clin Exp Dermatol* 26(2), 141
Dermatomyositis
(1994): Bloom BJ+, *J Rheumatology* 21, 2171
Erythema annulare centrifugum

(1985): Hudson LD, *J Am Acad Dermatol* 36, 129
(1982): Koralewski F, *Dermatosen* (German) 30, 125
(1967): Ashurst PJ, *Arch Dermatol* 95, 37
Erythema multiforme (<1%)
(1997): Rudolph R, Wyomissing, PA (from Internet) (observation)
Erythema nodosum
(1996): Jarrett P+, *Br J Dermatol* 134, 373 (chronic)
Erythroderma
(1990): Simoneaux PW, *Curr Concept Skin Dis* Winter, 15
(1985): Slagel GA+, *J Am Acad Dermatol* 12, 857
Exanthems (1–5%)
(2001): Werth V, *Dermatology Times* 18
(1995): Blumenthal HL, Beachwood, OH (personal case) (observation)
(1991): Ochsendorf FR+, *Hautarzt* (German) 42, 140
(1990): Simoneaux PW, *Curr Concept Skin Dis* Winter, 15
Exfoliative dermatitis
(1995): Blumenthal HL, Beachwood, OH (personal case) (observation)
(1986): Lavrijsen APM+, *Acta Derm Venereol* (Stockh) 66, 536
(1985): Slagel GA+, *J Am Acad Dermatol* 12, 857
(1980): Koranda FC, *J Am Acad Dermatol* 4, 650 (passim)
Fixed eruption (<1%)
Lichenoid eruption
(1990): Simoneaux PW, *Curr Concept Skin Dis* Winter, 15
(1980): Koranda FC, *J Am Acad Dermatol* 4, 650 (passim)
(1958): Savage J, *Br J Dermatol* 70, 181
(1948): Alving AS+, *J Clin Invest* 27, 56
Photosensitivity
(2002): Litt JZ, Beachwood, OH (personal observation)
(2001): Metayer I+, *Ann Dermatol Venereol* 128(6), 729 (4 cases)
(2000): Ainsworth GE, Salina, KS (from Internet) (observation)
(1991): Ochsendorf FR+, *Hautarzt* (German) 42, 140
(1982): van Weelden H, *Arch Dermatol* 118, 290
(1981): Journet M, *Union Med Can* (French) 110, 356
Phototoxicity
(2001): Metayer I+, *Ann Dermatol Venereol* 128(6), 729 (4 cases)
Pigmentation (1–10%)
(1991): Ochsendorf FR+, *Hautarzt* (German), 42, 140
(1982): Levy H, *S Afr Med J* 2, 735
(1980): Koranda FC, *J Am Acad Dermatol* 4, 650 (passim)
(1963): Tuffanelli D+, *Arch Dermatol* 88, 419
(1959): Dall JLC+, *BMJ* 1, 1387
Polymorphous light eruption
(1968): Reed WB+, *Arch Dermatol* 98, 327
Pruritus (>10%)
(2002): Litt JZ, Beachwood, OH (personal observation)
(2001): Silver B,Deerfield, IL (from Internet) (observation)
(1999): Holme SA+, *Acta Derm Venereol* (Stockh) 79, 333
(1995): Blumenthal HL, Beachwood, OH (personal case) (observation)
(1994): Fain O+, *Rev Med Interne* (French) 15, 433
(1991): Mnyika KS+, *J Trop Med Hyg* 94, 27 (47% incidence)
(1990): Abdulkadir SA+, *Trans Roy Soc Trop Med Hyg* 84, 898
(1990): Simoneaux PW, *Curr Concept Skin Dis* Winter, 15
(1984): Osifo NG, *Arch Dermatol* 120, 80
(1982): Spencer HC+, *BMJ* 285, 1703
(1969): Olatunde IA, *J Nigerian Med Assoc* 6, 23
(1964): Ekpechi OL+, *Arch Dermatol* 120, 80
Psoriasis (exacerbation)
(2001): Spencer L, Crawfordsville, IN (from Internet) (2 observations)
(2001): Thaler D, Monona, WI (from Internet) (exacerbation) (observation)
(1993): Potter B, *Cutis* 52, 229 (passim)
(1988): Nicolas J-F+, *Ann Dermatol Venereol* (French) 115, 289
(1985): Gray RG, *J Rheumatol* 12, 391
(1982): Abel EA+, *J Am Acad Dermatol* 15, 2007
(1982): Luzar MJ, *J Rheumatol* 9, 462
(1981): Olsen TG, *Ann Intern Med* 94, 546
(1966): Baker H, *Br J Dermatol* 78, 161
(1957): Cornbleet T+, *Arch Dermatol* 75, 286
Purpura
Pustular eruption
(1990): Lotem M+, *Acta Derm Venereol* (Stockh) 70, 250
Pustular psoriasis
(1996): Vine JE+, *J Dermatol* 23, 357
(1987): Friedman SJ, *J Am Acad Dermatol* 16, 1256
Rash (sic) (1–10%)
Stevens–Johnson syndrome
(2002): Leckie MJ+, *Rheumatology* (Oxford) 41(4), 473
Telangiectases
(2001): Vassallo C+, *Clin Exp Dermatol* 26(2), 141
Toxic epidermal necrolysis
(2002): Chavez JS, (Santiago) (Chile) March AAD Poster
(2001): Murphy M+, *Clin Exp Dermatol* 26(5), 457 (fatal)
Urticaria
(2002): Litt JZ, Beachwood, OH (personal case) (observation)
(1990): Simoneaux PW, *Curr Concept Skin Dis* Winter, 15
(1980): Koranda FC, *J Am Acad Dermatol* 4, 650 (passim)
Vasculitis

## Hair

Hair – alopecia
Hair – discoloration
(1999): Lecocq P+, *Presse Med* (French) 28, 741
Hair – pigmentation (bleaching) (1–10%)
(1991): Ochsendorf FR+, *Hautarzt* (German) 42, 140
(1985): Dupré A+, *Arch Dermatol* 121, 1164
(1980): Koranda FC, *J Am Acad Dermatol* 4, 650 (passim)
(1978): Dubois EL, *Semin Arthritis Rheum* 8, 33
(1976): Sams WM, *Int J Dermatol* 15, 99
(1965): Rook A, *Br J Dermatol* 77, 115

## Nails

Nails – discoloration
(1991): Zic JA+, *Arch Dermatol* 127, 1037
Nails – pigmentation
(2001): Vassallo C+, *Clin Exp Dermatol* 26(2), 141
(1980): Koranda FC, *J Am Acad Dermatol* 4, 650 (passim)
(1963): Tuffanelli D+, *Arch Dermatol* 88, 419

## Other

Death
(2001): Murphy M+, *Clin Exp Dermatol* 26(5), 457
Dysgeusia
(1996): Weber JC+, *Presse Med* (French) 25, 213
Gingival pigmentation
(1992): Veraldi S+, *Cutis* 49, 281
Lymphoproliferative disease
(1980): Schechter SL+, *Arthritis Rheum* 23, 256
Mucosal atrophy
(2001): Vassallo C+, *Clin Exp Dermatol* 26(2), 141
Myopathy
(1998): Richards AJ, *J Rheumatol* 25, 1642
(1969): Chapman RS+, *Br J Dermatol* 81, 217
Oral mucosal pigmentation
(1992): Veraldi S+, *Cutis* 49, 281
(1991): Zic JA+, *Arch Dermatol* 127, 1037
(1980): Koranda FC, *J Am Acad Dermatol* 4, 650 (passim)
(1971): Giansanti JS+, *Oral Surg* 31, 66
Oral mucosal ulceration
Oral pigmentation
(2001): Vassallo C+, *Clin Exp Dermatol* 26(2), 141
Porphyria
(1993): Potter B, *Cutis* 52, 229 (passim)
(1976): Baler GR, *Cutis* 17, 96
(1974): Kordac V+, *Br J Dermatol* 90, 95

(1962): Cripps DL+, *Arch Dermatol* 86, 575
(1959): Marsden CW, *Br J Dermatol* 71, 219
(1957): Davis MJ+, *Arch Dermatol* 75, 796
(1954): Linden IH+, *Calif Med* 81, 235
Stomatitis
(2001): Vassallo C+, *Clin Exp Dermatol* 26(2), 141
Stomatopyrosis
Tinnitus

# HYDROXYUREA

**Trade names:** Droxia (Bristol-Myers Squibb); Hydrea (Bristol-Myers Squibb); Mylocel
**Other common trade names:** *Litalir; Onco-Carbide*
**Indications:** Leukemia, malignant tumors
**Category:** Antineoplastic
**Half-life:** 3–4 hours
**Clinically important, potentially hazardous interactions with:** aldesleukin

### *Reactions*

## Skin

Acral erythema
(1993): Brincker H+, *Cancer Chemother Pharmacol* 32, 496 (edema and soreness)
(1992): Parodi A+, *G Ital Dermatol Venereol* (Italian) 127, 361 (fingers and toes)
(1991): Baack BR+, *J Am Acad Dermatol* 24, 457
(1989): Kampmann KK+, *Cancer* 63, 2482 (passim)
(1984): Sigal M+, *Ann Dermatol Venereol* (French) 111, 895 (band-like)
(1983): Silver FS+, *Ann Intern Med* 98, 675
Acral ulcers
(2001): Vassallo C+, *Clin Exp Dermatol* 26(2), 141
Acrodermatitis perstans
(2001): Eming SA+, *J Am Acad Dermatol* 45, 321
Acute febrile neutrophilic dermatosis (Sweet's syndrome)
(2002): Guennoc B+, *World Congress Dermatol* Poster 0102
Atrophy
(1997): Ena P+, *J Geriatr Dermatol* 5, 310
Baboon syndrome
(1999): Chowdhury MM+, *Clin Exp Dermatol* 24, 336
Band-like erythema
(1984): Sigal M+, *Ann Dermatol Venereol* (French) 111, 895 (fingers and toes)
Collodion-like skin
(1996): Gauthier O+, *Ann Dermatol Venereol (French)* 123, 727
Cutaneous side effects (sic)
(1998): Radaelli F+, *Am J Hematol* 58, 82
(1975): Kennedy BJ+, *Arch Dermatol* 111, 183 (35%)
(1973): Moschella SL+, *Arch Dermatol* 107, 363 (7%)
Dermatitis (sic) (dry, scaly)
(1984): Sigal M+, *Ann Dermatol Venereol* (French) 111, 895
(1975): Kennedy BJ+, *Arch Dermatol* 111, 183
Dermatomyositis
(2002): Dacey MJ+, Louisville, KY, March AAD Poster
(2001): Vassallo C+, *Clin Exp Dermatol* 26(2), 141
(2000): Kirby B+, *Clin Exp Dermatol* 25, 256
(1998): Suehiro M+, *Br J Dermatol* 139, 748
(1998): Velez A+, *Clin Exp Dermatol* 23, 94
(1997): Ena P+, *J Geriatr Dermatol* 5, 310
(1996): Bahadoran P+, *Br J Dermatol* 134, 1161
(1995): Senet P+, *Br J Dermatol* 133, 455
(1995): Weber L+, *Hautarzt* 46, 717
(1994): Kelly RI+, *Australas J Dermatol* 35, 61
(1994): Perrot JL+, *Ann Dermatol Venereol* (French) 121, 499
(1989): Richard M+, *J Am Acad Dermatol* 21, 797
(1984): Sigal M+, *Ann Dermatol Venereol* (French) 111, 895
Erythema multiforme (<1%)
Exanthems (1–10%)
(1992): Breathnach SM+, *Adverse Drug Reactions and the Skin* Blackwell, Oxford, 303 (passim)
Facial erythema (<1%)
(1975): Kennedy BJ+, *Arch Dermatol* 111, 183
Fixed eruption (<1%)
(1991): Boyd AS+, *J Am Acad Dermatol* 25, 518
(1976): Moschella SL, *Int J Dermatol* 15, 373
(1972): Hunter GA+, *Aust J Dermatol* 13, 93
(1969): Moschella SL+, *Arch Dermatol* 107, 363
Ichthyosis
(2002): Kumar B+, *Clin Exp Dermatol* 27(1), 8
(1997): Ena P+, *J Geriatr Dermatol* 5, 310
Keratoacanthoma
(2001): Vassallo C+, *Clin Exp Dermatol* 26(2), 141 (sun-exposed areas)
Keratoses
(1998): Salmon-Her V+, *Dermatology* 196, 274
(1995): Grange F+, *Ann Dermatol Venereol* (French) 122, 16
Leg edema
(2002): Kumar B+, *Clin Exp Dermatol* 27(1), 8
Lichen planus
(1998): Bohn J+, *J Eur Acad Dermatol Venereol* 10, 187 (ulcerative)
(1991): Renfro L+, *J Am Acad Dermatol* 24, 143 (ulcerative)
(1975): Kennedy BJ+, *Arch Dermatol* 111, 183 (atrophic)
Lichenoid acrodermatitis
(2001): Eming SA+, *J Am Acad Dermatol* 45(2), 321
Lichenoid eruption
(1997): Daoud MS+, *J Am Acad Dermatol* 36, 178
(1997): Ena P+, *J Geriatr Dermatol* 5, 310
Lupus erythematosus
(1994): Layton AM+, *Br J Dermatol* 130, 687
(1994): Layton AM+, *Br J Dermatol* 131, 581
Palmar–plantar keratoderma
(2001): Chaine B+, *Arch Dermatol* 137, 467 (2 cases)
(1997): Ena P+, *J Geriatr Dermatol* 5, 310 (plantar)
(1992): Breathnach SM+, *Adverse Drug Reactions and the Skin* Blackwell, Oxford, 303 (passim)
(1992): Parodi A+, *G Ital Dermatol Venereol* (Italian) 127, 361
(1989): Richard M+, *J Am Acad Dermatol* 21, 797 (passim)
(1984): Sigal M+, *Ann Dermatol Venereol* (French) 111, 895
Peripheral edema
(2002): Kumar B+, *Clin Exp Dermatol* 27(1), 8
Photosensitivity
(1992): Breathnach SM+, *Adverse Drug Reactions and the Skin* Blackwell, Oxford, 303 (passim)
Pigmentation (1–10%)
(2002): Kumar B+, *Clin Exp Dermatol* 27(1), 8 (58.6%)
(2001): Chaine B+, *Arch Dermatol* 137, 467 (29%)
(2001): O'Branski EE+, *J Am Acad Dermatol* 44, 859 (palmar creases) (2 patients; both had sickle cell anemia)
(1995): Weber L+, *Hautarzt* (German) 46, 717
(1993): Brincker H+, *Cancer Chemother Pharmacol* 32, 496
(1993): Gropper CA+, *Int J Dermatol* 32, 731
(1990): Majumdar G+, *BMJ* 300, 1468
(1989): Layton AM+, *Br J Dermatol* 121, 647
(1989): Richard M+, *J Am Acad Dermatol* 21, 797 (passim)
(1984): Sigal M+, *Ann Dermatol Venereol* (French) 111, 895 (band-like)
(1982): Jeanmougin M+, *Ann Dermatol Venereol* (French) 109, 169
(1975): Kennedy BJ+, *Arch Dermatol* 111, 183
(1972): Dahl MH+, *BMJ* 4, 585 (yellow-gray-brown)
(1966): Kennedy BJ+, *JAMA* 195, 162

Poikiloderma
(1997): Daoud MS+, *J Am Acad Dermatol* 36, 178
Pruritus (<1%)
(1995): Weber L+, *Hautarzt* 46, 717
(1992): Vosburgh E, *Am J Hematol* 41, 70
(1975): Kennedy BJ+, *Arch Dermatol* 111, 183
Psoriasis
(2002): Kumar B+, *Clin Exp Dermatol* 27(1), 8
Purpura
(1973): Moschella SL+, *Arch Dermatol* 107, 363
(1973): Roe LD+, *Arch Dermatol* 108, 426
Radiation recall (sic)
(1974): Levantine A+, *Br J Dermatol* 90, 239
(1964): Sears ME, *Cancer Chemother Rep* 40, 31
Rash (sic)
Squamous cell carcinoma
(2001): Vassallo C+, *Clin Exp Dermatol* 26(2), 141 (sun-exposed areas)
(2000): Bateman B, *Skin and Allergy News* August, 3 (observation)
Telangiectases
(1997): Daoud MS+, *J Am Acad Dermatol* 36, 178
(1995): Weber L+, *Hautarzt* (German) 46, 717
Ulceration
(2001): Chaine B+, *Arch Dermatol* 137, 467 (29%) (leg)
(2001): Olesen LH+, *Ugeskr Laeger* 163(49), 6908 (5 cases)
(2001): Young HS+, *Clin Exp Dermatol* 26(8), 664 (fatal)
(2000): Tarumoto T+, *Jpn J Clin Oncol* 30, 159 (heels)
(1999): Kato N+, *J Dermatol* 26, 56
(1999): Sirieix M-E+, *Arch Dermatol* 135, 818
(1999): Stagno F+, *Blood* 94, 1479
(1998): Best PJ+, *Ann Intern Med* 128, 29 (leg)
(1998): Disla E+, *Ann Intern Med* 129, 252
(1998): Kennedy BJ, *Ann Intern Med* 129, 252
(1998): Kido M+, *Br J Dermatol* 139, 1124
(1998): Liebschutz S+, *Rev Med Interne* (French) 19, 360 (malleolar)
(1998): Radaelli F+, *Am J Hematol* 58, 82 (hands)
(1998): Reichenberger F, *Schweiz Rundsch Med Praxis* (German) 87, 1370
(1998): Ruiz-Arguelles GL+, *Mayo Clin Proc* 73, 1125
(1998): Suehiro M+, *Br J Dermatol* 139, 748 (large leg ulcer)
(1998): Weinlich G+, *J Am Acad Dermatol* 39, 372 (painful) (legs) (2 cases)
(1997): Best PJ+, *Ann Int Med* 128, 29
(1997): Cox C+, *Ann Plastic Surg* 39, 546 (ankle)
(1997): Ena P+, *J Geriatr Dermatol* 5, 310 (malleolar squamous cell)
(1997): Glazier DB+, *Wounds* 9, 169
(1996): Callot-Mellot C+, *Arch Dermatol* 132, 1395
(1996): Esteve E+, *Ann Dermatol Venereol* (French) 123, 271
(1996): Iwama H+, *Gan To Kagaku Ryoho* (Japanese) 23, 937
(1995): Masuoka H+, *Rinsho Ketsueki* (Japanese) 36, 156
(1993): Nguyen TV+, *Cutis* 52, 217 (painful legs ulcers)
(1986): Montefusco E+, *Tumori* (Italian) 72, 317 (legs) (17 cases)
(1985): Stahl RL+, *Am J Med* 78, 869
(1984): Sigal M+, *Ann Dermatol Venereol* (French) 111, 895
Ulcers (genitalia)
(2001): Vassallo C+, *Clin Exp Dermatol* 26(2), 141
Urticaria
Vasculitis
(2001): Young HS+, *Clin Exp Dermatol* 26(8), 664
(1997): Reed BR, Denver, CO (from Internet) (observation)
(1992): Breathnach SM+, *Adverse Drug Reactions and the Skin* Blackwell, Oxford, 303 (passim)
(1989): Richard M+, *J Am Acad Dermatol* 21, 797 (passim)
(1976): Moschella SL, *Int J Dermatol* 15, 373
(1973): Moschella SL+, *Arch Dermatol* 107, 363
(1973): Roe LD+, *Arch Dermatol* 108, 426
Xerosis (1–10%)
(2002): Kumar B+, *Clin Exp Dermatol* 27(1), 8
(2001): Chaine B+, *Arch Dermatol* 137, 467 (6 cases)
(1995): Weber L+, *Hautarzt* (German) 46, 717
(1989): Richard M+, *J Am Acad Dermatol* 21, 797 (passim)
(1984): Sigal M+, *Ann Dermatol Venereol* (French) 111, 895
(1975): Kennedy BJ+, *Arch Dermatol* 111, 183

## Hair

Hair – alopecia (1–10%)
(2002): Kumar B+, *Clin Exp Dermatol* 27(1), 8 (diffuse)
(1992): Breathnach SM+, *Adverse Drug Reactions and the Skin* Blackwell, Oxford, 303 (passim)
(1989): Layton AM+, *Br J Dermatol* 121, 647
(1989): Richard M+, *J Am Acad Dermatol* 21, 797 (passim)
(1976): Bergstresser PR+, *Arch Dermatol* 112, 977
(1975): Kennedy BJ+, *Arch Dermatol* 111, 183

## Nails

Nails – atrophic
(1984): Daniel CR+, *J Am Acad Dermatol* 10, 250
(1984): Sigal M+, *Ann Dermatol Venereol* (French) 111, 895
(1975): Kennedy BJ+, *Arch Dermatol* 111, 183
Nails – dystrophy
(1992): Breathnach SM+, *Adverse Drug Reactions and the Skin* Blackwell, Oxford, 303 (passim)
(1989): Richard M+, *J Am Acad Dermatol* 21, 797 (passim)
Nails – onycholysis
(1992): Breathnach SM+, *Adverse Drug Reactions and the Skin* Blackwell, Oxford, 303 (passim)
(1989): Richard M+, *J Am Acad Dermatol* 21, 797 (passim)
Nails – pigmentation
(2002): Kumar B+, *Clin Exp Dermatol* 27(1), 8
(2001): Chaine B+, *Arch Dermatol* 137, 467 (9%)
(2001): O'Branski EE+, *J Am Acad Dermatol* 44, 859 (longitudinal bands) (patient had sickle cell anemia)
(1999): Hernández-Martin A+, *J Am Acad Dermatol* 40, 333
(1997): Ena P+, *J Geriatr Dermatol* 5, 310
(1996): Kwong YL, *J Am Acad Dermatol* 35, 275
(1995): Delmas-Marsalet B+, *Nouv Rev Fr Hematol* (French) 37, 205
(1989): Baran R+, *J Am Acad Dermatol* 21, 1165
Nails – pigmentation of lunula
(2002): Kumar B+, *Clin Exp Dermatol* 27(1), 8
Nails – pigmented bands
(1999): Hernández-Martin A+, *J Am Acad Dermatol* 40, 333
(1997): Cakir B+, *Int J Dermatol* 36, 234
(1994): Pirard C+, *Ann Dermatol Venereol* (French) 121, 106 (longitudinal)
(1993): Gropper CA+, *Int J Dermatol* 32, 731
(1992): Kelsey PR, *Clin Lab Haematol* 14, 337
(1991): Vomvouras S+, *J Am Acad Dermatol* 24, 1016
(1984): Sigal M+, *Ann Dermatol Venereol* (French) 111, 895
(1982): Jeanmougin M+, *Ann Dermatol Venereol* 109, 169

## Other

Death
(2001): Young HS+, *Clin Exp Dermatol* 26(8), 664
Glossitis
(2001): Vassallo C+, *Clin Exp Dermatol* 26(2), 141
Mucocutaneous eruption
(2002): Kumar B+, *Clin Exp Dermatol* 27(1), 8
Myositis
(1998): Ikeda K+, *Rinsho Ketsueki* (Japanese) 39, 676
Oral mucosal lesions
(1976): Bergstresser PR+, *Arch Dermatol* 112, 977
(1975): Kennedy BJ+, *Arch Dermatol* 111, 183
Oral mucosal pigmentation
(2002): Kumar B+, *Clin Exp Dermatol* 27(1), 8
Oral mucosal ulceration
(2001): Vassallo C+, *Clin Exp Dermatol* 26(2), 141

Oral pigmentation
(2002): Kumar B+, *Clin Exp Dermatol* 27(1), 8
(2001): Chaine B+, *Arch Dermatol* 137, 467 (29%)
Oral squamous cell carcinoma
(2001): Esteve E+, *Ann Dermatol Venereol* 128(8), 919
Oral ulceration
(2002): Kumar B+, *Clin Exp Dermatol* 27(1), 8
(1997): Norhaya MR+, *Singapore Med J* 38, 283
(1989): Richard M+, *J Am Acad Dermatol* 21, 797 (passim)
Scleral pigmentation
(2002): Kumar B+, *Clin Exp Dermatol* 27(1), 8
Stomatitis (>10%)
(1993): Brincker H+, *Cancer Chemother Pharmacol* 32, 496
(1992): Breathnach SM+, *Adverse Drug Reactions and the Skin* Blackwell, Oxford, 303 (passim)
(1989): Richard M+, *J Am Acad Dermatol* 21, 797 (passim)
Tongue pigmentation
(2001): Chaine B+, *Arch Dermatol* 137, 467 (29%)
(1997): Ena P+, *J Geriatr Dermatol* 5, 310
(1993): Gropper CA+, *Int J Dermatol* 32, 731
Tumors
(1998): Best PJ+, *Mayo Clin Proc* 73, 961 (multiple malignant)
(1998): De Simone C+, *Eur J Dermatol* 8, 114 (multiple squamous cell)
(1998): Salmon-Her V+, *Dermatology* 196, 274
(1993): Papi M+, *J Am Acad Dermatol* 28, 485 (on light-exposed areas)
(1992): Stasi R+, *Eur J Haematol* 48, 121

## HYDROXYZINE

**Trade names:** Atarax (Pfizer); Marax (Pfizer); Vistaril (Pfizer)
**Other common trade names:** *AH3 N; Anaxanil; Bobsule; Iremofar; Masmoran; Multipax; Otarex; Paxistil; Quiess; Rezine; Vamate*
**Indications:** Anxiety and tension, pruritus
**Category:** Antihistamine; anxiolytic and antiemetic
**Half-life:** 3–7 hours
**Clinically important, potentially hazardous interactions with: alcohol**, barbiturates, CNS depressants, narcotics, non-narcotic analgesics

### *Reactions*

#### Skin

Angioedema (<1%)
(1971): 9, 84
(1964): Welsh AL, *Med Clin North Am* 48, 459
(1958): Cohen AE+, *J Allergy* 29, 542
Contact dermatitis
(1997): Menne T, *Am J Contact Dermat* 8, 1
Diaphoresis
Edema (<1%)
Erythema multiforme (<1%)
(1959): Wright W, *JAMA* 171, 1642
Exanthems
(1964): Welsh AL, *Med Clin North Am* 48, 459
(1959): Wright W, *JAMA* 171, 1642
(1958): Cohen AE+, *J Allergy* 29, 542
Fixed eruption
(1997): Cohen HA+, *Ann Pharmacother* 31, 327 (penis)
(1996): Cohen HA+, *Cutis* 57, 431 (scrotum)
Flushing
(1998): Foster M+, *J Clin Dermatol* Winter, 7
Photosensitivity (<1%)
Purpura
Rash (sic) (<1%)
Urticaria
(1964): Welsh AL, *Med Clin North Am* 48, 459
(1959): Wright W, *JAMA* 171, 1642

#### Other

Hypersensitivity
(1978): Massoud N, *J Pediatr* 93, 308
Injection-site necrosis
(1995): Tokodi G+, *J Am Osteopath Assoc* 95, 609
Myalgia (<1%)
Priapism
(1994): Thavundayil JX+, *Neuropsychobiology* 30, 4
Xerostomia (10%)
(1998): Foster M+, *J Clin Dermatol* Winter, 7 (12.5%)
(1990): Kalivas J+, *J Allergy Clin Immunol* 86, 1014

## HYOSCYAMINE

**Synonyms:** Hyoscyamine sulfate; hyoscyamine sulfate
**Trade names:** A-Spas; Anaspaz (Ascher); Cytospaz; Donnamar; ED-SPAZ; Gastrosed; Hyco; Hycosol Sl; Hyospaz; Levbid (Schwarz Pharma); Levsin (Schwarz Pharma); Levsin/SL (Schwarz Pharma); Levsinex (Schwarz Pharma); Liqui-Sooth; Medispaz; Pasmex; Setamine; Spasdel
**Other common trade name:** *Duboisine, Egacene Durettes, Egazil, Peptard*
**Indications:** Treatment of gastrointestinal tract disorders caused by spasm, Adjunctive therapy for peptic ulcers, cystitis, Parkinsonism, biliary & renal colic
**Category:** Anticholinergic
**Duration of action:** 13–38 min
**Clinically important, potentially hazardous interactions with:** anticholinergics, arbutamine

### *Reactions*

#### Skin

Allergic reactions (sic)
Flushing
Hypohidrosis (>10%)
Photosensitivity (1–10%)
Rash (sic) (<1%)
Urticaria
Xerosis (>10%)

#### Other

Ageusia
Anaphylactoid reactions
Dysgeusia
Injection-site inflammation (>10%)
Xerostomia (>10%)

# IBRITUMOMAB

**Synonyms:** In-111 Zevalin; Y-90 Zevalin
**Trade name:** Zevalin (IDEC)
**Indications:** Non-Hodgkin's lymphoma
**Category:** Antineoplastic monoclonal antibody; radiopharmaceutical
**Half-life:** 30 hours

### *Reactions*

#### Skin

Allergic reactions (sic) (2%)
Angioedema (5%)
Chills (24%)
Diaphoresis (4%)
Ecchymoses (7%)
Flushing (6%)
Infections (sic) (29%)
Peripheral edema (8%)
Petechiae (3%)
Pruritus (9%)
Purpura (7%)
Rash (sic) (8%)
Urticaria (4%)

#### Other

Anaphylactoid reactions
Arthralgia (7%)
Arthritis (<1%)
Back pain (8%)
Cough (10%)
Death
Hypersensitivity
Infusion-site reactions (sic) (fatal)
Myalgia (7%)
Pain (13%)

# IBUPROFEN

**Trade names:** Advil (Wyeth); Genpril; Haltran; Medipren; Midol 220; Motrin (McNeil); Nuprin; Pamprin; Profen; Rufen; Trendar; Uni-Proc
**Other common trade names:** *Act-3; Actiprofen; Anco; Apsifen; Brufen; Ebufac; Lidifen; Proflex; Tabalom; Urem*
**Indications:** Arthritis, pain
**Category:** Nonsteroidal anti-inflammatory (NSAID); antipyretic
**Half-life:** 2–4 hours
**Clinically important, potentially hazardous interactions with:** aspirin, diuretics, methotrexate, NSAIDs, salicylates, tacrolimus, urokinase

### *Reactions*

#### Skin

Angioedema (<1%)
(1994): Halpern SM, *Arch Dermatol* 130, 259 (passim)
(1987): Shelley ED+, *J Am Acad Dermatol* 17, 1057
(1985): Bigby M+, *J Am Acad Dermatol* 12, 866
(1984): Stern RS+, *JAMA* 252, 1433
(1982): Bailin PL+, *Clinics in Rheumatic Diseases*, WB Saunders 8, 493 (passim)
Bullous eruption (<1%)
(1994): Halpern SM, *Arch Dermatol* 130, 259 (passim)
(1988): Laing VB+, *J Am Acad Dermatol* 19, 91
(1984): Stern R+, *JAMA* 252, 1433
Bullous pemphigoid
(1993): Fellner MJ, *Clin Dermatol* 11, 515
(1981): Pompeova L, *Cesk Dermatol* (Czech) 56, 256
Contact dermatitis (<1%)
(1993): Ophaswongse S+, *Contact Dermatitis* 29, 57
(1986): Veronesi S+, *Contact Dermatitis* 15, 103
(1985): Valsecchi R+, *Contact Dermatitis* 12, 286
Dermatitis herpetiformis
(1994): Tousignant J+, *Int J Dermatol* 33, 199
Diaphoresis
(1974): Regalado RG+, *J Int Med Res* 2, 115
Eczematous eruption (sic)
(1986): Veronesi S+, *Contact Dermatitis* 15, 103
Edema (<1%)
Erythema multiforme (<1%)
(1995): Lesko SM+, *JAMA* 273, 929
(1994): Halpern SM, *Arch Dermatol* 130, 259 (passim)
(1992): Breathnach SM+, *Adverse Drug Reactions and the Skin* Blackwell, Oxford, 186 (passim)
(1985): Bigby M+, *J Am Acad Dermatol* 12, 866
(1985): O'Brien WM+, *J Rheumatol* 12, 13
(1984): Stern R+, *JAMA* 252, 1433
(1978): Sternlieb P+, *N Y State J Med* 78, 1239
Erythema nodosum
(1994): Halpern SM, *Arch Dermatol* 130, 259 (passim)
Exanthems
(1994): Halpern SM, *Arch Dermatol* 130, 259 (passim)
(1994): Litt JZ, Beachwood, OH (personal case) (observation)
(1985): Bigby M+, *J Am Acad Dermatol* 12, 866
(1980): Shoenfeld Y+, *JAMA* 244, 547
(1979): Finch WR+, *JAMA* 241, 2616
(1978): Sonnenblick M+, *BMJ* 1, 619
(1975): Blechman WJ+, *JAMA* 233, 336 (3.4%)
(1974): Regalado RG+, *J Int Med Res* 2, 115 (0.86%)
(1973): Mills SB+, *BMJ* 4, 82 (>5%)
Fixed eruption (<1%)
(2001): Diaz Jara M+, *Pediatr Dermatol* 18, 66
(2000): Zabawski E, Longview, TX (from Internet) (observation)
(1998): Mahboob A+, *Int J Dermatol* 37, 833
(1996): Eichwald M, Redding, CA (from Internet) (observation)
(1994): Shelley WB+, *Cutis* 53, 282 (observation)
(1992): Breathnach SM+, *Adverse Drug Reactions and the Skin* Blackwell, Oxford, 186 (passim)
(1991): Kuligowski ME+, *Contact Dermatitis* 25, 259
(1990): Bharija SC+, *Dermatologica* 181, 237
(1985): Bigby M+, *J Am Acad Dermatol* 12, 866
(1984): Kanwar AJ+, *J Dermatol* 11, 383
(1984): Stern R+, *JAMA* 252, 1433
Flushing
Hot flashes (<1%)
Linear IgA bullous dermatosis
(2002): Au S+, (Vancouver) (Canada) March AAD Poster
Livedo reticularis
(1979): Finch WR+, *JAMA* 241, 2616
Lupus erythematosus
(1996): Vigouroux C+, *Rev Med Interne* (French) 14, 856
(1985): O'Brien WM+, *J Rheumatol* 12, 13
(1980): Bar-Sela S+, *J Rheumatol* 7, 379
(1978): Pereyo-Torrellas N, *Arch Dermatol* 114, 1097
(1978): Sonnenblick M+, *BMJ* 1, 619 (exacerbation)
Pemphigoid
(1988): Laing VB+, *J Am Acad Dermatol* 19, 91
Periorbital edema
(1979): Finch WR+, *JAMA* 241, 2616
Photoreactions

(1982): Bailin PL+, *Clinics in Rheumatic Diseases*, WB Saunders 8, 493

Photosensitivity
(1994): Berger TG+, *Arch Dermatol* 130, 609 (in HIV-infected) (5 cases)
(1994): Halpern SM, *Arch Dermatol* 130, 259 (passim)
(1992): Bergner T+, *J Am Acad Dermatol* 26, 114
(1990): Bergner T+, *J Allergy Clin Immunol* 85, 177
(1985): Bigby M+, *J Am Acad Dermatol* 12, 866

Pruritus (1–5%)
(1994): Halpern SM, *Arch Dermatol* 130, 259 (passim)
(1992): Breathnach SM+, *Adverse Drug Reactions and the Skin* Blackwell, Oxford, 186 (passim)
(1985): Bigby M+, *J Am Acad Dermatol* 12, 866 (1–5%)
(1979): Finch WR+, *JAMA* 241, 2616
(1975): Blechman WJ+, *JAMA* 233, 336 (1.8%)

Psoriasis (palms)
(1986): Ben-Chetrit E+, *Cutis* 38, 45 (exacerbation)
(1985): Bigby M+, *J Am Acad Dermatol* 12, 866

Purpura
(1969): Ward T, *BMJ* 4, 430

Rash (sic) (>10%)
(1974): Regalado RG+, *J Int Med Res* 2, 115

Stevens–Johnson syndrome (<1%)
(1994): Halpern SM, *Arch Dermatol* 130, 259 (passim)
(1978): Sternlieb P+, *N Y State J Med* 78, 1239

Toxic epidermal necrolysis (<1%)
(1994): Halpern SM, *Arch Dermatol* 130, 259 (passim)
(1980): Sternlieb P+, *Ann Intern Med* 92, 570

Urticaria (>10%)
(2001): Diaz Jara M+, *Pediatr Dermatol* 18, 66
(1994): Halpern SM, *Arch Dermatol* 130, 259 (passim)
(1993): Litt JZ, Beachwood, OH (personal case) (observation)
(1987): Shelley ED+, *J Am Acad Dermatol* 17, 1057
(1985): Bigby M+, *J Am Acad Dermatol* 12, 866
(1984): Stern RS+, *JAMA* 252, 1433
(1982): Bailin PL+, *Clinics in Rheumatic Diseases*, WB Saunders 8, 493 (passim)
(1975): Blechman WJ+, *JAMA* 233, 336 (0.2%)

Vasculitis
(2001): Davidson KA+, *Cutis* 67, 303 (bullous leukocytoclastic)
(1996): Peters F+, *J Rheumatol* 23, 2008
(1994): Halpern SM, *Arch Dermatol* 130, 259 (passim)
(1992): Breathnach SM+, *Adverse Drug Reactions and the Skin* Blackwell, Oxford, 186 (passim)
(1985): Bigby M+, *J Am Acad Dermatol* 12, 866
(1984): Stern R+, *JAMA* 252, 1433
(1982): Labbe A+, *Ann Dermatol Venereol* (French) 109, 995
(1978): Pereyo-Torrellas N, *Arch Dermatol* 114, 1097

Vesiculobullous eruption
(1992): Breathnach SM+, *Adverse Drug Reactions and the Skin* Blackwell, Oxford, 186 (passim)
(1988): Laing VB+, *J Am Acad Dermatol* 19, 91 (passim)

### Hair

Hair – alopecia (<1%)
(1985): O'Brien WM+, *J Rheumatol* 12, 13
(1979): Meyer HC, *JAMA* 242, 142

Hair – disorders (sic)
(1994): Halpern SM, *Arch Dermatol* 130, 259 (passim)

### Nails

Nails – disorder (sic)
(1994): Halpern SM, *Arch Dermatol* 130, 259 (passim)

Nails – onycholysis
(1982): Bailin PL+, *Clinics In Rheumatic Diseases*, WB Saunders 8, 493

### Other

Anaphylactoid reactions (<1%)
(2001): Verma S, Baroda, India (from Internet) (observation) (with acetaminophen)
(2000): Takahama H+, *J Dermatol* 27, 337
(1998): Menendez R+, *Ann Allergy Asthma Immunol* 80, 225
(1985): O'Brien WM+, *J Rheumatol* 12, 13
(1979): Finch WR+, *JAMA* 241, 2616

Aphthous stomatitis

DRESS syndrome
(2001): Descamps V+, *Arch Dermatol* 137, 301

Gingival ulceration (<1%)

Gynecomastia (<1%)

Hypersensitivity
(2001): McMahon AD+, *J Clin Epidemiol* 54(12), 1271
(1981): Ruppert GB+, *South Med J* 74, 241

Impaired wound healing
(1988): Proper SA+, *J Am Acad Dermatol* 18, 1173

Myopathy
(1987): Ross NS+, *JAMA* 257, 62

Oral lichenoid eruption
(1983): Hamburger J+, *BMJ* 287, 1258

Oral mucosal lesions
(1974): Regalado RG+, *J Int Med Res* 2, 115

Oral ulceration
(1974): Regalado RG+, *J Int Med Res* 2, 115

Paresthesias

Pseudolymphoma
(2001): Werth V, *Dermatology Times* 18

Pseudoporphyria
(2000): De Silva B+, *Pediatr Dermatol* 17, 480
(1992): Petersen CS+, *Ugeskr Laeger* (Danish) 154, 1713

Rhabdomyolysis
(1989): Menzies DG+, *Med Toxicol Adverse* 4(6), 468

Serum sickness
(1995): Lesko SM+, *JAMA* 273, 929

Stomatitis

Tinnitus

Xerostomia (<1%)

## IBUTILIDE

**Trade name:** Corvert (Pharmacia & Upjohn)
**Indications:** Atrial fibrillation and flutter
**Category:** Antiarrhythmic class III
**Half-life:** 2–12 hours

### *Reactions*

### Skin

Bullous eruption

Contact dermatitis
(1998): Dodds ES+, *Pharmacotherapy* 18, 880 (bullous)

# IDARUBICIN

**Synonyms:** 4-demethoxydaunorubicin; 4-DMDR
**Trade name:** Idamycin (Pharmacia & Upjohn)
**Other common trade name:** *Zavedos*
**Indications:** Acute myeloid leukemia
**Category:** Antineoplastic antibiotic
**Half-life:** 14–35 hours (oral)
**Clinically important, potentially hazardous interactions with:** aldesleukin

### *Reactions*

#### Skin
Acral erythema
(1993): Cohen PR, *Cutis* 51, 175
Bullous eruption (palms and soles)
Erythematous streaking (sic) (>10%)
Exanthems (<1%)
Radiation recall
(1995): Gabel C+, *Gynecol Oncol* 57, 266
Rash (sic) (>10%)
(1998): Stuart NS+, *Cancer Chemother Pharmacol* 21, 351
(1997): Maloney DG+, *J Clin Oncol* 15, 3266
Urticaria (>10%)
(1997): Maloney DG+, *J Clin Oncol* 15, 3266

#### Hair
Hair – alopecia (77%)
(2000): No author, *Prescrire Int* 9, 103
(1993): Ogawa M+, *Gan To Kaguku Ryoho* (Japanese) 20, 897
(1993): Ogawa M+, *Gan To Kaguku Ryoho* (Japanese) 20, 907
(1991): Hollingshead LM+, *Drugs* 42, 690
(1988): Gillies H+, *Cancer Chemother Pharmacol* 21, 261
(1986): Dodion P+, *Invest New Drugs* 4, 31
(1986): Lopez M+, *Invest New Drugs* 4, 39

#### Nails
Nails – pigmentary changes
(1997): Borecky Derrick J+, *Cutis* 59, 203

#### Other
Extravasation-site necrosis (>10%)
Injection-site urticaria
Mucositis (50%)
(2000): Creutzig U+, *Klin Padiatr* 212, 163
(1986): Dodion P+, *Invest New Drugs* 4, 31
Stomatitis (>10%)

# IFOSFAMIDE

**Trade name:** Ifex (Bristol-Myers Squibb)
**Other common trade names:** *Holoxan; Ifoxan; Mitoxana; Tronoxal*
**Indications:** Cancers, sarcomas, leukemias, lymphomas
**Category:** Antineoplastic; nitrogen mustard
**Half-life:** 4–15 hours
**Clinically important, potentially hazardous interactions with:** aldesleukin

### *Reactions*

#### Skin
Allergic reactions (sic) (1–10%)
Dermatitis (sic) (1–10%)
Pigmentation (1–10%)
(1994): Yule SM+, *Cancer* 73, 240
(1993): Teresi ME+, *Cancer* 71, 2873

#### Hair
Hair – alopecia (50–83%)
(1988): Negretti E+, *Tumori* (Italian) 74, 163 (100%)
(1971): Kunz W+, *Schweiz Med Wochenschr (German)* 101, 1151

#### Nails
Nails – ridging (1–10%)
(1994): Ben Dayan D+, *Acta Haematol* 91, 89

#### Other
Anaphylactoid reactions
Oral mucosal lesions
Phlebitis (2%)
Sialorrhea (<1%)
Stomatitis (<1%)

# IMATINIB

**Synonyms:** CGP57148; STI571
**Trade name:** Gleevec (Novartis)
**Other common trade name:** *Glivec*
**Indications:** Chronic myeloid leukemia
**Category:** Antineoplastic; tyrosine kinase inhibitor; signal transduction inhibitor
**Half-life:** 18 hours
**Clinically important, potentially hazardous interactions with:** amlodipine, anisindione, anticoagulants, atorvastatin, barbiturates, benzodiazepines, butabarbital, carbamazepine, chlordiazepoxide, clarithromycin, clonazepam, clorazepate, corticosteroids, cyclosporine, diazepam, dicumarol, erythromycin, ethotoin, felodipine, flurazepam, fluvastatin, fosphenytoin, isradipine, itraconazole, ketoconazole, lorazepam, lovastatin, mephenytoin, mephobarbital, midazolam, nicardipine, nifedipine, nimodipine, nisoldipine, oxazepam, pentobarbital, phenobarbital, phenytoin, pimozide, pravastatin, primidone, quazepam, rifampin, secobarbital, simvastatin, **St John's wort**, temazepam, warfarin

### *Reactions*

#### Skin
Edema (1–5%)
(2002): Tefferi A+, *Blood* 99(10), 3854
(2001): van Oosterom AT+, *Lancet* 358(9291), 1421
Night sweats (8–10%)
Periorbital edema
Peripheral edema
Petechiae (1–10%)
Pruritus (6–10%)
Rash (sic) (32–39%)
(2001): van Oosterom+, *Lancet* 358(9291), 1421

#### Other
Arthralgia (21–26%)
Myalgia (7–18%)
(2002): Tefferi A+, *Blood* 99(10), 3854
Myositis
(2002): Tefferi A+, *Blood* 99(10), 3854

## IMIPENEM/CILASTATIN

**Synonym:** imipemide
**Trade name:** Primaxin (Merck)
**Other common trade names:** *Tenacid; Tienam; Tienam 500; Zienam*
**Indications:** Various infections caused by susceptible organisms
**Category:** Carbapenem antibiotic
**Half-life:** 1 hour
**Clinically important, potentially hazardous interactions with:** cyclosporine, ganciclovir

### *Reactions*

#### Skin

Acute generalized exanthematous pustulosis (AGEP)
(1989): Escallier F+, *Ann Dermatol Venereol* (French) 116, 407
Allergic reactions (sic) (1–3%)
(1994): Pleasants RA+, *Chest* 106, 1124 (in patients with cystic fibrosis)
Angioedema (0.2%)
(1987): Clissold SP+, *Drugs* 33, 183
Candidiasis (0.2%)
Diaphoresis (0.2%)
Erythema multiforme (0.2%)
(1987): Clissold SP+, *Drugs* 33, 183
Exanthems (<1%)
(1989): Escallier F+, *Ann Dermatol Venereol* (French) 116, 407
(1987): Clissold SP+, *Drugs* 33, 183
(1985): Calandra GB+, *Am J Med* 78, 73 (1–5%)
Flushing (0.2%)
Pruritus (0.3%)
(1991): Machado ARL+, *J Allergy Clin Immunol* 87, 754
(1989): Escallier F+, *Ann Dermatol Venereol* (French) 116, 407
(1987): Clissold SP+, *Drugs* 33, 183
Pruritus vulvae (0.2%)
Pustular eruption
(1994): Spencer JM+, *Br J Dermatol* 130, 514
Rash (sic) (4%)
(1994): Grayson ML+, *Clin Infect Dis* 18, 683
Toxic epidermal necrolysis (0.2%)
Urticaria (0.2%)
(1991): Hantson P+, *BMJ* 302, 294
(1989): Escallier F+, *Ann Dermatol Venereol* (French) 116, 407
(1987): Clissold SP+, *Drugs* 33, 183
Vasculitis
(1997): Reiner MR+, *J Am Podiatr Med Assoc* 87, 245

#### Other

Dysgeusia (0.2%)
Glossitis (0.2%)
Hypersensitivity
(1988): Donowitz GR+, *N Engl J Med* 318, 490
Injection-site erythema (0.4%)
Injection-site pain
(1991): 29, 43
(1985): Calandra GB+, *Am J Med* 78, 73 (0.7%)
Injection-site phlebitis
(1991): 29, 43
(1988): Gould IM+, *Drugs Exp Clin Res* 14, 555
(1987): Clissold SP+, *Drugs* 33, 183 (2%)
(1985): Calandra GB+, *Am J Med* 78, 73 (3.8%)
Oral mucosal lesions
Paresthesias (0.2%)
Phlebitis (3%)
Sialorrhea (0.2%)
Thrombophlebitis (3.1%)
Tinnitus

## IMIPRAMINE

**Trade name:** Tofranil (Novartis)
**Other common trade names:** *Apo-Imipramine; Imidol; Imipramin; Impril; Novo-Pramine; Primonil; Pryleugan*
**Indications:** Depression
**Category:** Tricyclic antidepressant
**Half-life:** 6–18 hours
**Clinically important, potentially hazardous interactions with:** amprenavir, arbutamine, clonidine, epinephrine, fluoxetine, formoterol, guanethidine, isocarboxazid, linezolid, MAO inhibitors, phenelzine, quinolones, sparfloxacin, tranylcypromine

### *Reactions*

#### Skin

Acne
Allergic reactions (sic)
Angioedema (<1%)
(1971): Almeyda J, *Br J Dermatol* 84, 298
Ankle edema
Bullous eruption
(1977): Varma AJ+, *Arch Intern Med* 137, 1207 (passim)
Diaphoresis (1–25%)
(2002): Mavissakalian M+, *J Clin Psychopharmacol* 22(2), 155
(1990): Leeman CP, *J Clin Psychiatry* 51, 258
(1989): Butt MM, *J Clin Psychiatry* 50, 146
(1971): Almeyda J, *Br J Dermatol* 84, 298
(1962): Busfield BL+, *J Nerv Ment Dis* 134, 339 (25%)
(1961): Kiloh LG+, *BMJ* 1, 168
(1959): Mann AM+, *Can Psychiatr Assoc J* 4, 38
Edema
(1961): Kiloh LG+, *BMJ* 1, 168
Erythema
Exanthems (1–6%)
(1992): Breathnach SM+, *Adverse Drug Reactions and the Skin* Blackwell, Oxford, 197 (passim)
(1988): Warnock JK+, *Am J Psychiatry* 145, 425 (6%)
(1985): Walter-Ryan WG+, *JAMA* 254, 357
(1971): Almeyda J, *Br J Dermatol* 84, 298
(1968): Powell WJ+, *JAMA* 206, 642
(1959): Mann AM+, *Can Psychiatr Assoc J* 4, 38
Exfoliative dermatitis
(1992): Breathnach SM+, *Adverse Drug Reactions and the Skin* Blackwell, Oxford, 197 (passim)
(1971): Almeyda J, *Br J Dermatol* 84, 298
(1968): Powell WJ+, *JAMA* 206, 642
(1959): Mann AM+, *Can Psychiatr Assoc J* 4, 38
Fixed eruption (<1%)
(1978): Sehgal VN+, *Int J Dermatol* 17, 78
Flushing
(1961): Kiloh LG+, *BMJ* 1, 168
Lichen planus
(1971): Almeyda J, *Br J Dermatol* 84, 298
Lupus erythematosus
(1971): Almeyda J, *Br J Dermatol* 84, 298
Petechiae
Photoreactions
Photosensitivity (<1%)
(1985): Walter-Ryan WG+, *JAMA* 354, 357
(1971): Almeyda J, *Br J Dermatol* 84, 298
(1960): Gesensway D+, *Am J Psychiatry* 116, 1027

Pigmentation
(2002): Angel TA+, *Int J Dermatol* 41(6), 327 (slate gray) (photodistributed)
(1999): Ming ME+, *J Am Acad Dermatol* 40, 159 (4 cases)
(1991): Hashimoto K+, *J Am Acad Dermatol* 25, 357 (slate-gray)
(1990): Goldberg NC, *Dermatology Perspectives* 6, 8
(1988): Warnock JK+, *Am J Psychiatry* 145, 425
(1970): Hare PJ, *Br J Dermatol* 83, 420 ("visage mauve")
Pruritus
(1988): Warnock JK+, *Am J Psychiatry* 145, 425 (3%)
(1987): Pohl R+, *Am J Psychiatry* 144, 237
(1971): Almeyda J, *Br J Dermatol* 84, 298
(1968): Powell WJ+, *JAMA* 206, 642
(1961): Kiloh LG+, *BMJ* 1, 168
(1959): Mann AM+, *Can Psychiatr Assoc J* 4, 38
Purpura
(1988): Warnock JK+, *Am J Psychiatry* 145, 425
(1971): Almeyda J, *Br J Dermatol* 84, 298
(1971): Kosakova M, *Cesk Dermatol* (Czech) 46, 158
Rash (sic)
Urticaria
(1992): Breathnach SM+, *Adverse Drug Reactions and the Skin* Blackwell, Oxford, 197 (passim)
(1987): Pohl R+, *Am J Psychiatry* 144, 237
(1985): Burnett GB+, *South Med J* 78, 71
(1971): Almeyda J, *Br J Dermatol* 84, 298
(1961): Kiloh LG+, *BMJ* 1, 168
(1959): Mann AM+, *Can Psychiatr Assoc J* 4, 38
Vasculitis
(1992): Breathnach SM+, *Adverse Drug Reactions and the Skin* Blackwell, Oxford, 197 (passim)
Xerosis

### Hair

Hair – alopecia (<1%)
(1994): Friedman M, *J Fam Pract* 39, 114
(1991): Warnock JK+, *J Nerv Ment Dis* 179, 441
Hair – alopecia areata
(1987): Baral J+, *Int J Dermatol* 26, 198

### Nails

Nails – parrot beak nails
(1971): Kandil E, *J Med Liban* (French) 24, 433

### Other

Black tongue
Dysgeusia (>10%) (metallic taste)
(1961): Kiloh LG+, *BMJ* 1, 168
Galactorrhea (<1%)
(1964): Klein JJ+, *N Engl J Med* 271, 510
Glossitis
(1992): Breathnach SM+, *Adverse Drug Reactions and the Skin* Blackwell, Oxford, 197 (passim)
(1959): Delay J+, *Can Psychiatr Assoc J* 4, 100
Glossodynia
Gynecomastia (<1%)
(1964): Klein JJ+, *N Engl J Med* 271, 510
Hypogeusia
Mucous membrane desquamation
(1968): Powell WJ+, *JAMA* 206, 642
Oral mucosal lesions
(1971): Almeyda J, *Br J Dermatol* 84, 298
(1964): Pollack B+, *Am J Psychiatry* 121, 384
(1962): Busfield BL+, *J Nerv Ment Dis* 134, 339 (21%)
Oral ulceration
Paresthesias
Parkinsonism (1–10%)
Stomatitis
(1992): Breathnach SM+, *Adverse Drug Reactions and the Skin* Blackwell, Oxford, 197 (passim)
(1964): Pollack B+, *Am J Psychiatry* 121, 384
Tremors
Vaginitis
Xerostomia (>10%)
(2002): Mavissakalian M+, *J Clin Psychopharmacol* 22(2), 155
(1971): Almeyda J, *Br J Dermatol* 84, 298
(1962): Busfield BL+, *J Nerv Ment Dis* 134, 339 (21%)
(1961): Kiloh LG+, *BMJ* 1, 168
(1959): Mann AM+, *Can Psychiatr Assoc J* 4, 38

# IMIQUIMOD

**Trade name:** Aldara (3M)
**Indications:** External genital and perianal warts
**Category:** Immune response modifier (interferon inducer)
**Half-life:** N/A

## *Reactions*

### Skin

Bullous eruption
(2002): Chen TM+, *Dermatol Surg* 28, 344 (for BCCs)
Burning (9–31%)
(2001): Gollnick H+, *Int J STD AIDS* 12(1), 22
(1999): Perry CM+, *Drugs* 58(2), 375
(1998): Beutner KR+, *J Am Acad Dermatol* 38(2), 230 (31.3%)
Edema (12–17%)
Erosion (10–32%)
(1999): Perry CM+, *Drugs* 58(2), 375
(1998): Beutner KR+, *J Am Acad Dermatol* 38(2), 230 (10.4%)
Erythema (33–67%)
(2002): Chen TM+, *Dermatol Surg* 28, 344 (for BCCs)
(2001): Fife KH+, *Sex Transm Dis* 28(4), 226
(2001): Garland SM+, *Int J STD AIDS* 12(11), 722 (67%)
(2001): Gollnick H+, *Int J STD AIDS* 12(1), 22
(1999): Gilson RJ+, *AIDS* 13(17), 2397 (41.9%)
(1999): Perry CM+, *Drugs* 58(2), 375 (67%)
(1998): Beutner KR+, *J Am Acad Dermatol* 38(2), 230 (33.3%)
(1998): Edwards L+, *Arch Dermatol* 134(1), 25
Excoriations (18–25%)
(2001): Fife KH+, *Sex Transm Dis* 28(4), 226
(1999): Perry CM+, *Drugs* 58(2), 375
Flaking (18–25%)
(1999): Perry CM+, *Drugs* 58(2), 375 (67%)
Flu-like syndrome (1–3%)
Fungal infections (2–11%)
Induration (5%)
Irritation (sic)
(1998): Beutner KR+, *J Am Acad Dermatol* 38(2), 230 (16.7%)
Pain (2–8%)
(2001): Gollnick H+, *Int J STD AIDS* 12(1), 22
(1998): Beutner KR+, *J Am Acad Dermatol* 38(2), 230
Pigmentation
(2000): Geisse JK, *Dermatol Surg* 26, 579
Pruritus (22–67%)
(2001): Gollnick H+, *Int J STD AIDS* 12(1), 22
(1999): Perry CM+, *Drugs* 58(2), 375 (67%)
(1998): Beutner KR+, *J Am Acad Dermatol* 38(2), 230 (54.2%)
Scabbing (4%)
Tenderness (local)
(2002): Schroeder TL+, *J Am Acad Dermatol* 46(4), 545
(1998): Beutner KR+, *J Am Acad Dermatol* 38(2), 230 (12.5%)
Ulceration (5–10%)
(2002): Chen TM+, *Dermatol Surg* 28, 344 (for BCCs) (focal)

(2002): Emmet S, Solana Beach, CA (from Internet) (observation) (topical on lips)
(2001): Fife KH+, *Sex Transm Dis* 28(4), 226
(1998): Beutner KR+, *J Am Acad Dermatol* 38(2), 230 (10.4%)
Vesiculation (2–3%)
(2001): Fife KH+, *Sex Transm Dis* 28(4), 226

### Other

Aphthous stomatitis
(2002): Goldblum O, Pittsburgh, PA (from Internet) (observation) (topical on face and lips)
(2002): Kaufmann MD, Newyork, NY (from Internet) (observation) (topical on face)
Application-site reactions (sic)
(2001): Barba AR+, *Dermatol Online J* 7(1), 20
(2001): Gollnick H+, *Int J STD AIDS* 12, 22
(2000): Kagy MK+, *Dermatol Surg* 26(6), 577 (for BCCs)
Depression
(1998): Goldstein D+, *J Infect Dis* 178(3), 858 (oral intake)
Myalgia (1%)

## INAMRINONE

**Trade name:** Inocor (Sanofi)
**Other common trade names:** *Amcoral; Cartonic; Vestistol*
**Indications:** Congestive heart failure
**Category:** Positive inotropic agent
**Half-life:** 4.6 hours

#### *Reactions*

### Skin

None

### Other

Hypersensitivity
Injection-site burning (0.2%)

## INDAPAMIDE

**Trade name:** Lozol (Aventis)
**Other common trade names:** *Dapa-tabs; Fludex; Ipamix; Lozide; Naplin; Natrilix; Pamid*
**Indications:** Edema
**Category:** Oral antihypertensive sulfonamide* diuretic
**Half-life:** 14–18 hours
**Clinically important, potentially hazardous interactions with:** digoxin, lithium

#### *Reactions*

### Skin

Angioedema
(1994): Gales BJ+, *Am J Hosp Pharm* 51, 118
(1992): Spinler SA+, *Cutis* 50, 200
(1987): Stricker BHC+, *Br Med J Clin Res Ed* 295, 1313
Bullous eruption
Diaphoresis
Erythema multiforme
(1994): Gales BJ+, *Am J Hosp Pharm* 51, 118
(1987): Stricker BHC+, *Br Med J Clin Res Ed* 295, 1313
Exanthems
(1987): Stricker BHC+, *Br Med J Clin Res Ed* 295, 1313
Fixed eruption
(1998): De Barrio M+, *J Investig Allergol Clin Immunol* 8, 253
Flushing (<5%)
(1985): Chaignon M+, *Arch Mal Coeur Vaiss* (French) 78, 67
Necrotizing angiitis
Peripheral edema (<5%)
Photosensitivity (<1%)
Pruritus (<5%)
(1985): Kirsten R+, *Z Kardiol* (German) 74, 66
(1982): Brennan L+, *Clin Ther* 5, 121
Purpura
Rash (sic) (<5%)
(1988): Kandela D+, *BMJ* 296, 573
(1985): Kirsten R+, *Z Kardiol* (German) 74, 66
(1983): Slotkoff L, *Am Heart J* 106, 233
(1982): Brennan L+, *Clin Ther* 5, 121
Stevens–Johnson syndrome
(1992): Spinler SA+, *Cutis* 50, 200
Toxic epidermal necrolysis
(1993): Partanen J+, *Arch Dermatol* 129, 793
(1990): Black RJ+, *Br Med J Clin Res Ed* 301, 1280
(1987): Stricker BHC+, *Br Med J Clin Res Ed* 295, 1313
Urticaria (<5%)
(1987): Stricker BHC+, *Br Med J Clin Res Ed* 295, 1313
Vasculitis (<5%)

### Other

Anaphylactoid reactions
Paresthesias (<5%)
Xanthopsia
Xerostomia (<5%)
(1985): Kirsten R+, *Z Kardiol* (German) 74, 66
(1982): Brennan L+, *Clin Ther* 5, 121

***Note:** Indapamide is a sulfonamide and can be absorbed systemically. Sulfonamides can produce severe, possibly fatal, reactions such as toxic epidermal necrolysis and Stevens–Johnson syndrome

## INDINAVIR

**Trade name:** Crixivan (Merck)
**Indications:** HIV infection
**Category:** Antiretroviralviral; protease inhibitor*
**Half-life:** ~1.8 hours
**Clinically important, potentially hazardous interactions with:** alprazolam, chlordiazepoxide, clonazepam, clorazepate, delavirdine, diazepam, dihydroergotamine, ergot alkaloids, estazolam, fentanyl, flurazepam, halazepam, methysergide, midazolam, phenytoin, pimozide, quazepam, sildenafil, **St John's wort**, triazolam

#### *Reactions*

### Skin

Allergic reactions (sic)
(1998): Rijnders B+, *Clin Infect Dis* 26, 523
Buffalo hump
(2000): Calista D+, *Eur J Dermatol* 10, 292
Buffalo neck
(1999): Milpied-Homsi B+, *Ann Dermatol Venereol* (French) 126, 254
Cheilitis
(2001): Scully C+, *Oral Dis* 7, 205 (passim)
(2000): Bonfanti P+, *J Acquir Immune Defic Syndr* 23(3), 236
(2000): Calista D+, *Eur J Dermatol* 10, 292 (51.7%)
(2000): Fox PA+, *Sex Transm Infect* 76, 323

Contact dermatitis (<2%)
Dermatitis (sic) (<2%)
Diaphoresis (<2%)
Erythema multiforme
Exanthems
(1999): Fung HB+, *Pharmacotherapy* 19, 1328
Eyelid edema (<2%)
Flushing (<2%)
Folliculitis (<2%)
Herpes simplex (<2%)
Herpes zoster (<2%)
Pigmentation
Pruritus
(2000): Calista D+, *Eur J Dermatol* 10, 292 (11.9%)
(1999): Gajewski LK+, *Ann Pharmacother* 33, 17 (86%)
Pyogenic granuloma
(1998): Bouscarat F+, *N Engl J Med* 338, 1776 (great toes)
Rash (sic)
(1999): Gajewski LK+, *Ann Pharmacother* 33, 17 (67%)
Seborrhea (<2%)
Stevens–Johnson syndrome
(1998): Teira R+, *Scand J Infect Dis* 30, 634
Striae
(1999): Darvay A+, *J Am Acad Dermatol* 41, 467
Urticaria (<2%)
Vasculitis
(2001): Rachline A+, *Br J Dermatol* 143, 1112
Xerosis
(2000): Bonfanti P+, *J Acquir Immune Defic Syndr* 23(3), 236
(2000): Calista D+, *Eur J Dermatol* 10, 292 (11.9%)

## Hair

Hair – alopecia
(2000): Bonfanti P+, *J Acquir Immune Defic Syndr* 23(3), 236
(2000): Calista D+, *Eur J Dermatol* 10, 292 (11.9%)
(1999): Bouscarat F+, *N Engl J Med* 341, 618
(1998): d'Arminio Monforte A+, *AIDS* 12, 328

## Nails

Nails – ingrown
(2001): James CW+, *Ann Pharmacother* 35(7), 881 (with ritonavir)
(2000): Heim M+, *Haemophilia* 6, 191
(2000): Miot HA, Sao Paulo, Brazil (from internet) (observation)
Nails – paronychia
(2001): Colson AE+, *Clin Infect Dis* 32, 140
(2001): Garcia Garcia+, *Rev Clin Esp* 201(8), 455
(2000): Dauden E+, *Br J Dermatol* 142, 1063 (toes and finger)
(1998): Bouscarat F+, *N Engl J Med* 338, 1776 (great toes)
Nails – pyogenic granulomas
(2000): Calista D+, *Eur J Dermatol* 10, 292 (5.9%)

## Other

Aphthous stomatitis (<2%)
Bromhidrosis (<2%)
Bruxism (<2%)
Dysesthesia (<2%)
Dysgeusia (2.6%)
Foetor ex ore (halitosis) (<2%)
Gingivitis (<2%)
Gynecomastia
(2001): Manfredi R+, *Ann Pharmacother* 35, 438
(1998): Caeiro JP+, *Clin Infect Dis* 27, 1539
(1998): Lui A+, *Clin Infect Dis* 26, 1482
(1998): Toma E+, *AIDS* 12, 681
Hypesthesia (<2%)
Lipoatrophy
(2001): Lichtenstein KA+, *AIDS* 15(11), 1389
Lipodystrophy
(2002): Reid S, *Can Adv Drug Reaction Newsletter* 12, 5
(2000): Calista D+, *Eur J Dermatol* 10, 292 (14.3%)
(2000): Hartmann M+, *Hautarzt* (German) *51, 159*
(1999): Hermieu JF+, *Prog Urol* (French) 9, 537
(1999): Krautheim A, *Schweiz Rundsch Med Prax* (German) 88, 285
(1998): Miller KD+, *Lancet* 351, 871
(1998): Viraben R+, *AIDS* 12, F37
(1997): Herry I+, *Clin Infect Dis* 25, 937 (breast hypertrophy)
Lipomatosis
(2000): Calista D+, *Eur J Dermatol* 10, 292
(1997): Hengel RL+, *Lancet* 350, 1596 (benign symmetric)
Myalgia (<2%)
Paresthesias (<2%)
(2001): McMahon D+, *Antivir Ther* 6(2), 105
Porphyria (acute)
(2001): Schmutz JL+, *Ann Dermatol Venereol* 128(2), 184
(1999): Fox PA+, *AIDS* 16, 322
Tendinitis
(2002): Florence E+, *Ann Rheum Dis* 61(1), 82
Xerostomia (0.5%)

***Note:** Protease inhibitors cause dyslipidemia which includes elevated triglycerides and cholesterol and redistribution of body fat centrally to produce the so-called "protease paunch," breast enlargement, facial atrophy, and "buffalo hump"

# INDOMETHACIN

**Synonym:** indometacin
**Trade name:** Indocin (Merck)
**Other common trade names:** *Amuno; Apo-Indomethacin; Durametacin; Imbrilon; Indochron; Indolar SR; Indotec; Nu-Indo; Rhodacine; Vonum*
**Indications:** Arthritis
**Category:** Nonsteroidal anti-inflammatory (NSAID); antipyretic
**Half-life:** 4.5 hours
**Clinically important, potentially hazardous interactions with:** aldesleukin, aspirin, diflunisal, diuretics, methotrexate, NSAIDs, triamterene, urokinase

### *Reactions*

## Skin

Angioedema (<1%)
(1981): Juhlin L, *Br J Dermatol* 104, 369
(1966): Rothermich ND, *JAMA* 195, 531 (0.5%)
Bullous eruption (<1%)
(1986): Harrington CI+, *Br J Dermatol* 114, 265
(1969): Duperrat B+, *Bull Soc Franc Dermatol Syphiligr* (French) 76, 26
Contact dermatitis
(1999): Pulido Z+, *Contact Dermatitis* 41, 112
(1998): Ueda K+, *Contact Dermatitis* 39, 323
(1993): Goday-Bujan JJ+, *Contact Dermatitis* 28, 111
(1993): Ophaswongse S+, *Contact Dermatitis* 29, 57
(1987): Beller U+, *Contact Dermatitis* 17, 121
Cutaneous side effects (sic)
(1986): Bigby M+, *JAMA* 256, 3358 (0.21%)
Dermatitis herpetiformis (exacerbation)
(1986): Harrington CI+, *Br J Dermatol* 114, 265
(1985): Griffiths CEM+, *Br J Dermatol* 112, 443
Diaphoresis (<1%)
Ecchymoses (<1%)
Eczematous eruption (sic)

(1987): Beller U+, *Contact Dermatitis* 17, 121
Edema (3–9%)
(1978): Castles JJ+, *Arch Intern Med* 138, 362 (5.6%)
Erythema multiforme (<1%)
(1985): Ting HC+, *Int J Dermatol* 24, 58
Erythema nodosum (<1%)
(1982): Elizaga FV, *Ann Intern Med* 96, 383
Exanthems
(1978): Castles JJ+, *Arch Intern Med* 138, 362 (5.6%)
(1976): Arndt KA+, *JAMA* 235, 918 (0.4%)
(1975): Pasquariello G+, *Curr Med Res Opin* 3, 109 (1.8%)
(1973): Thorne N, *Practitioner* 211, 606
(1970): Almeyda J+, *Br J Dermatol* 83, 707
(1967): Boardman PL+, *Ann Rheum Dis* 26, 127 (1.7%)
(1967): *Clin Pharmacol Ther* 8, 11 (11%)
Exfoliative dermatitis (<1%)
(1983): O'Sullivan M+, *Br J Rheumatol* 22, 47
Fixed eruption
(1998): Mahboob A+, *Int J Dermatol* 37, 833
(1976): Mackie BS, *Arch Dermatol* 112, 122
Flushing (>1%)
Generalized eruption (sic)
(1966): Kern AB, *Arch Dermatol* 93, 239
Granulomas (plasma cell)
(1975): Shelley WB+, *Acta Derm Venereol* (Stockh) 55, 489
Hot flashes (<1%)
Lichen planus
(1983): Hamburger J+, *BMJ* 287, 1258
Pemphigus
Periorbital edema
(1970): Almeyda J+, *Br J Dermatol* 83, 707
(1966): Rothermich NO, *JAMA* 195, 531
Peripheral edema
Petechiae (>1%)
Photoreactions
(1984): Stern RS+, *JAMA* 252, 1433
Pruritus (1–10%)
(1973): Thorne N, *Practitioner* 211, 606
(1970): Almeyda J+, *Br J Dermatol* 83, 707
(1967): *Clin Pharmacol Ther* 8, 11 (5%)
Psoriasis
(1993): Shelley WB+, *Cutis* 51, 415 (observation)
(1989): Lazarova AZ+, *Clin Exp Dermatol* 14, 260 (from topical application)
(1987): Powles AV+, *Br J Dermatol* 117, 799
(1987): Sendagorta E+, *Dermatologica* 175, 300
(1986): Abel EA+, *J Am Acad Dermatol* 15, 1007
(1981): Katayama H+, *J Dermatol* (Tokio) 8, 323
(1980): Katayama H+, *Nippon Hifuka Gakkai Zasshi* (Japanese) 90, 1027
Purpura (<1%)
(1984): Camba L+, *Acta Hematol* 71, 350
(1974): Cuthbert MF, *Curr Med Res Opin* 2, 600
(1973): Thorne N, *Practitioner* 211, 606
(1970): Almeyda J+, *Br J Dermatol* 83, 707
(1968): Bartoletti L+, *Riv Crit Clin Med* (Italian) 68, 279
Pustular psoriasis
(1987): Sendagorta E+, *Dermatologica* 175, 300
Rash (sic) (>10%)
(1967): Boardman PL+, *Ann Rheum Dis* 26, 127
Reiter's syndrome (exacerbation)
(1989): Allegue F+, *Med Cutan Ibero Lat Am* (Spanish) 17, 113
Stevens–Johnson syndrome (<1%)
Toxic epidermal necrolysis (<1%)
(1996): Lear JT+, *Postgrad Med J* 72, 186
(1990): Roujeau JC+, *Arch Dermatol* 126, 37
(1989): Roth DE+, *Med Clin North Am* 73, 1275
(1986): Johnson VB+, *La Pharm* 45, 4
(1985): Heng MCY, *Br J Dermatol* 113, 597
(1983): O'Sullivan M+, *Br J Rheumatol* 22, 47
Urticaria
(1995): Gebhardt M+, *Z Rheumatol* (German) 54, 405
(1992): Shelley WB+, *Cutis* 50, 87 (observation)
(1985): O'Brien WM+, *J Rheumatol* 12, 13
(1981): Juhlin L, *Br J Dermatol* 104, 369
(1974): Mathews JI+, *Ann Intern Med* 80, 771
(1973): Thorne N, *Practitioner* 211, 606
(1970): Almeyda J+, *Br J Dermatol* 83, 707
Urticaria pigmentosa
(1968): Vissian L+, *Bull Soc Franc Dermatol Syphiligr* (French) 75, 591
Vasculitis (<1%)
(1988): Gamboa PM+, *Allergol Immunopathol Madr* (Spanish) 16, 53
(1985): Bigby M, *J Am Acad Dermatol* 12, 866
(1985): O'Brien WM+, *J Rheumatol* 12, 13
(1971): Marsh FP+, *Ann Rheum Dis* 30, 501
(1970): Almeyda J+, *Br J Dermatol* 83, 707

## Hair

Hair – alopecia (<1%)

## Nails

Nails – onycholysis

## Other

Ageusia
(1967): Boardman PL+, *Ann Rheum Dis* 26, 127
Anaphylactoid reactions (<1%)
Aphthous stomatitis
Gynecomastia (<1%)
Hypersensitivity (<1%)
Oral lichenoid eruption
(1983): Hamburger J+, *BMJ* 287, 1258
Oral mucosal lesions
(1967): Boardman PL+, *Ann Rheum Dis* 26, 127 (0.5%)
(1967): *Clin Pharmacol Ther* 8, 11 (7%)
Oral ulceration
(2000): Madinier I+, *Ann Med Interne (Paris)* (French) 151, 248
(1983): Hamburger J+, *BMJ* 287, 1258
(1975): Guggenheimer J+, *J Am Dent Assoc* 90, 632
(1967): Boardman PL+, *Ann Rheum Dis* 26, 127
Paresthesias (<1%)
Pseudolymphoma
(2000): Werth V, *Dermatology Times* 18
Pseudoporphyria
(2000): De Silva B+, *Pediatr Dermatol* 17, 480
Serum sickness
(1985): Ferraccioli G+, *Acta Haematol* 73, 45
Temporal arteritis
(1985): O'Brien WM+, *J Rheumatol* 12, 13
(1967): Easterbrook WM+, *Can Med Assoc J* 97, 296
Tinnitus
Tongue edema
(1967): Boardman PL+, *Ann Rheum Dis* 26, 127
Ulcerative stomatitis (<1%)
(1982): Bailin PL+, *Clin Rheum Dis* 8, 493 (passim)
Xerostomia

# INFLIXIMAB

**Trade name:** Remicade (Centocor)
**Indications:** Crohn's disease
**Category:** Monoclonal antibody; tumor necrosis factor alpha blocker
**Half-life:** 9.5 days

### *Reactions*

## Skin

Candidiasis (5%)
Chills (5–9%)
Edema
(1999): Lichenstein GR+, *Biologics in Clinical Practice Symposium*, Orlando, FL, May 19
Herpes simplex
(2001): Voigtländer C+, *Arch Dermatol* 137, 1571
Infections (sic) (21%)
(2001): Ouraghi A+, *Gastroenterol Clin Biol* 25(11), 949
(2001): Serrano MS+, *Ann Pharmacother* 35(7), 823
Lymphoma
(2001): Aithal GP+, *Aliment Pharmacol Ther* 15(8), 1101
(1992): Greenstein AJ+, *Cancer* 69, 1119
Necrotizing fasciitis
(2002): Chan AT+, *Postgrad Med J* 78(915), 47
Photosensitivity
(2002): Smith JG, Mobile, AL (from Internet) (observation) (2 cases)
Pruritus (5%)
(2001): Finkelstein RP, Stratford, NJ (from Internet) (observation)
(1999): Lichenstein GR+, *Biologics in Clinical Practice Symposium*, Orlando, FL, May 19
Psoriasis
(2001): Finkelstein RP, Stratford, NJ (from Internet) (observation)
Pustular eruption
(2002): Chan AT+, *Postgrad Med J* 78(915), 47
(2001): Finkelstein RP, Stratford, NJ (from Internet) (observation)
Rash (sic) (6%)
(2001): Serrano MS+, *Ann Pharmacother* 35(7), 823
(2000): Hyams JS+, *J Pediatr* 137(2), 192
(1999): Baert S+, *Int J Colorectal Dis* 14, 47
(1999): Lichenstein GR+, *Biologics in Clinical Practice Symposium* Orlando, FL, May 19
Skin disorders (sic)
(2001): Serrano MS+, *Ann Pharmacother* 35(7), 823
Ulceration (foot)
(2002): Conaghan P+, *Skin & Allergy News* June, 40
Urticaria
(1999): Lichenstein GR+, *Biologics in Clinical Practice Symposium*, Orlando, FL, May 19
(1997): Van Deventer SJH, *Clin Nutr* 16, 271

## Other

Anaphylactoid reactions
(2002): Diamanti A+, *J Pediatr* 140(5), 636
(2002): O'Connor M+, *Dig Dis Sci* 47(6), 1323
(2002): Sample C+, *Can J Gastroenterol* 16(3), 165
(2000): Soykan I+, *Am J Gastroenterol* 95(9), 2395
Arthralgia
(2002): Kugathasan S+, *Am J Gastroenterol* 97(6), 1408
(2002): Riegert-Johnson DL+, *Inflamm Bowel Dis* 8(3), 186
(2001): Serrano MS+, *Ann Pharmacother* 35(7), 823
Death
(2002): de' Clari F+, *Circulation* 105(21), E183
(2001): Lankarani KB, *J Clin Gastroenterol* 33(3), 255
(2001): Srinivasan R, *Am J Gastroenterol* 96, 2274 (neonatal)
Hypersensitivity
(2002): Riegert-Johnson DL+, *Inflamm Bowel Dis* 8(3), 186
(1999): Lichenstein GR+, *Biologics in Clinical Practice Symposium* Orlando, FL, May 19
(1997): Van Deventer SJH, *Clin Nutr* 16, 271
Infusion-site reactions (sic) (16%)
(2002): Kugathasan S+, *Am J Gastroenterol* 97(6), 1408
(1989): Morrison SL, *Hosp Prac* 24, 65
Myalgia (5%)
(2002): Kugathasan S+, *Am J Gastroenterol* 97(6), 1408
(2002): Riegert-Johnson DL+, *Inflamm Bowel Dis* 8(3), 186
(1999): Baert S+, *Int J Colorectal Dis* 14, 47
(1999): Lichenstein GR+, *Biologics in Clinical Practice Symposium* Orlando, FL, May 19
Oral mucosal reaction
(2002): Kugathasan S+, *Am J Gastroenterol* 97(6), 1408
Paresthesias (1–4%)
(2002): Conaghan P+, *Skin & Allergy News* June, 40
Tuberculosis
(2001): Keane J+, *N Engl J Med* 345(15), 1098 (70 cases)

# INH

(See ISONIAZID)

# INSULIN

**Trade names:** Humulin (Lilly); Iletin Lente (Lilly); Novolin R (Bristol-Myers Squibb); NPH (Lilly); Protamine (Lilly); Velosulin (Novo Nordisk)
**Other common trade names:** *Humalog; Huminsulin; Insuman; Monotard; Velosuline Humaine*
**Indications:** Diabetes
**Category:** Hypoglycemic
**Duration of action:** 5–28 hours
**Clinically important, potentially hazardous interactions with: alcohol**, ethanolamine, guanethidine, propranolol, vidarabine

**Note:** About 25% of patients with insulin allergy have a concomitant history of penicillin allergy

### *Reactions*

## Skin

Allergic reactions (sic) (local)
(1989): Zinman B, *N Engl J Med* 321, 363
(1988): Plantin P+, *Ann Dermatol Venereol* (French) 115, 813 (>5%)
(1985): Bruni B+, *Diabetes Care* 8, 201
(1984): Grammer LC+, *JAMA* 251, 1459
(1982): Carveth-Johnson AO+, *Lancet* 2, 1287
(1981): Hasche H+, *Dtsch Med Wochenschr* (German) 106, 1451
(1981): Kahn CB, *Handbook of Diabetes Mellitus* Garland STPM, 75
(1980): Jegasothy BV, *Int J Dermatol* 19, 139 (immediate and delayed) (10–56%)
(1979): Borsey DQ+, *Postgrad Med J* 55, 199
(1969): Aubert J+, *Rev Fr Allergol* (French) 9, 40
(1961): Hanauer L+, *Diabetes* 10, 105
(1939): Kern RA+, *JAMA* 113, 198
Angioedema
(1983): Grammer LC+, *J Allergy Clin Immunol* 71, 250
(1981): Kahn CB, *Handbook of Diabetes Mellitus* Garland STPM, 75

(1979): Lynfield Y+, *Arch Dermatol* 115, 591 (passim)
(1978): Galloway JA+, *Med Clin North Am* 62, 663
(1976): Lamkin N+, *J Allergy Clin Immunol* 58, 213
(1952): Dolger H, *Med Clin North Am* 36, 783

Bullous eruption
(1974): Haroon TS, *Scott Med J* 19, 257

Contact dermatitis
(1994): Goldfine AB+, *Curr Ther Endocrinol Metab* 5, 461
(1989): Geldof BA+, *Contact Dermatitis* 20, 384

Diaphoresis (1–10%)

Edema (1–10%)
(1981): Galloway JA+, *Diabetes Mellitus* Bowie 5, 117
(1979): Lawrence JR+, *BMJ* 2, 445

Exanthems
(1978): Galloway JA+, *Med Clin North Am* 62, 663

Flushing
(1961): Hanauer L+, *Diabetes* 10, 105

Granulomas (zinc)
(1989): Jordaan HF+, *Clin Exp Dermatol* 14, 227

Hyperkeratotic verrucous papules
(1989): Jordaan HF+, *Clin Exp Dermatol* 14, 277
(1986): Fleming MG+, *Arch Dermatol* 122, 1054 (resembling acanthosis nigricans)
(1969): Erickson L+, *JAMA* 209, 934

Keloid formation
(1970): Jelinek JE, *Year Book of Dermatology*, Chicago 5–35

Necrosis
(1974): Rohan P+, *Arch Dermatol Forsch* 250, (German) 121

Pallor (1–10%)

Pigmentation
(1970): Jelinek JE, *Year Book of Dermatology*, Chicago 5–35

Pigskin appearance (sic)
(1925): Lawrence RD, *Lancet* 1, 1125

Pruritus (1–10%)
(1981): Knick B, *Munch Med Wochenschr* (German) 123, 1197
(1925): Lawrence RD, *Lancet* 1, 1125
(1922): Banting FG+, *J Metab Res* 2, 547

Purpura
(1976): Lamkin N+, *J Allergy Clin Immunol* 58, 213
(1956): Constam GR, *Diabetes* 5, 121

Urticaria (1–10%)
(1996): Rowland-Payne CM+, *Br J Dermatol* 134, 184
(1995): Chng HH+, *Allergy* 50, 984
(1988): Plantin P+, *Ann Dermatol Venereol* (French) 115, 813
(1983): Grammer LC+, *J Allergy Clin Immunol* 71, 250
(1982): Mirouze J+, *Nouv Presse Med* (French) 11, 3121
(1982): Patterson R+, *JAMA* 248, 2637 (passim)
(1981): Kahn CB, *Handbook of Diabetes Mellitus* Garland STPM, 75
(1979): Levy WJ+, *Cleve Clin Q* 46, 155
(1979): Lynfield Y+, *Arch Dermatol* 115, 591 (passim)
(1978): Galloway JA+, *Med Clin North Am* 62, 663
(1978): Reisner C+, *BMJ* 2, 56
(1976): Lamkin N+, *J Allergy Clin Immunol* 58, 213
(1962): Arkins JA+, *J Allergy* 33, 69
(1952): Dolger H, *Med Clin North Am* 36, 783
(1925): Lawrence RD, *Lancet* 1, 1125
(1922): Banting FG+, *J Metab Res* 2, 547

Vasculitis
(2002): Mandrup-Poulsen T+, *Diabetes Care* 25(1), 242
(1983): Grammer LC+, *J Allergy Clin Immunol* 71, 250

Xanthomatosis
(1975): Vermeer BJ+, *Dermatologica* 151, 43

## Other

Anaphylactoid reactions (1–10%)
(1983): Grammer LC+, *J Allergy Clin Immunol* 71, 250
(1982): Patterson R+, *JAMA* 248, 2637 (passim)
(1981): Kahn CB, *Handbook of Diabetes Mellitus* Garland STPM, 75
(1979): Lynfield Y+, *Arch Dermatol* 115, 591 (passim)
(1978): Galloway JA+, *Med Clin North Am* 62, 663
(1976): Lamkin N+, *J Allergy Clin Immunol* 58, 213
(1952): Dolger H, *Med Clin North Am* 36, 783
(1925): Lawrence RD, *Lancet* 1, 1125

Dermal atrophy
(1978): Oakley WG+, *Diabetes and its Management*, Blackwell, 103

Dermal reactions (sic) (50%)
(1982): Patterson R+, *JAMA* 248, 2637 (passim)

Hypersensitivity
(1983): Berman BA+, *Cutis* 32, 320
(1982): deShazo RD+, *J Allergy Clin Immunol* 69, 229
(1974): Federlin K, *Dtsch Med Wochenschr* (German) 99, 535

Hypertrophic lipodystrophy
(1983): Johnson DA+, *Cutis* 32, 273

Injection-site calcification
(1995): Ullman HR+, *J Comput Assist Tomogr* 19, 657

Injection-site cancer (sic)
(1976): Sampson WI, *JAMA* 235, 374

Injection-site induration
(1983): White WB+, *Am J Med* 74, 909
(1981): Galloway JA+, *Diabetes Mellitus* Bowie 5, 117
(1979): Feinglos MN+, *Lancet* 1, 122 (due to zinc)
(1979): Lynfield Y+, *Arch Dermatol* 115, 591 (with erythema)
(1978): Galloway JA+, *Med Clin North Am* 62, 663

Injection-site pruritus
(1988): Plantin P+, *Ann Dermatol Venereol* (French) 115, 813
(1979): Lynfield Y+, *Arch Dermatol* 115, 591

Lipoatrophy (1–10%)
(1998): Murao S+, *Intern Med* 37, 1031
(1996): Logwin S+, *Diabetes Care* 19, 255
(1993): Chantelau E+, *Exp Clin Endocrinol* 101, 194
(1992): Igea JM+, *Allergol Immunopathol Madr* (Spanish) 20, 173
(1989): Gyimesi A+, *Orv Hetil* (Hungarian) 130, 2751
(1989): Zinman B, *N Engl J Med* 321, 363
(1988): McNally PG+, *Postgrad Med J* 64, 850
(1988): Perrot H, *Ann Dermatol Venereol* (French) 115, 523
(1983): Blickle JF+, *Presse Med* (French) 12, 2534
(1982): Levandoski LA+, *Diabetes Care* 5, 6
(1981): Jones GR+, *BMJ* 282, 190
(1981): Kahn CB, *Handbook of Diabetes Mellitus* Garland STPM, 75
(1980): Reeves WG+, *BMJ* 280, 1500
(1979): Asherov J+, *Diabete Metab* 5, 1
(1978): Aw TC+, *Singapore Med J* 19, 227
(1978): Galloway JA+, *Med Clin North Am* 62, 663
(1978): Oakley WG+, *Diabetes and its Management*, Blackwell, 103
(1978): Talantov VV, *Sov Med* (Russian) June, 104
(1977): Kumar O+, *Diabetes* 26, 296
(1976): Maaz E, *Z Gesamte Inn Med* (German) 31, 941
(1976): Whitley TH+, *JAMA* 235, 839
(1975): Jablonska S+, *Acta Derm Venereol* 55, 135
(1974): Talantov VV, *Sov Med* (Russian) 37, 80
(1974): Teuscher A, *Diabetologia* 10, 211
(1972): Bloom A, *BMJ* 4, 366

Lipodystrophy
(1990): Kohli V+, *Indian Pediatr* 27, 1120
(1988): Field LM, *J Am Acad Dermatol* 19, 570
(1988): Verbenko EV+, *Sov Med* (Russian) 3, 104
(1987): Goldman JM+, *Am J Med* 83, 195
(1985): Valenta LJ+, *Ann Intern Med* 102, 790
(1984): Campbell IW+, *Postgrad Med J* 60, 439
(1984): De Mattia G+, *Clin Ter* (Italian) 111, 169
(1984): Tebuev AM, *Pediatriia* (Russian) December 59
(1982): Levandoski LA+, *Diabetes Care* 5, 6

(1981): Libman E+, *Med Pregl* (Serbo-Croatian-Roman) 34, 49
(1981): Pisarskaia IV+, *Med Sestra* (Russian) 40, 54
(1979): Welk DS, *Nursing* 9, 42
(1978): da Cruz-Borges RC+, *Rev Bras Enferm* (Portuguese) 31, 252
(1974): Mehnert H, *Dtsch Med Wochenschr* (German) 99, 1274
(1973): Watson D+, *Med J Aust* 1, 248
(1972): Mehnert H, *Med Klin* (German) 67, 1384
(1971): Sapelkina LV+, *Pediatriia* (Russian) 50, 18
(1969): Todorovic M, *Med Pregl* (Serbo-Croatian-Cyrillic) 22, 177
(1968): Gleize J+, *Diabete* (French) 16, 281
(1968): Thosteson GC, *Mich Med* 67, 609
(1967): Hintz R, *Pol Tyg Lek* (Polish) 22, 828
(1967): Hintz R, *Pol Tyg Lek* (Polish) 22, 902
(1967): Jablonska S+, *Pol Tyg Lek* (Polish) 22, 977
(1965): Aubertin E+, *J Med Bord* (French) 142, 605

Lipohypertrophy (1–10%)
(1996): Hauner H+, *Exp Clin Endocrinol Diabetes* 104, 106
(1990): Schiazza L+, *J Am Acad Dermatol* 22, 148
(1989): Zinman B, *N Engl J Med* 321, 363
(1988): McNally PG+, *Postgrad Med J* 64, 850
(1987): Samadaei A+, *J Am Acad Dermatol* 17, 506
(1984): Young RJ+, *Diabetes Care* 7, 479
(1983): Johnson DA+, *Cutis* 32, 273
(1982): Mier A+, *BMJ* 285, 1539
(1969): Erickson L+, *JAMA* 209, 934

Panniculitis
(1988): Verbenko EV+, *Vestn Dermatol Venerol* (Russian) 1, 63

Paresthesias (1–10%)

Tremors (1–10%)

Tumors (nodules)
(1981): Galloway JA+, *Diabetes Mellitus*, Bowie 5, 117
(1978): Oakley WG+, *Diabetes and its Management*, Blackwell, 103
(1960): Oakley WG, *Br Med Bull* 16, 247

# INTERFERON BETA 1-A

**Synonym:** rIFN-b
**Trade name:** Avonex (Bioglan)
**Other common trade name:** *Rebif*
**Indications:** Multiple sclerosis
**Category:** Interferon; immunomodulator
**Half-life:** 10 hours

### *Reactions*

## Skin

Basal cell carcinoma (<1%)
Bullae
Cellulitis
Chills (21%)
(1998): Mohr DC+, *Mult Scler* 4(6), 487
Cold, clammy skin
Contact dermatitis
Diaphoresis
Ecchymoses
Erythema
(2000): Beghi E+, *Neurology* 54(2), 469 (local)
Exanthems
(2002): Beaudet LD, Trois-Rivieres, Quebec (from Internet) (observation)
Facial edema
Flu-like syndrome (61%)
(2000): Beghi E+, *Neurology* 54(2), 469
(2000): Gottberg K+, *Mult Scler* 6(5), 349
(1998): *Prescrire Int* 7(37), 142
(1998): Mohr DC+, *Mult Scler* 4(6), 487
Furunculosis
Genital pruritus
Herpes simplex (2–3%)
Herpes zoster (3)
Infections (sic) (11%)
Lipoma
Lupus erythematosus
(2000): Schmutz J+, *Ann Dermatol Venereol* 127(2), 237
(1998): Nousari HC+, *Lancet* 352(9143), 1825 (Subacute cutaneous)
Lymphadenopathy
Nevus (3%)
Pain (24%)
Petechiae
Photosensitivity (<1%)
Pigmentation
Pruritus
(2002): Beaudet LD, Trois-Rivieres, Quebec (from Internet) (observation)
Raynaud's phenomenon
(2000): De Broucker+, *Ann Med Interne* (Paris) 151(5), 424
Seborrhea
Spider angioma
Telangiectasia
Ulcer
Upper respiratory infection (31%)
Urticaria (5%)

## Hair

Hair – alopecia (4%)

## Other

Anaphylactoid reactions
(1999): Corona T+, *Neurology* 52(2), 425
Arthralgia (9%)
Bone pain
Death
(2000): Beghi E+, *Neurology* 54(2), 469
Depression
(1999): Mohr DC+, *Arch Neurol* 56(10), 1263
(1998): Mohr DC+, *Mult Scler* 4(6), 487
Gingival bleeding
Gingivitis
Hiccups
Hyperesthesia
Hypersensitivity (3%)
Injection-site atrophy
Injection-site burning
Injection-site ecchymoses (2%)
Injection-site edema
Injection-site hypersensitivity
Injection-site inflammation (3%)
Injection-site necrosis
(1999): Radziwill AJ+, *J Neurol Neurosurg Psychiatry* 67(1), 115
Injection-site purpura (2%)
Injection-site reactions (sic) (4%)
Mastodynia (7%)
Myalgia (34%)
Paresthesias
(1998): Mohr DC+, *Mult Scler* 4(6), 487
Peyronie's disease
Rhabdomyolysis
(2002): Lunemann JD+, *J Neurol Neurosurg Psychiatry* 72(2), 274
Tongue disorder (sic)
Toothache
Vaginitis (4%)
Xerostomia

# INTERFERONS, ALFA-2

**Synonyms:** IFLrA; IFN; rLFN-A; INF; INF-alpha-2
**Trade names:** Alferon N; Infergen (Amgen); Intron A (Schering); Rebetron (Schering); Roferon-A (Roche)
**Other common trade names:** *Green-Alpha; Introna; Introne; Laroferon; Roceron-A*
**Indications:** Chronic hepatitis C virus infection
**Category:** Biologic response modulator and antineoplastic
**Half-life:** 2 hours

**Note:** Many of the adverse reactions depend on the nature of the disease being treated. Either hairy cell leukemia [L] or AIDS-related Kaposi's sarcoma [K]

## *Reactions*

### Skin

Acne (1%)
Acral sclerosis
(2002): Saydam G+, *Acta Haematol* 107(1), 43
Acrocyanosis
(1998): Campo-Voegeli A+, *Dermatology* 196, 361
Angioedema
(2001): Ohmoto K, *Am J Gastroenterol* 96, 1311
Atrophie blanche
(2002): Bugatti L+, *Dermatology* 204(2), 154
Behçet's disease
(1995): Segawa F+, *J Rheumatol* 22, 1183
Bullous eruption
(2002): Pouthier D+, *Nephrol Dial Transplant* 17(1), 174
(1995): Chang LW+, *Cutis* 56, 144
(1993): Andry P+, *Ann Dermatol Venereol* (French) 120, 843
(1993): Parodi A+, *Dermatology* 186, 155
Candidiasis (1%)
Chills
(2002): Alpsoy E+, *Arch Dermatol* 138, 467
(2000): Cornejo P+, *Arch Dermatol* 136, 429
(2000): Shenefelt PD+, *Arch Dermatol* 136, 837
Contact dermatitis
(1995): Chang LW+, *Cutis* 56, 144
Cutaneous malignancy (sic)
(1991): Wagner RF+, *Arch Dermatol* 127, 272
Cutaneous necrosis
(1997): de Ledinghen V+, *Gastroenterol Clin Biol* 21, 523
(1995): Trautinger F+, *N Engl J Med* 333, 1222
(1991): Cnudde F+, *Int J Dermatol* 30, 147
(1989): Rasokat H+, *Dtsch Med Wochenschr* (German) 114, 458
Cutaneous reactions (sic)
(1996): Azagury M+, *Eur J Cancer* 32A, 1821 (severe)
Cutaneous vascular lesions (sic)
(1989): Dreno B+, *Ann Intern Med* 111, 95
Dermatitis herpetiformis
(1995): Dmochowski M+, *Postepy Dermatol* 12, 7
Dermatologic toxicity (sic)
(1993): Miglino M+, *Haematologica* 78, 411
Diaphoresis (22%) [L]; (7%) [K]
(1999): Angulo MP+, *Pediatr Cardiol* 20, 293 [L]
Discoloration (sic) (<1%)
Ecchymoses [L]
Eczematous eruption (sic)
(1999): Sookoian S+, *Arch Dermatol* 135, 999 ([K]) (with ribavirin)
(1989): Detmar U+, *Contact Dermatitis* 20, 149
Edema (11%) [L]
Erythema
(1999): Sookoian S+, *Arch Dermatol* 135, 999 (with ribavirin) (malar) ([K])
Erythema nodosum
(2001): Leveque L+, *Rev Med Interne* 22(12), 1248 (with ribavirin)
Exanthems
(2002): Farady KK, Austin, TX (with ribavirin) (from Internet) (observation)
(1994): Sollitto RB+, *Arch Dermatol* 130, 1194
(1994): Toyofuku K+, *J Dermatol* 21, 732
(1986): Quesada JR+, *Lancet* 1, 1466
Flu-like syndrome (sic) (>10%)
(2002): Alpsoy E+, *Arch Dermatol* 138, 467
(2002): Giuliani M+, *Arch Dermatol* 138, 535
Fungal infection (sic) (<1%)
Herpes simplex (1%)
(1995): Chang LW+, *Cutis* 56, 144
(1992): Breathnach SM+, *Adverse Drug Reactions and the Skin* Blackwell, Oxford, 322 (passim)
Hot flashes (sic) (1%)
Kaposi's sarcoma
(2002): Giuliani M+, *Arch Dermatol* 138(4), 535
(1993): Ariad S+, *South Afr Med J* 83, 430
Keratoses
(1994): Sollitto RB+, *Arch Dermatol* 130, 1194
Lichen myxedematosus
(1998): Rongioletti F+, *J Am Acad Dermatol* 38, 760
Lichen planus
(1999): Herstoff JK, Newport, RI (from Internet) (observation)
(1999): Sookoian S+, *Arch Dermatol* 135, 999 ([K]) (with ribavirin)
(1998): Dalekos GN+, *Eur J Gastroenterol Hepatol* 10, 933
(1995): Chang LW+, *Cutis* 56, 144
(1995): Fornaciari G+, *J Clin Gastroenterol* 20, 346
(1995): Hyrailles V+, *Gastroenterol Clin Biol* (French) 19, 833
(1993): Boccia S+, *Gastroenterology* 105, 1921
(1993): Heintges T+, *J Hepatol* 18, 129
(1993): Protzer U+, *Gastroenterology* 104, 903
Lichenoid eruption
(2002): Bohannon JS, Midlothian, VA (from Internet) (observation)
Linear IgA bullous dermatosis
(1993): Parodi A+, *Dermatology* 187, 155
(1990): Guillaume JC+, *Ann Dermatol Venereol* (French) 117, 899
Lupus erythematosus
(2001): Werth V, *Dermatology Times* 18
(1998): Garcia-Porrua C+, *Clin Exp Rheumatol* 16, 107
(1994): Flores A+, *Br J Rheumatol* 33, 787
(1994): Fritzler MJ, *Lupus* 3, 455
(1994): Sanchez Roman J+, *Med Clin (Barc)* (Spanish) 102, 198
(1992): Mehta ND+, *Am J Hematol* 41, 141
(1992): Tolaymat A+, *J Pediatr* 120, 429
(1991): Hess EV, *Curr Opin Rheumatol* 3, 809
(1991): Schilling JP+, *Cancer* 68, 1536
Lupus syndrome
(2002): Pouthier D+, *Nephrol Dial Transplant* 17(1), 174
Melanoma
(1988): Bork K+, *Dermatologica* 177, 249 (exacerbation)
Necrosis
(1998): Sickler JB+, *Am J Gastroenterol* 93, 463
(1995): Chang LW+, *Cutis* 56, 144
Nodules (sic) (painful)
(1995): Chang LW+, *Cutis* 56, 144
Pemphigus
(1995): Kirsner RS+, *Br J Dermatol* 132, 474
(1994): Niizeki H+, *Dermatology* 189 (Suppl), 129
Photosensitivity (<1%)
(1994): Sollitto RB+, *Arch Dermatol* 130, 1194

Pigmented purpuric dermatosis (capillaritis)
(2000): Gupta G+, *J Am Acad Dermatol* 43, 937
Pruritus (13%) [L]; (5%) [K]
(2002): Bohannon JS, Midlothian VA (from Internet) (observation)
(2001): Beaudet LD (from Internet) (observation)
(1994): Czarnetzki BM+, *J Am Acad Dermatol* 30, 500
(1992): Breathnach SM+, *Adverse Drug Reactions and the Skin* Blackwell, Oxford, 322 (passim)
Psoriasis
(2002): Oliveira-Soares+, *World Congress Dermatol* Poster, 0123 (aggravation in 3 cases)
(2001): Werth V, *Dermatology Times* 18
(2000): Taylor C+, *Postgrad Med J* 76, 365
(1996): Wolfer LU+, *Hautarzt* (German) 47, 124
(1995): Chang LW+, *Cutis* 56, 144
(1995): Wolfe JT+, *J Am Acad Dermatol* 32, 887
(1994): Matsuoka H+, *Rinsho Ketsueki* (Japanese) 35, 309
(1993): Cleveland MG+, *J Am Acad Dermatol* 29, 788
(1993): Garcia-Lora E+, *Dermatology* 187, 280
(1993): Georgetson MJ+, *Am J Gastroenterol* 88, 756
(1993): Pauluzzi P+, *Acta Derm Venereol* 73, 395
(1991): Funk J+, *Br J Dermatol* 125, 463
(1990): Fierlbeck G+, *Arch Dermatol* 126, 351 (at injection site)
(1990): Jucgla A+, *Arch Dermatol* 127, 910 (exacerbation)
(1990): Kowalzick L+, *Arch Dermatol* 126, 1515 (at injection site)
(1990): Kusec R+, *Dermatologica* 181, 170
(1989): Harrison P, *J Invest Dermatol* 93, 555
(1989): Hartmann F+, *Dtsch Med Wochenschr* (German) 114, 96 (exacerbation)
(1986): Quesada JR+, *Lancet* 1, 1466 (exacerbation)
Purpura
(2001): Toubai T+, *Nippon Naika Gakkai Zasshi* 90(7), 1330
Radiation recall
(2002): Thomas R+, *J Clin Oncol* 20(1), 355
Rash (sic) (44%) [L]; (11%) [K]
(1999): Sookoian S+, *Arch Dermatol* 135, 999 (with ribavirin) ([K])
Raynaud's phenomenon
(1996): Creutzig A+, *Ann Intern Med* 125, 423
(1994): Arslan M+, *J Intern Med* 235, 503
Reiter's syndrome (incomplete)
(1993): Cleveland MG+, *J Am Acad Dermatol* 29, 788
Sarcoidosis
(2002): Cogrel O+, *Br J Dermatol* 146(2), 320 (with ribavirin)
(2002): Li SD+, *J Gastroenterol* 37(1), 50
(2002): Wendling J+, *Arch Dermatol* 138, 546 (2 cases) (with ribavirin)
(2001): Leveque L+, *Rev Med Interne* 22(12), 1248 (with ribavirin)
(2001): Neglia V+, *J Cutan Med Surg* 5(5), 406
(2001): Ravenel JG+, *Am J Roentgenol* 177(1), 199
(1999): Pietropaoli A+, *Chest* 116, 569
(1993): Blum L+, *Rev Med Interne* (Paris) (French) 14, 1161
Seborrheic dermatitis
(1986): Quesada JR+, *Lancet* 1, 1466
Sjøgren's syndrome
(1994): Lunel F, *Gastroenterol Clin Biol* (French) 19, 442
Telangiectases
(1989): Dreno B+, *Ann Intern Med* 111, 95
Ulceration
(1992): Orlow SJ+, *Arch Dermatol* 128, 566
Urticaria (<3%) [K]
(1994): Czarnetzki BM+, *J Am Acad Dermatol* 30, 500
(1992): Breathnach SM+, *Adverse Drug Reactions and the Skin* Blackwell, Oxford, 322 (passim)
Vasculitis
(2001): Toubai T+, *Nippon Naika Gakkai Zasshi* 90(7), 1330
(2001): Werth V, *Dermatology Times* 18
(1998): Gordon AC+, *J Infect* 36, 229
(1996): Pateron D+, *Clin Exp Rheumatol* 14, 79
(1995): Chang LW+, *Cutis* 56, 144
(1992): Liet JM+, *Rev Med Interne* (French) 13, 169
(1983): Sangster G+, *Eur J Cancer Clin Oncol* 19, 1647
Vitiligo
(1997): Nouri K+, *Cutis* 60, 289
(1996): Le Gal F-A+, *J Am Acad Dermatol* 35, 650
(1996): Simsek H+, *Dermatology* 193, 65
(1995): Bernstein D+, *Am J Gastroenterol* 90, 1176
(1994): Scheibenbogen C+, *Eur J Cancer* 30A, 1209
Xerosis (17%) [L]; (22%) [K]

## Hair

Hair – alopecia (1–10%)
(2002): Alpsoy E+, *Arch Dermatol* 138, 467
(2001): Zucker DM+, *Gastroenterol Nurs* 24(4), 192 (with ribavirin)
(1997): Brehler R+, *J Am Acad Dermatol* 36, 983 (passim)
(1995): Chang LW+, *Cutis* 56, 144
(1994): Czarnetzki BM+, *J Am Acad Dermatol* 30, 500
(1992): Tosti A+, *Dermatology* 184, 124
(1989): Olsen EA+, *J Am Acad Dermatol* 20, 395
(1987): Werter MJBP, *Ned Tijdschr Geneeskd* (Dutch) 131, 2081
Hair – alopecia areata
(1999): Kernland KH+, *Dermatology* 198, 418
Hair – discoloration
(1996): Fleming CJ+, *Br J Dermatol* 135, 337
(1995): Bernstein D+, *Am J Gastroenterol* 90, 1176 (canities)
Hair – hypertrichosis
(1996): Ariyoshi K+, *Am J Hematol* 53, 50 (eyebrows)
(1990): Berglund EF+, *South Med J* 83, 363
(1984): Foon KA+, *N Engl J Med* 19, 1259 (eyelashes)

## Other

Ageusia
(2001): Manzano Alonso ML+, *Gastroenterol Hepatol* 24(8), 412
Anosmia
(2001): Manzano Alonso ML+, *Gastroenterol Hepatol* 24(8), 412
(1998): Maruyama S+, *Am J Gastroenterol* 93, 122
Aphthous stomatitis
(1998): Dalekos GN+, *Eur J Gastroenterol Hepatol* 10, 933
Arthralgia
(2001): Karim A+, *Am J Med Sci* 322(4), 233
(2001): Leveque L+, *Rev Med Interne* 22(12), 1248 (with ribavirin)
(2001): Zucker DM+, *Gastroenterol Nurs* 24(4), 192 (with ribavirin)
Depression
(2002): Bonaccorso S+, *J Clin Psychopharmacol* 22(1), 86
(2002): Castera L+, *Hepatology* 35(4), 978
(2002): Farah A, *J Clin Psychiatry* 63(2), 166
(2002): Herrine SK, *Ann Intern Med* 136(10), 747
(2001): Bonaccorso S+, *Psychiatry Res* 105(1), 45
(2001): Debien C+, *Encephale* 27(4), 308 (5–15%)
(2001): Kraus MR+, *N Engl J Med* 345(5), 375
(2001): Maes M+, *Mol Psychiatry* 6(4), 475
(2001): Malik UR+, *Cancer* 92(6), 1664
Dysgeusia (25%) (metallic taste) [K]
(1995): Chang LW+, *Cutis* 56, 144
Halo dermatitis
(1999): Krischer J+, *J Am Acad Dermatol* 40, 105
Hypersensitivity
(2001): Beckman DB+, *Allergy* 56(8), 806
Hypesthesia
Injection-site alopecia
(1999): Lang AM+, *Arch Dermatol* 135, 1127
Injection-site erythema
(1995): Chang LW+, *Cutis* 56, 144

Injection-site induration
(1997): Siegel M, New York, NY (from Internet) (observation)
(1995): Chang LW+, *Cutis* 56, 144
Injection-site necrosis
(1998): Krainick U+, *J Interferon Cytokine Res* 18, 823
(1997): Weinberg JM+, *Acta Derm Venereol* (Stockh) 77, 146
(1996): Konohana A+, *J Am Acad Dermatol* 35, 788
(1996): Kontochristopoulos G+, *J Hepatol* 25, 271
(1995): Shinohara K, *N Engl J Med* 333, 1222
(1994): Akiyama Y+, *Jpn J Dermatol* (Japanese) 104, 436
(1994): Tone T+, *Jpn J Dermatol* 104, 1047
(1993): Christian B+, *Presse Med* (French) 22, 783
(1993): Mihara K+, *Miyazakiikaishi* (Japanese) 17, 40
(1993): Nagai A+, *Int J Hematol* 58, 129
(1993): Oeda E+, *Am J Hematol* 44, 213
(1992): Orlow SJ+, *Arch Dermatol* 128, 566
(1991): Cnudde F+, *Int J Dermatol* 30, 147
(1989): Rasokat H+, *Dtsch Med Wochenschr* (German) 114, 158
Injection-site pruritus
(1989): Detmar U+, *Contact Dermatitis* 20, 149
Injection-site vasculitis
(1997): Christian MM+, *J Am Acad Dermatol* 37, 118
Lymphoma, malignant
(1994): Arico M+, *Blood* 83, 869
Myalgia (71%) [L]; (69%) [K]
(2002): Alpsoy E+, *Arch Dermatol* 138, 467
(2002): Herrine SK, *Ann Intern Med* 136(10), 747
(2001): Karim A+, *Am J Med Sci* 322(4), 233
(2000): Shenefelt PD+, *Arch Dermatol* 136, 837
(1999): Spieth K+, *Arch Dermatol* 135, 1035
(1997): Brehler R+, *J Am Acad Dermatol* 36, 983 (passim)
(1984): Foon KA+, *N Engl J Med* 19, 1259 (passim)
Myasthenia gravis
(2001): Weegink CJ+, *J Gastroenterol* 36(10), 723 (with ribavirin)
Myopathy
(1998): Dippel E, *Arch Dermatol* 134, 880 (4 patients)
Oral lichen planus
(1997): Kutting B+, *Br J Dermatol* 137, 836
(1997): Schlesinger TE+, *J Am Acad Dermatol* 36, 1023 (erosive)
(1995): Chang LW+, *Cutis* 56, 144
(1994): Papini M+, *Int J Dermatol* 33, 221
(1994): Perreard M+, *Gastroenterol Clin Biol* (French) 18, 1051
(1993): Sassigneux P+, *Gastroenterol Clin Biol* (French) 17, 764
Oral pemphigus
(2001): Marinho RT+, *Eur J Gastroenterol Hepatol* 13(7), 869
Oropharyngeal pemphigus
(2001): Marinho RT+, *Eur J Gastroenterol Hepatol* 13(7), 869
Paresthesias (12%) [L]; (8%) [K]
Parkinsonism
(2002): Sarasombath P+, *Hawaii Med J* 61(3), 48
Polyarteritis nodosa
(2001): *Drug & Ther Perspect* 17, 15
Polymyositis
(2002): Lee SW+, *J Korean Med Sci* 17(1), 141
Rhabdomyolysis
(2001): van Londen GJ+, *J Clin Oncol* 19(17), 3794
(1995): Anderlini P+, *Cancer* 76, 678
Sialopenia
Stomatitis (1–10%)
Tinnitus
Xerostomia (>10%)

# INTERLEUKIN-2

(See ALDESLEUKIN)

# IPODATE

**Trade names:** Bilivist (Berlex); Oragrafin (Bristol-Myers Squibb)
**Indications:** Cholecystography
**Category:** Cholecystographic contrast medium
**Half-life:** no data

### *Reactions*

## Skin
Allergic reactions (sic)
(1986): Bigby M+, *JAMA* 256, 3358 (2.78%)
Exanthems
Pruritus
Purpura
(1966): Stacher A, *Wien Klin Wochenschr* (German) 75, 820
Rash (sic)
Urticaria

## Other
Anaphylactoid reactions
Hypersensitivity
Serum sickness

# IPRATROPIUM

**Trade names:** Atrovent (Boehringer Ingelheim); Combivent (Boehringer Ingelheim); Duoneb
**Other common trade names:** *Alti-Ipratropium; Novo-Ipramide*
**Indications:** Bronchospasm
**Category:** Aerosol bronchodilator; anticholinergic
**Half-life:** 2 hours

Combivent is albuterol and ipratropium

### *Reactions*

## Skin
Contact dermatitis
(1988): Eedy DJ+, *Postgrad Med J* 64, 306
Exanthems
Flushing (<1%)
Miliaria profunda
(1990): Saurat JH+, *Pediatr Dermatol* 7, 325
Pruritus (<1%)
Rash (sic) (1.2%)
Urticaria (<1%)

## Hair
Hair – alopecia (<1%)

## Other
Anaphylactoid reactions
(1993): Bone WD+, *Chest* 103, 981
Dysgeusia (1%) (metallic taste)
(2002): Cuvelier A+, *Respir Care* 47(2), 159
(1980): Pakes GE+, *Drugs* 20, 237
Oral mucosal lesions (1–5%)
(1980): Pakes GE+, *Drugs* 20, 237
Oral mucosal ulceration (<1%)
(1987): High AS, *BMJ* 294, 375
(1986): Spencer PA, *BMJ* 292, 380
Paresthesias (<1%)
Stomatitis (<1%)
Trembling (1–10%)
Xerostomia (3.2%)
(1980): Pakes GE+, *Drugs* 20, 237

# IRBESARTAN

**Trade names:** Avalide (Bristol-Myers Squibb); Avapro (Bristol-Myers Squibb)
**Indications:** Hypertension
**Category:** Angiotensin II receptor antagonist; antihypertensive
**Half-life:** 11–15 hours

Avalide is irbesartan and hydrochlorothiazide (a sulfonamide)*

### *Reactions*

#### Skin
Chills (<1%)
Dermatitis (sic) (<1%)
Ecchymoses (<1%)
Edema (1–10%)
Erythema (<1%)
Facial edema (<1%)
Flushing (<1%)
Pemphigus herpetiformis (sic)
(2002): Viseux V+, *World Congress Dermatol* Poster, 0360
Pruritus (<1%)
Rash (sic) (1–10%)
Urticaria (<1%)

#### Other
Cough
(2002): Coca A+, *Clin Ther* 24(1), 126
Oral lesions (<1%)
Paresthesias (<1%)
Tremors (<1%)

***Note:** Avalide contains a sulfonamide which can be absorbed systemically. Sulfonamides can produce severe, possibly fatal, reactions such as toxic epidermal necrolysis and Stevens–Johnson syndrome

# IRINOTECAN

**Synonyms:** Camptothecin-11; CPT-11
**Trade name:** Camptosar (Pharmacia & Upjohn)
**Indications:** Metastatic colorectal carcinoma
**Category:** Antineoplastic
**Half-life:** 6–10 hours

### *Reactions*

#### Skin
Allergic reactions (sic)
(1997): Verschraegen CF+, *J Clin Oncol* 15, 625 (9%)
Chills (13.8%)
Diaphoresis (16%)
Edema (10.2%)
Flushing (11%)
Infections (sic)
(2001): Ulrich-Pur H+, *Ann Oncol* 12(9), 1269 (3%)
Pigmentation
Rash (sic) (12.8%)
(1997): Verschraegen CF+, *J Clin Oncol* 15, 625 (21%)

#### Hair
Hair – alopecia (60.5%)
(2001): Ulrich-Pur H+, *Ann Oncol* 12(9), 1269 (13%)
(1999): Takahashi Y+, *Gan To Kagaku Ryoho* (Japanese) 26, 1193
(1998): Berg D, *Oncol Nurs Forum* 25, 535
(1997): Verschraegen CF+, *J Clin Oncol* 15, 625 (48%)
(1996): Rougier P+, *Semin Oncol* 23, 34
(1995): Abigerges D+, *J Clin Oncol* 13, 210 (53%)
(1995): Catimel G+, *Ann Oncol* 6, 133
(1994): de Forni M+, *Cancer Res* 54, 4347
(1994): Sakata Y+, *Gan To Kagaku Ryoho* (Japanese) 21, 1039 (40%)
(1994): Taguchi T+, *Gan To Kagaku Ryoho* (Japanese) 21, 1017 (30%)
(1994): Taguchi T+, *Gan To Kagaku Ryoho* (Japanese) 21, 83 (61%)
(1992): Fukuoka M+, *J Clin Oncol* 10, 16 (4%)
(1991): Negoro S+, *Gan To Kagaku Ryoho* (Japanese) 18, 1013
(1991): Takeuchi S+, *Gan To Kagaku Ryoho* (Japanese) 18, 1681 (33%)
(1991): Takeuchi S+, *Gan To Kagaku Ryoho* (Japanese) 18, 579 (33%)
(1990): Taguchi T+, *Gan To Kagaku Ryoho* (Japanese) 17, 115

#### Other
Dysgeusia (metallic taste)
Mucositis (2%)
Oral ulceration
Sialorrhea
Stomatitis (12%)
(2002): Bass AJ+, *J Clin Oncol* 20(13), 2995
(2000): Adjei AA+, *J Clin Oncol* 18, 1116
(1997): Verschraegen CF+, *J Clin Oncol* 15, 625 (14%)
Thrombophlebitis (1–10%)

# ISOCARBOXAZID

**Trade name:** Marplan (Roche)
**Other common trade name:** *Enerzer*
**Indications:** Depression
**Category:** Monoamine oxidase (MAO) inhibitor; antidepressant and antipanic
**Half-life:** no data
**Clinically important, potentially hazardous interactions with:** amitriptyline, amoxapine, bupropion, citalopram, clomipramine, desipramine, doxepin, fluoxetine, fluvoxamine, imipramine, meperidine, nefazodone, nortriptyline, paroxetine, protriptyline, rizatriptan, sertraline, sibutramine, sumatriptan, trimipramine, **tryptophan**, venlafaxine, zolmitriptan

### *Reactions*

#### Skin
Diaphoresis
(1962): Busfield BL+, *J Nerv Ment Dis* 134, 339 (30%)
Exanthems (7%)
(1962): Busfield BL+, *J Nerv Ment Dis* 134, 339
Peripheral edema (1–10%)
Photosensitivity (4%)
(1962): Busfield BL+, *J Nerv Ment Dis* 134, 339
Pruritus (4%)
(1962): Busfield BL+, *J Nerv Ment Dis* 134, 339
Rash (sic)
Telangiectases

#### Other
Black tongue
Xerostomia (1–10%)
(1962): Busfield BL+, *J Nerv Ment Dis* 134, 339 (11%)

## ISOETHARINE

**Trade names:** Arm-a-Med; Beta-2; Bronkomed; Bronkometer (Sanofi); Bronkosol (Sanofi); Dey-Lute
**Other common trade names:** *Asthmalitan; Numotac*
**Indications:** Bronchial asthma
**Category:** Adrenergic agonist; bronchodilator; sympathomimetic
**Half-life:** no data

### *Reactions*

#### Skin
None

#### Other
Anaphylactoid reactions
(1982): Twarog FJ+, *JAMA* 248, 2030
Trembling (1–10%)
Tremors
Xerostomia (1–10%)

## ISONIAZID

**Synonym:** INH
**Trade names:** Rifamate (Aventis); Rifater (Aventis)
**Other common trade names:** *Cemidon; Diazid; Isotamine; Isozid; Nicotibine; Nicozid; PMS-Isoniazid; Tibinide*
**Indications:** Tuberculosis
**Category:** Tuberculostatic
**Half-life:** 1–4 hours
**Clinically important, potentially hazardous interactions with:** phenytoin, rifampin

### *Reactions*

#### Skin
Acne
(1988): Oliwiecki S+, *Clin Exp Dermatol* 13, 283
(1988): Yamanaka M+, *Kekkaku* (Japanese) 63, 11
(1982): Rosin MA+, *Southern Med J* 75, 81 (passim)
(1974): Cohen LK+, *Arch Dermatol* 109, 377
(1969): Lantis SH, *J Am Med Wom Assoc* 24, 305
(1959): Bereston ES, *J Invest Dermatol* 33, 427
Acute generalized exanthematous pustulosis (AGEP)
(1995): Moreau A+, *Int J Dermatol* 34, 263 (passim)
Angioedema (<1%)
(1989): Yagi S+, *Kekkaku* (Japanese) 64, 407
(1959): Bereston ES, *J Invest Dermatol* 33, 427
Bullous eruption
(1999): Scheid P+, *Allergy* 54, 294
Contact dermatitis
(1993): Meseguer J+, *Contact Dermatitis* 28, 110 (systemic)
(1986): Holdiness MR, *Contact Dermatitis* 15, 282
(1978): Ippen H, *Derm Beruf Umwelt* (German) 26, 57
Cutaneous side effects (sic)
(1985): Holdiness MR, *Int J Dermatol* 24, 280 (2%)
Cutis laxa
(1985): Koch SE+, *Pediatr Dermatol* 2, 282
Dermatomyositis
(1975): Fayolle J+, *Lyon Med* (French) 233, 135
Erythema multiforme (<1%)
(1988): Hira SK+, *J Am Acad Dermatol* 19, 451 (in AIDS patients)
(1976): Bomb BS+, *Tubercle* 57, 229
Exanthems
(1982): Rosin MA+, *Southern Med J* 75, 81 (passim)
(1979): Byrd RB+, *JAMA* 241, 1239 (0.9%)
(1963): Honeycutt WM+, *Arch Dermatol* 88, 190
(1959): Bereston ES, *J Invest Dermatol* 33, 427
Exfoliative dermatitis
(1985): Holdiness MR, *Int J Dermatol* 24, 280
(1982): Rosin MA+, *Southern Med J* 75, 81
(1969): Agrawal R, *BMJ* 4, 540
(1963): Abrahams I+, *Arch Dermatol* 87, 96
(1963): Honeycutt WM+, *Arch Dermatol* 88, 190
Flushing
(1953): Witbind E+, *Dis Chest* 23, 16 (>5%)
Herpes zoster
(1959): Bereston ES, *J Invest Dermatol* 33, 427
Keratoacanthoma
(1966): Randazzo SD, *G Ital Dermatol Minerva Dermatol* (Italian) 107, 1195
Lichenoid eruption
(2001): Sharma PK+, *J Dermatol* 28(12), 737
(1974): Haldar B, *Indian J Dermatol* 19(3), 71
Lupus erythematosus
(1994): Yung RL+, *Rheum Dis Clin North Am* 20, 61
(1992): Hofstra AH+, *Drug Metab Dispos* 20, 205
(1992): Rubin RL+, *J Clin Invest* 90, 165
(1992): Salazar-Pama M+, *Ann Rheum Dis* 51, 1085
(1992): Skaer TL, *Clin Ther* 14, 496
(1991): Gatenby PA, *Autoimmunity* 11, 61
(1990): Guleria R+, *Indian J Chest Dis Allied Sci* 32, 55
(1989): Ueda Y+, *Kekkaku* (Japanese) 64, 613
(1988): Jiang M, *Chung Kuo I Hsueh Ko Hsueh Yuan Hseuh Pao* (Chinese) 10, 379
(1988): Umeki S, *Kekkaku* (Japanese) 63, 713
(1986): Layer P+, *Dtsch Med Wochenschr* (German) 111, 1603
(1985): Cush JJ+, *Am J Med Sci* 290, 36
(1985): Holdiness MR, *Int J Dermatol* 24, 280
(1985): Kale SA, *Postgrad Med* 77, 231
(1985): Lovisetto P+, *Recenti Prog Med* (Ital) 76, 110
(1985): Stratton MA, *Clin Pharm* 4, 657
(1984): No Author, *Lancet* 2, 441
(1984): Sim E+, *Lancet* 2, 422
(1983): Escolar-Castellon F+, *Rev Clin Esp* (Spanish) 169, 209
(1982): Grunwald M+, *Dermatologica* 165, 172
(1982): Harmon CE+, *Clin Rheum Dis* 8, 121
(1981): Reidenberg MM, *Arthritis Rheum* 24, 1004
(1980): Agarwal MB+, *J Postgrad Med* 26, 263
(1980): Weinstein A, *Prog Clin Immunol* 4, 1
(1977): Dandavino R+, *Ann Med Interne Paris* (French) 128, 39
(1977): Seedat YK+, *S Afr Med J* 51, 335
(1976): Cohmen G, *Med Klin* (German) 71, 789
(1976): Dutt AK+, *Indian J Chest Dis Allied Sci* 18, 146
(1975): Laroche C+, *Sem Hop* (French) 51, 2515
(1974): Harpey JP, *Ann Allergy* 33, 256
(1974): *Med Lett Drugs Ther* 16, 34
(1974): McEwen J, *Lancet* 2, 1570
(1974): No Author, *Va Med Mon* 101, 299 (passim)
(1973): Alarcon-Segovia D, *Chest* 63, 299
(1973): Bar-On H, *Harefuah* (Hebrew) 84, 25
(1973): Blomgren SE, *Semin Hematol* 10, 345
(1973): Durand JP+, *Cah Med* (French) 14, 9
(1973): Godeau P+, *Ann Med Interne Paris* (French) 124, 181
(1972): Dorfmann H+, *Nouv Presse Med* (French) 1, 2907
(1972): Gaultier Cl+, *Ann Pédiatr Paris* (French) 19, 459
(1972): Goldman AL+, *Chest* 62, 71
(1972): Greenberg JH+, *JAMA* 222, 191
(1971): Delepierre F+, *Rev Tuberc Pneumol Paris* (French) 35, 397
(1970): No Author, *BMJ* 2, 192
(1970): Trad J+, *Sem Hop* (French) 46, 3013
(1969): Alarcon-Segovia D, *Mayo Clin Proc* 44, 664
(1967): Auquier L+, *Bull Mem Soc Med Hop Paris* (French) 118, 372

(1967): Hothersall TE+, *Scott Med J* 13, 245
(1967): Masel MA, *Med J Aust* 54, 738
(1967): Siegel M+, *Arthritis Rheum* 10, 407
(1963): Zingale SB+, *Arch Intern Med* 112, 63

Pellagra
(1999): Muratake T+, *Am J Psychiatry* 156, 660
(1987): Schmutz JL+, *Ann Derm Venereol* (French) 114, 569
(1983): Jorgensen J, *Int J Dermatol* 22, 44
(1981): Meyrick Thomas RH+, *BMJ* 283, 287
(1977): Comaish JS+, *Arch Dermatol* 113, 986
(1977): Harrington CI, *Practitioner* 218, 716
(1976): Comaish JS+, *Arch Dermatol* 112, 70
(1974): Cohen LK+, *Arch Dermatol* 109, 377
(1974): Forstrom L+, *Arch Dermatol* 110, 635
(1974): Schlenzka K+, *Dermatol Monatsschr* (German) 160, 848
(1972): Bjornstad RT, *Tidsskr Nor Laegeforen* (Norwegian) 92, 640
(1972): Harber LC+, *J Invest Dermatol* 58, 327
(1972): Jansen CT+, *Duodecim* 88, 928
(1969): Polano MK+, *Arch Belg Dermatol Syphiligr* (Dutch) 25, 345
(1967): Di Lorenzo PA, *Acta Derm Venereol* (Stockh) 47, 318
(1964): Aspinall DL, *BMJ* 2, 1177
(1959): Bereston ES, *J Invest Dermatol* 33, 427
(1958): Haynes WS, *East Afr Med J* 35, 171
(1956): Harrison RJ+, *BMJ* 2, 853
(1955): Wood MM, *Br J Tuberc Dis Chest* 49, 20
(1952): McConnell RB+, *Lancet* 2, 959

Photosensitivity
(1998): Lee AY+, *Photodermatol Photoimmunol Photomed* 14, 77 (lichenoid) (2 patients)
(1987): Schmutz JL+, *Ann Dermatol Venereol* (French) 114, 569
(1972): Kauppinen K, *Acta Derm Venereol* (Stockh) 52 (Suppl) 68
(1969): Kalivas J, *JAMA* 209, 1706

Pruritus
(1953): Witbind E+, *Dis Chest* 23, 16 (>5%)

Purpura
(1992): Breathnach SM+, *Adverse Drug Reactions and the Skin* Blackwell, Oxford, 159 (passim)
(1982): Rosin MA+, *Southern Med J* 75, 81 (passim)
(1980): Miescher PA+, *Clin Haematol* 9, 505
(1979): Byrd RB+, *JAMA* 241, 1239
(1965): Horowitz HI+, *Semin Hematol* 2, 287
(1964): Duncan JT, *Am Rev Respir Dis* 89, 103
(1959): Bereston ES, *J Invest Dermatol* 33, 427

Pustular eruption
(1993): Webster GF, *Clin Dermatol* 11, 541
(1985): Yamasaki R+, *Br J Dermatol* 112, 504 (subcorneal)

Rash (sic) (<1%)
(2000): Gordin F+, *JAMA* 283, 1445

Stevens–Johnson syndrome
(1976): Bomb BS+, *Tubercle* 57, 229
(1965): Ingle VN+, *Indian Pediatr* 2, 305

Striae
(1967): Hofer W, *Z Haut Geschlechtskr* (German) 42, 603

Systemic eczematous contact dermatitis
(1993): Meseguer J+, *Contact Dermatitis* 28, 110

Toxic epidermal necrolysis (<1%)
(1990): Nanda A+, *Arch Dermatol* 126, 125
(1983): Katoch K+, *Lepr India* 55, 133
(1976): Mital OP+, *Indian J Tuberc* 23, 32
(1974): Faye I+, *Bull Soc Med Afr Noire Lang Fr* (French) 19, 185 (fatal)
(1973): Sehgal VN+, *Indian J Chest Dis* 15, 57
(1967): Lowney ED+, *Arch Dermatol* 95, 359

Urticaria (1–5%)
(1992): Breathnach SM+, *Adverse Drug Reactions and the Skin* Blackwell, Oxford, 159 (passim)
(1982): Rosin MA+, *Southern Med J* 75, 81 (passim)
(1959): Bereston ES, *J Invest Dermatol* 33, 427
(1953): Cormia FE+, *Arch Dermatol* 68, 536 (4%)

Vasculitis
(1982): Rosin MA+, *Southern Med J* 75, 81 (passim)
(1963): Honeycutt WM+, *Arch Dermatol* 88, 190

### Hair

Hair – alopecia
(2001): Sharma PK+, *J Dermatol* 28(12), 737
(1996): FitzGerald JM+, *Lancet* 347, 472
(1978): Krivokhizh VN+, *Vestn Dermatol Venerol* (Russian) 3, 63

### Nails

Nails – onycholysis

### Other

Acute intermittent porphyria
Death
Gynecomastia
Hypersensitivity
(2001): Rebollo S+, *Contact Dermatitis* 45(5), 306
(1992): Dukes CS+, *Trop Geogr Med* 44, 308
(1969): Rykowska Z, *Gruzlica* (Polish) 37, 777
Injection-site irritation
Myopathy
(1989): Cronkright PJ+, *Ann Intern Med* 110, 945
Oral mucosal lesions
(1973): Parish LC+, *Int J Dermatol* 12, 324
(1971): *Med Lett* 13, 55 (1–5%)
Oral mucosal ulceration
Paresthesias
(1982): Porter IH, *Handbook of Clinical Neurology* 44, 648
Rhabdomyolysis
(2001): Panganiban LR+, *J Toxicol Clin Toxicol* 39(2), 143 (3%)
(1995): Blowey DL+, *Am J Emerg Med* 13(5), 543
Serum sickness
(1981): Simelaro J+, *J Am Osteopath Assoc* 80, 348
Tinnitus
Xerostomia

# ISOPROTERENOL

**Trade names:** Aerolone; Arm-a-Med; Isuprel (Sanofi); Medihaler-ISO (3M); Norisodrine (Abbott)
**Other common trade names:** *Isopro; Isuprel Mistometer; Isuprel Nebulimetro; Saventrine; Vapo-Iso*
**Indications:** Bronchospasm, ventricular arrhythmias
**Category:** Adrenergic bronchodilator; sympathomimetic
**Half-life:** 2.5–5 minutes

## *Reactions*

### Skin

Diaphoresis (1–10%)
Edema
Flushing (1–10%)
Pruritus
Rash (sic)
Urticaria

### Other

Oral mucosal lesions
(1969): Warth J+, *JAMA* 209, 417
Saliva discoloration (sic) (pinkish-red) (>10%)
Trembling
Tremors
Xerostomia (>10%)

## ISOSORBIDE

**Trade name:** Ismotic
**Indications:** Acute angle-closure glaucoma
**Category:** Osmotic diuretic
**Half-life:** 5–9.5 hours

### *Reactions*

#### Skin
Rash (sic) (<1%)

#### Other
Tinnitus

## ISOSORBIDE DINITRATE

**Synonyms:** ISD; ISDN
**Trade names:** Dilatrate-SR (Schwarz); Isordil (Wyeth-Ayerst); Sorbitrate (AstraZeneca)
**Other common trade names:** *Apo-ISDN; Cedocard; Coradur*
**Indications:** Angina pectoris
**Category:** Antianginal; vasodilator
**Half-life:** 4 hours (oral)
**Clinically important, potentially hazardous interactions with:** sildenafil

### *Reactions*

#### Skin
Ankle edema
(1981): Rodger JC, *BMJ* 283, 1365
Diaphoresis
Edema (<1%)
Flushing (>10%)
(1981): Rodger JC, *BMJ* 283, 1365 (passim)
Pallor
Peripheral edema

#### Other
Xerostomia

## ISOSORBIDE MONONITRATE

**Synonym:** ISMN
**Trade names:** Imdur (Schering-Plough); Ismo (Wyeth-Ayerst); Monoket (Schwarz)
**Indications:** Angina pectoris
**Category:** Antianginal; vasodilator
**Half-life:** ~4 hours
**Clinically important, potentially hazardous interactions with:** sildenafil

### *Reactions*

#### Skin
Ankle edema
(1981): Rodger JC, *BMJ* 283, 1365
Diaphoresis
Edema (<1%)
Flushing (>10%)
(1981): Rodger JC, *BMJ* 283, 1365 (passim)
Pruritus (<1%)
Rash (sic) (<1%)

#### Other
Hypesthesia (<1%)
Tooth disorder (sic) (<1%)

## ISOTRETINOIN

**Synonym:** 13-*cis*-retinoic acid
**Trade names:** Accutane (Roche); Amnesteem (Bertek)
**Other common trade names:** *Isotrex; Roaccutan; Roaccutane; Roacutan; Roacuttan*
**Indications:** Cystic acne
**Category:** Retinoid; inhibits sebaceous gland function
**Half-life:** 10–20 hours
**Clinically important, potentially hazardous interactions with:** acitretin, antacids, bexarotene, cholestyramine, co-trimoxazole, corticosteroids, **fish oil supplements**, minocycline, retinoids, tetracycline, vitamin A

### *Reactions*

#### Skin
Acne (fulminans)
(2002): Moroz B+, *World Congress Dermatol* Poster, 0119
(1997): Tan BB+, *Clin Exp Dermatol* 22, 26
(1996): Faverge B+, *Arch Pediatr* (French) 3, 188
(1993): Bottomley WW+, *Acta Derm Venereol* (Stockh) 73, 74
(1993): Lepagney ML+, *Ann Dermatol Venereol* (French) 120, 917
(1992): Choi EH+, *J Dermatol* 19, 378
(1992): Hagler J+, *Int J Dermatol* 31, 199
(1992): Jenkinson HA, *Br J Dermatol* 127, 62
(1991): Elias LM+, *J Dermatol* 18, 366
(1991): Joly P+, *Ann Dermatol Venereol* (French) 118, 369
(1989): Rotoli M+, *G Ital Dermatol Venereol* (Italian) 124, 120
(1988): Blanc D+, *Dermatologica* 177, 16
(1985): Kellett JK+, *BMJ* 290, 820
(1984): Darley CR+, *J R Soc Med* 77, 328
Bruising (sic)
(1993): Green C, *Br J Dermatol* 128, 465
Cellulitis (1–10%)
Cheilitis (>90%)
(2001): Önder M+, *J Dermatol Treat* 12, 115
(1999): Graham BS+, *Arch Dermatol* 349
(1997): Berger R, *The Schoch Letter* 47, 5
(1997): Goulden V+, *Br J Dermatol* 137, 106
(1988): Shalita AR+, *Cutis* 42, 10
(1976): Peck GL+, *Lancet* 2, 1172
Desquamation (palms and soles) (5%)
(1988): Shalita AR+, *Cutis* 42, 10
Diaphoresis
(2000): Popescu C, Bucharest, Romania (from Internet) (observation)
(1988): Rees JL+, *Br J Dermatol* 119, 79
(1987): Kiistala R+, *Acta Derm Venereol* 67, 331 (increased number of active sweat glands)
Edema (subcutaneous, recurrent)
(1999): Choquet-Kastylevsky G+, *Therapie* (French) 54, 263
(1999): Graham BS+, *Arch Dermatol* 135, 349
Eruptive xanthoma
(1983): Shalita AR+, *J Am Acad Dermatol* 9, 629
(1980): Dicken CH+, *Arch Dermatol* 116, 951
Erythema multiforme
(1988): Bigby M+, *J Am Acad Dermatol* 18, 543
Erythema nodosum

(1997): Tan BB+, *Clin Exp Dermatol* 22, 26
(1988): Bigby M+, *J Am Acad Dermatol* 18, 543
(1985): Kellett JK+, *BMJ* 290, 820

Exanthems
(1993): Litt JZ, Beachwood, OH (non-pruritic) (personal case) (observation)
(1988): Bigby M+, *J Am Acad Dermatol* 18, 543

Exfoliation (1–10%)

Facial cellulitis
(1994): Boffa MJ+, *J Am Acad Dermatol* 31, 800

Facial edema (1–10%)

Facial scarring
(1994): Katz BE+, *J Am Acad Dermatol* 30, 852

Fixed eruption
(1988): Bigby M+, *J Am Acad Dermatol* 18, 543

Flushing
(1998): Frederickson K (from Internet) (observation)
(1998): Gass M (from Internet) (2 observations)

Folliculitis
(1990): Hughes BR+, *Br J Dermatol* 122, 683

Fragility
(2000): *Prescrire Int* 7, 178 (from wax epilation)
(1997): Litt JZ, Beachwood, OH (lips from wax epilation) (2 personal cases) (observations)
(1997): Woollons A+, *Br J Dermatol* 137, 389
(1995): Holmes SC+, *Br J Dermatol* 132, 165

Granulation tissue
(1991): Rodland O+, *Tidsskr Nor Laegeforen* (Norwegian) 111, 2630
(1985): Miller RA+, *J Am Acad Dermatol* 5, 888
(1984): Robertson DB+, *Br J Dermatol* 111, 689

Herpes (sic)
(1990): Joly P+, *Ann Dermatol Venereol* (French) 117, 860

Keloid formation
(1999): Ginarte M+, *Int J Dermatol* 38, 228
(1997): Bernestein LJ+, *Arch Dermatol* 133, 111
(1994): Katz BE+, *J Am Acad Dermatol* 30, 852
(1988): Zachariae H, *Br J Dermatol* 118, 703

Keratolysis exfoliativa

Leucoderma
(1988): Bigby M+, *J Am Acad Dermatol* 18, 543

Lichenoid eruption
(2001): Boyd AS+, *Cutis* 68, 301

Melasma
(1998): Thaler D, Monona, WI (from internet) (observation)
(1997): Verros CD, Tripolis, Greece (from Internet) (observation)

Miliaria
(1986): Gupta AK+, *Cutis* 38, 275

Mycosis fungoides-like
(1985): Molin L+, *Acta Derm Venereol* 65, 69

Nummular eczema
(1987): Bettoli V+, *J Am Acad Dermatol* 16, 617

Pallor (1–10%)

Pemphigus
(1995): Georgala S+, *Acta Derm Venereol* 75, 413

Photosensitivity (>10%)
(1991): Auffret N+, *J Am Acad Dermatol* 23, 321
(1986): Ferguson J+, *Br J Dermatol* 115, 275
(1986): Wong RC+, *J Am Acad Dermatol* 14, 1095
(1985): Diffey BL+, *J Am Acad Dermatol* 12, 119
(1983): McCormack LS+, *J Am Acad Dermatol* 9, 273

Pigmentation
(1988): Bigby M+, *J Am Acad Dermatol* 18, 543

Pityriasis rosea
(1984): Helfman RJ+, *Cutis* 33, 297

Pruritus (1–5%)
(1994): Yee KC+, *Dermatology* 189, 117
(1988): Shalita AR+, *Cutis* 42, 10
(1976): Peck GL+, *Lancet* 2, 1172

Pyoderma gangrenosum
(2002): Moroz B+, *World Congress Dermatol* Poster
(1997): Gangaram HP+, *Br J Dermatol* 136, 636

Pyogenic granuloma
(1992): Hagler J+, *Int J Dermatol* 31, 199 (fatal)
(1988): Blanc D+, *Dermatologica* 177, 16
(1984): Robertson DB+, *Br J Dermatol* 111, 689
(1983): Campbell JP+, *J Am Acad Dermatol* 9, 708
(1983): Exner JH+, *Arch Dermatol* 119, 808
(1983): Spear KL+, *Mayo Clin Proc* 58, 509
(1983): Valentic JP+, *Arch Dermatol* 119, 871

Rash (sic)

Sebaceous casts (sic)
(2000): Agarwal S+, *Br J Dermatol* 143, 228 (nasolabial follicular)

Telangiectases
(1994): Thompson D, *The Schoch Letter* 44, 47 (#186) (observation)

Toxic epidermal necrolysis
(1994): Rosen T, *Arch Dermatol* 130, 260

Urticaria
(2000): Madnani N, Mumbai, India (from Internet) (observation)
(1988): Bigby M+, *J Am Acad Dermatol* 18, 543

Varicosities
(1994): Thompson D, *The Schoch Letter* 44, 47 (#186) (observation)

Vasculitis
(1990): Aractingi S+, *Lancet* 335, 362
(1989): Dwyer JM+, *Lancet* 2, 494
(1989): Reynolds P+, *Lancet* 2, 1216
(1987): Epstein EH, *Arch Dermatol* 123, 1124

Xerosis (>10%)
(1997): Berger R, *The Schoch Letter* 47, 5
(1988): Shalita AR+, *Cutis* 42, 10
(1976): Peck GL+, *Lancet* 2, 1172

## Hair

Hair – alopecia (16%)
(2000): Dintiman BJ, Fairfax, VA (from Internet) (4 observations)
(2000): Frederickson KS, Novalo, CA (from Internet) (observation)
(2000): Rehbein HM, Jacksonville, FL (from Internet) (2 observations)
(1998): Litt JZ, Beachwood, OH (personal case) (observation)
(1998): Thaler D, Monona, WI (from internet) (observation)
(1997): Berger R, *The Schoch Letter* 47, 5 (diffuse)
(1997): Thaler D, Monona, WI (from internet) (observation)
(1994): Shelley WB+, *Cutis* 53, 237 (observation)

Hair – hirsutism

Hair – pili torti (curly hair)
(2002): Spencer L, Crawforsville, IN (from Internet) (observation)
(1996): van der Pijl JW+, *Lancet* 348, 622
(1990): Bunker CB+, *Clin Exp Dermatol* 15, 143
(1985): Hays SB+, *Cutis* 25, 466

Hair – trichotillomania
(1990): Mahr G, *Psychosomatics* 31, 235

## Nails

Nails – fragility
(2001): Önder M+, *J Dermatol Treat* 12, 115

Nails – growth
(1994): Litt JZ, Beachwood, OH (personal case) (observation)

Nails – median canaliform dystrophy
(1997): Dharmagunawardena B+, *Br J Dermatol*
(1992): Bottomley WW+, *Br J Dermatol* 127, 447
(1988): Bigby M+, *J Am Acad Dermatol* 18, 543

Nails – onycholysis

(2001): Önder M+, *J Dermatol Treat* 12, 115
(1988): Bigby M+, *J Am Acad Dermatol* 18, 543

Nails – paronychia
(1998): Lepine EM, Rock Hill, SC (from Internet) (observation)
(1988): Bigby M+, *J Am Acad Dermatol* 18, 543
(1986): DeRaeve L+, *Dermatologica* 172, 278
(1984): Blumental G, *J Am Acad Dermatol* 10, 677

Nails – periungual hemorrhage
(1997): Leal G, Fortaleza, Brazil (from Internet) (observation)

### Other

Ageusia
(1996): Halpern SM+, *Br J Dermatol* 134(2), 378

Death

Dysgeusia
(1990): Heise E+, *Eur Arch Otorhinolaryngol* 247, 382

Galactorrhea
(1985): Larsen GK, *Arch Dermatol* 121, 450

Gynecomastia
(1994): Shelley WB+, *Cutis* 54, 149 (passim)
(1992): Fluckiger R, *Schweiz Rundsch Med Prax* (German) 81, 1370

Mucosal denudation of lips
(1999): Graham BS+, *Arch Dermatol* 349

Myalgia (>10%)
(1998): Heudes AM+, *Ann Dermatol Venereol* 125(2), 94

Myopathy
(1996): Fiallo P+, *Arch Dermatol* 132, 1521
(1986): Hodak E, *BMJ* 293, 425

Parosmia
(1990): Heise E+, *Eur Arch Otorhinolaryngol* 247, 382

Pseudoporphyria
(1993): Riordan CA+, *Clin Exp Dermatol* 18, 69

Pseudotumor cerebri
(1998): Sorkin MJ, Denver, CO (from Internet) (observation of 4 cases)
(1995): Lee AG, *Cutis* 55, 165
(1988): Roytman M+, *Cutis* 42, 399

Rhabdomyolysis
(2001): Trauner MA+, *Dermatology Online Journal* 5, 2
(2001): Zabawski E, Longwood, TX (from Internet) (observation)
(1998): Heudes AM+, *Ann Dermatol Venereol* 125(2), 94

Tinnitus

Xerostomia (>10%)
(1992): Breathnach SM+, *Adverse Drug Reactions and the Skin* Blackwell, Oxford, 259 (passim)

# ISOXSUPRINE

**Trade names:** Vasodilan (Bristol-Myers Squibb); Voxsuprine
**Other common trade names:** *Duvadilan; Isoxine; Sincen; Vasolan; Vasosuprina; Xuprin*
**Indications:** Peripheral vascular disease, Raynaud's phenomenon
**Category:** Peripheral vasodilator
**Half-life:** no data

## *Reactions*

### Skin

Allergic dermatitis (sic)
(1978): Horowitz JJ+, *Am J Obstet Gynecol* 131, 225

# ISRADIPINE

**Trade name:** DynaCirc (Novartis)
**Other common trade names:** *Dynacirc SRO; Lomir; Lomir SRO; Prescal; Vascal*
**Indications:** Hypertension
**Category:** Calcium channel blocker; antihypertensive
**Half-life:** 8 hours
**Clinically important, potentially hazardous interactions with:** epirubicin, imatinib

## *Reactions*

### Skin

Diaphoresis (<1%)

Edema (7.2%)
(1992): Lopez LM+, *Ann Pharmacother* 26, 789
(1992): Madias NE+, *Am J Hypertens* 5, 141
(1991): Eisner GM+, *Am J Hypertens* 4, 154S
(1991): Galloe AM+, *J Intern Med* 229, 447
(1991): Schachter M, *J Clin Pharm Ther* 16, 79
(1990): Vidt DG, *Cleve Clin J Med* 57, 677

Exanthems
(1993): Blumenthal HL, Beachwood, OH (personal case) (observation)
(1990): Fitton A+, *Drugs* 40, 31 (1.5%)

Flushing (2.6%)
(1992): Lopez LM+, *Ann Pharmacother* 26, 789
(1991): Galloe AM+, *J Intern Med* 229, 447
(1991): Schachter M, *J Clin Pharm Ther* 16, 79
(1990): Fitton A+, *Drugs* 40, 31 (10–15%)
(1990): Vidt DG, *Cleve Clin J Med* 57, 677
(1990): Welzel D+, *Drugs* 40 (Suppl 2), 60
(1990): Zubair M+, *Drugs* 40 (Suppl 2), 26 (7.8%)

Peripheral edema

Pruritus (<1%)
(1990): Zubair M+, *Drugs* 40 (Suppl 2), 26 (5.9%)

Rash (sic) (1.5%)

Urticaria (<1%)

### Other

Gingival hyperplasia (<1%)

Oral mucosal lesions
(1990): Zubair M+, *Drugs* 40 (Suppl 2), 26 (5.9%)

Paresthesias (<1%)

Xerostomia (<1%)

# ITRACONAZOLE

**Trade name:** Sporanox (Janssen)
**Other common trade names:** *Isox; Itranax; Sopronox; Sporacid; Sporal; Sporanox 15 D*
**Indications:** Onychomycosis, deep mycoses
**Category:** Antifungal
**Half-life:** 21 hours
**Clinically important, potentially hazardous interactions with:** alprazolam, amphotericin B, anisindione, antacids, atorvastatin, bosentan, cimetidine, clorazepate, dicumarol, didanosine, ethotoin, fosphenytoin, **grapefruit juice**, HMG-CoA reductase inhibitors, imatinib, lovastatin, mephenytoin, midazolam, phenytoin, pimozide, quinidine, rifampin, sildenafil, simvastatin, triazolam, vinblastine, vincristine, warfarin

## *Reactions*

### Skin

Acute generalized exanthematous pustulosis (AGEP)
(1997): Park YM+, *J Am Acad Dermatol* 36, 794
(1995): Heymann WR+, *J Am Acad Dermatol* 33, 130
Angioedema
(1996): Foong H, Malaysia (from Internet) (observation)
Cutaneous side effects (sic)
(1999): Gupta AK+, *Dermatology* 199, 248
(1997): Gupta AK+, *J Am Acad Dermatol* 36, 789
Edema (3.5%)
(1998): N Z Medicines Adverse Reactions Committee, (peripheral) (from Internet) (observation)
(1996): Tailor SA+, *Arch Dermatol* 132, 350 (peripheral) (with nifedipine)
(1994): Gupta AK+, *J Am Acad Dermatol* 30, 911
(1994): Rosen T, *Arch Dermatol* 130, 260
(1992): *Med Lett Drugs Ther* 34, 14
(1991): Diaz M+, *Chest* 100, 682
(1991): Sharkey PK+, *Antimicrob Agents Chemother* 35, 707
(1990): Denning DW+, *J Am Acad Dermatol* 23, 602 (2%)
(1990): Sharkey PK+, *J Am Acad Dermatol* 23, 577
(1990): Tucker RM+, *J Antimicrob Chemother* 26, 561
Eruption (sic)
(2000): Goto Y+, *Acta Derm Venereol* 80, 72
Erythema multiforme
(1998): Rademaker M+, *New Zealand Adverse Drug Reactions Committee*, April, 1998 (from Internet)
Exanthems
(1999): Burrow WH, Jackson, MS, (from Internet) (2 cases ) (observation)
(1999): Valentine MC, Everett, WA (from Internet) (2 cases) observation)
(1998): Litt JZ, Beachwood, OH (personal case) (observation)
(1997): Blumenthal HL, Beachwood, OH (personal case) (observation)
(1997): Danby FW, Kingston, Ontario (2 cases) (from Internet) (observation)
(1996): Degreef H, *Cutis* 58, 90
(1994): Litt JZ, Beachwood, OH (2 personal cases) (observation)
(1991): Smith DE+, *AIDS* 5, 1367
(1990): Roseeuw D+, *Clin Exp Dermatol* 15, 101 (2.6%)
(1990): Tucker RM+, *J Am Acad Dermatol* 23, 593 (3%)
Facial dermatitis (papular, id-like)
(1996): Thaler D, Monona, WI (2 cases) (from internet) (observation)
Fixed eruption
(1997): Perry S, *The Schoch Letter* 47, 19
(1994): Litt JZ, Beachwood, OH (personal case) (observation)
Flu-like syndrome
(2002): Faergemann J+, *Arch Dermatol* 138, 69
Peripheral edema (4%)
Photoreactions
(1996): Moreland A, *The Schoch Letter* 46, 19 (observation)
Phototoxicity
(1999): Gass M, Davis, CA (from Internet) (observation)
(1995): Epstein E Jr, *The Schoch Letter* 45, 28 (observation)
(1994): Milstein H, *The Schoch Letter* 44, 5 (observation)
Pruritus (2.5%)
(2002): Faergemann J+, *Arch Dermatol* 138, 69
(1997): Gupta AK+, *J Am Acad Dermatol* 36, 789
(1994): Gupta AK+, *J Am Acad Dermatol* 30, 911 (0.7%)
(1992): Cleary JD+, *Ann Pharmacother* 26, 502
(1992): Lavrijsen AP+, *Lancet* 340, 251
(1991): De Beule K+, *Curr Ther Res* 49, 814
(1990): Tucker RM+, *J Antimicrob Chemother* 26, 561
(1989): Grant SM+, *Drugs* 39, 877 (0.6%)
Purpura
(1997): Kramer KE+, *J Am Acad Dermatol* 37, 994
Rash (sic) (8.6%)
(1996): Odom R+, *J Am Acad Dermatol* 35, 110 (severe)
(1994): Gupta AK+, *J Am Acad Dermatol* 30, 911 (1.1%)
(1990): Sharkey PK+, *J Am Acad Dermatol* 23, 577
(1990): Tucker RM+, *J Am Acad Dermatol* 23, 593
(1990): Tucker RM+, *J Antimicrob Chemother* 26, 561
Skin eruptions (sic)
(1992): Cleary JD+, *Ann Pharmacother* 26, 502
Stevens–Johnson syndrome
Urticaria
(2002): Faergemann J+, *Arch Dermatol* 138, 69
(1999): Valentine MC, Everett, WA (from Internet) (observation)
(1997): Billon S, *The Schoch Letter* 47, 32 (observation)
(1996): Thaler D, Monona, WI (from internet) (observation)
(1994): Litt JZ, Beachwood, OH (personal case) (observation)
(1993): Litt JZ, Beachwood, OH (personal case) (observation)
(1992): Piepponen T+, *J Antimicrob Chemother* 29, 195
Vasculitis
(1996): Odom R+, *J Am Acad Dermatol* 35, 110

### Hair

Hair – alopecia
(1995): Litt JZ, Beachwood, OH (personal case) (observation)
(1992): de Gans J+, *AIDS* 6, 185
(1986): Moller Heilesen A, *BMJ* 293, 823

### Nails

Nails – beading
(1994): Donker PD+, *Clin Exp Dermatol* 19, 404
Nails – onychocryptosis
(1995): Arenas R+, *Int J Dermatol* 34, 138

### Other

Anaphylactoid reactions
Gynecomastia (<1%)
(1994): Gupta AK+, *J Am Acad Dermatol* 30, 911
Myalgia (1%)
Rhabdomyolysis
(2002): Vlahakos DV+, *Transplantation* 73(12), 1962
Serum sickness
(1998): Park H+, *Ann Pharmacother* 32, 1249
Tinnitus
Xerostomia
(1990): Tucker RM+, *J Am Acad Dermatol* 23, 593
(1990): Tucker RM+, *J Antimicrob Chemother* 26, 561

# IVERMECTIN

**Trade name:** Stromectol (Merck)
**Indications:** Various infections caused by susceptible helmintic organisms
**Category:** Antihelmintic antibiotic
**Half-life:** 16–35 hours
**Clinically important, potentially hazardous interactions with:** alprazolam, barbiturates, benzodiazepines, diazepam, midazolam, valproic acid

### *Reactions*

## Skin

Bullous eruption
(1993): Burnham GM, *Trans R Soc Trop Med Hyg* 87, 313
Bullous pemphigoid
(2001): Trindade P, Natal, Brazil (personal communication)
Burning
(1999): Editorial, *Arch Dermatol* 135, 705
Dermatitis (sic)
(1999): Editorial, *Arch Dermatol* 135, 705
Edema
(1998): Jaramillo-Ayerbe F+, *Arch Dermatol* 134, 143
(1995): Darge K+, *Trop Med Parasitol* 46, 206 (arms and legs) (10%)
(1993): Burnham GM, *Trans R Soc Trop Med Hyg* 87, 313
(1992): Chijioke CP+, *Trans R Soc Trop Med Hyg* 86, 284
(1992): Collins RC+, *Am J Trop Med Hyg* 47, 156 (facial) (31.8%)
(1992): Zea-Flores R+, *Trans R Soc Trop Med Hyg* 86, 663 (53%)
(1991): Bryan RT+, *Lancet* 337, 304
(1991): Guderian RH+, *Lancet* 337, 188 (leg)
Exanthems
(1993): Burnham GM, *Trans R Soc Trop Med Hyg* 87, 313
(1991): Whitworth JAG+, *Lancet* 337, 625 (1–5%)
(1990): Ette EI+, *Drug Intell Clin Pharm* 24, 426 (34%)
Facial edema (1.2%)
(1998): Jaramillo-Ayerbe F+, *Arch Dermatol* 134, 143
(1993): Burnham GM, *Trans R Soc Trop Med Hyg* 87, 313
Peripheral edema
Pruritus (2.8%–27.5%)
(1998): Jaramillo-Ayerbe F+, *Arch Dermatol* 134, 143
(1995): Darge K+, *Trop Med Parasitol* 46, 206
(1993): Burnham GM, *Trans R Soc Trop Med Hyg* 87, 313
(1993): Kar SK+, *Acta Trop* 55, 21
(1992): Chijioke CP+, *Trans R Soc Trop Med Hyg* 86, 284 (71.2%)
(1992): Collins RC+, *Am J Trop Med Hyg* 47, 156 (34%)
(1991): Bryan RT+, *Lancet* 337, 304
(1991): Whitworth JAG+, *Lancet* 337, 625 (8%)
(1990): Ette EI+, *Drug Intell Clin Pharm* 24, 426 (9.6%)
(1989): Guderian RH+, *Eur J Epidemiol* 5, 294 (4%)
Pustular eruption
Rash (sic) (0.9%)
(1998): Jaramillo-Ayerbe F+, *Arch Dermatol* 134, 143
(1993): Kar SK+, *Acta Trop* 55, 21
(1991): Bryan RT+, *Lancet* 337, 304 (93%)
(1991): Guderian RH+, *Lancet* 337, 188
(1991): Whitworth JAG+, *Lancet* 337, 625 (8%)
(1989): Guderian RH+, *Eur J Epidemiol* 5, 294 (4%)
Urticaria (0.9–22.7%)

## Other

Myalgia
(1995): Darge K+, *Trop Med Parasitol* 46, 206 (20%)
(1993): Kar SK+, *Acta Trop* 55, 21
Tremors

# KANAMYCIN

**Trade name:** Kantrex (Apothecon)
**Other common trade names:** *Kanamicina; Kanamycine; Kanamytrex; Kanescin; Kannasyn; Randikan*
**Indications:** Various infections caused by susceptible organisms
**Category:** Aminoglycoside antibiotic
**Half-life:** 2–4 hours
**Clinically important, potentially hazardous interactions with:** aldesleukin, atracurium, bumetanide, doxacurium, ethacrynic acid, furosemide, methoxyflurane, non-depolarizing muscle relaxants, pancuronium, polypeptide antibiotics, rocuronium, succinylcholine, torsemide, vecuronium

### *Reactions*

#### Skin

Burning
Edema (>10%)
Erythema (<1%)
Exanthems
Photosensitivity (<1%)
Pruritus (1–10%)
Rash (sic) (1–10%)
Systemic eczematous contact dermatitis
(1986): Holdiness MR, *Contact Dermatitis* 15, 282
Urticaria

#### Other

Hypersensitivity
Injection-site irritation
Injection-site pain (<1%)
Paresthesias
Phlebitis
Pseudotumor cerebri
Sialorrhea (<1%)
Tremors

# KAVA

**Scientific name:** *Piper methysticum*
**Other common names:** Ava; Awa; Intoxicating Pepper; Kava Kava; Kawa Kawa; Kew; Sakau; Tonga
**Family:** Piperaceae
**Other uses:** Epilepsy, psychosis, depression, sedative, headaches, migraines, colds, tuberculosis, rheumatism, cystitis, vaginal prolapse, leprosy, otitis, abscesses
**Clinically important, potentially hazardous interactions with:** alprazolam

"Products containing herbal extracts of kava have been implicated in cases of severe liver toxicity in Germany and Switzerland" says the FDA letter. "Approximatley 25 reports of [liver] toxicity associated with the use of products containing kava extracts have been reported in these countries. Serious adverse effects include hepatitis, cirrhosis and liver failure. At least one patient required a liver transplant." In both Switzerland and Germany, regulatory agencies have prohibited the sale of kava extract-containing products. The FDA is investigating whether the use of kava-containing dietary supplements poses a similar health hazard in the U.S., according to the letter. The agency has received several reports of serious injury allegedly associated with the use of kava-containing dietry supplements

**Note:** liver toxicity is a possibility and Kava has been banned in several European countries

### *Reactions*

#### Skin

Dermopathy (pellagra-like syndrome)
Lymphocytic inflammation of the dermis (sic)
Photosensitivity
Pigmentation (yellow)
Pruritus
Rash (sic)
Scaly rash (sic)
Seborrheic dermatitis
(2000): Caro I, *Skin & Aging* 80
Xerosis

#### Hair

Hair – pigmentation

#### Nails

Nails – pigmentation

#### Other

Hypersensitivity
(2000): Schmidt P+, *Contact Dermatitis* 42(6), 363
Mouth numbness (sic)
Parkinsonism

**Note:** Kava was discovered by Captain Cook, who named the plant "intoxicating pepper." In the South Pacific, kava is a popular social drink, similar to alcohol in Western societies

# KETAMINE

**Trade name:** Ketalar (Parke-Davis)
**Other common trade names:** *Calypsol; Ketalin; Ketanest; Ketolar; Petar*
**Indications:** Induction of anesthesia
**Category:** Anesthetic; sedative hypnotic
**Half-life:** 2–3 hours

### *Reactions*

#### Skin

Erythema
Exanthems
Pruritus
(2001): Burstal R+, *Anaesth Intensive Care* 29(3), 246
(2001): Subramaniam K+, *J Clin Anesth* 13(5), 339 (with morphine)
Rash (sic) (1–10%)

#### Other

Injection-site erythema
Injection-site pain (1–10%)
Sialorrhea (<1%)
(2001): Green SM+, *Pediatr Emerg Care* 17(4), 244
Tremors (>10%)

# KETOCONAZOLE

**Trade name:** Nizoral (Janssen)
**Other common trade names:** *Aquarius; Fungarest; Fungoral; Ketoderm; Ketoisidin; Nazoltec*
**Indications:** Fungal infections
**Category:** Imidazole antifungal
**Half-life:** initial: 2 hours; terminal: 8 hours
**Clinically important, potentially hazardous interactions with: alcohol**, almotriptan, alprazolam, amphotericin B, anisindione, anticoagulants, benzodiazepines, bosentan, chlordiazepoxide, cimetidine, clorazepate, cyclosporine, dicumarol, didanosine, dofetilide, gastric alkanizers, HMG-CoA reductase inhibitors, imatinib, midazolam, nevirapine, non-sedating antihistamines, pimozide, proton pump inhibitors, rifampin, ritonavir, saquinavir, sildenafil, sucralfate, tacrolimus, triazolam, vinblastine, vincristine, warfarin

## *Reactions*

### Skin

Allergic reactions (sic)
(1983): van Ketel WG, *Contact Dermatitis* 9, 313
Angioedema
(1994): Gonzalez-Delgado P+, *Ann Allergy* 73, 326
(1994): Gupta AK+, *J Am Acad Dermatol* 30, 677 (passim)
(1983): van Dijke CPH+, *BMJ* 287, 1673
Chills (1–3%)
Contact dermatitis
(1993): Lodi A+, *Contact Dermatitis* 29, 97
(1993): Valsecchi R+, *Contact Dermatitis* 29, 162
(1992): Santucci B+, *Contact Dermatitis* 27, 274
Eczema (generalized)
(1989): Garcia-Bravo B+, *Contact Dermatitis* 21, 346
Exanthems
(1985): Bradsher RW+, *Ann Intern Med* 103, 872 (2%)
(1985): Study Group, *Ann Intern Med* 103, 861 (9.7%)
(1984): Ford GP+, *Br J Dermatol* 111, 603 (5%)
(1984): Kahana M+, *Arch Dermatol* 120, 837
(1983): Dismukes WE+, *Ann Intern Med* 98, 13 (4%)
(1983): Rand R+, *Arch Dermatol* 119, 97
(1982): Heel RC+, *Drugs* 23, 1 (0.7%)
Exfoliative dermatitis
(1984): Parent D+, *Ann Dermatol Venereol* (French) 111,339
(1983): Rand R+, *Arch Dermatol* 119, 97
Fixed eruption
(1994): Gupta AK+, *J Am Acad Dermatol* 30, 677 (passim)
(1988): Bharija SC+, *Int J Dermatol* 27, 278
Jarisch–Herxheimer reaction
Photosensitivity
(1988): Mohamed KN, *Clin Exp Dermatol* 13, 54
Pigmentation
(1992): Gallais V+, *Ann Dermatol Venereol* (French) 119, 471
(1990): Poizot-Martin I+, *Int Conf AIDS* 6, 357
(1985): Tucker WS+, *JAMA* 253, 2413
Pruritus (1.5%)
(1994): Gupta AK+, *J Am Acad Dermatol* 30, 677 (passim)
(1988): Mohamed KN, *Clin Exp Dermatol* 13, 54 (passim)
(1985): Study Group, *Ann Intern Med* 103, 861 (9.7%)
(1983): Rand R+, *Arch Dermatol* 119, 97 (1.5%)
(1982): Heel RC+, *Drugs* 23, 1 (1.7%)
Purpura
(1994): Gupta AK+, *J Am Acad Dermatol* 30, 677 (passim)
(1982): Heel RC+, *Drugs* 23, 1
Rash (sic) (1–3%)
(1994): Gupta AK+, *J Am Acad Dermatol* 30, 677 (passim)
Urticaria (1–3%)
(1994): Gupta AK+, *J Am Acad Dermatol* 30, 677 (passim)
(1985): Bradsher RW+, *Ann Intern Med* 103, 872 (2%)
Vasculitis
(1982): Heel RC+, *Drugs* 23, 1
Xerosis
(1994): Gupta AK+, *J Am Acad Dermatol* 30, 677 (passim)
(1985): Study Group, *Ann Intern Med* 103, 861

### Hair

Hair – alopecia
(1994): Gupta AK+, *J Am Acad Dermatol* 30, 677 (passim)
(1990): Venturoli S+, *J Clin Endocrinol Metab* 71, 335
(1985): Study Group, *Ann Intern Med* 103, 861 (3.7%)
(1982): Heel RC+, *Drugs* 23, 1 (0.2%)
Hair – trichoptilosis
(1993): Aljabre SH, *Int J Dermatol* 32, 150

### Nails

Nails – pigmentation
(1985): Dreessen K, *Z Hautkr* (German) 60, 679 (black longitudinal bands)

### Other

Anaphylactoid reactions
(1994): Gupta AK+, *J Am Acad Dermatol* 30, 677 (passim)
(1983): van Dijke CPH+, *BMJ* 287, 1673
Death
(2001): Duman D+, *Am J Med* 111(9), 737
Gingival bleeding
(1994): Gupta AK+, *J Am Acad Dermatol* 30, 677 (passim)
(1983): Dismukes WE+, *Ann Intern Med* 98, 13
Gingival hyperplasia
(1988): Veraldi S+, *Int J Dermatol* 27, 730
Gynecomastia (1–3%)
(1994): Gupta AK+, *J Am Acad Dermatol* 30, 677 (passim)
(1993): Thompson DF+, *Pharmacotherapy* 13, 37
(1982): Moncada B, *J Am Acad Dermatol* 7, 557
(1981): DeFelice R+, *Antimicrob Agents Chemo* 19, 1073
Hypersensitivity
(1994): Gonzalez-Delgado P+, *Ann Allergy* 73, 326
(1992): Verschueren GL+, *Contact Dermatitis* 26, 47
(1989): Garcia-Bravo B+, *Contact Dermatitis* 21, 346
Myopathy
(1991): Garty BZ+, *Am J Dis Child* 145, 970
Oral hyperpigmentation
(1991): Poizot-Martin I+, *Presse Med* (French) 20, 632
(1989): Langford A+, *Oral Surg Oral Med Oral Pathol* 67, 301 (in HIV-infected patients)
Oral lichenoid eruption
(1993): Ficarra G+, *Oral Surg Oral Med Oral Pathol* 76, 460
(1986): Markitziu A+, *Mykosen* (German) 29, 317
Oral mucosal lesions
(1994): Gupta AK+, *J Am Acad Dermatol* 30, 677 (passim)
(1985): Study Group, *Ann Intern Med* 103, 861 (1–5%)
(1983): Dismukes WE+, *Ann Intern Med* 98, 13 (2%)
Paresthesias
(1994): Gupta AK+, *J Am Acad Dermatol* 30, 677 (passim)
Tongue pigmentation
(1982): Heel RC+, *Drugs* 23, 1

# KETOPROFEN

**Trade names:** Orudis (Wyeth-Ayerst); Oruvail (Wyeth-Ayerst)
**Other common trade names:** *Alrheumat; Alrheumun; Aneol; Bi-Profenid; Gabrilen Retard; Keduril; Novo-Keto; Rhodis; Rhovail*
**Indications:** Arthritis
**Category:** Nonsteroidal anti-inflammatory (NSAID); analgesic
**Half-life:** 1.5–4 hours
**Clinically important, potentially hazardous interactions with:** aspirin, methotrexate, probenecid

## *Reactions*

### Skin

Allergic reactions (sic) (<1%)
Angioedema (<1%)
(1978): Frith P+, *Lancet* 2, 847
Bullous eruption (<1%)
Contact dermatitis
(2001): Preisz K+, *Orv Hetil* 142(51), 2841
(1998): Baudot S+, *Therapie* (French) 53, 137
(1997): *Lakartidningen* (Swedish) 94, 2664
(1996): Jeanmougin M+, *Ann Dermatol Venereol* (French) 123, 251
(1996): Pigatto P+, *Am J Contact Dermat* 7, 220
(1995): Gebhardt M+, *Z Rheumatol* (German) 54, 405
(1995): Navarro LA+, *Contact Dermatitis* 32, 181
(1994): Mastrolonardo M+, *Contact Dermatitis* 30, 110
(1994): Oh VM, *BMJ* 309, 512
(1993): Ophaswongse S+, *Contact Dermatitis* 29, 57
(1990): Mozzanica N+, *Contact Dermatitis* 23, 336
(1990): Tosti A+, *Contact Dermatitis* 23, 112
(1990): Valsecchi R+, *Contact Dermatitis* 21, 345
(1989): Lanzarini M+, *Contact Dermatitis* 21, 51
(1989): Romaguera C+, *Contact Dermatitis* 20, 310
(1987): Mozzanica N, *Contact Dermatitis* 17, 325
(1985): Camarasa JG, *Contact Dermatitis* 12, 121
(1983): Angelini G+, *Contact Dermatitis* 9, 234
(1983): Valsecchi R+, *Contact Dermatitis* 9, 163
Cutaneous side effects (sic)
(1989): Le-Loet X, *Scand J Rheumatol* Suppl 83, 21 (0.7%)
Diaphoresis (<1%)
(1989): Roth DE+, *Med Clin North Am* 73, 1275
Eczematous eruption (sic) (<1%)
(1990): Tosti A+, *Contact Dermatitis* 23, 112
(1987): Mozzanica N, *Contact Dermatitis* 17, 325
Erythema multiforme (<1%)
Exanthems
(1975): Hingorani K+, *Curr Med Res Opin* 3, 407
Exfoliative dermatitis (<1%)
Facial edema (<1%)
Hot flashes (<1%)
Pemphigus (localized)
(2001): Kanitakis J+, *Acta Derm Venereol* 81(4), 304
Peripheral edema (1–3%)
Photocontact dermatitis
(2001): Milpied-Homsi B, *Presse Med* 30(12), 605 (from gel)
(2001): Sugiyama M+, *Am J Contact Dermat* 12(3), 180
(2000): Matsushita T+, *Photodermatol Photoimmunol Photomed* 17(1), 26 (from gel) (5 cases)
(1998): Baudot S+, *Therapie* (French) 53, 137
(1998): Le Coz CJ+, *Contact Dermatitis* 38, 245
(1997): Bastien M+, *Ann Dermatol Venereol* (French) 124, 523 (5 cases)
(1997): Leroy D+, *Photodermatol Photoimmunol Photomed* 13, 93
(1997): Mirande-Romero A+, *Contact Dermatitis* 37, 242 (connubial)
(1996): Jeanmougin M+, *Ann Dermatol Venereol* (French) 123, 251
(1995): Nabeya R+, *Contact Dermatitis* 32, 52
(1993): Ophaswongse S+, *Contact Dermatitis* 29, 57 (phototoxic and photoallergic)
(1992): Serrano G+, *J Am Acad Dermatol* 27, 204 (passim)
(1990): Black AK+, *Br J Dermatol* 123, 277
(1990): Mozzanica N+, *Contact Dermatitis* 23, 336
(1989): Roth DE+, *Med Clin North Am* 73, 1275
(1987): Cusano F+, *Contact Dermatitis* 17, 108
(1987): Cusano F+, *Contact Dermatitis* 27, 50
(1985): Alomar A, *Contact Dermatitis* 12, 112
(1985): Alomar A, *Contact Dermatitis* 12, 112
Photosensitivity (<1%)
Pigmentation (<1%)
Pruritus (1–10%)
(1975): Hingorani K+, *Curr Med Res Opin* 3, 407
Psoriasis
(1992): Shelley WB+, *Cutis* 51, 23 (observation)
Purpura (<1%)
(1989): Roth DE+, *Med Clin North Am* 73, 1275
Rash (sic) (>10%)
Stevens–Johnson syndrome (<1%)
Toxic epidermal necrolysis (<1%)
(1995): Tijhuis GJ+, *Dermatology* 190, 176
Urticaria (<1%)
(1978): Frith P+, *Lancet* 2, 847

### Hair

Hair – alopecia (<1%)
(1989): Roth DE+, *Med Clin North Am* 73, 1275

### Nails

Nails – onycholysis (<1%)
(1989): Roth DE+, *Med Clin North Am* 73, 1275

### Other

Acute intermittent porphyria
Anaphylactoid reactions (<1%)
(1985): O'Brien WM+, *J Rheumatol* 12, 13
(1978): Frith P+, *Lancet* 2, 847
Aphthous stomatitis
Dysgeusia (<1%)
Gynecomastia (<1%)
Myalgia (<1%)
Oral mucosal lesions
(1975): Hingorani K+, *Curr Med Res Opin* 3, 407
Oral mucosal numbness
(2001): Passali D+, *Clin Ther* 23(9), 1508
Oral mucosal paresthesias
(2001): Passali D+, *Clin Ther* 23(9), 1508
Paresthesias (<1%)
Pseudolymphoma
(2001): Werth V, *Dermatology Times* 18
Pseudoporphyria
(1992): Breathnach SM+, *Adverse Drug Reactions and the Skin* Blackwell, Oxford (passim)
(1987): Taylor BJ+, *N Z Med J* 100, 322
Sialorrhea (<1%)
Stomatitis (<1%)
Tinnitus
Xerostomia (<1%)
(2001): Passali D+, *Clin Ther* 23(9), 1508

# KETOROLAC

**Trade names:** Acular (Allergan); Toradol (Roche)
**Other common trade names:** *Dolac; Kelac; Ketonic; Nodine; Topadol; Torolac; Torvin*
**Indications:** Pain
**Category:** Nonsteroidal anti-inflammatory (NSAID)
**Half-life:** 2–8 hours
**Clinically important, potentially hazardous interactions with:** aspirin, methotrexate, probenecid, salicylates

### *Reactions*

## Skin

Allergic reactions (sic)
(2000): Reinhart DI, *Drug Saf* 22, 487
Angioedema
(1994): Shapiro N, *J Oral Maxillofac Surg* 52, 626
Cutaneous side effects (sic) (0.7%)
(1990): Buckley MMT+, *Drugs* 39, 86
Dermatitis (sic) (3–9%)
Diaphoresis (1–10%)
(1990): Buckley MMT+, *Drugs* 39, 86
Edema (3–9%)
Exanthems (3–9%)
(1990): Buckley MMT+, *Drugs* 39, 86
Excoriated papules
(1994): Shelley WB+, *Cutis* 53, 235 (observation)
Exfoliative dermatitis (<1%)
Flushing (<1%)
Pruritus (3–9%)
Purpura (>1%)
(1994): Shelley WB+, *Cutis* 54, 149 (palpable) (observation)
Rash (sic) (>1%)
Stevens–Johnson syndrome (<1%)
Toxic epidermal necrolysis (<1%)
Urticaria
(1990): Buckley MMT+, *Drugs* 39, 86

## Other

Anaphylactoid reactions (<1%)
Aphthous stomatitis (<1%)
(1990): Buckley MMT+, *Drugs* 39, 86
Dysgeusia
Hypersensitivity
(2000): Reinhart DI, *Drug Saf* 22, 487
Injection-site pain (1–10%)
Myalgia
Paresthesias
Stinging (from topical)
(2000): Shiuey Y+, *Ophthalmology* 107, 1512
Stomatitis (>1%)
Tinnitus
Tongue edema (<1%)
Xerostomia
(1990): Buckley MMT+, *Drugs* 39, 86

# KETOTIFEN

**Trade name:** Zaditor (CIBA Vision)
**Indications:** Allergic conjunctivitis
**Category:** Ophthalmic antihistamine $H_1$-blocker
**Half-life:** 22 hours

### *Reactions*

## Skin

Allergic reactions (sic) (1–10%)
Burning (1–10%)
Photosensitivity
Pityriasis rosea
(1985): Wolf R+, *Dermatologica* 171–355
Pruritus (1–10%)
Rash (sic) (1–10%)
Stinging (1–10%)

## Other

Xerophthalmia (1–10%)

# LABETALOL

**Trade names:** Normodyne (Schering); Normozide; Trandate (Faro)
**Other common trade names:** *Abetol; Amipress; Hybloc; Ipolab; Labrocol; Presolol; Salmagne*
**Indications:** Hypertension
**Category:** Alpha-adrenergic and beta-adrenergic blocker; antihypertensive
**Half-life:** 3–8 hours

Normozide is labetalol and hydrochlorothiazide

**Note:** Cutaneous side effects of beta-receptor blockaders are clinically polymorphous. They apparently appear after several months of continuous therapy. Atypical psoriasiform, lichen planus-like, and eczematous chronic rashes are mainly observed. (1983): Hödl St, *Z Hautkr* (German) 1:58, 17

### *Reactions*

## Skin

Angioedema
(1986): Ferree CE, *Ann Intern Med* 104, 729
Contact dermatitis
(1990): Bause GS+, *Contact Dermatitis* 23, 51
Cutaneous side effects (sic) (5.5%)
(1982): Waal-Manning HJ+, *Br J Clin Pharmacol* 13 (Suppl 1), 65S
(1978): No Author, *BMJ* 1, 987
Diaphoresis (<1%)
Eczematous eruption (sic)
Edema (<2%)
Exanthems
(1989): Goa KL+, *Drugs* 37, 583
(1984): Prichard BNC, *Drugs* 28 (Suppl 2), 51 (1–5%)
(1978): Branford WA+, *Practitioner* 221, 765
(1978): Finlay AY+, *BMJ* 1, 987
Exfoliative dermatitis
Facial edema
Flushing
(1978): Harris C, *Curr Med Res Opin* 5, 618 (19%)
Lichen planus (bullous)
(1978): Gange RW+, *BMJ* 1, 816
Lichenoid eruption
(1982): Bertani E+, *G Ital Dermatol Venereol* (Italian) 117, 229
(1980): Staughton R+, *Lancet* 2, 581
(1978): Branford WA+, *Practitioner* 221, 765
(1978): Finlay AY+, *BMJ* 1, 987
(1978): Savage RL+, *BMJ* 1, 987
Lupus erythematosus
(1984): Prichard BNC, *Drugs* 28 (Suppl 2), 51
(1981): Brown RC+, *Postgrad Med J* 57, 189
(1979): Griffiths ID+, *BMJ* 2, 496
Peripheral edema
Pigmentation (slate-gray)
(1978): Branford WA+, *Practitioner* 221, 765
Pityriasis rubra pilaris
(1978): Branford WA+, *Practitioner* 221, 765
(1978): Finlay AY+, *BMJ* 1, 987
Pruritus (1–10%)
(1984): Prichard BNC, *Drugs* 28 (Suppl 2), 51 (1–5%)
(1978): Finlay AY+, *BMJ* 1, 987
(1978): Harris C, *Curr Med Res Opin* 5, 618 (7.5%)
Psoriasis (exacerbation)
(1987): Savola J+, *BMJ* 295, 637 (induction)
(1986): Czernielewski J+, *Lancet* 1, 808
(1984): Arntzen N+, *Acta Derm Venereol* (Stockh) 64, 346
Purpura
(1978): Harris C, *Curr Med Res Opin* 5, 618
Rash (sic) (<1%)
Raynaud's phenomenon (<1%)
Urticaria
(1986): Ferree CE, *Ann Intern Med* 104, 729
Xerosis

## Hair

Hair – alopecia (reversible)
(1978): Finlay AY+, *BMJ* 1, 987

## Other

Anaphylactoid reactions
(1990): Bause GS+, *Contact Dermatitis* 23, 51
(1986): Ferree CE, *Ann Intern Med* 104, 729
Dysgeusia (1–10%)
(2000): Zervakis J+, *Physiol Behav* 68, 405
Hypersensitivity
Hypesthesia (1%)
Myopathy
(1989): Willis J+, *Ann Neurology* 26, 456
(1981): Teicher A+, *BMJ* 282, 1824
(1977): Bolli P+, *N Z Med J* 86, 557
(1976): Andersson O+, *Br J Clin Pharmacol* 3, 757
Paresthesias (7%)
(1984): Prichard BNC, *Drugs* 28 (Suppl 2), 51 (scalp) (6%)
(1977): Bailey RR, *Lancet* 2, 720 (tingling of scalp)
Peyronie's disease
(1979): Kristensen BO, *Acta Med Scand* 206, 511
Priapism
Scalp tingling
(1979): Coulter DM, *N Z Med J* 90, 397
(1977): Bailey RR, *Lancet* 2, 720
(1977): Hua AS+, *Lancet* 2, 295
Xerostomia

# LAMIVUDINE

**Synonym:** 3TC
**Trade names:** Combivir (GSK); Epivir (GSK)
**Indications:** HIV progression
**Category:** Antiretroviral; nucleoside reverse transcriptase inhibitor (NRTI)
**Half-life:** 5–7 hours

Combivir is lamivudine and zidovudine

### *Reactions*

## Skin

Angioedema
(1996): Kainer MA+, *Lancet* 348, 1519
Buffalo hump
(2000): Carr A+, *AIDS* 14, F25
Chills (1–10%)
Contact dermatitis
(2000): Smith KJ+, *Cutis* 65, 227
Exanthems
Pruritus
(2000): Smith KJ+, *Cutis* 65, 227
Rash (sic) (9%)
Urticaria
(1996): Kainer MA+, *Lancet* 348, 1519

## Hair

Hair – alopecia

(1994): Fong IW, *Lancet* 344, 1702

### Nails

Nails – ingrown toenails
(2001): James CW+, *Ann Pharmacother* 35(7), 881 (with ritonavir)
Nails – paronychia
(1998): Zerboni R+, *Lancet* 351, 1256

### Other

Anaphylactoid reactions
(1996): Kainer MA+, *Lancet* 348(9040), 1519
Gynecomastia
(2001): Manfredi R+, *Ann Pharmacother* 35(4), 438 (with savudine) (3 cases)
Myalgia (8%)
Paresthesias (>10%)
Rhabdomyolysis
(1997): Mendila M+, *Dtsch Med Wochenschr* 122(33), 1003

# LAMOTRIGINE

**Synonyms:** BW-430C; LTG
**Trade name:** Lamictal (GSK)
**Indications:** Epilepsy
**Category:** Anticonvulsant
**Half-life:** 24 hours

## *Reactions*

### Skin

Acne (1.3%)
Acute generalized exanthematous pustulosis (AGEP)
(2001): Wensween CA+, *Ned Tijdschr Geneeskd* 145(31), 1525
Angioedema (1–10%)
(2001): Hebert AA+, *J Clin Psychiatry* 62(suppl 14), 22 (~1%)
Anticonvulsant hypersensitivity syndrome
(2002): Metin A+, *World Congress Dermatol* Poster, 0116
Bullous eruption
(1997): Australian Adverse Drug Reactions Bulletin 16(1), February
Diaphoresis (<1%)
Ecchymoses (<1%)
Eczema (sic) (<1%)
Erythema (<1%)
(2001): Hebert AA+, *J Clin Psychiatry* 62(suppl 14), 22 (~10%)
Erythema multiforme
(1997): Australian Adverse Drug Reactions Bulletin 16(1), February
Exanthems (1–10%)
(2001): Hebert AA+, *J Clin Psychiatry* 62(suppl 14), 22 (~10%)
(1997): Australian Adverse Drug Reactions Bulletin 16(1), February
(1997): Hyson C+, *Can J Neurol Sci* 24, 245
(1996): Dooley J+, *Neurology* 46, 240 (7%)
(1996): Li LM+, *Arq Neuropsiquiatr* 54, 47
(1995): Brodie MJ, *Can J Neurol Sci* 23, S6 (<5%)
(1995): Fitton A+, *Drugs* 50, 691
(1995): Makin AJ+, *BMJ* 311, 292
(1995): Tavernor SJ+, *Seizure* 4, 67
(1994): Tavernor SJ+, *Epilepsia* 35, 72
Facial edema (<1%)
Fixed eruption
(2001): Hsiao C-J+, *Br J Dermatol* 144, 1289
Flu-like syndrome (sic) (7%)
Flushing (<1%)
Hot flashes (1–10%)
Lupus erythematosus
(1997): Mackay FJ+, *Epilepsia* 38, 881
Petechiae (<1%)
Photosensitivity
(1999): Borowitz SM, *Pediatric Pharmacotherapy* 5, 3
(1999): Bozikas V+, *Am J Psychiatry* 156, 2015
Pruritus (3.1%)
(2001): Hebert AA+, *J Clin Psychiatry* 62(suppl 14), 22 (~1%)
Rash (sic) (10%)
(2002): Anderson GD, *Epilepsia* 43(Suppl 3), 53 (10–20%)
(2001): Eisenberg E+, *Neurology* 57, 505
(2000): Besag FM+, *Seizure* 9, 282
(2000): Husain AM+, *South Med J* 93, 335
(2000): Jurynczyk J+, *Neurol Neurochir Pol* (Polish) 34, 43
(2000): Messenheimer JA+, *Drug Saf* 22, 303
(2000): Messenheimer JA+, *Epilepsia* 41, 488
(2000): Parmeggiani L+, *J Child Neurol* 15, 15
(1999): Faught E+, *Epilepsia* 40, 1135
(1999): Gericke CA+, *Epileptic Disord* 1, 159
(1999): Guberman AH+, *Epilepsia* 40, 985
(1999): Matsuo F, *Epilepsia* 40, S30
(1998): Buzan RD+, *J Clin Psychiatry* 59, 87 (re-challenged)
(1998): Messenheimer JA, *Can J Neurol Sci* 25, S14
(1997): Mackay FJ+, *Epilepsia* 38, 881
Stevens–Johnson syndrome (1–10%)
(2001): Hebert AA+, *J Clin Psychiatry* 62(suppl 14), 22 (~10%)
(2000): Popescu C, Bucharest, Romania (from Internet) (observation)
(2000): Yalcin B+, *J Am Acad Dermatol* 43, 898 (with valproic acid)
(1999): Bocquet H+, *Ann Dermatol Venereol* (French) 126, 46
(1999): Borowitz SM, *Pediatric Pharmacotherapy* 5, 3
(1999): Guberman AH+, *Epilepsia* 40, 985
(1999): Rzany B+, *Lancet* 353, 2190
(1998): *Drugs and Therapy Perspectives* 11, 11
(1998): Schlienger RG+, *Epilepsia* 39, S22
(1998): Zachariae CO+, *Ugeskr Laeger* (Danish) 160, 6656
(1997): Australian Adverse Drug Reactions Bulletin 16(1), February
(1997): Mackay FJ+, *Epilepsia* 38, 881
(1997): Sachs B+, *Dermatology* 195, 60
(1996): Dooley J+, *Neurology* 46, 240 (7%)
(1995): Campistol J+, *Rev Neurol* (Spanish) 23, 1236
(1995): Duval X+, *Lancet* 345, 1301
Toxic epidermal necrolysis
(2002): Wirtzer A, Sherman Oaks, CA (from Internet) (observation)
(2001): Hebert AA+, *J Clin Psychiatry* 62(suppl 14), 22 (~1%)
(2001): Wensween CA+, *Ned Tijdschr Geneeskd* 145(31), 1525
(2000): Bhushan M+, *Clin Exp Dermatol* 25, 349
(2000): Fernandez-Calvo C+, *Rev Neurol* 31(12), 1162
(1999): Bocquet H+, *Ann Dermatol Venereol* (French) 126, 46
(1999): Borowitz SM, *Pediatric Pharmacotherapy* 5, 3
(1999): *Actas Dermosifiliogr* (Spanish) 90, 612
(1999): Rzany B+, *Lancet* 353, 2190
(1998): *Drugs and Therapy Perspectives* 11, 11
(1998): Page RL+, *Pharmacotherapy* 18, 392 (fatal)
(1998): Schlienger RG+, *Epilepsia* 39, S22
(1998): Zachariae CO+, *Ugeskr Laeger* (Danish) 160, 6656
(1997): Australian Adverse Drug Reactions Bulletin 16(1), February
(1997): Chaffin JJ+, *Ann Pharmacother* 31, 720 (suspected)
(1997): Fogh K+, *Seizure* 6, 63
(1997): Vukelic D+, *Dermatology* 195, 307
(1996): Sachs B+, *Lancet* 348, 1597
(1996): Sullivan JR+, *Australas J Dermatol* 37, 208
(1996): Wadelius M+, *Lancet* 348, 1041
(1995): Duval X+, *Lancet* 345, 1301
(1995): Sterker M+, *Int J Clin Pharmacol Ther* 33, 595

Urticaria (<1%)
Xerosis (<1%)

### Hair

Hair – alopecia (1.3%)
Hair – hirsutism (<1%)

### Other

Anaphylactoid reactions
(1999): Borowitz SM, *Pediatric Pharmacotherapy* 5, 3
Death
Dysgeusia (<1%)
(2001): Avoni P+, *Neurology* 57(8), 1521 (3 cases)
Foetor ex ore (halitosis) (<1%)
Gingival hyperplasia (<1%)
Gingivitis (<1%)
Hypersensitivity (1–10%)
(2001): Hebert AA+, *J Clin Psychiatry* 62(suppl 14), 22
(2001): Lalanza J+, *Aten Primaria* 28(3), 213
(2000): Schaub N+, *Allergy* 55, 191
(1999): Borowitz SM, *Pediatric Pharmacotherapy* 5, 3
(1999): Brown TS+, *Pediatr Dermatology* 16, 46
(1999): Guberman AH+, *Epilepsia* 40, 985
(1999): Knowles SR+, *Drug Safety* 21, 489
(1999): Mylonakis E+, *Ann Pharmacol* 33, 557
(1998): Chapman MS+, *Br J Dermatol* 138, 710
(1998): Iannetti P+, *Epilepsia* 39, 502
(1998): Tugendhaft P+, *J Am Acad Dermatol* 38, 785 (phenytoin-like)
(1997): Jones D+, *J Am Acad Dermatol* 36, 1016 (phenytoin-like)
Hypesthesia (<1%)
Myalgia (>1%)
Oral ulceration (<1%)
Paresthesias (>1%)
Porphyria
(1996): Gregersen H+, *Ugeskr Laeger* (Danish) 158, 4091
Pseudolymphoma
(1998): Pathak P+, *Neurology* 50, 1509
Sialorrhea (<1%)
Stomatitis (<1%)
Tic disorder
(2000): Sotero de Menezes MA+, *Epilepsia* 41, 862
Tremors
(2000): Messenheimer JA+, *Drug Saf* 22, 303
Vaginal candidiasis (<1%)
Vaginitis (4.1%)
Xerostomia (1%)

## LANSOPRAZOLE

**Trade name:** Prevacid (TAP)
**Indications:** Active duodenal ulcer
**Category:** Gastric acid secretion (proton pump) inhibitor
**Half-life:** 2 hours
**Clinically important, potentially hazardous interactions with:** sucralfate

#### *Reactions*

### Skin

Acne (<1%)
Acute generalized exanthematous pustulosis (AGEP)
(1997): Dewerdt S+, *Acta Derm Venereol* (Stockh) 77, 250
Candidiasis (<1%)
Contact dermatitis
(2001): Vilaplana J+, *Contact Dermatitis* 44, 47 (with omeprazole)
Diaphoresis
(2000): Natsch S+, *Ann Pharmacother* 34, 474
Edema (<1%)
Erythroderma
(1999): Cockayne SE+, *Br J Dermatol* 141, 173
Exanthems
(1996): Blumenthal HL, Beachwood, OH (personal case) (observation)
(1996): Litt JZ, Beachwood, OH (personal case) (observation)
Facial edema
(2000): Natsch S+, *Ann Pharmacother* 34, 474
Lichenoid eruption
(2000): Bong JL+, *BMJ* 320, 283
Peripheral edema
(2001): Brunner G+, *Dig Dis Sci* 46(5), 993
Pruritus (3–10%)
(2000): Natsch S+, *Ann Pharmacother* 34, 474
Rash (sic) (3–10%)
Urticaria (<1%)
(2000): Gerson LB+, *Aliment Pharmacol* 14, 397 (1%)
(2000): Natsch S+, *Ann Pharmacother* 34, 474

### Hair

Hair – alopecia (<1%)
(2000): Litt JZ, Beachwood, OH (personal case) (observation)

### Other

Anaphylactoid reactions
(2000): Natsch S+, *Ann Pharmacother* 34, 474
Black tongue
(1997): Greco S+, *Ann Pharmacother* 31, 1548
Dysgeusia (<1%)
Foetor ex ore (halitosis) (<1%)
Glossitis
(1997): Greco S+, *Ann Pharmacother* 31, 1548
Gynecomastia (<1%)
(2000): Comas A+, *Med Clin (Barc)* (Spanish) 114, 397
Hypersensitivity
(1999): Baudot S, *Therapie* (French) 54, 491
Mastodynia (<1%)
Myalgia (<1%)
(1998): Smith JD+, *Ann Pharmacother* 32, 196 (with eosinophilia)
Paresthesias (<1%)
Stomatitis (<1%)
(1997): Greco S+, *Ann Pharmacother* 31, 1548
Xerostomia (<1%)

## LATANOPROST

**Trade name:** Xalatan (Pharmacia & Upjohn)
**Indications:** Glaucoma
**Category:** Prostaglandin ophthalmic; anti-glaucoma
**Half-life:** 17 minutes

#### *Reactions*

### Skin

Allergic reactions (sic) (1.1%)
Blepharitis (0.4%)
Ecchymoses (0.2%)
Eczema (sic) (0.7%)
Eyelid burning (1.1%)
Eyelid edema (1–4%)

(2001): Stewart WC+, *Am J Ophthalmol* 131(5), 631
Eyelid erythema (1–4%)
Eyelid pain (0.4%)
Eyelid pigment changes
(2001): Wand M+, *Arch Ophthalmol* 119(4), 614
Eyelid pigmentation
(2000): Kook MS+, *Am J Ophthalmol* 129, 804
Eyelid pruritus (1.7%)
Eyelid stinging (0.4%)
Facial rash
(1997): Rowe JA+, *Am J Ophthalmol* 124, 683
Herpes simplex (ocular)
(2001): Morales J+, *Am J Ophthalmol* 132(1), 114 (2 cases)
Local irritation
(1999): Hejkal TW+, *Semin Ophthalmol* 14, 114
Ocular erythema
(2001): Aung T+, *Am J Phthalmol* 131(5), 636
(2001): Stewart WC+, *Am J Ophthalmol* 131(5), 631
Ocular irritation
(2001): Aung T+, *Am J Ophthalmol* 131(5), 636
Pruritus (0.2%)
(1997): Crowe MA, Puyallup, WA (from Internet) (observation)
Rash (sic) (1–10%)

### Hair

Hair – eyelash hyperpigmentation
(1999): Hejkal TW+, *Semin Ophthalmol* 14, 114
(1998): Reynolds A+, *Eye* 12, 741
(1997): Johnstone MA, *Am J Ophthalmol* 124, 544
(1997): Wand M, *Arch Ophthalmol* 115, 1206
Hair – hypertrichosis
(2001): Demitsu T+, *J Am Acad Dermatol* 44, 721 (eyelashes) (77%)
(2001): Strober BE+, *Cutis* 67, 109 (eyelashes)
(1997): Johnstone MA, *Am J Ophthalmol* 124, 544

### Other

Conjuctival hyperemia
(2001): DuBiner H+, *Surv Opthalmol* 45(Suppl 4), S353–60
(2001): Gandolfi S+, *Adv Ther* 18(3), 110
Gynecomastia (0.2%)
Iris pigmentation increased
(2001): Netland PA+, *Am J Ophthalmol* 132(4), 472 (5.2%)
(2000): Alm A+, *Acta Ophthalmol Scand* 78, 71
(2000): Camras CB+, *J Glaucoma* 9, 95
(1999): Hejkal TW+, *Semin Ophthalmol* 14, 114
(1997): Bito LAZ, *Surv Ophthalmol* 41(Suppl 2), S1
(1997): Wistrand JP+, *Surv Ophthalmol* 41(Suppl 2), S129
Myalgia (1–10%)

# LAVENDER

**Scientific names:** *Lavandula angustifolia; Lavandula dentata; Lavandula latifolia; Lavandula pubescens; Lavandula spica; Lavandula vera*
**Other common names:** Alhucema; Common Lavender; English Lavender; French Lavender; Garden Lavender; Spanish Lavender; Spike Lavender; True Lavender
**Family:** Lamiaceae
**Purported indications:** Restlessness, insomnia, nervous stomach, loss of appetite
**Other uses:** Flatulence, colic spasms, giddiness, nervous headaches, migraines, toothaches, sprains, neuralgia, rheumatism, acne, pimples, sores, nausea and vomiting. Lavender products are used as flavor components, in pharmaceuticals, as fragrance ingredients in soaps and cosmetics, as an insect repellent

## *Reactions*

### Skin

Contact dermatitis
(1999): Coulson IH+, *Contact Dermatitis* 41(2), 111

# LEFLUNOMIDE

**Trade name:** Arava (Aventis)
**Indications:** Rheumatoid arthritis
**Category:** Immunosuppressant; antimetabolite
**Half-life:** 14–15 days

## *Reactions*

### Skin

Acne (1–10%)
Allergic reactions (sic) (2%)
(2000): Smolen JS+, *Rheumatology* (Oxford) 39 (Suppl 1), 48
(1999): Goldenberg MM, *Clin Ther* 21, 1837
(1997): Silva Junior HT+, *Am J Med Sci* 313, 289
(1995): Mladenovic V+, *Arthritis Rheum* 38, 1595
Bullous eruption
(2000): Lepine G, Rock Hill, SC, (from Internet) (observation) (occurred 6 months after starting drug)
Dermatitis (sic) (1–10%)
Diaphoresis (1–10%)
Eczema (sic) (2%)
Herpes infection (sic) (1–10%)
Infections (sic) (4%)
(2001): Cohen S+, *Arthritis Rheum* 44(9), 1984
Nodule (sic) (1–10%)
Peripheral edema (1–10%)
Pigmentation (1–10%)
Pruritus (4%)
Purpura (1–10%)
Rash (sic) (10%)
(2002): Sanders S+, *Am J Med Sci* 323(4), 190
(2001): Cohen S+, *Arthritis Rheum* 44(9), 1984
(2000): Emery P+, *Rheumatology* (Oxford) 39, 655
(2000): Nousari HC+, *Arch Dermatol* 136, 1204
(1999): Goldenberg MM, *Clin Ther* 21, 1837
(1999): Smolen JS+, *Lancet* 353, 259
(1997): Silva Junior HT+, *Am J Med Sci* 313, 289
(1995): Mladenovic V+, *Arthritis Rheum* 38, 1595
Squamous cell carcinoma

(2002): Shelly J (from Internet) (observation)
Stevens–Johnson syndrome
Subcutaneous nodule (sic) (1–10%)
Toxic epidermal necrolysis
Ulcer (1–10%)
Urticaria (<1%)
Vasculitis (1–10%)
Xerosis (2%)

### Hair

Hair – alopecia (10%)
(2002): Sanders S+, *Am J Med Sci* 323(4), 190
(2001): Cohen S+, *Arthritis Rheum* 44(9), 1984
(2000): Emery P+, *Rheumatology* (Oxford) 39, 655
(2000): Nousari HC+, *Arch Dermatol* 136, 1204
(2000): Smolen JS+, *Rheumatology* (Oxford) 39 (Suppl 1), 48
(1999): Goldenberg MM, *Clin Ther* 21, 1837
(1999): Smolen JS+, *Lancet* 353, 259 (8%)
(1997): Silva Junior HT+, *Am J Med Sci* 313, 289
(1995): Mladenovic V+, *Arthritis Rheum* 38, 1595
Hair – discoloration (1–10%)

### Nails

Nails – disorder (sic) (1–10%)

### Other

Anaphylactoid reactions (<1%)
Dysgeusia (1–10%)
Gingivitis (1–10%)
Myalgia (1–10%)
Oral candidiasis (3%)
Oral ulceration (3%)
Paresthesias (2%)
Stomatitis (3%)
Tendon rupture (1–10%)
Tooth disorder (sic) (1–10%)
Vaginal candidiasis (1–10%)
Xerostomia (1–10%)

## LETROZOLE

**Trade name:** Femara (Novartis)
**Indications:** Breast cancer
**Category:** Nonsteroidal aromatase inhibitor; antineoplastic
**Half-life:** ~2 days

#### *Reactions*

### Skin

Diaphoresis (<5%)
Exanthems (5%)
Hot flashes (6%)
Pruritus (2%)
Psoriasis (5%)
Rash (sic) (1–10%)
Vesicular eruptions (5%)

### Hair

Hair – alopecia (<5%)

## LEUCOVORIN

**Synonyms:** citrovorum factor; folinic acid
**Trade name:** Leucovorin
**Other common trade names:** *Antrex; Citrec; Lederfolin; Refolinin; Rescufolin; Rescuvolin*
**Indications:** Overdose of methotrexate
**Category:** Antidote; methotrexate toxicity prophylactic agent
**Half-life:** 15 minutes

#### *Reactions*

### Skin

Erythema (<1%)
Pruritus (<1%)
Rash (sic) (<1%)
Urticaria (<1%)

### Hair

Hair – alopecia
(2001): Madnani N, Mumbai, India (from Internet) (observation)

### Other

Anaphylactoid reactions (<1%)
Hypersensitivity

## LEUPROLIDE

**Synonym:** leuprorelin acetate
**Trade name:** Lupron (TAP)
**Other common trade names:** *Carcinil; Enantone; Lucrin; Procren Depot; Procrin; Tapros*
**Indications:** Prostate carcinoma, endometriosis
**Category:** Gonadotropin-releasing hormone
**Half-life:** 3–4 hours

#### *Reactions*

### Skin

Acne
Dermatitis (sic) (5%)
Diaphoresis
Ecchymoses (<5%)
Edema (1–10%)
Exanthems
Flushing
(1989): Crawford ED+, *N Engl J Med* 321, 419 (61%)
Hot flashes
(1993): Bressler LR+, *Ann Pharmacother* 27, 182
Lupus erythematosus
(1994): Fritzler MJ, *Lupus* 3, 455
Peripheral edema (12%)
(1989): Crawford ED+, *N Engl J Med* 321, 419 (4%)
Photosensitivity
Pigmentation (<5%)
Pruritus (<5%)
Purpura (<1%)
Rash (sic) (1–10%)
Stickiness
(2001): Sander HM, (Austin, TX ) (from Internet) (observation)
Urticaria
Xerosis (<5%)

### Hair
Hair – alopecia (<5%)
Hair – growth (sic) (<1%)

### Other
Dysgeusia (<5%)
Gynecomastia (7%)
Injection-site inflammation
(1989): Crawford ED+, *N Engl J Med* 321, 419 (2.1%)
Injection-site pruritus
(1989): Crawford ED+, *N Engl J Med* 321, 419 (2.1%)
Injection-site reactions
(2001): Fluker M+, *Fertil Steril* 75(1), 38 (24.4%)
Mastodynia (7%)
Myalgia (3%)
Paresthesias (<5%)
Thrombophlebitis (2%)
Vaginitis

# LEVALBUTEROL

**Synonym:** R-albuterol
**Trade name:** Xopenex (Sepracor)
**Indications:** Bronchospasm
**Category:** Beta-2 agonist
**Half-life:** 3.3–4.0 hours

## *Reactions*

### Skin
Chills (<2%)
Diaphoresis (<2%)
Flu-like syndrome (1–4%)
Ocular pruritus (<2%)
Viral infection (7–12%)

### Other
Cough (1–4%)
Hypersensitivity
Hypesthesia (<2%)
Leg cramps (~3%)
Myalgia (<2%)
Pain (1–3%)
Paresthesias (<2%)
Tremors (~7%)

# LEVAMISOLE

**Trade name:** Ergamisol (Janssen)
**Other common trade names:** *Ascaridil; Decaris; Detrax 40; Ketrax; Solaskil; Termizole*
**Indications:** Susceptible helmintic organism infections, colorectal carcinoma
**Category:** Antineoplastic adjunct; immune modulator and anthelmintic
**Half-life:** 2–6 hours
**Clinically important, potentially hazardous interactions with: alcohol**, aldesleukin

## *Reactions*

### Skin
Angioedema (<1%)
(1978): Multiple Authors, *Lancet* 2, 1007
Cutaneous side effects (sic)
(1978): Multiple Authors, *Lancet* 2, 1007 (20%)
Dermatitis (sic) (1–10%)
Edema (1–10%)
Erythema annulare
(1989): Lioté F+, *Rev Rhum Mal Ostéoartic* (French) 56, 11
Erythema multiforme
(1979): Hodinka L+, *Int Arch Allergy Appl Immunol* 58, 362
Exanthems
(1989): Lioté F+, *Rev Rhum Mal Ostéoartic* (French) 56, 11
(1980): Miller B+, *Arthritis Rheum* 23, 172 (>10%)
(1978): Multiple Authors, *J Rheumatol* 5 (Suppl 4), 5
(1978): Pinals RS, *J Rheumatol* 5 (Suppl 4), 71 (>5%)
(1978): Secher L+, *Acta Derm Venereol* 58, 372
(1978): Symoens J+, *Cancer Treat Rep* 62, 1721 (2.6%)
(1976): Rosenthal M+, *N Engl J Med* 295, 1204
Exfoliative dermatitis
Fixed eruption
(1994): Clavère P+, *Ann Dermatol Venereol* (French) 121, 238 (pigmented)
(1991): Thankappen TP+, *Int J Dermatol* 30, 867 (0.88%)
Hemorrhagic eruption (sic)
(1982): Papageorgiou P+, *J Clin Lab Immunol* 8, 121
Infections (sic) (1–10%)
Lichenoid eruption
(1980): Kirby JD+, *J R Soc Med* 73, 208
(1978): Multiple Authors, *Lancet* 2, 1007
(1978): Pinals RS, *J Rheumatol* 5 (Suppl 4), 71
Pemphigus
(1980): Mashkilleison NA, *Vestn Dermatol Venerol* (Russian) October 46
Pruritus (<1%)
(1992): Breathnach SM+, *Adverse Drug Reactions and the Skin* Blackwell, Oxford, 178 (passim)
(1989): Lioté F+, *Rev Rhum Mal Ostéoartic* (French) 56, 11
(1980): Kirby JD+, *J R Soc Med* 73, 208
(1978): Pinals RS, *J Rheumatol* 5 (Suppl 4), 71
(1978): Secher L+, *Acta Derm Venereol* 58, 372
Psoriasis
(1980): Kirby JD+, *J R Soc Med* 73, 208 (passim)
Purpura
(1999): Rongioletti F+, *Br J Dermatol* 140(5), 948
Rash (sic)
(1980): Husain Z+, *J Rheumatol* 7, 825
(1980): Kinsella PL+, *J Rheumatol* 7, 288
(1980): Miller B+, *Arthritis Rheum* 23, 172
(1979): Scherak O+, *Wien Klin Wochenschr* (German) 91, 758
(1978): Pinals RS, *J Rheumatol* 5 (Suppl 4), 71

(1978): Secher L+, *Acta Derm Venereol* 58, 372
(1978): Symoens J+, *Cancer Treat Rep* 62, 1721
(1977): Parkinson DR+, *Lancet* 2, 1129
Stevens–Johnson syndrome (<1%)
Urticaria (<1%)
(1992): Breathnach SM+, *Adverse Drug Reactions and the Skin* Blackwell, Oxford, 178 (passim)
(1989): Lioté F+, *Rev Rhum Mal Ostéoartic* (French) 56, 11
(1979): Hodinka L+, *Int Arch Allergy Appl Immunol* 58, 362
(1978): Pinals RS, *J Rheumatol* 5 (Suppl 4), 71
Vasculitis
(1999): Rongioletti F+, *Br J Dermatol* 140(5), 948
(1989): Lioté F+, *Rev Rhum Mal Ostéoartic* (French) 56, 11
(1983): Ferlazzo B+, *Boll Ist Sieroter Milan* (Italian) 62, 107
(1980): Huskisson EC, *Agents Actions* Suppl 7, 55
(1978): MacFarlane DG+, *BMJ* 1, 407
(1978): Multiple Authors, *Lancet* 2, 1007
(1978): Scheinberg MA+, *BMJ* 1, 408
Xerosis
(1980): Kirby JD+, *J R Soc Med* 73, 208

### Hair

Hair – alopecia (1–10%)
(1980): Kirby JD+, *J R Soc Med* 73, 208

### Other

Anaphylactoid reactions
Dysgeusia (1–10%) (metallic taste)
(1977): Runge LA+, *Arthritis Rheum* 20, 1445
(1977): Veys EM+, Willoughby DA+, *Perspectives in Inflammation*, Lancaster, England, MTP Press, W3 FU966 v3
Erosive lichen planus
(1980): Kirby JD+, *J R Soc Med* 73, 208 (passim)
Myalgia (1–10%)
Necrosis
(2002): Kumar B+, *Clin Exp Dermatol* 27(1), 8
(2002): Powell J+, *Clin Exp Dermatol* 27(1), 32
Oral mucosal lesions
(1989): Lioté F+, *Rev Rhum Mal Ostéoartic* (French) 56, 11 (2.1%)
(1980): Miller B+, *Arthritis Rheum* 23, 172 (>10%)
(1978): Multiple Authors, *J Rheumatol* 5 (Suppl 4), 5 (2.3%)
(1978): Multiple Authors, *Lancet* 2, 1007 (5.9%)
(1978): Symoens J+, *Cancer Treat Rep* 62, 1721 (0.3%)
Oral ulceration
(1978): Symoens J+, *Cancer Treat Rep* 62, 1721
Paresthesias (1–10%)
Parosmia (<1%)
Stomatitis (1–10%)
(1980): Kinsella PL+, *J Rheumatol* 7, 288
(1978): Multiple Authors, *Lancet* 2, 1007 (6%)

## LEVETIRACETAM

**Trade name:** Keppra (UCB Pharma)
**Indications:** Partial onset seizures
**Category:** Anticonvulsant
**Half-life:** 7 hours

#### *Reactions*

### Skin

Ecchymoses (<1%)
Flu-like syndrome (sic)
(2000): Cereghino JJ+, *Neurology* 55, 236
Fungal infection (>1%)
Infections (sic) (13%)
(2002): Boon P+, *Epilepsy Res* 48(1), 77
(2002): Glauser TA+, *Epilepsia* 43(5), 518
(2001): Nash EM+, *Am J Health Syst Pharm* 58(13), 1195
(2000): Cereghino JJ+, *Neurology* 55, 236
Rash (sic) (>1%)

### Other

Gingivitis (>1%)
Pain
(2002): Boon P+, *Epilepsy Res* 48(1), 77
Paresthesias (2%)

## LEVOBETAXOLOL

**Trade name:** Betaxon (Alcon)
**Other common trade name:** *L-betaxolol*
**Indications:** Chronic open-angle glaucoma, ocular hypertension
**Category:** beta-adrenergic blocker (ophthalmic); antiglaucoma agent
**Half-life:** 20 hours

#### *Reactions*

### Skin

Contact dermatitis
Dermatitis (sic) (<2%)
Infections (sic) (<2%)
Ocular transient discomfort (sic) (11%)
Psoriasis (<2%)
Rash (sic)
Xerosis

### Hair

Hair – alopecia (<2%)

### Other

Breast abscess (<2%)
Dysgeusia (<2%)
Tendinitis (<2%)
Tinnitus (<2%)

## LEVOBUNOLOL

**Trade names:** AKBeta; Betagan (Allergan)
**Other common trade names:** *AK-Beta; Bunolgan; Gotensin; Vistagan; Vistagen*
**Indications:** Glaucoma, ocular hypertension
**Category:** Ophthalmic beta adrenergic blocker
**Half-life:** no data*

#### *Reactions*

### Skin

Burning eyes
Contact dermatitis
(2001): Holdiness MR, *Am J Contact Dermat* 12(4), 217
(1999): Erdmann S+, *Contact Dermatitis* 41, 44
(1995): di Lernia V+, *Contact Dermatitis* 33, 57
(1995): Koch P, *Contact Dermatitis* 33, 140
(1995): Zucchelli V+, *Contact Dermatitis* 33, 66
(1993): van der Meeren HL+, *Contact Dermatitis* 28, 41
(1989): Schultheiss E, *Derm Beruf Umwelt* (German) 37, 185
Erythema
Lichen planus

(1995): Beckman KA+, *Am J Ophthalmol* 120, 530
Pruritus (<1%)
Rash (sic) (<1%)
Stinging eyes
Urticaria

### Hair

Hair – alopecia (1–10%)

### Other

Hypersensitivity

***Note:** Peak effect: 1–7 days

## LEVODOPA

**Synonym:** L-dopa
**Trade names:** Atamet (Athena); Sinemet (DuPont)
**Other common trade names:** *Brocadopa; Dopaflex; Doparl; Eldopal; Levodopa-Woelm*
**Indications:** Parkinsonism
**Category:** Antidyskinetic; antiparkinsonian
**Half-life:** 1–3 hours
**Clinically important, potentially hazardous interactions with:** MAO inhibitors, phenelzine, pyridoxine, selegiline, tranylcypromine

Sinemet is carbidopa and levodopa

#### *Reactions*

### Skin

Diaphoresis
(1995): Sage JI+, *Ann Neurol* 37, 120
Exanthems
(1976): Arndt KA+, *JAMA* 235, 918
(1970): Schwarz GA+, *Med Clin North Am* 54, 773
Flushing
Hot flashes
Hypomelanosis guttata
(2001): Mocci A, Panama City, Panama (from Internet) (observation)
Leukoplakia
Lupus erythematosus
(1985): Stratton MA, *Clin Pharm* 4, 657
(1979): Massarotti G+, *BMJ* 2, 553
Melanoma
(1997): Pfützner W+, *J Am Acad Dermatol* 37, 332
(1996): Kleinhans M+, *Hautarzt* (German) 47, 432
(1993): Weiner WJ+, *Neurology* 43, 674
(1992): Haider SA+, *Br J Ophthalmol* 76, 246
(1992): Sandyk R, *Int J Neurosci* 63, 137
(1989): Kande'l EI, *Zh Nevropatol Psikhiatr* (Russian) 89, 126
(1987): Morpurgo G+, *Eur J Cancer Clin Oncol* 23, 1213
(1985): Kochar AS, *Am J Med* 79, 119
(1985): Przybilla B+, *Acta Derm Venereol* (Stockh) 65, 556
(1985): Rampen FHJ, *J Neurol Neurosurg Psychiatry* 48, 585
(1984): Abramson DH+, *JAMA* 252, 1011
(1984): Rosin MA+, *Cutis* 33, 572
(1982): Van Rens GH+, *Ophthalmology* 89, 1464
(1980): Bernstein JE+, *Arch Dermatol* 116, 1041
(1980): Warner TF+, *J Cutan Pathol* 7, 50
(1979): Botteri A+, *Lakartidningen* (Swedish) 76, 316
(1979): Fermaglich J+, *JAMA* 241, 883
(1978): Fermaglich J, *Neurology* 28, 404
(1978): Sober AJ+, *JAMA* 240, 554
(1977): Fermaglich J+, *J Neurology* 215, 221
(1975): Pelfrene AF, *Nouv Presse Med* (French) 4, 1365
(1974): Happle R, *Fortschr* (German) 92, 1065
(1974): Liebermann AN+, *Neurology* 24, 340
(1973): Robinson E+, *Arch Pathol* 95, 213
(1972): Skibba JL+, *Arch Pathol* 93, 556
Pemphigus
(1986): Pisani M+, *G Ital Dermatol Venereol* (Italian) 121, 39
Purpura
(1976): Wanamaker WM+, *JAMA* 235, 2217
Rash (sic)
(1984): Goetz CG, *Clin Neuropharmacol* 7, 107
(1983): Goetz CG, *N Engl J Med* 309, 1387
Urticaria
Vitiligo
(1999): Sabate M+, *Ann Pharmacother* 33, 1228 (with tolcapone)

### Hair

Hair – alopecia
(1971): Marshall A+, *BMJ* 1, 407
Hair – repigmentation
(1989): Reynolds NJ+, *Clin Exp Dermatol* 14, 317
(1973): Grainger KM, *Lancet* 1, 97

### Nails

Nails – increased growth
(1984): Danial CR+, *J Am Acad Dermatol* 10, 250
(1973): Miller E, *N Engl J Med* 288, 916

### Other

Ageusia
Black cartilage
(1986): Connolly CE+, *Lancet* 1, 690
Bruxism
Chromhidrosis (1–10%)
Dysgeusia
Glossopyrosis
Paresthesias
Phlebitis
Priapism
Sialorrhea
Xerostomia (1–10%)

## LEVOFLOXACIN

**Trade name:** Levaquin (Ortho-McNeil)
**Indications:** Various infections caused by susceptible organisms
**Category:** Fluoroquinolone antibiotic
**Half-life:** 6–8 hours

#### *Reactions*

### Skin

Candidiasis (0.3%)
Diaphoresis (0.1%)
Edema (0.1%)
Erythema
(1992): Kanzaki H+, *Jpn J Antibiot* (Japanese) 45, 576
Erythema multiforme
Erythema nodosum (<3%)
Exanthems
(2000): Paily R, *J Dermatol* 27, 405
Exfoliative dermatitis
(2001): Sienkiewicz G, Johnson City, NY (from Internet) (observation)
Photosensitivity (<0.1%)
(2000): Boccumini LE+, *Ann Pharmacol* 34, 453

Phototoxicity
(2001): Carbon C, *Therapie* 56(1), 35
Pruritus (1.6%)
Purpura (<0.5%)
Rash (sic) (1.7%)
Stevens–Johnson syndrome
Toxic epidermal necrolysis
Urticaria (<0.5%)
(2001): Eisner J (from Internet) (presonal reaction)
Vasculitis
(2002): Drayton G, Los Angeles, CA (from Internet) (observation)

### Other

Anaphylactoid reactions
(2001): *Drug & Ther Perspect* 17, 15
Death
(2001): Spahr L+, *J Hepatol* 35(2), 308
Dysgeusia (0.2%)
Injection-site reactions (sic)
Myalgia (<0.5%)
Paresthesias
Seizures
(2001): Kushner JM+, *Ann Pharmacother* 35(10), 1194
Tendinitis
(2001): Carbon C, *Therapie* 56(1), 35
(2001): Emmet S, Solan Beach, CA (from Internet) (observatoin) (Achilles; long-lasting)
(2000): Casado Burgos E+, *Med Clin (Barc)* (Spanish) 114, 319
(1999): Lewis JR+, *Ann Pharmacother* 33(7), 792 (Achilles, bilateral)
Tendon rupture
(2001): Nuno Mateo FJ+, *Rev Clin Esp* 201(9), 539
Tremors
Vaginitis (1.8%)
Xerostomia (<1%)

## LEVOTHYROXINE

**Synonyms:** L-thyroxine sodium; $T_4$
**Trade names:** Eltroxin; Levo-T; Levothyroid (Forest); Levoxyl (Jones); Synthroid (Abbott)
**Other common trade names:** *Berlthyrox; Droxine; Eferox; Levo-T; Levothyrox; Thevier*
**Indications:** Hypothyroidism
**Category:** Synthetic thyroid hormone
**Half-life:** 6–7 days
**Clinically important, potentially hazardous interactions with:** dicumarol, oral anticoagulants, warfarin

#### *Reactions*

### Skin

Acne
Allergic reactions (sic)
Angioedema
(1991): Levesque H+, *Lancet* 338, 393
(1990): Pandya AG+, *Arch Dermatol* 126, 1238
Dermatitis herpetiformis
(1974): From E+, *Br J Dermatol* 91, 221
Diaphoresis (<1%)
Flushing
Nevi
(1976): Tofahrn J+, *Z Hautkr* (German) 51, 617 (eruption)
Pruritus
(1990): Pandya AG+, *Arch Dermatol* 126, 1238
Rash (sic)
Urticaria
(2000): Drayton GE, Los Angeles, CA (from Internet) (observation)
(1994): Magner J+, *Thyroid* 4, 341 (from the blue dye)
(1990): Pandya AG+, *Arch Dermatol* 126, 1238
(1966): Romanski B+, *Pol Med Sci Hist* 9, 92
Xerosis

### Hair

Hair – alopecia (<1%)

### Other

Hypersensitivity
Myalgia (<1%)
Pseudotumor cerebri (in infants)
Tremors

## LICORICE

**Scientific names:** *Glycyrrhiza glabra; Glycyrrhiza uralensis*
**Other common names:** Alcacuz; Alcazuz; Chinese Licorice; Gan Cao; Gan Zao; Glycyrrhiza; Licorice Root; Liquorice; Orozuz; Reglisse; Russian Licorice; Spanish Licorice; Subholz; Sweet Root
**Family:** Fabaceae; Leguminosae
**Purported indications:** Inflammation of the upper respiratory tract mucous membranes, gastric and duodenal ulcers, bronchitis, colic, dry cough, arthritis, lupus, hepatitis B and C, cholestatic liver disorders
**Other uses:** Increase fertility in women, prostate cancer (in combination with seven other herbs – PC-Spes), sore throats, malaria, tuberculosis, sores, abscesses, food poisoning, diabetes insipidus, contact dermatitis. Also used as a flavoring agent in foods, beverages and tobacco
**Clinically important, potentially hazardous interactions with:** hydrocortisone, oral contraceptives, prednisolone

#### *Reactions*

### Skin

Contact dermatitis
Edema
(2000): Olukoga A+, *J R Soc Health* 120(2), 83

### Other

Hypertension
(2001): Brouwers AJ+, *Ned Tijdschr Geneeskd* 145(15), 744
Myopathy
Rhabdomyolysis
(1997): Barrella M+, *Ital J Neurol Sci* 18(4), 217
(1995): Berlango Jimenez A+, *An Med Interna* 12(1), 33
(1992): Caradonna P+, *Ultrastruct Pathol* 16(5), 529
(1989): Achar KN+, *Aust N Z J Med* 19(4), 365
(1988): Maresca MC+, *Minerva Med* 79(1), 55 (3 cases)
(1983): Corsi FM+, *Ital J Neurol Sci* 4(4), 493
(1983): Heidemann HT+, *Klin Wochenschr* 61(6), 303
(1980): Cumming AM+, *Postgrad Med J* 56(657), 526
(1979): Mourad G+, *J Urol Nephrol* (Paris) 85(4), 315
(1970): Nielsen H, *Nord Med* 84(31), 999
(1970): Nielsen H+, *Ugeskr Laeger* 132(38), 1778
(1970): Tourtellotte CR+, *Calif Med* 113(4), 51
(1966): Geerling J, *Ned Tijdschr Geneeskd* 110(43), 1919
(1966): Gross EG+, *N Engl J Med* 274(11), 602

## LIDOCAINE

**Synonym:** lignocaine
**Trade names:** Anestacon (PolyMedica); ELA-Max (Ferndale); EMLA (AstraZeneca); Xylocaine (AstraZeneca)
**Other common trade names:** *Dentipatch; DermaFlex; Dilocaine; Lidodan; Lidoject-2; Octocaine; Xylocard*
**Indications:** Ventricular arrhythmias, topical anesthesia
**Category:** Anesthetic; antiarrhythmic
**Half-life:** terminal: 1.5–2 hours
**Clinically important, potentially hazardous interactions with:** amprenavir, antiarrhythmics, cimetidine

### *Reactions*

#### Skin

Angioedema
(1987): Bricker SR+, *Anaesthesia* 42, 323
(1961): Noble DS+, *Lancet* 2, 1436
(1961): Rajka G, *Allergie Asthma* (German) 7, 237
Bullous eruption
Contact dermatitis
(1996): Bassett IB+, *Australas J Dermatol* 37, 155
(1995): Thakur BK+, *J Allergy Clin Immunol* 95, 776
(1994): Hardwick N+, *Contact Dermatitis* 30, 245
(1993): Duggan M+, *Contact Dermatitis* 28, 190
(1993): Handfield-Jones SE+, *Clin Exp Dermatol* 18, 342
(1990): Black RJ+, *Contact Dermatitis* 23, 117
(1989): Budde J+, *Derm Beruf Umwelt* (German) 37, 181
(1986): Curley KR, *Arch Dermatol* 122, 924
(1985): Fernandes-de-Corres L+, *Contact Dermatitis* 12, 114
(1983): Nurse DS+, *Contact Dermatitis* 9, 513
(1979): Fregert S+, *Contact Dermatitis* 5, 185
(1979): Kernekamp AS+, *Contact Dermatitis* 5, 403
(1977): Turner TW, *Contact Dermatitis* 3, 210
Eczema (sic)
(1990): Huwyler T+, *Schweiz Monatsschr Zahnmed* (German) 100, 751
(1986): Curley KR, *Arch Dermatol* 122, 924
(1961): Rajka G, *Allergie Asthma* (German) 7, 237
Edema (<1%)
Erythema multiforme
(1987): Arrowsmith JB+, *Ann Intern Med* 107, 693
Exanthems
Exfoliative dermatitis
(1987): Arrowsmith JB+, *Ann Intern Med* 107, 693
(1975): Hoffmann H+, *Arch Dermatol* 111, 266
Fixed eruption
(1997): Garcia JC+, *J Investig Allergol Clin Immunol* 7, 127
(1996): Kawada A+, *Contact Dermatitis* 35, 375
Lupus erythematosus
(1988): Oliphant LD+, *Chest* 94, 427
Pigmentation
(1987): Curley RK+, *Br Dent J* 162, 113
Pruritus (<1%)
(1961): Rajka G, *Allergie Asthma* (German) 7, 237
Purpura
Rash (sic) (<1%)
Shivering (1–10%)
Stevens–Johnson syndrome
(1987): Arrowsmith JB+, *Ann Intern Med* 107, 693
Urticaria
(1980): Chin TM+, *Int J Dermatol* 19, 147
(1969): Aldrete JA+, *JAMA* 207, 356
(1961): Rajka G, *Allergie Asthma* (German) 7, 237

#### Other

Acute intermittent porphyria
Anaphylactoid reactions
(2001): Browne IM+, *Am J Obstet Gynecol* 185(5), 1253
(1999): Bircher AJ+, *Aust Dent J* 44, 64
(1984): Metzner HH+, *Dermatol Monatsschr* (German) 170, 648
(1980): Agathos M, *Contact Dermatitis* 6, 236
(1975): Tannenbaum H+, *J Allergy Clin Immunol* 56, 226
Death
(2002): Nisse P+, *Acta Clin Belg* Suppl 1, 51
Embolia cutis medicamentosa (Nicolau syndrome)
(1990): Wand A+, *Aktuel Dermatol* (German) 16, 128
Hypersensitivity
(1996): Bircher AJ+, *Contact Dermatitis* 34, 387
(1996): Whalen JD+, *Arch Dermatol* 132, 1256
(1975): Ravindranathan N, *Br Dent J* 138, 101
Injection-site pain
Injection-site phlebitis
Paresthesias (<1%)
Stomatitis
(1987): Arrowsmith JB+, *Ann Intern Med* 107, 693
Tinnitus
Tremors

## LINCOMYCIN

**Trade name:** Lincocin (Pharmacia & Upjohn)
**Other common trade names:** *Albiotic; Cillimicina; Cillimycin; Lincocine; Princol; Zumalin*
**Indications:** Various infections caused by susceptible organisms
**Category:** Macrolide antibiotic
**Half-life:** 2–11.5 hours

### *Reactions*

#### Skin

Allergic reactions (sic)
(1971): *Med Lett* 13, 55 (1–5%)
Angioedema
Contact dermatitis
(1991): Vilaplana J+, *Contact Dermatitis* 24, 225
(1985): Conde-Salazar L+, *Contact Dermatitis* 12, 59 (erythema multiforme-like)
Erythema multiforme
Exanthems
Exfoliative dermatitis
Photosensitivity
Pruritus
(1965): Kanee B, *Can Med Assoc J* 93, 220
Pruritus ani (<1%)
Purpura
(1973): Raff M, *Ann Intern Med* 78, 779
Rash (sic) (<1%)
Stevens–Johnson syndrome (<1%)
(1973): Pickering LK+, *JAMA* 223, 1392
Urticaria (<1%)
Vesiculobullous eruption

#### Other

Anaphylactoid reactions
Glossitis (<1%)
Injection-site erythema
(1990): Shen K, *Lancet* 336, 689
Oral mucosal lesions
Serum sickness
Stomatitis (<1%)
Tinnitus
Vaginitis (<1%)

# LINDANE

**Synonyms:** Hexachlorocyclohexane; Gamma Benzene Hexachloride
**Trade names:** Aphtiria; G-Well (Goldline); Hexicid; Kwell; Lorexane; Scabex
**Other common trade names:** *Benhex Cream; Bicide; Bio-Well; Davesol; Delice; Elentol; GAB; Gamabenceno; Gambex; Gamene; Gammalin; GBH; Herklin; Hexit; Jacutin; Kildane; Kwildane; Lencid; Locion-V; PMS-Lindane; Quellada; Sacbexyl; Sarconyl; Scabecid; Scabene; Scabi; Scabisan; Thinex; Varsan*
**Indications:** Scabies, pediculosis capitis, pediculosis pubis
**Category:** Topical scabicide; pediculicide
**Half-life:** 17–22 hours
**Clinically important, potentially hazardous interactions with:** oil-based hair dressings may increase toxic potential

### *Reactions*

## Skin

Adverse reactions (sic)
(2000): Hernandez Contreras N+, *Rev Cubana Med Trop* 52(3), 228 (2.54%)
(1999): Hall RC+, *Psychosomatics* 40(6), 513
(1995): Brown S+, *Clin Infect Dis* 20 (Suppl 1), S104
(1981): Rasmussen JE, *J Am Acad Dermatol* 5(5), 507
Bullous dermatosis
(1994): Bouree P+, *Bull Soc Fr Parasitol* 12, 75
Contact dermatitis
(1990): Andersen KE, *Occupational Skin Disease* 2nd ed, 73–88
(1983): Farkas J, *Derm Beruf Umwelt* (German) 31(6), 189
(1983): Fiumara NJ+, *Am Fam Physician* 28(1), 137
(1983): *AMA Drug Evaluations* 5th ed, 1850
Ecchymoses
Eczematous eruption
Erythema
(1987): Bowerman JG+, *Pediatr Infect Dis* 6(3), 252 (2.6%)
(1980): Smith DE+, *Cutis* 26(6), 618
Irritation (sic)
Lymphoma (non-Hodgkins)
(1998): Blair A+, *Am J Ind Med* 33(1), 82
Papulo-nodular lesions
(2000): Hashimoto K+, *J Dermatol* 27(3), 181
Pruritus
(2000): Hashimoto K+, *J Dermatol* 27(3), 181
(1999): Revenga Arranz F+, *Rev Clin Esp* 199(2), 101
(1998): Bowie C+, *Public Health* 112(4), 249
(1990): Schultz MW+, *Arch Dermatol* 126(2), 167
(1987): Bowerman JG+, *Pediatr Infect Dis* 6(3), 252 (2.6%)
Purpura
(1981): Fagan JE, *Pediatrics* 67, 310
Toxicity (sic)
(1999): Hall RC+, *Psychosomatics* 40(6), 513
Urticaria (0.16%)
(1996): Shuster J, *Hosp. Pharm* 31, 370
(1994): Fischer TF, *Ann Emerg Med* 24(5), 972

## Other

Death
(2000): Walker GJ+, *Cochrane Database Syst Rev* 3, CD00
(1996): Lewis RJ, *Sax's Dangerous Properties of Industrial Materials* 9th ed, 338
(1995): Aks SE+, *Ann Emerg Med* 26(5), 647
(1995): Surber C+, *Hautarzt* (German) 46(8), 528
(1994): Fischer TF, *Ann Emerg Med* 24(5), 972
(1989): Vercel M+, *Cah Anesthesiol* 37(7), 543
(1988): Sunder Ram Rao CV+, *Vet Hum Toxicol* 30(2), 132
(1985): *American Hospital Formulary Service-Drug Information* 85, 1601
(1984): Gosselin RE+, *Clinical Toxicology of Commercial Products* 5th ed, III–239
(1983): Davies JE+, *Arch Dermatol* 119(2), 142
(1982): Telch J+, *Can Med Assoc* 126(6), 662
(1982): Telch J+, *Can Med Assoc* 127(9), 821
(1980): Powell GM, *Cent Afr J Med* 26(7), 170
(1980): Rasmussen JE, *Arch Dermatol* 116(11), 1226
(1979): IARC, *Monographs on the Evaluation of the Carcinogenic Risk of Chemicals to Man* 20, 220
(1977): Wheeler M, *West J Med* 127, 518
(1970): Macnamara BG, *Br Med J* 3(722), 585
(1966): Sovljanski R+, *Med Pregl* 19(6), 349
Paresthesias
Pseudotumor cerebri
(1991): Verderber L+, *J Neurol Neurosurg Psychiatry* 54(12), 1123
(1976): Heuser M+, *Acta Univ Carol Med Monogr* 75, 133
Rhabdomyolysis
(1988): Sunder Ram Rao CV+, *Vet Hum Toxicol* 30(2), 132
(1984): Jaeger U+, *Vet Hum Toxicol* 26(1), 11
(1977): Munk ZM+, *Can Med Assoc* 117(9), 1050
Seizures
(2002): Simpson WM Jr+, *Am Fam Physician* 65(8), 1599
(2000): Cox R+, *J Miss Med Assoc* 41(8), 690
(2000): Nordt SP+, *J Emerg Med* 18(1), 51
(1995): Solomon BA+, *J Fam Pract* 40(3), 291
(1994): Fischer TF, *Ann Emerg Med* 24(5), 972
(1991): Ramchander V+, *West Indian Med J* 40(1), 41
(1991): Tenenbein M, *J Am Geriatr Soc* 39(4), 394
(1987): Friedman SJ, *Arch Dermatol* 123(8), 1056
(1984): Jaeger U+, *Vet Hum Toxicol* 26(1), 11
(1979): Pramanik AK+, *Arch Dermatol* 115(10), 1224
(1977): Munk ZM+, *Can Med Assoc J* 117(9), 1050

# LINEZOLID

**Trade name:** Zyvox (Pharmacia & Upjohn)
**Indications:** Various infections caused by susceptible organisms
**Category:** Oxazolidinone antibiotic
**Half-life:** 4–5 hours
**Clinically important, potentially hazardous interactions with:** amitriptyline, amoxapine, clomipramine, desipramine, dextromethorphan, doxepin, fluoxetine, fluvoxamine, imipramine, meperidine, nortriptyline, paroxetine, protriptyline, sertraline, sibutramine, trazodone, tricyclic antidepressants, trimipramine, venlafaxine

### *Reactions*

## Skin

Fungal infections (0.1–2%)
Pruritus
Rash (sic) (2%)

## Other

Candidal vaginitis (1–2%)
Dysgeusia (1–2%)
Oral candidiasis (<1%)
Serotonin syndrome
(2002): Wigen CL+, *Clin Infect Dis* 34(12), 1651
(2001): Lavery S+, *Psychosomatics* 42(5), 432
Tongue pigmentation (<1%)

# LIOTHYRONINE

**Synonym:** $T_3$ sodium
**Trade names:** Cytomel (Jones); Triostat (Jones)
**Other common trade names:** *Cynomel; T3; Tertroxin; Thyronine; Trijodthyronin BC N*
**Indications:** Hypothyroidism
**Category:** Synthetic thyroid hormone
**Half-life:** 16–49 hours
**Clinically important, potentially hazardous interactions with:** anticoagulants, dicumarol, warfarin

### *Reactions*

## Skin

Allergic reactions (sic)
Diaphoresis (<1%)
Rash (sic)
Urticaria
(1994): Magner J+, *Thyroid* 4, 341 (from the blue dye)
(1990): Pandya AG+, *Arch Dermatol* 126, 1238
(1966): Romanski B+, *Pol Med Sci Hist* 9, 92
Xerosis

## Hair

Hair – alopecia (<1%)

## Other

Hypersensitivity
Myalgia (<1%)
Phlebitis (1%)
Pseudotumor cerebri
Tremors

# LISINOPRIL

**Trade names:** Prinivil (Merck); Prinizide (Merck); Zestoretic (AstraZeneca); Zestril (AstraZeneca)
**Other common trade names:** *Acerbon; Alapril; Apo-Lisinopril; Carace; Coric; Prinil; Tensopril; Vivatec*
**Indications:** Hypertension
**Category:** Angiotensin-converting enzyme (ACE) inhibitor; antihypertensive
**Half-life:** 12 hours
**Clinically important, potentially hazardous interactions with:** amiloride, spironolactone, triamterene

Prinizide is lisinopril and hydrochlorothiazide; Zestoretic is lisinopril and hydrochlorothiazide

### *Reactions*

## Skin

Angioedema
(2001): Cohen EG+, *Ann Otol Rhinol Laryngol* 110(8), 701 (64 cases)
(1999): Guo X+, *J Okla State Med Assoc* 92, 71
(1999): Maestre ML+, *Rev Esp Anestesiol Reanim* (Spanish) 46, 88
(1999): Neutel JM+, *Am J Ther* 6, 161
(1997): Brown NJ+, *JAMA* 278, 232
(1997): Pavletic AJ, *J Am Board Fam Pract* 10, 370
(1996): Pillans PI+, *Eur J Clin Pharmacol* 51, 123
(1995): Bauwens LJ+, *Ned Tijdschr Geneeskd* (Dutch) 139, 674
(1995): Frontera Y+, *J Am Dent Assoc* 126, 217
(1995): Kuo DC+, *J Emerg Med* 13, 327 (uvular)
(1994): Krikorian RK+, *Chest* 106, 1922
(1993): Soo Hoo GW+, *West J Med* 158, 412
(1992): McElligott S+, *Ann Intern Med* 116, 426
(1992): Shelley WB+, *Cutis* 49, 391 (tongue) (observation)
(1990): Laher MS, *Drugs* 39 (Suppl 2), 55
(1990): McAreavey D+, *Drugs* 40, 326 (0.4%)
(1990): Orfan N+, *JAMA* 264, 1287
(1988): Lancaster SG+, *Drugs* 35, 646 (0.6%)
(1987): Rush JE+, *J Cardiovasc Pharmacol* 9, s99
Bullous eruption
(1988): Barlow RJ+, *Clin Exp Dermatol* 13, 117
Diaphoresis (<1%)
Edema (1%)
Erythema (1%)
Exanthems
(1990): Laher MS, *Drugs* 39 (Suppl 2), 55
(1990): McAreavey D+, *Drugs* 40, 326 (3.2%)
(1988): Barlow RJ+, *Clin Exp Dermatol* 13, 117
(1988): Lancaster SG+, *Drugs* 35, 646 (3.2%)
Facial edema (<1%)
Flushing (<1%)
(1997): Litt JZ, Beachwood, OH (personal case) (observation)
(1990): Laher MS, *Drugs* 39 (Suppl 2), 55
(1989): Healy LA+, *N Engl J Med* 321, 763
Lichenoid eruption
(1992): Shelley WB+, *Cutis* 50, 182 (observation)
Lupus erythematosus
Pemphigus
Pemphigus foliaceus
(2000): Ong CS+, *Australas J Dermatol* 41(4), 242
Peripheral edema (<1%)
(1988): Uretsky BF+, *Am Heart J* 116, 480
Photosensitivity (<1%)
Pruritus (1.2%)
(2000): Kalikhman ZM, (from Internet) (observation)
Purpura
(1993): Sztern B+, *Presse Med* (French) 22, 967
(1988): Barlow RJ+, *Clin Exp Dermatol* 13, 117
Rash (sic) (1.5%)
(1999): Horiuchi Y+, *J Dermatol* 26, 128
(1989): Giles TD+, *J Am Coll Cardiol* 13, 1240
(1988): Uretsky BF+, *Am Heart J* 116, 480
(1987): Bolzano K+, *J Cardiovasc Pharmacol* 9, s43
(1987): Rush JE+, *J Cardiovasc Pharmacol* 9, s99
Rosacea
(1999): Oakley A, Hamilton, New Zealand (from Internet) (observation)
Stevens–Johnson syndrome
Telangiectases
(1999): Oakley A, Hamilton, New Zealand (from Internet) (observation)
Toxic epidermal necrolysis
Ulceration (sic) (ischemic skin ulcer)
(1987): Rush JE+, *J Cardiovasc Pharmacol* 9, s99
Urticaria (<1%)
(1996): Pillans PI+, *Eur J Clin Pharmacol* 51, 123
(1989): Cameron HA+, *J Human Hypertension* 3, 177
Vasculitis (<1%)
(1988): Barlow RJ+, *Clin Exp Dermatol* 13, 117

## Hair

Hair – alopecia (<1%)

## Other

Anaphylactoid reactions (<1%)
Cough
(2001): Adigun AQ+, *West Afr J Med* 20(1), 46–7
(2001): Lee SC+, *Hypertension* 38(2), 166

Dysesthesia (<1%)
Dysgeusia
(1988): Uretsky BF+, *Am Heart J* 116, 480
Mastodynia (<1%)
Myalgia (0.5%)
Paresthesias (0.8%)
Tinnitus
Tremors
Xerostomia (<1%)

# LITHIUM

**Trade names:** Eskalith (GSK); Lithobid (Solvay); Lithonate (Solvay); Lithotabs (Solvay)
**Other common trade names:** *Carbolith; Duralith; Hynorex Retard; Lithicarb; Lithizine; Priadel; Teralithe*
**Indications:** Manic-depressive states
**Category:** Antidepressants; antipsychotic and antimanic
**Half-life:** 18–24 hours
**Clinically important, potentially hazardous interactions with:** acetazolamide, acitretin, bendroflumethiazide, benzthiazide, chlorothiazide, chlorthalidone, fluoxetine, haloperidol, hydrochlorothiazide, hydroflumethiazide, indapamide, meperidine, methotrexate, methyclothiazide, metolazone, olmesartan, polythiazide, quinethazone, rofecoxib, sibutramine, thiazides, trichlormethiazide, valdecoxib

**Note:** An excellent review of the cutaneous conditions associated with lithium can be found in (1983): Sarantidis D+, *Br J Psychiatry* 143, 42

## *Reactions*

### Skin

Acanthosis nigricans
(1979): Arnold HL+, *J Am Acad Dermatol* 1, 93
Acne
(2001): Oztas P+, *Ann Pharmacother* 35(7), 961
(1991): Srebrnik A+, *Cutis* 48, 65
(1986): Remmer HI+, *J Clin Psychiatry* 47, 48
(1985): Albrecht G, *Hautarzt* (German) 36, 77 (passim)
(1984): Lambert D+, *Ann Med Interne Paris* (French) 135, 637
(1983): Sarantidis D+, *Br J Psychiatry* 143, 42 (11%)
(1982): Deandrea D+, *J Clin Psychopharmacol* 2, 199
(1982): Heng MCY, *Arch Dermatol* 118, 246
(1982): Heng MCY, *Br J Dermatol* 106, 107
(1982): Lambert D+, *Ann Dermatol Venereol* (French) 109, 19
(1980): Vestergaard P+, *Acta Psychiatrica Scand* 62, 193
(1978): Oei TT+, *Ned Tijdschr Geneeskd* (Dutch) 122, 1302
(1977): Okrasinski H, *Dermatologica* 154, 251
(1977): Reiffers J+, *Dermatologica* 155, 155
(1975): Yoder FW, *Arch Dermatol* 111, 396
(1971): Kusumi Y, *Dis Nerv Syst* 32, 853
Angioedema
(1985): Berova N+, *Dermatol Venerol* (Sofia) (Bulgarian) 24, 23
(1982): Lambert D+, *Ann Dermatol Venereol* (French) 109, 19
Angular cheilitis
(1983): Sarantidis D+, *Br J Psychiatry* 143, 42 (1%)
Atopic dermatitis
(1983): Sarantidis D+, *Br J Psychiatry* 143, 42 (3%)
Bullous eruption
(1987): McWhirter JD+, *Arch Dermatol* 123, 1122
Cutaneous side effects (sic)
(1985): Berova N+, *Dermatol Venerol* (Sofia) (Bulgarian) 24, 23 (23%)
(1983): Sarantidis D+, *Br J Psychiatry* 143, 42 (up to one-third)
(1982): Lambert D+, *Ann Dermatol Venereol* (French) 109, 19
Darier's disease
(1995): Rubin MB, *J Am Acad Dermatol* 32, 674
(1990): Milton GP, *J Am Acad Dermatol* 23, 926 (exacerbation)
(1986): Clark RD Jr+, *Psychosomatics* 27, 800 (exacerbation)
Dermatitis (sic)
(1980): Aldoroty N+, *Am J Psychiatry* 137, 870
(1973): Kurtin SB, *JAMA* 223, 802
(1973): Ruiz-Maldonado R+, *JAMA* 224, 1534
(1972): Posey RE, *JAMA* 221, 1517
Dermatitis herpetiformis
(1985): Albrecht G, *Hautarzt* (German) 36, 77 (passim)
(1983): Sarantidis D+, *Br J Psychiatry* 143, 42
(1982): Heng MCY, *Arch Dermatol* 118, 246
Discoloration of fingers and toes (sic) (<1%)
Eczema (sic)
(1980): Vestergaard P+, *Acta Psychiatrica Scand* 62, 193
Edema
(1984): Lambert D+, *Ann Med Interne Paris* (French) 135, 637
(1975): Baldessarini RJ+, *Ann Intern Med* 83, 527
(1970): Demers R+, *JAMA* 214, 1845 (pretibial)
Erythema
(1996): Wakelin SH+, *Clin Exp Dermatol* 21, 296
Erythema multiforme
(1991): Balldin J+, *J Am Acad Dermatol* 24, 1015
Exanthems
(1985): Albrecht G, *Hautarzt* (German) 36, 77 (passim)
(1983): Sarantidis D+, *Br J Psychiatry* 143, 42
(1982): Deandrea D+, *J Clin Psychopharmacol* 2, 199
(1982): Lambert D+, *Ann Dermatol Venereol* (French) 109, 19
(1980): Meinhold JM+, *J Clin Psychiatry* 41, 395
(1975): Baldessarini RJ+, *Ann Intern Med* 83, 527
(1970): No Author, *Ann Intern Med* 73, 291
(1968): Callaway CL+, *Am J Psychiatry* 124, 1124
Exfoliative dermatitis
(1985): Albrecht G, *Hautarzt* (German) 36, 77 (passim)
(1983): Sarantidis D+, *Br J Psychiatry* 143, 42 (1%)
(1979): Kuhnley EJ+, *Am J Psychiatry* 136, 1340
Follicular keratosis (sic)
(1996): Wakelin SH+, *Clin Exp Dermatol* 21, 296
(1982): Lambert D+, *Ann Dermatol Venereol* (French) 109, 19
(1977): Reiffers J+, *Dermatologica* 155, 155
Folliculitis
(1985): Hogan DJ+, *J Am Acad Dermatol* 13, 245 (passim)
(1983): Sarantidis D+, *Br J Psychiatry* 143, 42
(1973): Kurtin SB, *JAMA* 223, 803
(1973): Rifkin A+, *Am J Psychiatry* 130, 1018
Hidradenitis suppurativa
(1997): Marinella MA, *Acta Derm Venereol* 77, 483
(1996): Blumenthal HL, Beachwood, OH (personal case) (observation)
(1995): Gupta AK+, *J Amer Acad Dermatol* 32, 382
(1981): Stamm T+, *Psychiatr Prax* (German) 8, 152
Hyperplasia (verrucous)
(1984): Frenk E, *Z Hautkr* (German) 2, 97
Ichthyosis
(1983): Sarantidis D+, *Br J Psychiatry* 143, 42 (1%)
(1977): Reiffers J+, *Dermatologica* 155, 155
Keratoderma
(1991): Labelle A+, *J Clin Psychopharmacol* 11, 149
Keratosis pilaris
(1985): Albrecht G, *Hautarzt* (German) 36, 77 (passim)
(1973): Rifkin A+, *Am J Psychiatry* 130, 1018
Lichen planus
(1994): Thompson DF+, *Pharmacotherapy* 14, 561
Lichen simplex chronicus
(1984): Shukla S+, *Am J Psychiatry* 141, 909
Linear IgA bullous dermatosis
(2002): Cohen LM+, *J Am Acad Dermatol* 46, S32 (passim)

(1996): Tranvan A+, *J Am Acad Dermatol* 35, 865
(1987): McWhirter JD+, *Arch Dermatol* 123, 1122
Lupus erythematosus
(1985): Stratton MA, *Clin Pharm* 4, 657
(1982): Shukla VR+, *JAMA* 248, 921
(1981): Hess EV, *Arthritis Rheum* 24, 6
Morphea
(1982): Lambert D+, *Ann Dermatol Venereol* (French) 109, 19
Mycosis fungoides
(2001): Francis GJ+, *J Am Acad Dermatol* 44, 308
Myxedema
(1981): Kvetny J+, *Ugeskr Laeger* (Danish) 143, 1323
(1979): Medley ES+, *J Fam Pract* 8, 855
(1978): Perrild H+, *BMJ* 1, 1108
(1973): Pousset G+, *Ann Endocrinol Paris* (French) 34, 454
(1973): Pousset G+, *Ann Endocrinol Paris* (French) 34, 549
(1972): Brandrup FO, *Ugeskr Laeger* (Danish) 134, 2710
(1972): Vestergaard PA+, *Lancet* 2, 427
(1972): Vestergaard PA+, *Ugeskr Laeger* (Danish) 134, 1282
(1972): Wiener JD, *JAMA* 220, 587
(1971): Luby ED+, *JAMA* 218, 1298
Papular eruption (elbows)
(1973): Kurtin SB, *JAMA* 223, 802
(1972): Posey RE, *JAMA* 221, 1517
Port-wine stain
(1987): Leung AK, *J Natl Med Assoc* 79, 877
Prurigo nodularis
(1983): Sarantidis D+, *Br J Psychiatry* 143, 42 (1%)
Pruritus (<1%)
(1985): Berova N+, *Dermatol Venerol* (Sofia) (Bulgarian) 24, 23 (1–5%)
(1984): Lambert D+, *Ann Med Interne Paris* (French) 135, 637
(1983): Sarantidis D+, *Br J Psychiatry* 143, 42
(1982): Lambert D+, *Ann Dermatol Venereol* (French) 109, 19
(1980): Vestergaard P+, *Acta Psychiatrica Scand* 62, 193
(1977): Reiffers J+, *Dermatologica* 155, 155
(1970): No Author, *Ann Intern Med* 73, 291
(1968): Callaway CL+, *Am J Psychiatry* 124, 1124
Psoriasis
(1996): Ockenfels HM+, *Arch Dermatol Res* 288, 173
(1994): Dorevitch A, *Harefuah* (Hebrew) 127, 228
(1993): Hermle L+, *Nervenarzt* (German) 64, 208
(1992): Abel EA, *Semin Dermatol* 11, 269
(1992): Hemlock C+, *Ann Pharmacother* 26, 211
(1992): Rudolph RI, *J Am Acad Dermatol* 26, 135
(1989): Sasaki T+, *J Dermatol* (Tokio) 16, 59 (exacerbation)
(1988): Koo E+, *Orv Hetil* (Hungarian) 129, 1699
(1988): Zirilli G+, *Minerva Psichiatr* (Italian) 29, 43
(1987): Gupta MA+, *Gen Hosp Psychiatry* 9, 157
(1986): Abel EA+, *J Am Acad Dermatol* 15, 1007 (exacerbation)
(1986): Ghadirian AM+, *J Clin Psychiatry* 47, 212
(1986): Holy B+, *Acta Univ Carol Med Praha* (Czech) 32, 217
(1986): Pande AC+, *J Clin Psychiatry* 47, 330 (exacerbation)
(1986): Segui-Montesinos J+, *Med Clin (Barc)* (Spanish) 86, 261
(1985): Albrecht G, *Hautarzt* (German) 36, 77 (passim)
(1984): Alvarez WA+, *Int J Psychosom* 31, 21
(1984): Farber EM+, *J Am Acad Dermatol* 10, 511
(1984): Fox BJ+, *J Assoc Military Dermatol* 10, 35 (exacerbation)
(1984): Lambert D+, *Ann Med Interne Paris* (French) 135, 637
(1984): Lin HN+, *Taiwan I Hsueh Hui Tsa Chih* (Chinese) 83, 1064
(1983): Hollander A, *Hautarzt* (German) 34, 487
(1983): Sarantidis D+, *Br J Psychiatry* 143, 42 (2%)
(1982): Deandrea D+, *J Clin Psychopharmacol* 2, 199
(1982): Heng MCY, *Arch Dermatol* 118, 246 (exacerbation)
(1982): Heng MCY, *Br J Dermatol* 106, 107 (exacerbation)
(1982): Lambert D+, *Ann Dermatol Venereol* (French) 109, 19 (exacerbation)
(1982): Pincelli C+, *G Ital Dermatol Venereol* (Italian) 117, 113
(1981): No Author, *Drug Ther Bull* 19, 68
(1980): Bakris GL+, *Int J Psychiatry Med* 10, 327
(1980): Thiers B, *J Am Acad Dermatol* 3, 101
(1979): Evans DL+, *Am J Psychiatry* 136, 1326
(1979): Lazarus GS+, *Arch Dermatol* 115, 1183
(1979): Skoven I+, *Arch Dermatol* 115, 1185 (exacerbation)
(1979): Umbert P+, *Actas Dermosifiliogr* (Spanish) 70, 623
(1978): Mobacken H+, *Br J Dermatol* 98, 597
(1978): Robak OH, *Tidsskr Nor Laegeforen* (Norwegian) 98, 566
(1978): Thormann J, *Ugeskr Laeger* (Danish) 140, 721
(1977): No Author, *Lakartidningen* (Swedish) 74, 2109
(1977): Reiffers J+, *Dermatologica* 155, 155 (exacerbation)
(1977): Skott AH+, *Br J Dermatol* 96, 445 (exacerbation)
(1977): Skott AH+, *Br J Psychiatry* 131, 223
(1976): Bakker JB+, *Psychosomatics* 17, 143 (exacerbation)
(1972): Carter TN, *Psychosomatics* 13, 325
Purpura
(1984): Lambert D+, *Ann Med Interne Paris* (French) 135, 637
(1982): Lambert D+, *Ann Dermatol Venereol* (French) 109, 19
Pustular eruption
(1993): Webster GF, *Clin Dermatol* 11, 541
(1982): White SW, *J Am Acad Dermatol* 7, 660 (palms and soles)
Pustular psoriasis
(1979): Evans DL+, *Am J Psychiatry* 136, 10
(1979): Skoven I+, *Arch Dermatol* 115, 1185
(1978): Lowe NJ+, *Arch Dermatol* 114, 1788
Rash (sic) (1–10%)
(1980): Bone S+, *Am J Psychiatry* 137:1, 103
Seborrheic dermatitis
(1984): Lambert D+, *Ann Med Interne Paris* (French) 135, 637
(1983): Sarantidis D+, *Br J Psychiatry* 143, 42
(1982): Lambert D+, *Ann Dermatol Venereol* (French) 109, 19
Subcorneal pustular dermatosis (Sneddon–Wilkinson)
(1988): Sterling GB+, *Cutis* 41, 165
Telangiectases
(1983): Brinkmann W+, *Z Hautkr* (German) 9, 681
Tinea versicolor
(1997): Fearfield LA+, *Clin Exp Dermatol* 22, 57
Toxicoderma
(1985): Lambert D, *Dermatologica* (French) 171, 209
Ulceration (lower extremities)
(1984): Lambert D+, *Ann Med Interne Paris* (French) 135, 637
(1975): Baldessarini RJ+, *Ann Intern Med* 83, 527
(1971): Kusumi Y, *Dis Nerv Syst* 32, 853
(1970): No Author, *Ann Intern Med* 73, 291
(1968): Callaway CL+, *Am J Psychiatry* 124, 1124
Urticaria
(1985): Berova N+, *Dermatol Venerol* (Sofia) (Bulgarian) 24, 23
(1984): Lambert D+, *Ann Med Interne Paris* (French) 135, 637
(1982): Lambert D+, *Ann Dermatol Venereol* (French) 109, 19
Vasculitis
(1994): Blumenthal HL, Beachwood, OH (personal case) (observation)
(1984): Lambert D+, *Ann Med Interne Paris* (French) 135, 637
(1982): Lambert D+, *Ann Dermatol Venereol* (French) 109, 19
(1970): *Ann Intern Med* 73, 291
Verrucous lesions (sic)
(1984): Frenk E, *Z Hautkr* (German) 59, 97
Warts
(1982): White SW, *Int J Dermatol* 21, 107
Xerosis
(1975): Hoxtell E+, *Arch Dermatol* 111, 1073

## Hair

Hair – alopecia
(2001): Francis GJ+, *J Am Acad Dermatol* 44, 308
(2000): Mercke Y+, *Ann Clin Psychiatry* 12, 35 (12–19%)
(1999): van dem Bent PM+, *Ned Tijdschr Geneeskd* (Dutch) 143, 990
(1998): Litt JZ, Beachwood, OH (personal case) (observation)
(1996): McKinney PA+, *Ann Clin Psychiatry* 8, 183 (10%)

(1991): Wagner KD+, *Psychosomatics* 32, 355
(1986): Ghadirian AM+, *J Clin Psychiatry* 47, 212
(1985): Albrecht G, *Hautarzt* (German) 36, 77 (passim)
(1984): Lambert D+, *Ann Med Interne Paris* (French) 135, 637
(1984): Mortimer PS+, *Int J Dermatol* 23, 603
(1983): Orwin A, *Br J Dermatol* 108, 503 (12%)
(1983): Shader RI, *J Clin Psychopharmacol* 3, 122
(1983): Yassa R+, *Can J Psychiatry* 28, 132
(1982): Dawber R+, *Br J Dermatol* 107, 125
(1982): Lambert D+, *Ann Dermatol Venereol* (French) 109, 19
(1982): Muniz CE+, *Psychosomatics* 23, 312
(1982): No Author, *Psychosomatics* 23, 563

Hair – alopecia areata
(1988): Silvestri A+, *Gen Hosp Psychiatry* 10, 46
(1983): Sarantidis D+, *Br J Psychiatry* 143, 42 (2%)
(1980): Vestergaard P+, *Acta Psychiatr Scand* 62, 193

Hair – brittle
(1970): No Author, *Ann Intern Med* 73, 291

Hair – changes in texture
(1985): McCreadle RG+, *Acta Psychiatr Scand* 72, 387

## Nails

Nails – Beau's lines (transverse nail bands)
(1988): Don PC+, *Cutis* 41, 20

Nails – dystrophy
(1988): Don PC+, *Cutis* 41, 20
(1982): Lambert D+, *Ann Dermatol Venereol* (French) 109, 19

Nails – onychomadesis
(1988): Don PC+, *Cutis* 41, 20

Nails – psoriasis
(1992): Rudolph RI, *J Am Acad Dermatol* 26, 135

## Other

Dysgeusia (>10%)

Geographic tongue
(1992): Patki AH, *Int J Dermatol* 31, 386

Gingival hyperplasia
(1968): Callaway CL+, *Am J Psychiatry* 124, 1124

Glossodynia

Lichenoid stomatitis
(1995): Menni S+, *Ann Dermatol Venereol* (French) 122, 91
(1991): Srebrnik A+, *Cutis* 48, 65
(1985): Hogan DJ+, *J Am Acad Dermatol* 13, 245

Oral ulceration
(2000): Madinier I+, *Ann Med Interne (Paris)* (French) 151, 248
(1985): Bar Nathan EA+, *Am J Psychiatry* 142, 1126
(1985): Hogan DJ+, *J Am Acad Dermatol* 13, 245

Parkinsonism
(2000): Muthane UB+, *J Neurol Sci* 176, 78

Pseudolymphoma
(1995): Magro CM+, *J Am Acad Dermatol* 32, 419

Pseudotumor cerebri (<1%)

Rhabdomyolysis
(1991): Bateman AM+, *Nephrol Dial Transplant* 6(3), 203
(1982): Unger J+, *Acta Clin Belg* 39, 216 (overdose)

Sialorrhea

Stomatitis
(1985): Bar Nathan EA+, *Am J Psychiatry* 142, 1126
(1978): Muniz CE+, *JAMA* 239, 2759

Stomatodynia
(1985): Bar Nathan EA+, *Am J Psychiatry* 142, 1126

Stutter
(2001): Netski AL+, *Ann Pharmacother* 35(7), 961

Tinnitus

Tremors

Vaginal ulceration
(1991): Srebrnik A+, *Cutis* 48, 65

Xerostomia (<1%)
(1980): Bone S+, *Am J Psychiatry* 137:1, 103

# LOMEFLOXACIN

**Trade name:** Maxaquin (Solvay)
**Other common trade names:** *Logiflox; Ontop*
**Indications:** Various infections caused by susceptible organisms
**Category:** Broad-spectrum fluoroquinolone antibacterial
**Half-life:** 4–6 hours
**Clinically important, potentially hazardous interactions with:** amiodarone, antacids, arsenic, bepridil, bismuth, bretylium, didanosine, disopyramide, erythromycin, NSAIDs, phenothiazines, procainamide, quinidine, sotalol, sucralfate, tricyclic antidepressants, zinc salts

### *Reactions*

## Skin

Allergic reactions (sic) (<1%)

Ankle edema

Chills (<1%)

Diaphoresis (<1%)
(1992): Crome P+, *Am J Med* 92 (Suppl 4A), 126S
(1992): Iravani A, *Am J Med* 92, 75S

Eczema (sic)

Edema (<1%)

Exanthems

Exfoliation (sic) (<1%)

Facial edema (<1%)

Flu-like syndrome (sic) (<1%)

Flushing (<1%)

Genital pruritus (sic)
(1992): Iravani A, *Am J Med* 92, 75S

Photosensitivity (2.4%)
(2000): Ferguson J+, *J Antimicrob Chemother* 45, 503
(1998): Arata J+, *Antimicrob Agents Chemother* 42, 3141
(1998): Kimura M+, *Contact Dermatitis* 38, 180
(1996): Young AR+, *J Photochem Photobiol B* 32, 165
(1994): Cohen JB+, *Arch Dermatol* 130, 805 (following tanning bed)
(1994): Correia O+, *Arch Dermatol* 130, 808 (bullous)
(1994): Lowe NJ+, *Clin Pharmacol Ther* 56, 587
(1994): Poh-Fitzpatrick MB, *Arch Dermatol* 130, 261
(1993): Tozawa K+, *Hinyokika Kiyo* (Japanese) 39, 801
(1992): Crome P+, *Am J Med* 92 (Suppl 4A), 126S
(1992): Iravani A, *Am J Med* 92, 75S
(1992): Kurumaji Y+, *Contact Dermatitis* 26, 5
(1992): Rizk E, *Am J Med* 92, 130S (2.4%)
(1990): LeBel M+, *Antimicrob Agents Chemother* 34, 1254

Phototoxicity
(2000): Traynor NJ+, *Toxicol Vitr* 14, 275
(1998): Martinez LJ+ *Photochem Photobiol* 67, 399

Pruritus (<1%)
(1992): Cox CE, *Am J Med* 92, 82S
(1992): Gotfried MH+, *Am J Med* 92, 108S
(1992): Kemper P+, *Am J Med* 92, 98S
(1992): Klimberg IW+, *Am J Med* 92, 121S
(1992): Mouton Y+, *Am J Med* 92, 87S
(1991): Wadworth AN+, *Drugs* 42, 1018

Purpura (<1%)

Pustular eruption
(1992): Mouton Y+, *Am J Med* 92, 87S

Rash (sic) (<1%)
(1992): Crome P+, *Am J Med* 92 (Suppl 4A), 126S
(1992): Gotfried MH+, *Am J Med* 92, 108S
(1992): Iravani A, *Am J Med* 92, 75S
(1992): Mouton Y+, *Am J Med* 92, 87S
(1991): Wadworth AN+, *Drugs* 42, 1018

Stevens–Johnson syndrome
Toxicoderma (sic)
(1991): Wadworth AN+, *Drugs* 42, 1018
Urticaria (<1%)
(1991): Wadworth AN+, *Drugs* 42, 1018
Vasculitis

### Other

Dysgeusia (<1%)
Hypersensitivity
(1991): Wadworth AN+, *Drugs* 42, 1018
Myalgia (<1%)
Paresthesias (<1%)
(1992): Crome P+, *Am J Med* 92 (Suppl 4A), 126S
Tendon rupture (many reports)
Tinnitus
Tongue pigmentation (<1%)
Tremors
Vaginal candidiasis
Vaginitis (<1%)
Xerostomia (<1%)
(1992): Mant TG, *Am J Med* 92, 26S

## LOMUSTINE

**Synonym:** CCNU
**Trade name:** CeeNU (Bristol-Myers Squibb)
**Other common trade names:** *Belustine; Cecenu; Lomeblastin; Lucostine; Lundbeck*
**Indications:** Brain tumors, lymphomas, melanoma
**Category:** Nitrosurea alkylating antineoplastic
**Half-life:** 16–72 hours
**Clinically important, potentially hazardous interactions with:** aldesleukin

#### *Reactions*

### Skin

Acral erythema
(1989): Oksenhendler E+, *Eur J Cancer Clin Oncol* 25, 1181
Flushing
(1992): Breathnach SM+, *Adverse Drug Reactions and the Skin* Blackwell, Oxford, 290
Neutrophilic eccrine hidradenitis
(1996): Shear NH+, *J Am Acad Dermatol* 35, 819
Rash (sic) (1–10%)

### Hair

Hair – alopecia (<1%)

### Other

Stomatitis (1–10%)

## LOPERAMIDE

**Trade names:** Imodium (McNeil); Maalox (Novartis)
**Other common trade names:** *Brek; Diar-Aid; Diarr-Eze; Diarstop-L; Imossel; Lop-Dia; Loperhoe; Maalox Anti-Diarrheal; Stopit; Vancotil*
**Indications:** Diarrhea
**Category:** Antidiarrheal
**Half-life:** 9–14 hours

#### *Reactions*

### Skin

Erythema nodosum
Exanthems
Pruritus
Rash (sic)
Urticaria

### Hair

Hair – alopecia
(1993): Litt JZ, Beachwood, OH (personal case) (observation)

### Other

Gingivitis
(1990): DuPont HL+, *Am J Med* 88, 20S
Hypersensitivity
Oral mucosal lesions (1.1%)
(1990): DuPont HL+, *Am J Med* 88, 20S
Xerostomia
(1990): DuPont HL+, *Am J Med* 88, 20S

## LORACARBEF

**Trade name:** Lorabid (Lilly)
**Other common trade name:** *Carbac*
**Indications:** Various infections caused by susceptible organisms
**Category:** Beta-lactam antibiotic (carbacephem)
**Half-life:** 60 minutes

#### *Reactions*

### Skin

Candidiasis
Erythema multiforme (<1%)
Pruritus (<1%)
Rash (sic) (1.2%)
Stevens–Johnson syndrome (<1%)
Urticaria (<1%)

### Other

Candidal vaginitis (1.3%)
Serum sickness (<1%)

# LORATADINE

**Trade names:** Claritin (Schering); Claritin-D (Schering)
**Other common trade names:** *Civeran; Claratyne; Claritine; Lisino; Lorastine; Velodan; Zeos*
**Indications:** Allergic rhinitis, urticaria
**Category:** $H_1$-receptor antihistamine and antiasthmatic
**Half-life:** 3–20 hours

### *Reactions*

## Skin

Angioedema (>2%)
(1989): Clissold SP+, *Drugs* 37, 42
Dermatitis (sic) (>2%)
Diaphoresis (>2%)
Erythema multiforme (>2%)
Exanthems
Fixed eruption
(2002): Ruiz-Genao DP+, *Br J Dermatol* 146(3), 528
Flushing (>2%)
Peripheral edema (>2%)
Photosensitivity (>2%)
Pruritus (>2%)
(1989): Barenholtz HA+, *Drug Intell Clin Pharm* 23, 445
Purpura (>2%)
Rash (sic) (>2%)
Urticaria (>2%)
(1992): Boner AL+, *Allergy* 47, 98
(1989): Clissold SP+, *Drugs* 37, 42
Xerosis (>2%)

## Hair

Hair – alopecia (>2%)
Hair – dry (sic) (>2%)

## Other

Anaphylactoid reactions (>2%)
Dysgeusia (>2%)
Gynecomastia (>2%)
Hypesthesia (>2%)
Mastodynia (1–10%)
Myalgia (>2%)
Paresthesias (>2%)
Sialorrhea (>2%)
Stomatitis (>2%)
Tinnitus
Vaginitis (>2%)
Xerostomia (>10%)
(1992): Monroe EW+, *Arzneimittelforschung* (German) 42, 1119
(1992): Olson OT+, *Arzneimittelforschung* (German) 42, 1227
(1990): Del Carpio J+, *J Allergy Clin Immunology* 84, 741
(1990): Irander K+, *Allergy* 45, 86
(1990): Simons FE, *Clin Exp Allergy* 20, 19
(1989): Barenholtz HA+, *Drug Intell Clin Pharm* 23, 445
(1989): Bruttman G+, *J Allergy Clin Immunology* 83, 411
(1988): Gutkowski A+, *J Allergy Clin Immunology* 81, 902

# LORAZEPAM

**Trade name:** Ativan (Wyeth-Ayerst)
**Other common trade names:** *Apo-Lorazepam; Durazolam; Laubeel; Merlit; Nu-Loraz; Punktyl; Tavor; Temesta; Titus*
**Indications:** Anxiety, depression
**Category:** Benzodiazepine anxiolytic; anticonvulsant; antiemetic
**Half-life:** 10–20 hours
**Clinically important, potentially hazardous interactions with: alcohol**, amprenavir, barbiturates, chlorpheniramine, clarithromycin, CNS depressants, efavirenz, erythromycin, esomeprazole, imatinib, MAO inhibitors, narcotics, nelfinavir, phenothiazines, valproate

### *Reactions*

## Skin

Dermatitis (sic) (1–10%)
Diaphoresis (>10%)
Erythema multiforme
(1991): Porteous DM+, *Arch Dermatol* 127, 741
Exanthems
Fixed eruption
(1988): Jafferany M+, *Dermatologica* 177, 386
Pruritus
Purpura
Rash (sic) (>10%)
Stevens–Johnson syndrome
(1991): Porteous DM+, *Arch Dermatol* 127, 741
Urticaria

## Hair

Hair – alopecia
Hair – hirsutism

## Other

Gingival lichenoid reaction
(1986): Colvard MD+, *Periodont Case Rep* 8, 69
Injection-site pain (>10%)
(1981): Ameer B+, *Drugs* 21, 161 (7–52%)
Injection-site phlebitis (>10%)
(1981): Clarke RSJ, *Drugs* 22, 26 (15%)
Paresthesias
Pseudolymphoma
(1995): Magro CM+, *J Am Acad Dermatol* 32, 419
Rhabdomyolysis
(1983): Cauana RJ+, *N C Med J* 44, 18 (with amitriptyline and perphenazine)
Sialopenia (>10%)
Sialorrhea (<1%)
(1978): Dodson ME+, *Br J Anaesth* 50, 1059
Tremors (1–10%)
Xerostomia (>10%)

# LOSARTAN

**Synonyms:** DuP 753; MK 594
**Trade names:** Cozaar (Merck); Hyzaar (Merck)
**Indications:** Hypertension
**Category:** Angiotensin II receptor antagonist; antihypertensive
**Half-life:** 2 hours

Hyzaar is losartan and hydrochlorothiazide

### *Reactions*

## Skin

Angioedema (<1%)
(2001): Chiu AG+, *Laryngoscope* 111(10), 1729 (3 cases)
(1999): Rivera JO, *Ann Pharmacother* 33, 933
(1999): Rupprecht R+, *Allergy* 54, 81
(1998): van Rijnsoever EW+, *Arch Intern Med* 158, 2063
(1996): Boxer M, *J Allergy Clin Immunol* 98, 471
(1996): *Med Sci Bull* 18, 6
(1995): Acker CG+, *N Engl J Med* 333, 1572
Dermatitis (sic) (<1%)
Diaphoresis (<1%)
Ecchymoses (<1%)
Edema (<1%)
Erythema (<1%)
Exanthems
Facial edema (<1%)
Flushing (<1%)
(1995): Ahmad S, *JAMA* 274, 1266
Photosensitivity (<1%)
Pruritus (<1%)
Purpura
(2001): Brouard M+, *Br J Dermatol* 145(2), 362
(1998): Bosch X, *Arch Intern Med* 158, 191
Rash (sic) (<1%)
Urticaria (<1%)
Xerosis (<1%)

## Hair

Hair – alopecia (<1%)

## Other

Ageusia
(2002): Ohkoshi N+, *Eur J Neurol* 9(3), 315
(1996): Schlienger RG+, *Lancet* 347, 471
Anaphylactoid reactions (<1%)
Aphthous stomatitis
(1998): Goffin E+, *Clin Nephrol* 50, 197
Dysgeusia (<1%)
(1998): Heeringa M+, *Ann Intern Med* 129, 72
Fetal death
(2001): Saji H+, *Lancet* 357(9253), 363
Hypesthesia (<1%)
Myalgia (1%)
Oral ulceration
(2000): Madinier I+, *Ann Med Interne (Paris)* (French) 151, 248
Paresthesias (<1%)
(1995): Ahmad S, *JAMA* 274, 1266
Pseudolymphoma
(1999): Goldstein E, Toronto, ON (from Internet) (observation)
(1997): Viraben R+, *Lancet* 350, 1366
Tremors (<1%)
Xerostomia (<1%)

# LOVASTATIN

**Trade names:** Advicor; Mevacor (Merck)
**Other common trade names:** *Apo-Lovastatin; Lovalip; Mevinacor; Mevinolin; Nergadan; Rovacor; Taucor*
**Indications:** Hypercholesterolemia
**Category:** Antihyperlipidemic; HMG-CoA reductase inhibitor
**Half-life:** 1–2 hours
**Clinically important, potentially hazardous interactions with:** azithromycin, azothromycin, bosentan, cholestyramine, clarithromycin, cyclosporine, erythromycin, fenofibrate, gemfibrozil, **grapefruit juice**, imatinib, itraconazole, tacrolimus, verapamil

### *Reactions*

## Skin

Erythema
Erythema multiforme
Exanthems
(1988): Henwood JM+, *Drugs* 36, 429 (5%)
(1988): Tobert JA+, *Am J Cardiol* 62 (Suppl), 28J (0.3%)
(1987): Havel RJ+, *Ann Intern Med* 107, 609 (1%)
Lupus erythematosus
(1993): Ahmad S, *Heart Dis Stroke* 2, 262
(1991): Ahmad S, *Arch Intern Med* 151, 1667
Pruritus (5.2%)
(1988): Tobert JA+, *Am J Cardiol* 62 (Suppl), 28J
Purpura
(1999): Stein EA+, *JAMA* 281, 137
Rash (sic) (5.2%)
(1993): Krasovec M+, *Dermatology* 186, 248
(1993): Merck Laboratories, *The Lovastatin Study Groups I through IV*, 153, 1079
Stevens–Johnson syndrome
(1998): Downs JR+, *JAMA* 279, 1615
Toxic epidermal necrolysis
Urticaria
Vasculitis

## Hair

Hair – alopecia (>1%)

## Other

Dysgeusia (0.8%)
Gynecomastia (1–10%)
(1999): Stein EA+, *JAMA* 281, 137
Hypersensitivity
Hyposmia
(1992): Weber R+, *Laryngorhinootologie* (German) 71, 483
Myalgia (2.4%)
Myopathy (1–10%)
(1995): Garnett WR, *Am J Health Syst Pharm* 52(15), 1639
(1990): Kogan AD+, *Postgrad Med J* 66, 294
(1989): Vaher VMG+, *Lancet* 2, 1098
Paresthesias (>1%)
Rhabdomyolysis
(2000): Davidson MH, *Curr Atheroscler Rep* 2(1), 14
(1999): Bottorff M, *Atherosclerosis* 147(Suppl 1), S23
(1999): Corsini A+, *Pharmacol Ther* 84, 413 (with either cyclosporine, mibefradil or nefazodone)
(1998): Reaven P+, *Ann Intern Med* 109, 597 (with nicotinic acid)
(1998): Tobert JA+, *Am J Cardiol* 62, 28J (with gemfibrozil)
(1998): Wong PW+, *South Med J* 91(2), 202 (with erythromycin)
(1997): Chu PH+, *Jpn Heart J* 38(4), 541
(1997): Grunden JW+, *Ann Pharmacother* 31(7), 859 (with azithromycin and clarithromycin)

(1997): Hermida Lazcano I+, *An Med Interne* 14, 488
(1997): Olbricht C+, *Clin Pharmacol Ther* 62(3), 311 (with cyclosporine)
(1996): Ballantyne CM+, *Am J Cardiol* 78(5), 532
(1995): Farmer JA+, *Baillieres Clin Endocrinol Metab* 9(4), 825
(1995): Garnett WR, *Am J Health Syst Pharm* 52(15), 1639 (with either cyclosporine, gemfibrozil or niacin)
(1994): Dallaire M+, *CMAJ* 150(12), 1991 (with danazol)
(1992): Hume AL, *Ann Pharmacother* 26(10), 1303
(1992): Wallace CS+, *Ann Pharmacother* 26(2), 190
(1990): Pierce LR+, *JAMA* 264(1), 71 (with gemfibrozil)
(1990): Tobert JA+, *Am J Cardiol* 65(Suppl), 23F
(1988): Tobert JA+, *Am J Cardiol* 62, 28J (with cyclosporine)

Stomatitis
Xerostomia (>1%)

# LOXAPINE

**Trade name:** Loxitane (Watson)
**Other common trade names:** *Desconex; Loxapac*
**Indications:** Psychoses
**Category:** Tricyclic antipsychotic; anxiolytic and antidepressant
**Half-life:** 12–19 hours (terminal)

### *Reactions*

## Skin

Cutaneous side effects (sic)
Dermatitis (sic)
(1992): Breathnach SM+, *Adverse Drug Reactions and the Skin* Blackwell, Oxford, 203 (passim)
Diaphoresis
Exanthems
Facial edema
Photosensitivity (<1%)
(1991): Anon, *Drug Ther Bull* 29, 41
Pigmentation (<1%)
Pruritus (<1%)
(1992): Breathnach SM+, *Adverse Drug Reactions and the Skin* Blackwell, Oxford, 203 (passim)
Purpura
Rash (sic) (1–10%)
Seborrhea
(1992): Breathnach SM+, *Adverse Drug Reactions and the Skin* Blackwell, Oxford, 203 (passim)
Urticaria

## Hair

Hair – alopecia

## Other

Galactorrhea (<1%)
Gynecomastia (1–10%)
Myopathy
(1984): Thase ME+, *J Clin Psychopharmacol* 4, 46
Paresthesias
Parkinsonism
Priapism (<1%)
Rhabdomyolysis
(1996): Meltzer HY+, *Neuropsychopharmacology* 15(4), 395
Xerostomia (>10%)

# MAPROTILINE

**Trade name:** Ludiomil (Novartis)
**Other common trade names:** *Delgian; Maprostad; Melodil; Mirpan; Nono-Maprotiline; Psymion; Retinyl*
**Indications:** Depression, anxiety
**Category:** Tetracyclic antidepressant
**Half-life:** 27–58 hours

### *Reactions*

## Skin

Acne
(1988): Warnock JK+, *Am J Psychiatry* 145, 425
(1985): Oakley AM+, *Aust N Z J Med* 15, 256
(1982): Ponte CD, *Am J Psychiatry* 139, 141
Diaphoresis
(1977): Pinder RM+, *Drugs* 13, 321 (3–8%)
Edema
Erythema
Erythema multiforme
(1990): Zukervar P+, *J Toxicol Clin Exp* 10, 169
Exanthems (1–5%)
(1988): Warnock JK+, *Am J Psychiatry* 145, 425
(1977): Pinder RM+, *Drugs* 13, 321 (3–9%)
(1976): Johnson NM+, *Lancet* 2, 1357 (4%)
Flushing
Ichthyosis
(1991): Niederauer HH+, *Hautarzt* (German) 42, 455
Petechiae
Photosensitivity
(1989): KochP+, *Derm Beruf Umwelt* (German) 37, 203
(1988): Warnock JK+, *Am J Psychiatry* 145, 425
Pruritus
Purpura
(1988): Warnock JK+, *Am J Psychiatry* 145, 425
Rash (sic) (>10%)
Stevens–Johnson syndrome
(1990): Zukervar P+, *J Toxicol Clin Exp* 10, 169
Urticaria
(1988): Warnock JK+, *Am J Psychiatry* 145, 425
(1976): Johnson NM+, *Lancet* 2, 1357 (4%)
Vasculitis
(1985): Oakley AM+, *Aust N Z J Med* 15, 256

## Hair

Hair – alopecia
(2000): Mercke Y+, *Ann Clin Psychiatry* 12, 35
(1991): Niederauer HH+, *Hautarzt* (German) 42, 455

## Other

Black tongue
Dysgeusia
Galactorrhea
Gynecomastia (<1%)
Parkinsonism
Sialorrhea
Stomatitis
Tinnitus
Tremors
Xerostomia (22%)
(1977): Pinder RM+, *Drugs* 13, 321 (30–40%)

# MARIHUANA

**Trade name:** Marihuana (Marijuana)
**Indications:** Nausea and vomiting, substance abuse drug
**Category:** Hallucinogen
**Half-life:** no data

**Note:** Marihuana is the popular name for the dried flowering leaves of the hemp plant, *Cannabis sativa*. It contains tetrahydrocannabinols. It is also known as "pot," "grass," "hashish," etc

### *Reactions*

## Skin

Allergic reactions (sic)
(2000): Perez JA, *J Emerg Med* 18, 260
Exanthems
Pruritus
Squamous metaplasia
(2000): Holdcroft A, *Br J Anaesth* 84(3), 419
Urticaria

## Other

Anaphylactoid reactions
(1971): Liskow B+, *Ann Intern Med* 75, 571

# MAZINDOL

**Trade names:** Mazanor (Wyeth-Ayerst); Sanorex (Novartis)
**Other common trade names:** *Diestet; Liofindol; Solucaps; Teronac*
**Indications:** Obesity
**Category:** Anorexiant (appetite suppressant)
**Half-life:** 10 hours
**Clinically important, potentially hazardous interactions with:** fluoxetine, fluvoxamine, MAO inhibitors, paroxetine, phenelzine, sertraline, tranylcypromine

### *Reactions*

## Skin

Diaphoresis
Edema
Exanthems
Rash (sic)
Urticaria

## Other

Dysgeusia
Paresthesias
Xerostomia

# MDMA*

**Trade name:** Ecstacy*
**Indications:** N/A
**Category:** Hallucinogenic 'designer drug'; recreational drug; psychotherapeutic
**Half-life:** N/A

### *Reactions*

## Skin

Acne
(1998): Wollina U+, *Dermatology* 197(2), 171 (2 cases)
Chills
Diaphoresis
(1999): Rochester JA+, *J Am Board Fam Pract* 12(2), 137
(1998): Weinmann W+, *Forensic Sci Int* 91(2), 91
(1988): Buchanan JF+, *Med Toxicol Adverse Drug Exp* 3(1), 1
Flushing
(1999): Rochester JA+, *J Am Board Fam Pract* 12(2), 137
Rash (sic)

## Other

Bruxism
(2001): Murray JB, *Psychol Rep* 88(3 Pt 1), 895
(1999): Milosevic A+, *Community Dent Oral Epidemiol* 27(4), 283
Death
(2001): Braback L+, *Lakartidningen* 98(8), 817 (after one pill)
(2001): Doyon S, *Curr Opin Pediatr* 13(2), 170
(2001): Murray JB, *Psychol Rep* 88(3 Pt 1), 895
(2001): Nielsen S+, *Ugeskr Laeger* 163(16), 2253
(2001): Vickrey V, *Mich Med* 100(6), 53
(2000): Carter N+, *Int J Legal Med* 113(3), 168
(2000): Weir E, *CMAJ* 162(13), 1843
(1999): de la Torre R+, *Lancet* 353(9152), 593
(1999): Fineschi V+, *Forensic Sci Int* 104(1), 65
(1999): Hedetoft C+, *Ugeskr Laeger* 161(50), 6907
(1999): Lind J+, *Lancet* 354(9196), 2167
(1999): Ramsey JD+, *Lancet* 354(9196), 2166
(1999): Schwab M+, *Lancet* 352(9142), 1751
(1999): Walubo A+, *Hum Exp Toxicol* 18(2), 119
(1998): Byard RW+, *Am J Forensic Med Pathol* 19(3), 261 (5 cases)
(1998): Henry JA+, *Lancet* 352(9142), 1751
(1998): Mueller PD+, *Ann Emerg Med* 32(3 Pt 1), 377
(1998): Weinmann W+, *Forensic Sci Int* 91(2), 91
(1997): Parr MJ+, *Med J Aust* 166(3), 136
(1997): Thomasius R+, *Fortschr Neurol Psychiatr* 65(2), 49
(1996): Burnat P+, *Presse Med* 25(26), 1208
(1996): Dowsett RP, *Med J Aust* 164(11), 700
(1996): Fineschi V+, *Int J Legal Med* 108(5), 272
(1996): McCauley JC, *Med J Aust* 164(1), 56
(1996): Milroy CM+, *J Clin Pathol* 49, 149
(1995): Nielsen JC+, *Ugeskr Laeger* 157(6), 724
(1995): Squier MV+, *J Neurol Neurosurg Psychiatry* 58(6), 756
(1994): Szukaj M, *Nervenarzt* 65(11), 802
(1993): Cregg MT+, *Ir Med J* 86(4), 118
(1992): Henry JA, *BMJ* 305, 5
(1992): Henry JA+, *Lancet* 340, 284
(1988): Buchanan JF+, *Med Toxicol Adverse Drug Exp* 3(1), 1
(1988): Suarez RV+, *Am J Forensic Med Pathol* 9(4), 339
(1987): Dowling GP+, *JAMA* 257(12), 1615 (5 cases)
Depression
(2000): Morgan ML, *Psychopharmacol* (Berl) 152(3), 230
(2000): Shannon M, *Pediatr Emerg Care* 16(5), 377
(1999): Rochester JA+, *J Am Board Fam Pract* 12(2), 137
(1998): Liberg JP+, *Tidsskr Nor Laegeforen* 118(28), 4384
(1998): Pennings EJ+, *Ned Tijdschr Geneeskd* 142(35), 1942
(1997): Williamson S+, *Drug Alcohol Depend* 44(2-3), 87
(1993): Cregg MT+, *Ir Med J* 86(4), 118
Jaw clenching
(2001): Murray JB, *Psychol Rep* 88(3 Pt 1), 895
(1999): Milosevic A+, *Community Dent Oral Epidemiol* 27(4), 283
Myalgia
Paresthesias
(2000): Yates KM+, *N Z Med J* 113(1114), 315
Parkinsonism
(1999): Mintzer S+, *N Engl J Med* (340(18) 1443
Priapism
(2000): Dubin N+, *Urology* 56(6), 1057
Rhabdomyolysis
(2001): Halachanova V+, *Mayo Clin Proc* 76(1), 112
(2001): Kalant H, *CMAJ* 165(7), 917
(1999): Fineschi V+, *Forensic Sci Int* 104(1), 65
(1999): Hedetoft C+, *Ugeskr Laeger* 161(50), 6907
(1999): Rochester JA+, *J Am Board Fam Pract* 12(2), 137
(1998): Liberg JP+, *Tidsskr Nor Laegeforen* 118(28), 4384
(1998): Ramcharan S+, *J Toxicol Clin Toxicol* 36(7), 727
(1997): Cunningham M, *Intensive Crit Care Nurs* 13(4), 216
(1997): Trkulja V+, *Lijec Vjesn* 119(5-6), 158
(1997): Tsatsakis AM+, *Vet Hum Toxicol* 39(4), 241
(1996): Ellis AJ+, *Gut* 38(3), 454 (8 cases)
(1996): Fineschi V+, *Int J Legal Med* 108(5), 272
(1996): Gouzoulis-Mayfrank E+, *Nervenarzt* 67(5), 369
(1996): Roebroek RM+, *Ned Tijdschr Geneeskd* 140(4), 205
(1995): Lehmann ED+, *Postgrad Med J* 71(833), 186
(1995): Nielsen JC+, *Ugeskr Laeger* 157(6), 724
(1995): Steidle B+, *Rofo Fortschr Geb Roentgenstr Neuen Bildgeb Verfahr* 163(4), 353
(1994): Forrest AR+, *Forensic Sci Int* 64(1), 57 (fatal)
(1992): Henry JA+, *Lancet* 340(8816), 384 (7 fatal)
(1992): Screaton GR+, *Lancet* 339(8794), 677
(1992): Singarajah C+, *Anaesthesia* 47(8), 686
Serotonin syndrome
(1997): Dinse H, *Anaesthetist* 46(8), 697
(1997): Huether G+, *J Neural Transm* 104(8-9), 771
Tremors
Xerostomia
(1999): Milosevic A+, *Community Dent Oral Epidemiol* 27(4), 283

***Note:** 3,4-Methylenedioxymethamphetamine

# MEADOWSWEET

**Scientific names:** *Filipendula ulmaria; Spiraea ulmaria*
**Other common names:** Bridewort; Dolloff; Dropwort; Filipendula; Lady of the Meadow; Meadow Queen; Meadow-Wart; Meadowsweet; Queen of the Meadow; Ulmaria
**Family:** Rosaceae
**Purported indications:** Colds, fevers
**Other uses:** Cough, bronchitis, dyspepsia, heartburn, peptic ulcer, gout, rheumatic disorders, diuretic

### *Reactions*

## Skin

Rash (sic)

## Other

Hypersensitivity

# MEBENDAZOLE

**Trade name:** Vermox (McNeil)
**Other common trade names:** *Amycil; Bantenol; Helminzole; Lomper; Mebensole; Mindol; Nemasol; Pantelmin; Revapole; Toloxim; Vermicol*
**Indications:** Parasitic worm infestations
**Category:** Anthelmintic
**Half-life:** 1–12 hours

### *Reactions*

#### Skin

Allergic reactions (sic)
(1979): Kern P+, *Tropenmed Parasitol* 30, 65 (2 in 7 patients)
Angioedema (<1%)
Exanthems
Pruritus (<1%)
Rash (sic) (<1%)
Stevens–Johnson syndrome
(2000): Ajonuma LC+, *Trop Doc* 30, 57
Urticaria

#### Hair

Hair – alopecia
(1992): Breathnach SM+, *Adverse Drug Reactions and the Skin* Blackwell, Oxford, 177 (passim)

#### Other

Xerostomia

# MECHLORETHAMINE

**Synonyms:** mustine; nitrogen mustard
**Trade name:** Mustargen (Merck)
**Other common trade names:** *Mustine; Mustine Hydrochloride Boots*
**Indications:** Hodgkin's disease, mycosis fungoides
**Category:** Antineoplastic
**Half-life:** <1 minute
**Clinically important, potentially hazardous interactions with:** aldesleukin, **vaccines**

### *Reactions*

#### Skin

Acanthosis nigricans
(1988): Schweitzer WJ+, *J Am Acad Dermatol* 19, 951
Allergic dermatitis (sic)
(1999): Estève E+, *Arch Dermatol* 135, 1349
Angioedema
(1981): Wilson KS+, *Ann Intern Med* 94, 823
Bullous eruption
(1990): Goday JJ+, *Contact Dermatitis* 22, 306
(1981): Weiss RB+, *Ann Intern Med* 94, 66
Cellulitis
(1981): Wilson KS+, *Ann Intern Med* 94, 823
Contact dermatitis
(1991): Sheehan MP+, *J Pediatr* 119, 317
(1988): Ramsay DL+, *J Am Acad Dermatol* 19, 684
(1986): Mauduit G+, *Br J Dermatol* 115, 82
(1985): Arrazola JM+, *Int J Dermatol* 24, 608
(1985): Zachariae H, *Int J Clin Pharmacol Res* 5, 193
(1984): Ramsay DL+, *Arch Dermatol* 120, 1585
(1984): Vonderheid EC, *Int J Dermatol* 23, 180
(1983): Bronner AK+, *J Am Acad Dermatol* 9, 645
(1983): Nusbaum BP+, *Arch Dermatol* 119, 117
(1983): Price NM+, *Cancer* 52, 2214
(1982): Price NM+, *Arch Dermatol* 118, 234
(1981): Halprin KM+, *Br J Dermatol* 105, 71
(1981): Shelley WB, *Acta Derm Venereol* 61, 161
(1979): Handler RM+, *Int J Dermatol* 18, 758
(1978): du Vivier A+, *BMJ* 2, 1300
(1978): Volden G+, *BMJ* 2, 865
(1977): Price NM+, *Br J Dermatol* 97, 547
(1977): Sanchez-Yus E+, *Actas Dermosifiliogr* (Spanish) 68, 39
(1977): Volden G+, *Tidsskr Nor Laegeforen* (Norwegian) 97, 1671
(1976): Grunnet E, *Br J Dermatol* 94, 101
(1976): Pariser DM+, *Arch Dermatol* 112, 1113
(1975): Constantine VS+, *Arch Dermatol* 111, 484
(1975): Mitchell JC+, *Contact Dermatitis* 1, 363
(1971): Mandy S+, *Arch Dermatol* 103, 272
(1970): Van Scott EJ+, *Arch Dermatol* 102, 507
Epidermal cysts
(1991): Smith SP+, *J Am Acad Dermatol* 25, 940
Erythema multiforme (<1%)
(1967): Brauer MJ+, *Arch Intern Med* 120, 499
Exanthems (<1%)
Fungal infection (sic)
(1981): Shelley WB, *Acta Derm Venereol* 61, 164
Herpes zoster (>10%)
Pigmentation
(1984): Vonderheid EC, *Int J Dermatol* 23, 180
(1983): Bronner AK+, *J Am Acad Dermatol* 9, 645
(1982): Price NM+, *Arch Dermatol* 118, 234
(1977): Price NM, *Arch Dermatol* 113, 1387
(1975): O'Doherty CS, *Lancet* 2, 365
(1973): Flaxman BA+, *J Invest Dermatol* 60, 321
(1970): Epstein E Jr+, *Arch Dermatol* 102, 504
(1970): Van Scott EJ+, *Arch Dermatol* 102, 507
Pruritus
(1981): Weiss RB+, *Ann Intern Med* 94, 66
(1981): Wilson KS+, *Ann Intern Med* 94, 823
Purpura
(1981): Weiss RB+, *Ann Intern Med* 94, 66
Rash (sic) (<1%)
Squamous cell carcinoma
(1991): Smith SP+, *J Am Acad Dermatol* 25, 940
(1982): Lee LA+, *J Am Acad Dermatol* 7, 590
(1978): du Vivier A+, *Br J Dermatol* 99, 61
Stevens–Johnson syndrome
(1997): Newman JM+, *J Am Acad Dermatol* 36, 112
Urticaria
(1981): Weiss RB+, *Ann Intern Med* 94, 66
(1981): Wilson KS+, *Ann Intern Med* 94, 823
(1973): Daughters D+, *Arch Dermatol* 107, 429
Xerosis
(1984): Vonderheid EC, *Int J Dermatol* 23, 180

#### Hair

Hair – alopecia (1–10%)

#### Other

Anaphylactoid reactions (1–10%)
(1983): Bronner AK+, *J Am Acad Dermatol* 9, 645
(1977): Sanchez-Yus E+, *Actas Dermosifiliogr* (Spanish) 68, 39
(1976): Grunnet E, *Br J Dermatol* 94, 101
(1973): Daughters D+, *Arch Dermatol* 107, 429
Dysgeusia (1–10%) (metallic taste)
Hypersensitivity (1–10%)
(1972): Zackheim HS+, *Arch Dermatol* 105, 702
Injection-site extravasation (1–10%)

(2000): Kassner E., *J Pediatr Oncon Nurs* 17, 135
Injection-site thrombophlebitis (1–10%)
(1989): Kerker BJ+, *Semin Dermatol* 8, 173
(1981): Wilson KS+, *Ann Intern Med* 94, 823
Tinnitus

# MECLIZINE

**Trade name:** Antivert (Pfizer)
**Other common trade names:** *Antrizine; Bonamine; Bonine; Dizmiss; Dramamine II; Dramine; Meni-D; Nico-Vert; Peremesin; Postadoxin; Postafen; Suprimal; Vergon*
**Indications:** Motion sickness
**Category:** Antiemetic and antivertigo; antihistamine $H_1$ blocker
**Half-life:** 6 hours
**Clinically important, potentially hazardous interactions with: alcohol**, barbiturates, chloral hydrate, ethchlorvynol, paraldehyde, phenothiazines, zolpidem

### *Reactions*

## Skin

Angioedema (<1%)
Exanthems
(2001): Litt JZ, Beachwood, OH (personal case) (observation)
Photosensitivity (<1%)
Rash (sic) (<1%)
Urticaria

## Other

Myalgia (<1%)
Paresthesias (<1%)
Tremors
Xerostomia (1–10%)

# MECLOFENAMATE

**Trade name:** Meclofenamate
**Other common trade names:** *Kyroxan; Melvon; Movens*
**Indications:** Arthritis
**Category:** Nonsteroidal anti-inflammatory (NSAID)
**Half-life:** 2 hours
**Clinically important, potentially hazardous interactions with:** methotrexate

### *Reactions*

## Skin

Angioedema (<1%)
(1984): Stern RS+, *JAMA* 252, 1433
Bullous eruption
Edema (>1%)
Erythema multiforme (<1%)
(1985): Bigby M+, *J Am Acad Dermatol* 12, 866
(1984): Stern RS+, *JAMA* 252, 1433
(1983): Harrington T, *J Rheumatol* 10, 169
Erythema nodosum (<1%)
Erythroderma
(1985): Bigby M+, *J Am Acad Dermatol* 12, 866
Exanthems (1–5%)
(1992): Breathnach SM+, *Adverse Drug Reactions and the Skin* Blackwell, Oxford, 190 (passim)
(1985): Bigby M+, *J Am Acad Dermatol* 12, 866 (3–9%)
(1984): Stern RS+, *JAMA* 252, 1433
(1978): Dresner AJ, *Curr Ther Res* 23, 107
Exfoliative dermatitis (<1%)
(1992): Breathnach SM+, *Adverse Drug Reactions and the Skin* Blackwell, Oxford, 190 (passim)
(1984): Stern RS+, *JAMA* 252, 1433
Fixed eruption (<1%)
(1992): Breathnach SM+, *Adverse Drug Reactions and the Skin* Blackwell, Oxford, 190 (passim)
(1985): Bigby M+, *J Am Acad Dermatol* 12, 866
(1984): Stern RS+, *JAMA* 252, 1433
Hot flashes (<1%)
Lupus erythematosus
Peripheral edema
Photosensitivity
(1985): Bigby M+, *J Am Acad Dermatol* 12, 866
(1984): Stern RS+, *JAMA* 252, 1433
Pruritus (1–10%)
(1992): Breathnach SM+, *Adverse Drug Reactions and the Skin* Blackwell, Oxford, 190 (passim)
(1985): Bigby M+, *J Am Acad Dermatol* 12, 866
(1984): Stern RS+, *JAMA* 252, 1433
Psoriasis (exacerbation)
(1983): Meyerhoff JO, *N Engl J Med* 309, 496
Purpura (>1%)
(1992): Breathnach SM+, *Adverse Drug Reactions and the Skin* Blackwell, Oxford, 190 (passim)
(1985): Bigby M+, *J Am Acad Dermatol* 12, 866
(1984): Stern RS+, *JAMA* 252, 1433
(1981): Rodriguez J, *Drug Intell Clin Pharm* 15, 999
Rash (sic) (3–9%)
(1984): Stern RS+, *JAMA* 252, 1433
Stevens–Johnson syndrome (<1%)
Toxic epidermal necrolysis (<1%)
Urticaria (>1%)
(1985): Bigby M+, *J Am Acad Dermatol* 12, 866
(1984): Stern RS+, *JAMA* 252, 1433
Vasculitis
(1992): Breathnach SM+, *Adverse Drug Reactions and the Skin* Blackwell, Oxford, 190 (passim)
(1985): Bigby M+, *J Am Acad Dermatol* 12, 866
(1984): Stern RS+, *JAMA* 252, 1433
Vesiculobullous eruption
(1992): Breathnach SM+, *Adverse Drug Reactions and the Skin* Blackwell, Oxford, 190 (passim)
(1984): Stern RS+, *JAMA* 252, 1433

## Hair

Hair – alopecia (<1%)

## Other

Aphthous stomatitis
(1996): Fetterman M, Hialeah, FL (from Internet) (observation)
Dysgeusia (<1%)
Hypersensitivity
(1993): Fernandez-Rivas M+, *Ann Allergy* 71, 515
Oral ulceration
Paresthesias (<1%)
Porphyria
Serum sickness
Stomatitis (1–3%)
Tinnitus
Xerostomia

# MEDROXYPROGESTERONE

**Trade names:** Amen (Carnrick); Curretab (Solvay); Cycrin (ESI Lederle); Depo-Provera (Pharmacia & Upjohn); Premphase (Wyeth-Ayerst); Prempro (Wyeth-Ayerst); Provera (Pharmacia & Upjohn)
**Other common trade names:** *Alti-MPA; Aragest 5; Clinofem; Gestapuran; Novo-Medrone; Perlutex; Progevera; Ralovera*
**Indications:** Secondary amenorrhea, renal or endometrial carcinoma
**Category:** Progestin; contraceptive; antineoplastic
**Half-life:** 30 days
**Clinically important, potentially hazardous interactions with:** acitretin, dofetilide

### *Reactions*

## Skin

Acne (1–5%)
(1974): Pochi PE, *Arch Dermatol* 109, 556
Allergic reactions (sic) (<1%)
Angioedema
Ankle edema
Chloasma (1–10%)
Diaphoresis (<1%)
(1990): Willemse PHB+, *Eur J Cancer* 26, 337 (31%)
Edema (>10%)
Erythema nodosum
(1974): Berant N, *Harefuah* (Hebrew) 87, 19
Exanthems
Flushing
(1990): Willemse PHB+, *Eur J Cancer* 26, 337 (12%)
Hemorrhagic eruption (sic)
Hot flashes
Melasma (1–10%)
Mucha–Habermann disease
(1973): Hollander A+, *Arch Dermatol* 107, 465
Photosensitivity
Pigmented purpuric eruption
(2000): Tsao H+, *J Am Acad Dermatol* 43, 308
Pruritus (1–10%)
Rash (sic) (1–5%)
Scleroderma (<1%)
Striae
(2000): Gupta M, *Br J Fam Plann* 26, 104
Urticaria
Xerosis (<1%)

## Hair

Hair – alopecia (1–5%)
Hair – hirsutism (<1%)
(1984): Delanoe D+, *Lancet* 1, 276

## Other

Anaphylactoid reactions (<1%)
Bromhidrosis (<1%)
Galactorrhea (<1%)
(1998): Cromwell P+, *J Adolesc Health* 23, 61
Gynecomastia (<1%)
Injection-site necrosis
(2000): Clark SM+, *Br J Dermatol* 143, 1356
Injection-site pain (>10%)
Mastodynia (1–5%)
Paresthesias (<1%)
Thrombophlebitis (1–10%)
Vaginitis (1–5%)

# MEFENAMIC ACID

**Trade name:** Ponstel (Parke-Davis)
**Other common trade names:** *Dysman; Lysalgo; Mefac; Mefic; Parkemed; Ponstan; Ponstyl*
**Indications:** Pain, dysmenorrhea
**Category:** Nonsteroidal anti-inflammatory (NSAID)
**Half-life:** 3.5 hours
**Clinically important, potentially hazardous interactions with:** methotrexate

### *Reactions*

## Skin

Angioedema (<1%)
Bullous pemphigoid
(1986): Shepherd AN+, *Postgrad Med J* 62, 67
Diaphoresis
Edema
Erythema multiforme (<1%)
(1990): Sowden JM+, *Clin Exp Dermatol* 15, 387
(1985): Ting HC+, *Int J Dermatol* 24, 587
Exanthems
(1992): Breathnach SM+, *Adverse Drug Reactions and the Skin* Blackwell, Oxford, 190 (passim)
Exfoliative dermatitis
(1992): Breathnach SM+, *Adverse Drug Reactions and the Skin* Blackwell, Oxford, 190 (passim)
Facial edema
Fixed eruption
(1998): Mahboob A+, *Int J Dermatol* 37, 833
(1992): Long CC+, *Br J Dermatol* 126, 409
(1991): Mohamed KN, *Aust N Z J Med* 21, 291
(1990): Sowden JM+, *Clin Exp Dermatol* 15, 387
(1986): Watson A+, *Australas J Dermatol* 27, 6
(1986): Wilson CL+, *BMJ* 293, 1243
Hot flashes (<1%)
Photosensitivity
(1997): O'Reilly FM+, American Academy of Dermatology Meeting, Poster #14
Pruritus (1–10%)
Purpura
Rash (sic) (>10%)
Stevens–Johnson syndrome (<1%)
(1991): Chan JC+, *Drug Safety* 6, 230
Toxic epidermal necrolysis (<1%)
(1991): Sakellariou G+, *Int J Artif Organs* 14, 634
(1990): Black AK+, *Br J Dermatol* 123, 277
Urticaria (<1%)
(1992): Breathnach SM+, *Adverse Drug Reactions and the Skin* Blackwell, Oxford, 190 (passim)
Vasculitis
(1980): Malik S+, *Lancet* 2, 746

## Other

Anaphylactoid reactions
(1985): O'Brien WM+, *J Rheumatol* 12, 13
Glossitis
Oral ulceration
Pseudoporphyria
(1998): O'Hagan AH+, *Br J Dermatol* 139, 1131
Sialorrhea
Xerostomia

## MEFLOQUINE

**Trade name:** Lariam (Roche)
**Other common trade names:** *Laricam; Mephaquin; Mephaquine*
**Indications:** Malaria
**Category:** Antimalarial
**Half-life:** 21–22 days

### *Reactions*

#### Skin

Erythema
(1992): Breathnach SM+, *Adverse Drug Reactions and the Skin* Blackwell, Oxford, 176 (passim)
Erythema multiforme
Exanthems
(1999): Smith HR+, *Clin Exp Dermatol* 24, 249 (30%)
Exfoliative dermatitis
(1993): Martin GJ+, *Clin Infect Dis* 16, 341
Facial dermatitis
(1991): Shlim DR, *JAMA* 266, 2560
Pruritus
(1999): Smith HR+, *Clin Exp Dermatol* 24, 249 (4–10%)
(1989): Sowunmi A+, *Lancet* 2, 313; 397
Psoriasis
(1998): Potasman I+, *J Travel Med* 5, 156
Rash (sic) (1–10%)
Stevens–Johnson syndrome
(1999): Smith HR+, *Clin Exp Dermatol* 24, 249
(1991): Van den Enden E+, *Lancet* 337, 683
Toxic epidermal necrolysis
(1999): Smith HR+, *Clin Exp Dermatol* 24, 249 (fatal)
(1997): McBride SR+, *Lancet* 349, 101
Urticaria
(1999): Smith HR+, *Clin Exp Dermatol* 24, 249
Vasculitis
(1999): Smith HR+, *Clin Exp Dermatol* 24, 249
(1995): White AC+, *Ann Intern Med* 123, 894
(1993): Scerri L+, *Int J Dermatol* 32, 517

#### Hair

Hair – alopecia (<1%)

#### Other

Death
Myalgia (1–10%)
Tinnitus

## MELATONIN

**Scientific name:** *N-acetyl-5-methoxytryptamine*
**Family:** None
**Purported indications:** Jet lag, sleep disorders, "shift-work" disorder, Alzheimer's disease, tinnitus, depressive disorders, migraine and cluster headaches, hypertension, hyperpigmentation, preventing osteoporosis, cancer of the breast, brain, lung and prostate
**Other uses:** Anti-aging; immune system enhancer, antioxidant, epilepsy. Skin protectant against sunburn

### *Reactions*

#### Skin

Fixed eruption
(1998): Bardazzi F+, *Acta Derm Venereol* 78(1), 69
Photosensitivity

## MELOXICAM

**Trade name:** Mobic (Abbott)
**Indications:** Osteoarthritis
**Category:** Nonsteroidal anti-inflammatory (NSAID)
**Half-life:** 15–20 hours

### *Reactions*

#### Skin

Allergic reactions (sic) (<2%)
Angioedema (<2%)
(2000): Quaratino D+, *Ann Allergy Asthma Immunol* 84, 613
Bullous eruption (<2%)
Edema (2–5%)
Erythema multiforme (<2%)
(1999): Nikas SN+, *Am J Med* 107, 532
Exanthems (<2%)
(2000): Quaratino D+, *Ann Allergy Asthma Immunol* 84, 613
Facial edema
(2000): Quaratino D+, *Ann Allergy Asthma Immunol* 84, 613
Hot flashes (<2%)
Photosensitivity (<2%)
Pruritus (<2%)
(2001): Bunyaratavej N+, *J Med Assoc Thai* 84(Suppl 2), S542 (2%)
Purpura (<2%)
Rash (sic) (1–3%)
(2001): Bunyaratavej N+, *J Med Assoc Thai* 84, S542 (2%)
Skin disorders (sic)
(1996): Huskisson EC+, *Br J Rheumatol* 35, 29 (18%)
Stevens–Johnson syndrome (<2%)
Toxic epidermal necrolysis (<2%)
(2002): Eastern J, North Caldwell, NJ (from Internet) (observation)
Urticaria (<2%)
(2000): Quaratino D+, *Ann Allergy Asthma Immunol* 84, 613
Vasculitis (<2%)

#### Other

Anaphylactoid reactions (<2%)
Dysgeusia (<2%)
Hypersensitivity
(2001): Nettis E+, *Allergy* 56(8), 803
Paresthesias (<2%)
Tremors (<2%)
Ulcerative stomatitis (<2%)
Xerostomia (<2%)

## MELPHALAN

**Trade name:** Alkeran (GSK)
**Indications:** Multiple myeloma, carcinomas
**Category:** Antineoplastic; nitrogen mustard
**Half-life:** 90 minutes
**Clinically important, potentially hazardous interactions with:** aldesleukin, PEG-interfeon alfa-2b

### *Reactions*

#### Skin

Angioedema
(1983): Bronner AK+, *J Am Acad Dermatol* 9, 645
(1981): Weiss RB+, *Ann Intern Med* 94, 66

Eccrine squamous syringometaplasia
(1997): Valks R+, *Arch Dermatol* 133, 873
Edema
Exanthems
(1981): Harvey HA+, *Ann Intern Med* 94, 542
(1981): Weiss RB+, *Ann Intern Med* 94, 66
(1978): Levine N+, *Cancer Treat Rev* 5, 67
(1969): Hoogstraten B+, *JAMA* 209, 251 (4%)
Petechiae
Pruritus (1–10%)
(1983): Bronner AK+, *J Am Acad Dermatol* 9, 645
Purpura
Rash (sic) (1–10%)
Scleroderma (localized)
(1998): Landau M+, *J Am Acad Dermatol* 39, 1011 (2 cases)
Urticaria
(1983): Bronner AK+, *J Am Acad Dermatol* 9, 645
(1981): Harvey HA+, *Ann Intern Med* 94, 542
(1981): Weiss RB+, *Ann Intern Med* 94, 66
Vasculitis (1–10%)
(1986): Hannedouche T+, *Ann Med Intern Paris* (French) 137, 57
Vesiculation (1–10%)

### Hair

Hair – alopecia (1–10%)
(1992): Zaun H+, *Hautarzt* (German) 43, 215
(1978): Levine N+, *Cancer Treat Rev* 5, 67

### Nails

Nails – Beau's lines (transverse nail bands)
(1992): Zaun H+, *Hautarzt* (German) 43, 215
(1983): James WD+, *Arch Dermatol* 119, 334
(1982): Jeanmougin M+, *Ann Dermatol Venereol* (French) 109, 169
(1977): Malacarne P+, *Arch Dermatol Res* 25, 81

### Other

Anaphylactoid reactions
(1983): Bronner AK+, *J Am Acad Dermatol* 9, 645
(1982): Dunagin WG, *Semin Oncol* 9, 14
Death
(2001): Sanchorawala V+, *Bone Marrow Transplant* 28(7), 637 (14%)
Gynecomastia
(2000): Cohen JD+, *Presse Med* 29(35), 1936
Hypersensitivity (1–10%)
(1992): Weiss RB, *Semin Oncol* 19, 458
Mucositis
(2002): Moreau P+, *Blood* 99(3), 731
Oral mucosal lesions
Oral mucositis
(2000): Wardley AM+, *Br J Haematol* 110, 292
Oral ulceration
Perfusion edema
(1995): Vrouenraets BC+, *Melanoma Res* 5, 425
Perfusion erythema
(1995): Vrouenraets BC+, *Melanoma Res* 5, 425
Stomatitis (1–10%)

## MEPACRINE

(See QUINACRINE)

## MEPERIDINE

**Trade names:** Demerol (Sanofi); Mepergan (Wyeth-Ayerst)
**Other common trade names:** *Dolantin; Dolestine; Dolosal; Opistan; Pethidine; Petidin*
**Indications:** Pain
**Category:** Narcotic agonist analgesic
**Half-life:** 3–4 hours
**Clinically important, potentially hazardous interactions with:** acyclovir, **alcohol**, amphetamines, barbiturates, CNS depressants, fluoxetine, furazolidone, general anesthetics, isocarboxazid, linezolid, lithium, MAO inhibitors, moclobemide, phenelzine, phenobarbital, phenothiazines, phenytoin, ritonavir, selegiline, sibutramine, SSRIs, tranquilizers, tranylcypromine, tricyclic antidepressants, **tryptophan**, valacyclovir

### *Reactions*

### Skin

Angioedema
(1960): Schoenfeld MR, *N Y State J Med* 60, 2591
Diaphoresis
Flushing
Herpes (sic)
(1986): Acalovschi I, *Anaesthesia* 41, 1271
Necrotizing angiitis
(1971): Halpern M+, *Am J Roentgenol Radium Ther Nucl Med* 111, 663
Pruritus
(1993): Riley RH, *Anaesth Intensive Care* 21, 474
(1984): Saissy JM, *Ann Fr Anesth Reanim* (French) 3, 402
(1960): Schoenfeld MR, *N Y State J Med* 60, 2591
Rash (sic) (<1%)
Toxic epidermal necrolysis
(1967): Caldwell IW+, *Br J Dermatol* 79, 287
Urticaria (<1%)
(2000): Anibarro B+, *Allergy* 55, 305

### Other

Cold microabscesses
(1978): Waisbren BA, *JAMA* 239, 1395
Embolia cutis medicamentosa (Nicolau syndrome)
(1995): Faucher L+, *Pediatr Dermatol* 12, 187
Injection-site erythema
(1993): Kundrotas L+, *Gastrointest Endosc* 39, 109
(1960): Schoenfeld MR, *N Y State J Med* 60, 2591
Injection-site pain (1–10%)
Injection-site scarring
(1994): Danielsen AG+, *Ugeskr Laeger* (Danish) 156, 162
Injection-site ulceration
(1994): Danielsen AG+, *Ugeskr Laeger* (Danish) 156, 162
Myopathy
(1968): Aberfeld DC+, *Arch Neurol* 19, 384
Tremors
Xerostomia (1–10%)

# MEPHENYTOIN

**Trade name:** Mesantoin (Novartis)
**Other common trade names:** *Epilan-Gerot; Epilanex*
**Indications:** Partial seizures
**Category:** Hydantoin anticonvulsant
**Half-life:** 7 hours (for the active metabolite: 95–144 hours)
**Clinically important, potentially hazardous interactions with:** chloramphenicol, cyclosporine, disulfiram, dopamine, imatinib, itraconazole

### *Reactions*

## Skin

Acne
(1951): Frankel AZ+, *Ohio State Med J* 47, 1013
Angioedema
(1951): Frankel AZ+, *Ohio State Med J* 47, 1013
Bullous eruption
(1948): Ruskin DB, *JAMA* 137, 1031
Cutaneous side effects (sic)
(1951): Frankel AZ+, *Ohio State Med J* 47, 1013 (10%)
Dermatomyositis
(1977): Zangemeister WH+, *Fortschr Neurol Psychiatr Grenzgeb* (German) 45, 501
Edema
Erythema multiforme
(1979): Pollack MA+, *Ann Neurol* 5, 262
(1951): Frankel AZ+, *Ohio State Med J* 47, 1013
(1951): Lindermayr W, *Hautarzt* (German) 2, 313
Exanthems
(1972): Levantine A+, *Br J Dermatol* 87, 646 (8–10%)
(1954): Dreyer R, *Dtsch Med Wochenschr* (German) 79, 1215
(1952): McArthur P, *Lancet* 1, 592 (5%)
(1951): Frankel AZ+, *Ohio State Med J* 47, 1013 (8.85%)
(1951): Lindermayr W, *Hautarzt* (German) 2, 313
Exfoliative dermatitis
(1951): Frankel AZ+, *Ohio State Med J* 47, 1013
Lupus erythematosus
(1989): Vivino FB+, *Arthritis Rheum* 32, 560
(1977): Zangemeister WH+, *Fortschr Neurol Psychiatr Grenzgeb* (German) 45, 501
(1976): Singsen BH+, *Pediatrics* 57, 529
(1968): Cochran M+, *Proc R Soc Med* 61, 656
(1967): Losada M+, *Rev Med Chil* (Spanish) 95, 380 (generalized)
(1965): Schütz E+, *Med Klin* (German) 60, 537
(1963): Jacobs JC, *Pediatrics* 32, 257
(1957): Lindquist T, *Acta Med Scand* 158, 131
(1957): Ruppli H+, *Schweiz Med Wochenschr* (German) 88, 1555
(1955): Capalbo EE+, *Rev Soc Argent Hemat* (Spanish) 5, 19
Pigmentation
(1964): Krebs A, *Schweiz Med Wochenschr* (German) 94, 748
(1964): Kuske H+, *Dermatologica* 129, 121
(1954): Dreyer R, *Dtsch Med Wochenschr* (German) 79, 1215 (Addison-like)
(1951): Hunter H+, *JAMA* 147, 744
Pruritus
(1954): Dreyer R, *Dtsch Med Wochenschr* (German) 79, 1215
Purpura
(1955): Capalbo EE+, *Rev Soc Argent Hemat* (Spanish) 5, 19
Scleroderma
(1990): May DG+, *Clin Pharmacol Ther* 28, 286
Stevens–Johnson syndrome
(1951): Frankel AZ+, *Ohio State Med J* 47, 1013
Toxic epidermal necrolysis
(1979): Pollack MA+, *Ann Neurol* 5, 262
(1976): Babala J+, *Acta Paediatr Acad Sci Hung* 17, 9
(1976): Nozickova M+, *Cesk Dermatol* (Czech) 51, 375
(1962): Walker J, *Med Proc* 8, 208
Urticaria
(1972): Levantine A+, *Br J Dermatol* 87, 646
(1951): Frankel AZ+, *Ohio State Med J* 47, 1013
(1951): Lindermayr W, *Hautarzt* (German) 2, 313

## Hair

Hair – alopecia

## Other

Gingival hyperplasia
Oral mucosal eruption
(1954): Dreyer R, *Dtsch Med Wochenschr* (German) 79, 1215
Polyarteritis nodosa
(1951): Frankel AZ+, *Ohio State Med J* 47, 1013
Stomatitis
(1996): Meloni G+, *Lancet* 347, 1691

# MEPHOBARBITAL

**Trade name:** Mebaral (Sanofi)
**Other common trade name:** *Prominal*
**Indications:** Epilepsy, anxiety
**Category:** Long-acting barbiturate; anticonvulsant; sedative
**Half-life:** 34 hours
**Clinically important, potentially hazardous interactions with: alcohol**, anticoagulants, antihistamines, brompheniramine, buclizine, chlorpheniramine, dicumarol, ethanolamine, imatinib, warfarin

### *Reactions*

## Skin

Angioedema (<1%)
Exanthems
Exfoliative dermatitis (<1%)
Purpura
Rash (sic) (<1%)
Stevens–Johnson syndrome (<1%)
Urticaria

## Other

Rhabdomyolysis
(1990): Larpin R+, *Presse Med* 19(30), 1403
Serum sickness
Thrombophlebitis (<1%)

# MEPROBAMATE

**Trade names:** Equanil (Wyeth-Ayerst); Miltown (Wallace)
**Other common trade names:** *Harmonin; Meditran; Meditrara; Meprate; Meprospan; Miltaun; Neuramate; Praol; Probamyl; Urbilat; Visanon*
**Indications:** Anxiety, insomnia
**Category:** Anxiolytic
**Half-life:** 10 hours

### *Reactions*

## Skin

Allergic reactions (sic)
(1955): Selling LS, *JAMA* 157, 1594 (1.1%)

Angioedema (<1%)
(1964): Welsh AL, *Med Clin North Am* 48, 459
(1958): Hollister LE, *Ann Intern Med* 49, 17
(1957): Bernstein C+, *JAMA* 163, 930
(1955): Selling LS, *JAMA* 157, 1594
Bullous eruption (<1%)
(1977): Varma AJ+, *Arch Intern Med* 137, 1208 (passim)
(1974): Tay C, *Asian J Med* 10, 223
Cutaneous side effects (sic)
(1972): Kauppinen K, *Acta Derm Venereol* (Stockh) 52 (Suppl), 68 (2%)
(1968): Montgomery DC+, *Can Med Assoc J* 99, 712 (2%)
Dermatitis (sic) (<1%)
Ecchymoses
Eczematous eruption (sic)
(1981): Edwards JG, *Drugs* 22, 495 (passim)
Erythema multiforme (<1%)
(1972): Kauppinen K, *Acta Derm Venereol* (Stockh) 52, 68
(1959): Wright W, *JAMA* 171, 1642
Erythema nodosum (<1%)
Exanthems
(1981): Edwards JG, *Drugs* 22, 495 (passim)
(1972): Kauppinen K, *Acta Derm Venereol* (Stockh) 52 (Suppl), 68
(1969): Savin JA, *Proc R Soc Med* 62, 349
(1967): Lockey SD, *Med Sci* 18, 43
(1966): Smith JW+, *Ann Intern Med* 65, 629 (2%)
(1965): Fellner MJ+, *Med Clin North Am* 49, 709
(1964): Welsh AL, *Med Clin North Am* 48, 459
(1959): Wright W, *JAMA* 171, 1642
(1958): Marcussen PV, *Acta Derm Venereol* (Stockh) 38, 398
(1957): Falk MS, *Arch Dermatol* 75, 437
(1956): Friedman HT+, *JAMA* 162, 628
Exfoliative dermatitis
Fixed eruption (<1%)
(1985): Kauppinen K+, *Br J Dermatol* 112, 575
(1984): Boyle J+, *BMJ* 289, 802
(1981): Edwards JG, *Drugs* 22, 495 (passim)
(1972): Kauppinen K, *Acta Derm Venereol* (Stockh) 52 (Suppl), 68
(1965): Gore HC+, *Arch Dermatol* 91, 627
Lupus erythematosus
(1957): Bernstein C+, *JAMA* 163, 930
Pemphigus
(1980): Godard W+, *Ann Dermatol Venereol* (French) 107, 1213
Pemphigus foliaceus
(1980): Godard W+, *Ann Dermatol Venereol* (French) 107, 1213
Peripheral edema (<1%)
Petechiae
(1956): Carmel WJ+, *N Engl J Med* 255, 770
Photosensitivity
(1957): Bernstein C+, *JAMA* 163, 930
Pityriasis rosea
(1959): Wright W, *JAMA* 171, 1642
Pruritus (<1%)
(1970): Savin JA, *Br J Dermatol* 83, 546
(1969): Savin JA, *Proc R Soc Med* 62, 349
(1964): Welsh AL, *Med Clin North Am* 48, 459
(1957): Falk MS, *Arch Dermatol* 75, 437
(1956): Carmel WJ+, *N Engl J Med* 255, 770
(1956): Friedman HT+, *JAMA* 162, 628
Purpura (<1%)
(1993): Pang BK+, *Ann Acad Med Singapore* 22, 870
(1985): Ambriz-Fernandez R+, *Rev Invest Clin* (Spanish) 37, 347
(1981): Edwards JG, *Drugs* 22, 495 (passim)
(1970): Savin JA, *Br J Dermatol* 83, 546
(1969): Peterkin GAG+, *Practitioner* 202, 117
(1969): Savin JA, *Proc R Soc Med* 62, 349
(1967): Lockey SD, *Med Sci* 18, 43
(1967): Peterson WC+, *Arch Dermatol* 95, 40
(1957): Bernstein C+, *JAMA* 163, 930
(1957): Falk MS, *Arch Dermatol* 75, 437
(1957): Levan NE, *Arch Dermatol* 75, 437
(1956): Carmel WJ Jr+, *N Engl J Med* 255, 770
(1956): Friedman HT+, *JAMA* 162, 628
Rash (sic) (1–10%)
Stevens–Johnson syndrome (<1%)
(1972): Kauppinen K, *Acta Derm Venereol* (Stockh) 52 (Suppl), 68
(1959): Wright W, *JAMA* 171, 1642
Toxic epidermal necrolysis (<1%)
(1969): Sander-Jensen K, *Tidsskr Nor Laegeforen* (Norwegian) 89, 398
Toxic erythema
(1974): Felix RH+, *Lancet* 1, 1017
Urticaria
(1981): Edwards JG, *Drugs* 22, 495 (passim)
(1972): Kauppinen K, *Acta Derm Venereol* (Stockh) 52 (Suppl), 68
(1967): Lockey SD, *Med Sci* 18, 43
(1966): Smith JW+, *Ann Intern Med* 65, 629 (2%)
(1964): Welsh AL, *Med Clin North Am* 48, 459
(1959): Wright W, *JAMA* 171, 1642
(1958): Hollister LE, *Ann Intern Med* 49, 17
(1957): Bernstein C+, *JAMA* 163, 930
(1956): Friedman HT+, *JAMA* 162, 628
(1955): Selling LS, *JAMA* 157, 1594
Vasculitis
(1964): Welsh AL, *Med Clin North Am* 48, 459
(1962): Schwank R, *Cesk Dermatol* 37, 6
(1959): Wright W, *JAMA* 171, 1642
(1958): von Marcussen P, *Acta Derm Venereol* (Stockh) 38 398
(1957): Bernstein C+, *JAMA* 163, 930
(1957): Falk MS, *Arch Dermatol* 75, 437
(1957): Levan NE, *Arch Dermatol* 75, 437
(1956): Carmel WJ+, *N Engl J Med* 255, 770

## Other

Acute intermittent porphyria
(1967): de Matteis F, *Pharmacol Rev* 19, 523
Anaphylactoid reactions
(1974): Felix RH+, *Lancet* 1, 1017
Gynecomastia
Hypersensitivity
Oral mucosal eruption
(1959): Wright W, *JAMA* 171, 1642
Oral ulceration
Paresthesias
Polyarteritis nodosa
(1962): Schwank R, *Cesk Dermatol* 37, 6
Porphyria
(1984): Magnus IA, *BMJ* 288, 1474
Rhabdomyolysis
(1992): Bertran F+, *Therapie* 47(5), 444
Stomatitis (<1%)
(1959): Brachfeld J+, *JAMA* 169, 1321
Xerostomia

# MERCAPTOPURINE

**Synonyms:** 6-mercaptopurine; 6-MP
**Trade name:** Purinethol (GSK)
**Other common trade names:** *Classen; Ismipur; Leukerin; Puri-Nethol*
**Indications:** Leukemias
**Category:** Antineoplastic; antimetabolite; immunosuppressant
**Half-life:** triphasic: 45 minutes; 2.5 hours; 10 hours
**Clinically important, potentially hazardous interactions with:** aldesleukin, allopurinol, mycophenolate, olsalazine, **vaccines**

### *Reactions*

## Skin

Acral erythema
(1991): Baack BR+, *J Am Acad Dermatol* 24, 457
Dermatitis (sic)
(1968): Moore GE+, *Cancer Chemother Abstr* 52, 655 (2%)
Edema
Exanthems
(1989): Present DH+, *Ann Intern Med* 111, 641 (0.5%)
Herpes zoster
(1999): Korelitz BI+, *Am J Gastroenterology* 94, 424
Lichenoid eruption
(1973): Beylot C+, *Bull Soc Fr Dermatol Syphiligr* (French) 80, 190
Lupus erythematosus
(1966): Lee SL+, *Arch Intern Med* 117, 620
Palmar–plantar erythema
(1986): Cox GJ+, *Arch Dermatol* 122, 1413
Pellagra
(1987): Schmutz JL+, *Ann Dermatol Venereol* (French) 114, 569
(1960): Ludwig GD+, *Clin Res* 8, 212
Petechiae
Photosensitivity
(1987): Schmutz JL+, *Ann Dermatol Venereol* (French) 114, 569
(1960): Ludwig GD+, *Clin Res* 8, 212
Pigmentation (1–10%)
Pruritus
Purpura
Radiation recall
(1975): Dreizen S+, *Postgrad Med* 58, 150
Rash (sic) (1–10%)
Toxic epidermal necrolysis
(1969): Amerio PL+, *G Ital Dermatol Venereol* (Italian) 110, 514
Urticaria
(1985): Sparling R+, *Clin Lab Haematol* 7, 184
Vasculitis
(1997): Andersen JM+, *Pharmacotherapy* 17, 173

## Hair

Hair – alopecia

## Nails

Nails – loss (sic)

## Other

Glossitis (<1%)
Lobular panniculitis
(1997): Andersen JM+, *Pharmacotherapy* 17, 173
Mucositis (1–10%)
Oral mucosal lesions
(1983): Bronner AK+, *J Am Acad Dermatol* 9, 645 (1–5%)
(1968): Moore GE+, *Cancer Chemother Abstr* 52, 655 (2%)
Serum sickness
(1997): Andersen JM+, *Pharmacotherapy* 17, 173
Stomatitis (1–10%)

# MESALAMINE

**Synonyms:** 5-aminosalicylic acid; 5-ASA; fisalamine; mesalazine
**Trade names:** Asacol (Procter & Gamble); Canasa; Pentasa (Shire); Rowasa (Solvay)
**Other common trade names:** *Asacolitin; Claversal; Mesalazine; Mesasal; Pentasa SR; Quintasa; Salofalk; Tidocol*
**Indications:** Ulcerative colitis
**Category:** Anti-inflammatory; bowel disease suppressant
**Half-life:** 0.5–1.5 hours

### *Reactions*

## Skin

Acne (1.2%)
Allergic reactions (sic) (<1%)
(1990): Boulain T+, *Gastroenterol Clin Biol* (French) 14, 288
(1989): Brogden RN+, *Drugs* 38, 500
Diaphoresis (3%)
Ecchymoses
Eczema (sic)
Edema (1.2%)
Erythema
(1990): Boulain T+, *Gastroenterol Clin Biol* 14, 288 (rectal)
Erythema nodosum
Exanthems
(1991): LeGros V+, *BMJ* 302, 970
(1988): Fardy JM+, *J Clin Gastroenterol* 10, 635
(1988): Gron I+, *Ugeskr Laeger* (Danish) 150, 32
Facial edema
(1990): Boulain T+, *Gastroenterol Clin Biol* 14, 288 (rectal application)
Folliculitis
(1996): Lizasoain J+, *Am J Gastroenterol* 91, 819
Kawasaki-like syndrome (sic) (<1%)
Lichen planus
(1991): Alstead EM+, *J Clin Gastroenterol* 13, 335
Lupus erythematosus
(1997): Timsit MA+, *Rev Rhum Engl Ed* 64, 586
(1992): Pent MT+, *BMJ* 305, 159
Mucocutaneous lymph node syndrome (Kawasaki syndrome)
(1991): Waanders H+, *Am J Gastroenterol* 86, 219
Peripheral edema (0.61%)
Photosensitivity
(1999): Horiuchi Y+, *Am J Gastroenterol* 94, 3386
Pruritus (1.2%)
Psoriasis
Pustuloderma
(2001): Gibbon KL+, *J Am Acad Dermatol* 45, S220–1
Pyoderma gangrenosum
Rash (sic) (3%)
(1992): Giaffer MH+, *Aliment Pharmacol Ther* 6, 51
(1992): Hautekeete ML+, *Gastroenterology* 103, 1925
(1991): Lesur G+, *Gastroenterol Clin Biol* (French) 15, 457
Urticaria
Vasculitis
(1994): Lim AG+, *BMJ* 308, 113
Xerosis

## Hair

Hair – alopecia (0.86%)
(1997): Timsit MA+, *Rev Rhum Engl Ed* 64, 586
(1995): Netzer P, *Schweiz Med Wochenschr* (German) 125, 2438
(1991): Hadjigogos K, *Ital J Gastroenterol* (Italian) 23, 257
(1989): Brogden RN+, *Drugs* 38, 500
(1982): Kutty PK+, *Ann Intern Med* 97, 785

### Nails
Nails – disorder (sic)

### Other
Dysgeusia
Hypersensitivity (<1%)
(2001): Safer L+, *Gastroenterol Clin Biol* 25(1), 104 (following severe allergic reaction to sulfasalazine)
(2001): Sule A+, *J Assoc Physicians India* 49, 1120
(1996): Aparicio J+, *Am J Gastroenterol* 91, 620
(1992): Hautekeete ML+, *Gastroenterology* 103, 1925
Myalgia (3%)
Oral candidiasis
Oral lichenoid eruption
(1991): Alstead EM+, *J Clin Gastroenterol* 13, 335
Oral ulceration
Paresthesias
Pseudotumor cerebri
(2001): Rottembourg D+, *J Pediatr Gastroenterol Nutr* 33(3), 337
Tinnitus

## MESNA

**Trade name:** Mesnex (Bristol-Myers Squibb)
**Other common trade names:** *Mexan; Uromitexan*
**Indications:** Hemorrhagic cystitis induced by ifosfamide
**Category:** Hemorrhagic cystitis prophylactic
**Half-life:** 24 minutes

#### *Reactions*

### Skin
Allergic reactions (sic)
(1991): D'Cruz D+, *Lancet* 338, 705
Angioedema
(1998): Leal G, Fortaleza, Brazil (from Internet) (observation)
(1992): Breathnach SM+, *Adverse Drug Reactions and the Skin* Blackwell, Oxford, 289
(1992): Zonzits E+, *Arch Dermatol* 128, 80
Erythema
(1992): Breathnach SM+, *Adverse Drug Reactions and the Skin* Blackwell, Oxford, 289
Exanthems
(1998): Leal G, Fortaleza, Brazil (from Internet) (observation)
(1992): Breathnach SM+, *Adverse Drug Reactions and the Skin* Blackwell, Oxford, 289
(1992): Zonzits E+, *Arch Dermatol* 128, 80
Fixed eruption
(1998): Leal G, Fortaleza, Brazil (from Internet) (observation) (2 patients)
(1992): Zonzits E+, *Arch Dermatol* 128, 80
Flushing
(1992): Breathnach SM+, *Adverse Drug Reactions and the Skin* Blackwell, Oxford, 289
Pruritus (<1%)
Rash (sic) (<1%)
Urticaria
(1998): Leal G, Fortaleza, Brazil (from Internet) (observation)
(1992): Breathnach SM+, *Adverse Drug Reactions and the Skin* Blackwell, Oxford, 289
(1992): Zonzits E+, *Arch Dermatol* 128, 80
(1988): Pratt CB+, *Drug Intell Clin Pharm* 22, 913

### Other
Dysgeusia (>17%)
Oral mucosal lesions
(1988): Pralt CB+, *Drug Intell Clin Pharm* 22, 913
Oral mucosal ulceration
(1992): Breathnach SM+, *Adverse Drug Reactions and the Skin* Blackwell, Oxford, 289

## MESORIDAZINE

**Trade name:** Serentil (Boehringer Ingelheim)
**Other common trade name:** *Mesorin*
**Indications:** Schizophrenia
**Category:** Phenothiazine antipsychotic
**Half-life:** 24–48 hours
**Clinically important, potentially hazardous interactions with:** antihistamines, arsenic, chlorpheniramine, dofetilide, piperazine, quinolones, sparfloxacin

#### *Reactions*

### Skin
Angioedema
Contact dermatitis
Eczema (sic)
Edema
Erythema
Exfoliative dermatitis
Flushing
Hypohidrosis (>10%)
Lupus erythematosus
Peripheral edema
Photosensitivity (1–10%)
Pigmentation (blue-gray) (<1%)
Pruritus
Rash (sic) (1–10%)
Seborrhea
Urticaria
Xerosis

### Hair
Hair – alopecia

### Other
Anaphylactoid reactions
Galactorrhea (<1%)
Gynecomastia
Hypertrophic papillae of tongue
Mastodynia (1–10%)
Paresthesias
Priapism (<1%)
Sialorrhea
Tremors
Xerostomia

## METAXALONE

**Trade name:** Skelaxin (Carnrick)
**Indications:** Muscle spasm
**Category:** Skeletal muscle relaxant
**Half-life:** 2–3 hours

#### *Reactions*

### Skin
Allergic dermatitis (sic) (<1%)

Fixed eruption
(2000): Mostow EN, Akron, OH (from Internet) (observation)
Pruritus
Rash (sic)
Urticaria

### Other

Anaphylactoid reactions (<1%)

## METFORMIN

**Trade names:** Glucophage (Bristol-Myers Squibb); Glucovance (Bristol-Myers Squibb)
**Other common trade names:** *Apo-Metformin; Diabex; Diaformin; Diformin; Gen-Metformin; Glucomet; Metforal; Metomin; Novo-Metformin*
**Indications:** Diabetes
**Category:** Antidiabetic
**Half-life:** 6.2 hours

Glucovance is metformin and glyburide

### *Reactions*

### Skin

Eczema (sic)
(1970): Lawson AAH+, *Lancet* 2, 437
Erythema (transient)
(1966): Berger W+, *Schweiz Med Wochenschr* (German) 96, 1335
(1966): Beurey J+, *Ann Dermatol Syphiligr* (French) 93,13
(1964): Puchegger R+, *Wien Klin Wochenschr* (German) 76, 335
Exanthems
Grinspan's syndrome*
(1990): Lamey PJ+, *Oral Surg Oral Med Oral Pathol* 70, 184
Lichenoid eruption
(1970): Lawson AAH+, Lancet 2, 437
Photosensitivity (1–10%)
Pruritus
(1964): Puchegger R+, *Wien Klin Wochenschr* (German) 76, 335
Purpura
(1966): Berger W+, *Schweiz Med Wochenschr* (German) 96, 1335
Rash (sic) (1–10%)
Urticaria (1–10%)
(1966): Berger W+, *Schweiz Med Wochenschr* (German) 96, 1335
(1966): Beurey J+, *Ann Dermatol Syphiligr* (French) 93,13
(1964): Puchegger R+, *Wien Klin Wochenschr* (German) 76, 335
Vasculitis
(1986): Klapholz L+, *BMJ* 293, 483

### Hair

Hair – alopecia
(1999): Smith JG, Mobile, AL (from Internet) (2 observations)
(1998): Klein AD, Statesboro, GA (from Internet) (observation)

### Other

Death
(2002): www.intellihealth.com (from Internet)
Dysgeusia (3%) (metallic taste)

***Note:** Grinspan's syndrome: the triad of oral lichen planus, diabetes mellitus, and hypertension

## METHADONE

**Trade name:** Dolophine (Roxane)
**Other common trade names:** *Eptadone; L-Polamidon; Mephenon; Metadon; Methadose; Physeptone*
**Indications:** Pain, narcotic addiction
**Category:** Narcotic analgesic; antitussive; suppressant (narcotic abstinence syndrome)
**Half-life:** 15–25 hours
**Clinically important, potentially hazardous interactions with:** diazepam, erythromycin, fluconazole

### *Reactions*

### Skin

Angioedema
Cellulitis
(1988): Naschitz JE+, *Harefuah* (Hebrew) 115, 271
Diaphoresis
(1973): Kreek MJ, *JAMA* 223, 665 (48%)
Edema (face)
Exanthems
Flushing
Pruritus (<1%)
Purpura
Rash (sic) (<1%)
Urticaria (<1%)

### Other

Death
(2001): Vormfelde SV+, *Pharmacopsychiatry* 34(6), 217
Injection-site burning
Injection-site induration
Injection-site pain (1–10%)
Rhabdomyolysis
(1990): Larpin R+, *Presse Med* 19(30), 1403
Tremors
(2001): Clark JD+, *Clin J Pain* 17(4), 375
Xerostomia (1–10%)

## METHAMPHETAMINE

**Trade name:** Desoxyn (Abbott)
**Indications:** Attention deficit disorder, obesity
**Category:** Central nervous system stimulant; 'recreational' drug
**Half-life:** 4–5 hours
**Clinically important, potentially hazardous interactions with:** fluoxetine, fluvoxamine, fluvoxamine, MAO inhibitors, paroxetine, phenelzine, sertraline, tranylcypromine

### *Reactions*

### Skin

Acaraphobia
(1971): Yaffee NS, *Arch Dermatol* 104, 687
Delusions of parasitosis
(1999): Gregg LJ, Tulsa, OK, (from Internet) (4 observations)
Diaphoresis (1–10%)
Lichenoid eruption
(1994): Deloach-Banta LJ, *Cutis* 53, 97
Pigmentation
(1971): Yaffee NS, *Arch Dermatol* 104, 687
Rash (sic) (<1%)

Toxic epidermal necrolysis
(2002): Yung A+, *Australas J Dermatol* 43(1), 35
Urticaria (<1%)

### Other

Dysgeusia
Polyarteritis nodosa
(1973): Koff RS+, *N Engl J Med* 288, 946
(1970): Citron BP+, *N Engl J Med* 283, 1003
Rhabdomyolysis
(1999): Richards JR+, *Am J Emerg Med* 17(7), 681 (43%)
(1998): Kolecki P, *Pediatr Emerg Care* 14(6), 385
(1998): Lan KC+, *J Formos Med Assoc* 97(8), 528
(1994): Chan P+, *J Toxicol Clin Toxicol* 32(2), 147 (8 cases) (3 fatal)
(1994): Sperling LS+, *Ann Intern Med* 121(12), 986
Tremors
Xerostomia (1–10%)

## METHANTHELINE

**Trade name:** Banthine (SCS)
**Other common trade name:** *Vagantin*
**Indications:** Duodenal ulcer
**Category:** Gastrointestinal anticholinergic and antispasmodic
**Half-life:** no data
**Clinically important, potentially hazardous interactions with:** anticholinergics, artbutamine

#### *Reactions*

### Skin

Exanthems
Exfoliative dermatitis
Flushing
Hypohidrosis
Urticaria
Xerosis

### Other

Ageusia
Anaphylactoid reactions
Dysgeusia
Sialopenia
Xerostomia

## METHAZOLAMIDE

**Trade name:** Methazolamide
**Indications:** Glaucoma
**Category:** Carbonic anhydrase inhibitor; sulfonamide diuretic
**Half-life:** ~14 hours

#### *Reactions*

### Skin

Exanthems (<1%)
(1998): Litt JZ, Beachwood, OH (personal case) (observation)
(1993): Gandham SB+, *Arch Ophthalmol* 111, 370
Photosensitivity
Pruritus
Purpura
Rash (sic)
Stevens–Johnson syndrome
(1998): Cotter JB, *Arch Ophthalmol* 116, 117
(1997): Shirato S+, *Arch Ophthalmol* 115, 550
(1995): Flach AJ+, *Ophthalmology* 102, 1677
Toxic epidermal necrolysis
Urticaria
(1993): Gandham SB+, *Arch Ophthalmol* 111, 370
Vasculitis

### Other

Anosmia (<1%)
Dysgeusia (>10%) (metallic taste)
Hypersensitivity (<1%)
Paresthesias (<1%)
Tinnitus
Trembling
Xerostomia (<1%)

## METHENAMINE

**Trade names:** Hiprex; Mandelamine (Warner Chilcott); Prosed (Star); Urex (3M); Urised (PolyMedica); Uroqid
**Other common trade names:** *Dehydral; Haiprex; Hip-Rex; Hipeksal; Hippramine; Reflux; Urasal; Urotractan*
**Indications:** Urinary tract infections
**Category:** Urinary tract antibacterial
**Half-life:** 3–6 hours

#### *Reactions*

### Skin

Edema
Erythema multiforme (<1%)
Exanthems
(1976): Arndt KA+, *JAMA* 235, 918 (0.6%)
(1968): *Med Lett* 10, 58
Fixed eruption (<1%)
(1961): Welsh AL, *Arch Dermatol* 84, 1004
Photosensitivity
(1994): Selvaag E+, *Photodermatol Photoimmunol Photomed* 10, 259
Pruritus (<1%)
Rash (sic) (3.5%)
Systemic eczematous contact dermatitis
Urticaria

### Other

Stomatitis

## METHICILLIN

**Trade name:** Staphcillin (Mead Johnson)
**Other common trade names:** *Estafcilina; Lucoperin; Mechicillin*
**Indications:** Various infections caused by susceptible organisms
**Category:** Penicillinase-resistant penicillin antibiotic
**Half-life:** 30 minutes
**Clinically important, potentially hazardous interactions with:** anticoagulants, cyclosporine, methotrexate, tetracyclines

#### *Reactions*

### Skin

Angioedema

Bullous eruption
(1976): Schiffer CA+, *Ann Intern Med* 85, 338
Ecchymoses
Erythema multiforme
(1969): Kaminska M+, *Pediatr Pol* (Polish) 44, 873
Erythema nodosum
Exanthems
(1980): Fields DA, *West J Med* 133, 521
(1978): Kancir LM+, *Arch Intern Med* 138, 909 (29%)
Exfoliative dermatitis
(1966): Hadida E+, *Bull Soc Fr Dermatol Syphiligr* (French) 73, 497
Hematomas
Jarisch–Herxheimer reaction
Pruritus
Purpura
Pustular psoriasis
(1966): Hadida E+, *Bull Soc Fr Dermatol Syphiligr* (French) 73, 497
Rash (sic) (1–10%)
Stevens–Johnson syndrome
Toxic epidermal necrolysis
Urticaria
Vasculitis

### Other

Anaphylactoid reactions
Black tongue
Dysgeusia
Glossitis
Glossodynia
Hypersensitivity
Injection-site pain
Oral candidiasis
Phlebitis (<1%)
Serum sickness (<1%)
Stomatitis
Stomatodynia
Vaginitis
Xerostomia

## METHIMAZOLE

**Synonym:** thiamazole
**Trade name:** Tapazole (Jones)
**Other common trade names:** *Strumazol; Thacapzol; Thiamazol; Thyrozol; Unimazole*
**Indications:** Hyperthyroidism
**Category:** Antithyroid agent
**Half-life:** 4–13 hours
**Clinically important, potentially hazardous interactions with:** anticoagulants, dicumarol, warfarin

### *Reactions*

### Skin

Cutaneous side effects (sic) (28% in high dosages)
(1972): Wiberg JJ+, *Ann Intern Med* 77, 414 (1–5%)
Edema (<1%)
Erythema nodosum
Exanthems
(1986): Shiroozu A+, *J Clin Endocrinol Metab* 63, 125 (5–15%)
(1972): Wiberg JJ+, *Ann Intern Med* 77, 414 (1–5%)
(1970): Amrhein JA+, *J Pediatr* 76, 54
(1951): Bartels EC+, *J Clin Endocrinol Metab* 11, 1057 (6%)
Exfoliative dermatitis
Fixed eruption
(1984): Chan HL, *Int J Dermatol* 23, 607
Lupus erythematosus (1–10%)
(1995): Kawachi Y+, *Clin Exp Dermatol* 20, 345
(1994): Sato-Matsumura KC+, *J Dermatol* 21, 501
(1987): Sakata S+, *Jpn J Med* 26, 373
(1981): Searles RP+, *J Rheumatol* 8, 498
(1981): Takuwa N+, *Endocrinol Jpn* 28, 663
(1973): Hung W+, *J Pediatr* 82, 852
(1970): Librik L+, *J Pediatr* 76, 64
Pigmentation
(2000): Drayton G, Los Angeles, CA (from Internet) (observation)
Pruritus (3–5%)
(1986): Shiroozu A+, *J Clin Endocrinol Metab* 63, 125 (2–3%)
(1972): Wiberg JJ+, *Ann Intern Med* 77, 414 (1–5%)
Purpura
(1972): Wiberg JJ+, *Ann Intern Med* 77, 414 (1%)
Rash (sic) (>10%)
Urticaria
(1972): Wiberg JJ+, *Ann Intern Med* 77, 414 (>5%)
(1970): Amrhein JA+, *J Pediatr* 76, 54
Vasculitis
(1995): Kawachi Y+, *Clin Exp Dermatol* 20, 345

### Hair

Hair – alopecia (<1%)

### Other

Ageusia (1–10%)
Aplasia cutis congenita
(1995): Vogt T+, *Br J Dermatol* 133, 994
(1992): Martinez-Frias ML+, *Lancet* 339, 742
(1985): Milham S, *Teratology* 32, 321
(1984): Bachrach LK+, *Can Med Assoc J* 130, 1264
Dysgeusia
Myalgia
Oral ulceration
Paresthesias (<1%)
Polyarteritis nodosa
Scalp defects (sic)
(1985): Milham S, *Teratology* 32, 321
Serum sickness
(1983): Van Kuyk M+, *Acta Clin Belg* (French) 38, 68
Sialadenitis

## METHOCARBAMOL

**Trade name:** Robaxin (Robins)
**Other common trade names:** *Carbametin; Carxin; Delaxin; Lumirelax; Marbaxin; Miowas; Ortoton; Robinax; Robomol; Trolar*
**Indications:** Muscle spasm, tetanus
**Category:** Skeletal muscle relaxant
**Half-life:** 1–2 hours

### *Reactions*

### Skin

Allergic reactions (sic) (1–10%)
Exanthems
Flushing (1–10%)
Pruritus
Rash (sic)
Urticaria

### Other

Anaphylactoid reactions
Dysgeusia
Injection-site pain (<1%)
Thrombophlebitis (<1%)

## METHOHEXITAL

**Trade name:** Brevital (Jones)
**Other common trade names:** *Brevimytal; Brietal; Brietal Sodium*
**Indications:** General anesthesia
**Category:** General anesthetic; barbiturate
**Half-life:** 4–8 minutes

### *Reactions*

### Skin

Angioedema
(1972): Driggs RL+, *J Oral Surg* 30, 906
(1972): Reichert EF+, *J Oral Surg* 30, 910
Erythema
Exanthems
(1972): Driggs RL+, *J Oral Surg* 30, 906
Rash (sic)
Urticaria
(1972): Driggs RL+, *J Oral Surg* 30, 906
(1972): Reichert EF+, *J Oral Surg* 30, 910

### Other

Anaphylactoid reactions
Injection-site edema
Injection-site pain (18%)
Injection-site phlebitis
(1981): Clark RSJ, *Drugs* 27, 26
Rhabdomyolysis
(1990): Larpin R+, *Presse Med* 19(30), 1403
Sialorrhea
Thrombophlebitis (<1%)
Tremors

## METHOTREXATE

**Synonyms:** amethopterin; MTX
**Trade name:** Rheumatrex (Lederle)
**Other common trade names:** *Farmitrexat; Lantarel; Ledertrexate; Maxtrex; Metex; Texate*
**Indications:** Carcinomas, leukemias, lymphomas, psoriasis, rheumatoid arthritis
**Category:** Anti-inflammatory; antiarthritic; antineoplastic and antimetabolite
**Half-life:** 3–10 hours
**Clinically important, potentially hazardous interactions with:** acitretin, aldesleukin, aminoglycosides, amiodarone, amoxicillin, ampicillin, aspirin, bacampicillin, bismuth, carbenicillin, chloroquine, cisplatin, cloxacillin, co-trimoxazole, dapsone, demeclocycline, diclofenac, dicloxacillin, etodolac, etretinate, fenoprofen, flurbiprofen, folic acid antagonists, haloperidol, ibuprofen, indomethacin, ketoprofen, ketorolac, lithium, magnesium trisalicylate, meclofenamate, mefenamic acid, methicillin, mezlocillin, minocycline, nabumetone, nafcillin, naproxen, NSAIDs, omeprazole, oxaprozin, oxytetracycline, paromomycin, penicillins, piperacillin, piroxicam, polypeptide antibiotics, probenecid, procarbazine, rofecoxib, salicylates, salsalate, sulfadiazine, sulfamethoxazole, sulfapyridine, sulfasalazine, sulfisoxazole, sulindac, tetracycline, ticarcillin, tolmetin, trimethoprim, **vaccines**

### *Reactions*

### Skin

Acne
Acral erythema
(1996): Hellier I+, *Arch Dermatol* 132, 590 (bullous variety)
(1989): Kampmann KK+, *Cancer* 63, 2482
(1983): Doyle LA+, *Ann Intern Med* 98, 611
Acute inflammation (sic) (reactivation)
(1969): Möller H, *J Invest Dermatol* 52, 437
Allergic reactions (sic)
(2000): Postovsky S+, *Med Pediatr Oncol* 35, 131
Bullous eruption
(1987): Chang JC, *Arch Dermatol* 123, 990
(1983): Reed KM+, *J Am Acad Dermatol* 8, 677
Burning (palms and soles)
(1978): McDonald CJ+, *Cancer Treat Rep* 62, 1009
Candidiasis
(1970): Baker H, *Br J Dermatol* 82, 65
Capillaritis
(1978): McDonald CJ+, *Cancer Treat Rep* 62, 1009
(1976): Jacobs SA+, *J Clin Invest* 57, 534
Carcinoma (sic)
(1971): Craig LR+, *Arch Dermatol* 103, 505
Cutaneous necrolysis (sic)
(1970): Baker H, *Br J Dermatol* 82, 65
Cutaneous side effects (sic)
(1997): Kasteler JS+, *J Am Acad Dermatol* 36, 67 (passim)
(1996): Furuya T+, *Rymachi* (Japanese) 36, 746
Dermatitis (sic)
(1996): Giordano N+, *Clin Exp Rheumatol* 14, 450
Ecchymoses
(1998): Roenigk HH+, *J Am Acad Dermatol* 38, 478
Eccrine squamous syringometaplasia
(1997): Valks R+, *Arch Dermatol* 133, 873
Epidermal necrosis (sic)
(1987): Harrison PV, *Br J Dermatol* 116, 867
(1983): Reed KM+, *J Am Acad Dermatol* 8, 677

(1982): Lawrence CM+, *Br J Dermatol* 107, 24
Erosion of psoriatic plaques (sic)
(1996): Pearce HP+, *J Am Acad Dermatol* 35, 835
(1988): Kaplan DL+, *Int J Dermatol* 27, 59
(1988): Shupack JL+, *JAMA* 259, 3594
(1987): Ng HW+, *BMJ* 295, 752
(1984): Lawrence CM+, *J Am Acad Dermatol* 11, 1059
(1983): Reed KM+, *J Am Acad Dermatol* 8, 677
(1969): McDonald CJ+, *Arch Dermatol* 100, 655
Erosions
(1996): Zackheim HS+, *J Am Acad Dermatol* 34, 626
Erythema (>10%)
Erythema multiforme
(1989): Taylor SW+, *Gynecol Oncol* 33, 376
(1978): Moe PJ+, *Acta Paediatr Scand* (French) 67, 265
Erythematous papules (sic)
(1999): Goerttler E+, *J Am Acad Dermatol* 40, 702 (4 cases)
Erythroderma
(2000): Alfaro J+, *Rev Med Chil* (Spanish) 128, 315
(1996): Zackheim HS+, *J Am Acad Dermatol* 34, 626
Exanthems (15%)
(1979): Stoller RG+, *Cancer Res* 39, 908
(1971): Hansen HH+, *Br J Cancer* 25, 298
Folliculitis
(1970): Baker H, *Br J Dermatol* 82, 65
Furunculosis
(1996): Zackheim HS+, *J Am Acad Dermatol* 34, 626
Herpes simplex
(1996): Vonderheid EC+, *J Am Acad Dermatol* 34, 470
Melanoma
(1984): Wemmer U, *Z Hautkr* (German) 59, 665
Nodules (sic)
(1998): Williams FM+, *J Am Acad Dermatol* 39, 359
(1996): Muzaffer MA+, *J Pediatr* 128, 698
(1996): Smith MD, *J Rheumatol* 23, 2004
(1995): Berris B+, *J Rheumatol* 22, 2359
(1995): Das SK+, *J Assoc Physicians India* 43, 651
(1994): Abu-Shakra M+, *J Rheumatol* 21, 934
(1994): Karam NE+ *J Rheumatol* 21, 1960
(1994): Smith MD, *J Rheumatol* 22, 1439
(1992): Kerstens PJSM+, *J Rheumatol* 19, 867
(1988): Segal R+, *Arthritis Rheum* 31, 1182
Nodulosis
(2001): Ahmed SS+, *Medicine* (Baltimore) 80(4), 271
Photosensitivity (5%)
(1996): Zackheim HS+, *J Am Acad Dermatol* 34, 626
(1994): Oliver F, *The Schoch Letter* 44, 6 (observation)
(1985): Neiman RA+, *J Rheumatol* 12, 354
(1969): Möller H, *J Invest Dermatol* 52, 437
(1969): Roenigk HH Jr+, *Arch Dermatol* 99, 86
(1965): Vogler WR+, *Arch Intern Med* 115, 285
Photosensitivity (recall)
(2002): Thami GP+, *Postgrad Med J* 78(916), 116
Pigmentation (1–10%)
Pruritus (1–5%)
(1998): Roenigk HH+, *J Am Acad Dermatol* 38, 478
Purpura
Radiation recall
(2001): Camidge DR, *Am J Clin Oncol* 24(2), 211
(2000): Kharfan Dabaja MA+, *Am J Clin Oncol* 23(5), 531
(1995): Guzzo C+, *Photodermatol Photoimmunol Photomed* 11, 55 (sunburn)
Radiodermatitis (reactivation)
Rash (sic) (1–3%)
(2000): Emery P+, *Rheumatology* (Oxford) 39(6), 655
(1995): Copur S+, *Anticancer Drugs* 6, 154
Scabies (reactivation)
(1975): Burrows D, *Br J Dermatol* 93, 219
Squamous cell carcinoma
(1989): Jensen DB+, *Acta Derm Venereol* (Stockh) 69, 274
(1971): Harris CC, *Arch Dermatol* 103, 501
Stevens–Johnson syndrome
(2000): Hani N+, *Eur J Dermatol* 10(7), 548
(1993): Cuthbert RJ+, *Ulster Med J* 62, 95
(1978): Moe PJ+, *Acta Paediatr Scand* (French) 67, 265
Sunburn (reactivation)
(2000): Khan AJ+, *Cutis* 66, 379
(1998): Roenigk HH+, *J Am Acad Dermatol* 38, 478
(1987): Westwick TJ+, *Cutis* 39, 49
(1986): Mallory SB+, *Pediatrics* 78, 514
(1981): Korossy KS+, *Arch Dermatol* 117, 310
Telangiectases
Toxic epidermal necrolysis (<1%)
(2000): Yang CH+, *Int J Dermatol* 39, 621 (with co-trimoxazole)
(1997): Primka EJ+, *J Am Acad Dermatol* 36, 815 (fatal)
(1970): Baker H, *Br J Dermatol* 82, 65
(1967): Lyell A, *Br J Dermatol* 79, 367
Ulceration
(2001): Del Pozo J+, *Eur J Dermatol* 11(5), 450 (knuckles)
(2000): Montero LC+, *J Rheumatol* 27(9), 2290
(1998): Ben-Amitai D+, *Ann Pharmacother* 32, 651
(1998): Roenigk HH+, *J Am Acad Dermatol* 38, 478 (of psoriatic lesions)
(1970): Baker H, *Br J Dermatol* 82, 65
Urticaria
(1998): Roenigk HH+, *J Am Acad Dermatol* 38, 478
(1995): al-Lamki Z+, *Med Pediatr Oncol* 24, 137
(1983): Bronner AK+, *J Am Acad Dermatol* 9, 645
Vasculitis (>10%)
(2000): Borcea A+, *Br J Dermatol* 143, 203 (urticarial)
(1998): Halevy S+, *J Eur Acad Dermatol Venereol* 10, 81
(1997): Torner O+, *Clin Rheumatol* 16, 108
(1995): Blanco R+, *Arthritis Rheum* 39, 1016
(1989): Fondevila CG+, *Br J Haematol* 72, 591
(1989): Jeurissen MEC+, *Clin Rheumatol* 8, 417
(1986): Navarro M+, *Ann Intern Med* 105, 471
(1984): Marks CR+, *Ann Intern Med* 100, 916

## Hair

Hair – alopecia (1–3%)
(2000): Emery P+, *Rheumatology* (Oxford) 39, 655
(1998): Roenigk HH+, *J Am Acad Dermatol* 38, 478
(1998): Zieglschmid ME+, *J Am Acad Dermatol* 38, 130
(1997): Kasteler JS+, *J Am Acad Dermatol* 36, 67 (passim)
(1996): Zackheim HS+, *J Am Acad Dermatol* 34, 626
(1995): Zieglschmid-Adams ME+, *J Am Acad Dermatol* 32, 754
(1989): Fehlauer CS+, *J Rheumatol* 16, 307
(1988): Weinblatt ME+, *Arthritis Rheum* 31 (Suppl), s115
(1982): Bachman DM, *Arthritis Rheum* 25, s65
(1982): Bertino JR, *Med Pediatr Oncol* 10, 401
(1971): Hansen HH+, *Br J Cancer* 25, 298
(1969): Roenigk HH Jr+, *Arch Dermatol* 99, 86 (6%)
Hair – pigmented bands
(1983): Wheeland RG+, *Cancer* 51, 1356

## Nails

Nails – discoloration
Nails – onycholysis
(1987): Chang JC, *Arch Dermatol* 123, 990
Nails – paronychia
(1983): Wantzin GL+, *Arch Dermatol* 119, 623
Nails – pigmentation
(1981): Nixon DW+, *Cutis* 27, 181

## Other

Anaphylactoid reactions (1–10%)
(1996): Alkins SA+, *Cancer* 77, 2123
(1995): Lobelle C+, *Pediatr Hematol Oncol* 12, 213

(1979): Gluck-Kuyt I+, *Cancer Treat Rep* 63, 797
(1978): Goldberg NH+, *Cancer* 41, 52
Death
Dysgeusia
(1988): Duhra P+, *Clin Exp Dermatol* 13, 126
Gingivitis (>10%)
Glossitis (>10%)
Gynecomastia
(1995): Finger DR+, *J Rheumatol* 22, 796
(1995): Thomas E+, *J Rheumatol* 22, 2189
(1983): Del Paine DW+, *Arthritis Rheum* 26, 691
Hodgkin's disease (nodular sclerosing)
(2000): Moseley AC+, *J Rheumatol* 27, 810
Malignant lymphoma
(1997): Kamel OW, *Arch Dermatol* 133, 903
(1996): Viraben R+, *Br J Dermatol* 135, 116
(1994): Zimmer-Galler I+, *Mayo Clin Proc* 69, 258
(1993): Kamel OW+, *N Engl J Med* 328, 1317
Mucositis
(2000): Alfaro J+, *Rev Med Chil* (Spanish) 128, 315
Myalgia
Oral mucositis
(1997): Plevova P+, *J Natl Cancer Inst* 89, 326
(1996): Moe PJ, *Pediatr Hematol Oncol* 13, 313
(1996): Rask C+, *Pediatr Hematol Oncol* 13, 359
(1996): Zackheim HS+, *J Am Acad Dermatol* 34, 626
(1979): Oliff A+, *Cancer Chemother Pharmacol* 2, 225
Oral ulceration
(2001): Litt JZ, Beachwood, OH (personal case) (observation) (severe)
(2001): Werth V, *Dermatology Times* 15
(2000): Madinier I+, *Ann Med Interne (Paris)* (French) 151, 248
(1986): Barrett AP, *J Periodontol* 57, 318
Peyronie's disease
(1992): Phelan MJI, *Br J Rheumatol* 31, 425
Porphyria cutanea tarda
(1983): Malina L+, *Z Hautkr* (German) 58, 241
Pseudolymphoma
(1997): Flipo RM+, *J Rheumatol* 24, 809
(1995): Delaporte E+, *Ann Dermatol Venereol* (French) 122, 521 (20 cases)
Stomatitis (3–10%)
(1998): Roenigk HH+, *J Am Acad Dermatol* 38, 478 (ulcerative)
(1998): Zieglschmid ME+, *J Am Acad Dermatol* 38, 130
(1997): Kasteler JS+, *J Am Acad Dermatol* 36, 67 (passim)
(1996): Vonderheid EC+, *J Am Acad Dermatol* 34, 470
(1995): Zieglschmid-Adams ME+, *J Am Acad Dermatol* 32, 754
(1994): Montecucco C+, *Arthritis Rheum* 37, 777
(1978): Moe PJ+, *Acta Paediatr Scand* (French) 67, 265
Tendinitis
(2001): Toverud EL+, *Med Pediatr Oncol* 37(2), 156 (Achilles; repeated)
Tinnitus

# METHOXSALEN

**Trade names:** 8-MOP (ICN); Oxsoralen (ICN)
**Other common trade names:** *Geroxalen; Meladinine; Oxsoralon; Puvasoralen; Ultra-MOP*
**Indications:** Psoriasis, vitiligo
**Category:** Repigmenting agent and antipsoriatic
**Half-life:** 1.1 hours
**Clinically important, potentially hazardous interactions with:** chloroquine, cyclosporine, fluroquinolones, phenothiazines, sulfonamides

## *Reactions*

### Skin
Acne
(1978): Nielsen EB+, *Acta Derm Venereol* (Stockh) 58, 374
Acute generalized exanthematous pustulosis (AGEP)
(2002): Morant C+, *Ann Dermatol Venereol* 129(2), 234
Basal cell carcinoma
(1996): Stern RS+, *J Pediatr* 129, 915
(1995): Gritiyarangsan P+, *Photodermatol Photoimmunol Photomed* 11, 174
Bowen's disease
(1979): Tam DW+, *Arch Dermatol* 115, 203
Bullous eruption (with UVA)
(1982): Stüttgen G, *Int J Dermatol* 21, 198
(1979): Abel EA+, *Arch Dermatol* 115, 988
(1977): Melski JW+, *J Invest Dermatol* 68, 328
(1976): Thomsen K+, *Br J Dermatol* 95, 568
Bullous pemphigoid
(1996): Perl S+, *Dermatology* 193, 245
Burning (1–10%)
(1982): Stüttgen G, *Int J Dermatol* 21, 198 (passim)
Burns
(1996): Geary P, *Burns* 22, 636
(1991): Boucaud C+, *Presse Med* (French) 20, 1945
Cancer (sic)
(1995): Halder RM+, *Arch Dermatol* 131, 734
(1984): Halprin KM+, *Natl Cancer Inst Monogr* 66, 185
(1979): Morgan RW, *N Engl J Med* 301, 554
(1979): Spellman CW, *N Engl J Med* 301, 554
(1979): Stern RS+, *N Engl J Med* 301, 555
(1976): Moller R+, *Arch Dermatol* 112, 1613 (multiple basal cell carcinomas)
Cheilitis (1–10%)
Contact dermatitis
(1994): Korffmacher H+, *Contact Dermatitis* 30, 283
(1991): Takashima A+, *Br J Dermatol* 124, 37
(1980): Weissmann I+, *Br J Dermatol* 102, 113
(1979): Saihan EM, *BMJ* 2, 20
Eczematous eruption (sic)
(1979): Saihan EM, *BMJ* 2, 20
Edema (1–10%)
Erythema (1–10%)
Exanthems
(2001): Ravenscroft J+, *J Am Acad Dermatol* 45, S2118–9
(1986): Gisslen P+, *Photodermatol* 3, 308
Exfoliative dermatitis
Freckles (1–10%)
(1995): Gritiyarangsan P+, *Photodermatol Photoimmunol Photomed* 11, 174
(1995): Pierard GE+, *Dermatology* 190, 338
(1984): Kietzmann E+, *Dermatologica* 168, 306
(1983): Kanerva L+, *Dermatologica* 166, 281
(1983): Kietzmann H+, *Ann Dermatol Venereol* (French) 110, 63

Granuloma annulare
(1979): Dorval JC+, *Ann Dermatol Venereol* (French) 106, 79
Herpes simplex
(1982): Stüttgen G, *Int J Dermatol* 21, 198
Herpes zoster
(1982): Stüttgen G, *Int J Dermatol* 21, 198
(1977): Roenigk HH+, *Arch Dermatol* 113, 1667
Hypopigmentation (1–10%)
Lupus erythematosus
(1985): Bruze M+, *Acta Derm Venereol* (Stockh) 65, 31
(1979): Eyanson S+, *Arch Dermatol* 115, 54
(1978): Millns J+, *Arch Dermatol* 114, 1177
Miliaria
Pemphigoid
(1978): Robinson JK, *Br J Dermatol* 99, 709
Photocontact dermatitis
(1998): Clark SM+, *Contact Dermatitis* 38, 289
(1991): Takashima A+, *Br J Dermatol* 124, 37
(1990): Cox NH+, *Clin Exp Dermatol* 15, 75
Photoreactions
(1992): Jeanmougin M+, *Ann Dermatol Venereol* (French) 119, 277
(1978): Plewig G+, *Arch Derm Res* 261, 201
(1968): Fulton JE+, *Arch Derm* 98, 445
Photosensitivity
(2001): Tanew A+, *J Am Acad Dermatol* 44, 638
(1991): Boucaud C+, *Presse Med* (French) 20, 1945
(1989): Cox NH+, *Photodermatol* 6, 96
Phototoxicity
(1997): Morison WL+, *J Am Acad Dermatol* 36, 183
(1993): Calzavara-Pinton PG+, *J Am Acad Dermatol* 28, 657
(1989): Morison WL, *Arch Dermatol* 125, 433 (topical)
(1985): Berakha GJ+, *Ann Plast Surg* 14, 458
(1984): Meffert H+, *Photodermatol* 1, 191
(1979): de Koning GA+, *Hautarzt* (German) 30, 27
(1979): Swanbeck G+, *Clin Pharmacol Ther* 25, 478
Pigmentation
(1989): Weiss E+, *Int J Dermatol* 28, 188
(1987): Bruce DR+, *J Am Acad Dermatol* 16, 1087
(1986): MacDonald KJS+, *Br J Dermatol* 114, 395
Porokeratosis (actinic)
(1988): Beiteke U+, *Photodermatology* 5, 274
(1985): Hazen PG+, *J Am Acad Dermatol* 12, 1077
(1980): Reymond JL, *Acta Derm Venereol* (Stockh) 60, 539
Prurigo
(1982): Stüttgen G, *Int J Dermatol* 21, 198 (passim)
Pruritus (>10%)
(1982): Stüttgen G, *Int J Dermatol* 21, 198 (passim)
Purpura
(1981): Barriere H+, *Nouv Presse Med* (French) 10, 337
Rash (sic) (1–10%)
Scleroderma
(1976): Duperrat B+, *Bull Soc Franc Dermatol Syphiligr* (French) 83, 79
Seborrheic dermatitis
(1983): Tegner E, *Acta Derm Venereol* (Stockh) Suppl 107, 5
Skin pain
(1987): Norris PG+, *Clin Exp Dermatol* 12, 403
(1983): Tegner E, *Acta Derm Venereol* (Stockh) Suppl 107, 5
Squamous cell carcinoma
(1998): Stern RS+, *Arch Dermatol* 134, 1582 (with UVA)
(1986): Kahn JR+, *Clin Exp Dermatol* 11, 398
(1979): Tam DW+, *Arch Dermatol* 115, 203
(1979): Verdich J, *Arch Dermatol* 115, 1338
Urticaria
(1994): Bech-Thomsen N+, *J Am Acad Dermatol* 31, 1063
Vasculitis
(1981): Barriere H+, *Presse Med* (French) 10, 37
Vitiligo
(1983): Tegner E, *Acta Derm Venereol* (Stockh) Suppl 107, 5
(1976): Duperrat B+, *Bull Soc Franc Dermatol Syphiligr* (French) 83, 79
Warts
(1982): Stüttgen G, *Int J Dermatol* 21, 198
Xerosis

## Hair

Hair – hypertrichosis
(1983): Rampen FHJ, *Br J Dermatol* 109, 657
(1967): Singh G+, *Br J Dermatol* 79, 501
(1959): Elliot JA, *J Invest Dermatol* 32, 311

## Nails

Nails – photo-onycholysis
(1990): Baran R+, *Ann Dermatol Venereol* (French) 117, 367
(1984): Balato N+, *Photodermatol* 1, 202
(1978): Rau RC+, *Arch Dermatol* 114, 448
(1977): Vella-Briffa D+, *BMJ* 2, 1150
(1977): Zala L+, *Dermatologica* 154, 203
Nails – pigmentation
(1990): Trattner A+, *Int J Dermatol* 29, 310
(1989): Weiss E+, *Int J Dermatol* 28, 188
(1986): MacDonald KJS+, *Br J Dermatol* 114, 395
(1982): Naik RPC+, *Int J Dermatol* 21, 275
(1979): Naik RP+, *Br J Dermatol* 100, 229

## Other

Anaphylactoid reactions
(2001): Legat FJ+, *Br J Dermatol* 145(5), 821
Lymphoproliferative disease
(1989): Aschinoff R+, *J Am Acad Dermatol* 21, 1134
Tumors (sic)
(1988): Gupta AK+, *J Am Acad Dermatol* 19, 67
(1987): Henseler T+, *J Am Acad Dermatol* 16, 108

# METHOXYFLURANE

**Trade name:** Penthrane (Astral)
**Indications:** Anesthesia
**Category:** Adjunct to provide anesthesia procedures hours in duration
**Half-life:** N/A
**Clinically important, potentially hazardous interactions with:** cisatracurium, demeclocycline, doxacurium, doxycycline, gentamicin, kanamycin, minocycline, neomycin, oxytetracycline, pancuronium, rapacuronium, streptomycin, tetracycline

### *Reactions*

## Skin

None

## Other

None

# METHSUXIMIDE

**Trade name:** Celontin (Parke-Davis)
**Other common trade name:** *Petinutin*
**Indications:** Absence (petit-mal) seizures
**Category:** Succinimide anticonvulsant
**Half-life:** 2–4 hours

### *Reactions*

## Skin

Acanthosis nigricans
(1972): Petko E+, *Arch Dermatol* 106, 918
Erythema multiforme
Exanthems
(1972): Petko E+, *Arch Dermatol* 106, 918
Exfoliative dermatitis (<1%)
Lupus erythematosus (>10%)
Periorbital edema
Pruritus
Purpura
Rash (sic)
Stevens–Johnson syndrome (>10%)
Urticaria (<1%)

## Hair

Hair – alopecia
Hair – hirsutism

## Other

Gingival hyperplasia
Oral ulceration

# METHYCLOTHIAZIDE

**Trade names:** Aquatensen (Wallace); Enduron (Abbott)
**Other common trade names:** *Enduron-M; Thiazidil; Urimor*
**Indications:** Hypertension
**Category:** Thiazide* diuretic; antihypertensive
**Half-life:** no data
**Clinically important, potentially hazardous interactions with:** digoxin, lithium

### *Reactions*

## Skin

Erythema multiforme
Exanthems
Photosensitivity (<1%)
Purpura
Rash (sic) (<1%)
Stevens–Johnson syndrome
Urticaria

## Other

Anaphylactoid reactions
Dysgeusia
Paresthesias (<1%)

***Note:** Methyclothiazide is a sulfonamide and can be absorbed systemically. Sulfonamides can produce severe, possibly fatal, reactions such as toxic epidermal necrolysis and Stevens–Johnson syndrome

# METHYLDOPA

**Trade names:** Aldoclor (Merck); Aldomet (Merck); Aldoril (Merck)
**Other common trade names:** *Amodopa; Densul; Dopamet; Equibar; Hydopa; Medimet; Nu-Medopa; Polinal; Presinol; Prodopa*
**Indications:** Hypertension
**Category:** Alpha-adrenergic inhibitor; antihypertensive
**Half-life:** 1.7 hours
**Clinically important, potentially hazardous interactions with:** ephedrine

Aldoril is methyldopa and hydrochlorothiazide

### *Reactions*

## Skin

Ankle edema
(1969): Varadi DP+, *Arch Intern Med* 124, 13
Cheilitis
(1973): Almeyda J+, *Br J Dermatol* 88, 313
Eczematous eruption (sic)
(1974): Church R, *Br J Dermatol* 91, 373
(1969): Peterkin GAG, *Practitioner* 202, 117 (keratotic – palms and soles)
(1965): Dollery CT, *Prog in Cardiovasc Dis* 8, 278
Edema
Erythema multiforme (<1%)
(1985): Ting HC+, *Int J Dermatol* 24, 587
(1975): Böttiger LE+, *Acta Med Scand* 198, 229
Erythema nodosum
(1978): Furhoff AK, *Acta Med Scand* 203, 425
Exanthems
(1986): Gidseg G, *South Med J* 79, 389
(1978): Furhoff AK, *Acta Med Scand* 203, 425
(1971): Perry HM+, *J Lab Clin Med* 78, 905 (3%)
Fixed eruption
(1974): Burry JN+, *Br J Dermatol* 91, 475
Granulomas
(1974): Wells JD+, *Ann Intern Med* 81, 701
Lichen planus
(1994): Thompson DF+, *Pharmacotherapy* 14, 561
(1979): Krebs A, *Hautarzt* (German) 30, 281
(1974): Burry JN+, *Br J Dermatol* 91, 475
Lichenoid eruption
(1986): Gonzalez JG+, *J Am Acad Dermatol* 15, 87
(1982): Brooks SL, *J Oral Med* 37, 42
(1982): Wiesenfeld D+, *Oral Surg Oral Med Oral Pathol* 54, 527
(1980): *Med J Aust* 2, 130
(1976): Burry JN, *Arch Dermatol* 112, 880 (ulcerative)
(1974): Holt PJA+, *BMJ* 3, 234
(1973): Almeyda J+, *Br J Dermatol* 88, 313
(1971): Almeyda J+, *Br J Dermatol* 85, 604
(1971): Stevenson CJ, *Br J Dermatol* 85, 600
Lupus erythematosus (<1%)
(1995): Sakurai Y+, *Nippon Naika Gakkai Zasshi* (Japanese) 84, 2069
(1992): Skaer TL, *Clin Ther* 14, 496
(1989): Nordstrom DM+, *Arthritis Rheum* 32, 205
(1985): Cush JJ+, *Am J Med Sci* 290, 36
(1985): Stratton MA, *Clin Pharm* 4, 657
(1983): Homberg JC+, *J Pharmacol* (French) 14, 61
(1982): Dupont A+, *BMJ* 2, 693
(1981): Harrington TM+, *Chest* 79, 696
(1977): Schubothe H+, *Immun Infekt* (German) 5, 142
(1974): Gustavsen WR, *Tidsskr Nor Laegeforen* (Norwegian) 94, 22

(1972): Dorfmann H+, *Nouv Presse Med* (French) 1, 2907
(1967): Sherman JD+, *Arch Intern Med* 120, 321
Papulo-vesicular eruption
(1977): Heid E+, *Ann Dermatol Venereol* (French) 104, 494
Peripheral edema (>10%)
Petechiae
(1978): Furhoff AK, *Acta Med Scand* 203, 425
Photosensitivity
(1988): Vaillant L+, *Arch Dermatol* 124, 326
(1973): Almeyda J+, *Br J Dermatol* 88, 313
Pigmentation
(1986): Brody HJ+, *Cutis* 38, 187
(1973): Almeyda J+, *Br J Dermatol* 88, 313
(1969): Varadi DP+, *Arch Intern Med* 124, 13
Pruritus
(1973): Almeyda J+, *Br J Dermatol* 88, 313
Purpura
(1971): Menohitharajah SM+, *BMJ* 1, 494
Rash (sic) (<1%)
Seborrheic dermatitis
(1974): Burry JN+, *Br J Dermatol* 91, 475
(1974): Church R, *Br J Dermatol* 91, 373
(1973): Church R, *Br J Dermatol* 89, 10
Stevens–Johnson syndrome
(1985): Ting HC+, *Int J Dermatol* 24, 587
Toxic epidermal necrolysis
Urticaria
(1986): Gidseg G, *S Med J* 79, 389
(1978): Furhoff AK, *Acta Med Scand* 203, 425
Vasculitis
(1989): Matteson EL+, *Arthritis Rheum* 32, 356

### Hair

Hair – alopecia

### Other

Acute intermittent porphyria
Black tongue (<1%)
(1986): Brody HJ+, *Cutis* 38, 137
Galactorrhea
(1963): Pettinger WA+, *BMJ* 1, 1460
Glossodynia
Gynecomastia (<1%)
Hypersensitivity
(1993): Wolf R+, *Ann Allergy* 71, 166
Myalgia
Oral lichenoid eruption
(1988): Zain RB+, *Dent J Malays* 10, 15
(1982): Brooks SL, *J Oral Med* 37, 42
Oral mucosal eruption
(1973): Almeyda J+, *Br J Dermatol* 88, 313
Oral ulceration
(1990): Espana A+, *Med Clin (Barc)* (Spanish) 94, 559 (lichenoid)
(1980): McLellan GH+, *Clin Prevent Dent* 2, 18
(1978): Hay KD+, *Br Dent J* 145, 195
(1974): Burry JN+, *Br J Dermatol* 91, 475
(1971): Stevenson CJ, *Br J Dermatol* 85, 600
(1967): Mackie BS, *Br J Dermatol* 79, 106 (LIP)
Paresthesias (<1%)
Parkinsonism
Xerostomia (1–10%)
(1969): Varadi DP+, *Arch Intern Med* 124, 13

# METHYLPHENIDATE

**Trade names:** Metadate CD (Celltech); Methylin (Mallinckrodt); Ritalin (Novartis)
**Other common trade names:** *Centedrin; Rilatine; Rubifen*
**Indications:** Attention deficit disorder, narcolepsy
**Category:** Central nervous system stimulant
**Half-life:** 2–4 hours
**Clinically important, potentially hazardous interactions with:** pimozide

## *Reactions*

### Skin

Angioedema
(1977): Sverd J+, *Pediatrics* 59, 115
(1972): Rothschild CJ+, *Can Med Assoc J* 106, 1064
Delusions of parasitosis
(1999): Eisner J (from Internet) (observation)
Diaphoresis
Edema (eyelids)
(1972): Rothschild CJ+, *Can Med Assoc J* 106, 1064
Eosinophilic syndrome
(1978): Wolf J+, *Ann Intern Med* 89, 224
Erythema multiforme
Exanthems
(1977): Sverd J+, *Pediatrics* 59, 115
Exfoliative dermatitis
(1977): Sverd J+, *Pediatrics* 59, 115
(1968): Weil AJ, *Ann Allergy* 26, 402
Fixed eruption
(1992): Cohen HA+, *Ann Pharmacother* 26, 1378 (scrotum)
Photosensitivity
(1977): Sverd J+, *Pediatrics* 59, 115
Pruritus
Purpura
(1978): Wolf J+, *Ann Intern Med* 89, 224
Rash (sic) (<1%)
Urticaria
(1977): Sverd J+, *Pediatrics* 59, 115
Vasculitis
(1977): Sverd J+, *Pediatrics* 59, 115

### Hair

Hair – alopecia

### Other

Bruxism
(2000): Gara L+, *J Child Adolesc Psychopharmacol* 10, 39 (with valproic acid)
Hypersensitivity (1–10%)
(1990): Calis KA+, *Clin Pharm* 9, 632
Injection-site abscess
(1976): Elenbaas RM+, *JACEP* 5, 977
Tourette's syndrome
Xerostomia
(1993): Pataki CS+, *J Am Acad Child Adolesc Psychiatry* 32, 1065

## METHYLTESTOSTERONE

**Trade names:** Android (ICN); Estratest (Solvay); Metandren; Oreton (ICN); Testred (ICN); Virilon (Star)
**Other common trade names:** *Androral; B; Enarmon; Teston; Testotonic ; Testovis; Viromone*
**Indications:** Hypogonadism, impotence, metastatic breast cancer
**Category:** Androgen; antineoplastic
**Half-life:** 2.5–3.5 hours
**Clinically important, potentially hazardous interactions with:** anticoagulants, cyclosporine, warfarin

### *Reactions*

#### Skin

Acanthosis nigricans
(1987): Shuttleworth D+, *Clin Exp Dermatol* 12, 288
Acne (>10%)
(1992): Fryand O+, *Acta Derm Venereol* 72, 148
(1990): Fuchs E+, *J Am Acad Dermatol* 23, 125
(1989): Fryand O+, *Tidsskr Nor Laegeforen* (Norwegian) 109, 239
(1989): Hartmann AA+, *Monatsschr Kinderheilkd* (German) 137, 466
(1989): Heydenreich G, *Arch Dermatol* 125, 571 (fulminans)
(1989): Scott MJ+, *Cutis* 44, 30
(1989): von Muhlendahl KE+, *Dtsch Med Wochenschr* (German) 114, 712
(1988): Traupe H+, *Arch Dermatol* 124, 414 (fulminans)
(1987): Kiraly CL+, *Am J Dermatopathol* 9, 515
(1984): Lamb DR, *Am J Sports Med* 12, 31
(1965): Kennedy BJ, *J Am Geriatr Soc* 13, 230
(1965): Rook A, *Br J Dermatol* 77, 115
Contact dermatitis
(1989): Holdiness MR, *Contact Dermatitis* 20, 3 (from patch)
Edema (>10%)
Exanthems
Flushing (1–5%)
(1965): Kennedy BJ, *J Am Geriatr Soc* 13, 230
Furunculosis
(1989): Scott MJ+, *Cutis* 44, 30
Lichenoid eruption
(1989): Aihara M+, *J Dermatol* (Tokio) 16, 330
Lupus erythematosus
(1978): Robinson HM, *Z Haut* (German) 53, 349
Pruritus
Psoriasis
(1990): O'Driscoll JB+, *Clin Exp Dermatol* 15, 68
Purpura
Seborrhea
Seborrheic dermatitis
(1989): Scott MJ+, *Cutis* 44, 30
Striae
(1989): Scott MJ+, *Cutis* 44, 30
Urticaria

#### Hair

Hair – alopecia
(1989): Scott MJ+, *Cutis* 44, 30
(1965): Kennedy BJ, *J Am Geriatr Soc* 13, 230
Hair – hirsutism (1–10%) (in females)
(1994): Castillo-Ceballos A+, *Med Clin (Barc)* (Spanish) 102, 78
(1991): Bates GW+, *Clin Obstet Gynecol* 34, 848
(1991): No Author, *Obstet Gynecol* 78, 474
(1991): Parker LU+, *Cleve Clin J Med* 58, 43
(1991): Urman B+, *Obstet Gynecol* 77, 595
(1989): Scott MJ+, *Cutis* 44, 30
(1974): Baron J, *Zentralbl Gynakol* (German) 96, 129
(1971): Fusi S+, *Folia Endocrinol* (Italian) 24, 412
(1965): Kennedy BJ, *J Am Geriatr Soc* 13, 230

#### Other

Anaphylactoid reactions
Gynecomastia (<1%)
Hypersensitivity (<1%)
Injection-site pain
Mastodynia (>10%)
Paresthesias
Priapism (>10%)
Stomatitis

## METHYSERGIDE

**Trade name:** Sansert (Novartis)
**Other common trade names:** *Deseril; Desernil; Deserril; Deseryl*
**Indications:** Vascular (migraine) headaches
**Category:** Vascular headache prophylactic; ergot alkaloid
**Half-life:** 10 hours
**Clinically important, potentially hazardous interactions with:** almotriptan, amprenavir, clarithromycin, delavirdine, efavirenz, erythromycin, indinavir, naratriptan, nelfinavir, ritonavir, rizatriptan, saquinavir, sibutramine, sumatriptan, troleandomycin, zolmitriptan

### *Reactions*

#### Skin

Collagenosis (sic)
(1973): Anker N, *Ugeskr Laeger* (Danish) 135, 2225
Exanthems
Flushing
(1964): Graham JR, *N Engl J Med* 270, 67 (0.8%)
Hypermelanosis
(1964): Graham JR, *N Engl J Med* 270, 67
Lupus erythematosus
(1968): Racouchot J+, *Bull Soc Franc Dermatol Syphiligr* (French) 75, 513
(1968): Racouchot J+, *Lyon Med* (French) 220, 1766
Orange-peel skin (sic)
(1964): Graham JR, *N Engl J Med* 270, 67 (1%)
Peripheral edema (1–10%)
Pruritus
Rash (sic) (1–10%)
Raynaud's phenomenon
Scleroderma
(1984): Garcia de Quesada FJ+, *Med Clin (Barc)* (Spanish) 82, 604
(1980): Graham JR, *Trans Am Clin Climatol Assoc* 92, 122
(1978): Goldberg NC+, *Arch Dermatol* 114, 550
Skin reactions (sic)
(1991): Mylecharane EJ, *J Neurol* 238, S45
Telangiectases
Urticaria

#### Hair

Hair – alopecia
(1991): Mylecharane EJ, *J Neurol* 238, S45
(1974): Sadjadpour K, *JAMA* 229, 639
(1964): Graham JR, *N Engl J Med* 270, 67 (1%)
(1964): Leyton N, *Lancet* 1, 830 (0.4%)

### Other

Hyperesthesia (<1%)
Myalgia
Paresthesias

## METOCLOPRAMIDE

**Trade name:** Reglan (Robins)
**Other common trade names:** *Apo-Metoclop; Duraclamid; Emex; Gastrocil; Gastronerton; Maxeran; Maxolon; Mygdalon; Primperan*
**Indications:** Gastroesophageal reflux
**Category:** Dopaminergic blocking agent; peristaltic stimulant; antiemetic
**Half-life:** 4–6 hours
**Clinically important, potentially hazardous interactions with:** sertraline, venlafaxine

#### *Reactions*

### Skin

Allergic reactions (sic)
 (1986): Bigby M+, *JAMA* 256, 3358
Angioedema
 (1983): Pinder RM+, *Drugs* 25, 451
 (1976): Pinder RM+, *Drugs* 12, 81
Diaphoresis
 (2002): Fisher AA+, *Ann Pharmacother* 36(1), 67
Exanthems
 (1983): Pinder RM+, *Drugs* 25, 451
 (1976): Arndt KA+, *JAMA* 235, 918 (0.4%)
 (1976): Pinder RM+, *Drugs* 12, 81
Flushing
Rash (sic) (1–10%)
Urticaria
 (1983): Pinder RM+, *Drugs* 25, 451
 (1976): Pinder RM+, *Drugs* 12, 81

### Other

Blue tongue
 (1989): Alroe C+, *Med J Aust* 150, 724
Galactorrhea
Gynecomastia
 (1997): Madani S+, *J Clin Gastroenterol* 24, 79
Mastodynia (1–10%)
Paresthesias
 (1997): du Bois A+, *Oncology* 54, 7
Parkinsonism
 (2002): Hoogendam A+, *Ned Tijdschr Geneeskd* 146(4), 175
Porphyria
 (1997): Gorchein A, *Lancet* 350, 1104
 (1981): Doss M+, *Lancet* 2, 91
Serotonin syndrome
 (2002): Fisher AA+, *Ann Pharmacother* 36(1), 67
 (2000): Vandermegel X+, *Rev Med Brux* 21(3), 161 (with sertaline)
Xerostomia (1–10%)

## METOLAZONE

**Trade names:** Mykrox (Medeva); Zaroxolyn (Medeva)
**Other common trade names:** *Barolyn; Diondel; Metenix 5; Normelan; Xuret*
**Indications:** Hypertension, edema
**Category:** Sulfonamide* diuretic; antihypertensive
**Half-life:** 6–20 hours
**Clinically important, potentially hazardous interactions with:** digoxin, lithium

#### *Reactions*

### Skin

Chills (1–10%)
Edema (<2%)
Exanthems
Exfoliative dermatitis
Necrotizing angiitis
Photosensitivity (<2%)
Pruritus (<2%)
Purpura (<1%)
Rash (sic) (<2%)
Stevens–Johnson syndrome
Toxic epidermal necrolysis
 (1991): Lacy JA, *Nutr Clin Pract* 6, 18
Urticaria (<2%)
Vasculitis
 (1991): Cox NH+, *Postgrad Med J* 67, 860
 (1982): Weinrauch LA+, *Cutis* 30, 83
Xerosis (<2%)

### Other

Anaphylactoid reactions (<2%)
Dysgeusia (<2%)
Paresthesias (<2%)
Tinnitus
Xanthopsia (<2%)
Xerostomia (<2%)

***Note:** Metolazone is a sulfonamide and can be absorbed systemically. Sulfonamides can produce severe, possibly fatal, reactions such as toxic epidermal necrolysis and Stevens–Johnson syndrome

## METOPROLOL

**Trade names:** Lopressor (Novartis); Toprol XL (AstraZeneca)
**Other common trade names:** *Beloc-Zoc; Betaloc; Betazok; Kenaprol; Mycol; Prolaken; Ritmolol; Seloken-Zok; Selozok*
**Indications:** Hypertension, angina pectoris
**Category:** Beta-adrenergic blocker; antihypertensive
**Half-life:** 3–4 hours
**Clinically important, potentially hazardous interactions with:** clonidine, epinephrine, verapamil

Lopressor HCT is metoprolol and hydrochlorothiazide

**Note:** Cutaneous side effects of beta-receptor blockaders are clinically polymorphous. They apparently appear after several months of continuous therapy. Atypical psoriasiform, lichen planus-like, and eczematous chronic rashes are mainly observed. (1983): Hödl St, *Z Hautkr* (German) 58, 17

#### *Reactions*

### Skin

Angioedema

(1994): Krikorian RK+, *Chest* 106, 1922
Diaphoresis
Eczematous eruption (sic)
(1981): Neumann HAM+, *Dermatologica* 162, 330
(1979): Neumann HAM+, *Lancet* 2, 745
Edema
Erythema multiforme
Exanthems
(1986): Benfield P+, *Drugs* 31, 376 (1.5%)
Exfoliative dermatitis
Hyperkeratosis (palms and soles)
Lichenoid eruption
(1988): Kardaun SH+, *Br J Dermatol* 118, 545
(1983): Hödl St, *Z Hautkr* (German) 58, 17
(1978): Savage RL+, *BMJ* 1, 987
Lupus erythematosus
(1981): Paladini G, *Int J Tissue React* 3, 95
Peripheral edema (1%)
Pigmentation
Pityriasis rubra pilaris
(1978): Finlay AY+, *BMJ* 1, 987
Prurigo
(1983): Hödl St, *Z Hautkr* (German) 58, 17
Pruritus (1–5%)
(1994): Shelley WB+, *Cutis* 53, 39 (scalp) (observation)
(1986): Benfield P+, *Drugs* 31, 376
Psoriasis (induction and aggravation of)
(2002): Litt JZ, Beachwood, OH (personal case) (observation) (induction of)
(1993): Litt JZ, Beachwood, OH (personal case) (observation)
(1988): Heng MCY+, *Int J Dermatol* 27, 619 (pustular, generalized)
(1987): Altomare GF+, *G Ital Dermatol Venereol* (Italian) 122, 531
(1986): Abel EA+, *J Am Acad Dermatol* 15, 1007
(1986): Czernielewski J+, *Lancet* 1, 808
(1984): Arntzen N+, *Acta Derm Venereol* (Stockh) 64, 346
(1981): Neumann HAM+, *Dermatologica* 162, 330
(1979): Neumann HAM+, *Lancet* 2, 745
Purpura
Rash (sic) (<5%)
Raynaud's phenomenon (<1%)
(1984): Eliasson K+, *Acta Med Scand* 215, 333
(1976): Marshall AJ+, *BMJ* 1, 1498
Scleroderma
(1980): Graham JR, *Trans Am Clin Climatol Assoc* 92, 122
Toxic epidermal necrolysis
Urticaria
Xerosis

### Hair
Hair – alopecia
(1981): Graeber CW+, *Cutis* 28, 633

### Nails
Nails – bluish
Nails – dystrophy
Nails – onycholysis
Nails – transverse depression (sic)
(1981): Graeber CW+, *Cutis* 28, 633

### Other
Dysgeusia
Gangrene (feet)
(1979): Gokal R+, *BMJ* 19, 837
Oculo-mucocutaneous syndrome
(1982): Cocco G+, *Curr Ther Res* 31, 362
Oral lichenoid eruption
Paresthesias
Peyronie's disease
(1981): Jones HA+, *Med J Aust* 2, 514
(1981): Neumann HAM+, *Dermatologica* 162, 330
(1981): Paladini G, *Int J Tissue React* 3, 95
(1979): Pryor JP+, *Lancet* 1, 331
(1977): Yudkin JS, *Lancet* 2, 1355
Polymyalgia
(1991): Snyder S, *Ann Intern Med* 114, 96
Scalp tingling
(1979): Coulter DM, *N Z Med J* 90, 397
Tinnitus

## METRONIDAZOLE

**Trade names:** Flagyl (Searle); Metrocream (Galderma); Metrogel (Galderma); Metrolotion (Galderma); Noritate (Dermik); Protostat; Satric
**Other common trade names:** *Arilin; Ariline; Asuzol; Clont; Fossyol; Milezzol; Nida Gel; Novo-Nidazol; Otrozol; Rozagel; Rozex; Trikacide; Zadstat*
**Indications:** Various infections caused by susceptible organisms, rosacea
**Category:** Antiprotozoal; anthelmintic and antibiotic
**Half-life:** 6–12 hours
**Clinically important, potentially hazardous interactions with: alcohol**, anisindione, anticoagulants, dicumarol, disulfiram, fluorouracil, warfarin

### *Reactions*

### Skin
Acute generalized exanthematous pustulosis (AGEP)
(1999): Watsky KL, *Arch Dermatol* 135, 93
(1994): Manders SM+, *Cutis* 54, 194 (with cefazolin)
Angioedema
(1978): Shevliakov LV, *Vestn Dermatol Venerol* (Russian) February, 49
Candidiasis (exacerbation)
(1977): Maize JC+, *Arch Dermatol* 113, 1457 (passim)
Contact dermatitis
(1997): Vincenzi C+, *Contact Dermatitis* 36, 116
Erythema
Exanthems
(1995): Litt JZ, Beachwood, OH (personal case) (observation)
(1977): Swami B+, *Curr Med Res Opin* 5, 152 (1–5%)
(1969): *Med Lett* 11, 27 (1–5%)
Fixed eruption
(2002): Short KA, (London) (England) March AAD Poster (4 recurrences)
(2002): Vila JB+, *Contact Dermatitis* 46(2), 122
(2002): Walfish AE+, *Cutis* 69, 207 (doxycycline, in the same patient, also produced a fixed eruption)
(2001): Gastaminza G+, *Contact Dermatitis* 44(1), 36
(1998): Mahboob A+, *Int J Dermatol* 37, 833
(1998): Thami GP+, *Dermatology* 196, 368
(1990): Gaffoor PMA+, *Cutis* 45, 242
(1990): Kanwar AJ+, *Dermatologica* 180, 277
(1990): Mishra D+, *Int J Dermatol* 29, 740
(1987): Shelley WB+, *Cutis* 39, 393
(1977): Naik RPC+, *Dermatologica* 155, 59
Flushing
(1992): Shelley WB+, *Advanced Dermatologic Diagnosis* WB Saunders, 582 (passim)
(1977): Maize JC+, *Arch Dermatol* 113, 1457 (passim)

Linear IgA bullous dermatosis
Pityriasis rosea
(1977): Maize JC+, *Arch Dermatol* 113, 1457
Pruritus (1–5%)
(2001): Gastaminza G+, *Contact Dermatitis* 44(1), 36
(1977): Maize JC+, *Arch Dermatol* 113, 1457 (passim)
(1977): Swami B+, *Curr Med Res Opin* 5, 152 (10%)
(1963): Foster SA+, *Am J Obstet Gynecol* 87, 1013
Rash (sic)
Toxic epidermal necrolysis
(1999): Egan CA+, *J Am Acad Dermatol* 40, 458
(1981): Titov RL, *Klin Med Mosk* (Russian) 59, 85
Urticaria
(1997): Blumenthal HL, Beachwood, OH (personal case) (observation)
(1977): Maize JC+, *Arch Dermatol* 113, 1457 (passim)
(1963): Foster SA+, *Am J Obstet Gynecol* 87, 1013

### Other

Acute intermittent porphyria
Disulfiram-type reaction
Dysgeusia (<1%) (metallic taste)
(1997): Palop Larrea V+, *Aten Primaria* (Spanish) 20, 524
Glossitis
(1987): Shelley WB+, *Cutis* 39, 393
Gynecomastia
(1985): Fagan TC+, *JAMA* 254, 3217
Hypersensitivity (<1%)
Injection-site vasculitis
Oral mucosal eruption
(1969): *Med Lett* 11, 27
Oral ulceration
Paresthesias
Serum sickness
(1983): Weart CW+, *South Med J* 76, 410
Stomatitis
(1987): Shelley WB+, *Cutis* 39, 393
Thrombophlebitis (<1%)
Tongue, furry (<1%)
(1987): Shelley WB+, *Cutis* 39, 393
(1977): Maize JC+, *Arch Dermatol* 113, 1457 (passim)
Vaginal candidiasis (<1%)
Xerostomia (<1%)

## MEXILETINE

**Trade name:** Mexitil (Boehringer Ingelheim)
**Other common trade names:** *Mexihexal; Mexilen; Mexitec*
**Indications:** Ventricular arrhythmias
**Category:** Antiarrhythmic (class I-b)
**Half-life:** 10–12 hours

### *Reactions*

### Skin

Acute generalized exanthematous pustulosis (AGEP)
(2001): Sasaki K+, *Eur J Dermatol* 11, 469
Diaphoresis (<1%)
Edema (3.8%)
Exanthems
(2001): Sasaki K+, *Eur J Dermatol* 11(5), 469
(1997): Higa K+, *Pain* 73, 97
(1996): Nagayama H+, *J Dermatol* 23, 899
(1992): Habot B+, *Harefuah* (Hebrew) 123, 462
(1991): Kikuchi K+, *Contact Dermatitis* 25, 70
(1988): Kardaun SH+, *Br J Dermatol* 118, 545
(1984): Ribera Pibernat M+, *Med Clin (Barc)* (Spanish) 83, 825
(1979): Habeler G+, *Dtsch Med Wochenschr* (German) 104, 1244
Exfoliative dermatitis (<1%)
Facial edema
(2001): Sasaki K+, *Eur J Dermatil* 11(5), 469
Hot flashes (<1%)
Lupus erythematosus (<1%)
Pruritus
(1997): Higa K+, *Pain* 73, 97
Purpura
Rash (sic) (3.8%)
Stevens–Johnson syndrome (<1%)
Urticaria
(1994): Yamazaki S+, *Br J Dermatol* 130, 538
(1988): Kardaun SH+, *Br J Dermatol* 118, 545
Xerosis (<1%)

### Hair

Hair – alopecia (<1%)

### Other

Dysgeusia (<1%)
(2000): Zervakis J+, *Physiol Behav* 68, 405
Paresthesias (3.8%)
Salivary changes (sic) (<1%)
Tinnitus
Trembling (1–10%)
Tremors (12.6%)
Xerostomia (2.8%)

## MEZLOCILLIN

**Trade name:** Mezlin (Bayer)
**Other common trade name:** *Baypen*
**Indications:** Various infections caused by susceptible organisms
**Category:** Beta-lactamase-sensitive penicillin antibiotic
**Half-life:** 0.8–1.0 hours
**Clinically important, potentially hazardous interactions with:** anticoagulants, cyclosporine, demeclocycline, doxycycline, methotrexate, minocycline, oxytetracycline, tetracycline

### *Reactions*

### Skin

Allergic reactions (sic)
(1994): Pleasants RA+, *Chest* 106, 1124 (in patients with cystic fibrosis)
Angioedema
Bullous eruption
Contact dermatitis
(1992): Keller K+, *Contact Dermatitis* 27, 348
Ecchymoses
Erythema multiforme
Erythema nodosum
Exanthems
Exfoliative dermatitis (<1%)
Hematomas
Jarisch–Herxheimer reaction
Pruritus
Rash (sic) (<1%)
Stevens–Johnson syndrome
Toxic epidermal necrolysis
Urticaria

Vasculitis

### Other

Anaphylactoid reactions
Black tongue
Dysgeusia
Glossitis
Glossodynia
Hypersensitivity
(1992): Keller K+, *Contact Dermatitis* 27, 348
Injection-site pain
Oral candidiasis
Phlebitis
Serum sickness (<1%)
Stomatitis
Stomatodynia
Thrombophlebitis
Vaginitis
Xerostomia

## MICONAZOLE

**Trade names:** Monistat (Ortho); Monistat-Derm (Ortho)
**Other common trade names:** *Aflorix; Aloid; Daktarin; Florid; Funcort; Fungoid Tincture; Micotef; Miracol; Monazole-7; Zole*
**Indications:** Fungal infections
**Category:** Imidazole antifungal
**Half-life:** initial: 40 minutes; terminal: 24 hours
**Clinically important, potentially hazardous interactions with:** anisindione, anticoagulants, dicumarol, vinblastine, vincristine, warfarin

### *Reactions*

### Skin

Angioedema
(1983): Stevens DA, *Drugs* 26, 347 (2.4%)
Bullous eruption
(1983): Stevens DA, *Drugs* 26, 347
Chills (>5%)
Contact dermatitis
(1996): Fernandez L+, *Contact Dermatitis* 34, 217
(1995): Goday JJ+, *Contact Dermatitis* 32, 370
(1991): Baes H, *Contact Dermatitis* 24, 89
(1988): Perret CM+, *Contact Dermatitis* 19, 75
(1988): Raulin C+, *Contact Dermatitis* 18, 76
(1984): Aldridge RD+, *Contact Dermatitis* 10, 58
(1983): Frenzel UH+, *Contact Dermatitis* 9, 74
(1982): Foged EK+, *Contact Dermatitis* 8, 284
(1979): Wade TR+, *Contact Dermatitis* 5, 168
(1977): Samsoen M+, *Contact Dermatitis* 3, 351
(1975): Degreef H+, *Contact Dermatitis* 1, 269
Erythema
Exanthems
(1987): Verhagen C+, *Eur J Haematol* 38, 225 (28%)
(1983): Stevens DA, *Drugs* 26, 347 (2.4%)
(1980): Heel RC+, *Drugs* 19, 7 (3–8%)
(1977): Fischer TJ+, *J Pediatr* 91, 815 (10%)
(1977): Sung JP+, *N Engl J Med* 297, 786 (87%)
Flushing (<1%)
(1983): Stevens DA, *Drugs* 26, 347
(1980): Heel RC+, *Drugs* 19, 7 (1–2%)
Pruritus (21%)
(1983): Stevens DA, *Drugs* 26, 347 (36%)
(1980): Heel RC+, *Drugs* 19, 7 (2–21%)
(1977): Fischer TJ+, *J Pediatr* 91, 815 (21%)
Purpura
(1980): Heel RC+, *Drugs* 19, 7 (3–8%)
Rash (sic) (9%)
Urticaria
(1983): Stevens DA, *Drugs* 26, 347 (2.4%)
Xanthomas
(1978): Barr RJ+, *Arch Dermatol* 114, 1544 (eruptive)

### Other

Anaphylactoid reactions
Injection-site pain (>10%)
(1980): Heel RC+, *Drugs* 19, 7 (0.5–2%)
Phlebitis (>5%)
(1983): Stevens DA, *Drugs* 26, 347 (35%)
(1980): Heel RC+, *Drugs* 19, 7 (6–28%)
(1977): Fischer TJ+, *J Pediatr* 91, 815 (79%)

## MIDAZOLAM

**Trade name:** Versed (Roche)
**Other common trade name:** *Dormicum*
**Indications:** Preoperative sedation
**Category:** Benzodiazepine; sedative-hypnotic; anesthetic
**Half-life:** 1–4 hours
**Clinically important, potentially hazardous interactions with:** amprenavir, carbamazepine, chlorpheniramine, cimetidine, clarithromycin, clorazepate, CNS depressants, delavirdine, dexamethasone, efavirenz, erythromycin, esomeprazole, fluconazole, fluoxetine, griseofulvin, imatinib, indinavir, itraconazole, ivermectin, ketoconazole, nelfinavir, nevirapine, phenobarbital, phenytoin, primidone, rifabutin, rifampin, ritonavir, saquinavir, **St John's wort**

### *Reactions*

### Skin

Angioedema
(1992): Yakel DL+, *Crit Care Med* 20, 307
Exanthems
Peripheral edema (<1%)
Pruritus (<1%)
(1989): Yates A+, *Anaesthesia* 44, 449
Rash (sic) (<1%)
Urticaria (<1%)

### Other

Anaphylactoid reactions (<1%)
Dysgeusia (<1%) (acid taste)
Injection-site pain (>10%)
(1984): Dundee JW+, *Drugs* 28, 519 (26%)
Injection-site reactions (sic) (>10%)
Localized flare reaction
(1993): Kundrotas L+, *Gastrointest Endosc* 39, 109
Paresthesias
Sialorrhea (<1%)

## MIDODRINE

**Trade name:** Pro-Amatine (Roberts)
**Other common trade names:** *Amatine; Gutron; Metligine; Midon*
**Indications:** Orthostatic hypotension, urinary incontinence
**Category:** Alpha agonist; vasopressor; antihypotensive
**Half-life:** ~3–4 hours

### *Reactions*

#### Skin
Chills (5%)
Erythema multiforme
Flushing (1–10%)
Piloerection
(1998): McClellan KJ+, *Drugs Aging* 12(1), 76
(1989): McTavish D+, *Drugs* 38(5), 757
Pruritus (12.2%)
(1998): McClellan KJ+, *Drugs Aging* 12(1), 76
(1993): Jankovic J+, *Am J Med* 95(1), 38 (scalp) (13.5%)
Rash (sic) (2.4%)
Xerosis (2%)

#### Other
Aphthous stomatitis
Hyperesthesia
Pain (5%)
Paresthesias (18.3%)
(1998): McClellan KJ+, *Drugs Aging* 12(1), 76
(1997): Cruz DN+, *Am J Kidney Dis* 30(6), 772
(1993): Jankovic J+, *Am J Med* 95(1), 38 (scalp) (13.5%)
Xerostomia (1–10%)

## MIFEPRISTONE

**Synonym:** RU-486
**Trade name:** Mifeprex (Danco)
**Indications:** Medical termination of intrauterine pregnancy
**Category:** Abortifacient; glucocorticoid antagonist
**Half-life:** ~20 hours

### *Reactions*

#### Skin
Chills (3%)
Infections (sic)
(2001): DeHart RM+, *Ann Pharmacother* 35(6), 707
Viral infections (4%)

#### Other
Vaginal bleeding (~100%)
Vaginitis (3%)

## MIGLITOL

**Trade name:** Glyset (Pharmacia & Upjohn)
**Indications:** Non-insulin dependent diabetes type II
**Category:** Antidiabetic (alpha-glucosidase inhibitor)
**Half-life:** ~2 hours

### *Reactions*

#### Skin
Rash (sic) (1–10%)

## MILK THISTLE*

**Scientific names:** *Carduus marainum; Silibum marianum*
**Other common names:** Cardui mariae fructus; Holy Thistle; Lady's Thistle; Marian Thistle; Mary Thistle; Silibum; Silymarin; St. Mary Thistle
**Family:** Asteraceae; Compositae
**Purported indications:** Dyspepsia, liver protectant, chronic hepatitis, loss of appetite
**Other uses:** Liver and gallbladder complaints, diseases of the spleen, supportive treatment for mushroom poisoning. Historically the fruit and seed are roasted for use as a coffee substitute

### *Reactions*

#### Skin
Adverse reaction (sic)
(1999): No Author, *Med J Aust* 170(5), 218
Allergic reactions (sic)
Diaphoresis
Urticaria
(1990): Mironets VI+, *Vrach Delo* 7, 86

***Note:** Fruit and seed as opposed to the "above-ground parts"

## MINOCYCLINE

**Trade names:** Arestin; Dynacin (Medicis); Minocin (Lederle)
**Other common trade names:** *Alti-Minocycline; Apo-Minocycline; Mestacine; Minoclir 50; Minogalen; Minomycin; Mynocine; Syn-Minocycline*
**Indications:** Various infections caused by susceptible organisms
**Category:** Tetracycline antibiotic
**Half-life:** 11–23 hours
**Clinically important, potentially hazardous interactions with:** acitretin, aluminum salts, amoxicillin, ampicillin, antacids, bacampicillin, bismuth, calcium, carbenicillin, cloxacillin, digoxin, iron salts, isotretinoin, magnesium salts, methotrexate, methoxyflurane, mezlocillin, nafcillin, oxacillin, penicillins, piperacillin, ticarcillin, vitamin A, zinc salts

### *Reactions*

#### Skin
Acute febrile neutrophilic dermatosis (Sweet's syndrome)
(1992): Thibault M-J+, *J Am Acad Dermatol* 27, 801
(1991): Mensing H+, *Dermatologica* 182, 43
Acute generalized exanthematous pustulosis (AGEP)

(1997): Yamamoto T+, *Acta Derm Venereol* (Stockh) 77, 168 (in a patient with pustular psoriasis)

Angioedema
(1997): Shapiro LE+, *Arch Dermatol* 133, 1224
(1994): Levy SB, Chapel Hill, NC (personal case) (reproducible) (observation)
(1993): Litt JZ, Beachwood, OH (personal case) (observation)

Candidiasis

Cellulitis
(1994): Kaufmann D+, *Arch Intern Med* 154, 1983
(1989): Andreano JM+, *J Am Acad Dermatol* 20, 934

Elastolysis
(2000): Ho NC+, *Am J Med* 109(4), 340

Eosinophilic pustular folliculitis (Ofuji's disease)
(1989): Andreano JM+, *J Am Acad Dermatol* 20, 934

Erythema multiforme
(1987): Shoji A+, *Arch Dermatol* 123, 18

Erythema nodosum
(1990): Bridges AJ+, *J Am Acad Dermatol* 22, 959

Erythroderma
(2002): Murray C+, *World Congress Dermatol* Poster, 0120

Exanthems
(1996): Knowles SR+, *Arch Dermatol* 132, 934
(1995): Karofsky PS+, *Arch Pediatr Adolesc Med* 149, 217
(1995): Litt JZ, Beachwood, OH (2 personal cases) (mother and daughter ) (observation)
(1994): Kaufmann D+, *Arch Intern Med* 154, 1983
(1975): Brogden RN+, *Drugs* 9, 251
(1973): Shelley WB+, *JAMA* 224, 125

Exfoliative dermatitis (<1%)
(1997): MacNeil M+, *J Am Acad Dermatol* 36, 347
(1996): Knowles SR+, *Arch Dermatol* 132, 934
(1989): Davies MG+, *BMJ* 298, 1523

Fixed eruption (<1%)
(1999): Correia O+, *Clin Exp Dermatol* 24, 137 (genital) (with doxycycline)
(1994): Chu P+, *J Am Acad Dermatol* 30, 802 (pigmentation)
(1992): Ridgway HB+, *Arch Dermatol* 128, 565
(1984): Bargman H, *J Am Acad Dermatol* 11, 900
(1983): LePaw MI, *J Am Acad Dermatol* 8, 263
(1978): Jolly HW+, *Arch Dermatol* 114, 1484
(1977): Shimizu Y+, *Jpn J Dermatol* 4, 73

Folliculitis
(1994): Kaufmann D+, *Arch Intern Med* 154, 1983 (pustular)
(1989): Andreano JM+, *J Am Acad Dermatol* 20, 934

Lichenoid eruption
(1993): Litt JZ, Beachwood, OH (personal case) (observation)

Livedo reticularis
(2000): Schlienger RG+, *Dermatology* 200, 223

Lupus erythematosus
(2002): Marai I+, *Harefuah* 141(2), 151
(2001): Balestero S+, *Int J Dermatol* 40, 475
(2001): Graham LE+, *Clin Rheumatol* 20(1), 67
(2001): Lawson TM+, *Rheumatology* (Oxford) 40(3), 329
(2000): Choi HK+, *Arthritis Rheum* 43, 2488
(2000): Colmegna I+, *J Rheumatol* 27, 1567
(2000): Dunphy J+, *Br J Dermatol* 142, 461
(2000): Schlienger RG+, *Dermatology* 200, 223 (57 cases)
(1999): Angulo JM+, *J Rheumatol* 26, 1420
(1999): Dadamessi I+, *Rev Med Interne* (French) 20, 930
(1999): Elkayam O+, *Semin Arthritis Rheum* 28, 392
(1999): Katz R, *Skin and Allergy News,* May, 13
(1999): Piette AM+, *Rev Med Interne* (French) 20, 869
(1999): Sturkenboom MC+, *Arch Intern Med* 159, 493
(1999): Thaler D, Monona, WI (from internet) (observation)
(1999): Tournigand C+, *Lupus* 8, 773
(1998): Akin E+, *Pediatrics* 101, 926
(1998): Angulo JM+, *Semin Arthritis Rheum* 28, 187
(1998): Blumenthal HL, Beachwood, OH (personal case) (observation)
(1998): Knights SE+, *Clin Exp Dermatol* 16, 587
(1997): Crosson J+, *J Am Acad Dermatol* 36, 867
(1997): Emery P+, *J Rheumatol* 24, 1850
(1997): Farver DK, *Ann Pharmacother* 31, 1160
(1997): Golstein PE+, *Am J Gastroenterol* 92, 143
(1997): Hoefnagel JJ+, *Ned Tijdschr Geneeskd* 141, 1424
(1997): Pointud P, *J Rheumatol* 24, 1851
(1997): Singer SJ+, *JAMA* 277, 295
(1997): Wilde JL+, *Arch Dermatol* 133, 1344
(1996): Gough A+, *BMJ* 312, 169 (18 cases)
(1996): Hewack J, *Gastroenterology* 110, A1211
(1996): Knowles SR+, *Arch Dermatol* 132, 934
(1996): Masson C+, *J Rheumatol* 23, 2160
(1995): Bulgen DY, *Br J Rheumatol* 34, 398
(1995): Gendi NS+, *Br J Rheumatol* 34, 584
(1995): Gordon P+, *Br J Dermatol* 132, 120
(1994): Byrne PA+, *Br J Rheumatol* 33, 674
(1994): Inoue CN+, *Eur J Pediatr* 153, 540
(1994): Quilty B+, *Br J Rheumatol* 33, 1197
(1992): Matsuura T+, *Lancet* 340, 1553
(1984): Alston LL, *The Schoch Letter* 34, #8, Item 110

Nodules (sic) (facial, blue-gray)
(1998): Dawe RS+, *Arch Dermatol* 134, 861

Petechiae
(2000): Warshaw E, Minneapolis, MN *The Schoch Letter* 50, February #16

Photosensitivity (1–10%)
(1996): Carrington PR, Little Rock, AR (from Internet) (observation) (from tanning bed)
(1996): Goulden V+, *Br J Dermatol* 134, 693
(1996): Uhlemann J, St. Charles, MO (from Internet) (observation)
(1996): Wegman A, Sydney, Australia (from Internet) (observation)
(1994): Litt JZ, Beachwood, OH (personal case) (observation)
(1990): Black AK+, *Br J Dermatol* 123, 277
(1985): Basler RSW, *Arch Dermatol* 121. 606
(1972): Frost P+, *Arch Dermatol* 105, 681

Phototoxicity
(2002): Sorkin M, Denver, CO (from Internet) (observation)
(2002): Zabawski E, Longview, TX (from Internet) (observation)

Pigmentation
(2002): Bloom E, Oakland, CA (from Internet) (observation) (shins)
(2002): Thaler D, Monona, WI (from Internet) (observation)
(2001): Assad SA+, *J Rheumatol* 28(3), 679 (extensive)
(2001): Bachelz H+, *Arch Dermatol* 137, 69 (grayish)
(2001): Bressack M, Merrillville, IN (from Internet) (observation) (bluish)
(2001): Ely H, Grass Valley, CA (from Internet) (observation)
(2001): Mocci A, Panama (from Internet) ('deep blue spots on face') (observation)
(2001): Werth V, *Dermatology Times* 18 (shins, ankles, arms)
(2000): Chave TA+, *Ann R Coll Surg Engl* 82(5), 348
(2000): Gregg LJ, Tulsa, OK (from Internet) (observation)
(2000): Joseph WS+, *J Am Podiatr Med Assoc* 90, 268
(2000): Mouton RW, Poster Exhibit at University of Vienna clinical dermatology meeting (bluish)
(2000): Ozog DM+, *Arch Dermatol* 136, 1133 (7 cases; all with pemphigus or pemphigoid)
(1999): Aylesworth RJ, Rhinelander, WI (from Internet) (observation)
(1999): Drayton GE, Los Angeles, CA (from Internet) (observation)
(1999): Frederickson K, Novalo, CA (from Internet) (observation)
(1999): Gregg LJ, Tulsa, OK (from Internet) (observation)
(1999): Johnston AM+, *N Engl J Med* 340, 1597

(1999): Koester GA, Edmond, OK (from Internet) (observation)
(1999): Lycka BAS,, Edmonton, Alberta (from Internet) (observation)
(1999): Messner E+, *J Clin Rheumatol* 5(5), 273
(1999): Pepper, M, Madison, WI, *The Schoch Letter* 49, 25 (linear purple streaks of back)
(1998): Eisen D+, *Drug Saf* 18, 431
(1998): Greve B+, *Lasers Surg Med* 22, 223
(1998): Karrer S+, *Hautarzt* (German) 49, 219
(1998): Morrow GL+, *Am J Ophthalmol* 125, 396
(1998): Patel K+, *Br J Dermatol* 185, 560
(1998): Wasel NR+, *J Cutan Med Surg* 3, 105
(1998): Wood B+, *Br J Dermatol* 139, 562
(1997): Hoefnagel JJ+, *Ned Tijdschr Geneeskd* 141, 1424
(1997): Houck HE+, *Arch Dermatol* 133, 15
(1997): Rademaker M, New Zealand (eyelids) (from Internet) (observation)
(1997): Smith KC, Niagara Falls, Ontario (from Internet) (observation)
(1997): Wilde JL+, *Arch Dermatol* 133, 1344
(1996): Collins P+, *Br J Dermatol* 135, 317
(1996): Fleming CJ+, *Br J Dermatol* 134, 784
(1996): Goulden V+, *Br J Dermatol* 134, 693
(1996): Hardman CM+, *Clin Exp Dermatol* 21, 244
(1996): Knoell AG+, *Arch Dermatol* 132, 1251
(1996): Korbol M+, *J Am Podiatr Med Assoc* 76, 87
(1996): Tsao H+, *Arch Dermatol* 132, 1250
(1995): Hung PH+, *J Fam Pract* 41, 183
(1995): Meyer AJ+, *Arch Dermatol* 131, 1447
(1995): Poskitt L+, *Br J Dermatol* 132, 784
(1994): Miralles ES+, *J Dermatol* 21, 965
(1994): Siller GM+, *J Am Acad Dermatol* 30, 350
(1993): Dwyer CM+, *Br J Dermatol* 129, 158
(1993): Okada N+, *Br J Dermatol* 129, 403
(1993): Pepine M+, *J Am Acad Dermatol* 28, 295
(1993): Schofield JK+, *Br J Gen Pract* 43, 173
(1992): Altman DA+, *J Cutan Pathol* 19, 340
(1992): Fakhfakh AC+, *Ann Dermatol Venereol* (French) 119, 975
(1992): Ridgway HB+, *Arch Dermatol* 128, 565 ("pseudo-mongolian")
(1991): Eedy DJ+, *Clin Exp Dermatol* 15, 55
(1991): Leffell D, *J Am Acad Dermatol* 24, 501
(1990): Bamberger N+, *Ann Dermatol Venereol* (French) 117, 299
(1990): Black AK+, *Br J Dermatol* 123, 277
(1990): Bridges AJ+, *J Am Acad Dermatol* 22, 959
(1989): Cataldo E+, *J Mass Dent Soc* 38, 5
(1989): Layton AM+, *J Dermatol Treatment* 1, 9
(1989): Okada N+, *Br J Dermatol* 121, 247
(1987): Angeloni VL+, *Cutis* 40, 229
(1987): Argenyi ZB+, *J Cutaneous Pathol* 14, 176
(1987): Zijdenbos AM+, *Ned Tijdschr Geneeskd* (Dutch) 131, 999
(1986): Prigent F+, *Ann Dermatol Venereol* (French) 113, 227
(1986): Shum DT+, *Arch Dermatol* 122, 18
(1985): Basler RSW, *Arch Dermatol* 121. 606
(1985): Basler RSW+, *J Am Acad Dermatol* 12, 577
(1985): Butler JM+, *Clin Exp Dermatol* 10, 432
(1985): Gordon G, *Arch Dermatol* 121, 618
(1985): Liu TTT+, *Cutis* 35, 254
(1984): Wolfe ID+, *Cutis* 33, 457
(1983): Verret JL+, *Ann Dermatol Venereol* (French) 110, 777
(1983): White SW+, *Arch Dermatol* 119, 1
(1982): Ridgway HA, *Br J Dermatol* 107, 95
(1981): Leroy JP+, *Ann Dermatol Venereol* (French) 108, 871
(1981): Sato S+, *J Invest Dermatol* 77, 264
(1980): Fenske NA+, *J Am Acad Dermatol* 3, 308
(1980): McGrae JD+, *Arch Dermatol* 116, 1262
(1980): Simons JJ+, *J Am Acad Dermatol* 3, 244
(1979): Sauer GC+, *Schoch Letter* 29, 3
(1975): Brogden RN+, *Drugs* 9, 251
(1972): Velasco JE+, *JAMA* 220, 1323

Pigmentation at sites of cutaneous inflammation
(1992): Altman DA+, *J Cutaneous Pathol* 19, 340 (in patients with bullous pemphigoid)
(1991): Eady DJ+, *Clin Exp Dermatol* 16, 55
(1991): Leffell DJ, *J Am Acad Dermatol* 24, 501
(1988): Serwatka LM, *J Assoc Military Derm* 14, 10
(1980): Fenske NA+, *JAMA* 244, 1103

Pruritus (<1%)
(2000): Bachelz H+, *Arch Dermatol* 137, 69
(1996): Goulden V+, *Br J Dermatol* 134, 693
(1996): Montemarano AD+, *J Am Acad Dermatol* 34, 253
(1973): Shelley WB+, *JAMA* 224, 125

Purpura
(2000): Warshaw E, Minneapolis, MN *The Schoch Letter* 50, February #16
(1995): Karofsky PS+, *Arch Pediatr Adolesc Med* 149, 217

Pustular eruption (generalized)
(1999): Antunes A+, *Ann Dermatol Venereol* 126, 518

Rash (sic) (<1%)
(2000): Bachelz H+, *Arch Dermatol* 137, 69
(2000): Schlienger RG+, *Dermatology* 200, 223
(1997): Shapiro LE+, *Arch Dermatol* 133, 1224
(1995): Karofsky PS+, *Arch Pediatr Adolesc Med* 149, 217
(1994): Kaufmann D+, *Arch Intern Med* 154, 1983
(1994): Sitbon O+, *Arch Intern Med* 154, 1633

Raynaud's phenomenon
(1996): Hewack J, *Gastroenterology* 110, A1211

Stevens–Johnson syndrome
(1996): Knowles SR+, *Arch Dermatol* 132, 934
(1987): Shoji A+, *Arch Dermatol* 123, 18

Urticaria
(2001): Bark J, Lexington, KY (from Internet) (observation)
(1997): Shapiro LE+, *Arch Dermatol* 133, 1224
(1996): Goulden V+, *Br J Dermatol* 134, 693
(1996): Knowles SR+, *Arch Dermatol* 132, 934
(1996): Ottuso P, *The Schoch Letter* 46, 37 Vero Beach, FL (from generic)
(1995): Wallis M, *The Schoch Letter* 45, 38 (from generic)
(1994): Litt JZ, Beachwood, OH (personal case) (observation)
(1993): Litt JZ, Beachwood, OH (2 personal cases) (observation)
(1990): Puyana J+, *Allergy* 45, 313
(1975): Brogden RN+, *Drugs* 9, 251

Vasculitis
(2001): Schaffer JV+, *J Am Acad Dermatol* 44, 198 (necrotizing)
(2000): Choi HK+, *Arthritis Rheum* 43, 2488
(1999): Elkayam O+, *Semin Arthritis Rheum* 28, 392
(1999): Schrodt BJ, *Skin and Allergy News* April, 22 (2 cases)
(1999): Schrodt BJ+, *South Med J* 92, 502
(1998): Merkel PA, *Curr Opin Rheumatol* 10, 45

## Hair

Hair – alopecia
(2000): Schlienger RG+, *Dermatology* 200, 223

## Nails

Nails – onycholysis

Nails – photo-onycholysis
(1987): Baran R+, *J Am Acad Dermatol* 17, 1012 (passim)
(1981): Kestel JL, *Cutis* 28, 53

Nails – pigmentation (<1%)
(2001): Gregg LJ, Tulsa, OK (from Internet) (observation)
(2001): Werth V, *Dermatology Times* 18
(1998): Morrow GL+, *Am J Ophthalmol* 125, 396
(1995): Hung PH+, *J Fam Pract* 41, 183
(1994): Mallon E+, *Br J Dermatol* 130, 794
(1989): Berger RS+, *J Am Acad Dermatol* 21, 1300 (3–5%)
(1988): Mooney E+, *J Dermatol Surg Oncol* 14, 1011
(1987): Angeloni VL+, *Cutis* 40, 229
(1985): Daniel CR III+, *Dermatol Clin* 3, 491 (longitudinal)

(1985): Liu TTT+, *Cutis* 35, 254
(1984): Wolfe ID+, *Cutis* 33, 457
(1982): Litt JZ, *Diagnosis* 4, 23

## Other

Anaphylactoid reactions (<1%)
(1996): Okano M+, *Acta Derm Venereol* (Stockh) 76, 164

Arthralgia
(2001): Emmet S, Solana Beach, CA (from Internet) (observation)

Black tongue
(1995): Katz J+, *Arch Dermatol* 131, 620
(1975): Brogden RN+, *Drugs* 9, 251

Conjuctival pigmentation
(1981): Brothers DM+, *Opthalmology* 88, 1212

Galactorrhea (black)
(1996): Hunt MJ+, *Br J Dermatol* 134, 943
(1985): Basler RSW+, *Arch Dermatol* 121, 417

Gingival pigmentation
(1989): Berger RS+, *J Am Acad Dermatol* 21, 1300 (8%)

Glossitis

Gynecomastia
(1995): Davies JP+, *Br J Clin Pract* 49, 179

Hypersensitivity*
(2002): Murray C+, *World Congress Dermatol* Poster, 0120
(2001): Bachelz H+, *Arch Dermatol* 137, 69
(2001): Colvin JH+, *Pediatr Dermatol* 18(4), 295
(2000): Gil P, *Ann Dermatol Venereol* 127(10), 841
(1999): Antunes A+, *Ann Dermatol Venereol* 126, 518
(1999): Clayton BD+, *Arch Dermatol* 135, 139
(1999): Lupton JR+, *Cutis* 64, 91 (infectious-mononucleosis-like)
(1999): Piette AM+, *Rev Med Interne* (French) 20, 869
(1998): Dutz J, Vancouver, Canada (from Internet) (observation)
(1998): Schlienger RG+, *Epilepsia* 39, S3 (passim)
(1997): Hoefnagel JJ+, *Ned Tijdschr Geneeskd* (Dutch) 141, 1424
(1997): MacNeil M+, *J Am Acad Dermatol* 36, 347
(1997): Shapiro LE+, *Arch Dermatol* 133, 1224
(1995): Parneix-Spake A+, *Arch Dermatol* 131, 490
(1994): Sitbon O+, *Arch Intern Med* 154, 1633
(1973): Shelley WB+, *JAMA* 224, 125

Myalgia
(1998): Matteson EL+, *J Rheumatol* 25, 1653

Oral mucosal pigmentation
(2002): Friedman IS+, *Dermatol Surg* 28(3), 205
(2001): Werth V, *Dermatology Times* 18

Oral pigmentation
(1998): Cockings JM+, *Aust Dent J* 43, 14
(1998): Morrow GL+, *Am J Ophthalmol* 125, 396
(1998): Patel K+, *Br J Dermatol* 185, 560
(1997): Eisen D, *Lancet* 349, 379
(1997): Smith KC, Niagara Falls, Ontario (from Internet) (observation) (blue on lips)
(1995): Odell EW+, *Oral Surg Oral Med Oral Pathol Oral Radiol Endod* 79, 459
(1994): Chu P+, *J Am Acad Dermatol* 30, 802
(1994): Siller GM+, *J Am Acad Dermatol* 30, 350
(1989): Berger RS+, *J Am Acad Dermatol* 21, 1300 (7%)
(1989): Regezi JA+, *Oral Pathology*, WB Saunders, 166
(1986): Beehner ME+, *J Oral Maxillofac Surg* 44, 582
(1985): Salman RA+, *J Oral Med* 40, 154
(1984): Fendrich P+, *Oral Surg Oral Med Oral Pathol 58*, 288

Oral ulceration
(2000): Schlienger RG+, *Dermatology* 200, 223

Paresthesias (<1%)
(1994): Blanchard L, *Schoch Letter* 44, #6 (observation)

Polyarteritis nodosa
(2001): Schaffer JV+, *J Am Acad Dermatol* 44, 198
(1999): Schrodt BJ+, *Pediatrics* 103, 503

Pseudo-mongolian spot (sic)
(1992): Ridgway HB+, *Arch Dermatol* 128, 565

Pseudotumor cerebri
(2002): Ang ERG+, *J Am Board Fam ract* 15, 229
(2001): Oswald J+, *Schweiz Rundsch Med Prax* 90(39), 1691
(2001): Weese-Mayer DE+, *Pediatrics* 108(2), 519
(2000): Frederickson KS, Novato, CA (from Internet) (observation)
(1998): Chiu AM+, *Am J Ophthalmol* 126, 116
(1990): Delaney RA+, *Mil Med* 156, A5
(1990): Shelley WB, *The Schoch Letter* 40, 27
(1980): Beran RG, *Med J Aust* 1, 323

Scleral pigmentation
(1998): Morrow GL+, *Am J Ophthalmol* 125, 396
(1985): Liu TT+, *Cutis* 35, 254

Serum sickness
(2001): Arch Dermatol 137, 100 (2 cases)
(1999): Elkayam O+, *Semin Arthritis Rheum* 28, 392
(1998): Martinez JA+, *Med Clin (Barc)* (Spanish) 111, 198
(1997): Blumenthal HL, Beachwood, OH (personal case) (observation)
(1997): Hoefnagel JJ+, *Ned Tijdschr Geneeskd* (Dutch) 141, 1424
(1997): Shapiro LE+, *Arch Dermatol* 133, 1224
(1997): Zabawski E, Dallas, TX (from Internet) (observation)
(1996): Harel L+, *Ann Pharmacother* 30, 481
(1996): Levenson T+, *Allergy Asthma Proc* 17, 79
(1990): Puyana J+, *Allergy* 45, 313

Teeth – pigmentation
(2001): Gregg LJ, Tulsa, OK (from Internet) (observation)

Tongue discoloration
(2000): Tanzi E+, *Arch Dermatol* 136, 427
(1995): Katz J+, *Arch Dermatol* 131, 620
(1995): Meyerson M+, *Oral Surg Oral Med Oral Pathol Oral Radiol Endod* 79, 180

Tongue pigmentation
(2002): Friedman IS+, *Dermatol Surg* 28(3), 205

Tongue pigmentation
(2002): Friedman IS+, *Dermatol Surg* 28(3), 205

Tooth discoloration (>10%) (primarily in children)
(2000): Bark JP, Lexington, KY (from Internet) (observation)
(2000): McKenna BE+, *Dent Update* 26, 160 (in an adult)
(2000): Thaler D, Monona, WI (from internet) (observation)
(1999): Cheek CC+, *J Esthet Dent* 11, 43
(1998): Dodd MA+, *Ann Pharmacother* 32, 887 (68-year-old woman)
(1998): Morrow GL+, *Am J Ophthalmol* 125, 396
(1998): Patel K+, *Br J Dermatol* 185, 560 (in an adult)
(1997): Bowles WK+, *J Esthet Dent* 9, 30
(1997): Smith KC, Niagara Falls, Ontario (from Internet) (observation)
(1995): Hung PH+, *J Fam Pract* 41, 183
(1994): Hofmann H, *Hautarzt* (German) 45, 803
(1991): Allegue F+, *Actas Dermo-Sif* (Spanish) 82, 43
(1989): Berger RS+, *J Am Acad Dermatol* 21, 1300 (3–5%)
(1989): Regezi JA+, *Oral Pathology*, WB Saunders, 166
(1989): Rosen T+, *J Am Acad Dermatol* 21, 569
(1988): Cale AE+, *J Periodontol* 59, 112
(1985): Poliak SC+, *JAMA* 254, 2930
(1984): Wolfe ID+, *Cutis* 33, 457
(1980): Caro I, *J Am Acad Dermatol* 3, 317
(1979): Basler RSW, *Arch Dermatol* 115, 1391

***Note:** The antiepileptic drug hypersensitivity syndrome is a severe, occasionally fatal, disorder characterized by any or all of the following: pruritic exanthems, toxic epidermal necrolysis, Stevens–Johnson syndrome, exfoliative dermatitis, fever, hepatic abnormalities, eosinophilia, and renal failure

# MINOXIDIL

**Trade names:** Minoxidil (Par); Rogaine (topical) (Pharmacia & Upjohn)
**Other common trade names:** *Alopexy; Apo-Gain; Hairgaine; Lonolox; Lonoten; Minoximen; Regaine*
**Indications:** Hypertension, androgenetic alopecia
**Category:** Antihypertensive; vasodilator
**Half-life:** 4.2 hours
**Clinically important, potentially hazardous interactions with: alcohol**, guanethidine

**Note:** For topical reaction patterns, I have added a bracket [T]

### *Reactions*

## Skin

Acne
(1985): Baral J, *J Am Acad Dermatol* 13, 1051 (scalp comedones)
Allergic contact dermatitis
(2002): Suzuki K+, *Am J Contact* 13(1), 45
Allergic reactions (sic) [T]
Ankle edema
Bullous eruption (<1%)
(1981): DiSantis DJ+, *Arch Intern Med* 141, 1515
(1978): Rosenthal T+, *Arch Intern Med* 138, 1856
Contact dermatitis (7.4%) [T]
(1998): Sanchez-Motilla J+, *Contact Dermatitis* 38, 283 (pustular)
(1995): Ebner H+, *Contact Dermatitis* 32, 316
(1992): Ruas E+, *Contact Dermatitis* 26, 57
(1992): Veraldi S+, *Contact Dermatitis* 26, 211
(1991): Wilson C+, *J Am Acad Dermatol* 24, 661
(1988): Alomar A+, *Contact Dermatitis* 18, 51
(1988): van Joost T, *Ned Tijdschr Geneeskd* (Dutch) 132, 1141
(1987): Valsecchi R+, *Contact Dermatitis* 17, 58
(1987): van der Willingen AH+, *Contact Dermatitis* 17, 44
(1985): Degreef H+, *Contact Dermatitis* 13, 194
(1985): Tosti A+, *Contact Dermatitis* 13, 275
Eczematous eruption (sic)
(1992): Ruas E+, *Contact Dermatitis* 26, 57
(1987): van der Willigen AH+, *Contact Dermatitis* 17, 44
Edema (>10%) [T]
(1977): Nawar T+, *Can Med Assoc J* 117, 1178
Erythema [T]
Erythema multiforme
(1981): DiSantis DJ+, *Arch Intern Med* 141, 1515
Erythroderma
(1988): Ackerman BH+, *Drug Intell Clin Pharm* 22, 703
Exanthems
(1988): Ackerman BH+, *Drug Intell Clin Pharm* 22, 703
(1981): Campese VM, *Drugs* 22, 257
(1981): DiSantis DJ+, *Arch Intern Med* 141, 1515
(1977): Nawar T+, *Can Med Assoc J* 117, 1178
Flushing [T]
Folliculitis [T]
(1996): Duvic M+, *J Am Acad Dermatol* 35, 74
Lupus erythematosus
(1987): Tunkel AR+, *Arch Intern Med* 147, 599
(1981): Mitas JA, *Arthritis Rheum* 24, 570
Peripheral edema (7%)
Pigmentation
Pruritus [T]
(1996): Duvic M+, *J Am Acad Dermatol* 35, 74
(1990): Colamarino R+, *Ann Intern Med* 113, 256
(1977): Nawar T+, *Can Med Assoc J* 117, 1178
Pyogenic granuloma
(1989): Baran R, *Dermatologica* 179(2), 76 (explosive, of the scalp)
Rash (sic) (<1%)
Seborrhea [T]
Stevens–Johnson syndrome (<1%)
(1981): DiSantis DJ+, *Arch Intern Med* 141, 1515
Sunburn (<1%)
Urticaria
Xerosis

## Hair

Hair – alopecia [T]
(1987): Olsen EA, *J Am Acad Dermatol* 16, 145
(1983): Ingles RM+, *Int J Dermatol* 22, 120
Hair – discoloration
(1989): Rebora A+, *J Am Acad Dermatol* 21, 1314
(1983): Ingles RM+, *Int J Dermatol* 22, 120 (red)
Hair – hirsutism (in women)
(1981): Campese VM, *Drugs* 22, 257 (100%)
(1973): Pettinger WA+, *N Engl J Med* 289, 167
Hair – hypertrichosis (80%)
(2002): Litt JZ, Beachwood, OH (personal case) (observation)
(1997): Peluso AM+, *Br J Dermatol* 136, 118
(1995): Veyrac G+, *Therapie* (French) 50, 474 (in an infant)
(1994): Gonzalez M+, *Clin Exp Dermatol* 19, 157 [T]
(1990): Miwa LJ+, *Drug Intell Clin Pharm* 24, 365
(1989): Rousseau C+, *Dermatologica* 179, 221
(1988): Toriumi DN+, *Arch Otolaryngol Head Neck Surg* 114, 918
(1985): Bencini PL+, *G Ital Dermatol Venereol* (Italian) 120, 137
(1985): Lorette G+, *Ann Dermatol Venereol* (French) 112, 527
(1984): Henkes J+, *Med Clin (Barc)* (Spanish) 83, 89
(1983): Ingles RM+, *Int J Dermatol* 22, 120
(1983): Wilkin JK+, *Cutis* 31, 61
(1981): Campese VM, *Drugs* 22, 257 (100%)
(1981): Nielsen PG, *Lakartidningen* (Swedish) 78, 1891
(1980): Feldman HA+, *Curr Ther Res* 27, 205
(1980): Ryckmanns F, *Hautarzt* (German) 31, 205
(1979): Burton JL+, *Br J Dermatol* 101, 593
(1979): Pierard GE+, *Dermatologica* (French) 158, 17.5
(1977): Earhart RN+, *South Med J* 70, 442
(1977): Nawar T+, *Can Med Assoc J* 117, 1178

## Other

Anaphylactoid reactions
(2001): Blumenthal HL, Beachwood, OH (observation)
Anosmia
(1993): Litt JZ, Beachwood, OH (personal case) (observation)
Dysgeusia [T]
(1993): Litt JZ, Beachwood, OH (personal case) (observation)
Gynecomastia
Mastodynia (<1%)
Paresthesias
Polymyalgia
(1990): Colamarino R+, *Ann Intern Med* 113, 256
Tendinitis [T]

# MIRTAZAPINE

**Trade name:** Remeron (Organon)
**Indications:** Depression
**Category:** Tetracyclic antidepressant; alpha-2 antagonist
**Half-life:** 20–40 hours

### *Reactions*

## Skin

Acne

Cellulitis
Chills
Diaphoresis
(1999): Leinonen E+, *Int Clin Psychopharmacol* 14, 329
Edema (1–10%)
Exfoliative dermatitis
Facial edema
Flu-like syndrome (sic) (1–10%)
(2000): Benkert O+, *J Clin Psychiatry* 61, 656
Herpes simplex
Peripheral edema (1–10%)
(2001): Kutscher EC+, *Ann Pharmacother* 35(11), 1494
Petechiae
Photosensitivity
Pruritus
Rash (sic) (1–10%)
Seborrhea
Ulcer
Xerosis

### Other

Ageusia
Aphthous stomatitis
Arthralgia
(2001): Jolliet P+, *Eur Psychiatry* 16(8), 503
(2000): Veyrac G+, *Therapie* 55(5), 652
Dysgeusia
Glossitis (1–10%)
Gynecomastia
Hypesthesia
Mastodynia
Myalgia (1–10%)
(2001): Jolliet P+, *Eur Psychiatry* 16(8), 503
Oral candidiasis
Paresthesias
(2001): Ribeiro L+, *Braz J Med Biol Res* 34(10), 1303
Parosmia
Phlebitis
Restless legs syndrome
(2002): Bahk WM+, *Psychiatry Clin Neurosci* 56(2), 209
Rhabdomyolysis
(1998): Retz W+, *Int Clin Psychopharmacol* 13(6), 277
Serotonin syndrome
(2002): Hernandez JL+, *Ann Pharmacother* 36(4), 641
(2001): Demers JC+, *Ann Pharmacother* 35(10), 1217 (with fluvoxamine)
(2001): Isbister GK+, *Ann Pharmacother* 35(12), 1674 (with fluvoxamine)
Sialorrhea
Stomatitis
Tendon rupture
Tongue discoloration
Tongue edema
Tremors (1–10%)
Vaginitis
Xerostomia (25%)
(1995): Montgomery SA, *Int Clin Psychopharmacol* 10, 37

# MISOPROSTOL

**Trade names:** Arthrotec (Searle); Cytotec (Searle)
**Other common trade name:** *Symbol*
**Indications:** Prevention of NSAID-induced ulcer
**Category:** Synthetic prostaglandin $E_1$ analogue; anti-ulcer agent
**Half-life:** 20–40 minutes

Arthrotec is diclofenac and misoprostol

## *Reactions*

### Skin

Dermatitis (sic)
Diaphoresis
Exanthems
(1987): Monk JP+, *Drugs* 33, 1
Rash (sic)
Shivering
(2001): Elsheikh A+, *Arch Gynecol Obstet* 265(4), 204 (17.3%)
(2001): Gulmezoglu AM+, *Lancet* 358, 689
(2001): Li YT+, *Zhonghua Yi Xue Za Zhi* (Taipei) 64(12), 721 (33%)
(1999): Lumbiganon P+, *Br J Obstet Gynaecol* 106, 304

### Hair

Hair – alopecia

### Other

Anaphylactoid reactions
Gingivitis
Gynecomastia
(1994): Garcia-Rodriguez LA+, *BMJ* 308, 503
Tinnitus

# MISTLETOE

**Scientific names:** American species *(Phoradendron serotinum, Phoradendron leucarpum, Phoradendron serontium, Phoradendron flavescens, Phoradendron tomentosum, Phoradendron macrophyllum, Phoradendron rubrum);* European species *(Viscum album)*
**Other common names:** All-heal; American Mistletoe; Birdlime Mistletoe; Devil's fuge; European Mistletoe; Folia Visci; Herbe de la Croix; Lignum Crucis; Stipites Visci; Visci albi herba; Viscum
**Family:** Loranthacae (Viscaceae)
**Purported indications:** (injected): Viscotoxins have cytotoxic and immune system-modulating effects. Immunomodulator in adjuvant tumor therapy.
**Other uses:** (as tincture): Abortifacient, arteriosclerosis, arthritis, asthma, common cold, depression, diabetes, epilepsy, hepatitis, headache, HIV infection, hypertension, hypotension, hysteria, labor pain, lumbago, metrorrhagia, muscle spasms, otitis, whooping cough.
Orally: European mistletoe is used for cancer, reducing side effects of chemotherapy and radiation therapy, high blood pressure, hemorrhoids, internal bleeding, gout, sleep disorders, headache, amenorrhea, diarrhea, chorea, liver and gallbladder conditions
**Clinically important, potentially hazardous interactions with:** bepridil, corticosteroids, digoxin, diltiazem, immunosuppressants, MAO inhibitors, verapamil

**Note:** Part Used: Dried or fresh young leafy twigs with flowers and fruits. Purified extracts injected intramuscularly, subcutaneously or given by intravenous infusion. Unless otherwise indicated, side effects listed are from injected preparations. The FDA considers *Viscum album* unsafe for human consumption

### *Reactions*

#### Skin

Adverse effects (sic)
(1999): Stein GM+, *Eur J Med Res* 4(5), 169
(1994): Stein G+, *Eur J Clin Phamacol* 47(1), 33

Allergic reactions (sic)
(2000): Büssing A, *Mistletoe: The Genus Viscum* Harwood Academic Publishers
(1994): Stein G+, *Eur J Clin Pharmacp;* 47(1), 33
(1991): Pichler WJ+, *Dtsch Med Wochenschr* (German) 116(35), 1333

Chills
(2000): Büssing A, *Mistletoe: The Genus Viscum* Harwood Academic Publishers
(1995): Murray MT, *The Healing Power of Herbs* 253 Prima Publishing

Dermatitis (sic)
(2000): Büssing A, *Mistletoe: The Genus Viscum* (Harwood Academic Publishers)

Edema of the lip
(1998): Hagenah W+, *Dtsch Med Wochenschr* (German) 123(34), 1001

Erythema
(2001): Hutt N+, *Allergol Immunopathol* (Madr) 29(5), 201
(1999): Stoss M+, *Arzneimittelforschung* 49(4), 366
(1999): van Wely+, *Am J Ther* 6(1), 37

Flu-like syndrome
(1999): Gorter RW+, *Altern Ther Health Med* 5(6), 37
(1999): van Wely+, *Am J Ther* 6(1), 37

Pruritus
(1999): Stoss M+, *Arzneimittelforschung* 49(4), 366

Subcutaneous nodes
(1998): Hagenah W+, *Dtsch Med Wochenschr* (German) 123(34), 1001

#### Other

Anaphylactoid reactions
(2001): Hutt N+, *Allergol Immunopathol* (Madr) 29(5), 201
(1996): Friess H+, *Anticancer Res* 16(2), 915 (28%)

Death (low incidence – accidental ingestion)
(1997): Krenzelok EP+, *Am J Emerg* 15(5), 516
(1996): Spiller HA+, *J Toxicol Clin Toxicol* 34(4), 405
(1995): Murray MT, *The Healing Power of Herbs* 253 Prima Publishing
(1986): Hall AH+, *Annals Emergency Med* 15, 1320

Gingivitis
(1999): Gorter RW+, *Altern Ther Health Med* 5(6), 37
(1999): van Wely+, *Am J Ther* 6(1), 37

Injection-site edema
(1999): Stoss M+, *Arzneimittelforschung* 49(4), 366

Injection-site inflammation
(1999): Stein GM+, *Eur J Med Res* 4(5), 169
(1999): Stoss M+, *Arzneimittelforschung* (German) 49(4), 366
(1998): Gorter RW+, *Am J Ther* 5(3), 181
(1998): Stoss M+, *Nat Immun* 16(5), 185
(1995): Murray MT, *The Healing Power of Herbs* 253 Prima Publishing
(1990): Kast A+, *Schweiz Rundsch Med Prax* (German) 79(10), 291

***Note:** The well-known mistletoe is an evergreen parasitic plant, growing on the branches of some tree species

****Note:** Shakespeare calls it "the baleful mistletoe," an illusion to the Scandinavian legend that Balder, the god of Peace, was slain with an arrow made of mistletoe

## MITHRAMYCIN

(See PLICAMYCIN)

## MITOMYCIN

**Synonyms:** mitomycin-C; MTC
**Trade name:** Mutamycin (Bristol-Myers Squibb)
**Other common trade names:** *Ametycine; Mitomycin; Mitomycin-C; Mitomycine*
**Indications:** Carcinomas
**Category:** Antineoplastic antibiotic
**Half-life:** 23–78 minutes
**Clinically important, potentially hazardous interactions with:** aldesleukin

### *Reactions*

#### Skin

Angioedema

Bullous eruption
(1984): Ritch PS+, *Cancer* 54, 32

Contact dermatitis
(1997): Gomez Torrrijos E+, *Allergy* 52, 687
(1993): Wahlberg JE+, *Lakartidningen* (Swedish) 90, 158
(1992): Vidal C+, *Dermatology* 184, 208
(1981): Nissenkorn I+, *J Urol* 126, 596

Dermatitis (sic)
(1990): Colver GB+, *Br J Dermatol* 122, 217
(1987): Sala F+, *G Ital Dermatol Venereol* (Italian) 122, 265
(1984): Neild VJ+, *J R Soc Med* 77, 610
(1975): *Med Lett* 17, 62

Edema

Erythema

Erythema multiforme
(1984): Spencer HJ, *J Surg Oncol* 26, 47

Exanthems
(1995): Echechipia S+, *Contact Dermatitis* 33, 432
(1987): Sala F+, *G Ital Dermatol Venereol* (Italian) 122, 265

Exfoliative dermatitis
(1987): Sala F+, *G Ital Dermatol Venereol* (Italian) 122, 265
(1985): Bencini PL+, *Int J Dermatol* 24, 472

Necrosis
(2000): Neulander EZ+, *J Urol* 164(4), 1306 (glans penis)

Palmar desquamation
(1981): Nissenkorn I+, *J Urol* 126, 596

Photosensitivity
(1981): Fuller B+, *Ann Intern Med* 94, 542

Pigmentation
(1989): Kerker BJ+, *Semin Dermatol* 8, 173

Pityriasis rosea
(1987): Sala F+, *G Ital Dermatol Venereol* (Italian) 122, 265

Pruritus (<1%)

Purpura

Rash (sic) (<1%)
(1981): Nissenkorn I+, *J Urol* 126, 596 (generalized)

Thrombocytopenic purpura

(2001): Medina PJ+, *Curr Opin Hematol* 8(5), 286
Ulceration
(1992): Ellsworth-Wolk J, *Oncol Nurs Forum* 19, 1554
Urticaria
(1981): Weiss RB+, *Ann Intern Med* 94, 66

### Hair
Hair – alopecia (1–10%)
(1975): *Med Lett* 17, 62

### Nails
Nails – pigmented bands (purple) (1–10%)

### Other
Injection-site cellulitis (>10%)
Injection-site extravasation
(2000): Kassner E, *J Pediatr Oncon Nurs* 17, 135
Injection-site necrosis (>10%)
(1987): Aizawa H+, *Acta Derm Venereol* (Stockh) 67, 364
(1987): Dufresne RG, *Cutis* 39, 197
(1987): Sala F+, *G Ital Dermatol Venereol* (Italian) 122, 265
Injection-site thrombophlebitis
Oral mucosal lesions
(1987): Sala F+, *G Ital Dermatol Venereol* (Italian) 122, 265
(1983): Bronner AK+, *J Am Acad Dermatol* 9, 645
(1978): Levine N+, *Cancer Treat Rev* 5, 67 (2–8%)
(1975): *Med Lett* 17, 62
Oral ulceration (1–10%)
(1984): Spencer HJ, *J Surg Oncol* 26, 47
Paresthesias (1–10%)
Stomatitis (>10%)
Thrombophlebitis (<1%)

## MITOTANE

**Synonym:** o,p'-DDD
**Trade name:** Lysodren (Bristol-Myers Squibb)
**Other common trade name:** *Opeprim*
**Indications:** Inoperable adrenocortical carcinoma
**Category:** Antiadrenal; antineoplastic
**Half-life:** 18–159 days
**Clinically important, potentially hazardous interactions with:** aldesleukin, spironolactone

### *Reactions*

### Skin
Acral erythema
(1991): Baack BR+, *J Am Acad Dermatol* 24, 457
(1974): Zühlke RL, *Dermatologica* 148, 90
Angioedema (<1%)
Cutaneous side effects (sic)
(1973): Lubitz JA+, *JAMA* 223, 1109 (13%)
(1966): Hutter AM+, *Am J Med* 41, 581 (17%)
Erythema multiforme
(1978): Levine N+, *Cancer Treat Rev* 5, 67
(1966): Hutter AM+, *Am J Med* 41, 581
Exanthems
(1973): Lubitz JA+, *JAMA* 223, 1109 (9%)
(1966): Hutter AM+, *Am J Med* 41, 581 (16%)
Flushing (1–10%)
Pigmentation
(1973): Lubitz JA+, *JAMA* 223, 1109
(1966): Hutter AM+, *Am J Med* 41, 581 (16%)
Pruritus
(1974): Zühlke RL, *Dermatologica* 148, 90
Rash (sic) (15%)
Urticaria
(1966): Hutter AM+, *Am J Med* 41, 581
Vasculitis (<1%)

### Hair
Hair – alopecia
(1973): Lubitz JA+, *JAMA* 223, 1109
(1966): Hutter AM+, *Am J Med* 41, 581 (16%)

### Other
Myalgia (1–10%)
Tremors (<1%)

## MITOXANTRONE

**Trade name:** Novantrone (Immunex)
**Indications:** Acute myelogenous leukemia, multiple sclerosis, prostate cancer
**Category:** parenteral; synthetic antineoplastic antibiotic
**Half-life:** median terminal: 75 hours
**Clinically important, potentially hazardous interactions with:** aldesleukin

### *Reactions*

### Skin
Allergic reactions (sic) (<1%)
Chills (1–10%)
Diaphoresis (1–10%)
Ecchymoses (7%)
Edema (>10%)
Erythema
Fungal Infection (>15%)
Infections (sic) (>66%)
Necrosis
Petechiae (>10%)
Pigmentation (bluish)
Purpura (>10%)
Rash (sic) (<1%)
Ulceration
Urticaria
Vitiligo
(2001): Schmid-Wendtner M-H+, *Lancet* 358, 1575

### Hair
Hair – alopecia (20–60%)

## MODAFINIL

**Trade name:** Provigil (Cephalon)
**Other common trade name:** *Alertec*
**Indications:** Narcolepsy
**Category:** Central nervous system stimulant; analeptic
**Half-life:** ~15 hours

### *Reactions*

### Skin
Allergic reactions (sic) (>1%)
Chills (2%)
Diaphoresis (>1%)
Ecchymoses (>1%)

Edema, generalized (>1%)
Erythema
Herpes simplex (1%)
Hot flashes
Pruritus (>1%)
Psoriasis (>1%)
Rash (sic) (>1%)
Xerosis (1%)

### Other

Dysgeusia (>1%)
Gingivitis (1%)
Myalgia (>1%)
Oral ulceration (1%)
Paresthesias (3%)
(2002): Nieves AV+, *Clin Neuropharmacol* 25(2), 111
Sialorrhea
Tooth disorder (sic) (>1%)
Tremors (1%)
Xerostomia (5%)

## MOEXIPRIL

**Trade names:** Uniretic (Schwarz); Univasc (Schwarz)
**Indications:** Hypertension
**Category:** Angiotensin converting enzyme (ACE) inhibitor; antihypertensive
**Half-life:** 1 hour
**Clinically important, potentially hazardous interactions with:** amiloride, spironolactone, triamterene

Uniretic is moexipril and hydrochlorothiazide

***Reactions***

### Skin

Angioedema (<1%)
(2001): Cohen EG+, *Ann Otol Rhinol Laryngol* 110(8), 701 (64 cases)
Diaphoresis (<1%)
Exanthems (1.6%)
Flushing (1.6%)
(1995): Drayer JIM+, *Am J Ther* 2, 525
Pemphigus (<1%)
Pemphigus foliaceus
(2000): Ong CS+, *Australas J Dermatol* 41(4), 242
Peripheral edema (1–10%)
(1995): Drayer JIM+, *Am J Ther* 2, 525
Photosensitivity (<1%)
Pruritus (1–10%)
Rash (sic) (1.6%)
Skin reactions (sic)
(1994): White WB+, *J Human Hypertens* 8, 917
Urticaria (<1%)

### Hair

Hair – alopecia (1–10%)

### Other

Anaphylactoid reactions (<1%)
Cough
(2001): Adigun AQ+, *West Afr J Med* 20(1), 46–7
(2001): Lee SC+, *Hypertension* 38(2), 166
Dysgeusia (<1%)
Myalgia (1.3%)
Xerostomia (<1%)

## MOLINDONE

**Trade name:** Moban (Endo)
**Indications:** Schizophrenia
**Category:** Antipsychotic
**Half-life:** 1.5 hours

***Reactions***

### Skin

Allergic reactions (sic)
Edema
Hypohidrosis (<1%)
Peripheral edema
Photosensitivity (<1%)
Pigmentation (<1%)
Pruritus (<1%)
Rash (sic) (<1%)

### Other

Galactorrhea (<1%)
Gynecomastia (1–10%)
Sialorrhea
Xerostomia (>10%)

## MONTELUKAST

**Trade name:** Singulair (Merck)
**Indications:** Asthma
**Category:** Antiasthmatic (leukotriene receptor antagonist)
**Half-life:** 2.7–5.5 hours

***Reactions***

### Skin

Allergic granulomatous angiitis (Churg–Strauss syndrome)
(2002): Alvarez-Fernandez JG+, *World Congress Dermatol* Poster, 0082
(2002): Hammer HB+, *Tidsskr Nor Laegeforen* 122(5), 484
(2002): Solans R+, *Thorax* 57(2), 183 (1 case)
(2001): Donohue J, *Chest* 119(2), 668
(2001): Hosker HS, *Thorax* 56(3), 244
(2001): Kalyoncu A+, *Allergol Immunopathol* (Madr) 29(5), 185
(2001): Lipworth BJ+, *Thorax* 56(3), 244
(2001): Mukhopadhyay A+, *Postgrad Med J* 56(5), 417
(2001): Sabio JM+, *Chest* 120(6), 2116
(2001): Weschler M Thorax, *Thorax* 56(5), 417
(2000): Price D, *Drugs* 59, 35 (passim)
(2000): Trujillo-Santos AJ+, *Med Clin* (Barc) 115(15), 599
(2000): Tuggey JM+, *Thorax* 55(9), 805
(2000): Villena V+, *Eur Resp J* 15, 626
(2000): Wechsler ME+, *Chest* 117. 708
Angioedema
(1998): Condrys P, Webster, NY (from Internet) (observation)
Erythema nodosum
(2000): Dellaripa PF+, *Mayo Clin Proc* 75(6), 643
Flu-like syndrome (sic) (1–10%)
Peripheral edema
(2000): Geller M, *Ann Intern Med* 132, 924
Rash (sic) (1.6%)
Urticaria (1.6%)
(1998): Jaffe P, Columbia, SC (from Internet) (observation)
(1998): Knorr B+, *JAMA* 279, 1181

### Other

Cough
(2001): Spector SL, *Ann Allergy Asthma Immunol* 86(6 Suppl 1), 18
Panniculitis
(2000): Dellaripa PF+, *Mayo Clin Proc* 75(6), 643

## MORICIZINE

**Trade name:** Ethmozine (Roberts)
**Indications:** Ventricular arrhythmias
**Category:** Antiarrhythmic; class I
**Half-life:** 3–4 hours

### *Reactions*

### Skin

Diaphoresis (2–5%)
Exanthems (<1%)
Periorbital edema (1–10%)
Pruritus (<2%)
Rash (sic) (<1%)
Urticaria (<2%)
Xerosis (<2%)

### Other

Dysgeusia (<2%)
Hypesthesia (2–5%)
Oral mucosal lesions
(1990): Fitton A+, *Drugs* 40, 138
Paresthesias (2–5%)
Thrombophlebitis (<2%)
Tinnitus
Tongue edema (<2%)
Xerostomia (2–5%)
(1990): Carnes CA+, *Drug Intell Clin Pharm* 24, 745 (2–5%)
(1990): Fitton A+, *Drugs* 40, 138 (2%)

## MORPHINE

**Trade names:** Astramorph; Duramorph; Infumorph; Kadian; MS Contin; MS/L; MS/S; MSIR Oral; OMS Oral; Oramorph SR; RMS; Roxanol
**Other common trade names:** *Anamorph; Astramorph; Contalgin; Epimorph; Morphine-HP; MOS; Moscontin; MS-IR; MST Continus; Sevredol; Statex*
**Indications:** Severe pain, acute myocardial infarction
**Category:** Narcotic analgesic
**Half-life:** 2–4 hours
**Clinically important, potentially hazardous interactions with:** buprenorphine, cimetidine, furazolidone, MAO inhibitors, pentazocine

### *Reactions*

### Skin

Diaphoresis
Edema
Exanthems
(1977): Voorhorst R+, *Ned Tijdschr Geneeskd* (Dutch) 121, 737
Flushing
Pallor
Peripheral edema
Pruritus (<1%)
(2002): Nakata K+, *J Clin Anesth* 14(2), 121
(2001): Charuluxananan S+, *Anesth Analg* 93(1), 162
(2001): Matsuda M+, *Masui* 50(10), 1096
(2001): Mercadante S+, *Support Care Cancer* 9(6), 467
(2001): Sakai T+, *Can J Anaesth* 48(8), 831
(2001): Subramaniam K+, *J Clin Anesth* 13(5), 339 (with ketamine)
(2000): Gunter JB+, *Paediatr Anaesth* 10, 167
(2000): Yeh HM+, *Anesth Analg* 91, 172
(1998): Thangaturai D+, *Anaesthesia* 43, 1055 (62%)
(1988): Gustafson LL+, *Drugs* 35, 597 (5–10%)
(1986): Attia J+, *Anesthesiology* 65, 590 (20%)
Rash (sic)

### Other

Death
(2002): Byard RW, *J Forensic Sci* 47(1), 202
Gynecomastia
Hypesthesia
Injection-site pain (>10%)
Rhabdomyolysis
(1985): Blain PG+, *Hum Toxicol* 4(1), 71
Trembling (1–10%)
Xerostomia (>10%)
(2002): Andersen G+, *Palliat Med* 16(2), 107
(1989): White JD+, *BMJ* 298, 1222 (75%)

## MOXIFLOXACIN

**Trade name:** Avelox (Bayer)
**Indications:** Various infections caused by susceptible organisms
**Category:** Fluoroquinolone antibiotic
**Half-life:** 12 hours
**Clinically important, potentially hazardous interactions with:** amiodarone, arsenic, bepridil, bretylium, disopyramide, erythromycin, phenothiazines, procainamide, quinidine, sotalol, tricyclic antidepressants

### *Reactions*

### Skin

Allergic reactions (sic)
Burning
Candidiasis (<1%)
Chills (<1%)
Diaphoresis (<1%)
Edema
Exanthems
(2000): Litt JZ, Beachwood, OH (personal case; no pruritus)
Fixed eruption
(2001): Litt JZ, Beachwood, OH (personal case)
Peripheral edema (<1%)
Photosensitivity (<1%)
(2000): Balfour JA+, *Drugs* 59, 115
(2000): Stein GE+, *Inf Med* 17, 564
(2000): Traynor NJ+, *Toxicol Vitr* 14, 275
Pruritus (<1%)
Rash (sic) (<1%)
(2001): Culley CM+, *Am J Health-Syst Pharm* 58, 379
Urticaria (<1%)
Xerosis (<1%)

### Other

Anaphylactoid reactions
(2001): Aleman A+, *J Allergy Clin Immunol* Feb, 107

Dysgeusia (>1%)
(2000): Stein GE+, *Inf Med* 17, 564
Glossitis (<1%)
Myalgia (<1%)
Paresthesias (<1%)
Stomatitis (<1%)
Tendinitis
Tendon rupture
Tremors (<1%)
Vaginitis (<1%)
(2000): Stein GE+, *Inf Med* 17, 564
Xerostomia (<1%)
(2001): Litt JZ, Beachwood, OH (personal case)

# MSM

**Scientific names:** *Dimethylsulfone; Methylsulfonylmethane*
**Other common names:** Crystalline DMSO; Dimethyl Sulfone; $DMSO_2$; Methyl Sulfonyl Methane; Methylsulfonyl Methane; OptiMSM; Sulfonyl Sulfur
**Purported indications:** Chronic pain, arthritis, joint inflammation, rheumatoid arthritis, osteoporosis, bursitis, tendinitis, tenosynovitis, muscle cramps scars, stretch marks, wrinkles, wounds, cuts, abrasions
**Other uses:** Relief of allergies, rhinitis, sinusitis, asthma, drug hypersensitivity, constipation, ulcers, diverticulosis, mood elevation, obesity, hypertension, elevated cholesterol, diabetes, Alzheimer's disease, chronic fatigue syndrome, autoimmune disorders (systemic lupus erythematosus), migraines, hangovers, and parasitic infections of the intestinal and urogenital tracts

### *Reactions*

## Skin

None

***Note:** MSM occurs naturally in green plants fruits, vegetables, and milk. It is destroyed by heat or dehydration

# MYCOPHENOLATE

**Synonym:** mycophenolate mofetil
**Trade name:** CellCept (Roche)
**Indications:** Prophylaxis of organ rejection
**Category:** Immunosuppressant
**Half-life:** 18 hours
**Clinically important, potentially hazardous interactions with:** antacids, azathioprine, basiliximab, cholestyramine, corticosteroids, cyclophosphamide, cyclosporine, daclizumab, mercaptopurine, mofetil, mycophenolate, tacrolimus, **vaccines**

### *Reactions*

## Skin

Acne (>10%)
Bullous eruption
(2000): Rault R, *Ann Intern Med* 133, 921 (hands)
Carcinoma (non-melanoma) (4%)
Dermatitis herpetiformis (aggravation)
(2002): Gladstone GC, Worcester, MA (personal correspondence)
Diaphoresis
Edema (12.2%)
Herpes simplex
(2000): Williams JV+, *Skin & Allergy News* September, 24
Infections (sic) (12–20%)
(2002): Bernabeu-Wittel M+, *Eur J Clin Microbiol Infect Dis* 21(3), 173
Peripheral edema (28.6%)
Pruritus
(2002): Gladstone GC, Worcester, MA (personal correspondence)
Rash (sic) (7.7%)
Toxiderma (sic)
(2002): Hafraoui S+, *Gastroenterol Clin Biol* 26(1), 17 (2 cases)

## Hair

Hair – alopecia
(2001): Zierhut M+, *Ophthalmologe* 98(7), 647

## Nails

Nails – onycholysis
(2000): Rault R, *Ann Intern Med* 133, 921

## Other

Arthralgia
(2002): Skelly MM+, *Inflamm Bowel Dis* 8(2), 93
Gingival hyperplasia
Gingivitis
Myalgia
Oral candidiasis (10.1%)
Oral ulceration
(2001): Garrigue V+, *Transplantation* 72(5), 968
Paresthesias
Thrombophlebitis (1–10%)
Thrombosis (deep vein)
(2001): Cherney DZI+, *Neph Dial Transp* 16, 1702
Tremors (11%)

## NABUMETONE

**Trade name:** Relafen (GSK)
**Other common trade names:** *Arthaxan; Consolan; Nabuser; Prodac; Relif; Relifex; Unimetone*
**Indications:** Arthritis
**Category:** Nonsteroidal anti-inflammatory (NSAID)
**Half-life:** 22.5–30 hours
**Clinically important, potentially hazardous interactions with:** methotrexate

### *Reactions*

#### Skin

Acne (<1%)
Angioedema (<1%)
(1990): Jenner PN, *Drugs* 40 (Suppl 5), 80
Bullous eruption (<1%)
Cutaneous side effects (sic)
(1991): Riccieri V+, *Clin Ter* (Italian) 137, 185
Diaphoresis (1–3%)
Edema (3–9%)
(1990): Munzel P+, *Drugs* 40 (Suppl 5), 62
Erythema
(1990): Alianti M+, *Clin Ter* (Italian) 133, 299
Erythema multiforme (<1%)
Exanthems (1.2%)
(1999): Litt JZ, Beachwood, OH (personal case) (observation)
(1988): Friedel HA+, *Drugs* 35, 504
Hot flashes (<1%)
Photosensitivity (<1%)
(1998): Litt JZ, Beachwood, OH (personal case) (observation)
(1994): Shelley WB+, *Cutis* 54, 70 (observation)
(1993): Litt JZ, Beachwood, OH (personal case) (observation)
(1989): Kaidbey KH+, *Arch Dermatol* 125, 783
(1988): Friedel HA+, *Drugs* 35, 504
Phototoxicity
(1989): Kaidbey KH+, *Arch Dermatol* 125, 783 and 824
Pruritus (3–9%)
(1999): Litt JZ, Beachwood, OH (personal case) (observation)
(1988): Friedel HA+, *Drugs* 35, 504
Rash (sic) (3–9%)
(1988): Friedel HA+, *Drugs* 35, 504
(1987): Jackson RE+, *Am J Med* 83, 115
(1987): Jenner PN+, *Am J Med* 83, 110
(1987): Mullen BJ, *Am J Med* 83, 70
Skin reactions (sic)
(1990): Fletcher AP, *Drugs* 40 (Suppl 5) 43
Stevens–Johnson syndrome (<1%)
(1997): Sienkiewicz G, Johnson City, NY (from Internet) (observation)
Toxic epidermal necrolysis (<1%)
Urticaria (<1%)
Vasculitis (necrotizing)
(1990): Willkins RF, *Drugs* 40 (Suppl 5), 34
Xerosis
(1987): Mullen BJ, *Am J Med* 83, 70

#### Hair

Hair – alopecia (<1%)
(1987): Mullen BJ, *Am J Med* 83, 70

#### Other

Anaphylactoid reactions (<1%)
Gingivitis (<1%)
Glossitis (<1%)
Myalgia
Oral ulceration
(1989): Lussier A+, *J Clin Pharmacol* 29, 225
Paresthesias (<1%)
Parkinsonism
Porphyria cutanea tarda (<1%)
Pseudolymphoma
(2001): Werth V, *Dermatology Times* 18
Pseudoporphyria
(2000): Antony F+, *Br J Dermatol* 142, 1067
(2000): Bergfeld W+, *Skin & Allergy News* December, 33
(1999): Aylesworth R, Rhinelander, WI (from Internet) (observation)
(1999): Krischer J+, *J Am Acad Dermatol* 40, 492
(1999): Magro CM+, *J Cutan Pathol* 26, 42
(1998): Varma S+, *Br J Dermatol* 138, 549
Sialorrhea
Stomatitis (1–3%)
Tinnitus
Xerostomia (1–3%)

## NADOLOL

**Trade name:** Corzide (Bristol-Myers Squibb)
**Other common trade names:** *Apo-Nadolol; Farmagard; Nadic; Solgol; Syn-Nadolol*
**Indications:** Hypertension, angina pectoris
**Category:** Beta-adrenergic blocker; antihypertensive; antianginal
**Half-life:** 10–24 hours
**Clinically important, potentially hazardous interactions with:** clonidine, epinephrine, verapamil

Corzide is nadolol and bendroflumethiazide*

**Note:** Cutaneous side effects of beta-receptor blockaders are clinically polymorphous. They apparently appear after several months of continuous therapy. Atypical psoriasiform, lichen planus-like, and eczematous chronic rashes are mainly observed. (1983): Hödl St, *Z Hautkr* (German) 58, 17

### *Reactions*

#### Skin

Bullous pemphigoid
(1984): Stage AH+, *Am J Obstet Gynecol* 150, 169
Diaphoresis (<1%)
(1980): Heel RC+, *Drugs* 20, 1 (0.6%)
Eczematous eruption (sic)
Edema (1–5%)
Erythema multiforme
Exanthems
(1980): Heel RC+, *Drugs* 20, 1 (0.4%)
Exfoliative dermatitis
Facial edema (<1%)
Hyperkeratosis (palms and soles)
Infiltrative dermatitis of the scalp (sic)
(1985): Shelley ED+, *Cutis* 35, 148
Lichenoid eruption
(1978): Savage RL+, *BMJ* 1, 987
Lupus erythematosus
Pityriasis rubra pilaris
(1978): Finlay AY+, *BMJ* 1, 987
Pruritus (1–5%)
Psoriasis
(1988): Gold MH+, *J Am Acad Dermatol* 19, 837 (aggravation of)
(1988): Heng MCY+, *Int J Dermatol* 27, 619

(1986): Czernielewski J+, *Lancet* 1, 808
(1984): Arntzen N+, *Acta Derm Venereol* (Stockh) 64, 346
Pustular eruption
(1991): Bernard P+, *Dermatologica* 182, 115
Rash (sic) (1–5%)
Raynaud's phenomenon (2%)
(1984): Eliasson K+, *Acta Med Scand* 215, 333
(1976): Marshall AJ+, *BMJ* 1, 1498
Toxic epidermal necrolysis
Urticaria
Xerosis

### Hair

Hair – alopecia
(1985): Shelley ED+, *Cutis* 35, 148

### Nails

Nails – bluish
Nails – dystrophy
Nails – onycholysis

### Other

Dysgeusia
Numbness (fingers and toes) (>5%)
Oculo-mucocutaneous syndrome
(1982): Cocco G+, *Curr Ther Res* 31, 362
Oral lichenoid eruption
Oral mucosal eruption
(1980): Heel RC+, *Drugs* 20, 1 (0.6%)
Paresthesias (>5%)
Peyronie's disease
(1979): Pryor JP+, *Lancet* 1, 331
Tinnitus
Xerostomia (<1%)
(1980): Heel RC+, *Drugs* 20, 1

***Note:** Bendroflumethiazide is a sulfonamide and can be absorbed systemically. Sulfonamides can produce severe, possibly fatal, reactions such as toxic epidermal necrolysis and Stevens–Johnson syndrome

## NAFARELIN

**Trade name:** Synarel (Searle)
**Other common trade name:** *Synarela*
**Indications:** Endometriosis
**Category:** Posterior pituitary hormone; gonadotropin inhibitor
**Half-life:** ~3 hours

#### *Reactions*

### Skin

Acne (>10%)
Chloasma (<1%)
Edema (1–10%)
Exanthems (<1%)
Flushing
(1990): Chrisp P+, *Drugs* 39, 523 (90%)
(1988): Henzl MR+, *N Engl J Med* 318, 485 (90%)
Hot flashes (>10%)
Pruritus (1–10%)
Rash (sic) (1–10%)
Seborrhea (1–10%)
Urticaria (1–10%)

### Hair

Hair – hirsutism (1–10%)

### Other

Gynecomastia (<1%)
Hypersensitivity (0.2%)
Mastodynia
Myalgia (>10%)
Paresthesias (<1%)
Vaginitis

## NAFCILLIN

**Trade name:** Nafcil (Apothecon)
**Other common trade name:** *Vigopen*
**Indications:** Various infections caused by susceptible organisms
**Category:** Penicillinase-resistant penicillin antibiotic
**Half-life:** 0.5–1.5 hours
**Clinically important, potentially hazardous interactions with:** anticoagulants, cyclosporine, demeclocycline, doxycycline, methotrexate, minocycline, oxytetracycline, tetracycline

#### *Reactions*

### Skin

Allergic reactions (sic)
(1994): Pleasants RA+, *Chest* 106, 1124 (in patients with cystic fibrosis)
Angioedema
Bullous eruption
Ecchymoses
Erythema multiforme
Exanthems
(1978): Kancir LM+, *Arch Intern Med* 138, 909 (10%)
Exfoliative dermatitis
Hematomas
Jarisch–Herxheimer reaction
Pruritus
Rash (sic) (<1%)
(2002): Maraqa NF+, *Clin Infect Dis* 34(1), 50 (32%)
Stevens–Johnson syndrome
Toxic epidermal necrolysis
Urticaria
Vasculitis

### Other

Anaphylactoid reactions
Black tongue
Dysgeusia
Glossitis
Glossodynia
Hypersensitivity (<1%)
Injection-site necrosis
(1987): Dufresne RG, *Cutis* 39, 197
(1980): Tilden SJ+, *Am J Dis Child* 134, 1046
Injection-site pain
Oral candidiasis
Serum sickness
Stomatitis
Stomatodynia
Thrombophlebitis (<1%)
Vaginitis
Xerostomia

# NALIDIXIC ACID

**Trade name:** NegGram (Sanofi)
**Other common trade names:** *Betaxina; Granexin; Mytacin; Nalidixin; Negram; Nogram; Youdix*
**Indications:** Various urinary tract infections caused by susceptible organisms
**Category:** Urinary tract anti-infective; quinolone antibiotic
**Half-life:** 6–7 hours
**Clinically important, potentially hazardous interactions with:** warfarin

### *Reactions*

#### Skin

Angioedema (<1%)
Bullous eruption (<1%)
(1981): Wolf A, *Z Hautkr* (German) 56, 109
(1970): Brehm G+, *Med Welt* (German) 11, 423
(1969): Birkett DA, *Br J Dermatol* 81, 342
(1969): Puissant A+, *Bull Soc Fr Dermatol Syphiligr* (French) 76, 84
(1968): Baes H, *Dermatologica* 136, 61
(1966): Burry JN+, *Med J Aust* 2, 243
Erythema multiforme (<1%)
(1971): Alexander S+, *Br J Dermatol* 84, 429
Exanthems (>5%)
(1971): Alexander S+, *Br J Dermatol* 84, 429
(1969): Atlas E+, *Ann Intern Med* 70, 713 (7%)
(1963): Barlow AM, *BMJ* 2, 1308 (3.5%)
(1963): Lishman IV+, *Br J Urol* 35, 116
(1962): Buchbinder M+, *Antimicrob Agents Chemother* 2, 308
Exfoliative dermatitis
(1971): Alexander S+, *Br J Dermatol* 84, 429
Lupus erythematosus
(1979): Rubinstein A, *N Engl J Med* 301, 1288
(1971): Alexander S+, *Br J Dermatol* 84, 429
Photoreactions
(1972): Jung EG, *Z Haut Geschlechtskr* (German) 47, 329
Photosensitivity (<1%)
(1997): O'Reilly FM+, American Academy of Dermatology Meeting, Poster #14
(1993): Wainwright NJ+, *Drug Saf* 9, 437
(1990): Bilsland D+, *Br J Dermatol* 123, 548
(1986): Ljunggren B+, *Photodermatol* 3, 26
(1985): Epstein JH+, *Drugs* 30, 42
(1982): Rosen K+, *Acta Derm Venereol* (Stockh) 62, 246
(1981): Boisvert A+, *Drug Intell Clin Pharm* 15, 126
(1981): Closas J+, *Rev Clin Esp* (Spanish) 162, 219
(1980): Stern RS+, *Arch Dermatol* 116, 1269
(1978): Fiocchi A+, *Minerva Pediatr* (Italian) 30, 585
(1974): Ramsay CA+, *Br J Dermatol* 91, 523
(1973): Ramsay CA, *Proc R Soc Med* 66, 747
(1971): Alexander S+, *Br J Dermatol* 84, 429
(1970): Luscombe HA, *Arch Dermatol* 101, 122
(1970): Neering KEHP, *Dermatologica* 141, 361
(1970): No Author, *Tidsskr Nor Laegeforen* (Norwegian) 90, 2100
(1970): Thivolet J+, *Bull Soc Fr Dermatol Syphiligr* (French) 77, 286
(1969): Garrett MH, *Med J Aust* 1, 83
(1968): Baes H, *Dermatologica* 136, 61
(1967): Haven E+, *Arch Belg Dermatol Syphiligr* (French) 23, 421
(1966): Mathew FH, *Med J Aust* 53, 243
(1965): Cahal DA, *BMJ* 1, 130
(1965): Elmes PC, *Prescrib J* 5, 12
(1965): Susskind W+, *BMJ* 1, 316
Phototoxic bullous eruption
(1978): Brauer GJ, *Am J Med* 58, 576
(1977): Hertzenberg S, *Tidsskr Nor Laegeforen* (Norwegian) 97, 792
(1976): Frodin T+, *Lakartidningen* (Swedish) 73, 3763
(1976): Klaasen CH+, *Ned Tijdschr Geneeskd* (Dutch) 120, 247
(1976): van Dijk E, *Ned Tijdschr Geneeskd* (Dutch) 120, 592
(1975): Brauner GJ, *Am J Med* 58, 576
(1974): Burry JN, *Arch Dermatol* 109, 263
(1974): Ramsay CA+, *Br J Dermatol* 91, 523
(1973): Louis P+, *Hautarzt* (German) 24, 445
(1969): Birkett DA, *Br J Dermatol* 81, 342
(1968): Baes H, *Dermatologica* 136, 61
(1966): Burry JN+, *Med J Aust* 2, 243
(1964): Zelickson AS, *JAMA* 190, 556
Pruritus (<1%)
(1971): Alexander S+, *Br J Dermatol* 84, 429
(1969): Atlas E+, *Ann Intern Med* 70, 713
Purpura
(1971): Alexander S+, *Br J Dermatol* 84, 429
Rash (sic) (<1%)
Toxic epidermal necrolysis
(1971): Alexander S+, *Br J Dermatol* 84, 429
Urticaria (<1%)
(1985): Goolamali SK, *Postgrad Med J* 61, 925
(1971): Alexander S+, *Br J Dermatol* 84, 429
(1966): Beaty HN+, *Ann Intern Med* 65, 641

#### Hair

Hair – alopecia
(1971): Alexander S+, *Br J Dermatol* 84, 429

#### Other

Acute intermittent porphyria
Anaphylactoid reactions
Arthralgia
(1972): Bailey RR+, *Can Med Assoc* 107, 604 (passim)
Paresthesias
Porphyria cutanea tarda
(1992): Shelley WB+, *Advanced Dermatologic Diagnosis* WB Saunders, 414 (passim)
(1983): Goldsman CI+, *Cleve Clin Q* 50, 151
Pseudoporphyria
(1990): Bilsland D+, *Br J Dermatol* 123, 547
(1984): Harber LC+, *J Invest Dermatol* 82, 207
Pseudotumor cerebri
(1998): Ryiaz A+, *J Indian Med Assoc* 96, 308

# NALOXONE

**Trade name:** Narcan (Endo)
**Other common trade names:** *Nalpin; Narcanti; Narcotan; Zynox*
**Indications:** Narcotic overdose
**Category:** Opioid (narcotic) antagonist
**Half-life:** 1–1.5 hours

### *Reactions*

#### Skin

Angioedema
(1982): Smitz S+, *Ann Intern Med* 97, 788
Diaphoresis (1–10%)
Exanthems
Pruritus
(1982): Smitz S+, *Ann Intern Med* 97, 788
Rash (sic) (1–10%)
Urticaria
(1982): Smitz S+, *Ann Intern Med* 97, 788

# NALTREXONE

**Trade names:** Revex (Baker Norton); ReVia (DuPont); Trexan
**Other common trade names:** *Antaxone; Celupan; Nalorex; Nemexin*
**Indications:** Substance abuse, opioid dependence, alcohol dependence
**Category:** Opioid antagonist
**Half-life:** 4 hours

### *Reactions*

## Skin

Acne (<1%)
Chills (<10%)
Diaphoresis
Edema (<1%)
Exanthems
(1988): Ganzalez JP+, *Drugs* 35, 192
Eyelid edema (<1%)
Herpes simplex (<1%)
Herpes zoster (<1%)
Hot flashes
Pruritus (<1%)
(1997): Sullivan JR+, *Australas J Dermatol* 38(4), 196
(1990): Abboud TK+, *Anesthesiol* 72, 233
Purpura
Rash (sic) (<10%)
(1988): Gonzalez JP+, *Drugs* 35, 192
Seborrhea (<1%)
Tinea pedis (<1%)

## Hair

Hair – alopecia (<1%)

## Other

Arthralgia (>10%)
(1997): Ciraulo AM+, *Drugs & Ther Perspect* 10, 5
Death (in ultrarapid detoxification)
Depression (<1%)
(1996): Berg BJ+, *Drug Saf* 15(4), 274
(1988): Gonzalez JP+, *Drugs* 35, 192
Myalgia
Phlebitis (<1%)
Rhabdomyolysis
(1999): Zaim S+, *Ann Pharmacother* 33(3), 312
Tinnitus
Tremors
Twitching
Xerostomia (<1%)

# NAPROXEN

**Trade name:** Naprosyn (Roche)
**Other common trade names:** *Aleve; Anaprox; Apranax; Dymenalgit; Flanax; Laraflex; Naprelan; Naprogesic; Napron X; Naprosyne; Naxen; Novo-Naprox; Nu-Naprox; Supradol; Synflex; Velsay*
**Indications:** Pain, arthritis
**Category:** Nonsteroidal anti-inflammatory (NSAID)
**Half-life:** 13 hours
**Clinically important, potentially hazardous interactions with:** methotrexate

### *Reactions*

## Skin

Angioedema (<1%)
(2000): Ghislain PD+, *Ann Med Interne (Paris)* 151, 227 (nuchal scalp)
(1984): Stern RS+, *JAMA* 252, 1433
Bullous eruption
(1996): Gonzalo-Garijo MA+, *Allergol Immunopathol Madr* (Spanish) 24, 89
(1990): Suarez SM+, *Arthritis Rheum* 33, 903
(1989): Rivers JK+, *Med J Aust* 151, 167
(1984): Stern RS+, *JAMA* 252, 1433
Cutaneous side effects (sic)
(1990): Todd PA+, *Drugs* 40, 91 (up to 9%)
(1985): Bigby M+, *J Am Acad Dermatol* 12, 866 (up to 5%)
(1974): Cuthbert MF, *Curr Med Res Opin* 2, 600 (5%)
Diaphoresis (<3%)
(1990): Todd PA+, *Drugs* 40, 91 (<3%)
(1985): Bigby M+, *J Am Acad Dermatol* 12, 866
(1982): Bailin PL+, *Clin Rheum Dis* 8, 493 (passim)
Ecchymoses (3–9%)
Edema (3–9%)
(1978): Castles JJ+, *Arch Intern Med* 138, 362 (1–5%)
Erythema multiforme (<1%)
(1985): Bigby M+, *J Am Acad Dermatol* 12, 866
(1984): Stern RS+, *JAMA* 252, 1433
Erythema nodosum
(1990): Todd PA+, *Drugs* 40, 91
Exanthems (>5%)
(1994): Shelley WB+, *Cutis* 55, 21 (observation)
(1990): Todd PA+, *Drugs* 40, 91
(1985): Bigby M+, *J Am Acad Dermatol* 12, 866 (1–5%)
(1984): Stern RS+, *JAMA* 252, 1433
(1979): Brogden RN+, *Drugs* 18, 241
(1978): Castles JJ+, *Arch Intern Med* 138, 362 (5.3%)
(1976): Dyer HR, *Ann Intern Med* 84, 221
(1975): Bowers DE+, *Ann Intern Med* 83, 470 (14%)
(1975): Brigden RN+, *Drugs* 9, 326
Exfoliative dermatitis
Facial scarring
(2001): Wallace CA+, *J Am Acad Dermatol* 45, 746 (in children)
Fixed eruption
(2002): Li H+, *Int J Dermatol* 41(2), 96
(2001): Gonzalo MA+, *Br J Dermatol* 144(6), 1291
(2000): Ozkaya-Bayazit E+, *Eur J Dermatol* 10, 288
(1998): Leal G, Fortaleza, Brazil (from internet) (observation)
(1996): Enta T, *Can Fam Physician* 42, 1099
(1996): Gonzalo-Garijo MA+, *Allergol Immunopathol Madr* (Spanish) 24, 89
(1991): Shelley WB+, *Cutis* 48, 368 (observation)
(1990): Black AK+, *Br J Dermatol* 123, 277 (observation)
(1990): Todd PA+, *Drugs* 40, 91
(1987): Habbema L+, *Dermatologica* 174, 184

(1985): Bigby M+, *J Am Acad Dermatol* 12, 866
(1984): Stern RS+, *JAMA* 252, 1433

Hot flashes (<1%)

Leg edema
(2002): Bandyopadhyay P+, *Int J Clin Pract* 56(2), 145

Lichen planus
(2002): Reed BR, Denver, CO (from Internet) (observation)
(1999): *Acta Derm Venereol* (Stockh) 79, 329 (bullous)
(1984): Heymann WR+, *J Am Acad Dermatol* 10, 299

Lichenoid eruption
(1996): Shelley WB+, *Cutis* 60, 20
(1990): Todd PA+, *Drugs* 40, 91
(1985): Bigby M+, *J Am Acad Dermatol* 12, 866

Linear IgA bullous dermatosis
(2000): Bouldin MB+, *Mayo Clin Proc* 75(9), 967

Lupus erythematosus
(1992): Parodi A+, *JAMA* 268, 51

Peripheral edema

Photodermatitis (bullous)
(1989): Rivers JK+, *Med J Aust* 151, 167

Photosensitivity (<1%)
(1999): Litt JZ, Beachwood, OH (personal case) (observation)
(1994): Berger TG+, *Arch Dermatol* 130, 609 (in HIV-infected)
(1991): Allen R+, *J Rheumatol* 18, 893
(1991): Lutzow-Holm C, *Tidsskr Nor Laegeforen* (Norwegian) 111, 2739
(1990): Suarez SM+, *Arthritis Rheum* 33, 903
(1990): Todd PA+, *Drugs* 40, 91
(1989): Kaidbey KH+, *Arch Dermatol* 125, 783
(1987): Sterling JC+, *Br J Rheumatol* 26, 210
(1986): Judd LE+, *Arch Dermatol* 122, 451
(1986): Mayou S+, *Br J Dermatol* 114, 519
(1986): Shelley WB+, *Cutis* 38, 169
(1986): Szczeklik A, *Drugs* 32 (Suppl 4), 148
(1985): Farr PM+, *Lancet* 1, 1166
(1983): Diffey BL+, *Br J Rheumatol* 22, 239

Phototoxicity
(1989): Kaidbey KH+, *Arch Dermatol* 125, 783

Pityriasis rosea
(1993): Yosipovitch G+, *Harefuah* (Hebrew) 124, 198; 247

Pruritus (3–9%)
(1990): Todd PA+, *Drugs* 40, 91 (1–5%)
(1985): Bigby M+, *J Am Acad Dermatol* 12, 866 (14%)
(1982): Bailin PL+, *Clin Rheum Dis* 8, 493 (passim)
(1978): Castles JJ+, *Arch Intern Med* 138, 362
(1975): Bowers DE+, *Ann Intern Med* 83, 470 (17%)

Pseudo-reactions (sic)
(1991): VanArsdel PP, *JAMA* 266, 3343

Purpura (<3%)
(1985): Bigby M+, *J Am Acad Dermatol* 12, 866
(1982): Bailin PL+, *Clin Rheum Dis* 8, 493 (passim)
(1979): Brogden RN+, *Drugs* 18, 241
(1975): Brogden RN+, *Drugs* 9, 326

Pustular eruption
(1989): Grattan CEH, *Dermatologica* 179, 57
(1986): Page SR+, *BMJ* 293, 510

Pyogenic granuloma
(1994): Shelley WB+, *Cutis* 53, 36 (observation)

Rash (sic) (3–9%)
(2002): Bandyopadhyay P+, *Int J Clin Pract* 56(2), 145
(1995): Knulst AC+, *Br J Dermatol* 133, 647

Stevens–Johnson syndrome (<1%)

Toxic epidermal necrolysis (<1%)
(1993): Correia O+, *Dermatology* 186, 32

Urticaria
(1985): Bigby M+, *J Am Acad Dermatol* 12, 866 (1–5%)
(1984): Stern RS+, *JAMA* 252, 1433
(1979): Brogden RN+, *Drugs* 18, 241
(1975): Brogden RN+, *Drugs* 9, 326

Vasculitis
(1996): Lossos IS+, *Harefuah* (Hebrew) 130, 600
(1992): Jahangiri M+, *Postgrad Med J* 68, 766
(1992): Veraguth AJ+, *Schweiz Med Wochenschr* (German) 122, 923
(1990): Todd PA+, *Drugs* 40, 91 (1–5%) (necrotizing venulitis)
(1989): Singhal PC+, *Ann Allergy* 63, 107
(1985): Bigby M+, *J Am Acad Dermatol* 12, 866
(1980): Mordes JP, *Arch Intern Med* 140, 985
(1979): Brogden RN+, *Drugs* 18, 241
(1979): Grennan DM+, *N Z Med J* 89, 48

Vesiculobullous eruption
(1984): Stern RS+, *JAMA* 252, 1433

## Hair

Hair – alopecia (<1%)
(1990): Todd PA+, *Drugs* 40, 91 (<1%)
(1989): Barter AC, *BMJ* 298, 325
(1989): Barth JH, *BMJ* 298, 675

## Other

Anaphylactoid reactions (<1%)

Aphthous stomatitis
(2001): Vincent L+, *Ann Dermatol Venereol* (French) 128(1), 57

Hypersensitivity
(2001): McMahon AD+, *J Clin Epidemiol* 54(12), 1271

Myalgia (<1%)

Oral ulceration
(2000): Madinier I+, *Ann Med Interne (Paris)* (French) 151, 248

Porphyria cutanea tarda
(1992): Shelley WB+, *Advanced Dermatologic Diagnosis* WB Saunders, 414 (passim)

Pseudolymphoma
(2001): Werth V, *Dermatology Times* 18

Pseudoporphyria
(2002): Haber H, Cleveland, OH (Cleveland Dermatological Society)
(2002): Schad SG+, *Hautarzt* 53(1), 51
(2001): Maerker JM+, *Hautarzt* 52(11), 1026
(2000): De Silva B+, *Pediatr Dermatol* 17, 480
(1999): Al-Khenaizan S+, *J Cutan Med Surg* 3, 162
(1995): Creemers MC+, *Scand J Rheumatol* 24, 185
(1995): Girschick HJ+, *Scand J Rheumatol* 24, 108
(1994): Lang BA+, *J Pediatr* 124, 639
(1992): Cox NH+, *Br J Dermatol* 126, 86
(1992): Petersen CS+, *Ugeskr Laeger* (Danish) 154, 1713
(1991): Allen R+, *J Rheumatol* 18, 893
(1990): Levy ML+, *J Pediatr* 117, 660
(1990): Sternberg A, *Acta Derm Venereol* 70, 354
(1990): Suarez SM+, *Arthritis Rheum* 33, 903
(1990): Todd PA+, *Drugs* 40, 91
(1989): Kaidbey KH+, *Arch Dermatol* 125, 783
(1988): Diffey BL+, *Clin Exp Dermatol* 13, 207
(1987): Burns DA, *Clin Exp Dermatol* 12, 296
(1987): Nicholls D, *N Z Med J* 100, 427
(1987): Shelley ED+, *Cutis* 40, 314
(1987): Sterling JC+, *Br J Rheumatol* 26, 210
(1987): Taylor BJ+, *N Z Med J* 100, 322
(1986): Judd LE+, *Arch Dermatol* 122, 451
(1986): Mayou S+, *Br J Dermatol* 114, 519
(1985): Farr PM+, *Lancet* 1, 1166
(1985): Howard AM+, *Lancet* 1, 819

Salivary gland enlargement
(1995): Knulst AC+, *Br J Dermatol* 133, 647

Stomatitis (<3%)

Tinnitus

Xerostomia

# NARATRIPTAN

**Trade name:** Amerge (GSK)
**Indications:** Acute migraine attacks
**Category:** Antimigraine; serotonin agonist
**Half-life:** 6 hours
**Clinically important, potentially hazardous interactions with:** dihydroergotamine, ergotamine, methysergide, rizatriptan, sibutramine, sumatriptan, zolmitriptan

### *Reactions*

## Skin

Acne (<1%)
Allergic reactions (sic) (<1%)
Atypical sensations (sic) (<1)%
Dermatitis (sic) (<1%)
Diaphoresis (<1%)
Edema (<1%)
Erythema (<1%)
Exanthems (<1%)
Folliculitis (<1%)
Photosensitivity (<1%)
Purpura (<1%)
Rash (sic) (<1%)
Urticaria (<1%)
Xerosis (<1%)

## Hair

Hair – alopecia (<1%)

## Other

Dysgeusia (<1%)
Hyperesthesia (<1%)
Hypesthesia (<1%)
Paresthesias (2%)
Photophobia (<1%)
Sialopenia (<1%)

# NATEGLINIDE

**Trade name:** Starlix (Novartis)
**Indications:** Type 2 diabetes
**Category:** Short-acting insulin secretagogue antidiabetic (phenylalanine derivative)
**Half-life:** 1.5 hours

### *Reactions*

## Skin

Exanthems
(2002): Danby FW, Manchester, NH (from Internet) (observation)
Flu-like syndrome (4%)
Rash (sic)

# NEBIVOLOL

**Trade name:** Nebilet (Menarini)
**Indications:** Hypertension
**Category:** Beta adrenergic blocking agent
**Half-life:** 8 hours

### *Reactions*

## Skin

None

## Other

Myalgia
Paresthesias
(1999): McNeely W+, *Drugs* 57, 633

# NEFAZODONE

**Trade name:** Serzone (Bristol-Myers Squibb)
**Indications:** Depression
**Category:** Phenylpiperazine antidepressant
**Half-life:** 2–4 hours
**Clinically important, potentially hazardous interactions with:** buspirone, isocarboxazid, MAO inhibitors, phenelzine, pimozide, selegiline, sibutramine, sumatriptan, tramadol, tranylcypromine, trazodone

### *Reactions*

## Skin

Acne (<1%)
Allergic reactions (sic) (<1%)
Burning (sic)
(2000): Lerner V+, *J Clin Psychiatry* 61, 216
Cellulitis (<1%)
Ecchymoses (<1%)
Eczema (sic) (<1%)
Exanthems (<1%)
Facial edema (<1%)
Flu-like syndrome (sic) (1–10%)
Flushing (4%)
Infections (sic) (8%)
Peripheral edema (3%)
Photosensitivity (<1%)
Pruritus (2%)
Rash (sic) (2%)
Urticaria (<1%)
Vesiculobullous eruption (<1%)
Xerosis (<1%)

## Hair

Hair – alopecia (<1%)
(1998): Rademaker M, Hamilton, New Zealand (from Internet) (observation)
(1997): Gupta S+, *J Fam Pract* 44, 20

## Other

Ageusia (<1%)
Dysgeusia (2%)
Foetor ex ore (halitosis) (<1%)
Gingivitis (<1%)
Glossitis (<1%)
Gynecomastia (<1%)

Hyperesthesia (<1%)
Mastodynia (1%)
Myalgia
Oral candidiasis (<1%)
Oral ulceration (<1%)
Paresthesias (4%)
(1999): Litt JZ, Beachwood, OH (personal case) (observation)
Priapism (<1%)
(1999): Brodie-Meijer CC+, *Int Clin Psychopharmacol* 14, 257 (clitoral)
Sialorrhea (<1%)
Stomatitis (<1%)
Vaginitis (2%)
Xerostomia (25%)

## NELFINAVIR

**Trade name:** Viracept (Agouron)
**Indications:** HIV infection
**Category:** Antiretroviral; protease inhibitor*
**Half-life:** 3.5–5 hours
**Clinically important, potentially hazardous interactions with:** benzodiazepines, chlordiazepoxide, clonazepam, clorazepate, diazepam, dihydroergotamine, ergot alkaloids, fentanyl, flurazepam, lorazepam, methysergide, midazolam, oral contraceptives, oxazepam, phenytoin, pimozide, quazepam, rifampin, sildenafil, **St John's wort**, temazepam

### *Reactions*

#### Skin
Allergic reactions (sic) (<1%)
Dermatitis (sic) (<1%)
Diaphoresis (<1%)
Exanthems
(1998): Bourezane Y+, *Clin Infect Dis* 27(5), 1321 (with indinavir)
Hyperhidrosis
(2000): Bonfanti P+, *J Acquir Immune Defic Syndr* 23(3), 236
Lichenoid reaction
(1998): Bourezane Y+, *Clin Infect Dis* 27(5), 1321
Palmar erythema
(1998): Bourezane Y+, *Clin Infect Dis* 27(5), 1321 (with indinavir)
Pruritus (<1%)
Rash (sic) (1–10%)
(2001): Abraham PE+, *Ann Pharmacother* 35(5), 553
(2000): Fortuny C+, *AIDS* 14, 335
Urticaria (<1%)
(1998): Demoly P+, *J Allergy Clin Immunol* 102(5), 875
Vasculitis
(1998): Bourezane Y+, *Clin Infect Dis* 27(5), 1321

#### Other
DRESS syndrome
(1998): Bourezane Y+, *Clin Infect Dis* 27, 1321
Gynecomastia
(2001): Manfredi R+, *Ann Pharmacother* 35(4), 438
Hypersensitivity
(1999): Demoly P+, *J Allergy Clin Immunol* 104 (2 Pt 1), 504
Myalgia (<1%)
Oral ulceration (<1%)
Paresthesias (<1%)
Perioral parasthesias
(2001): McMahon D+, *Antivir Ther* 6(2), 105

***Note:** Protease inhibitors cause dyslipidemia which includes elevated triglycerides and cholesterol and redistribution of body fat centrally to produce the so-called "protease paunch," breast enlargement, facial atrophy, and "buffalo hump"

## NEOMYCIN

**Trade name:** Neosporin (Warner-Lambert)
**Other common trade names:** *Gemicina; Myciguent; Neomicina; Neomycine Diamant; Neosulf; Nivemycin*
**Indications:** Various infections caused by susceptible organisms
**Category:** Aminoglycoside antibiotic
**Half-life:** 3 hours
**Clinically important, potentially hazardous interactions with:** aldesleukin, aminoglycosides, atracurium, bumetanide, doxacurium, ethacrynic acid, furosemide, methoxyflurane, pancuronium, polypeptide antibiotics, rocuronium, succinylcholine, torsemide, vecuronium

### *Reactions*

#### Skin
Allergic reactions (sic)
Angioedema
(1959): Pirilä V+, *Acta Derm Venereol* (Stockh) 39, 1470
Bullous eruption
Contact dermatitis
(2000): Hillen U+, *Hautarzt* 51, 239
(1999): Giordano-Labadie F+, *Contact Dermatitis* 40, 192 (2.6%) (in atopics)
(1999): Lestringant GG+, *Int J Dermatol* 38, 181 (5.1%)
(1998): Katsarou-Katsari A+, *J Eur Acad Dermatol Venereol* 11, 9
(1998): Kimura M+, *Contact Dermatitis* 39, 148
(1997): Dasaraju P+, *Clin Infect Dis* 25, 33
(1996): Sheretz EF, *Arch Dermatol* 132, 461
(1994): Fisher AA, *Cutis* 54, 300
(1993): Lipozencic J+, *Arh Hig Rada Toksikol* (Serbo-Croatian-Roman) 44, 173
(1991): Barros MA+, *Contact Dermatitis* 25, 156
(1991): Mariani R+, *Contact Dermatitis* 24, 227
(1990): Grandinetti PJ+, *J Am Acad Dermatol* 23, 646
(1990): Smith IM+, *Clin Otolaryngol* 15, 155
(1989): Guin JD+, *Cutis* 43, 564
(1989): Massone L+, *Contact Dermatitis* 21, 344
(1988): Shupp DL+, *Cutis* 42, 528
(1987): Abdul-Gaffoor PM, *Indian J Dermatol* 32, 102
(1986): Bajaj AK+, *Int J Dermatol* 25, 103
(1986): Baldinger J+, *Ann Ophthalmol* 18, 95
(1986): Rebandel P+, *Contact Dermatitis* 15, 92
(1985): Fisher AA, *Cutis* 35, 315
(1985): Fraki JE+, *Acta Otolaryngol Stockh* 100, 414
(1985): Frenzel U+, *Phlebologie* (French) 38, 389
(1985): Szarmach H+, *Przegl Dermatol* (Polish) 72, 521 (disseminated)
(1984): Menne T+, *Hautarzt* (German) 35, 319
(1983): Macdonald RH+, *Clin Exp Dermatol* 8, 249
(1982): Fisher AA, *Ann Allergy* 49, 97
(1981): Fisher AA+, *Cutis* 28, 491
(1981): Gordon W, *S Afr Med J* 59, 212
(1981): LeRoy R+, *Derm Beruf Umwelt* (German) 29, 168
(1980): Epstein E, *Contact Dermatitis* 6, 219
(1979): Leyden JJ+, *JAMA* 242, 1276
(1979): Prystowsky SD+, *Arch Dermatol* 115, 713
(1979): Prystowsky SD+, *Arch Dermatol* 115, 959
(1978): Durocher LP, *Can Med Assoc J* (French) 118, 162

(1978): Forstrom L+, *Contact Dermatitis* 4, 312
(1977): Shouji A, *Nippon Rinsho* (Japanese) 35, 210
(1977): Sinka L+, *Bratisl Lek Listy* (Slovak) 67, 59
(1976): Carruthers JA+, *Contact Dermatitis* 2, 269
(1976): Fisher AA+, *Cutis* 18, 637
(1974): Bandmann HJ+, *Internist Berl* (German) 15, 47
(1974): Malten KE+, *Phlebologie* (French) 27, 417
(1974): Peterkin GA, *J Laryngol Otol* 88, 15
(1973): Ebner H, *Wien Klin Wochenschr* (German) 85, 203
(1973): *BMJ* 1, 250
(1973): Naess K, *Tidsskr Nor Laegeforen* (Norwegian) 93, 2498
(1972): Hadida ME+, *J Med Lyon* (French) 53, 1093
(1972): Hattori S, *Nippon Ika Daigaku Zasshi* (Japanese) 39, 23
(1971): Bielicky T+, *Z Haut Geschlechtskr* (German) 46, 771
(1971): Epstein, E, *Arch Dermatol* 103, 562
(1971): Foussereau J+, *Bull Soc Fr Dermatol Syphiligr* (French) 78, 457
(1970): Bandmann HJ, *Munch Med Wochenschr* (German) 112, 1125
(1970): Bowczyc J+, *Przegl Dermatol* (Polish) 57, 763
(1970): Chilvers AS+, *Lancet* 1, 402
(1969): Matner T, *Hautarzt* (German) 20, 446
(1969): Novak M+, *Cesk Dermatol* (Czech) 44, 177
(1968): Bartova J, *Cesk Dermatol* (Czech) 43, 271
(1968): Hiemisch I+, *Z Haut Geschlechtskr* (German) 43, 49
(1968): Hjorth N+, *Br J Dermatol* 80, 163
(1967): *Med Lett Drugs Ther* 9, 71
(1967): Pirila V+, *Acta Derm Venereol* (Stockh) 47, 419
(1967): Schwank R, *Cesk Dermatol* 42, 341
(1966): Jensen OC+, *JAMA* 195, 131
(1966): Pirila V+, *Acta Derm Venereol* (Stockh) 46, 489
(1965): Kirton V+, *Lancet* 1, 138

Dermatitis (sic) (1–10%)
(1990): Bouffioux B+, *Nouv Dermatol* (French) 9, 25
(1959): Pirilä V+, *Acta Derm Venereol* (Stockh) 39, 1470

Eczematous eruption (sic)
(1969): Ekelund A+, *Acta Derm Venereol* (Stockh) 49, 422

Erythema multiforme
(1986): Fisher AA, *Cutis* 37, 158

Exanthems
(1990): Bouffioux B+, *Nouv Dermatol* (French) 9, 25

Fixed eruption
(1985): Gomez B+, *Allergol Immunopathol Madr* (Spanish) 13, 87

Pruritus

Rash (sic) (1–10%)

Toxic epidermal necrolysis
(1969): Muresan D+, *Viata Med* (Romanian) 16, 731
(1959): Catto JVF, *BMJ* 2, 544

Ulceration

Urticaria (1–10%)
(1959): Pirilä V+, *Acta Derm Venereol* (Stockh) 39, 1470

### Hair

Hair – alopecia

### Other

Anaphylactoid reactions
(1986): Goh CL, *Australian J Dermatol* 27, 125

Hypersensitivity
(2001): Le Coz CJ, *Ann Dermatol Venereol* 128(12), 1359

# NESIRITIDE

**Trade name:** Natrecor (Scios/Bayer)
**Indications:** Acutely decompensated congestive heart failure
**Category:** Human B-type natriuretic peptide; vasodilator
**Half-life:** 18 minutes

## *Reactions*

### Skin

Diaphoresis (>1%)
Pruritus (>1%)
Rash (sic) (>1%)

### Other

Back pain
Cough (>1%)
Leg cramps (>1%)
Paresthesias (>1%)
Phlebitis
Tremors (>1%)

# NEVIRAPINE

**Trade name:** Viramune (Roxane)
**Indications:** HIV infections
**Category:** Antiretroviral non-nucleoside reverse transcriptase inhibitor (NNRTI)
**Half-life:** 45 hours
**Clinically important, potentially hazardous interactions with:** ketoconazole, midazolam

## *Reactions*

### Skin

Exanthems
(2000): Barreiro P+, *AIDS* 14(14), 2153
(2000): Palacios Munoz R+, *Rev Clin Esp* (Spanish) 200(11), 635

Pruritus

Rash (sic) (<48%)
(2001): Barreiro P+, *Lancet* 356(9239), 392
(2001): Bersoff-Matcha SJ+, *Clin Infect Dis* 32(1), 124
(2001): Colebundrs R+, *Lancet* 357, 392
(2001): Wong KH+, *Clin Infect Dis* 33(12), 2096
(2000): Bardsley-Elliot A+, *Paediatr Drugs* 2(5), 373
(1999): Anton P+, *AIDS* 13, 524
(1998): Barner A+, *Lancet* 351, 1133
(1998): Bourezane Y+, *Clin Infect Dis* 27, 1321
(1998): Ho TT+, *AIDS* 12, 2082
(1996): Luzuriaga K+, *J Infect Dis* 174, 713
(1995): Havlir D+, *J Infect Dis* 171, 537 (48%)

Skin reactions (sic)
(2001): *MMWR* 49, 1153

Stevens–Johnson syndrome (<1%)
(2002): Dodi F+, *AIDS* 16(8), 1197 (2 cases)
(2001): Fagot JP+, *AIDS* 15(14), 1843
(2001): *MMWR* 49, 1153
(2001): Metry DW+, *J Am Acad Dermatol* 44, 354
(2001): Roujeau J-C+, *AIDS* 15, 1843
(2000): Bardsley-Elliot A+, *Paediatr Drugs* 2(5), 373
(2000): Garcia Fernandez D+, *Rev Clin Esp* (Spanish) 200, 179
(1999): Wetterwald E+, *Br J Dermatol* 140, 980 (SJS/TEN overlap syndrome)
(1998): McClain SA, SUNY Stony Brook, NY (from Internet) (observation)

(1998): Warren KJ+, *Lancet* 351–567
Toxic epidermal necrolysis
(2001): Fagot JP+, *AIDS* 15(14), 1843
(2001): Roujeau J-C+, *AIDS* 15, 1843
(1999): Descamps V+, *Lancet* 353, 1855
(1999): Phan TG+, *Australas J Dermatol* 40, 153
(1999): Wetterwald E+, *Br J Dermatol* 140, 980 (SJS/TEN overlap syndrome)

### Other

DRESS syndrome*
(2001): Claudio GA+, *Arch Intern Med* 161(20), 2501
(2000): Sissoko D+, *Presse Med* (French) 29, 1041
(1998): Bourezane Y+, *Clin Infect Dis* 27(5), 1321
Gingivitis (1–3%)
Hypersensitivity
(2001): Wit FW+, *AIDS* 15(18), 2423
(2000): Podzamczer D+, *AIDS* 14, 331
Lipodystrophy
(2000): Lewis RH+, *J Acquir Immune Defic Syndrom* 23, 355
(1999): Aldeen T+, *AIDS* 13, 865
Myalgia (1–10%)
Paresthesias (2%)
Ulcerative stomatitis (4%)

***Note:** The DRESS syndrome consists of "drug rash with eosinophilia and systemic symptoms"

## NIACIN

**Synonym:** nicotinic acid
**Trade names:** Advicor; Niacor (Upsher-Smith); Niaspan (Kos); Nicobid; Nicolar (Aventis); Nicotinex; Slo-Niacin (Upsher-Smith)
**Other common trade names:** *3; Apo-Nicotinamide; I*; IV; Nia-Bid; Niac; Niacels; Nicobion; Nicotinex; Nicovital; Pepeom Amide; Vitamin B*
**Indications:** Hyperlipidemia
**Category:** Antihyperlipidemic
**Half-life:** 45 minutes
**Clinically important, potentially hazardous interactions with:** atorvastatin

### *Reactions*

### Skin

Acanthosis nigricans
(1994): McKenney JM+, *JAMA* 271, 672
(1994): Stals H+, *Dermatology* 189, 203
(1993): Stone OJ, *Med Hypotheses* 40, 154
(1992): Coates P+, *Br J Dermatol* 126, 412
(1990): Audicana M+, *Contact Dermatitis* 22, 60
(1990): Brown G+, *N Engl J Med* 323, 1289 (8.3%)
(1989): Larmi E, *Int J Dermatol* 28, 609
(1989): Ylipieti S+, *Contact Dermatitis* 21, 105
(1981): Elgart ML, *J Am Acad Dermatol* 5, 709
(1974): Pedro S, *N Engl J Med* 29, 422
(1971): Curth HO, *Birth Defects* 7, 31
(1967): Branehog I+, *Lakartidningen* (Swedish) 64, 1449
(1964): Tromovitch TA+, *Arch Dermatol* 89, 222
Contact dermatitis
(1995): Bilbao I+, *Contact Dermatitis* 33, 435
Erythema
(1995): Fisher AA, *Cutis* 55, 132
Exanthems
(1997): Blumenthal HL, Beachwood, OH (personal case) (observation)
(1997): Litt JZ, Beachwood, OH (2 personal cases) (observation)
(1990): Brown G+, *N Engl J Med* 323, 1289 (2.8%)
Fixed eruption (<1%)
(1992): de la Hoz-Caballer B+, *Med Clin (Barc)* (Spanish) 98, 357
Flushing (1–10%)
(2002): Litt JZ, Beachwood, OH (personal case) (observation)
(1998): Capuzzi DM+, *Am J Cardiol* 82, 74U
(1998): Guyton JR+, *Am J Cardiol* 82, 737 (4.8%)
(1998): Knopp RH, *Am J Cardiol* 82, 24U
(1998): Morgan JM+, *Am J Cardiol* 82, 29U
(1997): Jungnickel PW+, *J Gen Intern Med* 12, 591
(1996): Crouse JR, *Coron Artery* 7, 321
(1996): Glen AI+, *Prostaglandins Leukot Essent Fatty Acids* 55, 9
(1994): Fivenson DP+, *Arch Dermatol* 130, 753
(1994): McKenney JM+, *JAMA* 271, 672
(1994): Sudan BJ, *Ann Pharmacother* 28, 1113
(1993): Fisher AA, *Cutis* 51, 225
(1992): Breathnach SM+, *Adverse Drug Reactions and the Skin* Blackwell, Oxford, 265 (passim)
(1992): Whelan AM+, *J Fam Pract* 34, 165 (passim)
(1989): Warady B+, *Perit Dial Int* 9, 81
(1988): Figge HL+, *Pharmacotherapy* 8, 287
(1985): Mooney E, *Int J Dermatol* 24, 549
(1977): Estep DL+, *Clin Toxicol* 11, 325
(1973): *Med Lett* 15, 102
(1973): Levy RI+, *Drugs* 6, 12
Ichthyosis
(1961): Berge KG+, *Am J Med* 31, 24
Keratoses, pigmented
(1974): Wittenborn JR+, *Adv Biochem Psychopharmacol* 9, 295
Pigmentation
(1992): Breathnach SM+, *Adverse Drug Reactions and the Skin* Blackwell, Oxford, 265 (passim)
Pruritus (1–5%)
(1997): Blumenthal HL, Beachwood, OH (personal case) (observation)
(1997): Jungnickel PW+, *J Gen Intern Med* 12, 591
(1994): Fivenson DP+, *Arch Dermatol* 130, 753
(1994): McKenney JM+, *JAMA* 271, 672
(1992): Breathnach SM+, *Adverse Drug Reactions and the Skin* Blackwell, Oxford, 265 (passim)
(1992): Whelan AM+, *J Fam Pract* 34, 165 (passim)
(1977): Estep DL+, *Clin Toxicol* 11, 325
(1973): *Med Lett* 15, 102
(1973): Levy RI+, *Drugs* 6, 12
Rash (sic) (<1%)
(1994): McKenney JM+, *JAMA* 271, 672
(1992): Breathnach SM+, *Adverse Drug Reactions and the Skin* Blackwell, Oxford, 265 (passim)
(1988): Figge HL+, *Pharmacotherapy* 8, 287
Scaling (sic)
(1992): Breathnach SM+, *Adverse Drug Reactions and the Skin* Blackwell, Oxford, 265 (passim)
Urticaria
(1995): Fisher AA, *Cutis* 55, 132
Xerosis

### Other

Anaphylactoid reactions
Burning mouth syndrome
(1988): Haustein UF, *Contact Dermatitis* 19, 225
Gingival pain
(1998): Leighton RF+, *Chest* 114, 1472
Myopathy
(1994): Gharavi AG+, *Am J Cardiol* 74, 841
(1989): Goldstein MR, *Am J Med* 87, 248
(1989): Litin SC+, *Am J Med* 86, 481
Paresthesias (1–10%)
(1997): Jungnickel PW+, *J Gen Intern Med* 12, 591

(1992): Whelan AM+, *J Fam Pract* 34, 165 (passim)
Tooth pain (sic)
(1998): Leighton RF+, *Chest* 114, 1472
Xerostomia

# NIACINAMIDE

**Synonyms:** nicotinamide; vitamin $B_3$
**Trade name:** Niacinamide
**Indications:** Prophylaxis and treatment of pellagra
**Category:** Water-soluble nutritional supplement
**Half-life:** 45 minutes
**Clinically important, potentially hazardous interactions with:** primidone

### *Reactions*

## Skin

Acanthosis nigricans
(1984): Papa CM, *Arch Dermatol* 120, 281
Pruritus (1–5%)
(1981): Zackheim HS+, *J Am Acad Dermatol* 4, 736
(1980): Bures FA, *J Am Acad Dermatol* 3, 530
Rash (sic)

## Other

Paresthesias (1–10%)

# NICARDIPINE

**Trade name:** Cardene (Wyeth-Ayerst)
**Other common trade names:** *Antagonil; Dagan; Loxen; Nicardal; Nicodel; Ranvil; Ridene; Rydene*
**Indications:** Angina, hypertension
**Category:** Calcium channel blocker; antianginal and antihypertensive; antimigraine
**Half-life:** 2–4 hours
**Clinically important, potentially hazardous interactions with:** epirubicin, imatinib

### *Reactions*

## Skin

Allergic reactions (sic)
Cutaneous side effects (sic)
(1993): Kitamura K+, *J Dermatol* 20, 279 (psoriasiform)
Edema (1%)
Erythromelalgia
(1989): Drenth JH, *BMJ* 298, 1582
(1989): Levesque H+, *BMJ* 298, 1252
Exanthems
Flushing (5.6%)
(1998): Knowles S+, *J Am Acad Dermatol* 38, 201 (passim)
(1990): Webster J+, *Br J Clin Pharmacol* 29, 587P
Peripheral edema (7.1%)
(1998): Knowles S+, *J Am Acad Dermatol* 38, 201 (passim)
(1990): Webster J+, *Br J Clin Pharmacol* 29, 587P (leg edema)
Rash (sic) (1.2%)
(1998): Knowles S+, *J Am Acad Dermatol* 38, 201 (passim)
(1985): Deedwania PC+, *Clin Pharmacol Ther* 37, 190
(1985): Gelman JS+, *Am J Cardiol* 56, 232
Urticaria
(1983): Brodmerkel GJ, *Ann Intern Med* 99, 415
(1983): Fisher JR+, *Ann Intern Med* 98, 671
(1982): Grunwald Z, *Drug Intell Clin Pharm* 16, 492

## Other

Gingival hyperplasia (<1%)
Myalgia (1%)
(1998): Knowles S+, *J Am Acad Dermatol* 38, 201 (passim)
Paresthesias (1%)
Parotitis
Tinnitus
Xerostomia (1.4%)

# NICOTINE*

**Trade names:** Habitrol Patch (Novartis); Nicoderm Patch (GSK); Nicorette Gum (GSK); Nicotrol Nasal Spray and Patch (McNeil); Polacrilex (GSK); Prostep Patch
**Other common trade names:** *Exodus; Nicabate; Nicolan; Nicorette Plus; Nicotinell-TTS; Nicotrans; Nikofrenon; Stubit*
**Indications:** Aid to smoking cessation
**Category:** Smoking deterrent
**Half-life:** varies with the delivery system*

### *Reactions*

## Skin

Contact dermatitis
(1993): Farm G, *Contact Dermatitis* 29, 214
Diaphoresis (1–3%)
Edema
Erythema (>10%)
Flushing
Pruritus (>10%)
Rash (sic)
Urticaria
Vasculitis
(1996): Van der Klauw MM+, *Br J Dermatol* 134, 361

## Other

Application-site burning
Application-site erythema
Application-site pruritus
Dysgeusia
Hypersensitivity (<1%)
Myalgia (1–10%)
Paresthesias
Sialorrhea (>10%)
Stomatitis (>10%)
Tinnitus
Tremors
Xerostomia (1–3%)

***Note:** Smoking cessation therapy has various delivery systems. These include: transdermal patches, chewing gum, nasal spray, inhaler, and oral forms

# NIFEDIPINE

**Trade names:** Adalat (Bayer); Procardia (Pfizer)
**Other common trade names:** *Adalate; Apo-Nifed; Aprical; Calcilat; Coracten; Corogal; Corotrend; Nifecor; Nu-Nifed; Pidilat*
**Indications:** Angina, hypertension
**Category:** Calcium channel blocker; antianginal and antihypertensive; antimigraine
**Half-life:** 2–5 hours
**Clinically important, potentially hazardous interactions with:** epirubicin, **grapefruit juice**, imatinib, rifampin, ritonavir

### *Reactions*

## Skin

Acute generalized exanthematous pustulosis (AGEP)
(1995): Moreau A+, *Int J Dermatol* 34, 263 (passim)
(1991): Roujeau J-C+, *Arch Dermatol* 127, 1333
Angioedema (<1%)
(1998): Knowles S+, *J Am Acad Dermatol* 38, 201 (passim)
(1989): Stern R+, *Arch Intern Med* 149, 829
Ankle edema
(1994): Mohammed KN, *Ann Pharmacother* 28, 967
(1991): Salmasi AM+, *Int J Cardiol* 30, 303
(1989): Williams SA+, *Eur J Clin Pharmacol* 37, 333
(1978): Bridgman JF, *BMJ* 276, 578
Bullous eruption
(1989): Stern R+, *Arch Intern Med* 149, 829
(1987): Alcalay J+, *Dermatologica* 175, 191
Chills (2%)
Cutaneous side effects (sic)
(1993): Kitamura K+, *J Dermatol* 20, 279 (psoriasiform)
Dermatitis (sic) (<2%)
Diaphoresis (<2%)
(1989): Stern R+, *Arch Intern Med* 149, 829
(1983): Lewis JG, *Drugs* 25, 196
Edema
(1983): Lewis JG, *Drugs* 25, 196
(1978): Bridgman JF, *BMJ* 276, 578 (erythematous, of legs)
Erysipelas
(1988): Leibovici V+, *Cutis* 41, 367
(1983): Lewis JG, *Drugs* 25, 196
Erythema
(1998): Knowles S+, *J Am Acad Dermatol* 38, 201 (passim)
(1992): Gonzalez-Castro U+, *Med Clin (Barc)* (Spanish) 98, 759
Erythema multiforme
(1998): Knowles S+, *J Am Acad Dermatol* 38, 201 (passim)
(1997): Springuel P, *Can Med Assoc J* 156, 90
(1989): Stern R+, *Arch Intern Med* 149, 829
(1986): Myrhed M+, *Acta Pharmacol Toxicol* 58, 133
Erythema nodosum
(1998): Knowles S+, *J Am Acad Dermatol* 38, 201 (passim)
(1989): Stern R+, *Arch Intern Med* 149, 829
Erythromelalgia (<0.5%)
(1989): Stern R+, *Arch Intern Med* 149, 829
(1987): Alcalay J+, *Dermatologica* 175, 191
(1983): Brodmerkel GJ, *Ann Intern Med* 99, 415
(1983): Fisher JR+, *Ann Intern Med* 98, 671
Exanthems
(1998): Knowles S+, *J Am Acad Dermatol* 38, 201 (passim)
(1995): Litt JZ, Beachwood, OH (personal case) (observation)
(1992): Parish LC+, *Cutis* 49, 113 (morbilliform)
(1989): Stern R+, *Arch Intern Med* 149, 829
(1987): Alcalay J+, *Dermatologica* 175, 191
(1985): Findlay GH, *S Afr Med J* 68, 176
(1983): Lewis JG, *Drugs* 25, 196 (1%)
(1982): Grunwald Z, *Drug Intell Clin Pharm* 16, 492
(1980): Antman E+, *N Engl J Med* 302, 1269 (1%)
Exfoliative dermatitis (<1%)
(1994): Mohammed KN, *Ann Pharmacother* 28, 967
(1993): Collins P, *Br J Dermatol* 129, 630 (passim)
(1989): Reynolds HJ+, *Br J Dermatol* 121, 401
(1989): Stern R+, *Arch Intern Med* 149, 829
(1984): Scoble JE+, *Clin Nephrol* 21, 302
Facial edema (1%)
Fixed eruption
(1993): Litt JZ, Beachwood, OH (personal case) (observation)
(1987): Alcalay J+, *Dermatologica* 175, 191
(1986): Alcalay J+, *BMJ* 292, 450
Flushing (3–25%)
(2001): Rudolph RI, Wyomissing, PA (from Internet) (observation)
(1992): Shelley WB+, *Advanced Dermatologic Diagnosis* WB Saunders, 582 (passim)
(1985): Aberg H+, *Drugs* 29 (Suppl 2), 117 (22%)
(1983): Lewis JG, *Drugs* 25, 196 (5–15%)
(1980): Antman E+, *N Engl J Med* 302, 1269 (11%)
Lichenoid eruption
(1989): Reynolds HJ+, *Br J Dermatol* 121, 401
(1988): Leibovici V+, *Cutis* 41, 367
(1984): Scoble JE+, *Clin Nephrol* 21, 302
Lupus erythematosus
(1998): Callen JP, Academy '98 Meeting
(1997): Crowson AN+, *Hum Pathol* 28, 67
Painful edema of extremities
(1985): Findlay GH, *S Afr Med J* 68, 176
(1982): Grunwald Z, *Drug Intell Clin Pharm* 16, 492
Pemphigoid nodularis
(2000): Ameen M+, *Br J Dermatol* 142, 575
Pemphigus foliaceus
(1993): Kim S-C+, *Acta Derm Venereol* (Stockh) 73, 210
Periorbital edema (1%)
(1985): Tordjman K+, *Am J Cardiol* 55, 1445
Peripheral edema (10–30%)
(2002): No author, *Medscape Primary Care 4*
(1996): Tailor SA+, *Arch Dermatol* 132, 350 (with itraconazole)
Photosensitivity
(1996): Seggev JS+, *J Allergy Clin Immunol* 97, 852
(1991): Zenarola P+, *Dermatologica* 182, 196
(1990): Guarrera M+, *Photodermatology* 7, 25
(1988): Zlotogorski A, *Dermatologica* 177, 249
(1986): Thomas SE+, *BMJ* 292, 992
Prurigo nodularis
(1992): Shelley WB+, *Cutis* 50, 179 (observation)
Pruritus (<2%)
(1998): Knowles S+, *J Am Acad Dermatol* 38, 201 (passim)
(1993): Collins P, *Br J Dermatol* 129, 630 (passim)
(1989): Stern R+, *Arch Intern Med* 149, 829
Purpura (<2%)
(1990): Regazzini R+, *Chron Derm* (Italian) 21, 225
(1989): Oren R+, *Drug Intell Clin Pharm* 23, 88
(1985): Findlay GH, *S Afr Med J* 68, 176
Rash (sic) (<3%)
(1998): Knowles S+, *J Am Acad Dermatol* 38, 201 (passim)
(1989): Stern R+, *Arch Intern Med* 149, 829
Stevens–Johnson syndrome
(1998): Knowles S+, *J Am Acad Dermatol* 38, 201 (passim)
(1993): Collins P, *Br J Dermatol* 129, 630 (passim)
(1989): Stern R+, *Arch Intern Med* 149, 829
Telangiectases
(1994): Shelley WB+, *Cutis* 53, 40 (observation)
(1993): Collins P, *Br J Dermatol* 129, 630 (photodistribution)
(1992): Tsele E+, *Lancet* 339, 365
Toxic epidermal necrolysis
(1998): Knowles S+, *J Am Acad Dermatol* 38, 201 (passim)
(1993): Collins P, *Br J Dermatol* 129, 630 (passim)

Ulcerations
(1999): Luca S+, *Minerva Cardioangiol* 47, 219
Urticaria (<1%)
(1999): Luca S+, *Minerva Cardioangiol* 47, 219 (legs)
(1998): Knowles S+, *J Am Acad Dermatol* 38, 201 (passim)
(1991): Zenarola P+, *Dermatologica* 182, 196
(1989): Stern R+, *Arch Intern Med* 149, 829
(1988): Toner M+, *Chest* 93, 1320
(1986): Myrhed M+, *Acta Pharmacol Toxicol* 58, 133
(1978): Bridgman JF, *BMJ* 276, 578
Vasculitis
(1989): Oren R+, *Drug Intell Clin Pharm* 23, 88
(1987): Alcalay J+, *Dermatologica* 175, 191
(1985): Brenner S+, *Harefuah* (Hebrew) 108, 139

### Hair

Hair – alopecia (1%)
(1998): Knowles S+, *J Am Acad Dermatol* 38, 201 (passim)
(1993): Collins P, *Br J Dermatol* 129, 630 (passim)
(1989): Reynolds HJ+, *Br J Dermatol* 121, 401
(1989): Stern R+, *Arch Intern Med* 149, 829
Hair – discoloration
(1989): Stern R+, *Arch Intern Med* 149, 829

### Nails

Nails – dystrophy
(1989): Stern R+, *Arch Intern Med* 149, 829

### Other

Dysgeusia (<1%)
Erythromyalgia
(1989): Stern R+, *Arch Intern Med* 149, 829
Gingival hyperplasia (>10%)
(2001): Uzel MI+, *J Periodontol* 72(7), 921
(2000): James JA+, *J Clin Periodontol* 27, 109 (with cyclosporine)
(1999): Ellis JS+, *J Periodontol* 70, 63 (6.3%)
(1998): Bokor-Bratic M+, *Med Pregl* (Serbo-Croatian [Roman]) 51, 445
(1998): Desai P+, *J Can Dent Assoc* 64, 263
(1998): Nakou M+, *J Periodontol* 69, 664
(1998): Nohl F+, *Ther Umsch* (German) 55, 573
(1997): Jackson C+, *N Y State Dent J* 63, 46
(1997): Slezak R, *J West Soc Periodontal Periodontal Abstr* 45, 105
(1997): Thomason JM+, *Clin Oral Investig* 1, 35
(1997): Westbrook P+, *J Periodontol* 68, 645
(1996): Abitbol TE+, *N Y State Dent J* 63, 34
(1996): Ciantar M, *Dent Update* 23, 374
(1996): Darbar UR+, *J Clin Periodontol* 23, 941
(1996): Deen-Duggins L+, *Quintessence Int* 27, 163 (4 cases)
(1996): Saito K+, *J Periodontol Res* 31, 545
(1995): Harel-Raviv M+, *Oral Surg Oral Med Oral Pathol Oral Radiol Endoc* 79, 715
(1995): Nery EB+, *J Periodontol* 66, 572
(1995): Ramsdale DR+, *Br Heart J* 73, 115
(1995): Silverstein LH+ *J Oral Implantol* 21, 116
(1995): Wynn RL, *Gen Dent* 43, 218
(1994): Henderson JS+ *Miss Dent Assoc J* 50, 12
(1994): Shelley WB+, *Cutis* 53, 282 (passim)
(1993): King GN+, *J Clin Periodontol* 20, 286
(1993): Morisaki I+, *J Periodontal Res* 28, 396
(1993): Steele RM+, *Arch Intern Med* 120, 663
(1992): Hancock RH+, *J Clin Periodontol* 19, 12
(1991): Nishikawa SJ+, *J Periodontol* 62, 30
(1991): Wynn RL, *Gen Dent* 39, 240
(1989): Veraldi S+, *Clin Exp Dermatol* 14, 93
(1988): Boisnic S+, *Ann Dermatol Venereol* (French) 115, 373
(1988): Zlotogorski A, *Dermatologica* 177, 249
(1986): Bencini PL+, *G Ital Dermatol Venereol* (Italian) 121, 29
(1986): Jones CM, *Br Dent J* 160, 416
(1985): Bencini PL+, *Acta Derm Venereol* (Stockh) 65, 362
(1985): Lucas RM+, *J Periodontol* 56, 211
(1984): Lederman D+, *Oral Surg Oral Med Oral Pathol* 57, 620
(1984): Ramon Y+, *Int J Cardiol* 5, 195
Gynecomastia (<1%)
(1995): Marcos-Olea JL+, *Aten Primaria* (Spanish) 16, 115
(1988): Zlotogorski A, *Dermatologica* 177, 249
(1986): Clyne CAC, *BMJ* 292, 380
Myalgia (<1%)
Paresthesias (<3%)
(1982): Macdonald JB, *BMJ* 285, 1744
Parosmia
Parotitis
Shakiness (sic) (2%)
Tinnitus
Tremors (2–8%)
Xerostomia (<3%)

## NIMODIPINE

**Trade name:** Nimotop (Bayer)
**Other common trade names:** *Admon; Periplum; Vasotop*
**Indications:** Subarachnoid hemorrhage
**Category:** Calcium channel blocker
**Half-life:** 3 hours
**Clinically important, potentially hazardous interactions with:** epirubicin, imatinib

#### *Reactions*

### Skin

Acne (<1%)
Acute generalized exanthematous pustulosis (AGEP)
(1999): Zabawski E+, Dallas, TX (from Internet) (observation)
Diaphoresis (<1%)
Edema (2%)
Exanthems (2.4%)
(1989): Langley MS+, *Drugs* 37, 669
Flushing (2.1%)
Peripheral edema
Pruritus (<1%)
Purpura
Rash (sic) (3%)

### Hair

Hair – alopecia
(1995): Daghfous R+, *Therapie* (French) 50, 590

## NISOLDIPINE

**Trade name:** Sular (AstraZeneca)
**Other common trade names:** *Baymycard; Syscor*
**Indications:** Hypertension
**Category:** Calcium channel blocker; antihypertensive
**Half-life:** 7–12 hours
**Clinically important, potentially hazardous interactions with:** epirubicin, imatinib

#### *Reactions*

### Skin

Acne (<1%)
Angioedema
Cellulitis (<1%)

Chills (<1%)
Cutaneous side effects (sic)
(1993): Kitamura K+, *J Dermatol* 20, 279
Diaphoresis (<1%)
Ecchymoses (<1%)
Exanthems (<1%)
(1988): Friedel HA+, *Drugs* 36, 682 (0.7%)
Exfoliative dermatitis (<1%)
Facial edema (<1%)
Flu-like syndrome (sic) (<1%)
Flushing
(1988): Friedel HA+, *Drugs* 36, 682 (13.21%)
Herpes simplex (<1%)
Herpes zoster (<1%)
Peripheral edema (22%)
(2001): Lenz TL+, *Pharmacotherapy* 21(8), 898 (4 cases) (with amlodipine)
Petechiae (<1%)
Photosensitivity
Pigmentation (<1%)
Pruritus (<1%)
Pustular eruption (<1%)
Rash (sic) (2%)
Ulceration (<1%)
Urticaria (<1%)
Xerosis (<1%)

### Hair

Hair – alopecia (<1%)

### Other

Dysgeusia (<1%)
Gingival hyperplasia (<1%)
Glossitis (<1%)
Gynecomastia (<1%)
Hypersensitivity
Hypesthesia (<1%)
Oral ulceration (<1%)
Paresthesias (<1%)
Tremors (<1%)
Vaginitis (<1%)
Xerostomia (<1%)

## NITROFURANTOIN

**Trade names:** Furadantin (Dura); Macrobid (Procter & Gamble); Macrodantin (Procter & Gamble)
**Other common trade names:** *Furadantina; Furadoine; Furalan; Furan; Furobactina; Infurin; Nephronex; Novo-Furan; Urofuran*
**Indications:** Various urinary tract infections caused by susceptible organisms
**Category:** Urinary tract antibiotic
**Half-life:** 20–60 minutes

### *Reactions*

### Skin

Acute febrile neutrophilic dermatosis (Sweet's syndrome)
(1999): Retief CR+, *Cutis* 63, 177
Angioedema
(1982): Penn RG+, *BMJ* 284, 1440
(1981): Chisholm JC+, *J Nat Med Assoc* 73, 59 (passim)
(1977): Delaney RA+, *Am J Pharm* 149, 26 (passim)
(1971): Koch-Weser J+, *Ann Intern Med* 128, 399 (0.1%)
Bullous eruption
Chills
Contact dermatitis
(1978): Novak M, *Cesk Dermatol* (Czech) 53, 128
(1974): Bleumink E+, *Hautarzt* (German) 25, 403
(1970): Laubstein H+, *Dermatol Monatsschr* (German) 156, 1
Eczematous eruption (sic)
(1977): Delaney RA+, *Am J Pharm* 149, 26 (passim)
(1976): Mitchell J+, *Modern Med* 44, 63
Erythema multiforme
(1990): Chan HL+, *Arch Dermatol* 126, 43
(1986): Chapman JA, *Ann Allergy* 56, 16
(1971): Koch-Weser J+, *Ann Intern Med* 128, 399 (0.1%)
Erythema nodosum
(1981): Chisholm JC+, *J Nat Med Assoc* 73, 59
Exanthems (1–5%)
(1984): Paver R+, *Current Ther* 25, 55
(1983): Swinyer LJ, *Dermatol Clin* 1, 417
(1980): Calderwood SB+, *Surgical Clin N Amer* 60, 65
(1980): Holmberg L+, *Am J Med* 69, 733 (28%)
(1976): Stubb S, *Acta Derm Venereol* (Stockh) 56 (Suppl 76), 16
(1974): Eggers B+, *Z Hautkr* (German) 49, 704
(1972): Kauppinen K, *Acta Derm Venereol* (Stockh) 52 (Suppl), 68
(1971): Bailey RR+, *Lancet* 2, 1112 (1%)
(1971): Koch-Weser J+, *Ann Intern Med* 128, 399 (1%)
Exfoliative dermatitis
(1984): Paver R+, *Current Ther* 25, 55
(1983): Swinyer LJ, *Dermatol Clin* 1, 417
(1972): Kauppinen K, *Acta Derm Venereol* (Stockh) 52 (Suppl), 68
Fixed eruption
(1985): Kauppinen K+, *Br J Dermatol* 112, 575
Flushing
Lupus erythematosus
(1986): Chapman JA, *Annals Allergy* 56, 16
(1985): Stratton MA, *Clin Pharm* 4, 657
(1981): Fleck RM, *Pennsylvania Med* 84, 36
(1975): Selroos O+, *Acta Med Scand* 197, 125
(1974): Back O+, *Lancet* 1, 930
Photosensitivity
(1987): Australian Drug Evaluation Committee, 61 (Oct 15)
Pruritus (<1%)
(1987): Australian Drug Evaluation Committee, 61 (Oct 15)
(1981): Chisholm JC+, *J Nat Med Assoc* 73, 59 (passim)
Purpura
(1984): Paver R+, *Current Ther* 25, 55
(1983): Swinyer LJ, *Dermatol Clin* 1, 417
Rash (sic) (<1%)
(1982): Penn RG+, *BMJ* 284, 1440
(1977): Takala J+, *Acta Med Scand* 202, 75
Reticular hyperplasia
(1966): Korting GW+, *Dermatol Wochenschr* (German) 152, 257
Stevens–Johnson syndrome
(1971): Koch-Weser J+, *Ann Intern Med* 128, 399
Toxic epidermal necrolysis
(1993): Stables GI+, *Br J Dermatol* 128, 357
(1984): Kauppinen K+, *Acta Derm Venereol* (Stockh) 64, 320
(1983): Swinyer LJ, *Dermatol Clin* 1, 417
(1967): Duperrat B+, *Bull Soc Fr Dermatol Syphiligr* (French) 74, 423 (fatal)
(1963): Oswald FH, *Ned Tijdschr Geneesk* (Danish) 107, 999
Urticaria
(1999): Litt JZ, Beachwood, OH (personal case) (observation)
(1996): Blumenthal HL, Beachwood, OH (personal case) (observation)
(1983): Griffin JP, *Practitioner* 227, 1283
(1983): Swinyer LJ, *Dermatol Clin* 1, 417
(1982): Schneider RE, *Clin Ther* 4, 390
(1978): Watson B+, *Br J Dermatol* 99, 183

(1977): McLundie S, *Ann Allergy* 38, 71
(1972): Kauppinen K, *Acta Derm Venereol* (Stockh) 52 (Suppl), 68
(1971): Koch-Weser J+, *Ann Intern Med* 128, 399 (0.4%)
(1969): Aaronson CM, *JAMA* 210, 557

### Hair

Hair – alopecia
(1983): No Author, *Lakartidningen* (Swedish) 80, 4040
(1983): Swinyer LJ, *Dermatol Clin* 1, 417
(1977): Delaney RA+, *Am J Pharm* 149, 26 (passim)
(1971): Coster C+, *Lakartidningen* (Swedish) 68, 3366
(1959): Johnson SH+, *J Urology* (Baltimore) 82, 162

### Nails

Nails – onycholysis
(1982): Penn RG+, *BMJ* 284, 1440

### Other

Anaphylactoid reactions
(1987): Australian Drug Evaluation Committee, 61 (Oct 15)
(1982): Penn RG+, *BMJ* 284, 1440
(1980): Calderwood SB+, *Surg Clin N Amer* 60, 65
Death
Galactorrhea
(1986): Auwaerter A+, *Krankenhausarzt* (German) 59, 766
Hypersensitivity
(1976): Fine SR, *Cutis* 17, 1171
Mastodynia
(1986): Auwaerter A+, *Krankenhausarzt* (German) 59, 766
Myalgia
Panniculitis, nodular nonsuppurative
(1987): Sanford RG+, *Arthritis Rheum* 30, 1076
Paresthesias (1–10%)
Tooth discoloration
Xerostomia
(1977): Takala J+, *Acta Med Scand* 202, 75

## NITROGLYCERIN

**Synonyms:** glyceryl trinitrate; nitroglycerol; NTG
**Trade names:**
Buccal tablets: Nitrogard
Lingual aerosol: Nitrolingual (First Horizon)
Oral capsules: Nitro-Bid; Nitrocap; Nitrocine; Nitroglyn; Nitrospan
Oral tablets: Klavikordal; Niong; Nitronet; Nitrong
Parenteral: Nitro-Bid; Nitroject; Nitrol; Nitrostat; Tridil
Sublingual tablets: Nitrostat
Topical ointment: Nitro-Bid; Nitrol; Nitrong; Nitrostat
Topical transdermal systems: Deponit; Minitran; Nitrocine; Nitrodisc; Nitrodur; Transderm-Nitro. (Various pharmaceutical companies.)
**Other common trade names:** *Cardinit; Corditrine; Lenitral; Nitradisc; Nitroglin; Suscard; Sustac*
**Indications:** Acute angina
**Category:** Antianginal; vasodilator; antihypertensive
**Half-life:** 1–4 minutes
**Clinically important, potentially hazardous interactions with:** alteplase, sildenafil

### *Reactions*

### Skin

Allergic reactions (sic) (<1%)
Angioedema
(1998): Rademaker M+, *New Zealand Adverse Drug Reactions Committee*, April, 1998 (from Internet)
Contact dermatitis (to topical systems) (<1%)
(2000): McKenna KE, *Contact Dermatitis* 42, 246
(1999): Machet L+, *Dermatology* 198, 106
(1994): de la Fuente-Prieto R+, *Ann Allergy* 72, 344
(1992): Torres V+, *Contact Dermatitis* 26, 53
(1991): Kanerva L+, *Contact Dermatitis* 24, 356
(1991): Laine R+, *Duodecim* (Finnish) 107, 41
(1990): Vaillant L+, *Contact Dermatitis* 23, 142
(1989): Carmichael AJ+, *Contact Dermatitis* 21, 113
(1989): Di Landro A+, *Contact Dermatitis* 21, 115
(1989): Holdiness MR, *Contact Dermatitis* 20, 3
(1988): Apted J, *Med J Aust* 148, 482
(1988): Niedner R, *Hautarzt* (German) 39, 761
(1987): Gupta AK+, *Arch Dermatol* 123, 295
(1987): Harari Z+, *Dermatologica* 174, 249
(1987): Topaz O+, *Ann Allergy* 59, 365
(1986): Schrader BJ+, *Pharmacotherapy* 6, 83
(1986): Weickel R+, *Hautarzt* (German) 37, 511
(1985): Fischer RG+, *South Med J* 78, 1523
(1984): Fisher AA, *Cutis* 34, 526
(1984): Letendre PW+, *Drug Intell Clin Pharm* 18, 69
(1984): Rosenfeld AS+, *Am Heart J* 108, 1061
(1983): Camarasa JG+, *Contact Dermatitis* 9, 320
(1979): Hendricks AA+, *Arch Dermatol* 115, 853
Cyanosis
Diaphoresis (<1%)
Eczematous eruption (sic)
(1989): Carmichael AJ+, *Contact Dermatitis* 21, 113
(1987): Topaz O+, *Ann Allergy* 59, 365
Edema
Erythema (to transdermal delivery system)
(1990): Hogan JD+, *J Am Acad Dermatol* 22, 811
Erythema multiforme
(2001): Silvestre JF+, *Contact Dermatitis* 45(5), 299
Erythroderma
(1972): Ryan FP, *Br J Dermatol* 87, 498
Exanthems
Exfoliative dermatitis (1–10%)
(1972): Ryan FP, *Br J Dermatol* 87, 498
Flushing (>10%)
(1992): Shelley WB+, *Advanced Dermatologic Diagnosis* WB Saunders, 582 (passim)
Pallor
Peripheral edema (<1%)
Purpura
(1989): Nishioka K+, *J Dermatol* 16, 220 (pigmented)
(1955): Shmushkovich J+, *Br J Dermatol* 67, 299
Rash (sic) (1–10%)
Rosacea (exacerbation)
(1980): Wilkin JK, *Arch Dermatol* 116, 598
Urticaria

### Other

Anaphylactoid reactions (from perianal application)
(1999): Pietroletti R+, *Am J Gastroenterol* 94, 292
Oral burning and tingling (from sublingual)
Xerostomia (<1%)

# NIZATIDINE

**Trade name:** Axid (Lilly)
**Other common trade names:** *Apo-Nizatidine; Calmaxid; Gastrax; Nizax; Nizaxid; Panaxid; Tazac; Zanizal*
**Indications:** Duodenal ulcer, gastroesophageal reflux disease (GERD)
**Category:** Histamine $H_2$-receptor antagonist and anti-ulcer
**Half-life:** 1–2 hours

### *Reactions*

## Skin

Acne (<1%)
Allergic reactions (sic) (<1%)
Contact dermatitis
Diaphoresis (1%)
(1988): Price AH+, *Drugs* 36, 521 (1%)
(1987): Cloud ML, *Scand J Gastroenterol* 22, 39
Edema
Exanthems
Exfoliative dermatitis
Pruritus (1.7%)
(1988): Price AH+, *Drugs* 36, 521
(1987): Cloud ML, *Scand J Gastroenterol* 22, 39
Rash (sic) (1.9%)
(1987): Cloud ML, *Scand J Gastroenterol* 22, 39
Urticaria (<1%)
(1988): Price AH+, *Drugs* 36, 521 (0.5%)
Vasculitis
Xerosis (<1%)

## Other

Gynecomastia
(1987): Cloud ML, *Scand J Gastroenterol* 22, 39
Myalgia (1.7%)
Paresthesias (<1%)
Pseudolymphoma
(1995): Magro CM+, *J Am Acad Dermatol* 32, 419
Serum sickness
Xerostomia (1.4%)

# NORFLOXACIN

**Trade names:** Chibroxin (Merck); Noroxin (Merck)
**Other common trade names:** *Barazan; Chibroxine; Chibroxol; Lexinor; Noroxine; Oranor; Utinor; Zoroxin*
**Indications:** Various urinary tract infections caused by susceptible organisms, conjunctivitis
**Category:** Broad-spectrum quinolone antibiotic
**Half-life:** 2.3–4 hours
**Clinically important, potentially hazardous interactions with:** amiodarone, arsenic, bepridil, bretylium, disopyramide, erythromycin, phenothiazines, procainamide, quinidine, sotalol, tricyclic antidepressants

### *Reactions*

## Skin

Angioedema
Bullous eruption
(1993): Ramsey B+, *Br J Dermatol* 129, 500
Contact dermatitis
(1998): Silvestre JF+, *Contact Dermatitis* 39, 83
Diaphoresis (<1%)
Edema
Erythema (sic) (<1%)
Erythema multiforme
Exanthems
(1988): Wolfson JS+, *Ann Intern Med* 108, 238
(1985): Holmes B+, *Drugs* 30, 482 (0.2%)
Exfoliative dermatitis
Fixed eruption
(1997): Fenandez-Rivas M, *Allergy* 52, 477
Photosensitivity
(1963): Oswald FH, *Ned Tijdschr Geneesk* (Dutch) 107, 999
Phototoxicity
(2000): Traynor NJ+, *Toxicol Vitr* 14, 275
(1998): Martinez LJ+, *Photochem Photobiol* 67, 399
(1994): Fujita H+, *Photodermatol Photoimmunol Photomed* 10, 202
(1993): Ferguson J+, *Br J Dermatol* 128, 285
Pruritus (<1%)
(1985): Holmes B+, *Drugs* 30, 482 (0.2%)
Pustular eruption
(1992): Allegue F+, *Med Clin (Barc)* (Spanish) 99, 274
Rash (sic) (<1%)
Stevens–Johnson syndrome
(1992): Kubo-Shimasaki A+, *Rinsho Ketsueki* (Japanese) 33, 823
Stinging (from ophthalmic solution)
Subcorneal pustular dermatosis (Sneddon–Wilkinson)
(1988): Shelley ED+, *Cutis* 42, 24
Toxic epidermal necrolysis
(1993): Correia O+, *Dermatology* 186, 32
Toxic pustuloderma
(1993): Tsuda S+, *Acta Derm Venereol* (Stockh) 73, 382 (passim)
Urticaria
Vasculitis

## Nails

Nails – photo-onycholysis
(1987): Baran R+, *J Am Acad Dermatol* 17, 1012
(1986): Baran R+, *Dermatologica* 173, 185

## Other

Anaphylactoid reactions
Dysgeusia (<1%) (bitter taste)
Myalgia
(2001): Guis S+, *J Rheumatol* 28, 1405
Paresthesias
Rhabdomyolysis
(2001): Guis S+, *J Rheumatol* 28, 1405
Stomatitis
Tendinitis
(1983): Bailey RR+, *N Z Med J* 96, 590
Tendon rupture (<1%)
Tinnitus
Vaginal candidiasis
Xerostomia (<1%)

# NORTRIPTYLINE

**Trade names:** Aventyl (Lilly); Pamelor (Novartis)
**Other common trade names:** *Allegron; Apo-Nortriptyline; Noritren; Norpress; Nortrilen; Paxtibi; Vividyl*
**Indications:** Depression
**Category:** Tricyclic antidepressant and antipanic
**Half-life:** 28–31 hours
**Clinically important, potentially hazardous interactions with:** amprenavir, arbutamine, clonidine, epinephrine, fluoxetine, formoterol, guanethidine, isocarboxazid, linezolid, MAO inhibitors, phenelzine, quinolones, sparfloxacin, tranylcypromine

### *Reactions*

## Skin
Acne
Allergic reactions (sic) (<1%)
Diaphoresis (1–10%)
Edema
Erythema
Exanthems
Flushing
Petechiae
Photosensitivity (<1%)
(1972): Macaione AS, *Bull Geisinger Med Cent* 24, 122
(1972): Richards DL+, *Adverse Drug Reactions*, Livingstone
Phototoxicity
Pruritus
Purpura
Rash (sic)
Urticaria
Vasculitis
Xerosis

## Hair
Hair – alopecia (<1%)

## Other
Acute intermittent porphyria
(1986): Krummel SJ+, *Drug Intell Clin Pharm* 20, 487
Black tongue
(1990): Vitiello B+, *Clin Pharm* 9, 421
Dysgeusia (>10%)
Galactorrhea (<1%)
Gynecomastia (<1%)
Paresthesias
Parkinsonism (1–10%)
Stomatitis
Tinnitus
Tongue edema
Tremors
Vaginitis
Xerostomia (>10%)
(2001): Pomara N+, *Prog Neuropsychopharmacol Biol Psychiatry* 25(5), 1035

# NYSTATIN

**Trade names:** Mycostatin (Bristol-Myers Squibb); Nystop (Paddock)
**Other common trade names:** *Biofanal; Candio-Hermal; Mestatin; Moronal; Nistaquim; Nyaderm; Nystacid; Nystan; Nystex; Oranyst; Pedi-Dri*
**Indications:** Candidiasis
**Category:** Antifungal (anti-candidal) antibiotic
**Half-life:** no data

### *Reactions*

## Skin
Acrodermatitis perstans (exacerbation)
(1971): Petrozzi JW+, *Arch Dermatol* 103, 442
Acute generalized exanthematous pustulosis (AGEP)
(1999): Przybilla B+, *Hautarzt* (German) 50, 136
(1998): Rosenberger A+, *Hautarzt* (German) 49, 492
(1997): Kuchler A+, *Br J Dermatol* 137, 808 (3 cases)
Contact dermatitis (<1%)
(1994): Fisher AA, *Cutis* 54, 300
(1993): Hills RJ+, *Contact Dermatitis* 28, 48
(1990): de Groot AC+, *Dermatologic Clinics* 8, 153
(1987): Lechner T+, *Mykosen* (German) 30, 143
(1985): Lang E+, *Contact Dermatitis* 12, 182
(1971): Chalmers D, *Arch Dermatol* 104, 437
(1971): Coskey RJ, *Arch Dermatol* 103, 228
(1971): Foussereau J+, *Bull Soc Fr Dermatol Syphiligr* (French) 78, 457
(1971): Wasilewski C, *Arch Dermatol* 104, 437
(1970): Wasilewski C, *Arch Dermatol* 102, 216
Dermatitis (sic)
(1991): Quirce S+, *Contact Dermatitis* 25, 197 (generalized)
Eczematous eruption (sic)
(1987): Lechner T+, *Mykosen* (German) 30, 143
(1971): Coskey RJ, *Arch Dermatol* 103, 228
Erythema multiforme
(1991): Garty BZ, *Arch Dermatol* 127, 741
Erythroderma
(1980): Pareek SS, *Br J Dermatol* 103, 679
Exanthems
(1991): Quirce S+, *Contact Dermatitis* 25, 197
Fixed eruption
(1980): Pareek SS, *Br J Dermatol* 103, 679
(1969): Kandil E, *Dermatologica* 139, 37
Pruritus
(1987): Lechner T+, *Mykosen* (German) 30, 143
Rash (sic)
Stevens–Johnson syndrome (<1%)
(1991): Garty BZ, *Arch Dermatol* 127, 741
Urticaria
Vulvovaginitis
(2001): Dan M, *Am J Obstet Gynecol* 185(1), 254

## Other
Hypersensitivity (<1%)
(2001): Barranco R+, *Contact Dermatitis* 45(1), 60
Tongue edema
(1991): Quirce S+, *Contact Dermatitis* 25, 197
Vaginitis
(2001): Dan M, *Am J Obstet Gynecol* 185(1), 254

## OCTREOTIDE

**Trade name:** Sandostatin (Novartis)
**Other common trade names:** *Sandostatina; Sandostatine*
**Indications:** Diarrhea
**Category:** Antidiarrheal; antihypotensive; growth hormone suppressant; antihypoglycemic; secretory inhibitor
**Half-life:** 1.5 hours

### *Reactions*

#### Skin

Allergic reactions (sic)
Cellulitis (1–4%)
Diaphoresis
Edema (1–10%)
Exanthems
(1990): Saltz L+, *Proc Am Soc Clin Oncol* 9, 97
Flushing (1–4%)
(2000): Caplin ME+, *Nucl Med Commun* 21, 97
Granulomas
(2001): Rideout DJ+, *Clin Nucl Med* 26, 650 (buttock)
Petechiae (1–4%)
Pruritus (1–4%)
Purpura (1–4%)
Rash (sic) (<1%)
Raynaud's phenomenon (1–4%)
Urticaria (1–4%)

#### Hair

Hair – alopecia (<1%)
(1995): Nakauchi Y+, *Endocr J* 42, 385
(1991): Jonsson A+, *Ann Intern Med* 115, 913

#### Other

Anaphylactoid reactions
Galactorrhea (1–4%)
Gynecomastia (1–4%)
Hyperesthesia (<1%)
Injection-site erythema (1%)
Injection-site granuloma
(2001): Rideout DJ+, *Clin Nucl Med* 26(7), 650
Injection-site local reaction (sic)
Injection-site pain (7.5%)
Thrombophlebitis (1–4%)
Vaginitis (1–4%)
Xerostomia

## OFLOXACIN

**Trade names:** Floxin (Ortho-McNeil); Ocuflox (Allergan)
**Other common trade names:** *Bactocin; Exocine; Flobasin; Floxan; Floxil; Floxstat; Oflocet; Oflocin; Tabrin; Taravid*
**Indications:** Various infections caused by susceptible organisms
**Category:** Broad-spectrum fluoroquinolone antibiotic
**Half-life:** 4–8 hours
**Clinically important, potentially hazardous interactions with:** amiodarone, arsenic, bepridil, bretylium, disopyramide, erythromycin, phenothiazines, procainamide, quinidine, sotalol, tricyclic antidepressants

### *Reactions*

#### Skin

Angioedema
(1987): Jüngst G+, *Drugs* 34 (Suppl 1), 144
(1987): Monk JP, *Drugs* 33, 346
Bullous eruption
Candidiasis (sic)
(1987): Jüngst G+, *Drugs* 34 (Suppl 1), 144
Chills (<1%)
Cutaneous side effects (sic) (0.4%)
(1988): Fostini R+, *Drug Exp Clin Res* 14, 393
(1987): Monk JP, *Drugs* 33, 346
Dermatitis (sic)
(2000): Litt JZ, Beachwood, OH (personal case) (observation)
(1987): Monk JP, *Drugs* 33, 346
Diaphoresis
Ecchymoses
Edema (<1%)
Erythema multiforme
Erythema nodosum
Exanthems
(1994): Shelley WB+, *Cutis* 54, 146 (observation)
(1994): Shelley WB+, *Cutis* 55, 22 (observation)
(1993): Litt JZ, Beachwood, OH (personal case) (observation)
(1987): Jüngst G+, *Drugs* 34 (Suppl 1), 144
(1987): Monk JP, *Drugs* 33, 346
(1986): Baran R+, *Dermatologica* 173, 185
Exfoliative dermatitis
Fixed eruption
(1996): Kawada A+, *Contact Dermatitis* 34, 427
(1994): Kawada A+, *Contact Dermatitis* 31, 182
Petechiae
Photosensitivity (<1%)
(1994): Fujita H+, *Photodermatol Photoimmunol Photomed* 10, 202
(1993): Scheife RT+, *Int J Dermatol* 32, 413
(1990): Przybilla G+, *Dermatologica* 181, 98
(1988): Halkin H, *Rev Infect Dis* 10 (Suppl 1), 258
(1987): Jensen T+, *J Antimicrob Chemother* 20, 585
(1987): Jüngst G+, *Drugs* 34 (Suppl 1), 144
(1986): Baran R+, *Dermatologica* 173, 185
Phototoxicity
(2000): Traynor NJ+, *Toxicol Vitr* 14, 275
(1998): Martinez LJ+, *Photochem Photobiol* 67, 399
Pigmentation
Pruritus (1–3%)
(2000): Litt JZ, Beachwood, OH (personal case) (observation)
(1987): Jüngst G+, *Drugs* 34 (Suppl 1), 144
(1987): Monk JP, *Drugs* 33, 346
Pruritus vulvae (1–3%)
Purpura
Rash (sic) (1–10%)

(1988): Kromann-Andersen B+, *J Antimicrob Chemother* 22 (Suppl C), 143
Stevens–Johnson syndrome
Toxic epidermal necrolysis
(2001): Melde LM, *Ann Pharmacother* 35, 1388
Toxic pustuloderma
(1993): Tsuda S+, *Acta Derm Venereol* (Stockh) 73, 382
Urticaria (<1%)
(1987): Jüngst G+, *Drugs* 34 (Suppl 1), 144
(1987): Monk JP, *Drugs* 33, 346
Vasculitis (<1%)
(1996): Pipek R+, *Am J Med Sci* 311, 82
(1989): Huminer D+, *BMJ* 299, 303
(1989): Pace JL+, *BMJ* 299, 658
(1987): Jüngst G+, *Drugs* 34 (Suppl 1), 144

### Nails

Nails – photo-onycholysis
(1987): Baran R+, *J Am Acad Dermatol* 17, 1012
(1986): Baran R+, *Dermatologica* 173, 185

### Other

Anaphylactoid reactions
(1987): Jüngst G+, *Drugs* 34 (Suppl 1), 144
(1987): Monk JP, *Drugs* 33, 346
Death
(2001): Melde SL, *Ann Pharmacother* 35(11), 1388
Dysgeusia (1–3%)
(1995): Dark DS+, *Infections in Medicine* October, 551
Hypersensitivity
(1999): Desai C+, *J Assoc Physicians India* 47, 349
Injection-site pain (1–10%)
Myalgia (<1%)
Oral mucosal eruption
(1987): Jüngst G+, *Drugs* 34 (Suppl 1), 144
(1987): Monk JP, *Drugs* 33, 346
Paresthesias (<1%)
Parosmia
Serum sickness
Tendon rupture (<1%)
Tinnitus
Tourette's syndrome
Vaginitis (1–10%)
Xerostomia (1–3%)

## OLANZAPINE

**Synonym:** LY170053
**Trade name:** Zyprexa (Lilly)
**Indications:** Psychotic disorders
**Category:** Benzodiazepine antipsychotic
**Half-life:** 21–54 hours

***Reactions***

### Skin

Angioneurotic edema
(2001): Biswasl PN+, *J Psychopharmacol* 15(4), 265
Candidiasis (<1%)
Contact dermatitis (<1%)
Diaphoresis (>1%)
Ecchymoses (>1%)
Eczema (sic) (<1%)
Edema
Exanthems (<1%)
Facial edema (<1%)
Neuroleptic malignant syndrome
(2002): Aboraya A+, *W V Med* 98(2), 63 (with risperidone)
(2002): Malyuk R+, *Int J Geriatr Psychiatry* 17(4), 326
(2001): Biswasl PN+, *J Psychopharmacol* 15(4), 265
(2001): Philibert RA+, *Psychosomatics* 42(6), 528
Peripheral edema (2%)
(2000): Yovtcheva SP+, *Gen Hosp Psychiatry* 22, 290
Photosensitivity (<1%)
Pigmentation (<1%)
Pruritus (>1%)
Pustular eruption
(1999): Adams BB+, *J Am Acad Dermatol* 41, 851
Rash (sic) (>1%)
(2001): Street JS+, *Int J Geriatr Psychiatry* 16(Suppl 1), S62
(1999): Green B, *Curr Med Res Opin* 15, 79 (2%)
Seborrhea (<1%)
Ulceration (<1%)
Urticaria (<1%)
Vesiculobullous eruption (2%)
Xerosis (<1%)

### Hair

Hair – alopecia (<1%)
(2000): Mercke Y+, *Ann Clin Psychiatry* 12, 35
Hair – hirsutism (<1%)

### Other

Akathisia
(2001): Ishigooka J+, *Psychiatry Clin Neurosci* 55(4), 353
Aphthous stomatitis (<1%)
Dysgeusia (<1%)
Galactorrhea
(2002): Kingsbury SJ+, *Am J Psychiatry* 159(6), 1061
Gingivitis (<1%)
Glossitis (<1%)
Hypersensitivity
(2001): Raz A+, *Am J Med Sci* 321(2), 156
Hypesthesia (<1%)
Myalgia (>1%)
(2001): Rosebraugh CJ+, *Ann Pharmacother* 35(9), 1020
Oral candidiasis (<1%)
Oral ulceration (<1%)
Parkinsonism (1–10%)
Priapism (<1%)
(2001): Compton MT+, *J Clin Psychiatry* 62(5), 363
(2001): Matthews SC+, *Psychosomatics* 42(3), 280
(2001): Songer DA+, *Am J Psychiatry* 158(12), 2087
(2000): Compton MT+, *Am J Psychiatry* 157, 659
(1999): Gordon M+, *J Clin Psychopharmacol* 19, 192
(1999): Green B, *Curr Med Res Opin* 15, 79 (0.1%)
(1998): Deirmenjian JM+, *J Clin Psychopharmacol* 18, 351
(1998): Heckers S+, *Psychosomatics* 39, 288
Rhabdomyolysis
(2001): Rosebraugh CJ+, *Ann Pharmacother* 35(9), 1020
(2000): Shuster J, *Nursing* 30(9), 87
(1999): Marcus EL+, *Ann Pharmacother* 33(6), 697
(1996): Meltzer HY+, *Neuropsychopharmacology* 15(4), 395
Sialorrhea (<1%)
(1998): Perkins DO+, *Am J Psychiatry* 155, 993
Stomatitis (<1%)
Tongue discoloration (<1%)
Tongue edema (<1%)
(1997): Litt JZ, Beachwood, OH (personal case) (observation)
Tremors (1–10%)
(2002): Tohen M+, *Arch Gen Psychiatry* 59(1), 62 (with lithium)
(2001): Ishigooka J+, *Psychiatry Clin Neurosci* 55(4), 353
Twitching (2%)

Vaginitis (>1%)
Xerostomia (13%)
(2002): Tohen M+, *Arch Gen Psychiatry* 59(1), 62 (with lithium)
(1999): Green B, *Curr Med Res Opin* 15, 79 (7%)
(1998): Bever KA+, *Am J Health Syst Pharm* 55, 1003

# OLMESARTAN

**Trade name:** Benicar (Sankyo)
**Indications:** Hypertension
**Category:** Angiotensin II receptor blocker
**Half-life:** ~13 hours
**Clinically important, potentially hazardous interactions with: ephedra**, **garlic**, **ginseng**, lithium

### *Reactions*

## Skin
Angioedema
Facial edema
Flu-like syndrome (>1%)
Peripheral edema (>0.5)
Rash (sic) (0.5%)
Upper respiratory infection (>1%)

## Other
Arthralgia (>0.5%)
Back pain (>1%)
Cough (0.7%)
Myalgia (>0.5%)
Pain (>0.5%)
Skeletal pain (>0.5%)

# OLOPATADINE

**Trade name:** Patanol (Alcon)
**Indications:** Pruritus due to allergic conjunctivitis
**Category:** Ophthalmic $H_1$ antagonist
**Half-life:** 3 hours

### *Reactions*

## Skin
Eyelid burning (<5%)
Eyelid edema (<5%)
Eyelid stinging (<5%)
Pruritus

## Other
Dysgeusia

# OLSALAZINE

**Trade name:** Dipentum (Pharmacia & Upjohn)
**Indications:** Ulcerative colitis
**Category:** Inflammatory bowel disease suppressant
**Half-life:** 0.9 hours
**Clinically important, potentially hazardous interactions with:** azathioprine, mercaptopurine

### *Reactions*

## Skin
Acne
(1990): Zinberg J+, *Am J Gastroenterol* 85, 562
Exanthems (0.4%)
(1994): Shelley WB+, *Cutis* 53, 240 (observation)
(1991): Wadworth AN+, *Drugs* 41, 647
Lupus erythematosus
(1997): Gunnarsson I+, *Scand J Rheumatol* 26, 65
Pallor
Pruritus (1.1%)
Rash (sic) (2.3%)
(1990): 28, 57
Urticaria (4.3%)
(1987): Meyers S+, *Gastroenterology* 93, 1255

## Other
Stomatitis (1%)
Tinnitus

# OMEPRAZOLE

**Trade name:** Prilosec (AstraZeneca)
**Other common trade names:** *Antra; Audazol; Gastroloc; Inhibitron; Logastric; Losec; Mopral; Omed; Ozoken; Parizac; Ulsen*
**Indications:** Duodenal ulcer, gastroesophageal reflux disease (GERD)
**Category:** Gastric acid secretion inhibitor; proton pump inhibitor; anti-ulcer
**Half-life:** 0.5–1 hour
**Clinically important, potentially hazardous interactions with:** methotrexate

### *Reactions*

## Skin
Allergic edema (sic)
(1989): Danish Omeprazole Study Group, *BMJ* 298, 645
Angioedema (<1%)
(2002): Odeh M+, *Postgrad Med J* 78(916), 114 (passim)
(1994): Bowlby HA+, *Pharmacotherapy* 14, 119
(1992): Haeney MR, *BMJ* 305, 870
Bullous eruption
(1995): Stenier C+, *Br J Dermatol* 133, 343
Bullous pemphigoid
(1991): Chosidow O+, *Ann Dermatol Venereol* (French) 118, 45
(1990): Joly P+, *Gastroenterol Clin Biol* (French) 14, 682
Burning (sic)
(1984): Blanchi A+, *Gastroenterol Clin Biol* (French) 8, 943
Contact dermatitis
(2002): Odeh M+, *Postgrad Med J* 78(916), 114 (passim)
Diaphoresis (<1%)
(1989): Delchier JC+, *Gut* 30, 1173
Eczema (sic)

(1985): Classen M+, *Dtsch Med Wochenschr* (German) 110, 628 (scalp)
Edema (1–10%)
(2000): Natsch S+, *Ann Pharmacother* 34, 474
Erythema (sic)
(1984): Blanchi A+, *Gastroenterol Clin Biol* (French) 8, 943
Erythema multiforme (<1%)
Erythema nodosum
(1996): Ricci RM+, *Cutis* 57, 434
Erythroderma
(1999): Cockayne SE+, *Br J Dermatol* 141, 173
Exanthems
(1991): Langman MSJ, *BMJ* 303, 481
Exfoliative dermatitis
(1998): Rebuck JA+, *Pharmacotherapy* 18, 877
(1995): Epelde-Gonzalo FD+, *Ann Pharmacother* 29, 82
Fixed eruption
(1999): Kepekci Y+, *Int J Clin Pharmacol Ther* 37, 307 (hands)
Furunculosis
(1998): West BC+, *Clin Infect Dis* 26, 1234
Lichen planus
(1997): Litt JZ, Beachwood, OH (personal case) (observation)
(1986): Pounder RE+, *Scand J Gastroenterol* 21, 108
(1984): Sharma BK+, *Gut* 25, 957
Lichen spinulosus
(2002): Odeh M+, *Postgrad Med J* 78(916), 114 (passim)
(1989): Lee ML+, *Med J Aust* 150, 410
Lichenoid eruption
(2000): Bong JL+, *BMJ* 320, 283
Lupus erythematosus
(1994): Sivakumar K+, *Lancet* 344, 619
Pemphigoid (exacerbation)
(1992): Cox NH, *Lancet* 340, 857
(1991): Chosidow D+, *Ann Dermatol Venereol* (French) 118, 45
Periorbital edema
(2000): Natsch S+, *Ann Pharmacother* 34, 474
Peripheral edema (<1%)
(2001): Brunner G+, *Dig Dis Sci* 46(5), 993
Pityriasis rosea
(1996): Buckley C, *Br J Dermatol* 135, 660
Pruritus (1–10%)
(2000): Natsch S+, *Ann Pharmacother* 34, 474
(1994): Bowlby HA+, *Pharmacotherapy* 14, 119
(1989): Danish Omeprazole Study Group, *BMJ* 298, 645
(1989): Lee ML+, *Med J Aust* 150, 410
(1987): Bertaccini G+, *Clin Ter* (Italian) 121, 201
(1987): Klinkenberg-Knol EC+, *Lancet* 1, 349
(1986): Bardhan KD+, *J Clin Gastroenterol* 8, 408
(1986): Rinetti M+, *Drugs Exp Clin Res* 12, 701
Psoriasis
(1984): Blanchi A+, *Gastroenterol Clin Biol* (French) 8, 943
Purpura
Rash (sic) (1.5%)
(2002): Odeh M+, *Postgrad Med J* 78(916), 114 (passim)
(1989): Delchier JC+, *Gut* 30, 1173
(1989): Lauritsen K+, *Aliment Pharmacol Ther* 3, 59
(1988): Hirschowitz BI+, *Gastroenterol* 94, A188
(1986): Bardhan KD+, *J Clin Gastroenterol* 8, 408
Stevens–Johnson syndrome (<1%)
Toxic epidermal necrolysis (<1%)
(2002): Odeh M+, *Postgrad Med J* 78(916), 114 (passim)
(1992): Cox NH, *Lancet* 340, 857
Urticaria (1–10%)
(2002): Odeh M+, *Postgrad Med J* 78(916), 114 (passim)
(1994): Bowlby HA+, *Pharmacotherapy* 14, 119
(1994): Schneider S+, *Gastroenterol Clin Biol* (French) 18, 534
(1993): Litt JZ, Beachwood, OH (personal case) (observation)
(1992): Haeney MR, *BMJ* 305, 870
Vasculitis
(2002): Odeh M+, *Postgrad Med J* 78(916), 114 (passim)
Xerosis (<1%)
(1988): Marks IN+, *S Afr Med J* (Suppl), 54

### Hair

Hair – alopecia (<1%)
(2002): Litt JZ, Beachwood, OH (observation)
(1999): Litt JZ, Beachwood, OH (2 personal cases) (observations)
(1997): Borum ML+, *Am J Gastroenterol* 92, 1576
(1994): Bowlby HA+, *Pharmacotherapy* 14, 119 (passim)
Hair – discoloration

### Other

Anaphylactoid reactions
(2000): Natsch S+, *Ann Pharmacother* 34, 474
(1999): Galindo PA+, *Ann Allergy Asthma Immunol* 82, 52
Dysesthesia (<1%)
Dysgeusia (1–10%)
(1996): Markitziu A+, *Scand J Gastroenterol* 31, 624
Gynecomastia
(2000): Hugues FC+, *Ann Med Interne (Paris)* (French) 151, 10 (passim)
(1998): N Z Medicines Adverse Reactions Committee, (from Internet) (observation) (3 cases)
(1995): Carvajal A+, *Am J Gastroenterol* 90, 1028
(1995): Durand JM+, *Ann Med Interne* (Paris) (French) 146, 195
(1994): Garcia-Rodriguez LA+, *BMJ* 308, 503
(1994): Lindquist M+, *BMJ* 305, 451
(1994): Pedrosa M+, *Med Clin (Barc)* (Spanish) 102, 435
(1991): Convens C+, *Lancet* 338, 1153
(1991): Santucci L+, *N Engl J Med* 324, 635
Myalgia (1–10%)
Oral candidiasis
(1995): Anderson PC, *Arch Dermatol* 131, 966
(1993): Mosimann F, *Transplantation* 56, 492
(1992): Larner AJ+, *Gut* 33, 860
Paresthesias (<1%)
(1986): Rinetti M+, *Drugs Exp Clin Res* 12, 701
(1984): Blanchi A+, *Gastroenterol Clin Biol* (French) 8, 943
Tinnitus
Tremors (<1%)
Xerostomia (1–10%)
(1985): Classen M+, *Dtsch Med Wochenschr* (German) 110, 628

## ONDANSETRON

**Trade name:** Zofran (GSK)
**Other common trade names:** *Emeset; Oncoden; Zofron*
**Indications:** Nausea and vomiting
**Category:** Antiemetic; serotonin antagonist
**Half-life:** 4 hours

#### *Reactions*

### Skin

Angioedema
Chills (5–10%)
Exanthems
Fixed eruption
(2000): Bernard S+, *Dermatology* 201, 184 (similar fixed eruption from acetaminophen)
(1995): Iglesias ME+, *Dermatology* 191, 270
Flushing
(1994): Ahn MJ+, *Am J Clin Oncol* 17, 150

Pruritus (5%)
Rash (sic) (<1%)
Urticaria

### Hair

Hair – alopecia

### Other

Anaphylactoid reactions
(2001): Weiss KS, *Arch Intern Med* 161(18), 2263
(1998): Ross AK+, *Anesth Analg* 87, 779
(1991): Milne RJ+, *Drugs* 41, 574
Dysgeusia
(2000): Robbins L, *Headache* 11, 275
Hypersensitivity (<1%)
(1996): Kataja V+, *Lancet* 347, 584
Injection-site burning
Injection-site erythema
Injection-site pain
Injection-site reactions (sic) (4%)
Paresthesias (2%)
Porphyria
(1992): DeWet M+, *S Afr Med J* 82, 480
Sialopenia (1–5%)
Xerostomia (1–10%)
(1994): Ahn MJ+, *Am J Clin Oncol* 17, 150
(1991): Milne RJ+, *Drugs* 41, 574

## ORAL CONTRACEPTIVES

**Trade names:** Alesse (Wyeth); Aviane (Organon); Brevicon (Searle); Demulen (Searle); Desogen (Organon); Enovid (Ortho); Estrostep (Warner Lambert); Evra (Organon); Genora; Intercon; Jenest (Ortho); Levlen (Berlex); Levlite (Berlex); Levora (Watson); Lo/Ovral (Wyeth); Loestrin (Warner Lambert); Lunelle (Pharmacia); Mircette (Organon); Modicon (Ortho); Necon (Watson); NEE; Nelova; Nordette (Wyeth); Norethin; Norinyl (Ortho); Norlestrin (Parke Davis); Ortho Tri-Cyclen (Ortho); Ortho-Cept (Ortho); Ortho-Cyclen (Ortho); Ortho-Novum (Ortho); Ovcon (BMS); Ovral (Wyeth); Tri-Levlen (Berlex); Tri-Norinyl (Watson); Triphasil (Wyeth); Trivora (Watson); Yasmin (Schering); Zovia
**Indications:** Prevention of pregnancy
**Clinically important, potentially hazardous interactions with:** anticonvulsants, **cigarette smoking**, danazol, efavirenz, **licorice**, nelfinavir, rifabutin, rifampin, ritonavir, **saw palmetto**, selegiline, theophylline, troleandomycin, tuberculostatics

#### *Reactions*

### Skin

Acanthosis nigricans
(1975): Curth HO, *Arch Dermatol* 111, 1069
Acne
(1987): Kovacs G+, *Australasian J Dermatol* 28, 86
(1984): van der Meeren HL+, *Ned Tijdschr Geneeskd* (Dutch) 128, 1333
(1981): Scholz C+, *Zentralbl Gynakol* (German) 103, 1158
(1979): Harrison PV+, *BMJ* 2, 495
(1979): Marghescu S, *Ther Ggw* (German) 118, 2230
(1978): Amann W, *ZFA Stuttgart* (German) 54, 1809
(1974): Woodward RK, *Arch Dermatol* 110, 812
(1972): Gibbs WP, *Arch Dermatol* 109, 912
(1972): Kligman AM, *Arch Dermatol* 105, 298
(1972): Olson RL+, *Arch Dermatol* 105, 928
(1971): Dugois P+, *Ann Dermatol Syphiligr Paris* (French) 98, 479
(1971): Jelinek JE, *Am Fam Physician* 4, 68
(1971): Peterson WC, *Minn Med* 54, 836
(1971): Prenen M+, *Arch Belg Dermatol Syphiligr* (French) 27, 253
(1970): Jelinek JE, *Arch Dermatol* 101, 181
(1969): Chanial G+, *Bull Soc Fr Dermatol Syphiligr* (French) 76, 125
(1969): Racouchot J+, *Bull Soc Fr Dermatol Syphiligr* (French) 76, 132
Acute febrile neutrophilic dermatosis (Sweet's syndrome)
(2002): Saez M+, *Dermatology* 204(1), 84
(1991): Tefany FJ+, *Aust J Dermatol* 32, 55
Angioedema
(2000): Bouillet L+, *Presse Med* (French) 29, 640
(1990): Borradori L+, *Dermatologica* 181, 78
(1967): Wolf RJ, *JAMA* 201, 982
Autoimmune progesterone dermatitis
(1981): Stone J+, *Int J Dermatol* 20, 50
Bullous eruption
(1981): Honeyman JF+, *Arch Dermatol* 117, 264
Candidiasis
(1983): Lebherz TB+, *Clin Ther* 5, 409
(1979): Marghescu S, *Ther Ggw* (German) 118, 1230
(1976): Aron-Brunetiere R, *Contracept Fertil Sex* (Paris) (French) 4, 175
(1971): Jelinek JE, *Am Fam Physician* 4, 68
(1970): Jelinek JE, *Arch Dermatol* 101, 181
(1969): Langer H, *Munch Med Wochenschr* (German) 111, 1748
(1968): Walsh H+, *Amer J Obstet Gynec* 101, 991
(1966): Catterall RD, *Lancet* 2, 830
(1966): Porter PS+, *Arch Dermatol* 93, 402
Chloasma
(1987): Kovacs G+, *Australasian J Dermatol* 28, 86
(1977): Smith AG+, *J Invest Dermatol* 68, 169
(1972): Ippen H, *Arch Dermatol Forsch* (German) 244, 500
(1972): Ippen H+, *Hautarzt* (German) 23, 21
(1972): Ippen H+, *Hautarzt* (German) 23, 235
(1971): Amblard P+, *Bull Soc Fr Dermatol Syphiligr* (French) 78, 561
(1969): Racouchot J+, *Bull Soc Fr Dermatol Syphiligr* (French) 76, 132
(1968): Carruthers R, *Practitioner* 200, 564
(1967): Basset H, *Bull Soc Fr Dermatol Syphiligr* (French) 74, 166
(1967): Carruthers R, *BMJ* 3, 307
(1967): Merklen FP+, *Bull Soc Fr Dermatol Syphiligr* (French) 74, 801
(1967): Quamina DB, *BMJ* 2, 638
(1966): Carruthers R, *Med J Aust* 2, 17
Cold urticaria
(1983): Burns MR+, *Ann Intern Med* 98, 1025
Dermatitis herpetiformis
(1972): Haim S+, *Dermatologica* 145, 199
Eczema (sic)
(1988): Edman B, *Acta Derm Venereol* 68, 402 (palmar)
Edema
Erythema
(1973): Delius L, *Dtsch Med Wochenschr* (German) 98, 1512 (flush-like)
Erythema multiforme
(1973): Naess K, *Tidsskr Nor Laegeforen* (Norwegian) 93, 2498
(1970): Savel H+, *Arch Dermatol* 101, 187
Erythema nodosum
(1981): Touboul JL+, *Nouv Presse Med* (French) 10, 712
(1980): Beaucaire G+, *Sem Hôp* (French) 56, 1426
(1980): Salvatore MA+, *Arch Dermatol* 116, 557
(1977): Bombardieri S+, *BMJ* 1, 1509
(1977): Taaffe A+, *BMJ* 2, 1353
(1976): Bernstein MZ+, *J Am Podiatry Assoc* 66, 417

(1976): Posternak F, *Rev Med Suisse Romande* (French) 96, 375
(1974): Berant N, *Harefuah* (Hebrew) 87, 19
(1974): Darlington LG, *Br J Dermatol* 90, 209
(1973): Elias PM, *Arch Dermatol* 108, 716
(1973): Kariher DH, *Obstet Gynecol* 42, 323
(1973): Stumbo WG, *J Ky Med Assoc* 71, 433
(1972): Kirby J+, *Obstet Gynecol* 40, 409
(1971): Jelinek JE, *Am Fam Physician* 4, 68
(1970): Jelinek JE, *Arch Dermatol* 101, 181
(1970): Savel H+, *Arch Dermatol* 101, 187
(1968): Baden HP+, *Arch Dermatol* 98, 634
(1967): Matz MH, *N Engl J Med* 276, 351

Exanthems
(1981): Scholz C+, *Zentralbl Gynakol* (German) 103, 1158

Fixed eruption
(1977): Coskey R, *Arch Dermatol* 113, 333

Fox-Fordyce disease
(1971): Jelinek JE, *Am Fam Physician* 4, 68

Herpes genitalis (sic)
(1981): Scholz C+, *Zentralbl Gynakol* (German) 103, 1158

Herpes gestationis
(1989): Kemper T+, *Akt Dermatol* (German) 15, 121
(1975): Kocsis M+, *Acta Derm Venereol* (Stockh) 55, 25
(1968): Morgan JK, *Br J Dermatol* 80, 456

Lichenoid eruption
(1977): Coskey R, *Arch Dermatol* 113, 333

Livedo racemosa (Sneddon's syndrome)
(1991): Berchtold B+, *Hautarzt* (German) 42, 328

Lupus erythematosus
(2001): Kakehasi AM+, *Arq Neuropsiquiatr* 59(3), 609
(1994): Hess EV+, *Curr Opin Rheumatology* 6, 474
(1994): Strom BL+, *Am J Epidemiol* 140, 632
(1993): Arden NK+, *Lupus* 2, 381
(1991): Furukawa F+, *J Dermatology* (Tokio) 18, 56
(1990): Franceschi S+, *Tumori* (Italian) 76, 439
(1990): Zanetti R+, *Int J Epidemiol* 19, 522
(1989): Beaumont V+, *Clin Physiol Biochem* 7, 263
(1989): Iskander MK+, *J Rheumatol* 16, 850
(1988): Mathur AK+, *J Rheumatology* 15, 1042
(1986): Asherson RA+, *Arthritis Rheum* 29, 1535
(1982): Jungers P+, *Arthritis Rheum* 25, 618
(1982): Jungers P+, *Nouv Presse Med* (French) 11, 3765
(1980): Garovich M+, *Arthritis Rheum* 23, 1396
(1975): Bielecka H, *Reumatologia* (Polish) 13, 223
(1974): Zurcher K+, *Dermatologica* 149, 321
(1973): Elias PM, *Arch Dermatol* 108, 716
(1972): Cordonnier V+, *J Sci Med Lille* (French) 90, 431
(1972): Dorfmann H+, *Nouv Presse Med* (French) 1, 2907
(1972): Tuffanelli DL, *Arch Dermatol* 106, 553
(1971): Chapel TA+, *Am J Obstet Gynecol* 110, 366
(1971): Cornet A+, *Ann Med Interne Paris* (French) 122, 1151
(1971): Laugier P+, *Bull Soc Fr Dermatol Syphiligr* (French) 78, 632
(1969): Rothfield NF, *Mayo Clin Proc* 44, 691
(1968): Dubois EL+, *Lancet* 2, 679
(1968): Pimstone BL, *Lancet* 1, 1153
(1968): Schleicher EM, *Lancet* 1, 821

Melanoma
(1992): Le MG+, *Cancer Causes Control* 3, 199
(1985): Bork K, *Hautarzt* (German) 36, 542
(1985): Gallagher RP+, *Br J Cancer* 52, 901
(1985): Green A+, *Med J Aust* 142, 446
(1985): Quencez E+, *Ann Dermatol Venereol* (French) 112, 341

Melasma
(1985): Lutfi RJ+, *J Clin Endocrinol Metab* 61, 28
(1981): Witkiewicz IM+, *Ned Tijdschr Geneeskd* (Dutch) 125, 609
(1970): Jelinek JE, *Arch Dermatol* 101, 181
(1968): *Northwest Med* 67, 251
(1967): Carruthers R, *BMJ* 3, 307
(1967): Resnick S, *JAMA* 199, 601
(1967): Resnick SS, *Trans N Engl Obstet Gynecol Soc* 21, 107
(1966): Resnick SS, *JAMA* 197, 25

Mucha–Habermann disease
(1973): Hollander A+, *Arch Dermatol* 107, 465

Perioral dermatitis
(1989): Ehlers G, *Hautarzt* (German) 20, 287
(1977): Kalkoff KW+, *Hautarzt* (German) 28, 74
(1975): Hornstein OP, *Internist Berl* (German) 16, 27
(1974): Buck A+, *Dtsch Med Wochenschr* (German) 99, 366
(1974): Reinken L+, *Int J Vitam Nutr Res* (German) 44, 75
(1972): Toyosi JO, *Hautarzt* (German) 23, 79
(1971): Kleine-Natrop HE, *Hautarzt* (German) 22, 508
(1969): Steigleder GK+, *Hautarzt* (German) 20, 288

Photosensitivity
(1994): Litt JZ, Beachwood, OH (personal case) (observation)
(1979): Marghescu S, *Ther Ggw* (German) 118, 1230
(1977): Roberts DT+, *Br J Dermatol* 96, 549
(1975): Horkay I+, *Arch Dermatol Res* 253, 53
(1973): Levantine A+, *Br J Dermatol* 89, 105
(1971): Elgart ML+, *Med Ann Dist Columbia* 40, 501
(1971): Jelinek JE, *Am Fam Physician* 4, 68
(1970): Jelinek JE, *Arch Dermatol* 101, 181
(1970): Mathison IW+, *Obstet Gynecol Surv* 25, 389
(1968): Erickson LR+, *JAMA* 203, 980
(1968): Oosterhuis WW, *Ned Tijdschr Geneeskd* (Dutch) 112, 2154

Pigmentation
(1981): Granstein RD+, *J Am Acad Dermatol* 5, 1
(1981): Scholz C+, *Zentralbl Gynakol* (German) 103, 1158
(1980): Hertz RS+, *J Am Dent Assoc* 100, 713
(1979): Marghescu S, *Ther Ggw* (German) 118, 1230
(1978): Harlap S, *Lancet* 2, 39
(1976): Aron-Brunetiere R, *Contracept Fertil Sex Paris* (French) 4, 175
(1972): Ippen H, *Arch Dermatol Forsch* (German) 244, 500
(1972): Leonhardi G, *Arch Dermatol Forsch* (German) 244, 495
(1971): Bazex A, *Rev Fr Gynecol Obset* (French) 66, 575
(1971): Dugois P+, *Ann Dermatol Syphiligr Paris* (French) 98, 479
(1971): Jelinek JE, *Am Fam Physician* 4, 68
(1971): Kleine-Natrop HE, *Dermatol Monatsschr* (German) 157, 549
(1970): Jelinek JE, *Arch Dermatol* 101, 181
(1969): Chanial G+, *Bull Soc Fr Dermatol Syphiligr* (French) 76, 125
(1968): Gotz H+, *Munch Med Wochenschr* (German) 110, 1913
(1968): Sotaniemi E+, *BMJ* 2, 120
(1967): No Author, *S Afr Med J* 41, 709
(1965): No Author, *BMJ* 5471, 1180

Polymorphous light eruption
(1989): Boonstra H+, *Photodermatol* 6, 55
(1988): Neumann R, *Photodermatol* 5, 40

Pruritus (<1%)
(1976): Medline A+, *Am J Gastroenterol* 65, 156
(1975): Gagnaire JC+, *Nouv Presse Med* (French) 4, 1105
(1971): Dugois P+, *Rev Fr Gynecol Obstet* (French) 66, 589
(1970): Dahl MG, *Trans St Johns Hosp Dermatol Soc* 56(1), 11
(1969): Baker H, *Br J Dermatol* 81, 946 (passim)

Psoriasis
(1981): Scholz C+, *Zentralbl Gynakol* (German) 103, 1158

Purpura
(1983): McShane PM+, *Am J Obstet Gynecol* 145, 762
(1971): Jelinek JE, *Am Fam Physician* 4, 68
(1970): Jelinek JE, *Arch Dermatol* 101, 181

Seborrhea
(1981): Scholz C+, *Zentralbl Gynakol* (German) 103, 1158 (seborrheic dermatitis)
(1979): Marghescu S, *Ther Ggw* (German) 118, 1230

(1969): Chanial G+, *Bull Soc Fr Dermatol Syphiligr* (French) 76, 125

Spider angiomas
(1970): Goldman L, *Lancet* 1, 108
(1970): Jelinek JE, *Arch Dermatol* 101, 181

Stevens–Johnson syndrome
(1972): O'Callaghan J+, *Med J Aust* 1, 695

Telangiectases
(1983): Wilkin JK+, *J Am Acad Dermatol* 8, 468
(1971): Jelinek JE, *Am Fam Physician* 4, 68
(1970): Goldman L, *Lancet* 2, 108
(1970): Jelinek JE, *Arch Dermatol* 101, 181
(1968): Gotz H+, *Munch Med Wochenschr* (German) 110, 1913
(1964): Kopera H+, *Int J Fertil* 9, 69

Urticaria
(1981): Scholz C+, *Zentralbl Gynakol* (German) 103, 1158
(1970): Meyer-de-Schmid JJ+, *Bull Soc Fr Dermatol Syphiligr* (French) 77, 158

Varicosities

## Hair

Hair – alopecia
(1989): Burke KE, *Postgrad Med* 85, 52
(1987): Kovacs G+, *Australasian J Dermatol* 28, 86
(1982): Hauser GA+, *Int J Tissue React* 4, 159
(1981): Scholz C+, *Zentralbl Gynakol* (German) 103, 1158
(1979): Marghescu S, *Ther Ggw* (German) 118, 1230
(1979): Price VH, *Int J Dermatol* 18, 95
(1978): Bergfeld W, *Cutis* 22, 190
(1978): Zaun H, *Dtsch Med Wochenschr* (German) 103, 240
(1974): Haim S, *Harefuah* (Hebrew) 86, 155
(1973): Levantine A+, *Br J Dermatol* 89, 549
(1973): No Author, *BMJ* 2, 499
(1973): Zaun H, *Z Geburtshilfe Perinatol* 177, 67
(1971): Dawber RP+, *BMJ* 4, 234
(1971): Prenen M+, *Arch Belg Dermatol Syphiligr* (French) 27, 253
(1970): Zaun H, *Dtsch Med Wochenschr* (German) 95, 1433
(1969): Chanial G+, *Bull Soc Fr Dermatol Syphiligr* (French) 76, 125
(1968): *BMJ* 1, 593
(1967): Cormia FE, *JAMA* 201, 635

Hair – alopecia areata
(1971): Jelinek JE, *Am Fam Physician* 4, 68
(1966): Orentreich N+, *BMJ* 5485, 483
(1965): *BMJ* 5470, 1124
(1965): Vallings R, *BMJ* 23, 1005

Hair – hirsutism
(1994): Burdova M+, *Ceska Gynekol* (Czech) 59, 62
(1987): Kovacs G+, *Australasian J Dermatol* 28, 86
(1981): Scholz C+, *Zentralbl Gynakol* (German) 103, 1158
(1979): Marghescu S, *Ther Ggw* (German) 118, 1230
(1973): Zaun H, *Hautarzt* (German) 24, 1
(1973): Zaun H, *Z Geburtshilfe Perinatol* (German) 177, 67
(1971): Dugois P+, *Ann Dermatol Syphiligr Paris* (French) 98, 479
(1971): Jelinek JE, *Am Fam Physician* 4, 68
(1971): Prenen M+, *Arch Belg Dermatol Syphiligr* (French) 27, 253
(1969): Chanial G+, *Bull Soc Fr Dermatol Syphiligr* (French) 76, 125
(1968): Gotz H+, *Munch Med Wochenschr* (German) 110, 1913
(1966): Carruthers R, *Med J Aust* 2, 17

## Nails

Nails – onycholysis
(1976): Byrne JPH+, *Postgrad Med J* 52, 535

## Other

Acute intermittent porphyria
(1979): Brinkmann OH+, *ZFA Stuttgart* (German) 55, 1227
(1978): Gerlis LS, *J Int Med Res* 6, 255
(1977): Tasic D+, *Med Pregl* (Serbo-Croatian) 30, 577
(1975): Schley G+, *Verh Dtsch Ges Inn Med* (German) 81, 1061
(1971): Contro L+, *Minerva Med* (Italian) 62, 2238

Application-site reactions
(2002): Sibai BM+, *Fertil Steril* 77(2 Suppl 2), S19 (patch) (92%)

Depression
(2001): Freeman MP, *JAMA* 286(6), 671

Galactorrhea
(1969): Friedman S+, *JAMA* 210, 1888

Gingival hyperplasia
(1967): Lindhe J+, *J Periodont Res* 2, 1
(1962): Sumner CF+, *J Periodont* 33, 344

Oral mucosal pigmentation
(1980): Hertz RS+, *J Am Dent Assoc* 100, 713 (gingival)

Porphyria cutanea prematura
(1977): Doss M, *Dtsch Med Wochenschr* (German) 102, 875
(1977): Leonhardi G+, *Dtsch Med Wochenschr* (German) 102, 160

Porphyria cutanea tarda
(2001): Emri G+, *Orv Hetil* 142(47), 2635
(1992): McKenna KE+, *Br J Dermatol* 127, 401
(1983): Doss M, *Dtsch Med Wochenschr* (German) 108, 1857
(1983): Zaumseil RP+, *Zentralbl Gynakol* (German) 105, 527
(1982): Zaumseil RP+, *Z Gesamte In Med* (German) 37, 703
(1981): Fiedler H+, *Dermatol Monatsschr* (German) 167, 481
(1979): Grossman ME+, *Am J Med* 67, 277
(1979): Willerson D+, *Ann Ophthalmol* 11, 409
(1977): Roberts DT+, *Br J Dermatol* 96, 549
(1976): Aron-Brunetiere R, *Contracept Fertil Sex Paris* (French) 4, 175
(1976): Byrne JPH+, *Postgrad Med J* 52, 536
(1976): Curtis P, *Br J Clin Pract* 30, 47
(1975): Austad WI+, *N Z Med J* 81, 8
(1974): Behm AR+, *Can Med Assoc J* 110, 1052
(1974): Le Reun M+, *Concours Med* (French) 96, 2697
(1974): Nuss A+, *Z Haut* (German) 49, 273
(1974): Vosmik F+, *Cesk Dermatol* (Czech) 49, 298
(1973): Constantinidis A+, *Minerva Ginecol* (Italian) 25, 192
(1973): Gajdos A+, *Nouv Presse Med* (French) 2, 1131
(1973): Gutzwiller P, *Dermatologia* (German) 146, 342
(1973): Palma-Carlos AG+, *Nouv Presse Med* (French) 1, 1996
(1973): Ruszczak Z+, *Wiad Lek* (Polish) 26, 2177
(1972): No Author, *BMJ* 3, 603
(1971): Goldswain PR+, *S Afr Med J* 25, 111
(1971): Jelinek JE, *Am Fam Physician* 4, 68
(1970): Roenigk HH+, *Arch Dermatol* 102, 260
(1969): Degos R+, *Ann Dermatol Syphiligr Paris* (French) 96, 5
(1967): Huber FB, *Schweiz Med Wochenschr* (German) 97, 1498

Porphyria variegata
(1975): Fowler CJ+, *BMJ* 1, 663
(1972): McKenzie AW+, *Br J Dermatol* 86, 453

Thrombophlebitis
(1967): Merklen FP+, *Bull Soc Fr Dermatol Syphiligr* (French) 74, 801

Tremors
(2001): Chetty M+, *Ther Drug Monit* 23(5), 556 (with chlorpromazine)

# ORLISTAT

**Trade name:** Xenical (Roche)
**Indications:** Obesity, weight reduction
**Category:** Lipase inhibitor
**Half-life:** 1–2 hours
**Clinically important, potentially hazardous interactions with:** cyclosporine

### *Reactions*

#### Skin
Dermatitis (sic)
Pedal edema
Rash (sic) (4.3%)
Xerosis

#### Other
Gingivitis (4.1%)
Myalgia (4.2%)
Tendinitis
Tooth disorder (sic) (4.3%)
Vaginitis (3.8%)

# ORPHENADRINE

**Trade names:** Banflex (Forest); Norflex (3M)
**Other common trade names:** *Biorfen; Biorphen; Disipal; Distalene; Flexojet; Flexon; Myolin; Norgesic; Opheryl; Orfenace; Prolongatum*
**Indications:** Painful musculoskeletal conditions
**Category:** Skeletal muscle relaxant
**Half-life:** 14 hours

### *Reactions*

#### Skin
Exanthems
Fixed eruption
(1998): Mahboob A+, *Int J Dermatol* 37, 833
Flushing (1–10%)
Pigment disorder (sic)
(1978): Rebhun J, *Ann Allergy* 40, 44
Pruritus
Rash (sic) (1–10%)
Urticaria

#### Other
Anaphylactoid reactions
Embolia cutis medicamentosa (Nicolau syndrome)
(1976): Brachtel R, *Med Klin* (German) 71, 504
Hypersensitivity
Paresthesias
Xerostomia

# OSELTAMIVIR

**Trade name:** Tamiflu (Roche)
**Indications:** Influenza infection
**Category:** Antiviral (neuraminidase inhibitor)
**Half-life:** 6–10 hours

### *Reactions*

#### Other
Cough
(2002): Bowles SK+, *J Am Geriatr Soc* 50(4), 608

# OXACILLIN

**Trade name:** Oxacillin
**Other common trade names:** *Bactocill; Bristopen; Prostaphlin; Stapenor*
**Indications:** Various infections caused by susceptible organisms
**Category:** Penicillinase-resistant penicillin antibiotic
**Half-life:** 23–60 minutes
**Clinically important, potentially hazardous interactions with:** anticoagulants, cyclosporine, demeclocycline, doxycycline, methotrexate, minocycline, oxytetracycline, tetracycline

### *Reactions*

#### Skin
Angioedema
Bullous eruption
(1974): Hadida E+, *Bull Soc Fr Dermatol Syphiligr* (French) 81, 87
Ecchymoses
Erythema multiforme
Erythema nodosum
Exanthems
(1978): Bruevich TS+, *Vestn Dermatol Venerol* (Russian) March, 74
(1974): Spitzy KH, *Acta Med Austriaca* (German) 2, 46
Exfoliative dermatitis
Hematomas
Jarisch–Herxheimer reaction
Necrosis
(1980): Tilden SJ+, *Am J Dis Child* 134, 1046
Pruritus
(1998): Siegfried EC+, *J Am Acad Dermatol* 39, 797 (passim)
Rash (sic) (<1%)
(2002): Maraqa NF+, *Clin Infect Dis* 34(1), 50 (22%)
Stevens–Johnson syndrome
(1982): Sukovatykh TN+, *Pediatriia* (Russian) May, 76
Toxic epidermal necrolysis
Urticaria
(1998): Siegfried EC+, *J Am Acad Dermatol* 39, 797 (passim)
Vasculitis
(2001): Koutkia P+, *Diagn Microbiol Infect Dis* 46(5), 993

#### Other
Anaphylactoid reactions (0.04%)
(1998): Siegfried EC+, *J Am Acad Dermatol* 39, 797 (passim)
Black tongue
Dysgeusia
Glossitis
Glossodynia
Hypersensitivity

Injection-site pain
Oral candidiasis
Phlebitis
Serum sickness (<1%)
Stomatitis
Stomatodynia
Thrombophlebitis
Tongue furry
Vaginitis
Xerostomia

# OXAPROZIN

**Trade name:** Daypro (Searle)
**Other common trade names:** *Deflam; Duraprox*
**Indications:** Arthritis
**Category:** Nonsteroidal anti-inflammatory (NSAID)
**Half-life:** 42–50 hours
**Clinically important, potentially hazardous interactions with:** methotrexate

### *Reactions*

## Skin

Angioedema (<1%)
Diaphoresis (<1%)
Ecchymoses (<1%)
Edema (<1%)
Erythema
Erythema multiforme (<1%)
(1986): Todd PA+, *Drugs* 32, 291
Exanthems
(1995): Litt JZ, Beachwood, OH (personal case) (observation)
(1994): Litt JZ, Beachwood, OH (personal case) (observation)
(1994): Shelley WB+, *Cutis* 54, 72 (eczematous eruption) (observation)
(1983): Hubsher JA+, *Clin Pharmacol Ther* 33, 267
Exfoliative dermatitis (<1%)
Fixed eruption
(1999): Blumenthal HL, Beachwood, OH (personal case) (observation)
Linear IgA dermatosis
(1999): Abate KL+, *Arch Dermatol* 135, 81–86 (off-center fold)
Photosensitivity (<1%)
Phototoxicity
(1995): Shelley WB+, *Cutis* 55, 143 (observation)
(1986): Todd PA+, *Drugs* 32, 291
Pruritus (1–10%)
(1994): Shelley WB+, *Cutis* 53, 284 (observation)
Purpura
Rash (sic) (>10%)
(1983): Kahn SB+, *J Clin Pharmacol* 23, 139
(1978): Jamar R+, *Curr Med Res Op* 5, 433
Stevens–Johnson syndrome (<1%)
(1998): Bell MJ+, *J Rheumatol* 25, 2027
Toxic epidermal necrolysis
(1999): Carucci JA+, *Int J Dermatol* 38, 233
(1999): Egan CA+, *J Am Acad Dermatol* 40, 458
(1998): Paul CD+, *J Burn Care Rehabil* 19, 321 (fatal)
Urticaria (<1%)
(1997): Hicks A, Houston, TX (from Internet) (observation) (Note: Person is not a physician)
Vasculitis
(1999): Reed BR, Denver, CO (from Internet) (observation)

## Hair

Hair – alopecia

## Other

Anaphylactoid reactions (<1%)
Death
Dysgeusia
Pseudolymphoma
(2001): Werth V, *Dermatology Times* 18
Pseudoporphyria
(1999): Al-Khenaizan S+, *J Cutan Med Surg* 3, 162
(1996): Ingrish G+, *Arch Dermatol* 132, 1519
(1996): Jaffe PG, Columbia, SC (from Internet) (observation)
Serum sickness (<1%)
Stomatitis (<1%)
Tinnitus

# OXAZEPAM

**Trade name:** Oxazepam
**Other common trade names:** *Adumbran; Apo-Oxazepam; Azutranquil; Durazepam; Murelax; Novoxapam; Oxpam; Praxiten; Serax; Serepax; Zapex*
**Indications:** Anxiety, depression
**Category:** Benzodiazepine antianxiety and sedative-hypnotic; anticonvulsant
**Half-life:** 3–6 hours
**Clinically important, potentially hazardous interactions with:** amprenavir, chlorpheniramine, clarithromycin, efavirenz, esomeprazole, imatinib, nelfinavir

### *Reactions*

## Skin

Dermatitis (sic) (1–10%)
Diaphoresis (>10%)
Edema
Erythema multiforme
(1986): McAlpine C, *BMJ* 293, 510
Exanthems
Fixed eruption
(1996): Krischer J, *Arch Dermatol* 132, 718
Pruritus
Purpura
Rash (sic) (>10%)
Toxic epidermal necrolysis
(2001): van der Meer JB+, *Clin Exp Dermatol* 26(8), 654
Urticaria

## Other

Paresthesias
Sialopenia (>10%)
Sialorrhea (1–10%)
Tongue, coated
Tremors
Xerostomia (>10%)

# OXCARBAZEPINE

**Synonym:** GP 47680
**Trade name:** Trileptal (Novartis)
**Indications:** Partial epileptic seizures
**Category:** Anticonvulsant
**Half-life:** 1–2.5 hours

### *Reactions*

## Skin

Acne
Allergy (sic) (2%)
(1994): Dam M, *Epilepsia* 35, S23
(1993): Beran RG, *Epilepsia* 34, 163
Angioedema
Contact dermatitis
Diaphoresis (3%)
Eczema
Edema (2%)
Erythema multiforme
Exanthems
(1999): Ruble R+, *CNS Drugs* 12, 215
Facial rash (sic)
Folliculitis
Genital pruritus
Hot flashes (2%)
Infections (sic) (2%)
Lupus erythematosus
Photosensitivity
Purpura (2%)
Rash (sic) (4%)
(1993): Friis ML+, *Acta Neurol Scand* 84, 224 (6%)
Sensitivity (sic)
(1991): Watts D+, *Neurol Neurosurg Psychiatry* 54, 376
Stevens–Johnson syndrome
Toxic epidermal necrolysis
Vitiligo

## Hair

Hair – alopecia

## Other

Dysgeusia (5%)
Gingival hyperplasia
Hypersensitivity
(2001): No authors, *Prescrire Int* 10(56), 170
Hypesthesia (3%)
Priapism
Stomatitis
Toothache (2%)
Tremors (4–6%)
Ulcerative stomatitis
Vaginitis (2%)
Xerostomia (3%)

# OXYBUTYNIN

**Trade name:** Ditropan (Alza)
**Other common trade names:** *Albert Oxybutynin; Cystrin; Dridase; Novitropan; Oxyban; Tropax*
**Indications:** Neurogenic bladder, urinary incontinence
**Category:** Urinary antispasmodic
**Half-life:** 1–2.3 hours
**Clinically important, potentially hazardous interactions with:** anticholenergics, arbutamine

### *Reactions*

## Skin

Allergic reactions (sic) (<1%)
(1993): Jonville AP+, *Arch Fr Pediatr* (French) 50, 27
(1992): Jonville AP+, *Therapie* (French) 47, 389
Erythema multiforme
(1992): Jonville AP+, *Therapie* (French) 47, 389
Flushing
Hot flashes (1–10%)
Hypohidrosis (>10%)
Pruritus
(2001): Ho C, *Issues Emerg Health Technol* 24, 1 (18%)
Rash (sic) (1–10%)
Urticaria
Xerosis
(1998): Arango Toro O+, *Actas Urol Esp* (Spanish) 22, 124 (6%)

## Other

Anhidrosis
Sialopenia
(1998): Arango Toro O+, *Actas Urol Esp* (Spanish) 22, 124 (42%)
(1995): Loesche WJ+, *J Am Geriatr Soc* 43, 401
Xerostomia (>10%)
(2002): Youdim K+, *Urology* 59(3), 428
(2001): Crandall C, *J Womens Health Gend Based Med* 10(8), 735
(2001): Davila GW+, *J Urol* 166(1), 140 (67–94%)
(2001): Harvey MA+, *Am J Obstet Gynecol* 185, 56
(2001): Ho C, *Issues Emerg Health Technol* 24, 1
(2000): Versi E+, *Obstet Gynecol* 95, 718
(1995): Loesche WJ+, *J Am Geriatr Soc* 43, 401

# OXYCODONE

**Trade names:** Endocodone; OxyContin (Purdue); OxyIR (Purdue); Percodan (Endo); Percolone (Endo); Percoset (Endo); Roxicodone (Roxane); Tylox (McNeil)
**Other common trade name:** *Supeudol*
**Indications:** Pain
**Category:** Narcotic analgesic
**Half-life:** 4.6 hours
**Clinically important, potentially hazardous interactions with:** cimetidine

Oxycodone is often combined with acetaminophen (Percoset, Roxicet, Tylox) or aspirin (Percodan, Roxiprin)

### *Reactions*

## Skin

Diaphoresis
Pruritus
(1999): Hale ME+, *Clin J Pain* 15, 179
(1999): Salzman RT+, *J Pain Symptom Manage* 18, 271

Rash (sic) (<1%)
Urticaria (<1%)

### Other

Injection-site pain (1–10%)
Xerostomia (1–10%)

## OXYTETRACYCLINE

**Trade name:** Terramycin (Pfizer)
**Other common trade names:** *Aknin; Cotet; Macocyn; Oxacycle; Oxitraklin; Oxy; Rorap; Terramycine; Uri-Tet*
**Indications:** Various infections caused by susceptible organisms
**Category:** Tetracycline antibiotic; antiprotozoal
**Half-life:** 6–10 hours
**Clinically important, potentially hazardous interactions with:** amoxicillin, ampicillin, antacids, bacampicillin, calcium, carbenicillin, cloxacillin, digoxin, methotrexate, methoxyflurane, mezlocillin, nafcillin, oxacillin, penicillins, piperacillin, ticarcillin

### *Reactions*

### Skin

Angioedema
Contact dermatitis
(1976): Moller H, *Contact Dermatitis* 2, 289
(1974): Bojs G+, *Berufsdermatosen* (German) 22, 202
(1969): Walczynski Z+, *Wiad Lek* (Polish) 22, 929
Exanthems
Exfoliative dermatitis (<1%)
Fixed eruption
(1985): Gomez B+, *Allergol Immunopathol Madr* (Spanish) 13, 87
(1981): Shukla SR, *Dermatologica* 163, 160
(1975): Giminez-Garcia RM+, *N Engl J Med* 292, 819
(1970): Delaney TJ, *Br J Dermatol* 83, 357
(1952): Dougherty JW, *Arch Dermatol* 65, 485
Lupus erythematosus
Photosensitivity (1–10%)
(1987): Santucci B+, *G Ital Dermatol Venereol* (Italian) 122, IL-LII
(1982): Hawk JL, *Clin Exp Dermatol* 7, 341
(1977): Ramsay CA, *Clin Exp Dermatol* 2, 255
(1963): Tromovitch TA+, *Ann Intern Med* 58, 529 (1–5%)
Pigmentation
Pruritus (<1%)
Purpura
(1975): Kounis NG, *JAMA* 231, 734
Pustular eruption
(1971): Stevanovic DN, *Br J Dermatol* 85, 134
Sensitivity (sic)
(1997): Rudzki E+, *Contact Dermatitis* 37, 136
Urticaria
Vasculitis

### Nails

Nails – pigmentation (<1%)

### Other

Anaphylactoid reactions (<1%)
Black tongue
(1954): No Author, *Lancet* 2, 179
Hypersensitivity (<1%)
Oral mucosal lesions
(1971): Merdi T+, *Czas Stomatol* (Polish) 24, 1309
Paresthesias (<1%)
Porphyria cutanea tarda
(1982): Hawk JL, *Clin Exp Dermatol* 7, 341
Pseudotumor cerebri (<1%)
Thrombophlebitis (<1%)
Tooth discoloration (>10%) (in children)

# PACLITAXEL

**Trade name:** Taxol (Bristol-Myers Squibb)
**Other common trade name:** *Paxene*
**Indications:** Metastatic carcinoma of the ovary
**Category:** Antineoplastic
**Half-life:** 5–17 hours

## *Reactions*

### Skin

Acral erythema
(1996): de Argila D+, *Dermatology* 192, 377
(1995): Zimmerman GC+, *Arch Dermatol* 131, 202

Allergic reactions (sic)
(2001): Ansell SM+, *Cancer* 91(8), 1543
(2001): Hurwitz CA+, *J Pediatr Hematol Oncol* 23(5), 277
(2001): Sakai H+, *Cancer Chemother Pharmacol* 48(6), 499 (with cisplatin)

Angioedema
(1990): Weiss RB+, *J Clin Oncol* 8, 1263

Cutaneous manifestations (sic)
(1995): Link CJ+, *Invest New Drugs* 13, 261

Cutaneous reactions (sic)
(2002): Feher O+, *Head Neck* 24(3), 228

Edema (21%)

Erythema
(2001): Robinson JB+, *Gynecol Oncol* 82(3), 550
(1995): Berghmans T+, *Support Care Cancer* 3, 203
(1995): Zimmerman GC+, *Arch Dermatol* 131, 202

Erythrodysesthesia
(1994): Zimmerman GC+, *J Natl Cancer Inst* 86, 557
(1993): Vukelja SJ+, *J Natl Cancer Inst* 85, 1423

Exanthems (<1%)
(1990): Weiss RB+, *J Clin Oncol* 8, 1263

Fixed eruption
(2000): Baykal C+, *Eur J Gynaecol Oncol* 21, 190
(1996): Young PC+, *J Am Acad Dermatol* 34, 313 (bullous)

Flushing (28%)
(2001): Robinson JB+, *Gynecol Oncol* 82(3), 550
(1990): Weiss RB+, *J Clin Oncol* 8, 1263

Infections (sic) (>10%)
(2001): Fidias P+, *Clin Cancer Res* 7(12), 3942 (8.8%)

Photosensitivity
(2000): Mermershtain W+, *Ann Oncol* 11(suppl 4), 28 (with trastuzumab) (3 cases)

Pruritus (<1%)
(2001): Robinson JB+, *Gynecol Oncol* 82(3), 550
(1995): Freilich RJ+, *J Natl Cancer Inst* 87, 933
(1990): Weiss RB+, *J Clin Oncol* 8, 1263

Purpura

Pustular eruption
(1997): Weinberg JM+, *Int J Dermatol* 36, 559

Radiation recall (<1%)
(1996): McCarty MJ+, *Med Pediatr Oncol* 27, 185
(1995): Phillips KA+, *J Clin Oncol* 13, 305
(1995): Schweitzer VG+, *Cancer* 76, 1069
(1994): Shenkier T+, *J Clin Oncol* 12, 439
(1993): Raghavan VT+, *Lancet* 341, 1354

Rash (sic) (12%)

Urticaria
(1990): Weiss RB+, *J Clin Oncol* 8, 1263

### Hair

Hair – alopecia (87 – 100%)
(2002): Iwamoto S+, *Gan To Kagaku Ryoho* 29(6), 917
(2002): Sehouli J+, *Gynecol Oncol* 85(2), 321 (with carboplatin)
(2001): Rohl J+, *Gynecol Oncol* 81(2), 201
(2001): Sakai H+, *Cancer Chemother Pharmacol* 48(6), 499 (with cisplatin)
(2000): Oettle H+, *Anticancer Drugs* 11(8), 635
(1997): Jiang Z+, *Chung Hua Chung Liu Tsa Chih* (Chinese) 19, 445
(1995): Lemenager M+, *Lancet* 346, 371
(1990): McGuire WP+, *Ann Intern Med* 111, 273 (total) (100%) (between days 14 and 21; reversible)

### Nails

Nails – disorders (sic)
(1998): Luftner D+, *Ann Oncol* 9, 1139

Nails – onycholysis
(2000): Hussain S+, *Cancer* 88, 2367 (5 cases)
(1999): Flory SM+, *Ann Pharmacother* 33, 584

Nails – pigmentation (2%)
(1998): Auvinet M+, *Rev Med Interne* (French) 19, 353

### Other

Anaphylactoid reactions
(1999): Smith ME, *Oncol Nurs Forum* 26, 516
(1997): Ciesielski-Carlucci C+, *Am J Clin Oncol* 20(4), 373 (with cisplatin)
(1995): Rowinsky EK+, *N Engl J* 332(15), 1004

Arthralgia
(2002): Hasegawa K+, *Gan To Kagaku Ryoho* 29(4), 569
(2001): Ansell SM+, *Cancer* 91(8), 1543
(2001): Ishikawa H+, *Int J Clin Oncol* 6(3), 128

Death
(2001): Fidias P+, *Clin Cancer Res* 7(12), 3942
(2001): Hurwitz CA+, *J Pediatr Hematol Oncol* 23(5), 277

Hypersensitivity (41%)
(2002): Denman JP+, *J Clin Oncol* 20(11), 2760
(2002): Kwon JS+, *Gynecol Oncol* 84(3), 420
(2002): Myers JS, *Clin J Oncol Nurs* 6(3), 177
(2001): Kintzel PE, *Ann Pharmacother* 35(9), 1114
(2001): Koppler H+, *Onkologie* 24(3), 283
(2001): Robinson JB+, *Gynecol Oncol* 82(3), 550 (with carboplatin)
(2001): Szebeni J+, *Int Immunopharmacol* 1(4), 721
(2001): Yamada Y+, *Ann Oncol* 12(8), 1133 (15%)
(1998): Borovik R+, *Harefuah* (Hebrew) 134, 605
(1998): Lokich J+, *Ann Oncol* 9, 573
(1998): Tsavaris NB+, *Cancer Chemother Pharmacol* 42, 509
(1995): Del Priore G+, *Gynecol Oncol* 56, 316
(1994): Uziely B+, *Ann Oncol* 5, 474
(1993): Peereboom DM+, *J Clin Oncol* 11, 885

Injection-site cellulitis (>10%)

Injection-site extravasation (>10%)
(1997): Herrington JD+, *Pharmacotherapy* 17, 163
(1995): Berghmans T+, *Support Care Cancer* 3, 203
(1995): Raymond E+, *Rev Med Interne* (French) 16, 141

Injection-site pain (>10%)

Injection-site reactions (sic) (13%)

Mucocutaneous toxicity (sic)
(1996): Payne JY+, *South Med J* 89, 542

Mucositis (>10%)
(2002): Feher O+, *Head Neck* 24(3), 228

Myalgia (60%)
(2002): Hasegawa K+, *Gan To Kagaku Ryoho* 29(4), 569
(2001): Ishikawa H+, *Int J Clin Oncol* 6(3), 128
(1999): Markman M+, *Gynecol Oncol* 72, 100
(1998): Savarese D+, *J Clin Oncol* 16, 3918
(1997): Jiang Z+, *Chung Hua Chung Liu Tsa Chih* (Chinese) 19, 445

Oral mucosal lesions
(1990): McGuire WP+, *Ann Intern Med* 111, 273 (3–8%)

Paresthesias (>10%)

Phantom limb pain
(2000): Khattab J+, *Mayo Clin Proc* 75, 740
Recall at site of prior extravasation
(1996): du Bois A+, *Gynecol Oncol* 60, 94
(1994): Meehan JL+, *J Natl Cancer Inst* 86, 1250
Stomatitis (39%)
(2001): Miglietta L+, *Oncology* 60(2), 116

# PALIVIZUMAB

**Trade name:** Synagis (MedImmune)
**Indications:** Prophylaxis of serious lower respiratory tract disease caused by RSV in pediatric patients
**Category:** Humanized monoclonal antibody
**Half-life:** 18 days

### *Reactions*

#### Skin
Eczema (sic) (>1%)
Erythema
Flu-like syndrome (>1%)
Fungal dermatitis (sic) (>1%)
Infections (sic)
Rash (sic) (25.6%)
Seborrhea (>1%)

#### Other
Anaphylactoid reactions
Injection-site bruising
(1999): Scott LJ+, *Drugs* 58, 305 (1–3%)
Injection-site edema
(1999): Scott LJ+, *Drugs* 58, 305 (1–3%)
Injection-site erythema
(1999): Scott LJ+, *Drugs* 58, 305 (1–3%)
(1998): *Pediatrics* 102, 531
Injection-site induration
(1999): Scott LJ+, *Drugs* 58, 305 (1–3%)
Injection-site pain (8.5%)
(1999): Scott LJ+, *Drugs* 58, 305 (1–3%)
Injection-site reactions (sic)
(1999): Sandritter T, *J Pediatr Health Care* 13, 191
Oral candidiasis (>1%)

# PAMIDRONATE

**Trade name:** Aredia (Novartis)
**Indications:** Hypercalcemia, Paget's disease
**Category:** Antidote (hypercalcemia)
**Half-life:** 1.6 hours

### *Reactions*

#### Skin
Angioedema (<1%)
Candidiasis
Edema (1%)
Exanthems
(1984): Mantalen CA+, *BMJ* 288, 828 (1.2%)
Flu-like syndrome
(2001): Body JJ, *Semin Oncol* 28(4 Suppl 11), 49
Rash (sic) (<1%)

#### Other
Dysgeusia (<1%)
Hypersensitivity (<1%)
Infusion-site reaction (4%)
(2001): Body JJ, *Semin Oncol* 28(4 Suppl 11), 49
Myalgia (1%)
Stomatitis (1%)

# PANCURONIUM

**Trade name:** Pavulon (Organon)
**Other common trade names:** *Alpax; Bromurex; Curon-B; Panconium; Panslan*
**Indications:** Anesthesia adjunct, neuromuscular blockade, muscle relaxant
**Category:** Nondepolarizing neuromuscular blockade
**Half-life:** 89–161 minutes
**Clinically important, potentially hazardous interactions with:** aminoglycosides, cyclopropane, enflurane, gentamicin, halothane, isoflurane, kanamycin, methoxyflurane, neomycin, piperacillin, streptomycin, tobramycin

### *Reactions*

#### Skin
Burning
Edema
Erythema
(1989): Patriarca G+, *Br J Anaesth* 62(2), 210
Flushing
Pruritus
Rash (sic)

#### Other
Anaphylactoid reactions
(1998): Sanchez-Guerrero IM+, *Eur J Anaesthesiol* 15(5), 613
(1990): Moneret-Vautrin DA+, *Br J Anaesth* 64(6), 743
(1989): Patriarca G+, *Br J Anaesth* 62(2), 210
(1986): Bonnet MC+, *Cah Anesthesiol* 34(3), 253
(1985): Conil C+, *Ann Fr Anesth Reanim* 4(2), 241
(1985): Galletly DC+, *Anaesthesia* 40(4), 329
(1985): Moneret-Vautrin DA+, *Anesth Analg* 64(9), 944
(1984): Mishima S+, *Anesth Analg* 63(9), 865
(1984): Pappagallo S+, *Minerva Anestesiol* 50(9), 481
Hypersensitivity
(1983): Nagao H+, *Br J Anaesth* 55(3), 253
Myalgia
Myopathy
(1994): Giostra E+, *Chest* 106(1), 210
(1993): De Smet, *Rev Neurol* 149(10), 573
(1993): Miyoshi T+, *Rinsho Shinkeigaku* 33(6), 620
Rhabdomyolysis
(1993): Clavelou P+, *Ann Fr Anesth Reanim* 12(3), 326
Sialorrhea

# PANTOPRAZOLE

**Trade name:** Protonix (Wyeth-Ayerst)
**Indications:** Esophagitis associated with gastroesophageal reflux disease (GERD)
**Category:** Proton pump (gastric acid secretion) inhibitor
**Half-life:** 1 hour

### *Reactions*

#### Skin
Abscess (<1%)
Acne (<1%)
Allergic reactions (sic) (<1%)
Angioedema (<1%)
Balanitis (<1%)
Contact dermatitis (<1%)
Diaphoresis (<1%)
(2000): Natsch S+, *Ann Pharmacother* 34, 474
Ecchymoses (<1%)
Eczema (<1%)
Edema (<1%)
Erythema multiforme (<1%)
Exanthems (<1%)
Facial edema (<1%)
Flu-like syndrome (sic) (1–10%)
Fungal infection (sic) (<1%)
Herpes simplex (<1%)
Herpes zoster (<1%)
Infections (sic) (1–10%)
Lichenoid eruption (<1%)
(2000): Bong JL+, *BMJ* 320, 283
Lupus erythematosus (discoid)
(2001): Correia O+, *Clin Exp Dermatol* 26(5), 455
Peripheral edema
(2001): Brunner G+, *Dig Dis Sci* 46(5), 993
(1994): Brunner G, *Aliment Pharmacol Ther* 8, 59
Photosensitivity
(2001): Correia O+, *Clin Exp Dermatol* 26(5), 455
Phototoxicity
(2001): Correia O+, *Clin Exp Dermatol* 26(5), 455
Pruritus (<1%)
(2000): Natsch S+, *Ann Pharmacother* 34, 474
Rash (sic) (<1%)
(2000): Avner DL, *Clin Ther* 22(10), 1169
(1992): Muller P+, *Z Gastroenterol* 30, 771
Stevens–Johnson syndrome (<1%)
Toxic epidermal necrolysis (<1%)
Ulceration (<1%)
Urticaria (<1%)
(2000): Natsch S+, *Ann Pharmacother* 34, 474
Xerosis (<1%)

#### Hair
Hair – alopecia (<1%)

#### Other
Anaphylactoid reactions (<1%)
(2002): Fardet L+, *Am J Gastroenterol* 97(6), 1578
(2002): Kaatz M+, *Allergy* 57(2), 184
(2000): Natsch S+, *Ann Pharmacother* 3(4), 474
Aphthous stomatitis (<1%)
Dysgeusia (<1%)
Foetor ex ore (halitosis) (<1%)
Gingivitis (<1%)
Glossitis (<1%)
Hypesthesia (<1%)
Mastodynia (<1%)
Myalgia (<1%)
Oral candidiasis (<1%)
Paresthesias (<1%)
Sialorrhea (<1%)
Stomatitis (<1%)
Thrombophlebitis (<1%)
Tongue edema
(2000): Natsch S+, *Ann Pharmacother* 34, 474
Tongue pigmentation (<1%)
Tremors (<1%)
Vaginitis (<1%)
Xerostomia (<1%)

# PANTOTHENIC ACID

**Trade name:** Dexol
**Indications:** Vitamin B complex malabsorption
**Category:** Water-soluble vitamin
**Half-life:** no data

### *Reactions*

#### Skin
Exanthems
Pruritus
Urticaria

# PAPAVERINE

**Trade names:** Genabid; Pavabid (Aventis); Pavatine
**Other common trade names:** *Angioverin; Genabid; Optenyl; Pameion; Papaverine 60; Papaverini; Pavagen; Pavased*
**Indications:** Peripheral and cerebral ischemia
**Category:** Peripheral vasodilator
**Half-life:** 0.5–2 hours

### *Reactions*

#### Skin
Diaphoresis (<1%)
Exanthems
Fixed eruption
(1994): Kirby KA+, *Urology* 43, 886
Flushing (<1%)
Pruritus (<1%)
Pyogenic granuloma
(1990): Summers JL, *J Urol* 143, 1227
Rash (sic)
Toxic epidermal necrolysis
(1989): Simochkina ZA+, *Vrach Delo* (Russian) October, 91
Urticaria

#### Other
Injection-site thrombophlebitis (<1%)
Priapism
(2001): Perimenis P+, *Urol Int* 66, 27 (5 cases)
(2001): Secil M+, *J Urol* 165(2), 416 (11.1%)
(1991): Schwarzer JU+, *J Urol* 146, 845
Xerostomia (<1%)

# PARA-AMINOSALICYLIC ACID (PAS)

(See AMINOSALICYLATE SODIUM)

# PARAMETHADIONE

**Trade name:** Paradione (Abbott)
**Indications:** Absence (petit-mal) seizures
**Category:** Anticonvulsant
**Half-life:** 12–24 hours

### *Reactions*

---

#### Skin

Acne
Erythema multiforme
(1972): Levantine A+, *Br J Dermatol* 87, 646
(1961): Leblanc JL+, *Can Med Assoc J* 85, 200
Exanthems
Exfoliative dermatitis
(1946): Lennox WG, *Am J Psychiatry* 103, 159
Lupus erythematosus
Pruritus

#### Hair

Hair – alopecia

#### Other

Bleeding gums
Oral mucosal eruption
(1946): Lennox WG, *Am J Psychiatry* 103, 159
Paresthesias

# PAROMOMYCIN

**Trade name:** Humatin (Parke-Davis)
**Other common trade names:** *Gabbroral; Gabroral; Humagel; Sinosid*
**Indications:** Intestinal amebiasis
**Category:** Broad spectrum antibacterial aminoglycoside amebicide
**Half-life:** N/A
**Clinically important, potentially hazardous interactions with:** methotrexate, succinylcholine

### *Reactions*

---

#### Skin

Exanthems (<1%)
Pruritus (<1%)

# PAROXETINE

**Trade name:** Paxil (GSK)
**Other common trade name:** *Aropax 20*
**Indications:** Depression
**Category:** Selective serotonin reuptake inhibitor (SSRI); antidepressant
**Half-life:** 21 hours
**Clinically important, potentially hazardous interactions with:** amphetamines, clarithromycin, dextroamphetamine, diethylpropion, erythromycin, isocarboxazid, linezolid, MAO inhibitors, mazindol, methamphetamine, phendimetrazine, phenelzine, phentermine, phenylpropanolamine, pseudoephedrine, selegiline, sibutramine, sumatriptan, sympathomimetics, tranylcypromine, trazodone, troleandomycin

### *Reactions*

---

#### Skin

Acne (<1%)
Allergic reactions (sic) (<1%)
Angioedema (<1%)
(1996): Mithani H+, *J Clin Psychiatry* 57, 486
Candidiasis
Contact dermatitis (<1%)
Cutaneous reactions (sic)
(1998): Beauquier B+, *Encephale* (French) 24, 62
Diaphoresis (11.2%)
(1998): Stein MB+, *JAMA* 280, 708
(1997): Litt JZ, Beachwood, OH (personal case) (observation)
(1992): Boyer WF+, *J Clin Psychiatry* 53, 61
(1991): Dechant KL+, *Drugs* 41, 225
(1990): Sindrup SH+, *Pain* 42, 135
(1985): Laursen AL+, *Acta Psychiatr Scand* 71, 249
Ecchymoses (<1%)
(1998): Cooper TA+, *Am J Med* 104, 197
Eczema (sic)
Edema (<1%)
Erythema multiforme
(2000): Altman, EA, New York, NY (from Internet) (observation)
Erythema nodosum (<1%)
Exanthems (<1%)
Facial edema (<1%)
Furunculosis (<1%)
Lymphedema
Melanoma (<1%)
Peripheral edema (<1%)
Photosensitivity (<1%)
(2001): Richard MA+, *Ann Dermatol Venereol* 128, 759
Pigmentation (<1%)
Pruritus (<1%)
(1991): Dechant KL+, *Drugs* 41, 225
Purpura (<1%)
Rash (sic) (1.7%)
Toxic epidermal necrolysis
(2000): Nelson RA+, Nashville, TN (Poster exhibit #16 from Academy 2000)
Urticaria (<1%)
Vasculitis
(2001): Margolese HC+, *Am J Psychiatry* 158, 497
Xerosis (<1%)

#### Hair

Hair – alopecia (<1%)
(2000): Umansky L+, *Harefuah* (Hebrew) 138, 547 ("massive")

### Other

Ageusia (<1%)
(1997): Litt JZ, Beachwood, OH (personal case) (observation)
Anosmia
(1997): Litt JZ, Beachwood, OH (personal case) (observation)
Aphthous stomatitis (<1%)
Bruxism (<1%)
(1996): Romanelli F+, *Ann Pharmacother* 30, 1246
Cough
(2000): Hamel H+, *Presse Med* (French) 29, 1045
Dysgeusia (2.4%)
(1998): Litt JZ, Beachwood, OH (personal case) (observation)
Galactorrhea
(2001): Morrison J+, *Can J Psychiatry* 46, 88
Gingivitis (<1%)
Glossitis (<1%)
Myalgia (1.7%)
Myopathy (1–10%)
Oral ulceration
Paresthesias (3.8%)
Priapism
(1996): Bertholon F+, *Ann Med Psychol Paris* (French) 154, 145
Serotonin syndrome
(1999): Cavallazzi LO+, *Arq Neuropsiq* 57(3B), 886
Sialorrhea (<1%)
Stomatitis (<1%)
Tinnitus
Tongue edema (<1%)
(1996): Mithani H+, *J Clin Psychiatry* 57, 486
Tremors (1–10%)
Vaginal candidiasis (<1%)
Vaginitis
Xerostomia (18.1%)
(1998): Stein MB+, *JAMA* 280, 708
(1992): Boyer WF+, *J Clin Psychiatry* 53, 61
(1992): Claghorn JL, *J Clin Psychiatry* 53, 33
(1992): Fabre LF, *J Clin Psychiatry* 53, 40
(1992): Shrivastava RK+, *J Clin Psychiatry* 53, 48
(1992): Smith WT+, *J Clin Psychiatry* 53, 36
(1991): Dechant KL+, *Drugs* 1, 225
(1991): Dunbar GC+, *Br J Psychiatry* 159, 394
(1990): Cohn JB+, *Psychopharmacol Bull* 26, 185
(1990): Sindrup SH+, *Pain* 42, 135

## PC-SPES

**Scientific name:** See *note*.
**Other common names:** See note
**Purported indications:** Prostate cancer (PC stands for Prostate Cancer, SPES is Latin for 'hope'), to decrease serum prostate-specific antigen (PSA)
**Other uses:** Lymphoma, Leukemia, Breast cancer, Melanoma

#### *Reactions*

### Skin

Allergic reactions (sic)
(2000): Small EJ+, *J Clinical Oncol* 18, 3595
Facial edema
Hot flashes
Leg edema
(1999): Porterfield H, *Mol Urol* 3, 333
Pitting edema
(1999): Moyad MA+, *Urology* 54, 319

### Hair

Hair – hypotrichosis
(1999): Moyad MA+, *Urology* 54, 319

### Other

Gynecomastia (90%)
(2000): De La Taille A+, *J Urol* 164, 1229
(2000): Small EJ+, *J Clinical Oncol* 18, 3595
(1999): Moyad MA+, *Urology* 54, 319
Leg cramps (30%)
(2000): Small EJ+, *J Clinical Oncol* 18, 3595
Mastodynia
(2000): De La Taille A+, *J Urol* 164, 1229
(1999): Moyad MA+, *Urology* 54, 319
(1999): Porterfield H, *Mol Urol* 3, 333
(1998): DiPaola RS+, *N Engl J Med* 339, 785 (100%)
Nipple tenderness (80%)
(2000): De La Taille A+, *J Urol* 164, 1229
Thrombophlebitis
Tongue edema

**Note:** PC-SPES is a combination product containing eight Chinese herbs. Each capsule contains Da Quing Ye (*Isatis indigotica*); Licorice (*Glycyrrhiza glabral*): San-Qi Ginseng (*Panax pseudoginseng*); Reishi Mushroom (*Ganoderma lucidum*); Baikal Skullcap (*Scutellaria baicalensis*); Chrysanthemum (*Dendrathema morifolium*); Rabdosia rubescens; Saw Palmetto (*Serenoa repens*). Manufactured by BotanicLab Inc.

PC-SPES has been withdrawn in the USA

## PEG-INTERFERON ALFA-2B

**Trade name:** PEG-Intron (Schering)
**Indications:** Chronic hepatitis C
**Category:** Interferon immunomodulator
**Half-life:** ~40 hours
**Clinically important, potentially hazardous interactions with:** ACE inhibitors, melphalan, warfarin, zidovudine

#### *Reactions*

### Skin

Abscess (~1%)
Angioedema (~1%)
Dermatitis (sic) (7%)
Diaphoresis (6%)
Flu-like syndrome (46%)
Flushing (6%)
Pruritus (12%)
Psoriasis (~1%)
Purpura
Rash (sic) (6%)
Urticaria (~1%)
Viral infection (11%)
Xerosis (11%)

### Hair

Hair – alopecia (22%)

### Other

Anaphylactoid reactions (~1%)
Cough (6%)
Depression (16–29%)
Dysgeusia (1–10%)
Hypersensitivity (~1%)
Injection-site pain (2%)

Musculoskeletal pain (56%)
Myalgia (38–42%)
(2001): Perry CM+, *Drugs* 61(15), 2263
Pain (12%)
Rigors (23–45%)

# PEMIROLAST

**Trade name:** Alamast (Santen)
**Other common trade name:** *Alegysal*
**Indications:** Pruritus of allergic conjunctivitis
**Category:** Mast cell stabilizer; antiallergic ophthalmic
**Half-life:** 4.5 hours

### Reactions

**Skin**
Allergy (sic)
Dry eyes (sic)
Flu-like syndrome (10–25%)
Ocular burning
Ocular discomfort (<5%)

**Other**
Back pain (<5%)

# PEMOLINE

**Trade name:** Cylert (Abbott)
**Other common trade names:** *Betanamin; Tradon*
**Indications:** Attention deficit disorder, narcolepsy
**Category:** Central nervous system stimulant; anorexiant
**Half-life:** 9–14 hours
**Clinically important, potentially hazardous interactions with:** pimozide

### Reactions

**Skin**
Exanthems (<1%)
(1992): Zürcher K and Krebs A, *Cutaneous Drug Reactions* Karger, 280
Rash (sic) (>10%)

**Other**
Parkinsonism
Rhabdomyolysis
(1988): Briscoe JG+, *Med Toxicol Adverse Drug Exp* 3(1), 72
Tourette's syndrome

# PENBUTOLOL

**Trade name:** Levatol (Schwarz)
**Other common trade names:** *Betapresin; Betapressin*
**Indications:** Hypertension
**Category:** Beta-adrenergic blocker; antihypertensive
**Half-life:** 5 hours
**Clinically important, potentially hazardous interactions with:** clonidine, epinephrine, verapamil

**Note:** Cutaneous side effects of beta-receptor blockaders are clinically polymorphous. They apparently appear after several months of continuous therapy. Atypical psoriasiform, lichen planus-like, and eczematous chronic rashes are mainly observed. (1983): Hödl St, *Z Hautkr* (German) 1:58, 17

### Reactions

**Skin**
Allergic reactions (sic)
(1985): Marone C+, *Curr Med Res Opin* 9, 417 (1–5%)
Ankle edema
Diaphoresis (1.6%)
Exanthems
(1985): Marone C+, *Curr Med Res Opin* 9, 417 (1–5%)
Flushing
(1985): Marone C+, *Curr Med Res Opin* 9, 417 (1–5%)
Peripheral edema
Pruritus
Psoriasis
Purpura
Rash (sic)

**Hair**
Hair – alopecia

**Nails**
Nails – bluish

**Other**
Dysgeusia
Paresthesias
Peyronie's disease

# PENICILLAMINE

**Trade names:** Cuprimine (Merck); Depen (Wallace)
**Other common trade names:** *Artamin; D-Penamine; Distamine; Kelatin; Pendramine*
**Indications:** Wilson's disease, rheumatoid arthritis
**Category:** Antidote; chelating agent and antirheumatic
**Half-life:** 1.7–3.2 hours
**Clinically important, potentially hazardous interactions with:** aluminum hydroxide, antacids, ascorbic acid, bone marrow suppressants, chloroquine, cytotoxic agents, **food**, gold, hydroxychloroquine, iron, magnesium, primaquine, probenecid

**Note:** For excellent reviews of many of the cutaneous manifestations caused by penicillamine see (1983): Levy RS+, *J Am Acad Dermatol* 8, 548 and (1981): Sternlieb I+, *J Rheumatol* 8 (Suppl 7), 149

### Reactions

**Skin**
Anetoderma
(1977): Davis W, *Arch Dermatol* 113, 976
Atrophy
(1982): Bailin PL+, *Clin Rheum Dis* 8, 493 (passim)
Bullous eruption
(1996): Bialy-Golan A+, *J Am Acad Dermatol* 35, 732 (passim)
(1982): Fulton RA+, *Br J Dermatol* 107 (Suppl 22), 95
(1977): Stewart WM+, *Ann Dermatol Venereol* (French) 104, 542
Bullous pemphigoid
(1998): Weller R+, *Ann Pharmacother* 32, 1368
(1996): Weller R+, *Clin Exp Dermatol* 21, 121
(1989): Rasmussen HB+, *J Cutan Pathol* 16, 154
(1987): Brown MD+, *Arch Dermatol* 123, 1119
(1986): Gall Y+, *Ann Dermatol Venereol* (French) 113, 55

Contact dermatitis
(1993): De Moor A+, *Contact Dermatitis* 29, 155 (eyedrops)
(1990): Coenraads PJ+, *Contact Dermatitis* 23, 371
Cutis laxa
(2000): Werth V, *Dermatology Times* 18
(1994): Amichai B+, *Isr J Med Sci* 30, 667
(1983): Harpey JP+, *Lancet* 2, 858
(1983): Levy RS+, *J Am Acad Dermatol* 8, 548
(1982): Bailin PL+, *Clin Rheum Dis* 8, 493 (passim)
(1979): Linares A+, *Lancet* 2, 43
(1979): Walshe JM, *Lancet* 2, 144
(1977): Solomon L+, *N Engl J Med* 296, 54
Dermatomyositis
(1992): Kolsi R+, *Rev Rhum Mal Osteoartic* (French) 59, 341
(1991): Wilson CL+, *Int J Dermatol* 30, 148
(1987): Carroll CG+, *J Rheumatol* 14, 995
(1983): Doyle DR+, *Ann Intern Med* 98, 327
(1983): Levy RS+, *J Am Acad Dermatol* 8, 548
(1983): Lund HI+, *Scand J Rheumatol* 12, 350
(1982): Bailin PL+, *Clin Rheum Dis* 8, 493 (passim)
(1981): Major GA, *J R Soc Med* 74, 393
(1980): Wojnarowska F, *J R Soc Med* 73, 884
(1979): Simpson NB+, *Acta Derm Venereol* (Stockh) 59, 543
(1978): Petersen J+, *Scand J Rheumatol* 7, 113
(1977): Fernandes L+, *Ann Rheum Dis* 36, 94
Dermopathy
(1987): Dootson G+, *Clin Exp Dermatol* 12, 66
Discoid lupus erythematosus
(1978): Appelboom T+, *Scand J Rheumatol* 7, 64
Ecchymoses
Edema (1–10%)
(1999): Hsu HL+, *Taiwan Erh Ko I Hsueh Tsa Chih* 40, 448 (lip)
Ehlers–Danlos syndrome
(1982): Bailin PL+, *Clin Rheum Dis* 8, 493 (passim)
(1982): Yung CW+, *J Am Acad Dermatol* 6, 317 (passim)
Elastosis perforans serpiginosa
(2001): Danby FW, Manchester, NH (from Internet) (observation)
(2000): Hill VA+, *Br J Dermatol* 142, 560
(2000): Werth V, *Dermatology Times* 18
(1994): Amichai B+, *Isr J Med Sci* 30, 667
(1994): Ratnavel RC+, *Dermatology* 189, 81
(1994): Wilhelm KP+, *Hautarzt* (German) 45, 45
(1989): Sahn EE+, *J Am Acad Dermatol* 20, 279
(1988): van Joost T+, *Ned Tijdschr Geneeskd* (Dutch) 132, 501
(1986): Price RG+, *Am J Dermatopathol* 8, 314
(1985): Meyrick-Thomas RHM+, *Clin Exp Dermatol* 10, 386
(1984): Venencie PY+, *Ann Med Interne (Paris)* (French) 135, 642
(1983): Levy RS+, *J Am Acad Dermatol* 8, 548
(1983): Rosenblum GA, *J Am Acad Dermatol* 8, 718
(1982): Bailin PL+, *Clin Rheum Dis* 8, 493 (passim)
(1982): Essigman WK, *Ann Rheum Dis* 41, 617
(1982): Gloor M+, *Hautarzt* (German) 33, 291
(1982): Raymond JL+, *J Cutan Pathol* 9, 352
(1981): Bardach H+, *Wien Klin Wochenschr* (German) 93, 117
(1979): Bardach H, *Hautarzt* (German) 30, 449
(1977): Abel M, *Arch Dermatol* 113, 1303
(1977): Kirsch N+, *Arch Dermatol* 113, 630
(1973): Pass F+, *Arch Dermatol* 108, 713
Epidermal inclusion cysts
(1967): Katz R, *Arch Dermatol* 95, 196
Epidermolysis bullosa
(1982): Bailin PL+, *Clin Rheum Dis* 8, 493 (passim)
(1982): Yung CW+, *J Am Acad Dermatol* 6, 317 (passim)
(1967): Beer WE+, *Br J Dermatol* 79, 123
Erythema multiforme (1–5%)
Erythema nodosum (<1%)
(1983): Grauer JL+, *Presse Med* (French) 12, 1997
Exanthems
(1999): Hsu HL+, *Taiwan Erh Ko I Hsueh Tsa Chih* 40, 448
(1983): Levy RS+, *J Am Acad Dermatol* 8, 548
(1982): Bailin PL+, *Clin Rheum Dis* 8, 493 (passim)
(1982): Egeland T+, *J Oral Pathol* 11, 183
(1981): Walshe JM, *J Rheumatol 8* (Suppl 7), 155
(1980): Stein HB+, *Ann Intern Med* 92, 24
(1979): Hill HFH, *Scand J Rheumatol* 28, 94
Exfoliative dermatitis
Facial edema
(1996): Bialy-Golan A+, *J Am Acad Dermatol* 35, 732 (passim)
Flushing
(1996): Bialy-Golan A+, *J Am Acad Dermatol* 35, 732 (passim)
Fragility (sic)
(1981): Shaw M+, *Clin Exp Dermatol* 6, 429
Graft-versus-host reaction
(1998): Jappe U+, *Hautarzt* (German) 49, 126 (passim)
Guillain–Barré syndrome
(1984): Knezevic W+, *Aust N Z J Med* 14, 50
Lathyrism
(1992): Godar JM+, *Arch Dermatol* 128, 977
Lichen planus
(1994): Thompson DF+, *Pharmacotherapy* 14, 561
(1986): Weismann K+, *Ugeskr Laeger* (Danish) 148, 456
(1981): Powell FC+, *Lancet* 2, 525
(1979): Krebs A, *Hautarzt* (German) 30, 281
Lichenoid eruption
(1983): Levy RS+, *J Am Acad Dermatol* 8, 548
(1983): Powell FC+, *J Am Acad Dermatol* 9, 540
(1982): Bailin PL+, *Clin Rheum Dis* 8, 493 (passim)
(1982): Powell FC+, *Br J Dermatol* 107, 616
(1981): Seehafer JR+, *Arch Dermatol* 117, 140
(1981): Van Hecke E+, *Arch Dermatol* 117, 676
(1975): Van de Staak WJBM+, *Dermatologica* 150, 372
Lupus erythematosus
(2000): Lin HC+, *J Microbiol Immunol Infect* 33, 202
(1996): Bialy-Golan A+, *J Am Acad Dermatol* 35, 732 (passim)
(1995): Barthel HR+, *Dtsch Med Wochenschr* (German) 120, 1253
(1994): Borg AA, *Clin Rheumatol* 13, 522
(1994): Fritzler MJ, *Lupus* 3. 455
(1994): Yung RL+, *Rheum Dis Clin North Am* 20, 61
(1993): Donnelly S+, *Br J Rheumatol* 32, 251
(1992): Rubin RL+, *J Clin Invest* 90, 165
(1992): Skaer TL, *Clin Ther* 14, 496
(1991): Chin GL+, *J Rheumatol* 18, 947
(1991): Weinstein A, *Arthritis Rheum* 34, 1343
(1990): Enzenauer RJ+, *Arthritis Rheum* 33, 1582
(1990): Suda M+, *Nippon Jinzo Gakkai Shi* (Japanese) 32, 1235
(1990): Tsankov NK+, *Int J Dermatol* 29, 571
(1987): Lopez-Guerra N+, *Med Clin (Barc)* (Spanish) 88, 552
(1985): Kalina P+, *Bratisl Lek Listy* (Slovak) 84, 336
(1985): Lovisetto P+, *Recenti Prog Med* (Italian) 76, 110
(1985): Stratton MA, *Clin Pharm* 4, 657
(1984): Clerc C+, *Ann Dermatol Venereol* (French) 135, 420
(1983): Levy RS+, *J Am Acad Dermatol* 8, 548
(1982): Bailin PL+, *Clin Rheum Dis* 8, 493 (passim)
(1982): Chalmers A+, *Ann Intern Med* 97, 659
(1982): Egeland T+, *J Oral Pathol* 11, 183
(1982): Yung CW+, *J Am Acad Dermatol* 6, 317 (passim)
(1981): Hughes GR+, *Arthritis Rheum* 24, 1070
(1981): Thorvaldsen J, *Dermatologia* 162, 277
(1981): Walshe JM, *J Rheumatol* Suppl 7, 155
(1979): Burns DA+, *Clin Exp Dermatol* 4, 389
(1978): Appelboom T+, *Scand J Rheumatol* 7, 64
(1978): Harkcom TM+, *Ann Intern Med* 89, 1012
(1975): Lee SL+, *Semin Arthritis Rheum* 5, 83
(1974): Crouzet J+, *Ann Med Interne Paris* (French) 125, 71
(1974): Harpey JP, *Ann Allergy* 33, 256

(1972): Oliver T+, *JAMA* 220, 588
(1971): Boudin G+, *Ann Med Interne Paris* (French) 122, 269
(1971): Caille B+, *Ann Med Interne Paris* (French) 122, 255
(1971): Harpey JP+, *Ann Med Interne Paris* (French) 122, 261
(1971): Harpey JP+, *Lancet* 1, 292 (letter)

Morphea
(1989): Liddle BJ, *Ann Rheum Dis* 48, 963
(1981): Bernstein RM+, *Ann Rheum Dis* 40, 42

Papular lesions at site of trauma
(1985): Thomas RHM+, *Clin Exp Dermatol* 10, 386

Pemphigoid
(1989): Marti-Huguet T+, *Arch Ophthalmol* 107, 1115
(1986): Peyri J+, *J Am Acad Dermatol* 14, 681 (cicatricial)
(1985): Lever LR+, *Br J Dermatol* 113, 88
(1985): Shuttleworth D+, *Br J Dermatol* 113, 89
(1985): Shuttleworth D+, *Clin Exp Dermatol* 10, 392 (cicatricial)
(1985): Velthuis PJ+, *Br J Dermatol* 112, 615

Pemphigus
(2000): Shapiro M+, *J Am Acad Dermatol* 42, 297
(1999): Jan V+, *Ann Dermatol Venereol* (French) 126, 153
(1997): Brenner S+, *J Am Acad Dermatol* 36, 919
(1997): Haimowitz JE+, PA, American Academy of Dermatology Meeting (SF) (gross and microscopic)
(1995): Ciompi ML+, *Rheumatol Int* 15, 95
(1993): Brenner S+, *Clin Dermatol* 11, 501
(1993): Jones E+, *J Am Acad Dermatol* 28, 655
(1992): Bauer-Vinassac D+, *Scand J Rheumatol* 21, 17
(1991): Korman NJ+, *J Invest Dermatol* 96, 273
(1990): Black AK+, *Br J Dermatol* 123, 277
(1990): Wouters EA+, *Acta Clin Belg* (French) 45, 15
(1989): Civatte J, *Dermatol Monatsschr* (German) 175, 1
(1988): Blanken R+, *Acta Derm Venereol* (Stockh) 68, 456
(1988): Buckley C+, *Ir J Med Sci* 157, 267
(1987): Enjolras O+, *Ann Dermatol Venereol* (French) 114, 25
(1987): Kind P+, *Hautarzt* (German) 38, 548
(1987): Walton S+, *Clin Exp Dermatol* 12, 275
(1986): Civatte J, *Bull Soc Fr Dermatol Syphiligr* (French) 170, 1057
(1986): Dijkstra JW, *J Am Acad Dermatol* 14, 687
(1986): Peyri J+, *J Am Acad Dermatol* 14, 681
(1986): Steen VD+, *Ann Intern Med* 104, 699
(1986): Tholen S, *Z Hautkr* (German) 61, 719
(1985): Ho VC+, *J Rheumatol* 12, 583
(1985): Piette-Brion B+, *Dermatologica* (French) 170, 297
(1985): Velthuis PJ+, *Br J Dermatol* 112, 615
(1984): Hashimoto K+, *Arch Dermatol* 120, 762
(1984): Venencie PY+, *Ann Med Interne (Paris)* (French) 135, 642
(1983): Doutre MS+, *Rev Rhum Mal Osteoartic* (French) 50, 167
(1983): Kaplan RP+, *Clin Dermatol* 1, 42
(1983): Levy RS+, *J Am Acad Dermatol* 8, 548
(1983): Tinozzi CC, *G Ital Dermatol Venereol* (Italian) 118, 45
(1982): Barety M+, *Therapie* (French) 37, 471
(1982): Benito-Urbino S+, *Rev Clin Esp* (Spanish) 166, 249
(1982): Fye KH+, J *Rheumatol* 9, 331
(1982): Ruocco V+, *Arch Dermatol Res* 274, 123
(1982): Ruocco V+, *Dermatologica* 164, 236
(1982): Yung CW+, *J Am Acad Dermatol* 6, 317 (pemphigus syndrome)
(1982): Zone J+, *JAMA* 247, 2705
(1981): Livden JK+, *Scand J Rheumatol* 10, 95
(1981): Santa-Cruz DJ+, *Am J Dermatopathol* 3, 85
(1981): Troy JL+, *J Am Acad Dermatol* 4, 547
(1981): Trunnell TN+, *Cutis* 27, 402 (pemphigus-like)
(1980): Chouyet B+, *Dermatologica* (French) 160, 297
(1980): Trau H+, *Arch Dermatol* 116, 721
(1979): Delcambre B+, *Lille Med* (French) 24, 283
(1979): Hill HF, *Scand J Rheumatol Suppl* 28, 94
(1978): Christoph R+, *Med Welt* (German) 29, 1761
(1977): Marsden RA+, *Proc R Soc Med* 70, 103
(1977): Stewart WM+, *Ann Dermatol Venereol* (French) 104, 542
(1976): Cairns RJ, *Proc R Soc Med* 69, 384
(1976): Colliard H+, *Rev Stomatol Chir Maxillofac* (French) 77, 741
(1976): Davies MG+, *Arch Dermatol* 112, 1308
(1976): From E+, *Dermatologica* 152, 358
(1976): Tan SG+, *Br J Dermatol* 95, 99 (pemphigus-like)
(1975): Asboe-Hansen G, *Acta Derm Venereol* 55, 461
(1975): Benveniste M+, *Nouv Presse Med* (French) 4, 3125
(1975): Hewitt J+, *BMJ* 3, 371
(1971): Hewitt J+, *Ann Med Interne Paris* (French) 122, 1003
(1969): Degos R+, *Bull Soc Fr Dermatol Syphiligr* (French) 76, 751

Pemphigus erythematodes (Senear–Usher)
(1990): Willemsen MJ+, *Int J Dermatol* 29, 193
(1985): Amerian ML+, *Int J Dermatol* 24, 16
(1985): Gibson LE+, *J Am Acad Dermatol* 12, 883
(1984): Amerian ML+, *J Am Acad Dermatol* 10, 215
(1982): Yung CW+, *J Am Acad Dermatol* 6, 317
(1980): Keilhauer A+, *Z Hautkr* (German) 55, 948
(1979): Thorvaldsen J, *Dermatologica* 159, 167
(1978): Fellner MJ+, *Int J Dermatol* 17, 308
(1977): Scherak O+, *BMJ* 1, 838

Pemphigus foliaceus
(2000): Elston DM+, *Cutis* 66, 375
(2000): Werth V, *Dermatology Times* 18
(1999): Toth GG+, *Br J Dermatol* 141, 583
(1998): Brenner S+, *J Am Acad Dermatol* 39, 137
(1997): McGovern TW+, *Arch Dermatol* 133, 499
(1997): Peñas PF+, *J Am Acad Dermatol* 37, 121
(1995): Brenner S+, American Academy of Dermatology Meeting, New Orleans (observation)
(1993): Zillikens D+, *Hautarzt* (German) 44, 167
(1986): Kohn SR, *Arch Dermatol* 122, 17 (fatal)
(1985): Bahmer FA+, *Arch Dermatol* 121, 665
(1984): Knezevic W+, *Aust N Z J Med* 14, 50
(1983): Brenner S+, *Harefuah* (Hebrew) 104, 94
(1982): Kohn SR, *Dermatologic Capsule and Comment* 4, 11
(1981): Matkaluk RM+, *Arch Dermatol* 117, 156
(1977): Kristensen JK+, *Acta Derm Venereol* (Stockh) 57, 69
(1976): Marsden RA+, *BMJ* 2, 1423

Pemphigus herpetiformis
(1988): Weltfriend S+, *Hautarzt* (German) 39, 587
(1980): Morioka S+, *J Dermatol* 7, 425
(1977): Marsden RA+, *Br J Dermatol* 97, 451

Pemphigus vulgaris
(2000): Werth V, *Dermatology Times* 18

Peripheral edema (1–10%)

Pruritus (44–50%)
(1982): Bailin PL+, *Clin Rheum Dis* 8, 493 (passim)
(1982): Yung CW+, *J Am Acad Dermatol* 6, 317 (passim)

Pseudoxanthoma elasticum
(2000): Werth V, *Dermatology Times* 18
(1998): Coatesworth AP+, *J Clin Pathol* 51, 169
(1992): Bolognia JL+, *Dermatology* (Basel) 184, 12
(1992): Narron GH+, *Ann Plast Surg* 29, 367
(1991): Buckley C+, *Clin Exp Dermatol* 16, 310
(1990): Dalziel KL+, *Br J Dermatol* 123, 305
(1988): Burge S+, *Clin Exp Dermatol* 13, 255
(1987): Dootson G+, *Clin Exp Dermatol* 12, 66
(1986): Light N+, *Br J Dermatol* 114, 381
(1985): Bentley-Phillips B, *J R Soc Med* 78, 787
(1985): Meyrick-Thomas RH+, *Clin Exp Dermatol* 10, 386

Psoriasis
(1987): Forgie JC+, *BMJ* 294, 1101
(1986): Daunt SON+, *Br J Rheumatol* 25, 74
(1983): Levy RS+, *J Am Acad Dermatol* 8, 548
(1981): Sternlieb I+, *J Rheumatol* 8, 149

Purpura
(1983): Trice JM+, *Arch Intern Med* 143, 1487
(1982): Bailin PL+, *Clin Rheum Dis* 8, 493 (passim)

(1982): Speth PA+, *J Rheumatol* 9, 812
(1964): Sternlieb I+, *JAMA* 189, 748

Rash (sic) (44–50%)
(2000): Shannon MW+, *Ann Pharmacother* 34, 15
(1991): Barash J+, *Clin Exp Rheumatol* 9, 541
(1982): Kean WF+, *J Am Geriatr Soc* 30, 94
(1982): Smith PJ+, *Br Med J (Clin Res Ed)* 285, 595

Scleroderma
(1991): Bourgeois P+, *Baillieres Clin Rheumatol* 5, 13
(1987): Miyagawa S+, *Br J Dermatol* 116, 95
(1981): Bernstein RM+, *Ann Rheum Dis* 40, 42

Sjøgren's syndrome
(1996): Bialy-Golan A+, *J Am Acad Dermatol* 35, 732 (passim)

Stevens–Johnson syndrome
(1996): Kammler H-J, Jena, Germany (from Internet) (observation)

Toxic epidermal necrolysis (<1%)
(1984): Chan HL, *J Am Acad Dermatol* 10, 973
(1981): Ward K+, *Ir J Med Sci* 150, 252

Urticaria (44–50%)
(1983): Levy RS+, *J Am Acad Dermatol* 8, 548
(1979): Hill HFH, *Scand J Rheumatol* 28, 94

Vasculitis
(1998): Merkel PA, *Curr Opin Rheumatol* 10, 45
(1986): Gall Y+, *Ann Dermatol Venereol* (French) 113, 55
(1983): Banfi G+, *Nephron* 33, 56
(1983): Curran JJ+, *J Rheumatol* 10, 344
(1982): Bailin PL+, *Clin Rheum Dis* 8, 493 (passim)
(1974): Hill HFH, *Curr Med Res Opin* 2, 573

Vesicular eruptions
(1992): Godar JM+, *Arch Dermatol* 128, 977

Wrinkling (sic)
(1983): Levy RS+, *J Am Acad Dermatol* 8, 548

Xerosis
(1982): Yung CW+, *J Am Acad Dermatol* 6, 317 (passim)

## Hair

Hair – alopecia
(1983): Levy RS+, *J Am Acad Dermatol* 8, 548
(1981): Sternlieb I+, *J Rheumatol* 8 (Suppl 7), 149

Hair – hirsutism
(1990): Rose BI+, *J Reprod Med* 35, 43
(1983): Levy RS+, *J Am Acad Dermatol* 8, 548

## Nails

Nails – dystrophy
(1987): Brown MD+, *Arch Dermatol* 123, 1119 (passim)

Nails – elkonyxis (punched-out appearance of the nail at lunulae)
(1989): Bjellerup M, *Acta Derm Venereol* (Stockh) 69, 339

Nails – leukonychia
(1967): Thivolet J+, *Bull Soc Fr Dermatol* (French) 75, 61

Nails – longitudinal ridges
(1967): Thivolet J+, *Bull Soc Fr Dermatol* (French) 75, 61

Nails – onychoschizia
(1989): Bjellerup M, *Acta Derm Venereol* (Stockh) 69, 339

Nails – yellow nail syndrome
(1991): Ichikawa Y+, *Tokai J Exp Clin Med* 16, 203
(1989): Bjellerup M, *Acta Derm Venereol* (Stockh) 69, 339
(1983): Ilchyshyn A+, *Acta Derm Venereol* (Stockh) 63, 534
(1979): Lubach D+, *Hautarzt* (German) 30, 547

## Other

Ageusia (12%)
(1982): Yung CW+, *J Am Acad Dermatol* 6, 317 (passim)

Aphthous stomatitis
(1983): Levy RS+, *J Am Acad Dermatol* 8, 548

Benign mucous membrane pemphigoid
(1985): Shuttleworth D+, *Clin Exp Dermatol* 10, 392
(1977): Pegum JS+, *BMJ* 1, 1473

Bromhidrosis
(1996): Bialy-Golan A+, *J Am Acad Dermatol* 35, 732 (passim)

Death

Dermatopathy with lymphangiectases
(1989): Goldstein JB+, *Arch Dermatol* 125, 92

Dysgeusia (metallic taste)
(1996): Bialy-Golan A+, *J Am Acad Dermatol* 35, 732 (passim)
(1983): Levy RS+, *J Am Acad Dermatol* 8, 548
(1982): Kean WF+, *J Am Geriatr Soc* 30, 94
(1980): Stein HB+, *Ann Intern Med* 92, 24

Gingivitis

Glossitis
(1967): Thivolet J+, *Bull Soc Fr Dermatol* (French) 75, 61

Gynecomastia
(1994): Desautels JE, *Can Assoc Radiol J* 45, 143 (gigantism)
(1985): Kahl LE+, *J Rheumatol* 12, 990
(1982): Reid DM+, *BMJ* 285, 1083

Hypersensitivity
(1999): Hsu HL+, *Taiwan Erh Ko I Hsueh Tsa Chih* 40, 448
(1994): Chan CY+, *Am J Gastroenterol* 89, 442

Hypogeusia (25–33%)
(1968): Keiser HR+, *JAMA* 203, 381
(1967): Henkin RI+, *Lancet* 2, 1268

Mucocutaneous reactions (sic)
(1982): Halla JT+, *Am J Med* 72, 423

Mucosal lesions (pemphigus-like)
(1981): Eisenberg E+, *Oral Surg Oral Med Oral Pathol* 51, 409
(1978): Hay KD+, *Oral Surg Oral Med Oral Pathol* 45, 385

Mucosal ulceration
(1981): Eisenberg E+, *Oral Surg* 51, 409

Oral lichenoid eruption
(1984): Blasberg B+, *J Rheumatol* 11, 348

Oral ulceration
(2000): Madinier I+, *Ann Med Interne (Paris)* (French) 151, 248
(1996): Bialy-Golan A+, *J Am Acad Dermatol* 35, 732 (passim)
(1982): Egeland T+, *J Oral Pathol* 11, 183
(1980): Stein HB+, *Ann Intern Med* 92, 24
(1964): Sternlieb I+, *JAMA* 189, 748

Polymyositis
(1996): Bialy-Golan A+, *J Am Acad Dermatol* 35, 732 (passim)
(1991): Santos JC+, *Clin Exp Dermatol* 16, 76
(1978): Petersen J+, *Scand J Rheumatol* 7, 113

Serum sickness
(1996): Bialy-Golan A+, *J Am Acad Dermatol* 35, 732 (passim)

Stomatitis
(1996): Bialy-Golan A+, *J Am Acad Dermatol* 35, 732 (passim)
(1982): Yung CW+, *J Am Acad Dermatol* 6, 317 (passim)
(1981): Sternlieb I+, *J Rheumatol* 8 (Suppl 7), 149 (passim)
(1980): Stein HB+, *Ann Intern Med* 92, 24
(1968): Thivolet J+, *Bull Soc Fr Dermatol Syphiligr* (French) 75. 61

Tinnitus

# PENICILLINS

**Generic names:**

**Amoxicillin**

Trade names: Amoxil; Augmentin; Larotid; Polymox; Trimox; Wymox

**Ampicillin**

Trade names: Omnipen; Olycillin; Principen; Unasyn

**Azlocillin**

Trade names: Azlin

**Bacampicillin**

Trade name: Spectrobid

**Carbenicillin**

Trade name: Geopen

**Cloxacillin**

Trade names: Cloxapen; Tegopen

**Cyclacillin**

Trade name: none

**Dicloxacillin**

Trade names: Dycil; Dynapen; Pathocil

**Methicillin**

Trade name: Staphcillin

**Mexlocillin**

Trade name: Mezlin

**Nafcillin**

Trade name: Unipen

**Oxacillin**

Trade names: Bactocill; Prostaphlin

**Penicillin G**

Trade names: Bicillin; Crysticillin; Megacillin; Wycillin

**Penicillin V**

Trade names: Beepen; Betapen; Ledercillin; Pen Vee K; V-Cillin; etc.

**Piperacillin**

Trade name: Pipracil

**Ticarcillin**

Trade name: Ticar (Various pharmaceutical companies.)

**Indications:** Various infections caused by susceptible organisms

**Category:** Antibiotic

**Half-life:** varies

**Clinically important, potentially hazardous interactions with:** anisindione, anticoagulants, cyclosporine, demeclocycline, dicumarol, doxycycline, methotrexate, minocycline, oxytetracycline, tetracyclines

**Note:** "Patients with a history of penicillin allergy are about ten times more likely than the general population to experience a potentially fatal reaction to subsequent therapy with most other haptenating drugs." The degradation products of penicillin can bind with tissue or serum proteins to form an immunogenic complex that can elicit an immune response

## *Reactions*

### Skin

Acral numbness
(1997): Takahashi H, *J Dermatol* 24, 50

Acute generalized exanthematous pustulosis (AGEP)
(1995): Gebhardt M+, *Contact Dermatitis* 33, 204
(1995): Moreau A+, *Int J Dermatol* 34, 263 (passim)
(1994): Manders SM+, *Cutis* 54, 194
(1991): Roujeau J-C+, *Arch Dermatol* 127, 1333

Allergic reactions (sic)
(2000): Lee CE+, *Arch Intern Med* 160, 2819
(2000): Li JT+, *Mayo Clin Proc* 75, 902
(1984): Cameron W+, *Ann Allergy* 53, 455
(1984): Jolivet M+, *Union Med Can* (French) 113, 842

Angioedema
(1988): Van Arsdel PP Jr, *JAMA* 260, 2572
(1978): Girard JP, *Contact Dermatitis* 4, 309
(1968): Rosenblum AH, *J Allergy* 42, 309

Baboon syndrome
(1999): Panhans-Gross A+, *Contact Dermatitis* 41, 352

Bullous pemphigoid
(1992): Shelley WB+, *Advanced Dermatologic Diagnosis* WB Saunders, 414 (passim)
(1988): Alcalay J+, *J Am Acad Dermatol* 18, 345

Contact dermatitis
(1991): Rudzki E+, *Contact Dermatitis* 25, 192
(1990): Pecegueiro M, *Contact Dermatitis* 23, 190

Contact urticaria
(1985): Rudzki E+, *Contact Dermatitis* 13, 192
(1983): Fisher AA, *Cutis* 32, 314
(1978): Girard JP, *Contact Dermatitis* 4, 309

Cutis laxa
(1971): Reed WB+, *Arch Dermatol* 103, 661

Dermatitis (sic)
(1984): Beckerman A+, *Int J Dermatol* 23, 149

Diaphoresis

Eczematous eruption (sic)

Erythema annulare centrifugum
(1978): Gupta HL+, *J Indian Med Assoc* 65, 307
(1964): Shelley WB, *Arch Dermatol* 90, 54

Erythema multiforme
(2000): Ibia EO+, *Arch Dermatol* 136, 849
(1990): Garcia JJ+, *Clin Exp Allergy* 20 (Suppl 1), 121
(1990): Staretz LR+, *JADA* 121, 436
(1985): Huff JC, *Dermatologic Clinics* 3(1), 141
(1983): Ansel J+, *Arch Dermatol* 119, 1006

Erythema nodosum

Exanthems
(2000): Ibia EO+, *Arch Dermatol* 136, 849
(2000): Schnyder B+, *Hautarzt* (German) 51, 46
(1995): Romano A+, *Allergy* 50, 113
(1986): de Haan P+, *Allergy* 41, 75
(1976): Lackner F+, *Int J Clin Pharmacol Biopharm* (German) 13, 90
(1976): Richter G, *Dermatol Monatsschr* (German) 162, 533
(1974): Spitzy KH, *Acta Med Austriaca* (German) 2, 46
(1970): Baer RL+, *Br J Dermatol* 83, 37
(1970): Fellner MN+, *J Invest Dermatol* 55, 390

Exfoliative dermatitis
(1986): Wengrower D+, *Respiration* 50, 301

Fixed eruption
(1993): Inadomi T+, *Eur J Dermatol* 3, 674
(1980): Haustein UF, *Dermatol Monatsschr* (German) 166, 680
(1979): Pasricha JS, *Br J Dermatol* 100, 183
(1975): Coskey RJ+, *Arch Dermatol* 111, 791
(1970): Dennison WL+, *Arch Dermatol* 101, 594
(1951): Canizares O, *Arch Dermatol* 63, 800

Jarisch–Herxheimer reaction (<1%)
(2002): Whitley LS, Washington, DC (March AAD Poster)
(1977): Pareek SS, *Br J Vener Dis* 53, 389

Linear IgA bullous dermatosis
(1998): Wakelin SH+, *Br J Dermatol* 138, 310
(1994): Kuechle MK+, *J Am Acad Dermatol* 30, 187
(1993): Combemale P+, *Ann Dermatol Venereol* (French) 120, 847

Lupus erythematosus

Pemphigoid
(1988): Alcalay J+, *J Am Acad Dermatol* 18, 345

Pemphigus
(1997): Brenner S+, *J Am Acad Dermatol* 36, 919
(1991): Escallier F+, *Ann Dermatol Venereol* (French) 118, 381
(1988): Duhra P+, *Br J Dermatol* 118, 307
(1987): Brenner S+, *J Am Acad Dermatol* 17, 514
(1987): Seidenbaum M+, *Drug Intell Clin Pharm* 21, 1012

(1984): Ruocco V+, *Arch Dermatol Res* 274, 123
(1980): Fellner MJ, *Int J Dermatol* 9, 392
(1979): Ruocco V+, *Dermatologica* 159, 266
Pityriasis rosea
Pruritus
(1995): Litt JZ, Beachwood, OH (personal case) (observation)
(1970): Baer RL+, *Br J Dermatol* 83, 37
Purpura
Pustular psoriasis
(1987): Katz M+, *J Am Acad Dermatol* 17, 918
(1976): Lindgren S+, *Acta Derm Venereol* (Stockh) 56, 139
(1971): Ryan TJ+, *Br J Dermatol* 85, 407
(1969): Hadida E+, *Bull Soc Fr Dermatol Syphiligr* (French) 76, 1095
(1969): Privat Y+, *Bull Soc Fr Dermatol Syphiligr* (French) 76, 505
Rash (sic) (<1%)
Stevens–Johnson syndrome
(1997): Shoji T+, *J Am Acad Dermatol* 37, 337
(1996): Kammler H-J, Jena, Germany (from Internet) (observation)
(1993): Leenutaphong V+, *Int J Dermatol* 32, 428
(1983): Herold M+, *Ethiop Med J* 21, 227
(1983): Sullivan M, *Dent Health London* 22, 10
(1971): Nava-Negrete A, *Alergia* (Spanish) 19, 29
Toxic epidermal necrolysis
(1993): Leenutaphong V+, *Int J Dermatol* 32, 428
(1983): Herold M+, *Ethiop Med J* 21, 227
(1983): Tagami H+, *Arch Dermatol* 119, 910
(1982): Herold M+, *Z Gesamte Inn Med* (German) 37, 706
(1979): Frontera-Izquierdo P+, *An Esp Pediatr* 12, 703
(1977): Ghosh JS, *Arch Dermatol* 113, 1162
(1972): Carli-Basset C+, *Sem Hôp* (French) 48, 497
(1969): Pustovaia AI+, *Vestn Dermatol Venerol* (Russian) 43, 73
(1966): Ulcova I+, *Cesk Pediatr* (Czech) 21, 923
Toxic erythema
(1995): Rademaker M, *N Z Med J* 108, 165 (with vancomycin)
Urticaria
(2001): Torres MJ+, *Allergy* 56(9), 850
(2000): Ibia EO+, *Arch Dermatol* 136, 849
(1988): Sorensen HT+, *Ugeskr Laeger* (Danish) 150, 2913
(1982): Boonk WJ+, *Br J Dermatol* 106, 183
(1971): Van Hecke E, *Ann Dermatol Syphiligr* (Paris) (French) 98, 147
(1970): Baer RL+, *Br J Dermatol* 83, 37
(1968): Rosenblum AH, *J Allergy* 42, 309
Vasculitis
Vesicular eruptions

## Hair

Hair – alopecia
(1977): Pareek SS, *Br J Vener Dis* 53, 389

## Other

Anaphylactoid reactions
(2001): Garvey LH+, *Acta Anaesthesiol Scand* 45(10), 1204
(2001): Kruszewski J+, *Wiad Lek* 54, 116 (recurrent)
(2001): Torres MJ+, *Allergy* 56(9), 850
(2000): Xi-Moy S+, *Anesthesiology* 93, 280
(1999): Dunn AB+, *J Reprod Med* 44, 381
(1993): van der Klauw MM+, *Br J Clin Pharmacol* 35, 400
(1977): Matveikov GP+, *Antibiotiki* (Russian) 22, 813
(1976): Kraus SJ+, *Cutis* 17, 765
(1972): Kelle L+, *Z Arztl Fortbild* (Jena) (German) 66, 538
(1969): Idsoe O+, *Schweiz Med Wochenschr* (German) 99, 1221 (151 deaths)
(1968): Bowszyc J, *Przegl Dermatol* (Polish) 55, 307
(1968): Rosenblum AH, *J Allergy* 42, 309
(1967): Fellner MJ+, *Arch Dermatol* 96, 687
(1953): Feinberg S+, *JAMA* 152, 114
Black tongue
Death
(2002): Gerber N+, *Otolaryngol Head Neck Surg* 126(3), 321
Dysgeusia
Embolia cutis medicamentosa (Nicolau syndrome)
(2002): Poletti E+, *World Congress Dermatol* Poster, 0124
(1998): Saputo V+, *Pediatr Med Chir* (Italian) 20, 105
(1966): Deutsch J, *Dtsch Gesundheitw* (German) 21, 2433
Glossitis
Hypersensitivity (<1%)
(1998): Romano A, *Clin Exp Allergy* 28 (Suppl 4), 29
(1995): Bircher AJ, *Curr Probl Dermatol* 22, 31
(1988): Weiss ME+, *Clin Allergy* 18, 515
(1977): Reznikova ZT+, *Pediatriia* (Russian) April, 25
(1969): Leonhardi G+, *Hautarzt* (German) 20, 21
Injection-site aseptic necrosis
Injection-site reactions (sic) (1–10%)
(1990): Shen K, *Lancet* 336, 689
Injection-site urticaria
Lipoatrophy
(2000): Kuperman-Beade M+, *Pediatr Dermatol* 17, 302
Oral candidiasis (>10%)
Oral ulceration
(1990): Staretz LR+, *JADA* 121, 436
Serum sickness
(2001): Tatum AJ+, *Ann Allergy Asthma Immunol* 86(3), 330 (3 cases)
(2000): Ibia EO+, *Arch Dermatol* 136, 849
(1990): Heckbert SR+, *Am J Epidemiol* 132, 336
(1980): Brandslund I+, *Haemostasis* 9, 193
(1967): Fellner MJ+, *Arch Dermatol* 96, 687
(1967): Fellner MJ+, *J Invest Dermatol* 48, 384
Stomatitis
Thrombophlebitis (<1%)
Tongue, furry
Xerostomia

# PENTAGASTRIN

**Trade name:** Peptavlon (Wyeth-Ayerst)
**Other common trade name:** *Gastrodiagnost*
**Category:** Diagnostic aid (gastric function)
**Half-life:** 10 minutes

### *Reactions*

## Skin

Angioedema
(1985): Arnved J+, *Lancet* 2, 1068
(1975): Wastell C+, *BMJ* 1, 334
Diaphoresis
Exanthems
(1975): Wastell C+, *BMJ* 1, 334
Flushing
(1975): Wastell C+, *BMJ* 1, 334
Pruritus
(1975): Wastell C+, *BMJ* 1, 334
Purpura
(1985): Arnved J+, *Lancet* 2, 1068
Rash (sic)
Urticaria

## Other

Hypersensitivity
Injection-site pain
Paresthesias

## PENTAMIDINE

**Trade names:** NebuPent (Fujisawa); Pentam-300 (Fujisawa)
**Other common trade name:** *Pentacarinat*
**Indications:** *Pneumocystis carinii* infection, trypanosomiasis
**Category:** Antiprotozoal antibiotic
**Half-life:** 9.1–13.2 hours (IM); 6.5 hours (IV)
**Clinically important, potentially hazardous interactions with:** sparfloxacin

**Note:** The rate of adverse side effects is increased in patients with AIDS

### *Reactions*

#### Skin

Bullous eruption
(1970): Wang JJ+, *J Pediatr* 77, 311
Cutaneous side effects (sic)
(1989): Berger TG+, *Ann Intern Med* 110, 1035
Edema
Erythema
Exanthems
(1992): Breathnach SM+, *Adverse Drug Reactions and the Skin* Blackwell, Oxford, 179 (passim)
(1990): Leoung GS+, *N Engl J Med* 323, 769 (0.25%)
(1990): Monk JP+, *Drugs* 39, 741
(1990): Soo Hoo GW+, *Ann Intern Med* 113, 195 (1–5%)
(1989): Berger TG+, *Ann Intern Med* 110, 1035
(1988): Leen CLS+, *Lancet* 2, 1250
(1988): Sattler FR+, *Ann Intern Med* 109, 280 (15%)
(1987): Goa KL+, *Drugs* 33, 242 (1.5%)
(1984): Gordon FM+, *Ann Intern Med* 100, 495 (3%)
(1984): Kovacs JA+, *Ann Intern Med* 100, 663 (6%)
Jarisch–Herxheimer reaction (<1%)
(1987): Goa KL+, *Drugs* 33, 242
Pruritus
(1989): Berger TG+, *Ann Intern Med* 110, 1035
(1988): Leen CLS+, *Lancet* 2, 1250
Purpura
Rash (sic) (31–47%)
(1993): Dohn M+, *Int Conf AIDS* 9, 372
(1988): Leen CL+, *Lancet* 2, 1250
(1984): Gordin FM+, *Ann Intern Med* 100, 495
(1974): Walzer PD+, *Ann Intern Med* 80, 83 (1.5%)
Stevens–Johnson syndrome (0.2%)
Toxic epidermal necrolysis
(1988): Leen CLS+, *Lancet* 2, 1250 (passim)
(1987): Goa KL+, *Drugs* 33, 242
(1985): Heng MCY, *Br J Dermatol* 113, 597
Ulceration
(1985): Gottlieb JR+, *Plast Reconstr Surg* 76, 630
Urticaria
(1993): Belsito DV, *Contact Dermatitis* 29, 158 (contact)
(1992): Breathnach SM+, *Adverse Drug Reactions and the Skin* Blackwell, Oxford, 179 (passim)
(1988): Leen CLS+, *Lancet* 2, 1250
Vasculitis
Xerosis

#### Other

Ageusia
Anosmia
Dysgeusia (1.7%) (metallic taste)
Gingivitis
Injection-site calcification
(1987): Goa KL+, *Drugs* 33, 242
Injection-site cutaneous reaction (sic) (>10%)
(1992): Jones RS+, *Clin Infect Dis* 15, 561
Injection-site irritation
(1996): Andersen JM, *Am J Health Syst Pharm* 53, 185
(1996): Herrero-Ambrosio A+, *Am J Health Syst Pharm* 53, 2881
Injection-site ulceration
(1991): Bolognia JL, *Dermatologica* 183, 221
Myalgia (<5%)
Phlebitis
Rhabdomyolysis
(1985): Sensakovic JW+, *Arch Intern Med* 145(12), 2247
Xerostomia

## PENTAZOCINE

**Trade name:** Talwin (Sanofi)
**Other common trade names:** *Fortral; Fortwin; Liticon; Ospronim; Pentafen; Sosegon; Susevin; Talacen*
**Indications:** Pain
**Category:** Narcotic; analgesic; sedative
**Half-life:** 2–3 hours
**Clinically important, potentially hazardous interactions with:** cimetidine, morphine

### *Reactions*

#### Skin

Cellulitis
(1992): Breathnach SM+, *Adverse Drug Reactions and the Skin* Blackwell, Oxford, 212 (passim)
Dermatitis (sic)
Diaphoresis
Exanthems
(1987): Pedragosa R+, *Arch Dermatol* 123, 297
Facial edema
Flushing
(1973): Brogden RN+, *Drugs* 5, 6
Generalized eruption (sic)
(1992): Breathnach SM+, *Adverse Drug Reactions and the Skin* Blackwell, Oxford, 212 (passim)
Pigmentation (surrounding ulcers)
(1990): Furner BB, *J Am Acad Dermatol* 694 (passim)
Pruritus (<1%)
Rash (sic) (1–10%)
Scleroderma
(2000): D'Cruz D, *Toxicol Lett* 112 and 421
(1991): Bourgeois P+, *Baillieres Clin Rheumatol* 5, 13
Sclerosis (sic)
(1980): Palestine RF+, *J Am Acad Dermatol* 2, 47
(1974): Beckner TF, *JAMA* 227, 1383
(1973): Brogden RN+, *Drugs* 5, 6 (widespread)
Toxic epidermal necrolysis (<1%)
(1987): Pedragosa R+, *Arch Dermatol* 123, 297 (passim)
(1973): Hunter AAJ+, *Br J Dermatol* 88, 287
Tricotropism (sic)
(1987): Pedragosa R+, *Arch Dermatol* 123, 297 (passim)
Ulceration
(1992): Breathnach SM+, *Adverse Drug Reactions and the Skin* Blackwell, Oxford, 212 (passim)
(1990): Furner BB, *J Am Acad Dermatol* 694
(1980): Palestine RF+, *J Am Acad Dermatol* 2, 47
(1979): Padilla RS+, *Arch Dermatol* 115, 975 (punched-out ulcers)
(1974): Winfield JB+, *South Med J* 67, 292
(1973): Winfield JB+, *JAMA* 226, 189

Urticaria

### Other

Dysgeusia
Embolia cutis medicamentosa (Nicolau syndrome)
(1983): Bockers M+, *Med Welt* (German) 34, 1450
Fibrous myopathy
(1976): Johnson KR+, *Arthritis Rheum* 19, 923
(1975): Oh SJ+, *JAMA* 231, 271
Injection-site calcification
(1991): Magee KL+, *Arch Dermatol* 127, 1591
(1986): Hertzman A+, *J Rheumatol* 13, 210
Injection-site fibrosis
(1979): Padilla RS+, *Arch Dermatol* 115, 975
Injection-site granulomas and induration
(1982): Menon PA, *J Assoc Military Dermatol* 2, 65
(1972): Agache P+, *Bull Soc Fr Dermatol Syphiligr* (French) 79, 37
(1971): Schlicher JE+, *Arch Dermatol* 104, 90
Injection-site induration and ulcers
(1996): Bellman B+, *Arch Dermatol* 132, 1365
(1996): Gillum P, Oklahoma City, OK (from Internet) (observation)
(1984): Choucair AK+, *Neurology* 34, 524
(1983): Adams EM+, *Arch Intern Med* 143, 2203
(1977): Cosman A+, *Plast Reconstr Surg* 59, 255
(1977): Schiff BL+, *JAMA* 238, 1542
(1974): Seymour R+, *Am Surg* 40, 671
(1973): Hönigsmann H+, *Hautarzt* (German) 24, 128
(1971): Parks DL+, *Arch Dermatol* 104, 231
Injection-site pain
Injection-site pigmentation
(1980): Palestine RF+, *J Am Acad Dermatol* 2, 47
Lipogranulomas
(1973): Hönigsmann H, *Dermatol Monatsschr* (German) 159, 146
Myofibrosis
(1999): Jain A+, *J Dermatol* 26, 368
Panniculitis (chronic)
(1992): Breathnach SM+, *Adverse Drug Reactions and the Skin* Blackwell, Oxford, 212 (passim)
Paresthesias
Phlebitis
(1992): Breathnach SM+, *Adverse Drug Reactions and the Skin* Blackwell, Oxford, 212 (passim)
Soft tissue calcification
(1990): Furner BB, *J Am Acad Dermatol* 694 (passim)
Tinnitus
Xerostomia (1–10%)

## PENTOBARBITAL

**Trade name:** Nembutal (Abbott)
**Other common trade names:** *Medinox Mono; Mintal; Nova Rectal; Pentobarbitone; Prodromol; Sombutol*
**Indications:** Insomnia, sedation
**Category:** Hypnotic and sedative barbiturate; anticonvulsant
**Half-life:** 15–50 hours
**Clinically important, potentially hazardous interactions with: alcohol**, anticoagulants, antihistamines, brompheniramine, buclizine, chlorpheniramine, dicumarol, ethanolamine, imatinib, warfarin

#### *Reactions*

### Skin

Acne
Angioedema (<1%)
Bullous eruption
(1970): Groeschel D+, *N Engl J Med* 283, 409
Erythema multiforme
(1975): Böttiger LE, *Acta Med Scand* 198, 229
Exanthems
(1943): Davison TC, *Curr Res Anesth Analg* 22, 52
Exfoliative dermatitis (<1%)
(1944): Potter JK+, *Ann Intern Med* 21, 1041
Fixed eruption
(1970): Savin JA, *Br J Dermatol* 83, 546
Herpes simplex (activation)
Lupus erythematosus
(1967): Williams DI, *Proc R Soc Med* 60, 299
(1951): Grant Peterkin GA, *Edinb Med J* 58, 41
Necrosis
(1972): Almeyda J+, *Br J Dermatol* 86, 313
Photoreactions
(1939): Stryker GV, *J Mo Med Assn* 36, 484
Photosensitivity
Pruritus
Purpura
(1946): Grant Peterkin GA, *BMJ* 2, 52
Rash (sic) (<1%)
Stevens–Johnson syndrome (<1%)
Toxic epidermal necrolysis
(1973): Stüttgen G, *Br J Dermatol* 88, 291
Urticaria
Vasculitis

### Other

Hypersensitivity
Injection-site pain (1–10%)
Injection-site reactions (sic) (<1%)
Oral ulceration
Porphyria
(1968): Lang PA+, *Tex Rep Biol Med* 26, 525
Porphyria variegata
Rhabdomyolysis
(1990): Larpin R+, *Presse Med* 19(30), 1403
Thrombophlebitis (<1%)

## PENTOSAN

**Synonym:** PPS
**Trade name:** Elmiron (Alza)
**Indications:** Bladder pain, interstitial cystitis
**Category:** Urinary analgesic
**Half-life:** 4.8 hours

#### *Reactions*

### Skin

Allergic reactions (sic) (<1%)
Ecchymoses
Photosensitivity (<1%)
Pruritus (<1%)
Purpura (<1%)
Rash (sic) (1–10%)
Urticaria (<1%)

### Hair

Hair – alopecia (1–10%)

### Other

Gingival bleeding (<1%)
Oral ulceration (<1%)

## PENTOSTATIN

**Trade name:** Nipent (SuperGen)
**Indications:** Hairy-cell leukemia
**Category:** Antineoplastic; antimetabolite
**Half-life:** 5–15 hours
**Clinically important, potentially hazardous interactions with:** aldesleukin

### *Reactions*

#### Skin

Acne (<3%)
Allergic reactions (sic) (>10%)
Bullous eruption (3–10%)
Candidiasis (<3%)
Contact dermatitis (<3%)
Dermatitis (sic) (<1%)
Diaphoresis (3–10%)
Ecchymoses (3–10%)
Eczema (sic) (3–10%)
Erythema
Erythroderma
(1999): Ghura HS+, *BMJ* 319, 549
Exanthems (3–10%)
(1997): Greiner D+, *J Am Acad Dermatol* 36, 950
(1989): O'Dwyer PJ+, *Cancer Chemother Pharmacol* 23, 173
Exfoliative dermatitis (<3%)
Facial edema (<3%)
Flushing (<3%)
Herpes simplex (3–10%)
Herpes zoster (3–10%)
Peripheral edema (3–10%)
Petechiae (3–10%)
Photosensitivity (<3%)
Pigmentation (3–10%)
Pruritus (3–10%)
Psoriasis (<3%)
Purpura (<3%)
(1999): Leach JW+, *Am J Hematol* 61, 268
Rash (sic) (26%)
Reactivation of pruritus and erythema of preexisting keratoses (sic)
(1989): Kerker BJ+, *Semin Dermatol* 8, 173
(1985): Camisa C+, *J Am Acad Dermatol* 12, 1108
Seborrhea (3–10%)
Skin disorder (sic) (17%)
Urticaria (<1%)
Xerosis (3–10%)

#### Hair

Hair – alopecia (<3%)

#### Other

Anaphylactoid reactions (<3%)
Dysgeusia (<3%)
Gingivitis (<3%)
Gynecomastia (<3%)
Injection-site hemorrhage (<3%)
Injection-site inflammation (<3%)
Leukoplakia (<3%)
Myalgia (>10%)
Paresthesias (3–10%)
Stomatitis (1–10%)
Thrombophlebitis (3–10%)
Tinnitus
Vaginitis (<3%)

## PENTOXIFYLLINE

**Trade names:** Pentoxil (Upsher-Smith); Trental (Aventis)
**Other common trade names:** *Apo-Pentoxifylline; Artal; Azupentat; Elorgan; Hemovas; Pentoxi; Pexal; Torental*
**Indications:** Peripheral vascular disease, intermittent claudication
**Category:** Blood viscosity reducing agent
**Half-life:** 0.4–0.8 hours

### *Reactions*

#### Skin

Allergic reactions (sic)
(1986): Bigby M+, *JAMA* 256, 3358
Angioedema (<1%)
(1994): Samlaska CP+, *J Am Acad Dermatol* 30, 603 (passim)
Diaphoresis
Edema (<1%)
Exanthems
Flushing
(1987): Ward A+, *Drugs* 34, 50 (2%)
(1976): 14, 59
Pruritus (<1%)
(1994): Samlaska CP+, *J Am Acad Dermatol* 30, 603 (passim)
Purpura
Rash (sic) (<1%)
Urticaria

#### Nails

Nails – brittle (<1%)

#### Other

Dysgeusia (<1%)
Dysphagia
(1997): Fetterman M, Miami, FL (from Internet) (observation)
(1997): Puritz E, Smithtown, NY (from Internet) (observation)
Paresthesias
(1994): Samlaska CP+, *J Am Acad Dermatol* 30, 603 (passim)
Serum sickness
(1986): Panwalker AP+, *Drug Intell Clin Pharm* 20, 953
Sialorrhea (<1%)
Tremors
Xerostomia (<1%)
(1994): Samlaska CP+, *J Am Acad Dermatol* 30, 603 (passim)

## PERGOLIDE

**Trade name:** Permax (Athena)
**Other common trade names:** *Celance; Parkotil; Pergolide*
**Indications:** Parkinsonism
**Category:** Antiparkinsonian; dopamine receptor agonist; ergot alkaloid
**Half-life:** 27 hours

### *Reactions*

#### Skin

Acne
Chills (1–10%)
Diaphoresis (2.1%)
Discoloration (sic)
Edema (1.6%)

Erythromelalgia
(1989): Horn TD+, *Arch Dermatol* 125, 1512
(1984): Monk BE+, *Br J Dermatol* 111, 97 (on shins)
Exanthems
Facial edema (1.1%)
(1993): Garcia-Escrig M+, *Medicina Clinica* (Spanish) 101, 275
Flu-like syndrome (sic) (1–10%)
Peripheral edema (1–10%)
Pruritus
Rash (sic) (3.2%)
Seborrhea
Ulceration
Urticaria
Vasculitis
(1989): Horn TD+, *Arch Dermatol* 125, 1512
Xerosis

### Hair

Hair – alopecia
Hair – hirsutism

### Other

Dysgeusia (1.6%)
Gingivitis (<1%)
Mastodynia
Myalgia (<1%)
Paresthesias (1.6%)
Priapism
Tinnitus
Tremors (1–10%)
Xerostomia (1–10%)

## PERINDOPRIL

**Trade name:** Aceon (Solvay)
**Other common trade names:** *Acertil; Coversum; Coversyl; Prexum*
**Indications:** Hypertension
**Category:** Angiotensin-converting enzyme (ACE) inhibitor; antihypertensive
**Half-life:** 1.5–3 hours

### *Reactions*

### Skin

Angioedema (<1%)
(2001): Cohen EG+, *Ann Otol Rhinol Laryngol* 110(8), 701 (64 cases)
(1998): Lapostolle F+, *Am J Cardiol* 81, 523 (lingual)
Chills (<1%)
Cutaneous reactions (sic) (1.3%)
(1993): Desche P+, *Am J Cardiol* 71, 61E
Diaphoresis (0.3–1%)
Ecchymoses (0.3–1%)
Edema (3.9%)
Erythema (0.3–1%)
Exanthems
Facial edema (<1%)
Herpes simplex (0.3–1%)
Palmar–plantar pustulosis
(1995): Eriksen JG+, *Ugeskr Laeger* (Danish) 157, 3335
Pemphigus foliaceus
(2000): Ong CS+, *Australas J Dermatol* 41(4), 242
Pruritus (1–10%)
Psoriasis (<1%)
Purpura (<0.1%)
Rash (sic) (1–10%)
(1991): Dratwa M+, *J Cardiovasc Pharmacol* 18, S40
Xerosis (0.3–1%)

### Other

Anaphylactoid reactions (<1%)
(1998): Speirs C+, *Br J Clin Pharmacol* 46, 63
Cough
(2001): Adigun AQ+, *West Afr J Med* 20(1), 46–7
(2001): Lee SC+, *Hypertension* 38(2), 166
Dysgeusia (<1%)
Myalgia (<1%)
Paresthesias (2.3%)
Vaginitis (0.3–1%)
Xerostomia (0.3–1%)

## PERPHENAZINE

**Trade names:** Etrafon (Schering); Triavil (Lotus); Trilafon (Schering)
**Other common trade names:** *Apo-Perphenzine; Decentan; Fentazin; Leptopsique; Peratsin; Perphenan; Trilifan Retard; Triomin*
**Indications:** Psychotic disorders, nausea and vomiting
**Category:** Phenothiazine antipsychotic and antiemetic
**Half-life:** 9 hours
**Clinically important, potentially hazardous interactions with:** sparfloxacin

Etrafon and Triavil are combinations of perphenazine and amitriptyline

### *Reactions*

### Skin

Angioedema
Contact dermatitis
Diaphoresis
Eczema (sic)
Erythema
Exanthems
(1976): Arndt KA+, *JAMA* 235, 918
(1959): Wright W, *JAMA* 171, 1642
Exfoliative dermatitis
Lupus erythematosus
(1988): Steen VD+, *Arthritis Rheum* 31, 923
(1986): Gupta MA+, *J Am Acad Dermatol* 14, 638
(1978): Gold MS+, *J Nerv Ment Dis* 166, 442
(1971): Fabius AJM+, *Acta Rheum Scand* 17, 137
Peripheral edema
Photosensitivity
Pigmentation (blue-gray) (<1%)
Pruritus
Purpura
Rash (sic) (1–10%)
Seborrhea
Urticaria
(1959): Wright W, *JAMA* 171, 1642
Xerosis

### Other

Anaphylactoid reactions
Galactorrhea (black) (<1%)
(1985): Basler RSW+, *Arch Dermatol* 121, 418

Gynecomastia
Mastodynia (1–10%)
Parkinsonism
Priapism (<1%)
Pseudolymphoma
(1995): Magro CM+, *J Am Acad Dermatol* 32, 419
Rhabdomyolysis
(1983): Caruana RJ+, *N C Med J* 44, 18 (with lorazepam and amitriptyline)
Sialorrhea
Tinnitus
Xerostomia

## PHENAZOPYRIDINE

**Trade names:** Baridium; Geridium; Prodium; Pyridiate; Pyridium (Parke-Davis)
**Other common trade names:** *Azodine; Eridium; Phenazo; Pyronium; Sedural; Urodine; Urogesic; Urohman; Uropyridin*
**Indications:** Urinary urgency, dysuria
**Category:** Urinary analgesic
**Half-life:** no data

### *Reactions*

#### Skin
Allergic reactions (sic)
(1986): Bigby M+, *JAMA* 256, 3358 (0.88%)
Edema
Exanthems
(1976): Arndt KA+, *JAMA* 235, 918 (0.6%)
Pigmentation (<1%)
(1974): Eybel CE+, *JAMA* 228, 1027 (blue-gray; orange-yellow)
(1970): Alano FA+, *Ann Intern Med* 72, 89
Pruritus
Rash (sic) (<1%)

#### Nails
Nails – lemon-yellow
(1997): Amit G+, *Ann Intern Med* 127, 1137

#### Other
Anaphylactoid reactions

## PHENDIMETRAZINE

**Trade names:** Bontril (Carnrick); Prelu-2 (Roxane)
**Other common trade name:** *Obesan-X*
**Indications:** Obesity
**Category:** Appetite suppressant
**Half-life:** 5–12.5 hours
**Clinically important, potentially hazardous interactions with:** fluoxetine, fluvoxamine, MAO inhibitors, paroxetine, phenelzine, sertraline, tranylcypromine

### *Reactions*

#### Skin
Diaphoresis
Flushing
Urticaria

#### Other
Dysgeusia
Xerostomia

## PHENELZINE

**Trade name:** Nardil (Parke-Davis)
**Other common trade name:** *Nardelzine*
**Indications:** Depression
**Category:** Monoamine oxidase (MAO) inhibitor; antidepressant and antipanic
**Half-life:** no data
**Clinically important, potentially hazardous interactions with:** amitriptyline, amoxapine, amphetamines, bupropion, citalopram, clomipramine, cyproheptadine, desipramine, dextroamphetamine, dextromethorphan, diethylpropion, dopamine, doxepin, entacapone, ephedrine, epinephrine, fluoxetine, fluvoxamine, **ginseng**, levodopa, mazindol, meperidine, methamphetamine, nefazodone, nortriptyline, paroxetine, phendimetrazine, phentermine, phenylephrine, protriptyline, pseudoephedrine, rizatriptan, sertraline, sibutramine, sumatriptan, sympathomimetics, tramadol, tricyclic antidepressants, trimipramine, **tryptophan**, venlafaxine, zolmitriptan

### *Reactions*

#### Skin
Angioedema
(1962): Busfield BL+, *J Nerv Ment Dis* 134, 339
Ankle edema
(1977): Dunleavy DLF, *BMJ* 1, 1353
(1970): Kelly D+, *Br J Psychiatry* 116, 387
Diaphoresis
(1985): Levy AB+, *Can J Psychiatry* 30, 434
Edema
Exanthems
Lupus erythematosus
(1978): Swartz C, *JAMA* 239, 2693
Peripheral edema (1–10%)
Photosensitivity
(1988): Case JD+, *Photodermatology* 5, 101
(1962): Busfield BL+, *J Nerv Ment Dis* 134, 339 (13%)
Pruritus (13%)
(1962): Busfield BL+, *J Nerv Ment Dis* 134, 339
Rash (sic)
Telangiectases
Urticaria

#### Other
Black tongue
Glossitis
(1992): Zürcher K+, *Cutaneous Drug Reactions*, Karger, Basel (passim)
Parkinsonism
Priapism
Rhabdomyolysis
(1984): Linden CH+, *Ann Emerg Med* 13(12), 1137
Tremors
Twitching
Xerostomia (1–10%)
(1962): Busfield BL+, *J Nerv Ment Dis* 134, 339 (20%)

# PHENINDAMINE

**Trade name:** Nolahist (Carnrick)
**Indications:** Allergic rhinitis, urticaria, angioedema
**Category:** $H_1$-receptor antihistamine and appetite stimulant
**Half-life:** no data

### *Reactions*

## Skin

Angioedema
Dermatitis (sic)
Diaphoresis
Erythema
Flushing
Lupus erythematosus
Photosensitivity
Purpura
Rash (sic)
Urticaria

## Other

Xerostomia

# PHENOBARBITAL

**Synonyms:** phenobarbitone; phenylethylmalonylurea
**Trade names:** Barbita; Luminal (Sanofi); Solfoton (ECR)
**Other common trade names:** *Alepsal; Barbilixir; Barbital; Gardenal; Luminaletten; Phenaemal; Phenobarbitone*
**Indications:** Insomnia, seizures
**Category:** Sedative-hypnotic and anticonvulsant barbiturate
**Half-life:** 2–6 days
**Clinically important, potentially hazardous interactions with: alcohol**, anticoagulants, antihistamines, brompheniramine, buclizine, chlorpheniramine, dicumarol, ethanolamine, fluconazole, imatinib, meperidine, midazolam, warfarin

### *Reactions*

## Skin

Acne
(1992): Hesse S+, *Ann Dermatol Venereol* (French) 119, 655
Acute generalized exanthematous pustulosis (AGEP)
(1996): Wolkenstein P+, *Contact Dermatitis* 35, 234
Allergic reactions (sic)
(1987): Pigatto PD, *Contact Dermatitis* 16, 279
(1979): Montowska L+, *Pol Tyg Lek* (Polish) 34, 2029
Angioedema (<1%)
Bullous eruption
(1990): Dunn C+, *Cutis* 45, 43 (in coma)
(1970): Groeschel D+, *N Engl J Med* 283, 409
(1965): Beveridge GW+, *BMJ* 1, 835
(1940): Moss RE+, *Arch Dermatol* 46, 386
(1925): Birch CA, *Brit J Child Dis* 22, 280
Depigmentation
(1992): Mion N+, *Ann Dermatol Venereol* (French) 119, 927
Edema
Erythema multiforme
(1994): Shelley WB+, *Cutis* 53, 162 (observation)
(1994): Stewart MG+, *Otolaryngol Head Neck Surg* 111, 236
(1990): Salomon D+, *Br J Dermatol* 123, 797
(1988): Shear NH+, *J Clin Invest* 82, 1826
(1986): Palomeque A+, *An Esp Pediatr* (Spanish) 34, 328
(1975): Böttiger LE, *Acta Med Scand* 198, 229
(1940): Moss RE+, *Arch Dermatol* 46, 386
Erythroderma
(1993): Sakai C+, *Intern Med* 32, 182
Exanthems
(2001): Hebert AA+, *J Clin Psychiatry* 62 (suppl 14), 22
(1997): Hyson C+, *Can J Neurol Sci* 24, 245
(1988): Shear NH+, *J Clin Invest* 82, 1826
(1986): Savich RD+, *Ill Med J* 169, 232
(1984): Fernandez de Corres L+, *Contact Dermatitis* 11, 319
(1979): Rudzki E, *Przegl Dermatol* (Polish) 66, 415
(1952): Sneddon IB+, *BMJ* 1, 1276
(1943): Davison TC, *Curr Res Anesth Analg* 22, 52
(1940): Moss RE+, *Arch Dermatol* 46, 386
(1925): Birch CA, *Brit J Child Dis* 22, 280
Exfoliative dermatitis (<1%)
(1993): Sakai C+, *Intern Med* 32, 182
(1986): Savich RD+, *Ill Med J* 169, 232
(1976): Weisburst M+, *South Med J* 69, 126
(1950): Welton DG, *JAMA* 143, 232
(1944): Potter JK+, *Ann Intern Med* 21, 1041
(1940): Moss RE+, *Arch Dermatol* 46, 386
Fixed eruption
(1998): Mahboob A+, *Int J Dermatol* 37, 833
(1989): Shiohara T+, *Arch Dermatol* 125, 1371
(1987): Savchak VI, *Vestn Dermatol Venerol* (Russian) 6, 62
(1979): Pasricha JS, *Br J Dermatol* 100, 183
(1974): Kuokkanen K, *Int J Dermatol* 13, 4 (genitalia and mucous membranes)
(1970): Savin JA, *Br J Dermatol* 83, 546
(1967): Schulz KH+, *Z Haut Geschlechtskr* (German) 42, 561
Graft-versus-host reaction
(1998): Jappe U+, *Hautarzt* (German) 49, 126 (passim)
Herpes simplex (activation)
Lupus erythematosus
(1967): Williams DI, *Proc R Soc Med* 60, 299
(1951): Grant Peterkin GA, *Edinb Med J* 58, 41
Necrosis
(1972): Almeyda J+, *Br J Dermatol* 86, 313
Pellagra
(1982): Stadler R+, *Hautarzt* (German) 33, 276
Pemphigus
(1986): Dourmishev AL+, *Dermatologica* 173, 256
Photoreactions
(1939): Stryker GV, *J Mo Med Assn* 36, 484
Photosensitivity
Pruritus
(1994): Sigl B, *Hautarzt* (German) 45, 409
Purpura
(1952): Sneddon IB+, *BMJ* 1, 1276
(1946): Grant Peterkin GA, *BMJ* 2, 52
Pustules (generalized)
(1991): Kleier RS+, *Arch Dermatol* 127, 1361
Rash (sic) (<1%)
Stevens–Johnson syndrome (<1%)
(1999): Duncan KO, *J Am Acad Dermatol* 40, 493 (at sites of radiation therapy)
(1999): Rzany B+, *Lancet* 353, 2190
(1995): Labandiera-Garcia J, *An Med Interna* (Spanish) 12, 569
(1995): Wolkenstein P+, *Arch Dermatol* 131, 544
(1994): Koukoulis A+, *An Med Interna* (Spanish) 11, 311
(1993): Leenutaphong V+, *Int J Dermatol* 32, 428
(1992): Lleonart R+, *Med Clin (Barc)* (Spanish) 99, 474
(1985): Avery JK, *J Tenn Med Assoc* 78, 764
(1985): de Rego JA+, *Hillside J Clin Psychiatry* 7, 141
(1982): Brahams D, *Lancet* 2, 1474
(1982): Oles KS+, *Clin Pharm* 1, 565
(1971): Adeloye A+, *Ghana Med J* 10, 56
Toxic epidermal necrolysis

(2000): Devidal R+, *Therapie* 55, 225 (2 cases)
(1999): Rzany B+, *Lancet* 353, 2190
(1996): Blum L+, *J Am Acad Dermatol* 34, 1088
(1995): Wolkenstein P+, *Arch Dermatol* 131, 544
(1994): Errani A+, *Br J Dermatol* 131, 586
(1994): Shelley WB+, *Cutis* 53, 162 (observation)
(1993): Correia O+, *Dermatology* 186, 32
(1993): Leenutaphong V+, *Int J Dermatol* 32, 428
(1989): Dominguez-Perez F+, *Rev Esp Anestesiol Reanim* (Spanish) 36, 350
(1988): Shear NH+, *J Clin Invest* 82, 1826
(1987): Teillac D+, *Arch Fr Pediatr* (French) 44, 583
(1985): de Rego JA+, *Hillside J Clin Psychiatry* 7, 141
(1984): Chan HL, *J Am Acad Dermatol* 10, 973
(1975): Deviller G+, *Union Med Can* (French) 104, 399
(1975): Giallorenzi AF+, *Oral Surg Oral Med Oral Pathol* 40, 611
(1973): Stüttgen G, *Br J Dermatol* 88, 291
(1966): Campos EC de+, *An Bras Dermatol* (Portuguese) 41, 165
(1966): Haraszti A+, *Orv Hetil* (Hungarian) 107, 2133 (fatal)
(1966): Kaczorowska-Hanke H+, *Przegl Dermatol* (Polish) 53, 197

Toxicoderma (sic)
(1998): Arima M+, *Jpn Circ J* 62, 132

Urticaria
(1940): Moss RE+, *Arch Dermatol* 46, 386

Vasculitis

## Hair

Hair – depigmentation
(1992): Mion N+, *Ann Dermatol Venereol* (French) 119, 927

## Nails

Nails – hypoplasia
(1991): Thakker JC+, *Indian Pediatr* 28, 73
(1990): Holder M+, *Monatsschr Kinderheilkr* (German) 138, 34

## Other

Acute intermittent porphyria
(2001): Sykes RM, *Seizure* 10(1), 64

Death

DRESS syndrome
(2001): Lachgar T+, *Allerg Immunol (Paris* (Paris) 33(4), 173
(1997): Descamps V+, *Br J Dermatol* 137, 605

Hypersensitivity (<1%)*
(2002): Metin A+, *World Congress Dermatol* Poster, 0116
(1999): Moss DM+, *J Emerg Med* 17, 503
(1998): Chapman MS+, *Br J Dermatol* 138, 710
(1998): Schlienger RG+, *Epilepsia* 39, S3 (passim)
(1997): Morkunas AR+, *Crit Care Clin* 13, 727
(1992): Nagata T+, *Jpn J Clin Oncol* 22, 421
(1984): Fonseca JC+, *Med Cutan Ibero Lat Am* (Spanish) 12, 187

Hypoplasia of phalanges
(1991): Thakker JC+, *Indian Pediatr* 28, 73
(1990): Holder M+, *Monatsschr Kinderheilkr* (German) 138, 34

Injection-site bullous eruption
(1987): Haroun M+, *Cutis* 39, 233

Injection-site pain (>10%)

Injection-site thrombophlebitis (>10%)

Oral ulceration

Porphyria cutanea tarda
(1966): Ziprkowski L+, *Isr J Med Sci* 2, 338

Porphyria variegata

Rhabdomyolysis
(1990): Larpin R+, *Presse Med* 19(30), 1403

Xerostomia
(1952): Sneddon IB+, *BMJ* 1, 1276

***Note:** The antiepileptic drug hypersensitivity syndrome is a severe, occasionally fatal, disorder characterized by any or all of the following: pruritic exanthems, toxic epidermal necrolysis, Stevens–Johnson syndrome, exfoliative dermatitis, fever, hepatic abnormalities, eosinophilia, and renal failure

# PHENOLPHTHALEIN

**Trade names:** Agoral; Alophen; Caroid; Correctol; Doxidan; Espotabs; Evac-U-Gen; Ex-Lax; Feen-A-Mint; Medilax; Modane; Phenolax; Prulet; Trilax
**Other common trade names:** *Bom-Bon; Bonomint; Darmol; Easylax; Purganol; Ruguletts*
**Indications:** Constipation
**Category:** Laxative
**Half-life:** no data

### *Reactions*

## Skin

Angioedema
(1972): Grillat JP+, *Rev Fr Allergie* (French) 12, 351

Bullous eruption
(1974): Magill M+, *Med J Aust* 1, 771

Diaphoresis

Erythema annulare (sic)
(1972): Grillat JP+, *Rev Fr Allergie* (French) 12, 351

Erythema multiforme
(1992): Breathnach SM+, *Adverse Drug Reactions and the Skin* Blackwell, Oxford, 344
(1972): Shelley WB+, *Br J Dermatol* 86, 118

Exanthems
(1972): Grilliat JP+, *Rev Fr Allergol* (French) 12, 351
(1969): Török H, *Dermatol Int* 8, 57

Exfoliative dermatitis
(1973): Nicolis GD+, *Arch Dermatol* 108, 788

Fixed eruption
(1997): Blumenthal HL, Beachwood, OH (personal case) (observation)
(1993): Zanolli MD+, *Pediatrics* 91, 1199
(1991): Smoller BR+, *J Cutan Pathol* 18, 13
(1990): Gaffoor PMA+, *Cutis* 45, 242
(1987): Stroud MB+, *Arch Dermatol* 123, 1227
(1986): Kanwar AJ+, *Dermatologica* 172, 315
(1985): Kauppinen K+, *Br J Dermatol* 112, 575
(1984): Chan HL, *Int J Dermatol* 23, 607
(1978): Sehgal VN+, *Int J Dermatol* 17, 78
(1972): Hunziker N, *Rev Med Suisse Romande* (French) 92, 237
(1972): Louis P, *Z Haut Geschlechtskr* (German) 47, 387
(1972): Shelley WB+, *Br J Dermatol* 86, 118 (bullous)
(1972): Wyatt E+, *Arch Dermatol* 106, 671
(1970): Savin JA, *Br J Dermatol* 83, 546
(1969): Török H, *Dermatol Int* 8, 57
(1967): Schulz KH+, *Z Haut Geschlechtskr* (German) 42, 561
(1964): Browne SG, *BMJ* 2, 1041

Lupus erythematosus
(1992): Breathnach SM+, *Adverse Drug Reactions and the Skin* Blackwell, Oxford, 344

Perianal irritation

Pigmentation
(1973): Levantine A+, *Br J Dermatol* 89, 105

Pruritus
(1972): Grillat JP+, *Rev Fr Allergie* (French) 12, 351

Stevens–Johnson syndrome
(1972): Monnat A, *Schweiz Med Wochenschr* (French) 102, 1876

Toxic epidermal necrolysis
(1997): Artymowicz RJ+, *Ann Pharmacother* 31, 1157
(1986): Kar PK+, *J Indian Med Assoc* 84, 189
(1973): Björnberg A, *Acta Dermatol Venereol* (Stockh) 53, 149

(1973): Khamadullin LG, *Vestn Dermatol Venerol* (Russian) 47, 67
(1972): Monnat A, *Schweiz Med Wochenschr* (French) 102, 1876
(1967): Lowney ED+, *Arch Dermatol* 95, 359
(1966): Témime P+, *Bull Soc Fr Dermatol Syphiligr* (French) 73, 305
(1961): Browne SG+, *BMJ* 1, 550
(1957): Lang R+, *S Afr Med J* 31, 713

Urticaria
(1972): Grillat JP+, *Rev Fr Allergie* (French) 12, 351

### Nails

Nails – discoloration of lunulae
(1984): Daniel CR+, *J Am Acad Dermatol* 10, 250

### Other

Oral mucosal fixed eruption
Oral mucosal pigmentation
Oral mucosal ulceration

## PHENOXYBENZAMINE

**Trade name:** Dibenzyline (GSK)
**Other common trade names:** *Dibenyline; Dibenzyran*
**Indications:** Pheochromocytoma
**Category:** Alpha-adrenergic blocking agent; antihypertensive
**Half-life:** 24 hours
**Clinically important, potentially hazardous interactions with:** epinephrine

#### *Reactions*

### Skin

Contact dermatitis
(1975): MitchellJC+, *Contact Dermatitis* 1, 363
Reactions (sic)
(1973): Alexander SL+, *Lancet* 1, 317

### Other

Priapism
(1974): Funderburk SJ+, *N Engl J Med* 290, 630
Xerostomia (1–10%)

## PHENSUXIMIDE

**Trade name:** Milontin (Parke-Davis)
**Indications:** Petit mal seizures
**Category:** Anticonvulsant
**Half-life:** 5–12 hours

#### *Reactions*

### Skin

Erythema multiforme (<1%)
Lupus erythematosus
Periorbital edema
Pruritus
Purpura
(1980): Miescher PA+, *Clin Haematol* 9, 505
Rash (sic)
Stevens–Johnson syndrome

### Hair

Hair – alopecia
Hair – hirsutism

### Other

Acute intermittent porphyria
Gingival hyperplasia
Oral ulceration

## PHENTERMINE

**Trade names:** Adipex-P (Gate); Fastin (GSK); Ionamin (Medeva)
**Other common trade names:** *Behapront; Diminex; Minobese-Forte; Panbesy; Panbesyl; Redusa; Umine; Zantryl*
**Indications:** Obesity
**Category:** Appetite suppressant (anorexiant)
**Half-life:** 19–24 hours
**Clinically important, potentially hazardous interactions with:** fluoxetine, fluvoxamine, MAO inhibitors, paroxetine, phenelzine, sertraline, tranylcypromine

#### *Reactions*

### Skin

Diaphoresis (<1%)
Peripheral edema
Peripheral vasculopathy (sic)
(1999): Jefferson HJ+, *Nephrol Dial Transplant* 14, 1761
Purpura
Rash (sic)
Raynaud's phenomenon
(1990): Aeschlimann A+, *Scand J Rheumatol* 19, 87
Urticaria

### Hair

Hair – alopecia (<1%)

### Other

Dysgeusia
Myalgia (<1%)
Tremors
Xerostomia

## PHENTOLAMINE

**Trade name:** Regitine (Novartis)
**Other common trade names:** *Regitin; Rogitene; Rogitine*
**Indications:** Hypertensive episodes in pheochromocytoma
**Category:** Alpha-adrenergic blocking agent; antihypertensive; diagnostic aid for pheochromocytoma
**Half-life:** 19 minutes

#### *Reactions*

### Skin

Flushing (1–10%)

### Other

Priapism

## PHENYLEPHRINE

**Trade names:** AK-Dilate; Isopto Frin; L-Phrine; Neo-Synephrine; Prefrin; Sinarest; Vicks Sinest
**Other common trade names:** *Dionephrine; Novahistine; Prefrin Liquifilm*
**Indications:** Nasal congestion, glaucoma, hypotension
**Category:** Alpha-adrenergic agonist; mydriatic ophthalmic agent
**Half-life:** 2.5 hours
**Clinically important, potentially hazardous interactions with:** epinephrine, furazolidone, MAO inhibitors, phenelzine, tranylcypromine

### *Reactions*

#### Skin

Contact dermatitis
(1999): Resano A+, *J Invest Allergol Clin Immunol* 9, 55 (blepharoconjunctivitis)
(1998): Rafael M+, *Contact Dermatitis* 39, 143 (blepharoconjunctivitis)
(1998): Thomas P+, *Contact Dermatitis* 38, 41 (blepharoconjunctivitis)
(1998): Wigger-Alberti W+, *Allergy* 53, 217 (blepharoconjunctivitis)
(1997): Mancuso G+, *Contact Dermatitis* 36, 110
(1997): Marcos ML+, *Contact Dermatitis* 37, 189
(1997): Moreno-Ancillo M+, *Ann Allergy Asthma Immunol* 78, 569 (periorbital)
(1997): Ockenfels HM+, *Dermatology* 195, 119 (periorbital)
(1995): Thomas P+, *Contact Dermatitis* 32, 249
(1993): Wilkinson SM+, *Contact Dermatitis* 29, 100
(1991): Anibarro B+, *Contact Dermatitis* 25, 323 (blepharoconjunctivitis)
(1991): Bardazzi F+, *Contact Dermatitis* 24, 56
(1991): Okamoto H+, *Cutis* 47, 357
(1990): Zucchi A+, *G Ital Dermatol Venereol* (Italian) 125, 155
(1986): Ducombs G+, *Contact Dermatitis* 15, 107
(1984): Camarasa JG, *Contact Dermatitis* 10, 182
(1983): Hanna C+, *Am J Ophthalmol* 95, 703
(1983): Rarber KA, *Contact Dermatitis* 9, 274 (periorbital)
(1979): De Vita L+, *Minerva Pediatr* (Italian) 31, 535
(1979): Mathias CG+, *Arch Ophthalmol* 97, 286
Pallor
Periorbital edema
(1998): Blum A+, *Hautarzt* (German) 49, 651
Stinging (from nasal or ophthalmic preparations) (1–10%)

#### Other

Hypersensitivity
(1991): Quirce Gancedo S+, *Med Clin (Barc)* (Spanish) 96, 317
Injection-site reactions
Paresthesias
Tremors

## PHENYLPROPANOLAMINE

**Synonym:** PPA
**Trade names:** Acutrim; BC Cold Powder; Control; Dex-a-Diet; Dexatrim; Diet Gum; Genex; Maigret-50; Phenoxine; Phenyldrine; Prolamine; Propagest; Propandrine; Rhindecon; Spray-U-Thin; St. Joseph Aspirin-Free Cold Tablets; Stay Trim; Unitrol; Westrim
**Indications:** Nasal decongestion, anorexiant
**Category:** Adrenergic agonist; anorexiant; decongestant; sympathomimetic
**Half-life:** 3–4 hours
**Clinically important, potentially hazardous interactions with:** ephedrine, fluoxetine, fluvoxamine, furazolidone, paroxetine, tranylcypromine

### *Reactions*

#### Skin

Fixed eruption
(2000): Heikkila H+, *Br J Dermatol* 142(4), 845
Pallor

#### Other

Death
(1984): Logie AW+, *Br Med J* 289(6445), 591
(1983): Mueller SM, *N Engl J* 308(11), 653
Depression
Rhabdomyolysis
(1983): Blewitt GA+, *JAMA* 249(22), 3017
(1983): Hampel G+, *Hum Toxicol* 2(2), 197
(1983): Rumpf KW+, *JAMA* 250(16), 2112
(1982): Swenson RD+, *JAMA* 248(10), 1216
Tremors
Xerostomia

## PHENYTOIN

**Synonyms:** diphenylhydantoin; DPH; phenytoin sodium
**Trade names:** Dilantin (Parke-Davis); Phenytek (Bertek)
**Other common trade names:** *Di-Hydran; Diphenylan; Epanutin; Fenytoin; Phenhydan; Pyoredol; Zentropil*
**Indications:** Grand mal seizures
**Category:** Hydantoin anticonvulsant; antiarrhythmic
**Half-life:** 7–42 hours (dose dependent)
**Clinically important, potentially hazardous interactions with:** amprenavir, calcium, chloramphenicol, cimetidine, clorazepate, cyclosporine, delavirdine, diazoxide, disulfiram, dopamine, fluconazole, fluoxetine, **ginkgo biloba**, imatinib, indinavir, isoniazid, itraconazole, meperidine, midazolam, nelfinavir, **primrose**, ritonavir, **sage**, saquinavir, sucralfate

An excellent overview of cutaneous reactions to phenytoin can be found in (1988): Silverman AK+, *J Am Acad Dermatol* 18, 721

**Note:** About 19% of patients receiving phenytoin develop skin reactions (1983): Rapp RP+, *Neurosurg* 13, 272. They typically develop 10 to 14 days following the start of treatment

### *Reactions*

#### Skin

Acne
(1993): Shah M+, *Eur J Dermatol* 3, 576
(1990): Grunwald MH+, *Int J Dermatol* 29, 559

(1983): Greenwood R+, *Br Med J Clin Res Ed* 287, 1669
(1980): Stankler L+, *Br J Dermatol* 103, 453 (neonatal)
(1977): Frentz G, *Ugeskr Laeger* (Danish) 139, 338
(1972): Jenkins RB+, *N Engl J Med* 287, 148
(1964): Fegeler F, *Arch Klin Exp Derm* (German) 219, 335

Acute generalized exanthematous pustulosis (AGEP)
(2001): Burrow W, Jackson, MS (from Internet) (observation)
(1995): Moreau A+, *Int J Dermatol* 34, 263 (passim)

Angioedema
(1992): Schlaifer D+, *Eur J Hematol* 48, 274
(1967): Coleman WP, *Med Clin North Am* 51, 1073

Bullous eruption
(1988): Baird BJ+, *Int J Dermatol* 27, 170

Dermatomyositis
(1998): Dimachkie MM+, *J Child Neurol* 13, 577

Eosinophilic fasciitis
(1980): Buchanan RR+, *J Rheumatol* 7, 733

Epidermal necrosis
(2001): Bravo F, Lima, Peru (from Internet) (observation)

Epidermolysis bullosa
(1982): Bergfeld WF+, *J Am Acad Dermatol* 7, 275

Erythema multiforme
(2001): Bravo F, Lima, Peru (from Internet) (observation)
(1999): Marinella MA, *Ann Pharmacother* 33, 748
(1999): Micali G+, *Pharmacotherapy* 19, 223 (with cranial irradiation)
(1995): Rodriguez-Castellanos M+, *Arch Dermatol* 131, 620
(1990): Giroud M+, *Therapie* (French) 45, 23
(1988): Delattre JY+, *Neurology* 38, 194
(1988): Shear NH+, *J Clin Invest* 82, 1826
(1986): Green ST, *Clin Neuropharmacol* 9, 561
(1985): Tucker MS+, *J Am Osteopath Assoc* 85, 511
(1972): Almeyda J+, *Br J Dermatol* 87, 646
(1967): Coleman WP, *Med Clin North Am* 51, 1073

Erythroderma
(1996): Chopra S+, *Br J Dermatol* 134, 1109
(1991): Yamashina T+, *Nippon Shokakibyo Gakkai Zasshi* (Japanese) 88, 1269
(1983): Lillie MA+, *Arch Dermatol* 119, 415
(1966): Fischbeck R+, *Dtsch Gesundheitsw* (German) 21, 1273

Exanthems
(2000): Cohen AD+, *Isr Med Assoc J* 1, 95
(1997): Hyson C+, *Can J Neurol Sci* 24, 245
(1996): Leong KP+, *Asian Pac J Allergy Immunol* 14, 65 (71.4%)
(1992): Tone T+, *J Dermatol* 19, 27
(1991): Pelekanos J+, *Epilepsia* 32, 554
(1988): Shear NH+, *J Clin Invest* 82, 1826
(1984): Chadwick D+, *J Neurol Neurosurg Psychiatry* 47, 642 (6%)
(1983): Rapp RP+, *Neurosurgery* 13, 272
(1978): Wilson JT+, *BMJ* 1, 1583
(1975): Weedon AP, *Aust NZ J Med* 5, 561
(1970): Robinson HM+, *Arch Dermatol* 101, 462
(1969): Levene G+, *Br J Dermatol* 81, 712
(1967): Coleman WP, *Med Clin North Am* 51, 1073

Exfoliative dermatitis
(1997): Westhoven GS+, *Arch Dermatol* 133, 494
(1996): Leong KP+, *Asian Pac J Allergy Immunol* 14, 65 (2.4%)
(1996): Sigurdsson V+, *J Am Acad Dermatol* 35, 53
(1989): Danno K+, *J Dermatol* (Tokio) 16, 392
(1985): Matson JR+, *Hum Pathol* 16, 94
(1983): Rapp RP+, *Neurosurgery* 13, 272
(1972): Almeyda J+, *Br J Dermatol* 87, 646
(1963): Beerman H+, *Arch Dermatol* 87, 783
(1958): Chaiken BH+, *N Engl J Med* 242, 897
(1956): Gropper AL, *N Engl J Med* 254, 522
(1948): Van Wyck JJ+, *Arch Intern Med* 81, 605
(1942): Ritchie EB+, *Arch Dermatol* 46, 856

Fixed eruption
(1997): Chan HL+, *J Am Acad Dermatol* 36, 259
(1988): Baird BJ+, *Int J Dermatol* 27, 170 (bullous)
(1963): Goldstein N+, *Arch Dermatol* 87, 612

Heel pad thickening
(1975): Kattan KR, *AJR* 124, 52

Lichen planus
(1991): MacLeod SP+, *Br Dent J* 171, 237

Lichenoid eruption
(1992): Tone T+, *J Dermatol* 19, 27

Linear IgA bullous dermatosis
(2002): Cohen LM+, *J Am Acad* 46(2), S32 (passim)
(1998): Acostamadiedo JM+, *J Am Acad Dermatol* 38, 352
(1994): Kuechle MK+, *J Am Acad Dermatol* 30, 187

Lupus erythematosus
(1993): Drory VE+, *Clin Neuropharmacol* 16, 19 (passim)
(1988): Jiang M, *Chung Kuo I Hsueh Ko Hsueh Yuan Hsueh Pao* (Chinese) 10, 379
(1985): Lovisetto P+, *Recenti Prog Med* (Italian) 76, 84
(1984): Wollina U, *Z Gesamte Int Med* (German) 39, 69
(1982): Gleichman H, *Arthritis Rheum* 25, 1387
(1977): Rybicka K+, *Pol Tyg Lek* (Polish) 32, 1269
(1976): Singsen BH+, *Pediatrics* 57, 529
(1974): Harpey JP, *Ann Allergy* 33, 256
(1970): Okuda M+, *Naika* (Japanese) 26, 989
(1967): Siegel M+, *Arthritis Rheum* 10, 407
(1966): Lee SL+, *Arch Intern Med* 117, 620
(1963): Goldstein N+, *Arch Dermatol* 87, 612
(1963): Jacobs JC, *Pediatrics* 32, 257
(1962): Benton JW+, *JAMA* 180, 115

Lymphoma (<1%)
(1985): Wolf R+, *Arch Dermatol* 121, 1181
(1978): Wilden JN+, *J Clin Pathol* 31, 761
(1975): Bichel J, *Acta Med Scand* 198, 327
(1975): Li FP+, *Cancer* 36, 1359
(1970): Anthony JJ, *Arch Neurol* 22, 450

Mycosis fungoides
(1991): Rijlaarsdam U+, *J Am Acad Dermatol* 24(2 Pt 2), 216 (with carbamazepine)
(1990): Souteyrand P+, *Curr Probl Dermatol* 19, 176
(1985): Wolf R+, *Arch Dermatol* 121, 1181
(1982): Rosenthal CH+, *Cancer* 49, 2305

Pellagra

Pemphigus
(1988): Seghal VN+, *Int J Dermatol* 27, 258

Pigmentation
(1964): Kuske H+, *Dermatologica* 129, 121

Pruritus
(1997): Litt JZ, Beachwood, OH (personal case) (observation)
(1985): Rubinstein N+, *Int J Dermatol* 24, 54
(1967): Coleman WP, *Med Clin North Am* 51, 1073
(1963): Beerman H+, *Arch Dermatol* 87, 783

Pseudoacanthosis nigricans
(1972): Petko E+, *Arch Dermatol* 106, 918

Purple glove syndrome (sic)
(2000): Schmutz J+, *Ann Dermatol Venereol* (French) 127, 548
(2000): Yoshikawa H+, *J Child Neurol* 15(11), 762
(1998): Cadenbach A+, *Dtsch Med Wochenschr* (German) 123, 318
(1994): Helfaer MA+, *J Neurosurg Anesthesiol* 6, 48

Purpura
(1975): Targan SR+, *Ann Intern Med* 83, 227 (fulminans)
(1967): Coleman WP, *Med Clin North Am* 51, 1073
(1963): Beerman H+, *Arch Dermatol* 87, 783
(1962): Weintraub RM+, *JAMA* 180, 528

Pustular eruption
(1993): O'Brien TJ+, *Australas J Dermatol* 34, 128
(1991): Kleier RS, *Arch Dermatol* 127, 1361
(1978): Stanley J+, *Arch Dermatol* 114, 1350

Rash (sic) (1–10%)

(2001): Aihara M+, *Br J Dermatol* 144, 1231
(1999): Mamon HJ+, *Epilepsia* 40, 341 (with cranial radiation)
(1987): Maguire JH+, *Br J Clin Pharmacol* 24, 554

Reticular hyperplasia
(1975): Wasik F+, *Hautarzt* (German) 26, 273
(1966): Korting GW+, *Dermatol Wochenschr* (German) 152, 257

Rhinophyma
(2000): Jaramillo MJ+, *Br J Plast Surg* 53(6), 521

Scleroderma
(1974): Kashiwazaki S+, *Ryumachi* (Japanese) 14, 220

Sezary syndrome
(1994): Doyle MF+, *Acta Hematol* 92, 204

Sjøgren's syndrome
(1996): Chakravarty K+, *Br J Rheumatol* 35, 1033

Stevens–Johnson syndrome
(2001): Eralp Y+, *Am J Clin Oncol* 24(4), 347
(2000): Madnani NA, Mumbai, India (from Internet) (observation)
(1999): Khafaga YM+, *Acta Oncol* 38, 111 (with cranial irradiation)
(1999): Ruble R+, *CNS Drugs* 12, 215
(1999): Rzany B+, *Lancet* 353, 2190
(1996): Cockey G+, *Am J Clin Oncol* 19, 32 (with irradiation of brain)
(1996): Leong KP+, *Asian Pac J Allergy Immunol* 14, 65 (14.3%)
(1995): Borg M+, *Australas Radiol* 39, 42 (with irradiation of brain)
(1995): Cockey GH+, *Am J Clin Oncol* 19, 32
(1995): Wolkenstein P+, *Arch Dermatol* 131, 544
(1994): Marti J+, *An Med Interna* (Spanish) 11, 621
(1993): Janinis J+, *Eur J Cancer* 29A, 478 (with cranial irradiation)
(1993): Leenutaphong V+, *Int J Dermatol* 32, 428
(1993): Schlienger RG+, *Schweiz Rundsch Med Prax* (German) 82, 888
(1992): Tone T+, *J Dermatol* 19, 27
(1989): Kelly DF+, *Neurosurgery* 25, 976
(1988): Delattre JY+, *Neurology* 38, 194 (with cranial irradiation)
(1988): Shear NH+, *J Clin Invest* 82, 1826
(1985): Burge SM+, *J Am Acad Dermatol* 13, 665
(1985): de Rego JA+, *Hillside J Clin Psychiatry* 7, 141
(1985): Maiche A+, *Lancet* 2, 45 (with radiation therapy)
(1982): Oles KS+, *Clin Pharm* 1, 565
(1978): Assaad D+, *Can Med Assoc* 118, 154
(1976): Marg E, *Psychiatr Neurol Med Psychol Leipz* (German) 28, 436
(1971): Greenberg LM+, *Ann Ophthalmol* 3, 137
(1970): Rudner EJ, *Arch Dermatol* 102, 561

Toxic dermatitis (sic)
(1978): Huijgens PC+, *Acta Haematol* 59, 31

Toxic epidermal necrolysis
(2000): Cohen AD+, *Isr Med Assoc J* 1, 95 (2 patients)
(2000): Moussala M+, *J Fr Ophtalmol* (French) 23, 229
(1999): Cohen AD+, *Isr Med Assoc J* 1, 95 (2 cases)
(1999): Egan CA+, *J Am Acad Dermatol* 40, 458 (3 cases)
(1999): Ruble R+, *CNS Drugs* 12, 215
(1999): Rzany B+, *Lancet* 353, 2190
(1997): Jester BA+, American Academy of Dermatology Meeting (SF), Poster #163
(1997): Sapadin A+, American Academy of Dermatology Meeting (SF), Poster #111 (with radiation)
(1996): Creamer JD+, *Clin Exp Dermatol* 21, 116
(1996): Frangogiannis NG+, *South Med J* 89, 1001
(1996): Leong KP+, *Asian Pac J Allergy Immunol* 14, 65 (2.4%)
(1995): Pion IA+, *N Engl J Med* 333, 1609
(1993): Janinis J+, *Eur J Cancer* 29A, 478
(1993): Leenutaphong V+, *Int J Dermatol* 32, 428
(1992): Tone T+, *J Dermatol* 19, 27
(1991): Rowe JE+, *Int J Dermatol* 30, 747
(1989): Kelly DF+, *Neurosurgery* 25, 976
(1989): Renfro L+, *Int J Dermatol* 28, 441
(1988): Dreyfuss DA+, *Ann Plast Surg* 20, 146
(1987): Birchall N+, *J Am Acad Dermatol* 16, 368
(1985): Burge SM+, *J Am Acad Dermatol* 13, 665
(1985): Muhar U, *Pediatr Dermatology* 3, 54
(1985): Sherertz EF+, *J Am Acad Dermatol* 12, 178
(1984): Chan HL, *J Am Acad Dermatol* 10, 973
(1984): Smith DA+, *J Am Acad Dermatol* 10, 106 (followed by universal depigmentation)
(1983): Schmidt D+, *Epilepsia* 24, 440 (fatal)
(1982): Peterson KA+, *Md State Med J* 31, 53
(1981): Spechler SJ+, *Ann Intern Med* 95, 455
(1979): Gately LE+, *Ann Intern Med* 91, 59
(1979): Lyell A, *Br J Dermatol* 100, 69
(1978): Assaad D+, *Can Med Assoc* 118, 154
(1975): Giallorenzi AF+, *Oral Surg Oral Med Oral Pathol* 40, 611
(1975): Schopf E+, *Z Hautkr* (German) 50, 865
(1968): Rodriguez-Adrados J+, *Rev Clin Esp* (Spanish) 110, 267
(1967): Coleman WP, *Med Clin North Am* 51, 1073
(1967): Vandvik IH, *Tidsskr Nor Laegeforen* (Norwegian) 87, 1068

Urticaria
(1995): Rodriguez-Castellanos M+, *Arch Dermatol* 131, 620
(1967): Coleman WP, *Med Clin North Am* 51, 1073
(1951): Jones DP, *BMJ* 1, 64

Vasculitis
(1999): Holt P, *N Z Med J* 112, 100
(1996): Leong KP+, *Asian Pac J Allergy Immunol* 14, 65 (2.4%)
(1996): Parry RG+, *Nephrol Dial Transplant* 11, 357
(1993): Drory VE+, *Clin Neuropharmacol* 16, 19 (passim)
(1983): Yermakov VM+, *Hum Pathol* 14, 182
(1967): Hass P, *Wiener Klin Wochenschr* (German) 75, 56

Warts
(1998): Kayal JD+, *Cutis* 61, 101

## Hair

Hair – alopecia
(1984): Smith DA+, *J Am Acad Dermatol* 10, 106
(1973): Levantine A+, *Br J Dermatol* 89, 549

Hair – hirsutism
(1989): Backman K+, *Scand J Dent Res* 97, 222
(1989): Vivard P+, *Ann Dermatol Venereol* (French) 116, 562
(1972): Leng JJ+, *Pediatr Clin North Am* 19, 681
(1972): Levantine A+, *Br J Dermatol* 87, 646
(1970): Herberg KP, *South Med J* 70, 19

Hair – hypertrichosis
(2001): Oakley A, Hamilton, NZ (from Internet) (observation)
(1989): Rousseau C+, *Dermatologica* 179, 221

## Nails

Nails – disorders
(1981): Krebs A, *Schweiz Rundsch Med Prax* (German) 70, 1951

Nails – hypoplasia
(1991): D'Souza SW+, *Arch Dis Child* 66, 320
(1981): Johnson RB+, *J Am Acad Dermatol* 5, 191
(1978): Prakash P+, *Indian Pediatr* 15, 866

Nails – malformation
(1975): Hanson JW+, *J Pediatrics* 87, 285

Nails – onychopathy
(1988): Verdeguer JM+, *Pediatr Dermatol* 5, 56

Nails – pigmentation
(1981): Johnson RB+, *J Am Acad Dermatol* 5, 191

## Other

Acromegaloid features
(1972): Lefebvre EB+, *N Engl J Med* 286, 1301

Acute intermittent porphyria
(1989): Herrick AL+, *Br J Clin Pharmacol* 27, 491

Ageusia
(1998): Henkin RI, *Lancet* 352, 68
(1998): Zeller JA+, *Lancet* 351, 1101

Coarse facies (sic)

(1973): Falconer MA+, *Lancet* 2, 1112
(1972): Lefebvre EB+, *Med Intell* 286, 1301

Death

Digital malformations
(1981): Johnson RB+, *J Am Acad Dermatol* 5, 191
(1978): Prakash P+, *Indian Pediatr* 15, 866
(1974): Barr M+, *J Pediatr* 84, 254 (hypoplasia)

Fetal hydantoin syndrome*
(1998): Ozkinay F+, *Turk J Pediatr* 40, 273 (2 siblings)
(1994): Buehler BA+, *Neurol Clin*, 12, 741
(1989): Nanda A+, *Pediatr Dermatol* 6, 130
(1989): Nanda A+, *Pediatr Dermatol* 6, 66
(1988): Verdeguer JM+, *Pediatr Dermatol* 5, 56
(1983): Tomsick RS, *Cutis* 32, 535
(1981): Nagy R, *Arch Dermatol* 117, 593

Gingival hyperplasia (>10%)
(2001): Uzel MI+, *J Periodontol* 72(7), 921
(1999): Kamali F+, *J Periodontal Res* 34, 145
(1999): Wood WH, San Jose, CA (from Internet) (observation)
(1998): Desai P+, *J Can Dent Assoc* 64, 263
(1998): Garzino-Demo P+, *Minerva Somatol* (Italian) 47, 387
(1998): Mattson JS+, *J Am Dent Assoc* 129, 78
(1998): Meraw SJ+, *Mayo Clin Proc* 73, 1196
(1997): Iacopino AM+, *J Periodontol* 68, 73
(1997): Mattioli A, *Minerva Stomatol* (Italian) 46, 525
(1997): Newland JR, *J Gt House Dent Soc* 69, 3
(1997): Silverstein LH+, *Gen Dent* 45, 371
(1996): Hayakawa I+, *Quintessence Int* 27, 235
(1996): Saito K+, *J Periodontol Res* 31, 545
(1995): Moghadam BKH+, *Cutis* 56, 46 (passim)
(1993): Lipton JM+, *J Indiana Dent Assoc* 72, 18
(1991): Hassell TM+, *Crit Rev Oral Biol Med* 2, 103
(1990): Hall WB, *Compendium* (Suppl) 14, 502
(1989): Backman K+, *Scand J Dent Res* 97, 222
(1989): Dooley G+, *J N Z Soc Periodontol* 68, 19
(1987): Norris JF+, *Int J Dermatol* 26, 602
(1987): Stinnett E+, *J Am Dent Assoc* 114, 814
(1976): Hassell TM+, *Proc Nat Acad Sci* 73, 2909
(1975): Angelopoulos AP, *J Can Dent Assoc* 2, 102

Gynecomastia
(1998): Ikeda A+, *J Neurol Neurosurg Psychiatry* 65, 803

Hypersensitivity syndrome**
(2002): Metin A+, *World Congress Dermatol* Poster, 0116
(2001): Aihara M+, *Br J Dermatol* 144, 1231
(2001): Bessmertny O+, *Ann Pharmacother* 35(5), 533
(2001): Klassen BD+, *Epilepsia* 42(3), 433
(2001): Nashed MH+, *Pharmacotherapy* 21(4), 502
(2000): Cohen AD+, *Isr Med Assoc J* 1, 95
(2000): Colombo-Arnet E, *Schweiz Rundsch Med Prax* (German) 89, 675
(2000): Lynfield Y, Brooklyn, NY (from Internet) (observation)
(2000): Moore SJ+, *J Med Genet* 37, 489
(2000): Troger U+, *Int J CLin Pharmacol Ther* 38(9), 452
(1999): Hamer HM+, *Seizure* 8, 190
(1999): Moss DM+, *J Emerg Med* 17, 503
(1999): Quinones MD+, *Allergy* 54, 83 (fatal)
(1998): Galindo Bonilla PA+, *J Investig Allergol Clin Immunol* 8, 186
(1997): Morkunas AR+, *Crit Care Clin* 13, 727
(1997): Tennis P+, *Neurology* 49, 542
(1996): Chopra S+, *Br J Dermatol* 134, 1109
(1996): Conger LA+, *Cutis* 57, 223
(1994): Potter T+, *Arch Dermatol* 130, 856
(1993): Handfield-Jones SE+, *Br J Dermatol* 129, 175
(1984): Fonseca JC+, *Med Cutan Ibero Lat Am* (Portuguese) 12, 187
(1983): Rapp RP+, *Neurosurgery* 13, 272
(1978): Stanley J+, *Arch Dermatol* 114, 1350
(1975): Weedon AP, *Aust N Z J Med* 5, 561
(1973): Cohen BL+, *Clin Pediatr Phila* 12, 622
(1973): Sisca TS, *Am J Hosp Pharm* 30, 446

Injection-site necrosis
(1995): Hunt SJ, *Am J Dermatopathol* 17, 399
(1993): Hayes AG+, *J Am Acad Dermatol* 28, 360

Injection-site pain

Lymphadenopathy
(1971): Oates R+, *Med J Australia* 2/58, 371

Lymphoproliferative disease
(1992): Schlaifer D+, *Eur J Hematol* 48, 274

Mucocutaneous eruption
(1992): Tone T+, *J Dermatol* 19, 27
(1979): Pollack MA+, *Ann Neurol* 5, 262

Mucocutaneous lymph node syndrome
(1979): Anderson VM+, *Cutis* 23, 493

Myopathy
(1986): Engel JN+, *Am J Med* 81, 928
(1983): Harney J+, *Neurology* 33, 790

Oral ulceration

Paresthesias (<1%)
(1995): Rodriguez-Castellanos M+, *Arch Dermatol* 131, 620

Periarteritis nodosa
(1967): Haas P, *Wiener Klin Wochenschr* (German) 75, 56
(1948): Van Wyk JJ+, *Arch Intern Med* 81, 605

Peyronie's disease

Polyfibromatosis
(1979): Pierard GE+, *Br J Dermatol* 100, 335

Polymyositis
(1983): Harney J+, *Neurology* 33, 790

Porphyria
(1980): Fuchs T+, *Int J Biochem* 12, 955

Porphyria cutanea tarda
(1996): Ruggian JC+, *J Am Soc Nephrol* 7, 397

Pseudolymphoma (<1%)
(2002): Lifshitz AY, Israel (from Internet) (observation) (solitary in infant)
(1998): Cooke LE+, *Clin Pharm* 7, 153
(1997): Gigli GL+, *Int J Neurosci* 87, 181
(1995): Wolkenstein P+, *Arch Dermatol* 131, 544
(1993): Sigal M+, *Ann Dermatol Venereol* (French) 120, 175
(1992): Braddock SW+, *J Am Acad Dermatol* 27, 337
(1992): D'Incan M+, *Arch Dermatol* 128, 1371
(1992): Harris DW+, *Br J Dermatol* 127, 403
(1988): Cooke LE+, *Clin Pharm* 7, 153
(1988): Silverman AK+, *J Am Acad Dermatol* 18, 721
(1985): Brodell RT, *Dermatol Clin* 3, 719
(1983): Rapp RP+, *Neurosurgery* 13, 272
(1982): Rosenthal CJ+, *Cancer* 49, 2305
(1981): Adams JD, *Australas J Dermatol* 22, 28
(1980): Vellucci A+, *Clin Ter* (Italian) 94, 229
(1977): Charlesworth EN, *Arch Dermatol* 113, 477
(1977): Halevy S+, *Dermatologica* 155, 321
(1971): Oates RK+, *Med J Aust* 2, 371
(1968): Gams RA+, *Ann Intern Med* 69, 557
(1968): Schreiber MM+, *Arch Dermatol* 97, 297

Rhabdomyolysis
(1989): Korman LB+, *Clin Pharm* 8(7), 514
(1986): Engel JN+, *Am J Med* 81, 928

Serum sickness
(1981): Menitove JE+, *Am J Hematol* 10, 277
(1975): Zidar BL+, *Am J Med* 58, 704

Thrombophlebitis (<1%)

***Note:** The fetal hydantoin syndrome (FHS) – children whose mothers receive phenytoin during pregnancy are born with FHS. The main features of this syndrome are mental and growth retardation, unusual facies, digital and nail hypoplasia, and coarse scalp hair. Occasionally neonatal acne will be present

**Note: The phenytoin hypersensitivity reaction (also known as the anticonvulsant hypersensitivity syndrome) is described in detail in (1978): Stanley J+, *Arch Dermatol* 114, 1350. The salient features of this reaction, which characteristically occur within the first 2 to 4 weeks of phenytoin therapy, are fever, generalized tender lymphadenopathy, hepatitis, leukocytosis, and a widespread, pruritic, irregular eruption consisting of ill-defined patches of macular erythema. Periorbital edema is common. The mucous membranes are frequently involved with erythema of the oral mucosa and pharynx. Papules, vesicles and pustules occasionally develop

# PHYTONADIONE

**Synonyms:** phylloquinone; phytomenadione; vitamin $K_1$
**Trade names:** AquaMEPHYTON (Merck); Konakion; Mephyton (Merck); Phytomenadione; Vitamin K1 (Abbott)
**Other common trade names:** *Kaywan; Vitak*
**Indications:** Coagulation disorders
**Category:** Fat-soluble nutritional supplement and antihemorrhagic
**Half-life:** 2–4 hours
**Clinically important, potentially hazardous interactions with:** warfarin

## *Reactions*

### Skin

Allergic reactions (sic)
(1999): Wong DA+, *Australas J Dermatol* 40, 147
(1990): Pigatto PD+, *Contact Dermatitis* 22, 307

Contact dermatitis
(1999): Drayton G, Los Angeles, CA (from Internet) (observation)
(1995): Bruynzeel I+, *Contact Dermatitis* 32, 78
(1995): Guy C+, *Therapie* (French) 50, 483
(1988): Dinis A+, *Contact Dermatitis* 18, 170
(1982): Camarasa JG+, *Contact Dermatitis* 8, 268
(1980): Romaguera C+, *Contact Dermatitis* 6, 355
(1979): Romaguera C+, *Actas Dermosifilogr* (Spanish) 70, 215

Diaphoresis (<1%)

Eczematous plaques
(1992): Lee MM+, *Arch Dermatol* 128, 257
(1988): Sanders MN+, *J Am Acad Dermatol* 19, 699

Erythema (annular)
(1986): Kay MH+, *Cutis* 37, 445

Exanthems
(1987): Finkelstein H+, *J Am Acad Dermatol* 16, 540

Flushing

Rash (sic)

Scleroderma
(1995): Morell A+, *Int J Dermatol* 34, 201
(1994): Guidetti MS+, *Contact Dermatitis* 31, 45
(1992): Fitzpatrick JE, *Dermatol Clin* 10, 19
(1989): Pujol RM+, *Cutis* 43, 365
(1988): Brunskill NJ+, *Clin Exp Dermatol* 13, 276
(1987): Finkelstein H+, *J Am Acad Dermatol* 16, 540
(1985): Janin-Mercier A+, *Arch Dermatol* 121, 1421
(1982): Rommel A+, *Ann Pediatr Paris* (French) 29, 64
(1981): Jean-Pastor MJ+, *Therapie* (French) 36, 369
(1975): Texier L+, *Bull Soc Fr Derm Syphiligr* (French) 82, 448
(1972): Texier L+, *Ann Dermatol Syphiligr Paris* (French) 99, 363
(1972): Texier L+, *Bord Med* (French) 5, 700

Urticaria
(1993): Ford G, *J Paediatr Child Health* 29, 241
(1988): Sanders MN+, *J Am Acad Dermatol* 19, 699
(1987): Mosser C+, *Ann Dermatol Venereol* (French) 114, 243
(1964): Piguet B+, *Bull Mem Soc Med Hop Paris* (French) 118, 1337

Vasculitis
(1964): Piguet B+, *Bull Mem Soc Med Hop Paris* (French) 118, 1337

### Other

Anaphylactoid reactions (<1%)
(2001): Riegert-Johnson DL+, *Bone Marrow Transplant* 28(12), 1176

Dysgeusia (<1%)

Hypersensitivity (<1%)
(1998): Keogh GC+, *Cutis* 61, 81 (eczematous)

Injection-site eczematous eruption
(1996): Moreau-Cabarrot A+, *Ann Dermatol Venereol* (French) 123, 177
(1995): Keltz M+, American Academy of Dermatology Meeting, New Orleans (observation)
(1994): Giudetti MS+, *Contact Dermatitis* 31, 45
(1989): Allue-Bellosta L+, *Rev Clin Esp* (Spanish) 185, 217
(1988): Joyce JP+, *Arch Dermatol* 124, 27
(1988): Tsuboi R+, *J Am Acad Dermatol* 18, 386
(1987): Finkelstein H+, *J Am Acad Dermatol* 16, 540
(1978): Bullen AW+, *Br J Dermatol* 98, 561
(1978): Robinson JW+, *Arch Dermatol* 114, 1790
(1970): Anekoji K, *Chiryo* (Japanese) 52, 1577
(1970): Honda M+, *Hifuka no Rinsho* (Japanese) 12, 295

Injection-site erythema
(1995): Keltz M+, American Academy of Dermatology Meeting, New Orleans (observation)
(1993): Lemlich G+, *J Am Acad Dermatol* 28, 345
(1992): Breathnach SM+, *Adverse Drug Reactions and the Skin* Blackwell, Oxford, 265 (passim)

Injection-site indurated plaques (Texier's syndrome) (<1%)
(2001): Jaffe PG, Columbia SC (from Internet) (observation)
(1999): Chung JY+, *Cutis* 63, 33 (2 cases)
(1996): Bourrat E+, *Ann Dermatol Venereol* (French) 123, 634 (6 cases)
(1996): Pang BK+, *Australas J Dermatol* 37, 44
(1995): Keltz M+, American Academy of Dermatology Meeting, New Orleans (observation)
(1994): Shelley WB+, *Cutis* 52, 203 (passim)
(1993): Lemlich G+, *J Am Acad Dermatol* 28, 345
(1993): Long CC+, *BMJ* 307, 336
(1992): Tuppal R+, *J Am Acad Dermatol* 27, 105
(1989): Pujol RM+, *Cutis* 43, 365
(1988): Brunskill NJ+, *Clin Exp Dermatol* 13, 276
(1988): Joyce JP+, *Arch Dermatol* 124, 27
(1988): Tsuboi R+, *J Am Acad Dermatol* 18, 386
(1977): Heydenreich G, *Br J Dermatol* 97, 697
(1976): Barnes HM+, *Br J Dermatol* 95, 653
(1972): Bazex A+, *Bull Soc Fr Dermatol Syphiligr* (French) 79, 578
(1972): Misson R+, *Bull Soc Fr Dermatol Syphiligr* (French) 79, 581

# PILOCARPINE

**Trade names:** Adsorbocarbine; Akarpine; I-Pilopine; Isopto Carpine; Ocu-Carpine; Pilopine HS; Pilostat; Salagen; Storzine
**Other common trade names:** *Diocarpine; Isopto Pilocarpine; Liocarpina; Miocarpine; Pilo Grin; Pilogel; Pilopt; Sno Pilo; Spersacarpine; Vistacarpin*
**Indications:** Glaucoma, miosis induction, xerostomia
**Category:** Cholinergic parasympathomimetic agent
**Half-life:** no data
**Clinically important, potentially hazardous interactions with:** galantamine

### *Reactions*

#### Skin

Burning (1–10%)
(1996): Rattenbury JM+, *Ann Clin Biochem* 33, 456
Chills
Contact dermatitis
(2001): Holdiness MR, *Am J Contact Dermat* 12(4), 217
(1993): Cusano F+, *Contact Dermatitis* 29, 99
(1991): Helton J+, *Contact Dermatitis* 25, 133
(1991): Ortiz FJ+, *Contact Dermatitis* 25, 203
Diaphoresis (<1%)
Edema (4%)
Flushing
Photocontact dermatitis
(1991): Helton J+, *Contact Dermatitis* 25, 133
Pruritus
Rash (sic)
Stinging (1–10%)
Urticaria
(1997): LeGrys VA+, *Pediatr Pulmonol* 24, 296

#### Other

Dysgeusia (2%)
Hypersensitivity (1–10%)
Myalgia (1%)
Ocular cicatricial pemphigoid
(2000): Plotkin A+, *Arch Dermatol* 136, 113
Sialorrhea (<1%)

# PIMECROLIMUS

**Synonym:** ASM981
**Trade name:** Elidel (Novartis)
**Indications:** Atopic dermatitis
**Category:** Macrolactam ascomycin; calcineurin inhibitor
**Half-life:** N/A

### *Reactions*

#### Skin

Flu-like syndrome
Herpes simplex (1.2%)
Infections (sic) (5.4%)
Molluscum contagiosum (1.2%)
Upper respiratory infection (19.4%)

#### Other

Application-site burning (8–26%)
Application-site irritation (0.9%)
Application-site pruritus (0.6%)
Application-site reaction (sic) (2.1%)

# PIMOZIDE

**Trade name:** Orap (Gate)
**Other common trade names:** *Frenal; Neurap; Pimodac*
**Indications:** Tourette's syndrome, schizophrenia
**Category:** Antipsychotic and antidyskinetic (Tourette's syndrome); neuroleptic agent
**Half-life:** 50 hours
**Clinically important, potentially hazardous interactions with:** amphetamines, azithromycin, azole antifungals, clarithromycin, dirithromycin, erythromycin, fluoxetine, **grapefruit juice**, imatinib, indinavir, itraconazole, ketoconazole, methylphenidate, nefazodone, nelfinavir, pemoline, phenothiazines, protease inhibitors, quinidine, ritonavir, saquinavir, sparfloxacin, tricyclic antidepressants, troleandomycin, voriconazole, zileuton

### *Reactions*

#### Skin

Diaphoresis
Exanthems
Facial edema (1–10%)
Periorbital edema
Photosensitivity
(1991): Opler LA+, *J Clin Psychiatry* 52, 221
Pigmentation
(1991): Opler LA+, *J Clin Psychiatry* 52, 221
Pruritus
Rash (sic) (8.3%)
Urticaria

#### Other

Death
(2001): Glassman AH+, *Am J Psychiatry* 158(11), 1774
Dysgeusia
Galactorrhea
Gynecomastia (>10%)
Myalgia (2.7%)
Sialorrhea (13.8%)
(1987): Shapiro AK+, *Pediatrics* 79, 1032
Tremors
Xerostomia (>10%)
(1991): Opler LA+, *J Clin Psychiatry* 52, 221
(1990): Sandor P+, *J Clin Psychopharmacol* 10, 197
(1987): Shapiro AK+, *Pediatrics* 79, 1032

# PINDOLOL

**Trade name:** Visken (Novartis)
**Other common trade names:** *Alti-Pindolol; Apo-Pindol; Barbloc; Durapindol; Gen-Pindolol; Nonspi; Pinbetol; Pinden; Syn-Pindol; Vypen*
**Indications:** Hypertension
**Category:** Beta-adrenergic blocker; antihypertensive
**Half-life:** 3–4 hours
**Clinically important, potentially hazardous interactions with:** clonidine, epinephrine, verapamil

**Note:** Cutaneous side effects of beta-receptor blockaders are clinically polymorphous. They apparently appear after several months of continuous therapy. Atypical psoriasiform, lichen planus-like, and eczematous chronic rashes are mainly observed. (1983): Hödl St, *Z Hautkr* (German) 1:58, 17

### *Reactions*

#### Skin

Diaphoresis (2%)
Eczematous eruption (sic)
Edema (6%)
Erythema multiforme
Exanthems
Exfoliative dermatitis
Hyperkeratosis (palms and soles)
Lichenoid eruption
(1978): Savage RL+, *BMJ* 1, 987
(1976): Palatsi R, *Ann Clin Res* 8, 239
Lupus erythematosus
(1979): Bensaid J+, *BMJ* 1, 1603
Peripheral edema
Pityriasis rubra pilaris
(1978): Finlay AY+, *BMJ* 1, 987
Pruritus (1–5%)
(1976): Palatsi R, *Ann Clin Res* 8, 239
Psoriasis
(1986): Abel EA+, *J Am Acad Dermatol* 15, 1007
(1986): Czernielewski J+, *Lancet* 1, 808
(1984): Arntzen N+, *Acta Derm Venereol* (Stockh) 64, 346
(1976): Bonerandi JJ+, *Ann Dermatol Syphiligr* (Paris) (French) 103, 604
(1976): Palatsi R, *Ann Clin Res* 8, 239
Purpura
Rash (sic) (1–10%)
Raynaud's phenomenon
(1984): Eliasson K+, *Acta Med Scand* 215, 333
(1976): Marshall AJ+, *BMJ* 1, 1498
Toxic epidermal necrolysis
Urticaria
Xerosis

#### Hair

Hair – alopecia

#### Nails

Nails – dystrophy
Nails – onycholysis

#### Other

Dysgeusia
Myalgia
Myopathy
(1980): Uusitupa M+, *BMJ* 1, 183
Oculo-mucocutaneous syndrome
(1982): Cocco G+, *Curr Ther Res* 31, 362
Oral lichenoid eruption
Paresthesias (3%)
Peyronie's disease
(1979): Pryor JP+, *Lancet* 1, 331

## PIOGLITAZONE

**Trade name:** Actos (Takeda)
**Indications:** Type 2 diabetes
**Category:** Thiazolidinedione antidiabetic
**Half-life:** 3–7 hours

### *Reactions*

#### Skin

Edema (4.8%)

#### Other

Myalgia (5.4%)
Tooth disorder (sic) (2.3%)

## PIPERACILLIN

**Trade names:** Pipracil (Lederle); Zosyn (Lederle)
**Other common trade names:** *Avocin; Ivacin; Picillin; Pipcil; Piperilline; Pipril; Piprilin; Pitamycin*
**Indications:** Various infections caused by susceptible organisms
**Category:** Beta-lactamase-sensitive penicillin antibiotic
**Half-life:** 0.6–1.2 hours
**Clinically important, potentially hazardous interactions with:** anticoagulants, atracurium, cisatracurium, demeclocycline, dicumarol, doxacurium, doxycycline, methotrexate, minocycline, non-depolarizing muscle relaxants, oxytetracycline, pancuronium, rapacuronium, reteplase, tetracyclines

Zosyn is piperacillin and tazobactam

### *Reactions*

#### Skin

Allergic reactions (sic) (2–4%)
(1994): Pleasants RA+, *Chest* 106, 1124 (in patients with cystic fibrosis)
(1984): Holmes B+, *Drugs* 28, 375
Angioedema
Bullous eruption
Candidiasis
Ecchymoses
Edema
Erythema nodosum
Exanthems
(1993): Warrington RJ+, *J Allergy Clin Immunol* 92, 626
(1985): Mead GM+, *Lancet* 2, 499 (56%)
(1985): No Author, *Lancet* 2, 723
(1984): Holmes B+, *Drugs* 28, 375
Exfoliative dermatitis
Jarisch–Herxheimer reaction (<1%)
Pruritus
Purpura
(2000): Yata Y+, *Ann Hematol* 79(10), 593
Radiation recall
(2001): Krishnan RS+, *J Am Acad Dermatol* 44, 1045 (with tobramycin & ciprofloxacin)
Rash (sic) (1%)
Stevens–Johnson syndrome
(1995): Cheriyan S+, *Allergy Proc* 16, 85
Toxic epidermal necrolysis
Urticaria
(1995): Moscato G+, *Eur Respir J* 8, 467

(1984): Holmes B+, *Drugs* 28, 375
Vasculitis
Vesicular eruptions

### Other

Anaphylactoid reactions (<1%)
Glossodynia
Hypersensitivity (<1%)
(2002): Romano A+, *Allergy* 57(5), 459
(1998): Cabanes R+, *Allergy* 53, 819
Injection-site pain (2%)
(1984): Holmes B+, *Drugs* 28, 375
Injection-site phlebitis (2%)
(1984): Holmes B+, *Drugs* 28, 375
Oral candidiasis
Serum sickness
Stomatodynia
Thrombophlebitis (<1%)
Tinnitus
Vaginitis

## PIRBUTEROL

**Trade name:** Maxair (3M)
**Other common trade names:** *Exirel; Spirolair; Zeisin Autohaler*
**Indications:** Asthma, bronchospasm
**Category:** Bronchodilator; $beta_2$-adrenergic agonist
**Half-life:** 2–3 hours

### *Reactions*

### Skin

Edema
Pruritus
Purpura (<1%)
Rash (sic)

### Hair

Hair – alopecia

### Other

Dysgeusia (1–10%)
Glossitis
Paresthesias (<1%)
Trembling (>10%)
Xerostomia

## PIROXICAM

**Trade name:** Feldene (Pfizer)
**Other common trade names:** *Antiflog; Apo-Piroxicam; Baxo; Doblexan; Felden; Larapam; Nu-Pirox; Rogal; Sotilen; Zunden*
**Indications:** Arthritis
**Category:** Nonsteroidal anti-inflammatory (NSAID); analgesic
**Half-life:** 50 hours
**Clinically important, potentially hazardous interactions with:** methotrexate, ritonavir

### *Reactions*

### Skin

Angioedema (<1%)
(1987): Gerber D, *Drug Intell Clin Pharm* 21, 707 (passim)
Bullous dermatosis
(1985): Guillaume JC+, *Ann Dermatol Venereol* (French) 112, 807
Contact allergy
(2001): Trujillo MJ+, *Allergol Immunopathol* (Madr) 29(4), 133 (with thimerosal)
Contact dermatitis
(1995): Valsecchi R+, *Contact Dermatitis* 32, 63
(1993): Ophaswongse S+, *Contact Dermatitis* 29, 57
(1993): Valsecchi R+, *Contact Dermatitis* 29, 167
(1992): Green C+, *Contact Dermatitis* 27, 261 (to the gel)
(1990): Serrano G+, *J Am Acad Dermatol* 23, 479
Cutaneous side effects (sic) (46.9%)
(1987): Gerber D, *Drug Intell Clin Pharm* 21, 707 (passim)
Diaphoresis (<1%)
(1987): Gerber D, *Drug Intell Clin Pharm* 21, 707 (passim)
Dyshidrosis
(1985): Braunstein BL, *Cutis* 35, 485
Ecchymoses (<1%)
Edema (>1%)
Erythema (<1%)
Erythema annulare centrifugum
(1985): Hogan DJ+, *J Am Acad Dermatol* 13, 840
Erythema multiforme (<1%)
(1987): Gerber D, *Drug Intell Clin Pharm* 21, 707 (passim)
(1986): Penso D, *J Am Acad Dermatol* 14, 275
(1986): Stern RS, *J Am Acad Dermatol* 14, 276
(1985): Bigby M+, *J Am Acad Dermatol* 12, 866
(1985): Guillaume JC+, *Ann Dermatol Venereol* (French) 112, 807
(1985): O'Brien WM+, *J Rheumatol* 12, 13
(1984): Brogden RN+, *Drugs* 28, 292
(1984): Duro JC+, *J Rheumatol* 11, 554
(1984): Stern RS+, *JAMA* 252, 1433
(1982): Bertail MA, *Ann Dermatol Venereol* (French) 109, 261
(1982): Faure M, *Ann Dermatol Venereol* (French) 109, 255
Erythroderma
(1993): Sangla I+, *Rev Neurol Paris* (French) 149, 217
(1985): Guillaume JC+, *Ann Dermatol Venereol* (French) 112, 807
Exanthems (>5%)
(1994): Litt JZ, Beachwood, OH (personal case) (observation)
(1987): Gerber D, *Drug Intell Clin Pharm* 21, 707 (passim)
(1985): Bigby M+, *J Am Acad Dermatol* 12, 866 (2.4%)
(1985): Guillaume JC+, *Ann Dermatol Venereol* (French) 112, 807
(1984): Brogden RN+, *Drugs* 28, 292 (0.8%)
(1984): Stern RS+, *JAMA* 252, 1433
(1982): Faure M+, *Ann Dermatol Venereol* (French) 109, 255
(1979): Dessain P+, *J Int Med Res* 7, 335
Exfoliative dermatitis (<1%)
(1987): Gerber D, *Drug Intell Clin Pharm* 21, 707 (passim)
Fixed eruption
(1998): Leal G, Fortaleza, Brazil (from Internet) (observation) (2 cases)
(1995): Ordoqui E+, *Allergy* 50, 741
(1994): Ordoqui E+, *J Allergy Clin Immunology* 93, 242
(1993): Gastaminza G+, *Contact Dermatitis* 28, 43
(1993): No Author, *Dermatology* 186, 164
(1990): de la Hoz B+, *Int J Dermatol* 29, 672
(1990): Stubb S+, *J Am Acad Dermatol* 22, 1111
(1989): Shiohara T+, *Arch Dermatol* 125, 1371
(1989): Valsecchi R+, *J Am Acad Dermatol* 21, 1300
Hot flashes (<1%)
Lichenoid eruption
(1993): Veraldi S+, *Eur J Dermatol* 3, 156
(1992): Vaillant L+, *Ann Dermatol Venereol* (French) 119, 936
(1985): Guillaume JC+, *Ann Dermatol Venereol* (French) 112, 807

(1984): Stern RS+, *JAMA* 252, 1433
Linear IgA bullous dermatosis
(2001): Plunkett RW+, *J Am Acad Dermatol* 45(5), 691
(1998): Camilleri M+, *J Eur Acad Dermatol Venereol* 10, 70
Lupus erythematosus
(1991): Roura M+, *Dermatologica* 182, 56
Pemphigus
(1985): Guillaume JC+, *Ann Dermatol Venereol* (French) 112, 807
(1983): Martin RL, *N Engl J Med* 309, 795
Pemphigus foliaceus
(1984): Brogden RN+, *Drugs* 28, 292
Peripheral edema
Petechiae (<1%)
Photocontact dermatitis
(1992): Torinuki W, *Tohoku J Exp Med* 167, 267
Photodermatitis
(2001): Trujillo MJ+, *Allergol Immunopathol* (Madr) 29(4), 133 (with thimerosal)
Photoreactions (<1%)
(1995): Gebhardt M+, *Z Rheumatol* (German) 54, 405
(1994): Sassolas B+, *Clin Exp Dermatol* 19, 189
(1989): Sunohara A, *Photodermatol* 6, 188
Photosensitivity
(1998): Valentine M, Everett, WA (from Internet) (observation)
(1998): Varela P+, *Acta Med Port* (Portugese) 11, 997
(1998): Varela P+, *Contact Dermatitis* 38, 229
(1996): Stingeni L+, *Contact Dermatitis* 34, 60
(1995): Gebhardt M+, *Z Rheumatol* (German) 54, 405
(1995): Mammen L+, *Am Fam Physician* 52, 575
(1993): Hariya T+, *J Dermatol Sci* 5, 165
(1993): Youn JI+, *Clin Exp Dermatol* 18, 52
(1992): Goncalo M+, *Contact Dermatitis* 27, 287
(1992): Izekawa Z+, *J Invest Dermatol* 98, 918
(1992): Serrano G+, *J Am Acad Dermatol* 26, 545
(1991): de Castro JL+, *Contact Dermatitis* 24, 187
(1991): Roura M+, *Dermatologica* 182, 56
(1990): Black AK+, *Br J Dermatol* 123, 277
(1990): Serrano G+, *J Am Acad Dermatol* 23, 479
(1989): Cirne de Castro JL+, *J Am Acad Dermatol* 20, 706
(1989): De la Cuadra J+, *Contact Dermatitis* 21, 349
(1989): Kaidbey KH+, *Arch Dermatol* 125, 783
(1987): Figueiredo A+, *Contact Dermatitis* 17, 73
(1987): Gerber D, *Drug Intell Clin Pharm* 21, 707 (passim)
(1987): Halasz CL, *Cutis* 39, 37
(1987): Magana-Garcia M+, *Rev Invest Clin* (Spanish) 39, 177
(1987): Morison WL+, *J Am Acad Dermatol* 17, 698
(1986): Kochevar IE+, *Arch Dermatol* 122, 1283
(1986): McKerrow KJ+, *J Am Acad Dermatol* 15, 1237
(1985): Bigby M+, *J Am Acad Dermatol* 12, 866
(1985): Braunstein BL, *Cutis* 35, 485
(1985): Guillaume JC+, *Ann Dermatol Venereol* (French) 112, 807
(1985): Serrano G+, *J Am Acad Dermatol* 11, 113
(1985): Weigand DA, *J Am Acad Dermatol* 12, 373
(1984): Brogden RN+, *Drugs* 28, 292
(1984): Stern RS+, *JAMA* 252, 1433
(1983): Diffey BL+, *Br J Rheumatol* 22, 239
(1983): Fjellner B, *Acta Derm Venereol* (Stockh) 63, 557
(1982): Faure M+, *Ann Dermatol Venereol* (French) 109, 255
Pruritus (1–10%)
(1987): Gerber D, *Drug Intell Clin Pharm* 21, 707 (passim)
(1984): Brogden RN+, *Drugs* 28, 292
(1984): Stern RS+, *JAMA* 252, 1433
(1979): Dessain P+, *J Int Med Res* 7, 335
Purpura (<1%)
(1987): Gerber D, *Drug Intell Clin Pharm* 21, 707 (passim)
(1984): Brogden RN+, *Drugs* 28, 292
Rash (sic) (>10%)
Stevens–Johnson syndrome (<1%)
(1995): Katoh N+, *J Dermatol* 22, 677
(1985): Guillaume JC+, *Ann Dermatol Venereol* (French) 112, 807
Toxic dermatitis (sic)
(1991): Chosidow O+, *Ann Dermatol Venereol* (French) 118, 903
Toxic epidermal necrolysis (<1%)
(2002): Correia O+, *Arch Dermatol* 138, 29 (two cases)
(1996): Blum L+, *J Am Acad Dermatol* 34, 1088
(1993): Correia O+, *Dermatology* 186, 32
(1990): Black AK+, *Br J Dermatol* 123, 277
(1987): Gerber D, *Drug Intell Clin Pharm* 21, 707 (passim)
(1987): Guillaume JC+, *Arch Dermatol* 123, 1166
(1986): Penso D+, *J Am Acad Dermatol* 14, 275 (letter)
(1986): Szczeklik A, *Drugs* 32 (Suppl 4), 148
(1985): Coscojuela C+, *Med Cutan Ibero Lat Am* (Spanish) 13, 291
(1985): Guillaume JC+, *Ann Dermatol Venereol* (French) 112, 807
(1982): Faure M+, *Ann Dermatol Venereol* (French) 109, 255
Urticaria (<1%)
(1987): Gerber D, *Drug Intell Clin Pharm* 21, 707 (passim)
(1985): Serrano G+, *J Am Acad Dermatol* 11, 113
(1984): Stern RS+, *JAMA* 252, 1433
(1982): Torras H+, *Med Cutan Ibero Lat Am* (Spanish) 10, 351
Vasculitis (<1%)
(1985): Bigby M+, *J Am Acad Dermatol* 12, 866
(1985): Guillaume JC+, *Ann Dermatol Venereol* (French) 112, 807
(1984): Stern RS+, *JAMA* 252, 1433
Vesicular eruptions (<1%)
(1986): Stern RS, *J Am Acad Dermatol* 14, 276 (letter)
(1984): Stern RS+, *JAMA* 252, 1433

## Hair

Hair – alopecia
(1987): Gerber D, *Drug Intell Clin Pharm* 21, 707
(1985): Bigby M+, *J Am Acad Dermatol* 12, 866
(1984): Stern RS+, *JAMA* 252, 1433

## Nails

Nails – onycholysis

## Other

Anaphylactoid reactions (<1%)
Aphthous stomatitis
(2001): Vincent L+, *Ann Dermatol Venereol* 128(1), 57
(1991): Siegel MA+, *J Am Dent Assoc* 122, 75
Buccal ulceration
(1987): Gerber D, *Drug Intell Clin Pharm* 21, 707 (passim)
Death
(2002): Correia O+, *Arch Dermatol* 138, 29
Paresthesias
(1987): Gerber D, *Drug Intell Clin Pharm* 21, 707
Pseudoporphyria
(2000): De Silva B+, *Pediatr Dermatol* 17, 480
Serum sickness (<1%)
Stomatitis (>1%)
Tinnitus
Xerostomia (<1%)

## PLICAMYCIN

**Synonym:** mithramycin
**Trade name:** Mithracin (Bayer)
**Other common trade name:** *Mithraline*
**Indications:** Paget's disease, malignant testicular tumors
**Category:** Antineoplastic; antihypercalcemic; antihypercalciuric; bone resorption inhibitor
**Half-life:** I hour
**Clinically important, potentially hazardous interactions with:** aldesleukin

### *Reactions*

#### Skin
Bleeding tendency (5–12%)
Ecchymoses
(1970): Kennedy BJ, *Am J Med* 49, 494
Exanthems
Flushing (1–10%)
(1983): Bronner AK+, *J Am Acad Dermatol* 9, 645
(1982): Dunagin WG, *Semin Oncol* 9, 14
(1970): Kennedy BJ, *Am J Med* 49, 494 (35%)
Petechiae 1-(1–10%)
Purpura
(1970): Kennedy BJ, *Am J Med* 49, 494 (10%)
Seborrheic keratoses (inflammation of)
(1987): Johnson TM+, *J Am Acad Dermatol* 17, 192
Toxic epidermal necrolysis
(1978): Purpora D+, *N Engl J Med* 299, 1412

#### Other
Dysgeusia (metallic taste)
Injection-site cellulitis (1–10%)
Injection-site erythema (1–10%)
Injection-site pain (1–10%)
Oral mucosal lesions
(1989): Kerker BJ+, *Semin Dermatol* 8, 173 (1–5%)
(1970): Kennedy BJ, *Am J Med* 49, 494 (15%)
Stomatitis (>10%)

## POLYTHIAZIDE

**Trade names:** Minizide (Pfizer); Renese (Pfizer)
**Other common trade names:** *Drenusil; Nephril*
**Indications:** Hypertension, edema
**Category:** Thiazide* diuretic; antihypertensive
**Half-life:** no data
**Clinically important, potentially hazardous interactions with:** digoxin, lithium

Minizide is prazosin and polythiazide

### *Reactions*

#### Skin
Exanthems
Photosensitivity (<1%)
Purpura
Rash (sic) (<1%)
Urticaria
Vasculitis

#### Other
Paresthesias

***Note:** Polythiazide is a sulfonamide and can be absorbed systemically. Sulfonamides can produce severe, possibly fatal, reactions such as toxic epidermal necrolysis and Stevens–Johnson syndrome

## POTASSIUM IODIDE

**Synonyms:** KI; Lugol's solution; strong iodine solution
**Trade names:** Kie (Laser); Pima (Fleming); SSKI (Upsher Smith); Thyroid-Block
**Other common trade names:** *Jodatum; Jodid; Kalium*
**Indications:** Hyperthyroidism
**Category:** Antihyperthyroid; thyroid inhibitor; antifungal; expectorant
**Half-life:** no data
**Clinically important, potentially hazardous interactions with:** ACE inhibitors, potassium-sparing diuretics, spironolactone, triamterene

### *Reactions*

#### Skin
Acne (1–10%)
Angioedema (1–10%)
(1979): Curd JG+, *Ann Intern Med* 91, 853
Bullous pemphigoid
(1994): Piletta P+, *Br J Dermatol* 131, 145
Dermatitis herpetiformis
(1989): Zone JJ+, *Immunol Ser* 46, 565
Diaphoresis
Exanthems
(1981): Farkas J, *Dermatol Monatsschr* (German) 167, 579
Iododerma
(1996): Alpay K+, *Pediatr Dermatol* 13, 51
(1990): Soria C+, *J Am Acad Dermatol* 22, 418 (vegetating)
(1989): Romanenko VN+, *Vestn Dermatol Venerol* (Russian) 12, 60
(1987): O'Brien TJ, *Australas J Dermatol* 28, 119
(1986): Raznatovskii IM+, *Vestn Dermatol Venerol* (Russian) 10, 71
(1985): Stone OJ, *Int J Dermatol* 24, 565
(1985): Wilkin JK+, *Cutis* 36, 335
(1981): Huang TY+, *Ann Allergy* 46, 264
(1978): Jezova J, *Cesk Dermatol* (Czech) 53, 240
(1978): Labohm EB, *Ned Tijdschr Geneeskd* (Dutch) 122, 1291 (vegetating)
(1974): Dienhart KJ, *N Engl J Med* 290, 521 (suppurative ulcerating)
(1973): Khan F+, *N Engl J Med* 289, 1018 (suppurative ulcerating)
(1971): Werbitt W, *J Am Osteopath Assoc* 70, 460
Lupus erythematosus
(1979): Curd JG+, *Ann Intern Med* 91, 853
Purpura
Pustular psoriasis
(1967): Shelley WB, *JAMA* 201, 1009
Rash (sic)
Systemic eczematous contact dermatitis
Urticaria (1–10%)
(1979): Curd JG+, *Ann Intern Med* 91, 853
Vasculitis
(1987): Eeckhout E+, *Acta Derm Venereol* (Stockh) 67, 362
(1981): Zone JJ, *Arch Dermatol* 117, 758
(1979): Curd JG+, *Ann Intern Med* 91, 853

### Other
Dysgeusia (1–10%) (metallic taste)
Gingival pain
Paresthesias
Serum sickness
Sialorrhea
Stomatodynia

## PRAMIPEXOLE

**Trade name:** Mirapex (Boehringer Ingelheim)
**Indications:** Parkinsonism
**Category:** Antiparkinsonian
**Half-life:** ~8 hours

#### *Reactions*

### Skin
Allergic reactions (sic) (>1%)
Diaphoresis (>1%)
Edema (5%)
Peripheral edema (5%)
(2000): Tan EK+, *Arch Neurol* 57, 729
Pruritus (>1%)
Rash (sic) (>1%)
Skin disorders (sic) (2%)

### Other
Dysgeusia (>1%)
Hyperesthesia (3%)
Myalgia (>1%)
Paresthesias (>1%)
Sialorrhea (>1%)
Tooth disease (>1%)
Twitching (sic) (2%)
Xerostomia (7%)
(1998): Dooley M+, *Drugs Aging* 12, 495

## PRAVASTATIN

**Trade name:** Pravachol (Bristol-Myers Squibb)
**Other common trade names:** *Elisor; Lipostat; Pravasin; Pravasine; Selectin; Selektine; Selipran*
**Indications:** Hypercholesterolemia
**Category:** Antihyperlipidemic; HMG-CoA reductase inhibitor
**Half-life:** ~2–3 hours
**Clinically important, potentially hazardous interactions with:** azithromycin, clarithromycin, cyclosporine, erythromycin, gemfibrozil, imatinib

#### *Reactions*

### Skin
Allergic reactions (sic)
(1994): de Boer EM+, *Contact Dermatitis* 30, 238
Angioedema
Dermatomyositis
(1992): Schalke BB+, *N Engl J Med* 327, 649
Eczematous eruption (generalized)
(1993): Krasovec M+, *Dermatology* 186, 248
Erythema multiforme
Exanthems
Flu-like syndrome (sic)
Flushing
(1990): Wiklund O+, *J Intern Med* 228, 241
Lichenoid eruption
(1998): Keough GC+, *Cutis* 61, 98
(1997): Anthony JL, Montgomery, AL (from Internet) (observation)
Lupus erythematosus
Photosensitivity
Pruritus
(1992): Yoshimura N+, *Transplantation* 53, 94
(1991): Malini PL+, *Clin Ther* 13, 500
Purpura
Rash (sic) (1–10%)
(1992): Betteridge DJ+, *BMJ* 304, 1335
(1992): Jungnickel PW+, *Clin Pharm* 11, 677
(1991): Crepaldi G+, *Arch Intern Med* 151, 146
(1991): *Med Lett Drugs Ther* 33, 18
(1991): McTavish D+, *Drugs* 42, 65
(1991): Raasch RH, *Drug Intell Clin Pharm* 25, 388
(1990): Hunninghake DB+, *Atherosclerosis* 85, 81 (3.4%)
Stevens–Johnson syndrome
Toxic epidermal necrolysis
Urticaria
Vasculitis

### Hair
Hair – alopecia
(1999): Oakley A, Hamilton, New Zealand (from Internet) (observation)
Hair – broken-off patches of scalp hair (sic) (greenish)
(1998): Fixler R, Cincinnati, OH (personal communication) (observation)

### Other
Anaphylactoid reactions
Dysgeusia (<1%)
Gynecomastia
(1999): Aerts J+, *Presse Med* (French) 28, 787
Hypersensitivity
Myalgia (2.7%)
(2001): Rehbein H, Jacksonville, FL (from Internet) (observation)
Myopathy
(1995): Garnett WR, *Am J Health Syst Pharm* 52(15), 1639
(1992): Schalke BB+, *N Engl J Med* 327, 649
Paresthesias
Porphyria cutanea tarda
(1994): Perrot JL+, *Ann Dermatol Venereol* (French) 121, 817
Rhabdomyolysis
(2002): Sica DA+, *Am J Geriatr Cardiol* 11(1), 48
(2002): Sica DA+, *Curr Opin Nephrol Hypertens* 11(2), 123
(2001): Borrego FJ+, *Nefrologia* 21(3), 309
(1996): Ballantyne CM+, *Am J Cardiol* 78(5), 532
(1995): Farmer JA+, *Baillieres Clin Endocrinol Metab* 9(4), 825
(1995): Garnett WR, *Am J Health Syst Pharm* 52(15), 1639 (with either cyclosporine, erythromycin, gemfibrozil or niacin)
(1992): Raimondeau J+, *Presse Med* 21(14), 663 (with fenofibrate)
Stomatitis

# PRAZEPAM

**Trade name:** Centrax (Parke-Davis)
**Other common trade names:** *Centrac; Demetrin; Lysanxia; Prazene; Sedapran; Trepidan*
**Indications:** Anxiety, depression
**Category:** Benzodiazepine sedative-hypnotic; anxiolytic and antidepressant; anticonvulsant
**Half-life:** 30–100 hours

### *Reactions*

#### Skin
Ankle edema
Dermatitis (sic) (1–10%)
Diaphoresis (>10%)
Exanthems
Facial edema
Pruritus
Purpura
Rash (sic) (>10%)
Urticaria

#### Hair
Hair – alopecia
Hair – hirsutism

#### Other
Gingivitis
Paresthesias
Sialopenia (>10%)
Sialorrhea (1–10%)
Xerostomia (>10%)

# PRAZIQUANTEL

**Trade name:** Biltricide (Bayer)
**Other common trade names:** *Cisticid; Distocide; Flukacide; Kalcide; Prazite; Tecprazin; Teniken*
**Indications:** Helmintic infections
**Category:** Anthelmintic
**Half-life:** 0.8–1.5 hours

### *Reactions*

#### Skin
Diaphoresis (1–10%)
Edema
(1995): Stelma FF+, *Am J Trop Med Hyg* 53, 167
Pruritus (<1%)
Rash (sic) (<1%)
Urticaria (<1%)
(1996): Jaoko WG+, *East Afr Med J* 73, 499
(1995): Stelma FF+, *Am J Trop Med Hyg* 53, 167

# PRAZOSIN

**Trade names:** Minipress (Pfizer); Minizide (Pfizer)
**Other common trade names:** *Alti-Prazosin; Apo-Prazo; Duramipress; Eurex; Hypovase; Nu-Prazo; Peripress; Pratisol; Pressin*
**Indications:** Hypertension
**Category:** Alpha-adrenergic blocker; antihypertensive
**Half-life:** 2–4 hours
**Clinically important, potentially hazardous interactions with:** epinephrine

Minizide is prazosin and polythiazide

### *Reactions*

#### Skin
Angioedema
(1983): Ruzicka T+, *Lancet* 1, 473
Diaphoresis (<1%)
(1977): Lahon HFJ+, *Excerpta Med Int Congr* 431, 26
(1975): Pitts NE, *Postgraduate Medicine, Prazosin Clinical Symposium Proceedings* 20
Edema (1–4%)
(1975): Pitts NE, *Postgraduate Medicine, Prazosin Clinical Symposium Proceedings* 20
Exanthems (1–5%)
(1977): Lahon HFJ+, *Excerpta Med Int Congr* 431, 26 (0.7%)
Lichen planus (<1%)
Lichenoid eruption
Lupus erythematosus
(1979): Marshall AJ+, *BMJ* 1, 165
(1979): Wilson JD+, *Clin Pharmacol Ther* 26, 209
Pruritus (<1%)
(1975): Pitts NE, *Postgraduate Medicine, Prazosin Clinical Symposium Proceedings* 20
Rash (sic) (1–4%)
(1983): Stanaszek WF+, *Drugs* 25, 339
(1975): Pitts NE, *Postgraduate Medicine, Prazosin Clinical Symposium Proceedings* 20
Urticaria
(1983): Ruzicka T+, *Lancet* 1, 473

#### Hair
Hair – alopecia (<1%)

#### Other
Anaphylactoid reactions
(1983): Ruzicka T+, *Lancet* 1, 473
Myopathy
(1977): Tomlinson IW+, *BMJ* 1, 1319
Paresthesias (<1%)
Priapism (<1%)
(1980): Burke JR+, *Med J Aust* 1, 382
(1975): Pitts NE, *Postgraduate Medicine, Prazosin Clinical Symposium Proceedings* 20
Tinnitus
Xerostomia (1–4%)
(1983): Stanaszek WF+, *Drugs* 25, 339
(1977): Lahon HFJ+, *Excerpta Med Int Congr* 431, 26 (5.6%)
(1975): Pitts NE, *Postgraduate Medicine, Prazosin Clinical Symposium Proceedings* 20

# PRIMAQUINE

**Synonym:** prymaccone
**Trade name:** Primaquine (Sanofi)
**Other common trade names:** *Neo-Quipenyl; Palum*
**Indications:** Malaria
**Category:** Antiprotozoal; antimalarial
**Half-life:** 4–10 hours
**Clinically important, potentially hazardous interactions with:** penicillamine

### *Reactions*

#### Skin
Angioedema
(1970): Stevenson DD+, *JAMA* 212, 624
Exanthems
(1976): Arndt KA+, *JAMA* 235, 918 (5%)
Pallor
Pruritus (<1%)
Psoriasis
(1963): Kirschenbaum MB, *JAMA* 185, 1044
Urticaria
(1970): Stevenson DD+, *JAMA* 212, 624

# PRIMIDONE

**Trade name:** Mysoline (Elan)
**Other common trade names:** *Midone; Mylepsin; PMS Primidone; Prysoline; Sertan*
**Indications:** Seizures
**Category:** Anticonvulsant; barbiturate
**Half-life:** 10–12 hours
**Clinically important, potentially hazardous interactions with: alcohol**, anticoagulants, antihistamines, brompheniramine, buclizine, chlorpheniramine, dicumarol, ethanolamine, imatinib, midazolam, niacinamide, warfarin

### *Reactions*

#### Skin
Acne
Allergic reactions (sic)
(1984): Steffan MA+, *Contact Dermatitis* 10, 184
Erythema multiforme (<1%)
(2002): Krivo JM, Franklin Square, NY (from Internet) (observation)
(1979): Pollack MA+, *Ann Neurol* 5, 262
(1975): Böttiger LE+, *Acta Med Scand* 198, 229
Exanthems (1–5%)
(1980): Marghescu S+, *Fortschr Med* (German) 98, 723
Exfoliative dermatitis
Lupus erythematosus (<1%)
(1993): Drory VE+, *Clin Neuropharmacol* 16, 19 (passim)
(1977): Schubothe H+, *Verh Dtsch Ges Inn Med* (German) 83, 727
(1972): Levantine A+, *Br J Dermatol* 87, 646 (passim)
(1966): Ahuja GK+, *JAMA* 198, 201
Rash (sic) (<1%)
Toxic epidermal necrolysis
(1985): Muhar U+, *Pediatr Dermatol* 3, 54
(1979): Pollack MA+, *Ann Neurol* 5, 262
(1973): Stüttgen G, *Br J Dermatol* 88, 291
(1970): Hermann WA, *Dermatologica* 141, 366
Urticaria
(1984): Steffan MA+, *Contact Dermatitis* 10, 184

#### Other
Acute intermittent porphyria
Gingival hyperplasia
Hypersensitivity*
(2002): Krivo JM, Franklin Square, NY (from Internet) (observation)
(1998): Schlienger RG+, *Epilepsia* 39, S3 (passim)
Mucocutaneous syndrome
(1975): Böttiger LE+, *Acta Med Scand* 198, 229
Rhabdomyolysis
(1990): Larpin R+, *Presse Med* 19(30), 1403

***Note:** The antiepileptic drug hypersensitivity syndrome is a severe, occasionally fatal, disorder characterized by any or all of the following: pruritic exanthems, toxic epidermal necrolysis, Stevens–Johnson syndrome, exfoliative dermatitis, fever, hepatic abnormalities, eosinophilia, and renal failure

# PROBENECID

**Trade names:** Benemid (Merck); Col-Benemid (Merck); Probalan
**Other common trade names:** *Bencid; Benecid; Benuryl; Panuric; Procid; Solpurin; Urocid*
**Indications:** Gouty arthritis
**Category:** Uricosuric
**Half-life:** 6–12 hours (dose-dependent)
**Clinically important, potentially hazardous interactions with:** amphotericin B, benzodiazepines, ertapenem, ketoprofen, ketorolac, methotrexate, NSAIDs, penicillamine, salicylates, sulfonamides

### *Reactions*

#### Skin
Allergic reactions (sic)
Dermatitis (sic)
Erythema multiforme
(1985): Ting HC+, *Int J Dermatol* 24, 587
Exanthems
Flushing (1–10%)
Pruritus (1–10%)
Rash (sic) (1–10%)
Urticaria (1–5%)

#### Hair
Hair – alopecia

#### Other
Anaphylactoid reactions (<1%)
Gingivitis (1–10%)
Hypersensitivity
(1998): Myers KW+, *Ann Allergy Asthma Immunol* 80, 416 (in AIDS)

# PROCAINAMIDE

**Trade names:** Procan (Parke-Davis); Procanbid (Monarch); Pronestyl (Bristol-Myers Squibb); Rhythmin
**Other common trade names:** *Amisalen; Biocoryl; Procan SR; Promine; Ritmocamid*
**Indications:** Ventricular arrhythmias
**Category:** Antiarrhythmic class I-A
**Half-life:** 2.5–4.5 hours
**Clinically important, potentially hazardous interactions with:** arsenic, ciprofloxacin, enoxacin, gatifloxacin, lomefloxacin, moxifloxacin, norfloxacin, ofloxacin, quinolones, sparfloxacin

## *Reactions*

### Skin

Angioedema (<1%)
(1985): Ponte CD+, *Drug Intell Clin Pharm* 19, 139
Chills (<1%)
Dermatitis (sic)
(1985): Gorsulowsky DC+, *J Am Acad Dermatol* 12, 245 (6%)
Eczematous eruption (sic)
Exanthems (1–5%)
(1999): Numata T+, *Sangyo Ika Daigaku Zasshi* (Japanese) 21, 235
(1985): Gorsulowsky DC+, *J Am Acad Dermatol* 12, 245 (8%)
(1984): Christensen DJ+, *Ann Intern Med* 100, 918
(1973): Kosowski BD+, *Circulation* 47, 1204 (5%)
(1972): Blomgren SE+, *Am J Med* 52, 338
Flushing (<1%)
Lichen planus
(1988): Sherertz EF, *Cutis* 42, 51
Lupus erythematosus (>10%)
(1998): Kameda H+, *Br J Rheumatol* 37, 1236
(1998): Ohtani Y+, *Nihon Kokyuki Gakkai Zasshi* (Japanese) 36, 535
(1997): Yung R+, *Arthritis Rheum* 40, 1436
(1996): Miyasaka N, *Intern Med* 35, 527
(1995): Finger DR+, *J Rheumatol* 22, 574
(1995): Muramatsu M+, *Nippon Naika Gakkai Zasshi* (Japanese) 84, 1736
(1995): Panine VV+, American Academy of Dermatology Meeting, New Orleans (observation)
(1995): Rubin RL+, *J Immunol* 154, 2483
(1994): Cohen MG, *J Rheumatol* 21, 578
(1993): McDonald E+, *Hosp Pract Off ED* 28, 95
(1992): Klimas NG+, *Am J Med Sci* 303, 99
(1992): Rubin RL, *Clin Biochem* 25, 223
(1992): Rubin RL+, *J Clin Invest* 90, 165
(1992): Skaer TL, *Clin Ther* 14, 496
(1992): Stevens MB, *Hosp Pract Off Ed* 27, 27
(1990): Pauls JD+, *Mol Immunol* 27, 701
(1989): Adams LE+, *J Lab Clin Med* 113, 482
(1989): Asherson RA+, *Ann Rheum Dis* 48, 232
(1989): Mohindra SK+, *Crit Care Med* 17, 961
(1989): Nichols CJ+, *Ophthalmology* 96, 1535
(1989): Turgeon PW+, *Ophthalmology* 96, 68
(1989): Vivino FB+, *Arthritis Rheum* 32, 560
(1988): Agudelo CA+, *J Rheumatol* 15, 1431
(1988): Forrester J+, *J Rheumatol* 15, 1384
(1988): Hess E, *N Engl J Med* 318, 1460
(1988): No Author, *J Tenn Med Assoc* 81, 579
(1988): Sheretz EF, *Cutis* 42, 51
(1988): Totoritis MC+, *N Engl J Med* 318, 1431
(1988): Uetrecht JP, *Chem Res Toxicol* 1, 133
(1987): Craft JE+, *Arthritis Rheum* 30, 689
(1987): Shoenfeld Y+, *J Clin Immunol* 7, 410
(1986): Harle JR+, *Ann Med Interne Paris* (French) 137, 599
(1986): Jackson C+, *Clin Exp Rheumatol* 4, 290
(1986): Reidenberg MM+, *Angiology* 37, 968
(1986): Rubin RL+, *Am J Med* 80, 999
(1986): Vitas B+, *Lijec Vjesn* (Serbo-Croatian-Roman) 108, 137
(1986): Weisbart RH+, *Ann Intern Med* 104, 310
(1985): Amadio P+, *Ann Intern Med* 102, 419
(1985): Cush JJ+, *Am J Med Sci* 290, 36
(1985): Epstein A+, *Arthritis Rheum* 28, 158
(1985): Gorsulowsky DC+, *J Am Acad Dermatol* 12, 245 (>5%)
(1985): Kale SA, *Postgrad Med* 77, 231
(1985): Lovisetto P+, *Recenti Prog Med* (Italian) 76, 110
(1985): Rubin RL+, *Clin Immunol Immunopathol* 36, 49
(1985): Stratton MA, *Clin Pharm* 4, 657
(1985): Totoritis MC+, *Postgrad Med* 78, 149
(1984): Browning CA+, *Am J Cardiol* 53, 376
(1984): Goldberg SK+, *Am J Med* 76, 146
(1984): Tan EM+, *Allergy Clin Immunol* 74, 631
(1984): Wollina U, *Z Gesamte Inn Med* (German) 39, 69
(1982): Chokron R+, *Nouv Presse Med* (French) 11, 2568
(1982): Gupta AK+, *Indian J Dermatol* 27, 112
(1982): Harmon CE+, *Clin Rheum Dis* 8, 121
(1982): Hess EV, *Arthritis Rheum* 25, 857
(1982): Tannen RH+, *Immunol Commun* 11, 33
(1981): Edwards RL+, *Arch Intern Med* 141, 1688
(1981): Gonzalez ER, *JAMA* 246, 1634
(1981): Hess EV, *Arthritis Rheum* 24, vi
(1981): Reidenberg MM, *Arthritis Rheum* 24, 1004
(1981): Schoen RT+, *Am J Med* 71, 5
(1981): Sheikh TK+, *Am J Clin Pathol* 75, 755
(1981): Tan EM+, *Arthritis Rheum* 24, 1064
(1981): Uetrecht JP+, *Arthritis Rheum* 24, 994
(1980): Ahmad S, *Circulation* 61, 865
(1980): Chubick A, *Adv Intern Med* 26, 467
(1980): Dixon JA+, *J Rheumatol* 7, 544
(1980): Seligmann H+, *Harefuah* (Hebrew) 99, 166
(1980): Weinstein A, *Prog Clin Immunol* 4, 1
(1979): Bernstein RE, *Lancet* 2, 1076
(1979): Bluestein HG+, *Lancet* 2, 816
(1979): Foucar E+, *J Clin Lab Immunol* 2, 79
(1979): Hoff BH, *Chest* 75, 107
(1979): McLain DA+, *Arthritis Rheum* 22, 305
(1979): Sonnhag C+, *Acta Med Scand* 206, 245
(1979): Stec GP+, *Ann Intern Med* 90, 799
(1979): Stein HB+, *J Rheumatol* 6, 543
(1978): Jones WN+, *Ariz Med* 35, 16
(1978): Kaplan AI+, *Chest* 73, 875
(1978): Nick J+, *Ann Med Interne Paris* (French) 129, 259
(1978): Robinson HM, *Z Hautkr* (German) 53, 349
(1978): Wierzchowiecki M+, *Pol Arch Med Wewn* (Polish) 59, 197
(1978): Woosley RL+, *N Engl J Med* 298, 1157
(1978): Zeide MS+, *Clin Orthop* 134, 290
(1977): Bell WR+, *Arch Intern Med* 137, 1471
(1977): Carel RS+, *Chest* 72, 670
(1977): Healey LA, *Med Times* 105, 87
(1977): Homma M, *Nippon Rinsho* (Japanese) 35, 1330
(1977): Kahn MF+, *Sem Hôp* (French) 53, 2201
(1977): Sahenk Z+, *Ann Neurol* 1, 378
(1977): Schubothe H+, *Immun Infekt* 5, (German) 142
(1977): Schubothe H+, *Verh Dtsch Ges Inn Med* (German) 83, 727
(1977): Warner WA, *Ariz Med* 34, 172
(1977): Weiss RB, *W V Med J* 73, 101
(1976): Cohmen G, *Med Klin* (German) 71, 789
(1976): Demay-Wechsler P, *Rev Stomatol Chir Maxillofac* (French) 77, 727
(1976): Levo Y+, *Ann Rheum Dis* 35, 181
(1976): No Author, *Johns Hopkins Med J* 138, 289
(1976): Utsinger PD+, *Ann Intern Med* 84, 293

(1976): Whittle TS+, *Arch Pathol Lab Med* 100, 469
(1975): Dubois EL, *J Rheumatol* 2, 204
(1975): Falko JM+, *Ann Intern Med* 83, 832
(1975): Ghose MK, *Am J Med* 58, 581
(1975): Henningsen NC+, *Acta Med Scand* 198, 475 (>5%)
(1975): Lee SL+, *Semin Arthritis Rheum* 5, 83
(1975): Novack MA+, *JAMA* 232, 1269
(1975): Sunder SK+, *Am J Cardiol* 36, 960
(1974): Artinian B+, *Can Med Assoc J* 110, 314
(1974): Bareis RJ, *S D J Med* 27, 19
(1974): Frislid K+, *Tidsskr Nor Laegeforen* (Norwegian) 94, 1926
(1974): Harpey JP, *Ann Allergy* 33, 256
(1974): McEwen J, *Lancet* 2, 1570
(1974): No Author, *Med Lett Drugs Ther* 16, 34
(1974): No Author, *Va Med Mon* 101, 299
(1974): Winfield JB+, *Arthritis Rheum* 17, 325
(1974): Winfield JB+, *Arthritis Rheum* 17, 97
(1973): Auerbach RC+, *Radiology* 109, 287
(1973): Blomgren SE+, *Semin Hematol* 10, 345
(1973): Durand JP+, *Can Med* (French) 14, 9
(1973): Kosowski BD+, *Circulation* 47, 1204 (>5%)
(1973): Manigand G+, *Sem Hop* (French) 49, 3207
(1973): Rosenberg DS+, *South Med J* 66, 1294
(1973): Sokol SA, *J Maine Med Assoc* 64, 54
(1973): Swarbrick ET+, *Rheumatol Phys Med* 12, 94
(1972): Anastassiades TP+, *Can Med Assoc J* 107, 312
(1972): Blomgren SE+, *Am J Med* 52, 338
(1972): Donlan CJ+, *Chest* 61, 685
(1972): Dorfmann H+, *Nouv Presse Med* (French) 1, 2967
(1972): Hope RR+, *Med J Aust* 2, 298 (>5%)
(1972): Rasmussen K, *Tidsskr Nor Laegeforen* (Norwegian) 92, 709
(1972): Swarbrick ET+, *Br Heart J* 34, 284
(1971): Dabrowska B+, *Kardiol Pol* (Polish) 14, 316
(1971): Maxon HR+, *Mil Med* 136, 617
(1971): Sawaya J, *J Med Liban* (French) 24, 59
(1971): Wehr KL+, *N C Med J* 32, 56
(1970): Baker H+, *Br J Dermatol* 82, 320
(1970): Heymans G+, *Acta Cardiol* (French) 25, 404
(1970): Hopkins BE, *Med J Aust* 2, 734
(1970): Merwe JP van de, *Ned Tijdschr Geneeskd* (Dutch) 114, 105
(1970): Sheldon PJ+, *Ann Rheum Dis* 29, 236
(1970): Waagstein F, *Nord Med* (Swedish) 83, 468
(1970): Whittingham S+, *Australas Ann Med* 19, 358
(1969): Alarcon-Segovia D, *Mayo Clin Proc* 44, 664
(1969): Atkins CJ+, *Proc R Soc Med* 62, 197
(1969): Byrd RB+, *Dis Chest* 55, 170
(1969): Dubois EL, *Medicine* (Baltimore) 48, 217
(1969): Fellner MJ+, *Arch Belg Dermatol Syphiligr* (French) 25, 417
(1969): Gunther R+, *Dtsch Med Wochenschr* (German) 94, 2338
(1969): No Author, *JAMA* 208, 525
(1969): Russel AS+, *Ann Rheum Dis* 28, 328
(1968): Cohen AI+, *Ariz Med* 25, 565
(1968): Hunt WH, *Tex Med* 64, 54
(1968): Lappat EJ+, *Am J Med* 45, 846
(1968): Mehta BR, *Hawaii Med J* 28, 120
(1968): Petersen BN+, *Ugeskr Laeger* (Danish) 130, 2131
(1968): Puech P+, *Arch Mal Coeur Vaiss* (French) 61, 1550
(1968): Rutherford BD, *N Z Med J* 68, 235
(1967): Compton-Smith RN+, *Br J Clin Pract* 21, 248
(1967): Fakhro AM+, *Am J Cardiol* 20, 367 (>5%)
(1967): McDevitt DG+, *BMJ* 3, 780
(1967): Sanford HS+, *Dis Chest* 51, 172
(1966): Alarcon-Segovia D, *Rev Invest Clin* (Spanish) 18, 445
(1966): London BL+, *Am Heart J* 72, 806
(1966): Oster ZH, *Isr J Med Sci* 2, 354
(1966): Prockop LD, *Arch Neuron* 14, 326
(1965): Carabia AG+, *J Tenn Med Assoc* 58, 287
(1965): Paine R, *JAMA* 194, 23
(1962): Ladd AT, *N Engl J Med* 267, 1357

Pruritus (<1%)
Purpura
(1984): Christensen DJ+, *Ann Intern Med* 100, 918
(1976): Bluming AZ+, *JAMA* 236, 2521
(1966): Stoffer RP, *J Kans Med Soc* 67, 20
Rash (sic) (<1%)
Sjøgren's syndrome
(1968): Taylor JA, *Lancet* 1, 978
Urticaria (1–5%)
(1988): Knox JP+, *Cutis* 42, 469
Vasculitis
(1988): Knox JP+, *Cutis* 42, 469
(1984): Ekenstam E+, *Arch Dermatol* 120, 484
(1968): Dolan DL, *Mo Med* 65, 365
(1967): Rosin JM, *Am J Med* 42, 625

### Other

Dysgeusia (3–4%) (bitter taste)
(2000): Zervakis J+, *Physiol Behav* 68, 405
Myalgia (<1%)
Myopathy (<1%)
(1986): Lewis CA+, *BMJ* 292, 593
(1968): Taylor JA, *Lancet* 1, 978
Oral mucosal eruption
(1985): Gorsulowsky DC+, *J Am Acad Dermatol* 12, 245 (2%)
Tremors (<1%)

## PROCARBAZINE

**Trade name:** Matulane (Sigma-Tau)
**Other common trade name:** *Natulan*
**Indications:** Hodgkin's disease, lymphomas
**Category:** Antineoplastic
**Half-life:** 60 minutes
**Clinically important, potentially hazardous interactions with:** aldesleukin, methotrexate

### *Reactions*

### Skin

Allergic reactions (sic) (<1%)
Angioedema
(1976): Glovsky MM+, *J Allergy Clin Immunol* 57, 134
Dermatitis (sic) (<1%)
Diaphoresis
Edema
Exanthems
(1980): Andersen E+, *Scand J Haematol* 24, 149 (9%)
(1972): Jones SE+, *Cancer* 29, 498
(1966): Witte S+, *Schweiz Med Wochenschr* (German) 96, 93 (2%)
(1965): Brunner KW+, *Ann Intern Med* 63, 69 (4%)
(1965): Todd IDH, *BMJ* 1, 628
Exfoliative dermatitis
(1976): Glovsky MM+, *J Allergy Clin Immunol* 57, 134
Fixed eruption
(1988): Giguere JK+, *Med Pediatr Oncol* 16, 378
Flu-like syndrome (sic) (<1%)
Flushing
(1966): Witte S+, *Schweiz Med Wochenschr* (German) 96, 93
(1965): Todd IDH, *BMJ* 1, 628
Herpes zoster
Petechiae

Photosensitivity
Pigmentation (1–10%)
Pruritus (<1%)
(1965): Brunner KW+, *Ann Intern Med* 63, 69
Purpura
Rash (sic)
Toxic epidermal necrolysis
(1980): Andersen E+, *Scand J Haematol* 24, 149
(1969): Guerrin J+, *Rev Med Dijon* (French) 4, 523
Urticaria
(1980): Andersen E+, *Scand J Haematol* 24, 149 (9%)
(1976): Glovsky MM+, *J Allergy Clin Immunol* 57, 134
(1972): Jones SE+, *Cancer* 29, 498

### Hair

Hair – alopecia (1–10%)
(1970): Stolinsky DC+, *Cancer* 26, 984
(1965): Todd IDH, *BMJ* 1, 628

### Other

Disulfiram-like reaction** (<1%)
Gynecomastia
Hypersensitivity (2%)
(1972): Jones SE+, *Cancer* 29, 498
Myalgia (<1%)
Oral mucosal lesions
(1983): Bronner AK+, *J Am Acad Dermatol* 9, 645 (1–5%)
(1970): Stolinsky DC+, *Cancer* 26, 984
Paresthesias (>10%)
Stomatitis (>10%)
Xerostomia

***Note:** Disulfiram-like reactions include headache, respiratory difficulties, nausea, vomiting, sweating, thirst, hypotension, and flushing

## PROCHLORPERAZINE

**Trade name:** Compazine (GSK)
**Other common trade names:** *Edisylate; Novamin; Novomit; Pasotomin; Prorazin; Stella; Stemetil; Tementil; Vertigon*
**Indications:** Psychotic disorders
**Category:** Phenothiazine antipsychotic and antiemetic
**Half-life:** 23 hours
**Clinically important, potentially hazardous interactions with:** antihistamines, arsenic, chlorpheniramine, dofetilide, piperazine, quinolones, sparfloxacin

#### *Reactions*

### Skin

Diaphoresis
Eczema (sic)
Erythema
Exanthems
(1959): Wright W, *JAMA* 171, 1642
Exfoliative dermatitis
Fixed eruption (<1%)
(1984): Reilly GD+, *Acta Derm Venereol* (Stockh) 64, 270
Hypohidrosis (>10%)
Lupus erythematosus
Peripheral edema
Photosensitivity (1–10%)
(1997): O'Reilly FM+, American Academy of Dermatology Meeting, Poster #14
(1988): Rasmussen HB+, *Ugeskr Laeger* (Danish) 150, 930
(1964): Hartman DL+, *Skin* 3, 198
Phototoxicity
Pigmentation (<1%) (blue-gray)
Pruritus (1–10%)
Purpura
(1965): Horowitz HI+, *Semin Hematol* 2, 287
Rash (sic) (1–10%)
Seborrhea
Toxic epidermal necrolysis
(1986): Mérot Y+, *Arch Dermatol* 122, 455
(1975): Benini G+, *Minerva Anestesiol* (Italian) 41, 314
Urticaria
Xerosis

### Other

Anaphylactoid reactions (1–10%)
Blue tongue (sic)
(1989): Alroe C+, *Med J Aust* 150, 724
Galactorrhea (<1%)
Gynecomastia (1–10%)
Lip ulceration
(1984): Reilly GD+, *Acta Derm Venereol* (Stockh) 64, 270
Mastodynia
Parkinsonism
Priapism (<1%)
Sialorrhea
Tremors
Xerostomia (>10%)

## PROCYCLIDINE

**Trade name:** Kemadrin (GSK)
**Other common trade names:** *Apricolin; Kemadren; Onservan; Procyclid*
**Indications:** Parkinsonism
**Category:** Anticholinergic; antidyskinetic; antiparkinsonian
**Duration of action:** 4 hours
**Clinically important, potentially hazardous interactions with:** anticholinergics, arbutamine

#### *Reactions*

### Skin

Hypohidrosis (>10%)
Photosensitivity (1–10%)
Rash (sic) (<1%)
Urticaria
Xerosis (>10%)

### Other

Xerostomia (>10%)

# PROGESTINS

**Generic names:**
**Hydroxyprogesterone**
Trade names: Delta-Lutin; Duralutin; Hylutin; Pro-Depo; Prodrox
**Medroxyprogesterone**
Trade names: Amen; Curretab; Cycrin; Provera
**Megestrol**
Trade name: Megace
**Norethindrone**
Trade names: Aygestin; Micronor; Norlutin; Norlutate; Nor-QD
**Norgestrol**
Trade name: Ovrette
**Progesterone**
Trade names: Gesterol 50; Progestaject (Various pharmaceutical companies.)

**Category:** Progestin; antineoplastic; contraceptive (systemic)
**Clinically important, potentially hazardous interactions with:** acitretin, dofetilide

### *Reactions*

## Skin

Acne
(1995): Freeman EW+, *JAMA* 274, 51
Acute generalized exanthematous pustulosis (AGEP)
(1998): Kuno Y+, *Acta Derm Venereol* 78, 383
Angioedema
Ankle edema
Autoimmune dermatitis
(1991): Freychet F+, *Ann Dermatol Venereol* (French) 118, 551
(1990): Teelucksingh S+, *J Intern Med* 227, 143
(1985): Katayama I+, *Br J Dermatol* 112, 487
(1984): Anderson RH, *Cutis* 33, 490
(1978): Linse R+, *Dermatol Monatsschr* (German) 164, 656
(1974): Hipkin LJ, *BMJ* 3, 575
(1971): Farah FS+, *J Allergy Clin Immunol* 48, 257 (urticarial)
(1967): Tromovitch TA+, *Calif Med* 106, 211 (urticarial)
Autoimmune progesterone dermatitis
(1997): Shahar E+, *Int J Dermatol* 36, 708
Dermatitis (sic)
(2001): Izu K+, *J UOEH* 23(4), 431
(1974): Hipkin LJ, *BMJ* 3, 575
(1964): Shelley WB+, *JAMA* 190, 35
Diaphoresis
(1990): Willemse PHB+, *Eur J Cancer* 26, 337 (31%)
Edema
Erythema multiforme
(1985): Wojnarowska F+, *J R Soc Med* 78, 407
Erythema nodosum
Exanthems
Flushing
(1990): Willemse PHB+, *Eur J Cancer* 26, 337 (12%)
Hemorrhagic eruption (sic)
Melasma
Pruritus
Rash (sic)
Telangiectases
(1970): Aram H+, *Acta Derm Venereol* 50, 302
Urticaria
(1995): Shelley WB+, *Cutis* 55, 282 (observation)
(1994): Shelley WB+, *Cutis* 55, 21 (observation)
(1994): Yee KC+, *Br J Dermatol* 130, 121

## Hair

Hair – alopecia
Hair – hirsutism

## Other

Anaphylactoid reactions
Galactorrhea
Gynecomastia (painful)

# PROMAZINE

**Trade name:** Sparine (Wyeth-Ayerst)
**Other common trade names:** *Liranol; Prazine; Protactyl; Savamine; Talofen*
**Indications:** Psychotic disorders, schizophrenia
**Category:** Phenothiazine antipsychotic; antiemetic
**Half-life:** 24 hours
**Clinically important, potentially hazardous interactions with:** sparfloxacin

### *Reactions*

## Skin

Dermatitis (sic)
Edema
Exanthems
(1974): Rothstein E, *N Engl J Med* 290, 521
Hypohidrosis (>10%)
Photoreactions
Photosensitivity (1–10%)
(1964): Hartman DL+, *Skin* 3, 198
Phototoxicity
(1985): Chignell CF+, *Environ Health Perspect* 64, 103
(1985): Motten AG+, *Photochem Photobiol* 42, 9
Pigmentation (<1%) (slate-gray)
Purpura
Rash (sic) (1–10%)
Urticaria
Xerosis

## Other

Galactorrhea (<1%)
Gynecomastia
Mastodynia (1–10%)
Parkinsonism
Priapism (<1%)
Xerostomia

# PROMETHAZINE

**Trade names:** Anergan (Forest); Phenazine; Phenergan (Wyeth-Ayerst)
**Other common trade names:** *Atosil; Bonnox; Closin; Goodnight; Histantil; Pentazine; Prometh-50; Prothiazine; Pyrethia*
**Indications:** Allergic rhinitis, urticaria
**Category:** Phenothiazine $H_1$-receptor antihistamine and antiemetic; antivertigo and sedative-hypnotic
**Half-life:** 10–14 hours
**Clinically important, potentially hazardous interactions with:** antihistamines, arsenic, chlorpheniramine, dofetilide, piperazine, quinolones, sparfloxacin

### *Reactions*

#### Skin

Allergic reactions (sic) (<1%)
Angioedema (<1%)
Bullous eruption (<1%)
Chills
Contact dermatitis
(1997): Varela P, Porto, Portugal (from Internet) (observation)
(1970): Pirila V, *Allerg Asthma Leipz* (German) 16, 15 (endogenic)
(1968): Periss Z, *Lijec Vjesn* (Serbo-Croat) 90, 15
(1955): Sidi I+, *J Invest Dermatol* 24, 345
Dermatitis (sic)
Diaphoresis
Eczematous eruption (sic)
(1955): Sidi E+, *J Invest Dermatol* 24, 345
Erythema multiforme
(1986): Dikland WJ+, *Pediatr Dermatol* 3, 135
(1986): Fisher AA, *Cutis* 37, 158
Exanthems
(1967): Lockey SD, *Med Sci* 18, 43
Fixed eruption
(1984): Chan HL, *Int J Dermatol* 23, 607
Flushing
Jaundice
Lupus erythematosus
(1971): Fabius AJM+, *Acta Rheumatol Scand* 17, 137
(1965): Grupper C+, *Bull Soc Fr Dermatol Syphiligr* (French) 72, 714
Photoreactions
Photosensitivity (<1%)
(1997): Varela P, Porto, Portugal (from Internet) (observation)
(1991): Bergner T+, *J Allergy Clin Immunol* 87, 278
(1988): Menz J+, *J Am Acad Dermatol* 18, 1044
(1982): Rosen K+, *Acta Derm Venereol* 62, 246
(1982): Torinuki W+, *Tohoku J Exp Med* 138, 223
(1974): Tay C, *Asian J Med* 10, 223
(1970): Leong YO, *Acta Rheumatol Scand* 17, 137
(1969): Kalivas J, *JAMA* 209, 1706
(1967): Lockey SD, *Med Sci* 18, 43
(1964): Hartman DL+, *Skin* 3, 198
(1961): Stevanovic DV, *Br J Dermatol* 73, 233
(1960): Newell RGD, *BMJ* 2, 359
(1957): Epstein S+, *J Invest Dermatol* 29, 319
Pigmentation
Purpura
(1967): Lockey SD, *Med Sci* 18, 43
(1965): Horowitz HI+, *Semin Hematol* 2, 287
Rash (sic) (<1%)
(1991): Blanc VF+, *Can J Anaesth* 38, 54
Stevens–Johnson syndrome
(1972): Monnat A, *Schweiz Med Wochenschr* (German) 102, 1876
Systemic eczematous contact dermatitis
Toxic epidermal necrolysis (<1%)
(1972): Monnat A, *Schweiz Med Wochenschr* (German) 102, 1876
(1959): Messaritakis J, *Ann Paediatr* (German) 207, 236
Urticaria
(1994): Myers P+, *Arch Ophthalmol* 112, 734
(1988): Mills PJ, *Anaesthesia* 43, 66 (with temazepam)
(1967): Lockey SD, *Med Sci* 18, 43

#### Other

Anaphylactoid reactions
(1988): Mills PJ, *Anaesthesia* 43, 66 (with temazepam)
Embolia cutis medicamentosa (Nicolau syndrome)
(1995): Faucher L+, *Pediatr Dermatol* 12, 187
Galactorrhea
Gynecomastia
Hypersensitivity
(1996): Palop V+, *Aten Primaria* (Spanish) 18, 47
Injection-site reactions
Mastodynia
Myalgia (<1%)
Oral ulceration
(1967): Mackie BS, *Br J Dermatol* 79, 106
Paresthesias (<1%)
Parkinsonism
Priapism
Tinnitus
Xerostomia (1–10%)
(1991): Blanc VF+, *Can J Anaesth* 38, 54

# PROPAFENONE

**Trade name:** Rythmol (Abbott)
**Other common trade names:** *Arythmol; Norfenon; Normorytmin; Rythmex; Rytmonorm*
**Indications:** Ventricular arrhythmias
**Category:** Antiarrhythmic class I C
**Half-life:** 10–32 hours
**Clinically important, potentially hazardous interactions with:** digoxin, ritonavir

### *Reactions*

#### Skin

Acne (1%)
Diaphoresis (1%)
Edema (<1%)
Exanthems
(1975): Harron DWG+, *Drugs* 34, 617
Flushing (<1%)
Lupus erythematosus (<1%)
(1986): Guindo J+, *Ann Intern Med* 104, 589
(1975): Harron DWG+, *Drugs* 34, 617
Pruritus (<1%)
Purpura (<1%)
Rash (sic) (1–3%)
Urticaria

#### Hair

Hair – alopecia (<1%)

#### Other

Dysgeusia (3–23%)
(2000): Zervakis J+, *Physiol Behav* 68, 405
Oral mucosal lesions

(1975): Harron DWG+, *Drugs* 34, 617 (>5%)
Paresthesias (<1%)
Parosmia (<1%)
Tinnitus
Tremors (<1%)
Xerostomia (2%)

# PROPANTHELINE

**Trade name:** Propantheline
**Other common trade names:** *Bropantil; Corrigast; Ercoril; Ercotina; Norproban; Propantel*
**Indications:** Peptic ulcer
**Category:** Gastrointestinal anticholinergic; antispasmodic
**Half-life:** 1.6 hours
**Clinically important, potentially hazardous interactions with:** anticholinergics, arbutamine, digoxin

### *Reactions*

## Skin

Allergic reactions (sic)
Contact dermatitis
(1996): Jansen T+, *Dtsch Med Wochenschr* (German) 121, 41
(1983): Przybilla B+, *Hautarzt* (German) 34, 459 (from antiperspirant)
(1982): Gall H+, *Derm Beruf Umwelt* (German) 30, 55 (from antiperspirant)
(1976): Agren-Jonsson S+, *Contact Dermatitis* 2, 79 (from antiperspirant)
(1975): Hannuksela M, *Contact Dermatitis* 1, 244
(1975): Osmundsen PE, *Contact Dermatitis* 1, 251
Diaphoresis (>10%)
Exanthems
Hypohidrosis
Rash (sic) (<1%)
Urticaria
Xerosis (>10%)

## Other

Ageusia
Anaphylactoid reactions
Dysgeusia
Sialopenia
Xerostomia (>10%)

# PROPOFOL

**Trade name:** Diprivan (AstraZeneca)
**Indications:** Induction and maintenance of anesthesia
**Category:** General anesthetic; sedative
**Half-life:** initial: 40 minutes; terminal: 3 days

### *Reactions*

## Skin

Allergic reactions (sic)
(1988): Jamieson V+, *Anaesthesia* 43, 70
Edema (<1%)
Exanthems
(1987): Boittiaux P+, *Ann Fr Anesth Reanim* (French) 6, 324 (6.6%)
(1987): Coursange F+, *Ann Fr Anesth Reanim* (French) 6, 258 (6.6%)
Fixed eruption (1%)
Flushing (>1%)
Pruritus (>1%)
(1987): Coursange F+, *Ann Fr Anesth Reanim* (French) 6, 258
Rash (sic) (5%)
Raynaud's phenomenon
(1999): Gilston A, *Anaesthesia* 54, 307
Urticaria
(1988): Aitken HA, *Anaesthesia* 43, 170
(1987): Coursange F+, *Ann Fr Anesth Reanim* (French) 6, 258

## Hair

Hair – color change (sic)
(1994): Motsch J+, *Eur J Anaesthesiol* 11, 499 (passim)
(1992): Bublin JG+, *J Clin Pharm Ther* 17, 297

## Other

Anaphylactoid reactions (1–10%)
(2001): Girgis Y, *Anaesthesia* 56(10), 1016
(2001): Knoarzewski W+, *Anaesthesia* 56(5), 497 (fatal) (with fentanyl)
(2001): Lewis S+, *Anaesthesia* 56(11), 1128
(2001): Tsai MH+, *J Formos Med Assoc* 100(6), 424
(2000): Ducart AR+, *J Cardiothorac Vasc Anesth* 14(2), 200
Cough
(2001): Aly EE, *Anaesthesia* 56(10), 1016
Death
(2001): Girgis Y, *Anaesthesia* 56(10), 1016
Dysgeusia (<1%)
Injection-site erythema (<1%)
Injection-site pain (>10%)
(2001): Gupta S+, *Anaesthesia* 56(10), 1016
(2001): Larsen B+, *Anaesthesist* 50(11), 842
(2001): Larsen R+, *Anaesthesist* 50(9), 676
(2001): Liljeroth E+, *Acta Anaesthesiol Scand* 45(7), 839
(2001): Tsubokura H+, *Masui* 50(11), 1196
(2000): Levecque JP+, *Can J Anaesth* (French) 47, 291
(2000): Picard P+, *Anesth Analg* 90, 963
(2000): Pickford A+, *Pediatr Anaesth* 10, 129
(1998): Nathanson MH+, *Anaesthesia* 53, 608
(1998): Ozturk E+, *Anesthesiology* 89, 1041
(1998): Tan CH+, *Anaesthesia* 53, 468
(1988): Langley MS+, *Drugs*
Injection-site pruritus (<1%)
Myalgia (>1%)
Phlebitis
Sialorrhea (>1%)
Tinnitus
Twitching (1–10%)
Xerostomia (<1%)

# PROPOLIS

**Scientific name:** *Propolis*
**Other common names:** Bee Glue; Bee Propolis; Hive Dross; Propolis Balsam; Propolis Resin; Propolis Wax; Russian Penicillin
**Family:** None
**Purported indications:** Tuberculosis, bacterial and fungal infections, protozoal infections, nasopharyngeal carcinoma, improving immune response, duodenal ulcer
**Other uses:** *Helicobacter pylori* infection, common cold, wound cleansing, mouth rinse, genital herpes. Used as an ingredient in cosmetics

### *Reactions*

## Skin

Allergic reactions (sic)
(1988): Slezak R, *Prakt Zubn Lek* 36(7), 208
Allergy (sic)
(1996): Bellagrandi S+, *J Am Acad Dermatol* 35(4), 644 (in HIV-positive patient)
(1988): Hausen BM+, *Contact Dermatitis* 19(4), 296
(1987): Blanken R+, *Ned Tijdschr Geneeskd* 131(26), 1121
(1987): Rudzki E+, *Przegl Dermatol* 19(4), 296
Cheilitis
(1996): Bellegrandi S+, *J Am Acad Dermatol* 35, 644
Contact dermatitis
(2002): Lieberman HD+, *J Am Acad Dermatol* 46, S30
(2001): Teraki Y+, *Br J Dermatol* 144(6), 1277 (granulomatous)
(2000): Tumova L+, *Ceska Slov Farm* 49(6), 285
(1998): Burdock GA, *Food Chem Toxicol* 36(4), 347
(1998): Downs AM+, *Contact Dermatitis* 38(6), 359 (occupational)
(1998): Thomas P+, *Arch Dermatol* 134(4), 511
(1997): Silvani S+, *Contact Dermatitis* 37(1), 48 (in patients with psoriasis)
(1990): Hegyi E+, *Hautarzt* 41(12), 675 (0.64%)
(1990): Raton JA+, *Contact Dermatitis* 22(3), 183
(1988): Schuler TM+, *Hautarzt* 39(3), 139 (6 patients)
(1987): Angelini G+, *Contact Dermatitis* 17(4), 251 (in psoriasis)
(1987): Cirasino L+, *Contact Dermatitis* 16(2)
(1987): Frosch PJ, *Z Haut* 62(23), 1631
(1987): Hausen BM+, *Contact Dermatitis* 17(3), 163
(1987): Kleinhaus D, *Contact Dermatitis* 17(3), 187 (airborne)
(1987): Trevisan G+, *Contact Dermatitis* 16(1), 48
(1985): Ayala F+, *Contact Dermatitis* 12(3), 181
(1985): Machackova J, *Contact Dermatitis* 13(1), 43
(1985): Tosti A+, *Contacr Dermatitis* 12(4), 227
(1984): Bedello PG+, *G Ital Deramtol Venereol* 119(6), 431
(1984): Pincelli C+, *Contact Dermatitis* 11(1), 49
(1983): Kokelj F+, *Contact Dermatitis* 9(6), 518
(1983): Melli MC+, *Contact Dermatitis* 9(5), 427 (in a bee-keeper)
(1983): Monti M+, *Contact Dermatitis* 9(2), 163 (occupational and cosmetic)
(1983): Rudzki E+, *Contact Dermatitis* 9(1), 40
(1983): Takahashi M+, *Contact Dermatitis* 9(6) (from honeybee royal jelly)
(1982): Monti M+, *G Ital Dermatol Venereol* 117(2), 119
(1982): Proserpio G, *G Ital Dermatol Venereol* 117(5), 316
(1975): Camarasa G, *Contact Dermatitis* 1(2), 124 (from beeswax)
Dermatitis (sic)
(1985): Rudzki E+, *Contact Dermatitis* 13(3), 198
(1984): Valsecchi R+, *Contact Dermatitis* 11(5), 317
Erythroderma
(2001): Horiuchi Y, *Br J Dermatol* 145, 691
Sensitivity (sic)
(1988): Nakamura T, *Contact Dermatitis* 18(5), 313
(1987): Young E, *Contact Dermatitis* 16(1), 49
(1980): Bogdaszewska-Czabanowska J+, *Przegl Dermatol* 67(6), 747
(1979): Grzywa Z+, *Przegl Dermatol* 66(6), 709

## Other

Hypersensitivity (sic)
(1987): Rudzki E+, *Pol Tyg Lek* (Polish) 42(2), 40
(1984): Tosti A+, *G Ital Dermatol Venereol* 119(5)
(1977): Peterson HO, *Contact Dermatitis* 3, 278
Mucositis
(1990): Hay KD+, *Oral Surg Oral Med Oral Pathol* 70, 584
Oral ulceration
(1990): Hay KD+, *Oral Surg Oral Med Oral Pathol* 70, 584
Stomatitis
(1996): Bellegrandi S+, *J Am Acad Dermatol* 35, 644

# PROPOXYPHENE

**Trade names:** Darvocet-N (Lilly); Darvon (Lilly); Darvon Compound (Lilly)
**Other common trade names:** *Algafan; Antalvic; Develin; Dolotard; Doloxene; Liberan; Parvon*
**Indications:** Pain
**Category:** Narcotic analgesic
**Half-life:** 8–24 hours
**Clinically important, potentially hazardous interactions with: alcohol**, alprazolam, ritonavir, warfarin

Darvocet is propoxyphene and acetaminophen; Darvon Compound is propoxyphene and aspirin

### *Reactions*

## Skin

Diaphoresis
Exanthems
(1976): Arndt KA+, *JAMA* 235, 918
Facial edema
Flushing
Pruritus
Rash (sic) (<1%)
Urticaria (<1%)

## Other

Ano-recto-vaginal ulcerations
(1984): Laplanche G+, *Ann Dermatol Venereol* (French) 111, 347 (from suppositories)
Injection-site nodules (sic)
(1987): Pedragosa R+, *Arch Dermatol* 123, 297
Injection-site pain (1–10%)
Trembling
Xerostomia (1–10%)

# PROPRANOLOL

**Trade names:** Inderal (Wyeth-Ayerst); Inderide (Wyeth-Ayerst)
**Other common trade names:** *Acifol; Apsolol; Betabloc; Cinlol; Detensol; Inderalici; Inderex; Novo-Pranol; Prosin; Sinal; Tesnol*
**Indications:** Hypertension, angina pectoris
**Category:** Beta-adrenergic blocker; antianginal; antihypertensive; antiarrhythmic class II
**Half-life:** 2–6 hours
**Clinically important, potentially hazardous interactions with:** cimetidine, clonidine, epinephrine, haloperidol, insulin, terbutaline, verapamil

Inderide is propranolol and hydrochlorothiazide

**Note:** Cutaneous side effects of beta-receptor blockaders are clinically polymorphous. They apparently appear after several months of continuous therapy. Atypical psoriasiform, lichen planus-like, and eczematous chronic rashes are mainly observed. (1983): Hödl St, *Z Hautkr* (German) 58, 17

## *Reactions*

### Skin

Acne
(1973): Almeyda J+, *Br J Dermatol* 88, 313
Angioedema
(1983): Hannaway PJ+, *N Engl J Med* 308, 1536
Bullous eruption
(1979): Faure M+, *Ann Dermatol Venereol* (French) 106, 161
Contact dermatitis
(1994): Valsecchi R+, *Contact Dermatitis* 30, 177 (occupational)
(1990): Rebandel P+, *Contact Dermatitis* 23, 199
Diaphoresis
Eczematous eruption (sic)
(1981): van Joost T+, *Arch Dermatol* 117, 600
(1979): Faure M+, *Ann Dermatol Venereol* (French) 106, 161
Edema
Erythema multiforme
(1969): Pimstone B+, *S Afr Med J* 43, 1203
Exanthems
(1976): Jensen HA+, *Acta Med Scand* 199, 363
(1974): Greenblatt DJ+, *Drugs* 7, 118. (0.8%)
(1973): Almeyda J+, *Br J Dermatol* 88, 313
(1966): Stephen SA+, *Am J Cardiol* 18, 463 (0.4%)
Exfoliative dermatitis
(1976): Jensen HA+, *Acta Med Scand* 199, 363
Flushing
(1973): Almeyda J+, *Br J Dermatol* 88, 313
(1966): Stephen SA+, *Am J Cardiol* 18, 463
Hyperkeratosis (palms and soles)
Lichenoid eruption
(1991): Massa MC+, *Cutis* 48, 41
(1980): Hawk JLM, *Clin Exp Dermatol* 5, 93
(1976): Cochran REI+, *Arch Dermatol* 112, 1173
Lupus erythematosus
(1982): Hughes GRV, *BJM* 284, 1358
(1976): Harrison T+, *Postgrad Med* 59, 241
Necrosis
Pemphigus
(1982): Ruocco V+, *Arch Dermatol Res* 274, 123
(1980): Godard W+, *Ann Dermatol Venereol* (French) 107, 1213
Peripheral edema
Peripheral skin necrosis (sic)
(1979): Gokal R+, *BMJ* 1, 721
(1979): Hoffbrand BI, *BMJ* 1, 1082
Photosensitivity
(1979): Faure M+, *Ann Dermatol Venereol* (French) 106, 161
Phototoxicity
(1992): Shelley WB+, *Cutis* 50, 182 (observation)
Pruritus
(1973): Almeyda J+, *Br J Dermatol* 88, 313
Psoriasis
(1993): Halevy S+, *J Am Acad Dermatol* 29, 504
(1992): Raychaudhuri SP+, *J Am Acad Dermatol* 27, 787
(1990): Halevy S+, *Arch Dermatol Res* 283, 472
(1988): Heng MCY+, *Int J Dermatol* 27, 619
(1987): Altomare GF+, *G Ital Dermatol Venereol* (Italian) 122, 531
(1987): Savola J+, *BMJ* 295, 637
(1986): Abel EA+, *J Am Acad Dermatol* 15, 1007
(1986): Czernielewski J, *Lancet* 1, 808 (exacerbation)
(1984): Arntzen K+, *Acta Derm Venereol* (Stockh) 64, 346
(1983): Kaur S+, *Indian Heart J* 35, 181
(1979): Faure M+, *Ann Dermatol Venereol* (French) 106, 161
(1979): Halevy S+, *Cutis* 24, 95
(1976): Enger E, *Tidsskr Nor Laegeforen* (Norwegian) 96, 1103
(1976): Jensen HA+, *Acta Med Scand* 199, 363
(1976): Wadskov S+, *Ugeskr Laeger* (Danish) 138, 784
(1975): Padfield PL+, *BMJ* 1, 626
Purpura
(1966): Harris A, *Am J Cardiol* 18, 431
Pustular psoriasis
(1988): Heng MCY+, *Int J Dermatol* 27, 619
(1985): Hu C-H+, *Arch Dermatol* 121, 1326
Rash (sic) (1–10%)
Raynaud's phenomenon
(1976): Marshall AJ+, *BMJ* 1, 1498 (59%)
Sclerosis
(1980): Graham JR, *Trans Am Clin Climatol Assoc* 92, 122
Stevens–Johnson syndrome
(1990): Zukervar P+, *J Toxicol Clin Exp* (French) 10, 169
(1989): Mukul+, *J Assoc Physicians India* 37, 797
Systemic erythematous eruption (sic)
(1975): Felix RH+, *BMJ* 1, 626
Toxic epidermal necrolysis
(1977): van Ketel WG+, *Ned Tijdschr Geneeskd* (Dutch) 121, 1475
Toxicoderma
(1981): Danilov LN, *Vestn Dermatol Venerol* (Russian) January 42
Urticaria
(1983): Hannaway PJ+, *N Engl J Med* 308, 1536
(1983): Oliver R, *Cent Afr J Med* 29, 91
(1975): Seides SF+, *Chest* 67, 496
Xerosis

### Hair

Hair – alopecia
(1994): Friedman M, *J Fam Pract* 39, 114
(1983): Hödl ST, *Z Hautkr* (German) 58, 17.
(1982): England JRF+, *Aust Fam Physician* 11, 225
(1979): Hilder RJ, *Cutis* 24, 63
(1977): Scribner MD, *Arch Dermatol* 113, 1303
(1973): Martin CM+, *Am Heart J* 86, 236
Hair – alopecia areata
(2001): Vinson RP, El Paso, TX (from Internet) (observation) (from a single dose)

### Nails

Nails – discoloration
(1976): Jensen HA+, *Acta Med Scand* 199, 363
Nails – onycholysis
(1983): Hödl ST, *Z Hautkr* (German) 58, 17.
Nails – pitting (psoriasiform)
(1976): Jensen HA+, *Acta Med Scand* 199, 363
Nails – thickening

(1983): Hödl ST, *Z Hautkr* (German) 58, 17.
(1979): Faure M+, *Ann Dermatol Venereol* (French) 106, 161

### Other

Anaphylactoid reactions
(1983): Hannaway PJ+, *N Engl J Med* 308, 1536
Cheilostomatitis (sic)
(1977): Tangsrud SE+, *BMJ* 2, 1385
Dupuytren's contracture
(1966): Coupland WW, *Med J Aust* 2, 137
Dysgeusia
(2000): Zervakis J+, *Physiol Behav* 68, 405
Myalgia
Myopathy
(1980): Uuisitupa M+, *BMJ* 1, 183
Oral ulceration
(1980): Hawk JLM, *Clin Exp Dermatol* 5, 93
Paresthesias
Peyronie's disease
(1981): Neumann HAM+, *Dermatologica* 162, 330
(1979): Pryor JP+, *Lancet* 1, 824
(1977): Osborne DR, *Lancet* 1, 1111
(1977): Wallis AA+, *Lancet* 2, 980
(1977): Yudkin JS, *Lancet* 2, 1355 (passim)
(1966): Coupland WW, *Med J Aust* 2, 137
Serum sickness
(1983): Yen MC+, *Postgrad Med* 74, 291
Tongue pigmentation
(1975): Raleigh F, *Drug Intell Clin Pharm* 9, 455
Xerostomia

## PROPYLTHIOURACIL

**Trade name:** Propylthiouracil (Lederle)
**Other common trade names:** *Propacil; Propycil; Propyl-Thyracil; Tiotil*
**Indications:** Hyperthyroidism
**Category:** Antithyroid
**Half-life:** 1–5 hours
**Clinically important, potentially hazardous interactions with:** anticoagulants, dicumarol, warfarin

### *Reactions*

### Skin

Acne
(1980): Vasily DB+, *JAMA* 243, 458
Angioedema
(1980): Vasily DB+, *JAMA* 243, 458
(1970): Amrhein JA+, *J Pediatr* 76, 54 (1%)
(1965): Shelley WB, *Arch Dermatol* 91, 165
Dermatitis (sic)
(1993): Elias AN+, *J Am Acad Dermatol* 29, 78
Edema (<1%)
Erythema nodosum
(1985): Keren G+, *Isr J Med Sci* 21, 62
Exanthems
(1987): Wing SS+, *Can Med Assoc J* 136, 121
(1982): Gammeltoft M+, *Acta Dermatol Venereol* (Stockh) 62, 171 (3–5%)
(1980): Vasily DB+, *JAMA* 243, 458
(1972): Wiberg JJ+, *Ann Intern Med* 77, 414
(1970): Amrhein JA+, *J Pediatr* 76, 54
Exfoliative dermatitis (<1%)
Lichenoid eruption
(1967): Coleman WP, *Med Clin North Am* 51, 1073
Lupus erythematosus (1–10%)
(1994): Sato-Matsumura KC+, *J Dermatol* 21, 501
(1992): Skaer TL, *Clin Ther* 14, 496
(1991): Alarcon-Segovia D+, *Baillieres Clin Rheumatol* 5, 1
(1989): Horton RC+, *Lancet* 2, 568
(1987): Wing SS+, *Can Med Assoc J* 136, 121 (20% ANA)
(1985): Bulvik S+, *Harefuah* (Hebrew) 109, 13
(1983): Berkman EM+, *Transfusion* 23, 135
(1981): Searles RP+, *J Rheumatol* 8, 498
(1981): Takuwa N+, *Endocrinol Jpn* 28, 663
(1973): Hung W+, *J Pediatr* 82, 852
(1970): Amrhein JA+, *J Pediatr* 76, 54
(1966): Faber V+, *Acta Med Scand* 179, 257
(1964): Best MM+, *J Ky Med Assoc* 62, 47
Photosensitivity
(1997): Ohtsuka M+, *Eur Resp J* 10, 1405
Pigmentation
Pruritus (<1%)
(1980): Vasily DB+, *JAMA* 243, 458
Purpura
(1987): Wing SS+, *Can Med Assoc J* 136, 121
(1962): Walzer RA, *Arch Dermatol* 86, 826
Pyoderma gangrenosum
(1999): Darben T+, *Australas J Dermatol* 40, 144
Rash (sic) (>10%)
Rosacea
(1980): Vasily DB+, *JAMA* 243, 458
Skin reaction (sic)
(1982): Pacini F+, *J Endocrinol Invest* 5, 403
Ulceration
(1987): Wing SS+, *Can Med Assoc J* 136, 121
Urticaria (<1%)
(1980): Vasily DB+, *JAMA* 243, 458
(1970): Amrhein JA+, *J Pediatr* 76, 54
Vasculitis (<1%)
(2000): Lopez-Marina V+, *Med Clin (Barc)* (Spanish) 114, 398
(1998): Harper L+, *Nephrol Dial Transplant* 13, 455
(1998): Merkel PA, *Curr Opin Rheumatol* 10, 45
(1998): Miller RM+, *Australas J Dermatol* 39, 96
(1997): Kitahara T+, *Clin Nephrol* 47, 336
(1997): Yarman S+, *Int J Clin Pharm Ther* 35, 282
(1993): Dolman KM+, *Lancet* 342, 651
(1992): Stankus SJ+, *Chest* 102, 1595
(1992): Wolf D+, *Cutis* 49, 253
(1987): Carrasco MD+, *Arch Intern Med* 147, 1677
(1987): Wing SS+, *Can Med Assoc J* 136, 121
(1986): Gleisner A+, *Rev Child Pediatr* (Spanish) 57, 64
(1985): Cox NH+, *Clin Exp Dermatol* 10, 292
(1982): Gammeltoft M+, *Acta Dermatol Venereol* (Stockh) 62, 171
(1982): Reidy TJ+, *South Med J* 75, 1297
(1980): Vasily DB+, *JAMA* 243, 458
(1979): Houston BD+, *Arthritis Rheum* 22, 925
(1978): Griswold WR+, *West J Med* 128, 543
(1973): Hung W+, *J Pediatr* 82, 852
(1965): McCombs RP, *JAMA* 194, 1059
(1965): Shelley WB, *Arch Dermatol* 91, 165
(1962): Walzer RA, *Arch Dermatol* 86, 826
Vesicular eruptions (in newborn)
(1980): Vasily DB+, *JAMA* 243, 458
(1977): Caplan RH+, *Wis Med J* 76, S88

### Hair

Hair – alopecia (<1%)
(1997): Ohtsuka M+, *Eur Resp J* 10, 1405
(1980): Vasily DB+, *JAMA* 243, 458
(1951): Clarke MLB, *JAMA* 147, 1711
Hair – depigmentation
(1980): Vasily DB+, *JAMA* 243, 458

### Other

Ageusia (1–10%)
Dysgeusia (1–10%) (metallic taste)
(1993): Elias AN+, *J Am Acad Dermatol* 29, 78
Hypersensitivity
(1999): Chastain MA+, *J Am Acad Dermatol* 41, 757
(1991): Fong PC+, *Horm Res* 35, 132
(1963): Walzer RA+, *JAMA* 184, 743
Myalgia
Oral mucosal lesions
(1970): Amrhein JA+, *J Pediatr* 76, 54
Oral ulceration
(1979): Houston BD+, *Arthritis Rheum* 22, 925
(1970): Amrhein JA+, *J Pediatr* 76, 54
Paresthesias (<1%)

# PROTAMINE

**Trade name:** Protamine Sulfate (Lilly)
**Indications:** Heparin overdose
**Category:** Heparin antagonist
**Duration of action:** 2 hours

## *Reactions*

### Skin

Angioedema
(1991): Roelofse JA+, *Anesth Prog* 38, 99
Exanthems
(1989): Weiss ME+, *N Engl J Med* 320, 886
Flushing (<1%)
Urticaria
(1989): Weiss ME+, *N Engl J Med* 320, 886

### Other

Anaphylactoid reactions
(1991): Roelofse JA+, *Anesth Prog* 38, 99
(1988): Oswald-Mammosser M+, *Rev Fr Allergol* (French) 28, 173
Death
(2002): Kimmel SE+, *Anesth Analg* 94(6), 1402
Hypersensitivity (<1%)

# PROTEASE INHIBITORS*

**Generic names:**
**Amprenavir**
Trade name: Agenerase
**Indinavir**
Trade name: Crixivan
**Nelfinavir**
Trade name: Viracept
**Ritonavir**
Trade name: Norvir
**Saquinavir**
Trade names: Invirase; Fortovase
**Indications:** HIV infection
**Half-life:** varies
**Clinically important, potentially hazardous interactions with:** pimozide, rifampin

## *Reactions*

### Skin

Acute generalized exanthematous pustulosis (AGEP)
(1998): Aquilina C+, *Arch Intern Med* 158, 2160
Angiolipomas
(2002): Dauden E+, *AIDS* 16(5), 805
Striae
(1999): Darvay A+, *J Am Acad Dermatol* 41, 467

### Nails

Nails – ingrown
(2000): Miot HA, Sao Paulo, Brazil (from Internet) (observation)
Nails – paronychia
(2000): Panse I+, *Br J Dermatol* 142, 496

### Other

Buffalo hump
(2000): Carr A+, *AIDS* 14, F25
(1998): De Luca A+, *Lancet* 352, 320
(1998): Dieleman JP+, *Ned Tijdschr Geneeskd* (Dutch) 142, 2856 (3 patients)
(1998): Lo JC+, *Lancet* 351, 867 (8 patients)
(1998): Saint-Marc T+, *Lancet* 352, 319
(1998): Schindler JT+, *Ann Intern Med* 129, 164
Buffalo neck
(1999): Milpied-Homsi B+, *Ann Dermatol Venereol* (French) 126, 254
Bull neck (sic)
(1998): Meinrenken S, *Dtsch Med Wochenschr* (German) 123, A9
Fat distribution abnormality
(1999): Mann M+, *Aids Patient Care* 13, 287
(1998): Ho TT+, *Lancet* 351, 1736
(1998): Mishriki YY, *Postgrad Med* 104, 45 ("bulging belly")
(1998): Wurtz R, *Lancet* 351, 1735
Hypersensitivity
(1997): Bonfanti P+, *AIDS* 11, 1301
Lipoatrophy
(2000): Carr A+, *AIDS* 14, F25
(2000): Panse I+, *Br J Dermatol* 142, 496
Lipodystrophy
(2001): Allan DA+, *Int J STD AIDS* 12(8), 532
(2001): Djokic M+, *Vojnosanit Pregl* 58(4), 433
(2000): Behrens GM+, *MMM Fortschr Med* (German) 142, 68
(2000): Hartmann M+, *Hautarzt* (German) 51, 159
(2000): Lyon DE+, *J Assoc Nurses AIDS Care* 11, 36
(2000): Panse I+, *Br J Dermatol* 142, 496
(2000): Paparizos VA+, *AIDS* 14, 903
(2000): Reus S+, *An Med Interna* (Spanish) 17, 123
(1999): Ponce-de-Leon S+, *Lancet* 353, 1244

(1999): Yanovski JA+, *J Clin Endocrinol Metab* 84, 1925
(1998): Carr A+, *AIDS* 12, F51
(1998): Carr A+, *N Engl J Med* 339, 1296
(1998): Dieleman JP+, *Ned Tijdschr Geneeskd* (Dutch) 142, 2856 (3 patients)
(1998): Fischer T+, *Dtsch Med Wochenschr* (German) 123, 1512
(1998): *Drugs and Ther Perspect* 12, 11
(1998): Lipsky J, *Lancet* 351, 847
(1998): Miller KD+, *Lancet* 351, 871 (indinavir)

**Note:** Protease inhibitors cause dyslipidemia which includes elevated triglycerides and cholesterol and redistribution of body fat centrally to produce the so-called "protease paunch," breast enlargement, facial atrophy, and "buffalo hump"

***Note:** Please see individual generic drugs for more references

# PROTRIPTYLINE

**Trade name:** Vivactil (Merck)
**Other common trade names:** *Concordin; Triptil*
**Indications:** Depression
**Category:** Tricyclic antidepressant and antinarcolepsy adjunct
**Half-life:** 54–92 hours
**Clinically important, potentially hazardous interactions with:** amprenavir, arbutamine, clonidine, epinephrine, formoterol, guanethidine, isocarboxazid, linezolid, MAO inhibitors, phenelzine, quinolones, sparfloxacin, tranylcypromine

### *Reactions*

## Skin

Acne
Allergic reactions (sic) (<1%)
Angioedema
Dermatitis (sic) (3%)
(1967): Gilbert MM, *Int J Neuropsychiatry* 3, 36
Diaphoresis (1–10%)
Edema
Erythema
Exanthems
Flushing
Petechiae
Photosensitivity (<1%)
(1972): Bruinsma W, *Dermatologica* 145, 377
Phototoxicity
(1980): Kochevar IE, *Toxicol App Pharmacol* 54, 258
Pruritus (1–5%)
(1967): Gilbert MM, *Int J Neuropsychiatry* 3, 36
Purpura
Rash (sic)
Urticaria
Vasculitis
Xerosis

## Hair

Hair – alopecia (<1%)

## Other

Black tongue
Death
Dysgeusia (>10%)
Galactorrhea (<1%)
Glossitis
Gynecomastia (<1%)
Oral mucosal eruption
Paresthesias
Parkinsonism (1–10%)
Rhabdomyolysis
(1974): Greenblatt DJ+, *JAMA* 229(5), 556 (overdose) (fatal)
Stomatitis
Tinnitus
Tremors
Xerostomia (>10%)

# PSEUDOEPHEDRINE

**Trade names:** Actifed; Afrinol; Allerid; Cenafed; Decofed; Drixoral; Entex; Novafed; Seldane-D; Sudafed; Trinalin
**Other common trade names:** *Balminil; Eltor 120; Maxiphed; Robidrine*
**Indications:** Nasal congestion
**Category:** Nasal decongestant; sympathomimetic; adrenergic agonist
**Half-life:** 9–16 hours
**Clinically important, potentially hazardous interactions with:** bromocriptine, fluoxetine, fluvoxamine, furazolidone, MAO inhibitors, paroxetine, phenelzine, sertraline, tranylcypromine

### *Reactions*

## Skin

Angioedema
(1997): Rademaker M, Hamilton, New Zealand (3 personal cases) (observation)
(1993): Cavanah DK+, *Ann Intern Med* 119, 302
Baboon syndrome
(2000): Sanchez TS+, *Contact Dermatitis* 42, 312
Contact dermatitis
(1998): Downs AM+, *Contact Dermatitis* 39, 33
Dermatitis (sic)
(1998): Vega F+, *Allergy* 53, 218
Diaphoresis (1–10%)
Eczematous eruption (sic)
(1991): Tomb RR+, *Contact Dermatitis* 24, 86
Exanthems
(1995): Rochina A+, *J Invest Allergol Clin Immunol* 5, 235
(1994): Shelley WB+, *Cutis* 52, 203 (observation)
(1993): Cavanah DK+, *Ann Intern Med* 119, 302 (generalized)
(1978): Frankland AW, *Practitioner* 211, 828
Exfoliative dermatitis
(1993): Cavanah DK+, *Ann Intern Med* 119, 302
Fixed eruption
(2001): Cowen E, *Dermatology Online Journal* 7, 23C
(2001): Cowen E, *Dermatology Online Journal* 7, 24C (disseminated bullous)
(1998): Anibarro B+, *Allergy* 53, 902
(1998): Hindioglu U+, *J Am Acad Dermatol* 38, 499 (non-pigmenting solitary)
(1998): Litt JZ, Beachwood, OH (personal case) (observation)
(1998): Vidal C+, *Ann Allergy Asthma Immunol* 80, 309 (non-pigmenting)
(1997): Garcia Ortiz JC+, *Allergy* 52, 229 (non-pigmenting)
(1996): Alanko K+, *J Am Acad Dermatol* 35, 647
(1996): Quan MB+, *Int J Dermatol* 35, 367 (non-pigmenting)
(1994): Hauken M, *Ann Intern Med* 120, 442
(1994): Krivda SJ+, *J Am Acad Dermatol* 31, 291 (non-pigmenting)
(1994): Shelley WB+, *Cutis* 53, 116 (observation)
(1994): Shelley WB+, *Cutis* 54, 240 (observation)
(1988): Camisa C, *Cutis* 41, 339

(1987): Shelley WB+, *J Am Acad Dermatol* 17, 403 (non-pigmenting)
(1968): Brownstein MH, *Arch Dermatol* 97, 115

Pallor

Pseudo-scarlatina (sic)
(1988): Taylor BJ+, *Br J Dermatol* 118, 827

Systemic contact dermatitis
(1991): Tomb RR+, *Contact Dermatitis* 24, 86

Toxic erythema
(1999): Oakley A, (from Internet) (2 observations)

Toxic shock syndrome
(1994): Shelley WB+, *Cutis* 52, 203 (observation)
(1993): Cavanah DK+, *Ann Intern Med* 119, 302

Urticaria
(1997): Rademaker M, Hamilton, New Zealand (3 personal cases) (observation)
(1994): Shelley WB+, *Cutis* 54, 375 (observation)

### Other

Tinnitus
Trembling
Tremors
Xerostomia

## PSORALENS

**Trade names:** 8-MOP (ICN); Oxsoralen (ICN); Trisoralen (ICN)
**Indications:** Vitiligo
**Category:** Repigmenting agents
**Half-life:** 2 hours

### *Reactions*

### Skin

Acne
(1978): Nielsen EB+, *Acta Derm Venereol* (Stockh) 58, 374

Basal cell carcinoma
(2002): Katz KA+, *J Invest Dermatol* 118(6), 1038
(1999): Hannuksela-Svahn A+, *J Am Acad Dermatol* 40, 694

Blistering (sic)
(1993): Sheehan MP+, *Br J Dermatol* 129, 431 (PUVA)
(1991): No Author, *Ned Tijdschr Geneeskd* (Dutch) 135, 1764

Bowen's disease
(1979): Hofmann C+, *Br J Dermatol* 101, 685

Bullous pemphigoid (with UVA)
(1996): George PM, *Photodermatol Photoimmunol Photomed* 11, 185
(1996): Perl S+, *Dermatology* 193, 245
(1994): Fryer EJ+, *J Am Acad Dermatol* 30, 651 (passim)
(1989): Weber PJ+, *Arch Dermatol* 125, 690
(1985): Grunwald MH+, *J Am Acad Dermatol* 13, 224
(1982): Stüttgen G, *Int J Dermatol* 21, 198
(1979): Abel EA+, *Arch Dermatol* 115, 988
(1978): Robinson JK, *Br J Dermatol* 99, 709
(1977): Melski JW+, *J Invest Dermatol* 68, 328
(1976): Thomsen K+, *Br J Dermatol* 95, 568

Burning (1–10%)
(1996): Nettelblad H+, *Burns* 22, 633
(1982): Stüttgen G, *Int J Dermatol* 21, 198 (passim)

Burns
(2000): Al-Qattan MM, *Burns* 26 (children)

Cheilitis (1–10%)

Contact dermatitis
(1994): Korffmacher H+, *Contact Dermatitis* 30, 283
(1991): Takashima A+, *Br J Dermatol* 124, 37
(1990): Fleming D+, *Allergy Proc* 11, 125
(1990): Moller H, *Photodermatol Photoimmunol Photomed* 7, 43
(1979): Saihan EM, *BMJ* 2, 20

Eczematous eruption (sic)
(1994): Korffmacher H+, *Contact Dermatitis* 30, 283
(1979): Saihan EM, *BMJ* 2, 20

Edema (1–10%)

Erythema
(2000): Yeo UC+, *Br J Dermatol* 142, 733

Folliculitis

Freckles (1–10%)
(1993): Sheehan MP+, *Br J Dermatol* 129, 431 (PUVA)
(1984): Kietzmann E+, *Dermatologica* 168, 306
(1983): Kanerva L+, *Dermatologica* 166, 281
(1983): Kietzmann H+, *Ann Dermatol Venereol* (French) 110, 63
(1978): Bleehen SS, *Br J Dermatol* 99, 20

Granuloma annulare
(1979): Dorval JC+, *Ann Dermatol Venereol* (French) 106, 79

Herpes simplex
(1993): Sheehan MP+, *Br J Dermatol* 129, 431 (PUVA)
(1982): Stüttgen G, *Int J Dermatol* 21, 198

Herpes zoster
(1982): Stüttgen G, *Int J Dermatol* 21, 198
(1977): Roenigk HH+, *Arch Dermatol* 113, 1667

Hypopigmentation (1–10%)

Keratoacanthoma
(1979): Hofmann C+, *Br J Dermatol* 101, 685

Lichen planus
(1980): Dupre A+, *Ann Dermatol Venereol* (French) 107, 557

Lupus erythematosus
(1991): Lehmann P, *J Am Acad Dermatol* 24, 515 (discoid)
(1985): Bruze M+, *Acta Derm Venereol* (Stockh) 65, 31
(1979): Domke HF+, *Arch Dermatol* 115, 642
(1979): Eyanson S+, *Arch Dermatol* 115, 54 (systemic)
(1978): Millns J+, *Arch Dermatol* 114, 1177

Melanoma
(1999): Lindelof B, *Drug Saf* 20, 289
(1994): Reseghetti A+, *Dermatology* 189, 75
(1980): Forrest JB+, *J Surg Oncol* 13, 337

Miliaria

Pemphigoid
(1980): Lutowiecka-Wranicz A+, *Przegl Dermatol* (Polish) 67, 641

Pemphigus vulgaris
(1994): Fryer EJ+, *J Am Acad Dermatol* 30, 651

Photocontact dermatitis
(1998): Clark SM+, *Contact Dermatitis* 38, 289
(1991): Takashima A+, *Br J Dermatol* 124, 37
(1990): Moller H, *Photodermatol Photoimmunol Photomed* 7, 43
(1982): Kavli G+, *Acta Derm Venereol* 62, 435
(1982): Weiss W+, *Dermatol Monatsschr* (German) 168, 116
(1981): Bleehen SS, *Br J Dermatol* 105, 23

Photoreactions
(1978): Plewig G+, *Arch Dermatol Res* 261, 201

Photosensitivity
(2001): Tanew A+, *J Am Acad Dermatol* 44, 638
(1986): Jeanmougin M, *Biochimie* (French) 68, 891
(1986): Lerman S, *Ophthalmology* 93, 304
(1986): Morliere P, *Biochimie* (French) 68, 849
(1982): Haudenschild-Falb E+, *Ther Umsch* (German) 39, 178
(1980): Dupre A+, *Ann Dermatol Venereol* (French) 107, 557
(1980): Heidbreder G, *Z Hautkr* (German) 55, 84

Phototoxicity
(2001): Snellman E+, *Br J Dermatol* 144, 490
(2001): Voss A+, *Arch Dermatol* 137, 383 (fatal)
(1997): Morison WL, *Arch Dermatol* 133, 1609
(1997): Morison WL+, *J Am Acad Dermatol* 36, 183
(1997): Neumann NJ+, *Acta Derm Venereol* 77, 385
(1990): Ljunggren B, *Arch Dermatol* 126, 1334

(1989): Morison WL, *Arch Dermatol* 125, 433 (topical)
(1986): Lowe NJ, *Br J Dermatol* 115, 86
(1986): Toback AC+, *Dermatol Clin* 4, 223
(1983): Kavli G+, *Contact Dermatitis* 9, 257
(1980): Barth J+, *Z Arztl Fortbild Jena* (German) 74, 789
(1980): Kornhauser A, *Ann N Y Acad Sci* 346, 398
(1980): Wolska H+, *Przegl Dermatol* (Polish) 67, 439

Phytophotodermatitis
(1998): Adams SP, *Can Fam Physician* 44, 503
(1994): Finkelstein E+, *Int J Dermatol* 33, 116
(1993): Leopold JC+, *Am J Dis Child* 147, 311
(1985): Lembo G+, *Photodermatol* 2, 119
(1984): Goitre M, *G Ital Dermatol Venereol* (Italian) 119, 435
(1983): Heskel NS+, *Contact Dermatitis* 9, 278

Pigmentation
(1994): Burrows NP+, *Clin Exp Dermatol* 19, 380
(1993): Poskitt BL+, *J R Soc Med* 86, 665
(1990): Trattner A+, *Int J Dermatol* 29, 310
(1989): Weiss E+, *Int J Dermatol* 28, 188
(1987): Bruce DR+, *J Am Acad Dermatol* 16, 1087
(1986): MacDonald KJS+, *Br J Dermatol* 114, 395
(1985): Rodighiero G, *Farmaco Prat* 40, 173
(1983): Farber EM+, *Arch Dermatol* 119, 426
(1981): No Author, *Br Med J Clin Red Ed* 283, 335

Porokeratosis (actinic)
(1988): Beiteke U+, *Photodermatology* 5, 274
(1985): Hazen PG+, *J Am Acad Dermatol* 12, 1077
(1980): Reymond JL, *Acta Derm Venereol* (Stockh) 60, 539

Prurigo
(1982): Stüttgen G, *Int J Dermatol* 21, 198 (passim)

Pruritus (>10%)
(1990): Roelandts R+, *Photodermatol Photoimmunol Photomed* 7, 141
(1982): Stüttgen G, *Int J Dermatol* 21, 198 (passim)
(1979): Jordan WP, *Arch Dermatol* 115, 636

Psoriasis

Rash (sic) (1–10%)

Rosacea
(1989): McFadden JP+, *Br J Dermatol* 121, 413

Scleroderma
(1976): Duperrat B+, *Bull Soc Franc Dermatol Syphiligr* (French) 83, 79

Seborrheic dermatitis
(1983): Tegner E, *Acta Derm Venereol* (Stockh) Suppl 107, 5

Skin pain
(1993): Burrows NP+, *Br J Dermatol* 129, 504
(1987): Norris PG+, *Clin Exp Dermatol* 12, 403
(1983): Tegner E, *Acta Derm Venereol* (Stockh) Suppl 107, 5

Squamous cell carcinoma
(2002): Katz KA+, *J Invest Dermatol* 118(6), 1038
(1986): Kahn JR+, *Clin Exp Dermatol* 11, 398

Urticaria
(1994): Bech-Thomsen N+, *J Am Acad Dermatol* 31, 1063

Vasculitis
(1981): Barriere H+, *Presse Med* (French) 10, 37

Vitiligo
(1983): Tegner E, *Acta Derm Venereol* (Stockh) 107 (Suppl), 5
(1976): Duperrat B+, *Bull Soc Franc Dermatol Syphiligr* (French) 83, 79

Warts
(1982): Stüttgen G, *Int J Dermatol* 21, 198

## Hair

Hair – hypertrichosis
(1992): Shelley WB+, *Advanced Dermatologic Diagnosis* WB Saunders, 725 (passim)
(1983): Rampen FHJ, *Br J Dermatol* 109, 657
(1967): Singh G+, *Br J Dermatol* 79, 501
(1959): Elliot JA, *J Invest Dermatol* 32, 311

## Nails

Nails – photo-onycholysis
(1979): Warin AP, *Arch Dermatol* 115, 235
(1978): Ortonne JP+, *Ann Dermatol Venereol* (French) 105, 887

Nails – pigmentation
(1990): Trattner A+, *Int J Dermatol* 29, 310
(1989): Weiss E+, *Int J Dermatol* 28, 188
(1986): MacDonald KJS+, *Br J Dermatol* 114, 395
(1982): Naik RPC+, *Int J Dermatol* 21, 275

## Other

Anaphylactoid reactions
(2001): Legat FJ+, *Br J Dermatol* 145(5), 821

Lymphoproliferative disease
(1989): Aschinoff R+, *J Am Acad Dermatol* 21, 1134

Tumors (for the most part malignant)
(1995): Weinstock MA+, *Arch Dermatol* 131, 701
(1994): Altman JS+, *J Am Acad Dermatol* 31, 505
(1994): Lever LR+, *Clin Exp Dermatol* 19, 443 (malignant)
(1994): Lewis FM+, *Lancet* 344, 1157
(1993): Lindelof B+, *Br J Dermatol* 129, 39
(1990): Young AR, *J Photochem Photobiol* B 6, 237
(1989): Hannuksela M+, *J Am Acad Dermatol* 21, 813
(1989): Stern RS+, *Carcinog Compr Surv* 11, 85
(1988): Gupta AK+, *J Am Acad Dermatol* 19, 67
(1987): Henseler T+, *J Am Acad Dermatol* 16, 108
(1983): Farber EM+, *Arch Dermatol* 119, 426
(1983): Shafrir A, *Harefuah* (Hebrew) 104, 364
(1981): No Author, *Br Med J Clin Red Ed* 283, 335
(1980): Brown FS+, *J Am Acad Dermatol* 2, 393
(1980): Halprin KM, *J Am Acad Dermatol* 2, 334
(1980): Halprin KM, *J Am Acad Dermatol* 2, 432
(1978): Bridges BA, *Clin Exp Dermatol* 3, 349

# PYRAZINAMIDE

**Trade names:** Pyrazinamide (Lederle); Rifater (Aventis)
**Other common trade names:** *Braccopril; Dipimide; Isopas; Lynamide; Pirilene; Pyrazide; Rozide; Tebrazid; Zinastat*
**Indications:** Tuberculosis
**Category:** Antibacterial; antitubercular
**Half-life:** 9–10 hours
**Clinically important, potentially hazardous interactions with:** rifampin

### *Reactions*

## Skin

Acne (<1%)

Erythema multiforme
(1996): Perdu D+, *Allergy* 51, 340

Exanthems
(1990): Goday J+, *Contact Dermatitis* 22, 181

Fixed eruption
(1990): Goday J+, *Contact Dermatitis* 22, 181

Flushing

Pellagra
(1983): Jorgensen J, *Int J Dermatol* 22, 44

Photoallergic reaction
(2001): Maurya V+, *Int J Tuberc Lung Dis* 5(11), 1075

Photodermatitis (<1%)
(1999): Choonhakarn C+, *J Am Acad Dermatol* 40, 645 (lichenoid)

Pruritus (<1%)

Purpura

Rash (sic) (<1%)

(2000): Gordin F+, *JAMA* 283, 1445
(1998): Olivier C+, *Arch Pediatr* (French) 5, 289
(1998): Radal M+, *Rev Mal Respir* (French) 15, 305 (3 cases)
Urticaria

### Other

Acute intermittent porphyria
(1976): Treece GL+, *Am Rev Respir Dis* 113, 233
Death
(2002): Medinger A, *Chest* 121(5), 1710 (with rifampin)
(2001): No authors, *Can Commun Dis Rep* 27(13), 114 (with rifampin)
(2001): No authors, *JAMA* 286(12), 1445 (with rifampin)
(2001): No authors, *MMWR Morb Mortal Wkly Rep* 50(34), 733 (with rifampin)
Hypersensitivity
Myalgia (1–10%)
Oral mucosal lesions
Porphyria cutanea tarda (<1%)
Tinnitus

## PYRIDOXINE

**Synonym:** vitamin $B_6$
**Trade names:** Hexabetalin (Lilly); Nestrex
**Other common trade names:** *B(6)-Vicotrat; Beesix; Benadon; Godabion B6; Hexa-Betalin*
**Indications:** Pyridoxine deficiency
**Category:** Water-soluble nutritional supplement and antidote
**Half-life:** 15–20 days
**Clinically important, potentially hazardous interactions with:** levodopa

#### *Reactions*

### Skin

Acne
(1991): Sherertz EF, *Cutis* 48, 119
(1976): Braun-Falco O+, *MMW Münch Med Wochenschr* (German) 118, 155
(1964): Fegeler F, *Arch Klin Exp Dermatol* (German) 219, 335
Allergic reactions (sic) (<1%)
Bullous eruption
(1984): Ruzicka T+, *Hautarzt* (German) 35, 197
Contact dermatitis
(2001): Bajaj AK+, *Contact Dermatitis* 44(3), 184 (occupational)
(1990): Camarasa JG+, *Contact Dermatitis* 23, 115
(1985): Yoshikawa K+, *Contact Dermatitis* 12, 55
(1983): Fujita M+, *Contact Dermatitis* 9, 61
Fixed eruption
(1972): Kuokkanen K, *Acta Allergol* 27, 407
Photoreactions
(1996): Tanaka M+, *J Dermatol* 23, 708
Photosensitivity
(2001): Bajaj AK+, *Contact Dermatitis* 44(3), 184 (occupational)
(1998): Murata Y+, *J Am Acad Dermatol* 39, 314 (2 cases)
Purpura
Rosacea fulminans
(2001): Jansen T+, *J Eur Acad Dermatol Venereol* 15(5), 484
Toxic epidermal necrolysis
(1980): Andriushchenko OM+, *Klin Med Mosk* (Russian) 58, 101
Vasculitis
(1984): Ruzicka T+, *Hautarzt* (German) 35, 197
Vesicular eruptions
(1986): Friedman MA+, *J Am Acad Dermatol* 14, 915

### Hair

Hair – pigmentation
(1972): Shelley WB+, *Arch Dermatol* 106, 228

### Other

Hypersensitivity
(1969): Zheltakov MM+, *Vestn Dermatol Venerol* (Russian) 43, 62
Injection-site burning
Injection-site stinging
Paresthesias (<1%)
Porphyria cutanea tarda
(1992): Shelley WB+, *Advanced Dermatologic Diagnosis* WB Saunders, 414 (passim)
Pseudoporphyria
(1984): Baer RL+, *J Am Acad Dermatol* 10, 527

## PYRILAMINE

**Trade name:** Triaminic (Novartis)
**Indications:** Allergic rhinitis
**Category:** $H_1$-receptor antihistamine
**Half-life:** no data

#### *Reactions*

### Skin

Angioedema
Dermatitis (sic)
Diaphoresis
Flushing
Lupus erythematosus
Photosensitivity
Purpura
Rash (sic)
Urticaria

### Other

Anaphylactoid reactions
Gynecomastia
Paresthesias
Stomatitis
Tinnitus
Xerostomia

## PYRIMETHAMINE

**Trade names:** Daraprim (GSK); Fansidar (Roche)
**Other common trade names:** *Erbaprelina; Malocide; Pirimecidan*
**Indications:** Malaria
**Category:** Antimalarial
**Half-life:** 80–95 hours
**Clinically important, potentially hazardous interactions with:** dapsone

Fansidar is pyrimethamine and sulfadoxine

#### *Reactions*

### Skin

Acute generalized exanthematous pustulosis (AGEP)
(1995): Moreau A+, *Int J Dermatol* 34, 263 (passim)
Angioedema

(1992): Breathnach SM+, *Adverse Drug Reactions and the Skin* Blackwell, Oxford, 176 (passim)

Bullous eruption
(1992): Breathnach SM+, *Adverse Drug Reactions and the Skin* Blackwell, Oxford, 176 (passim)
(1989): Caumes E+, *Presse Med* (French) 18, 1708

Dermatitis (sic) (<1%)

Erythema multiforme (<1%)
(1993): Sturchler D+, *Drug Saf* 8, 160
(1991): Porteous DM+, *Arch Dermatol* 127, 740 (in HIV+ patients)
(1987): Hellgren U+, *Br Med J Clin Res Ed* 295, 365
(1986): Miller KD+, *Am J Trop Med Hyg* 35, 451

Exanthems
(2002): Thong BY+, *Ann Allergy Asthma Immunol* 88(5), 527 (with dapsone)
(1989): Ortel B+, *Dermatologica* 178, 39 (papular)
(1987): Groth H+, *Schweiz Rundsch Med Prax* (German) 76, 570

Exfoliative dermatitis
(1987): Elsas T+, *Tidsskr Nor Laegeforen* (Norwegian) 107, 1231
(1986): Langtry JA+, *Br Med J Clin Res Ed* 292, 1107

Fixed eruption
(1988): Tham SN+, *Singapore Med J* 29, 300

Lichenoid eruption
(1989): Zain RB, *Southeast Asian J Trop Med Public Health* 20, 253 (oral)
(1980): Cutler TP, *Clin Exp Dermatol* 5, 253

Lymphoma
(1997): Costello JM+, *N Z Med J* 86, 430

Photosensitivity (>10%)
(1992): Breathnach SM+, *Adverse Drug Reactions and the Skin* Blackwell, Oxford, 176 (passim)
(1989): Ortel B+, *Dermatologica* 178, 39
(1974): Craven SA, *BMJ* 2, 556

Pigmentation (<1%)
(1991): Poizot-Martin I+, *Presse Med* (French) 20, 632
(1990): Poizot-Martin I+, *Int Conf AIDS* 6, 357
(1977): Costello JM+, *N Z Med J* 86, 430
(1965): TenPas A+, *Am J Med Sciences* 249, 448

Pruritus
(1987): Groth H+, *Schweiz Rundsch Med Prax* (German) 76, 570

Purpura
(1965): TenPas A+, *Am J Med Sciences* 249, 448

Pustular eruption
(1973): Macmillan AL, *Dermatologica* 146, 285 (generalized)

Rash (sic) (<1%)

Stevens–Johnson syndrome (1–10%)
(1995): Caumes E+, *Clin Infect Dis* 21, 656
(1993): Schlienger RG+, *Schweiz Rundsch Med Prax* (German) 82, 888
(1993): Sturchler D+, *Drug Saf* 8, 160
(1992): Breathnach SM+, *Adverse Drug Reactions and the Skin* Blackwell, Oxford, 176 (passim)
(1991): Porteous DM+, *Arch Dermatol* 127, 740 (in HIV+ patients)
(1990): Thiel HJ+, *Klin Monatsbl Augenheilkd* (German) 197, 142
(1989): Ortel B+, *Dermatologica* 178, 39
(1989): Phillips-Howard PA+, *Lancet* 2, 803
(1988): Mimoun G+, *Bull Soc Ophtalmol Fr* (French) 88, 961
(1987): Hellgren U+, *Br Med J Clin Res Ed* 295, 365
(1987): Lenox-Smith I, *J Infect* 14, 90 (fatal)
(1987): Lyn PC+, *Med J Aust* 146, 335
(1986): Bamber MG+, *J Infect* 13, 31 (fatal)
(1986): Gascon-Brustenga J+, *Med Clin (Barc)* (Spanish) 87, 821
(1986): Miller KD+, *Am J Trop Med Hyg* 35, 451
(1985): Adams SJ+, *Postgrad Med J* 61, 263
(1985): Clareus BW+, *Lakartidningen* (Swedish) 82, 4211
(1983): Ligthelm RJ+, *Ned Tijdschr Geneeskd* (Dutch) 127, 1735
(1982): Hornstein OP+, *N Engl J Med* 307, 1529

Toxic dermatitis (sic)
(1995): Piketty C+, *Presse Med* (French) 24, 1710

Toxic epidermal necrolysis (<1%)
(1998): Moussala M+, *J Fr Ophtalmol* (French) 21, 72
(1998): Schmidt-Westhausen A+, *Oral Dis* 4, 90
(1995): Caumes E+, *Clin Infect Dis* 21, 656
(1993): Sturchler D+, *Drug Saf* 8, 160
(1992): Breathnach SM+, *Adverse Drug Reactions and the Skin* Blackwell, Oxford, 176 (passim)
(1991): Kimura S+, *Jpn J Med* 30, 553
(1990): Ward DJ+, *Burns* 16, 97
(1988): *Morb Mortal Wkly Rep* 37, 571
(1988): Phillips-Howard PA+, *Br Med J Clin Res Ed* 296, 1605
(1988): Raviglione MC+, *Arch Intern Med* 148, 2683 (fatal)
(1987): Hellgren U+, *Br Med J Clin Res Ed* 295, 365
(1986): Miller KD+, *Am J Trop Med Hyg* 35, 451

Urticaria

Vasculitis

## Hair

Hair – alopecia

## Other

Anaphylactoid reactions (<1%)

Death

Dysgeusia

Glossitis (<1%) (atrophic)

Hypersensitivity (>10%)
(2002): Thong BY+, *Ann Allergy Asthma Immunol* 88(5), 527 (with dapsone)

Lymphoproliferative disease
(1977): Costello JM+, *N Z Med J* 86, 430

Tinnitus

Xerostomia (<1%)

# QUAZEPAM

**Trade name:** Doral (Wallace)
**Other common trade names:** *Oniria; Pamerex; Quazium; Quiedorm; Selepam; Temodal*
**Indications:** Insomnia
**Category:** Benzodiazepine sedative-hypnotic; antidepressant
**Half-life:** 25–41 hours
**Clinically important, potentially hazardous interactions with:** amprenavir, chlorpheniramine, clarithromycin, efavirenz, esomeprazole, imatinib, indinavir, nelfinavir, ritonavir

### *Reactions*

#### Skin
Dermatitis (sic) (1–10%)
Diaphoresis (>10%)
Pruritus
(1991): Roth T+, *J Clin Psychiatry* 52 Suppl 38–41
Purpura
Rash (sic) (>10%)
(1991): Roth T+, *J Clin Psychiatry* 52 Suppl 38–41
Urticaria

#### Hair
Hair – alopecia
Hair – hirsutism

#### Other
Dysgeusia
Oral ulceration
Paresthesias
Sialopenia (>10%)
Sialorrhea (1–10%)
Xerostomia (1–5%)
(1991): Roth T+, *J Clin Psychiatry* 52 Suppl 38–41

# QUETIAPINE

**Trade name:** Seroquel (AstraZeneca)
**Indications:** Psychotic disorders, schizophrenia
**Category:** Antipsychotic
**Half-life:** ~6 hours

### *Reactions*

#### Skin
Angioedema
(1999): Drayton G, Los Angeles, CA (from Internet) (observation) (patient is also allergic to sulfa)
Candidiasis (<1%)
Diaphoresis (1–10%)
Edema
Facial edema (<1%)
Neuroleptic malignant syndrome
(2002): Bourgeois JA+, *J Neuropsychiatry Clin neurosci* 14(1), 87
(2002): Sing KJ+, *Am J Psychiatry* 159(1), 149
Photosensitivity (<1%)
Rash (sic) (4%)
Xerosis (<1%)

#### Other
Bruxism (<1%)
Gingivitis (<1%)
Glossitis (<1%)
Myalgia (<1%)
Oral ulceration (<1%)
Paresthesias (1%)
Priapism
(2001): Pais VM+, *Urology* 58(3), 462
Sialorrhea (<1%)
Stomatitis (<1%)
Thrombophlebitis (<1%)
Tongue edema (<1%)
Xerostomia (7%)
(2001): Mullen J+, *Clin Ther* 23(11), 1839 (14.5%)
(2000): Matheson AJ+, *CNS Drugs* 14(2), 157

# QUINACRINE

**Trade name:** Atabrine (Sanofi)
**Other common trade name:** *Atabil*
**Indications:** Various infections caused by susceptible helminths
**Category:** Anthelmintic; antimalarial
**Half-life:** 4–10 hours

### *Reactions*

#### Skin
Contact dermatitis
Erythema dyschromicum perstans
(1970): Tolman MM, *Arch Dermatol* 102, 113
Erythematous plaques
(1981): Bauer F, *J Am Acad Dermatol* 4, 239
Exanthems
(1981): Bauer F, *J Am Acad Dermatol* 4, 239 (eczematous) (80%)
(1963): Nagy E+, *Dermatologica* (German) 126, 13 (1.4%)
(1955): Alexander HL, *Reactions with Drug Therapy* Philadelphia, WB Saunders
(1953): Zeller F, *Hautarzt* (German) 4, 384
Exfoliative dermatitis
(1981): Bauer F, *J Am Acad Dermatol* 4, 239 (8%)
(1967): Lockey SD, *Med Sci* 18, 43
(1955): Alexander HL, *Reactions with Drug Therapy* Philadelphia, WB Saunders
Fixed eruption
(1967): Lockey SD, *Med Sci* 18, 43
(1964): Browne SG, *BMJ* 2, 1041
(1961): Welch AL+, *Arch Dermatol* 84, 1004
(1955): Alexander HL, *Reactions with Drug Therapy* Philadelphia, WB Saunders
Hypomelanosis
(1967): Lockey SD, *Med Sci* 18, 43
Keratoderma
(1978): Bauer F, *Aust J Dermatol* 19, 9
Lichenoid eruption
(1981): Bauer F, *J Am Acad Dermatol* 4, 239 (12%)
(1979): Callaway JL, *J Am Acad Dermatol* 1, 456
(1978): Bauer F, *Aust J Dermatol* 19, 9
(1971): Almeyda J+, *Br J Dermatol* 85, 604
(1964): Baker H, *Br J Dermatol* 76, 186
(1963): Nagy E+, *Dermatologica* (German) 126, 13 (1.4%)
(1955): Alexander HL, *Reactions with Drug Therapy* Philadelphia, WB Saunders
Ochronosis
(1976): Egorin MJ+, *JAMA* 236, 385
(1976): Tuffanelli DL, *JAMA* 236, 2491
Photosensitivity
(1997): Hindson C, *The Schoch Letter* 47, 53

Pigmentation
(1982): Sokol RJ+, *Pediatrics* 69, 232 (yellow)
(1981): Koranda FC, *J Am Acad Dermatol* 4, 650
(1981): Zuehlke RL+, *Int J Dermatol* 20, 57
(1979): Leigh IM+, *Br J Dermatol* 101, 147
(1978): Bauer F, *Aust J Dermatol* 19, 9
(1969): *Med Lett* 11, 27 (yellowish)
Pruritus (<1%)
Squamous cell carcinoma
(1979): Callaway JL, *J Am Acad Dermatol* 1, 456
(1978): Bauer F, *Aust J Dermatol* 19, 9
Urticaria
(1969): *Med Lett* 11, 27 (1–5%)
(1955): Alexander HL, *Reactions with Drug Therapy* Philadelphia, WB Saunders

### Hair

Hair – alopecia
(1981): Bauer F, *J Am Acad Dermatol* 4, 239 (eczematous) (80%)
(1978): Bauer F, *Aust J Dermatol* 19, 9

### Nails

Nails – changes (sic)
(1978): Bauer F, *Aust J Dermatol* 19, 9
Nails – nail bed pigmentation (blue-gray)
(2000): Kleinegger CL+, *Oral Surg Oral Med Oral Pathol Oral Radiol Endod* 90, 189
Nails – pigmentation
(1969): *Med Lett* 11, 27
Nails – pigmentation (ala nasi) (blue-gray)
(2000): Kleinegger CL+, *Oral Surg Oral Med Oral Pathol Oral Radiol Endod* 90, 189

### Other

Oral mucosal pigmentation
(2000): Kleinegger CL+, *Oral Surg Oral Med Oral Pathol Oral Radiol Endod* 90, 189
Oral pigmentation
(1970): Brynolf I, *Sven Tandlak Tidskr* (Swedish) 63, 585

# QUINAPRIL

**Trade name:** Accupril (Parke-Davis)
**Other common trade names:** *Accuprin; Accupro; Acuitel; Acupril; Asig; Korec; Quinazil*
**Indications:** Hypertension
**Category:** Angiotensin-converting enzyme (ACE) inhibitor; antihypertensive and vasodilator
**Half-life:** 1–2 hours
**Clinically important, potentially hazardous interactions with:** amiloride, spironolactone, triamterene

## *Reactions*

### Skin

Angioedema (<1%)
(2001): Cohen EG+, *Ann Otol Rhinol Laryngol* 110(8), 701 (64 cases)
(1997): Sigler C+, *Arch Dermatol* 113, 972
(1996): Boxer M, *J Allergy Clin Immunol* 98, 471
(1995): Maier C, *Anaesthesist* (German) 44, 875
(1994): Cosano L+, *Med Clin (Barc)* (Spanish) 102, 275
(1993): Mendez-Mora JL+, *Med Clin (Barc)* (Spanish) 101, 76
(1992): Materson BJ, *Am J Cardiol* 69, 46C
(1989): Sedman AJ+, *Angiology* 40 (4 Pt 2), 360
Ankle edema
(1992): Bahena JH+, *Clin Ther* 14, 527
Bullous eruption
(1998): Sienkiewicz G, Johnson City, NY (from Internet) (observation)
Diaphoresis (<1%)
(1991): Morant J+, *Arzneimittel-Kompendium der Schweiz* (German) Basel, Documed, 1990
(1989): Frank GJ+, *Angiology* 40 (4 Pt 2), 405
(1989): Maclean D, *Angiology* 40 (4 Pt 2), 370
Edema
(1989): Frank GJ+, *Angiology* 40 (4 Pt 2), 405
(1989): Frank GJ, *Cardiology* 76 (Suppl 2), 56
Exanthems
(1991): Morant J+, *Arzneimittel-Kompendium der Schweiz* (German) Basel, Documed, 1990
Exfoliative dermatitis (<1%)
Facial edema (sic)
(1989): Sedman AJ+, *Angiology* 40 (4 Pt 2), 360
Flushing (<1%)
Pemphigus (<1%)
Pemphigus foliaceus
(2000): Ong CS+, *Australas J Dermatol* 41(4), 242
Pemphigus vulgaris
(2000): Ong CS+, *Australas J Dermatol* 41(4), 242
Peripheral edema (<1%)
(1991): Wadworth AN+, *Drugs* 41, 378
Photosensitivity (<1%)
(1989): Maclean D, *Angiology* 40 (4 Pt 2), 370
Pruritus (<1%)
(1991): Cetnarowski-Cropp AB, *Drug Intell Clin Pharm* 25, 499
(1991): Morant J+, *Arzneimittel-Kompendium der Schweiz* (German) Basel, Documed, 1990
(1990): Frishman WH, *Clin Cardiol* 13 (Suppl 7), VII19
(1990): Swartz RD+, *J Clin Pharmacol* 30, 1136
(1989): Frank GJ+, *Angiology* 40 (4 Pt 2), 405
(1989): Frank GJ, *Cardiology* 76 (Suppl 2), 56
(1989): Maclean D, *Angiology* 40 (4 Pt 2), 370
Rash (sic) (1.2%)
(1992): Materson BJ, *Am J Cardiol* 69, 46C
(1989): Frank GJ+, *Angiology* 40 (4 Pt 2), 405
(1989): Frank GJ, *Cardiology* 76 (Suppl 2), 56
(1989): Maclean D, *Angiology* 40 (4 Pt 2), 370
(1989): Taylor SH, *Angiology* 40 (4 Pt 2), 382
Urticaria (<1%)
Vasculitis (<1%)

### Hair

Hair – alopecia (<1%)

### Other

Cough
(2002): Culy CR+, *Drugs* 62(2), 339 (2–4%)
(2001): Adigun AQ+, *West Afr J Med* 20(1), 46–7
(2001): Lee SC+, *Hypertension* 38(2), 166
Dysgeusia
(1991): Cetnarowski-Cropp AB, *Drug Intell Clin Pharm* 25, 499
(1989): Taylor SH, *Angiology* 40 (4 Pt 2), 382
Hypersensitivity
Myalgia (1.5%)
Paresthesias (<1%)
Xerostomia (<1%)

# QUINESTROL

**Trade name:** Estrovis (Parke-Davis)
**Indications:** Atrophic vaginitis, menopausal symptoms
**Category:** Estrogen
**Half-life:** 120 hours

### *Reactions*

**Skin**

Angioedema
 (1970): Aitken DA+, *BMJ* 2, 177
Chloasma (<1%)
Edema (<1%)
Erythema
Melasma (<1%)
Peripheral edema (>10%)
Photosensitivity
Rash (sic) (<1%)
Urticaria
 (1970): Aitken DA+, *BMJ* 2, 177

**Other**

Acute intermittent porphyria
Gynecomastia (>10%)
Mastodynia (>10%)
Thrombophlebitis

# QUINETHAZONE

**Trade name:** Hydromox (Lederle)
**Other common trade name:** *Aquamox*
**Indications:** Hypertension, edema
**Category:** Sulfonamide* diuretic and antihypertensive
**Half-life:** no data
**Clinically important, potentially hazardous interactions with:** digoxin, lithium

### *Reactions*

**Skin**

Bullous eruption (<1%)
 (1966): Miller RC+, *Arch Dermatol* 93, 346
Exanthems
 (1966): Miller RC+, *Arch Dermatol* 93, 346
Photoreactions
Photosensitivity (<1%)
 (1969): Kalivas J, *JAMA* 209, 1706
 (1966): Miller RC+, *Arch Dermatol* 93, 346
Pruritus
 (1969): Kalivas J, *JAMA* 209, 1706
Purpura
Rash (sic) (<1%)
Urticaria
Vasculitis

**Other**

Hypersensitivity
Paresthesias
Xanthopsia
Xerostomia

***Note:** Quinethazone is a sulfonamide and can be absorbed systemically. Sulfonamides can produce severe, possibly fatal, reactions such as toxic epidermal necrolysis and Stevens–Johnson syndrome

# QUINIDINE

**Trade names:** Cardioquin (Purdue Frederick); Cin-Quin; Quinaglute (Berlex); Quinalan; Quinidex (Robins); Quinora
**Other common trade names:** *Cardine; Gluquine; Kinidin; Quinate; Quini Durules*
**Indications:** Tachycardia, atrial fibrillation
**Category:** Antiarrhythmic class I-A
**Half-life:** 6–8 hours
**Clinically important, potentially hazardous interactions with:** amiloride, amiodarone, amprenavir, anisindione, anticoagulants, arsenic, ciprofloxacin, delavirdine, dicumarol, digoxin, enoxacin, gatifloxacin, itraconazole, lomefloxacin, moxifloxacin, norfloxacin, ofloxacin, pimozide, quinolones, ritonavir, sparfloxacin, verapamil, voriconazole, warfarin

### *Reactions*

**Skin**

Acne
 (1981): Burkhart CG, *Arch Dermatol* 117, 603
Acute generalized exanthematous pustulosis (AGEP)
 (1995): Moreau A+, *Int J Dermatol* 34, 263 (passim)
 (1991): Roujeau J-C+, *Arch Dermatol* 127, 1333
Allergic reactions (sic)
 (1986): Bigby M+, *JAMA* 256, 3358 (1.34%)
Angioedema (<1%)
Bullous eruption
Contact dermatitis
 (1985): Fowler JF, *Contact Dermatitis* 13, 280
 (1981): Wahlberg JE+, *Contact Dermatitis* 7, 27 (occupational)
 (1965): Fernstrom AI, *Acta Derm Venereol* 45, 129
Cutaneous side effects (sic)
 (1977): Cohen IS+, *Prog Cardiovasc Dis* 20, 151 (1%)
Eczematous eruption (sic)
Erythema multiforme
 (1989): Alanko K, *Acta Derm Venereol* (Stockh) 69, 223
Exanthems
 (1990): Lou CP+, *Postgrad Med J* 66, 406
 (1985): Bruce S+, *J Am Acad Dermatol* 12, 332
 (1982): Holt RJ, *Drug Intell Clin Pharm* 16, 615
 (1980): Harrison DC+, *Am Heart J* 100, 1046 (16.6%)
 (1976): Arndt KA+, *JAMA* 235, 918 (generalized) (1.2%)
 (1976): Geltner D+, *Gastroenterology* 70, 650 (0.8%)
Exfoliative dermatitis (<1%)
 (1996): Sigurdsson V+, *J Am Acad Dermatol* 35, 53
 (1987): Bellogini GC+, *Minerva Cardioangiol* (Italian) 35, 457
 (1985): Bruce S+, *J Am Acad Dermatol* 12, 332
 (1965): Gouffault J+, *Sem Hôp* (French) 41, 1350
 (1951): Taylor DR+, *JAMA* 145, 641
Exudative dermatitis (sic)
 (1942): Goldschlag F, *Med J Australia* 2, 501
Fixed eruption
 (1960): Engelhardt AW, *Hautarzt* (German) 11, 49
Flushing (<1%)
 (1991): Ross EV+, *J Assoc Military Dermatol* XVII (1), 16
 (1985): Bruce S+, *J Am Acad Dermatol* 12, 332
Granuloma annulare
 (1991): Ross EV+, *J Assoc Military Dermatol* XVII (1), 16
Lichen planus
 (1994): Thompson DF+, *Pharmacotherapy* 14, 561
 (1985): Bruce S+, *J Am Acad Dermatol* 12, 332 (passim)
 (1985): Rebondy JP+, *Ann Dermatol Venereol* (French) 112, 989
 (1980): Maltz BL+, *Int J Dermatol* 19, 96
 (1967): Anderson TE, *Br J Dermatol* 79, 500
 (1967): Sarkany I, *Br J Dermatol* 79, 123

(1954): Wechsler HL, *Arch Dermatol* 69, 741

Lichenoid eruption
(1988): de Larrard G+, *Ann Dermatol Venereol* (French) 115, 1172
(1987): Jeanmougin M+, *Ann Dermatol Venereol* (French) 114, 1397 (photosensitive)
(1982): Berger TC+, *Cutis* 29, 595
(1981): Haim S+, *Harefuah* (Hebrew) 101, 310
(1976): Gammer S+, *Cutis* 17, 72
(1968): Pegum JS, *Br J Dermatol* 80, 343

Livedo reticularis (<1%)
(1989): Manzi S+, *Arch Dermatol* 125, 417 (photosensitive)
(1985): Bruce S+, *J Am Acad Dermatol* 12, 332 (photosensitive)
(1977): Cohen IS+, *Prog Cardiovasc Dis* 20, 151
(1974): de Groot WP+, *Dermatologica* 148, 371 (photosensitive)
(1973): Marion DF+, *Arch Dermatol* 108, 100 (photosensitive)

Lupus erythematosus (<1%)
(1996): Rich MW, *Postgrad Med* 100, 299
(1995): Alloway JA+, *Semin Arthritis Rheum* 24, 315
(1994): Yung RL+, *Rheum Dis Clin North Am* 20, 61
(1992): Rubin RL, *Clin Biochem* 25, 223
(1992): Rubin RL+, *J Clin Invest* 90, 165
(1992): Skaer TL, *Clin Ther* 14, 496
(1991): Alarcon-Segovia D+, *Baillieres Clin Rheumatol* 5, 1
(1991): Tebas P+, *Rev Clin Esp* (Spanish) 189, 123
(1989): Cohen MG, *Geriatric Med Today* 8, 95
(1988): Cohen MG+, *Ann Intern Med* 108, 369
(1988): Schmid FR, *Ann Intern Med* 109, 247
(1988): Webb J+, *Med J Aust* 149, 53
(1987): Sukenik S+, *Isr J Med Sci* 23, 1232
(1986): Bar-El Y+, *Am Heart J* 111, 1209
(1985): Amadio P+, *Ann Intern Med* 102, 419
(1985): Gastineau DA+, *Arch Intern Med* 145, 1926
(1985): Krainin MJ+, *Arch Intern Med* 145, 1740
(1985): Lavie CJ+, *Arch Intern Med* 145, 446
(1985): McCormack GD+, *Semin Arthritis Rheum* 15, 73
(1985): Rebondy JP+, *Ann Dermatol Venereol* (French) 112, 989
(1985): Stratton MA, *Clin Pharm* 4, 657
(1984): West SG+, *Ann Intern Med* 100, 840
(1982): Chagnon A+, *Nouv Presse Med* (French) 11, 2020
(1981): Barrier J+, *Nouv Presse Med* (French) 10, 2991
(1978): Robinson HM, *Z Hautkr* (German) 53, 349
(1977): Cohen IS+, *Prog Cardiovasc Dis* 20, 151
(1977): Tweed JM, *N Z Med J* 86, 40
(1976): Yudis M+, *JAMA* 235, 2000
(1974): Donoho CR+, *Arthritis Rheum* 17, 322
(1973): Hanauer LB, *Ann Intern Med* 78, 308
(1973): Marion DF+, *Arch Dermatol* 108, 100
(1972): Anderson FP+, *Conn Med* 36, 84
(1970): Kendall MJ+, *Postgrad Med J* 46, 729

Palmar–plantar keratoderma
(1988): De Larrard G+, *Ann Dermatol Venereol* (French) 115, 1172

Photoreactions
(1991): Schürer NY+, *Hautarzt* (German) 42, 158
(1990): Fertin C+, *Nouv Dermatol* (French) 9, 446
(1986): Jeanmougin M+, *Ann Dermatol Venereol* (French) 113, 985
(1976): Gammer S+, *Cutis* 17, 72

Photosensitivity (<1%)
(1992): Schürer NY+, *Photodermatol Photoimmunol Photomed* 9, 78
(1989): Rosen C, *Semin Dermatol* 8, 149
(1988): De Larrard G+, *Ann Dermatol Venereol* (French) 115, 1172
(1987): Bonnetblanc JM+, *Ann Dermatol Venereol* (French) 114, 957 (lichenoid)
(1987): Ferguson J+, *Br J Dermatol* 117, 631
(1987): Wolf R+, *Dermatologica* 174, 285 (lichenoid and eczematous)
(1986): Ljunggren B+, *Photodermatol* 3, 26
(1985): Armstrong RB+, *Arch Dermatol* 121, 525
(1985): Bonnetblanc JM+, *Ann Dermatol Venereol* (French) 112, 671
(1985): Rebondy JP+, *Ann Dermatol Venereol* (French) 112, 989
(1984): Fisher DA, *Arch Dermatol* 120, 298
(1983): Lang PS, *J Am Acad Dermatol* 9, 124
(1983): Marx JL+, *Arch Dermatol* 119, 39
(1982): Berger TC+, *Cutis* 29, 595 (lichenoid)
(1976): Bogoch ER+, *Arch Dermatol* 112, 559
(1976): Pariser RJ+, *Arch Dermatol* 112, 1610
(1975): Pariser DM+, *Arch Dermatol* 111, 1440

Pigmentation (<1%)
(1996): Conroy EA+, *Cutis* 57, 425
(1996): Messina JL+, *J Geriatr Dermatol* 4, 198
(1995): Rippis G+, American Academy of Dermatology Meeting, New Orleans (observation)
(1986): Mahler R+, *Arch Dermatol* 122, 1062

Pruritus (<1%)
(1985): Bruce S+, *J Am Acad Dermatol* 12, 332 (passim)
(1982): Holt RJ, *Drug Intell Clin Pharm* 16, 615
(1976): Geltner D+, *Gastroenterology* 70, 650 (0.8%)

Psoriasis (<1%)
(1998): Smith KC, Niagara Falls, Canada (from Internet) (observation)
(1993): Brenner S+, *Arch Dermatol* 129, 1331
(1986): Abel EA+, *J Am Acad Dermatol* 15, 1007
(1983): Harwell WB, *J Am Acad Dermatol* 9, 278
(1977): Cohen IS+, *Prog Cardiovasc Dis* 20, 151 (with erythroderma)
(1973): Almeyda J+, *Br J Dermatol* 88, 313 (with erythroderma)

Purpura
(1993): Kaufman DW+, *Blood* 82, 2714
(1991): Salom IL, *JAMA* 266, 1220 (letter)
(1988): Reid DM+, *Ann Intern Med* 108, 206
(1981): Barrier J+, *Nouv Presse Med* (French) 10, 2991
(1981): Conri C+, *Nouv Presse Med* (French) 7, 3361
(1980): Miescher PA+, *Clin Haematol* 9, 505
(1976): Geltner D+, *Gastroenterology* 70, 650 (1.4%)
(1976): Khaleeli AA, *BMJ* 2, 562
(1962): Weintraub RM+, *JAMA* 180, 528
(1959): Bishop RC+, *Ann Intern Med* 50, 1227
(1958): Shaftel N+, *Angiology* 9, 34
(1956): Bolton FG, *Blood* 11, 547
(1956): Freedman AL+, *J Lab Clin Med* 48, 205

Pustular eruption
(1951): Taylor DR+, *JAMA* 145, 641

Rash (sic) (1–10%)

Subcorneal pustular dermatosis (Sneddon–Wilkinson)
(1983): Halevy S+, *Acta Derm Venereol* (Stockh) 63, 441

Toxic epidermal necrolysis
(2000): Adornato MC, *N Y State Dent J* 66, 38
(1974): Callaway JL+, *Arch Dermatol* 109, 909

Urticaria (<1%)
(1985): Bruce S+, *J Am Acad Dermatol* 12, 332

Vasculitis (<1%)
(1990): Zax RH+, *Arch Dermatol* 126, 69
(1989): Cohen MG, *Geriatric Med Today* 8, 99
(1988): Quin J+, *Med J Aust* 148, 145 (allergic granulomatous)
(1985): Shalit M+, *Arch Intern Med* 145, 2051

### Hair

Hair – alopecia
(1988): de Larrard G+, *Ann Dermatol Venereol* (French) 115, 1172

### Other

Dysgeusia (>10%) (bitter taste)

Hypersensitivity
(1966): Martt JM+, *Mo Med* 63, 908

Lymphoproliferative disease
(1987): Gay RG+, *Am J Med* 82, 143
Myalgia (<1%)
Oral mucosal eruption
(1988): De Larrard G+, *Ann Dermatol Venereol* (French) 115, 1172
(1958): Shaftel N+, *Angiology* 9, 34
Oral mucosal pigmentation
(1988): Birek C+, *Oral Surg Oral Med Oral Pathol* 66, 59
Oral ulceration
Polymyalgia
(1995): Alloway JA+, *Semin Arthritis Rheum* 24, 315
Porphyria
(1971): Sayag J+, *Bull Soc Franc Dermatol Syphiligr* (French) 78, 664
Pseudoporphyria
(1992): Petersen CS+, *Ugeskr Laeger* (Danish) 154, 1713
Sicca syndrome (<1%)
(1983): Naschitz JE+, *J Toxicol Clin Toxicol* 20, 367
Tinnitus
Tremors (2%)

# QUININE

**Trade names:** Formula-Q; Legatrin (Columbia); M-KYA; Q-Vel; Quiphile (Geneva)
**Other common trade names:** *Adaquin; Chinine; Genin; Quinate; Quinoctal; Quinsan; Quinsul*
**Indications:** Malaria, nocturnal leg cramps
**Category:** Antiprotozoal and antimyotonic
**Half-life:** 8–14 hours
**Clinically important, potentially hazardous interactions with:** anisindione, anticoagulants, dicumarol, warfarin

### *Reactions*

## Skin

Acne
(1981): Burkhart CC, *Arch Dermatol* 117, 603
(1967): Hitch JM, *JAMA* 200, 879
Acral erythema
(2000): Abreu-Gerke L+, *Hautarzt* 51(5), 332
Acral necrosis
(2000): Abreu-Gerke L+, *Hautarzt* 51(5), 332
Angioedema (<1%)
Bullous eruption
Contact dermatitis
(1994): Dias M+, *Contact Dermatitis* 30, 121
(1994): Isaksson M+, *Acta Derm Venereol* 74, 286
(1994): Tapadinhas C+, *Contact Dermatitis* 31, 127 (from hair lotion)
(1978): Calnan CD+, *Contact Dermatitis* 4, 58
(1978): Hardie RA+, *Contact Dermatitis* 4, 121 (occupational)
(1961): Calnan CD+, *BMJ* 2, 1750
Diaphoresis
Eczematous eruption (sic)
Erythema
Erythema multiforme (<1%)
(2000): Abreu-Gerke L+, *Hautarzt* 51(5), 332 (passim)
(1967): Coleman WP, *Med Clin North Am* 51, 1073
Exanthems (1–5%)
(2000): Abreu-Gerke L+, *Hautarzt* 51(5), 332 (passim)
(1969): Török H, *Dermatol Int* 8, 57
Exfoliative dermatitis
(1975): Jarratt M+, *Arch Dermatol* 111, 132
(1974): Callaway JL+, *Arch Dermatol* 109, 909
Facial edema
Fixed eruption
(2000): Litt JZ, Beachwood, OH (personal case) (observation)
(1993): Litt JZ, Beachwood, OH (from quinine water) (personal case) (observation)
(1990): Gaffoor PMA+, *Cutis* 45, 242 (passim)
(1974): Kuokkanen K, *Int J Dermatol* 13, 4
(1970): Savin JA, *Br J Dermatol* 83, 546
(1967): Kogoj F, *Med Glas* (Serbo-Croatian-Roman) 21, 351
(1961): Welsh AL+, *Arch Dermatol* 84, 1004
(1960): Engelhardt AW, *Hautarzt* (German) 11, 49
Flushing (<1%)
Lichen planus
(1994): Litt JZ, Beachwood, OH (personal case) (observation)
(1986): Dawson TAJ, *Clin Exp Dermatol* 11, 670
(1986): Meyrick-Thomas RH+, *Clin Exp Dermatol* 11, 97 (photosensitive distribution)
(1979): Krebs A, *Hautarzt* (German) 30, 281
Lichenoid eruption
(1995): Dawson TA, *BMJ* 310, 738
(1989): Tan SV+, *Clin Exp Dermatol* 14, 335
(1987): Ferguson J+, *Br J Dermatol* 117, 631
Livedo racemosa (photosensitive)
(1988): Diffey BL+, *Br J Dermatol* 118, 679
(1974): de Groot WP+, *Dermatologica* 148, 371
(1973): Marion DF, *Arch Dermatol* 108, 100
Lupus erythematosus
(1996): Rosa-Re D+, *Ann Rheum Dis* 55, 559
Ochronosis
(1986): Bruce S+, *J Am Acad Dermatol* 15, 357
Photoreactions
Photosensitivity
(2000): Abreu-Gerke L+, *Hautarzt* 51(5), 332 (passim)
(1998): Rademaker M, Hamilton, New Zealand (from Internet) (observation)
(1995): Dawson TA, *BMJ* 310, 738
(1995): Delmas A+, *Presse Med* (French) 24, 1707
(1994): Isaksson M+, *Acta Derm Venereol* 74, 286
(1994): Litt JZ, Beachwood, OH (personal case) (observation)
(1994): Okun MM+, *Clin Exp Dermatol* 19, 246 (mycosisfungoides-like)
(1994): Wagner GH+, *Br J Dermatol* 131, 734 (from tonic water)
(1992): Fitzpatrick JE, *Dermatol Clin* 10, 19
(1992): Ljunggren B+, *Contact Dermatitis* 26, 1
(1990): Guzzo C+, *Photodermatol Photoimmunol Photomed* 7, 166
(1988): Diffey BL+, *Br J Dermatol* 118, 679
(1987): Ferguson J+, *Br J Dermatol* 117, 631
(1986): Dawson TAJ, *Clin Exp Dermatol* 11, 670 (lichenoid)
(1986): Ljunggren B+, *Arch Dermatol* 122, 909
(1986): Ljunggren B+, *Photodermatol* 3, 26
(1984): Jeanmougin M+, *Ann Dermatol Venereol* (French) 11, 565
(1978): Calnan CD+, *Contact Dermatitis* 4, 58
(1975): Johnson BE+, *Br J Dermatol* 93 (Suppl 11), 21
(1969): Kalivas J, *JAMA* 209, 1706
Pigmentation
(1999): Rosen T+, Houston, TX (personal case) (observation)
(1994): Litt JZ, Beachwood, OH (personal case) (observation)
(1986): Bruce S+, *J Am Acad Dermatol* 15, 357 (from injections)
(1986): Mahler R+, *Arch Dermatol* 122, 1062
(1964): Dummett CO, *J Oral Ther Pharmacol* 1, 106
(1963): Tuffanelli D+, *Arch Dermatol* 88, 419
Pruritus (<1%)
(2000): Abreu-Gerke L+, *Hautarzt* 51(5), 332 (passim)
Psoriasis
(1998): Smith KC, Niagara Falls, Canada (from Internet) (observation)
Purpura

(2000): Abreu-Gerke L+, *Hautarzt* 51(5), 332 (passim)
(1993): Kaufman DW+, *Blood* 82, 2714
(1985): Ambriz-Fernandez R+, *Rev Invest Clin* (Spanish) 37, 347
(1980): Miescher PA+, *Clin Haematol* 9, 505
(1969): Török H, *Dermatol Int* 8, 57
(1967): Belkin CA, *Ann Intern Med* 66, 583
(1967): Helmly RB+, *Arch Intern Med* 120, 59
(1965): Horowitz HI+, *Semin Hematol* 2, 287
(1962): Weintraub RM+, *JAMA* 180, 528
(1952): Lincoln RB+, *Am Pract* 3, 42
(1946): Schrager J+, *Am J Med Sci* 212, 54

Rash (sic) (<1%)
(1993): Siderov J, *J Am Geriatr Soc* 41, 498

Stevens–Johnson syndrome
(1986): Gascon-Brustenga J+, *Med Clin (Barc)* (Spanish) 87, 821
(1967): Coleman WP, *Med Clin North Am* 51, 1073

Thrombocytopenic purpura
(2001): Medina PJ+, *Curr Opin Hematol* 8(5), 286

Toxic epidermal necrolysis (<1%)
(1975): Jarratt M+, *Arch Dermatol* 111, 132
(1974): Callaway JL+, *Arch Dermatol* 109, 909 (tonic water)

Urticaria
(2000): Abreu-Gerke L+, *Hautarzt* 51(5), 332 (passim)
(1969): Török H, *Dermatol Int* 8, 57

Vasculitis
(1992): Price EJ+, *Br J Clin Pract* 46, 138
(1991): Harland CC+, *BMJ* 302, 295
(1990): Mathur S+, *BMJ* 300, 613
(1968): Rockl H+, *Munch Med Wochenschr* (German) 110, 2549
(1952): Lincoln RB+, *Am Pract* 3, 42

Vitiligo
(1998): Rademaker M, Hamilton, New Zealand (from Internet) (observation) (following photosensitivity)

### Nails

Nails – photo-onycholysis
(1989): Tan SV+, *Clin Exp Dermatol* 14, 335

### Other

Hypersensitivity (<1%)
(1998): Schattner A, *Am J Med* 104–488

Oral mucosal eruption
(1964): Dummett CO, *J Oral Ther Pharmacol* 1, 106

Oral ulceration

Porphyria
(1971): Sayag J+, *Bull Soc Franc Dermatol Syphiligr* (French) 78, 664

Tinnitus

# QUINUPRISTIN/DALFOPRISTIN

**Synonyms:** pristinamycin; RP59500
**Trade name:** Synercid (Aventis)
**Indications:** Serious life-threatening bacterial infections
**Category:** Streptogramin antibiotic
**Half-life:** 1.3–1.5 hours

## *Reactions*

### Skin

Allergic reactions (sic) (<1%)
Candidiasis (<1%)
Diaphoresis (<1%)
Exanthems (<1%)
Peripheral edema (<1%)
Pruritus (1.5%)
Rash (sic) (2.5%)
(2001): Allington DR+, *Clin Ther* 23(1), 24 (2.5–4.6%)
Ulceration (<1%)
Urticaria (<1%)

### Other

Anaphylactoid reactions (<1%)

Arthralgia
(2001): Allington DR+, *Clin Ther* 23(1), 24
(2001): Manzella JP, *Am Fam Physician* 64(11), 1863
(2001): Olsen KM+, *Clin Infect Dis* 32(4), 83
(2000): Delgado G+, *Pharacotherapy* 20(12), 1469

Infusion-site edema (17.3%)
(2001): Allington DR+, *Clin Ther* 23(1), 24

Infusion-site inflammation (42%)
(2001): Allington DR+, *Clin Ther* 23(1), 24

Infusion-site pain (40%)
(2001): Allington DR+, *Clin Ther* 23(1), 24
(2000): Delgado G+, *Pharmacotherapy* 20(12), 1469

Infusion-site reactions (sic) (13.4%)

Myalgia (<1–5%)
(2001): Allington DR+, *Clin Ther* 23(1), 24
(2001): Manzella JP, *Am Fam Physician* 64(11), 1863
(2001): Olsen KM+, *Clin Infect Dis* 32(4), 83
(2000): Delgado G+, *Pharacotherapy* 20(12), 1469

Oral candidiasis (<1%)
Paresthesias (<1%)
Phlebitis (<1%)
Stomatitis (<1%)

Thrombophlebitis (2.4%)
(2001): Allington DR+, *Clin Ther* 23(1), 24

Tremors (<1%)
Vaginitis (<1%)

## RABEPRAZOLE

**Synonym:** pariprazole
**Trade name:** Aciphex (Janssen)
**Indications:** Gastroesophageal reflux disease (GERD)
**Category:** Proton pump (gastric acid secretion) inhibitor
**Half-life:** 1–2 hours

### *Reactions*

#### Skin
Allergic reactions (sic) (<1%)
Chills (<1%)
Diaphoresis (<1%)
Ecchymoses (<1%)
Edema
Eruptions (sic) (<1%)
Facial edema (<1%)
Herpes zoster (<1%)
Peripheral edema (<1%)
Photosensitivity (<1%)
Pigmentation (<1%)
Pruritus (<1%)
Psoriasis (<1%)
Purpura
Rash (sic) (<1%)
Urticaria (<1%)
Xerosis (<1%)

#### Hair
Hair – alopecia (<1%)

#### Other
Gingivitis (<1%)
Glossitis (<1%)
Gynecomastia (<1%)
Myalgia (<1%)
Oral ulceration
Paresthesias (<1%)
Stomatitis (<1%)
Thrombophlebitis (<1%)
Tremors (<1%)
Twitching (<1%)
Xerostomia (<1%)

## RALOXIFENE

**Synonym:** Keoxifene
**Trade name:** Evista (Lilly)
**Indications:** Osteoporosis
**Category:** Selective estrogen receptor modulator
**Half-life:** 27.7 hours
**Clinically important, potentially hazardous interactions with:** cholestyramine

### *Reactions*

#### Skin
Diaphoresis (3.1%)
Edema
Flu-like syndrome (sic) (~2%)
Hot flashes (24.6%)
(2001): Seeman E, *J Bone Miner Metab* 19, 65 (406%)
(2000): Eriksen EF, *Ugeskr Laeger* (Danish) 162, 4182
(2000): Snyder KR+, *Am J Health Syst Pharm* 57, 1669
(1999): Ettinger B+, *JAMA* 282, 637 (10%)
(1999): Scott JA+, *Am Fam Physician* 60, 1131
(1998): Walsh BW+, *JAMA* 279, 1445 (22%)
Infections (sic) (~2%)
Peripheral edema (3.3%)
(2000): Eriksen EF, *Ugeskr Laeger* (Danish) 162, 4182
(1999): Cummings SR+, *JAMA* 281, 2189
(1999): Ettinger B+, *JAMA* 282, 637 (5%)
Rash (sic) (5.5%)
Vitiligo
(2002): Litt JZ, Beachwood, OH (personal case) (observation) (after 3 weeks of raloxifene, patient developed leukoderma over exposed areas of chest and forearms after sun exposure)

#### Other
Leg cramps
(2001): Seeman E, *J Bone Miner Metab* 19, 65 (2–4%)
Mastodynia (4.4%)
(1999): Cummings SR+, *JAMA* 281, 2189
(1998): Walsh BW+, *JAMA* 279, 1445 (4%)
Myalgia (7.7%)
Vaginitis (4.3%)

## RAMIPRIL

**Trade name:** Altace (Monarch)
**Other common trade names:** *Delix; Hytren; Pramace; Quark; Ramace; Triatec; Tritace; Unipril*
**Indications:** Hypertension
**Category:** Angiotensin-converting enzyme (ACE) inhibitor; antihypertensive and vasodilator
**Half-life:** 3–17 hours
**Clinically important, potentially hazardous interactions with:** amiloride, spironolactone, triamterene

### *Reactions*

#### Skin
Acne
(1987): Predel HG+, *Am J Cardiol* 59, 143D
Angioedema (0.3%)
(2002): Kaur S+, *J Dermatol* 29(6), 336
(2001): Cohen EG+, *Ann Otol Rhinol Laryngol* 110(8), 701 (64 cases)
(1995): Epeldo-Gonzalo F+, *Ann Pharmacother* 29, 431
(1990): Todd PA+, *Drugs* 39, 110
Dermatitis (sic) (<1%)
Diaphoresis (<1%)
(1988): Zabludowski J+, *Curr Med Res Opin* 11, 93
(1987): Walter U+, *Am J Cardiol* 59, 125D
Dry feeling on face (sic)
(1987): Fukiyama K+, *Am J Cardiol* 59, 121D
Edema (<1%)
(1990): Todd PA+, *Drugs* 39, 110
Erythema (sic) (circumscribed)
(1987): Predel HG+, *Am J Cardiol* 59, 143D
Erythema multiforme (<1%)
Exanthems
(1990): Todd PA+, *Drugs* 39, 110
Flushing
(1988): Zabludowski J+, *Curr Med Res Opin* 11, 93
(1987): Kaneko Y+, *Am J Cardiol* 59, 86D
Lichen planus pemphigoides
(1997): Ogg GS+, *Br J Dermatol* 136, 412

Pemphigus (<1%)
(1996): Vignes S+, *Br J Dermatol* 135, 657
Pemphigus foliaceus
(2000): Ong CS+, *Australas J Dermatol* 41(4), 242
Photosensitivity (<1%)
(2000): Wagner SN+, *Contact Dermatitis* 43(4), 245 (with hydrochlorothiazide)
(1994): Shelley WB+, *Cutis* 53, 39 (observation)
(1993): Shelley WB+, *Cutis* 52, 81 (observation)
Pruritus (<1%)
(1990): Todd PA+, *Drugs* 39, 110
(1987): Predel HG+, *Am J Cardiol* 59, 143D
(1987): Walter U+, *Am J Cardiol* 59, 125D
Purpura (<1%)
Rash (sic) (<1%)
(1990): Janka HU+, *Arzneimittelforschung* (German) 40, 432
(1990): Todd PA+, *Drugs* 39, 110
(1987): Ball SG+, *Am J Cardiol* 59, 23D
(1987): Walter U+, *Am J Cardiol* 59, 125D
Urticaria (<1%)
Vasculitis (<1%)

### Hair

Hair – alopecia (1–10%)

### Other

Ageusia (<1%)
Anaphylactoid reactions (<1%)
Cough
(2001): Adigun AQ+, *West Afr J Med* 20(1), 46–7
(2001): Lee SC+, *Hypertension* 38(2), 166
Dysgeusia (<1%)
(1990): Todd PA+, *Drugs* 39, 110
Hypersensitivity (<1%)
Paresthesias (<1%)
(1987): Walter U+, *Am J Cardiol* 59, 125D
Sialorrhea (<1%)
Tinnitus
Tremors (<1%)
Xerostomia (<1%)

## RANITIDINE

**Trade name:** Zantac (GSK)
**Other common trade names:** *Apo-Ranitidine; Axoban; Azantac; Nu-Ranit; Raniben; Raniplex; Ranisen; Sostril; Zantab; Zantac-C; Zantic*
**Indications:** Duodenal ulcer
**Category:** Histamine $H_2$-receptor antagonist; antiulcer drug
**Half-life:** 2.5 hours
**Clinically important, potentially hazardous interactions with:** alfentanil, fentanyl

**Note:** Ranitidine is present in mother's milk in relatively large amounts. It is thought that gynecomastia develops as a result of ranitidine blocking the androgen receptors at the end organs

### *Reactions*

### Skin

Acute generalized exanthematous pustulosis (AGEP)
(1996): Sawhney RA+, *Int J Dermatol* 35, 826
Angioedema (<1%)
Contact dermatitis
(1988): Romaguera C+, *Contact Dermatitis* 18, 177
(1987): Alomar A+, *Contact Dermatitis* 17, 54
(1984): Goh CL+, *Contact Dermatitis* 4, 252
(1983): Rycroft RJ, *Contact Dermatitis* 9, 456 (occupational)
Eczematous eruption (sic)
(1992): Juste S+, *Contact Dermatitis* 27, 339
(1988): Romaguera C+, *Contact Dermatitis* 18, 177
Erythema multiforme
Exanthems
(1993): Devuyst O+, *Acta Clin Belg* 48, 109
(1989): Grant SM+, *Drugs* 37, 801
(1988): Haboubi N+, *Br Med J Clin Res Ed* 296, 897
(1984): Khandheria BK, *JAMA* 253, 3252
Fixed eruption
(1990): Black AK+, *Br J Dermatol* 123, 277
Lichenoid eruption
(1996): Horiuchi Y+, *J Dermatol* 23, 510
Lupus erythematosus
(1999): Crowson AN+, *J Cutan Pathol* 26, 95 (subacute cutaneous)
Photosensitivity
(2000): Kondo S+, *Dermatology* 201, 71
(1995): Todd P+, *Clin Exp Dermatol* 20, 146
Pruritus (<1%)
(1985): Classen M+, *Dtsch Med Wochenschr* (German) 110, 628
Psoriasis
(1991): Andersen M, *Ugeskr Laeger* (Danish) 153, 132
Purpura
(1989): Gafter U+, *Gastroenterol* 84, 560
(1987): Gafter U+, *Ann Intern Med* 106, 477
Pustular eruption
Rash (sic) (1–10%)
(1988): Haboubi N+, *Br Med J Clin Res Ed* 296, 897
Stevens–Johnson syndrome
(2001): Lin C-C+, *Gastroenterol Hepatol* 16, 481
Toxic epidermal necrolysis
(2000): Velez A+, *J Am Acad Dermatol* 42, 305
(1995): Miralles ES+, *J Am Acad Dermatol* 32, 133
Urticaria
(1997): Sancho Calabuig A+, *Aten Primaria* 20, 396
(1989): Grant SM+, *Drugs* 37, 801
(1984): Khandheria BK, *JAMA* 253, 3252
(1983): Picardo M+, *Contact Dermatitis* 4, 327
Vasculitis
(1988): Haboubi N+, *BMJ* 296, 897
Xerosis

### Hair

Hair – alopecia
(1995): Shelley WB+, *Cutis* 55, 148 (observation)

### Other

Anaphylactoid reactions
(1993): Lazaro M+, *Allergy* 48, 385
(1993): Powell JA+, *Anaesth Intensive Care* 21, 702
Dysgeusia
(1985): Classen M+, *Dtsch Med Wochenschr* (German) 110, 628
Gynecomastia (>1%)
(1994): Garcia-Rodriguez LA+, *BMJ* 308, 503
(1984): Bianchi Porro G+, *It J Gastroenterol* (Italian) 16, 56
(1982): Tosi S+, *Lancet* 2, 160
Hypersensitivity
(1996): Gonzalo-Garijo MA+, *Allergy* 51, 659
Injection-site burning
Injection-site pain
Myalgia
Porphyria
(1988): Bhadoria DP+, *J Assoc Physicians India* 36, 295
(1988): Pratap D+, *J Assoc Physicians India* 36, 237
(1988): Tripathi SK, *J Assoc Physicians India* 36, 680
Pseudolymphoma
(1995): Magro CM+, *J Am Acad Dermatol* 32, 419

# RAPACURONIUM

**Trade name:** Raplon (Organon)
**Indications:** To facilitate tracheal intubation
**Category:** Anesthesia; adjunct; nondepolarizing neuromuscular blocking agent
**Half-life:** ~22 Days
**Clinically important, potentially hazardous interactions with:** aminoglycosides, cyclopropane, enflurane, halothane, isoflurane, methoxyflurane, piperacillin

### *Reactions*

#### Skin

Diaphoresis (~1%)
Edema (~1%)
Erythema
(1999): Abouleish EI+, *Br J Anaesth* 83, 862
Exanthems (>1%)
Flushing
Non-inflammatory swelling (sic)
Peripheral edema (~1%)
Pruritus
Purpura (~1%)
Rash (sic) (~1%)
Urticaria (~1%)

#### Other

Hypesthesia (~1%)
Injection-site pain (~1%)
Injection-site reactions (sic) (~1%)
(1999): Onrust SV+, *Drugs* 58, 887
Myalgia (~1%)
Sialorrhea (~1%)
(2000): Meakin GH+, *Anesthesiology* 92, 1002
Thrombophlebitis (~1%)
Tooth disorder (sic) (~1%)

# RED CLOVER

**Scientific name:** *Trifolium pratense*
**Other common names:** Coumestrol; Cow Clover; Cowgrass; Meadow Clover; Menoflavon (Pascoe); Pavine Clover; Phytoestrogen; Promensil (Novogen); Purple Clover; Three-Leaved Grass; Trefoil; Trifolium Flower; Wild Clover
**Family:** Leguminosae
**Purported indications:** Alternative to HRT for treatment of menopausal symptoms such as hot flashes, muscle spasms, hypercholesterolemia, breast pain, osteoporosis
**Other uses:** Diuretic, expectorant, mild antispasmodic, sedative, blood purifier, bladder infections, liver disorders. Ointment for acne, eczema, psoriasis and other rashes

### *Reactions*

#### Skin

Mutagen
(2001): Domon OE+, *Mutat Res* 474(1), 129

**Note:** Red clover contains phytoestrogens that bind to estrogen and progesterone receptors, potentially adversely affecting breast tissue

# REPAGLINIDE

**Trade name:** Prandin (Novo Nordisk)
**Indications:** Non-insulin dependent diabetes type II
**Category:** Antidiabetic
**Half-life:** 1 hour

### *Reactions*

#### Skin

Allergy (sic) (2%)

#### Other

Anaphylactoid reactions (<1%)
Paresthesias (3%)
Tooth disorder (sic)

# RESERPINE

**Trade names:** Resa; Ser-Ap-Es (Novartis); Serpalan; Serpasil (Ciba); Serpatabs
**Other common trade names:** *Anserpin; Inerpin; Novo-Reserpine; Reserfia; Sedaraupin; Serpasol; Tionsera*
**Indications:** Hypertension
**Category:** Nondiuretic antihypertensive; *Rauwolfia* alkaloid
**Half-life:** 50–100 hours

Ser-Ap-Es is reserpine, hydralazine and hydrochlorothiazide

### *Reactions*

#### Skin

Ankle edema
Bullous eruption
(1994): Watanabe S+, *Reg Anesth* 19, 59 (following intravenous block)
Edema
Exanthems
Flushing
Lupus erythematosus (exacerbation)
(1963): Rivero I+, *Arthritis Rheum* 6, 293
Peripheral edema (1–10%)
Pruritus
Purpura
Rash (sic) (<1%)
Toxic epidermal necrolysis
(1979): Kats GL+, *Vrach Delo* (Russian) November, 97
Urticaria

#### Other

Gynecomastia
Parkinsonism
Sialorrhea
Xerostomia (>10%)

# RETEPLASE

**Synonyms:** recombinant plasminogen activator; r-PA
**Trade name:** Retavase (Centocor)
**Indications:** Acute myocardial infarction
**Category:** Tissue plasminogen activator; thrombolytic agent
**Half-life:** 13–16 minutes
**Clinically important, potentially hazardous interactions with:** abciximab, aspirin, bivalirudin, dipyridamole, piperacillin, salicylates

### *Reactions*

## Skin
Allergic reactions (sic) (<1%)
Bleeding
Ecchymoses
Purpura

## Other
Anaphylactoid reactions (<1%)
Injection-site bleeding (1–10%)

# RIBAVIRIN

**Synonyms:** RTCA; tribavirin
**Trade names:** Rebetol; Rebetron (Schering); Virazole (ICN)
**Other common trade names:** *Viramid; Virazid*
**Indications:** Respiratory syncytial viral infections
**Category:** Antiviral (against respiratory syncytial virus [RSV])
**Half-life:** 24 hours
**Clinically important, potentially hazardous interactions with:** zidovudine

Rebetron is interferon and ribavirin

### *Reactions*

## Skin
Erythema multiforme
(1960): Heijer A+, *Acta Derm Venereol* (Stockh) 40, 35
Exanthems
(2002): Farady KK, Austin, TX* (from Internet) (observation)
(1990): Janai HK+, *Pediatr Infect Dis J* 9, 209 (0.5%)
Flu-like syndrome (sic) (10%)*
Grover's disease
(2000): Antunes I+, *Br J Dermatol* 142, 1257
Herpes simplex (activation)
Photosensitivity
(2002): Castillo R+, *World Congress Dermatol* Poster, 0091
(1999): Stryjek-Kaminska D+, *Am J Gastroenterol* 94, 1686
Pruritus (>10%)*
(1999): Stryjek-Kaminska D+, *Am J Gastroenterol* 94, 1686
Rash (sic) (<10%)*
(2001): Karim A+, *Am J Med Sci* 322(4), 233
Sarcoidosis
(2002): Cogrel O+, *Br J Dermatol* 146(2), 320 *
(2002): Wendling J+, *Arch Dermatol* 138, 546 * (2 cases)
Urticaria
(1999): Stryjek-Kaminska D+, *Am J Gastroenterol* 94, 1686

## Hair
Hair – alopecia (>10%)*
(2001): Zucker DM+, *Gastroenterol Nurs* 24(4), 192 (with interferon alpha)

## Other
Arthralgia
(2001): Zucker DM+, *Gastroenterol Nurs* 24(4), 192 *
Cough
(2001): Karim A+, *Am J Med Sci* 322(4), 233
Depression
(2001): Karim A+, *Am J Med Sci* 322(4), 233
Dysgeusia (1–10%)*
Myalgia (>10%)*

***Note:** The reaction patterns with an asterisk occurred while receiving combination therapy with interferon alpha 2-B

# RIBOFLAVIN

**Synonyms:** Lactoflavin; Vitamin $B_2$; Vitamin G
**Trade name:** Riobin
**Indications:** Riboflavin deficiency
**Category:** Water-soluble nutritional supplement
**Half-life:** 66–84 minutes

### *Reactions*

## Skin
Acne
(1964): Fegeler F, *Arch Klin Exp Dermatol* (German) 219, 335
Allergic reactions (sic)
(1975): Soloshenko EN+, *Sov Med* (Russian) October, 141
Angioedema
(1972): Kuokkanen K, *Acta Allergol* 27, 407
Ichthyosis
(1985): Spirov G+, *Dermatol Venereol* (Sofia) 24, 50
Urticaria
(1972): Kuokkanen K, *Acta Allergol* 27, 407

## Other
Anaphylactoid reactions
(2001): Ou LS+, *Ann Allergy Asthma Immunol* 87(5), 430

# RIFABUTIN

**Trade name:** Mycobutin (Pharmacia & Upjohn)
**Indications:** Prevention of disseminated *Mycobacterium avium* infection
**Category:** Antitubercular antibiotic
**Half-life:** 45 hours
**Clinically important, potentially hazardous interactions with:** amiodarone, anisindione, anticoagulants, corticosteroids, cyclosporine, dapsone, dicumarol, midazolam, oral contraceptives, ritonavir, tacrolimus, voriconazole

### *Reactions*

## Skin
Lupus erythematosus
(1997): Berning SE+, *Lancet* 349, 1521
Pigmentation
(1995): Smith JF+, *Clin Infect Dis* 21, 1515
Rash (sic) (11%)
Urticaria

## Other
Ageusia
(1993): Morris JT+, *Ann Intern Med* 119, 171

Discolored sputum (sic)
Dysgeusia (3%)
Myalgia (2%)
Paresthesias (<1%)
Polyarthalgia-arthritis syndrome
(2000): Curino C+, *Presse Med* 29(28), 1563

# RIFAMPIN

**Synonym:** rifampicin
**Trade names:** Rifadin (Aventis); Rimactane (Geneva)
**Other common trade names:** *Abrifam; Corifam; Ramicin; Rifaldin; Rifamed; Rimpin; Rimycin; Rofact*
**Indications:** Tuberculosis
**Category:** Tuberculostatic and antileprotic antibiotic
**Half-life:** 3–5 hours
**Clinically important, potentially hazardous interactions with:** amiodarone, amprenavir, anisindione, antacids, anticoagulants, atovaquone, corticosteroids, cyclosporine, dapsone, delavirdine, dicumarol, digoxin, halothane, imatinib, isoniazid, itraconazole, ketoconazole, midazolam, nelfinavir, nifedipine, oral contraceptives, protease inhibitors, pyrazinamide, ritonavir, saquinavir, tacrolimus, triazolam, voriconazole, warfarin

## *Reactions*

### Skin

Acne
(1990): Mimouni A+, *Drug Intell Clin Pharm* 24, 947
(1985): Holdiness MR, *Int J Dermatol* 24, 280
(1974): Nwokolo U, *BMJ* 3, 473 (1–5%) (only men)
Allergic reactions (sic)
(1973): Nessi R+, *Scand J Respir Dis* 84, 15
Angioedema
(1989): Holdiness MR, *Med Toxicol Adv Drug Exp* 4, 444 (72%)
Bullous eruption (<1%)
Contact dermatitis
(1991): Guerra L+, *Contact Dermatitis* 25, 328
(1986): Holdiness MR, *Contact Dermatitis* 15, 282
(1986): Milpied B+, *Contact Dermatitis* 14, 252
Contact urticaria
(1987): Grob JJ+, *Contact Dermatitis* 16, 284
Cutaneous side effects (sic)
(1985): Holdiness MR, *Int J Dermatol* 24, 280 (5%)
Diaphoresis (1–10%)
Erythema multiforme (<1%)
(1990): Mimouni A+, *Drug Intell Clin Pharm* 24, 947
(1988): Hira SK+, *J Am Acad Dermatol* 19, 451 (in AIDS patients)
(1979): Nigam P+, *Lepr India* 51, 249
(1977): Nyirenda R+, *BMJ* 2, 1189
Exanthems (1–5%)
(1998): Zimmerli W+, *JAMA* 279, 1537
(1989): Wurtz RM+, *Lancet* 1, 955 (in AIDS patients)
(1985): Holdiness MR, *Int J Dermatol* 24, 280
(1976): Mangi RJ, *N Engl J Med* 294, 113 (3%)
(1971): Esposito R+, *Lancet* 2, 491 (1–5%)
(1971): Poole G+, *BMJ* 3, 343 (1–5%)
Exfoliative dermatitis
(1987): Goldin HM+, *Ann Intern Med* 107, 789
Facial edema
Fixed eruption
(2001): Goel A+, *Indian J Lepr* 73(2), 159 (bullous, necrotizing)
(2000): Jaiswal AK+, *Lepr Rev* 71, 217
(1998): John SS, *Lepr Rev* 69, 397
(1993): Pavithran K, *Indian J Lepr* 65, 339
(1990): Mimouni A+, *Drug Intell Clin Pharm* 24, 947
(1985): Naik RPC+, *Indian J Lepr* 57, 648
Flushing
(1995): Hoss DM+, *Arch Dermatol* 131, 647
(1993): Tsankov NK+, *Int J Dermatol* 32, 401 (passim)
(1990): Mimouni A+, *Drug Intell Clin Pharm* 24, 947
(1985): Holdiness MR, *Int J Dermatol* 24, 280
(1982): Girling DJ, *Drugs* 23, 56 (5%)
(1976): Mangi RJ, *N Engl J Med* 294, 113 (7%)
(1972): Girling HM+, *BMJ* 1, 765
(1971): Girling DJ+, *BMJ* 4, 231
Linear IgA bullous dermatosis
(2002): Cohen LM+, *J Am Acad Dermatol* 46, S32 (passim)
(1994): Kuechle MK+, *J Am Acad Dermatol* 30, 187
Lupus erythematosus
(2001): Patel GK+, *Clin Exp Dermatol* 26(3), 260
Pemphigus
(1995): Hoss DM+, *Arch Dermatol* 131, 647
(1993): Tsankov NK+, *Int J Dermatol* 32, 401 (passim)
(1987): Honeybourne D+, *Br J Clin Pract* 41, 937
(1986): Miyagawa S+, *Br J Dermatol* 114, 729 (exacerbation)
(1984): Lee CW+, *Br J Dermatol* 111, 619 (foliaceus)
(1982): Ruocco V+, *Arch Dermatol Res* 274, 123
(1976): Gange RW+, *Br J Dermatol* 95, 445
Pruritus (<1%)
(1995): Hoss DM+, *Arch Dermatol* 131, 647
(1995): Walker-Renard P, *Ann Pharmacother* 29, 267
(1993): Tsankov NK+, *Int J Dermatol* 32, 401 (passim)
(1989): Holdiness MR, *Med Toxicol Adv Drug Exp* 4, 444 (62%)
(1987): Goldin HM+, *Ann Intern Med* 107, 789
(1972): Girling HM+, *BMJ* 1, 765
(1971): Girling DJ+, *BMJ* 4, 231
Purpura
(1980): Miescher PA+, *Clin Haematol* 9, 505
(1972): Girling HM+, *BMJ* 1, 765 (0.5–1%)
(1971): Esposito R+, *Lancet* 2, 491
(1971): Girling DJ+, *BMJ* 4, 231 (0.5–1%)
(1971): Poole G+, *BMJ* 3, 343
(1970): Blajckman MA+, *BMJ* 3, 24
Rash (sic) (1–5%)
(2000): Gordin F+, *JAMA* 283, 1445
(1995): Chaisson RE, *Infections in Medicine* 12, 48
Red man syndrome
(1995): Dayavathi+, *J Assoc Physicians India* 43, 724
(1992): Gupta M+, *Indian Pediatr* 29, 1315
(1989): Holdiness MR, *Med Toxicol Adv Drug Exp* 4, 444
(1988): Gross DJ+, *Cutis* 42, 175 (red/orange person syndrome)
(1986): Bolan G+, *Pediatrics* 77, 633
(1980): Meisel S+, *Ann Intern Med* 92, 262
(1975): Newton RW+, *Scott Med J* 20, 55
Stevens–Johnson syndrome
(1994): Marfatia YS, *Arch Dermatol* 130, 1074 (passim)
(1993): Tsankov NK+, *Int J Dermatol* 32, 401 (passim)
(1988): Hira SK+, *J Am Acad Dermatol* 19, 451 (in AIDS patients)
(1977): Nyirenda R+, *BMJ* 2, 1189
Toxic epidermal necrolysis
(1996): Blum L+, *J Am Acad Dermatol* 34, 1088
(1994): Marfatia YS, *Arch Dermatol* 130, 1074 (passim)
(1990): Prazuck T+, *Scand J Infect Dis* 22, 629
(1987): Guillaume JC+, *Arch Dermatol* 123, 1166
(1987): Okano M+, *J Am Acad Dermatol* 17, 303
Urticaria
(1997): Sharma VK+, *Lepr Rev* 68, 331
(1987): Gupta CM+, *Lepr Rev* 58, 308
(1985): Holdiness MR, *Int J Dermatol* 24, 280
(1972): Girling HM+, *BMJ* 1, 765
(1971): Girling DJ+, *BMJ* 4, 231
Vasculitis
(1995): Hoss DM+, *Arch Dermatol* 131, 647

(1990): Chan CH+, *Tubercle* 71, 297
(1989): Iredale JP+, *Chest* 96, 215

### Hair

Hair – alopecia areata
(2001): McMillen R+, *J Am Acad Dermatol* 44(1), 142 (in 2 sisters)

### Other

Anaphylactoid reactions
(1999): Garcia F+, *Allergy* 54, 527 (to topical)
(1999): Magnan A+, *J Allergy Clin Immunol* 103, 954
(1998): Erel F+, *Ann Allergy Asthma Immunol* 81, 257
(1995): Cardot E+, *J Allergy Clin Immunol* 95, 1
(1989): Piazza I, *Allergologia* 12, 96 (suppl)
(1989): Wurtz RM+, *Lancet* 1, 955 (in AIDS patients)
Death
(2002): Medinger A, *Chest* 121(5), 1710 (with pyrazinamide)
(2001): No authors, *Can Commun Dis Rep* 27(13), 114 (with pyrazinamide)
(2001): No authors, *JAMA* 286(12), 1445 (with pyrazinamide)
(2001): No authors, *MMWR Morb Mortal Wkly Rep* 50(34), 733 (with pyrazinamide)
Glossodynia
Injection-site erythema
(1988): Fan-Havard P+, *Clin Pharm* 7, 616
Mucosal bleeding (sic)
(1971): Poole G+, *BMJ* 3, 343
Myalgia
Myopathy
Oral mucosal eruption
(1971): Poole G+, *BMJ* 3, 343
Porphyria
(1985): Holdiness MR, *Int J Dermatol* 24, 280
(1982): Igual JP+, *Presse Med* (French) 11, 2846
Porphyria cutanea tarda
(1980): Millar JW, *Br J Dis Chest* 74, 405
Serum sickness
(1994): Parra FM+, *Ann Allergy* 73, 123
Stomatitis (<1%)

## RIFAPENTINE

**Trade name:** Priftin (Aventis)
**Indications:** Tuberculosis
**Category:** Antitubercular antibiotic
**Half-life:** 14–17 hours
**Clinically important, potentially hazardous interactions with:** amiodarone, anisindione, anticoagulants, corticosteroids, cyclosporine, dicumarol, ritonavir, tacrolimus, warfarin

#### *Reactions*

### Skin

Acne (1–10%)
Peripheral edema (<1%)
Pigmentation (<1%)
Pruritus (1–10%)
Purpura (<1%)
Rash (sic) (1–10%)
Urticaria (<1%)

## RILUZOLE

**Synonym:** Rilutek (Aventis)
**Indications:** Amyotrophic lateral sclerosis (ALS)
**Category:** Amyotrophic lateral sclerosis (ALS) agent
**Half-life:** no data

#### *Reactions*

### Skin

Candidiasis
Cellulitis
Chills
Eczema (sic) (1.6%)
Edema
Exfoliative dermatitis
Facial edema
Granulomas (sic)
Peripheral edema (3%)
Petechiae
Photosensitivity
Pruritus
Purpura

### Hair

Hair – alopecia (1%)

### Other

Dysgeusia
Glossitis
Gum hemorrhage
Hypesthesia
Injection-site reactions (sic)
Mastodynia
Oral candidiasis (0.6%)
Paresthesias
Phlebitis (1%)
Stomatitis (1%)
Tongue discoloration
Tooth disorder (sic) (1%)
Vaginal candidiasis
Xerostomia (3.5%)

## RIMANTADINE

**Trade name:** Flumadine (Forest)
**Other common trade name:** *Ruflual*
**Indications:** Various infections caused by influenza virus
**Category:** Oral antiviral
**Half-life:** 25–30 hours

#### *Reactions*

### Skin

Edema (pedal) (1–10%)
Rash (sic) (<1%)
(1989): Hayden FG+, *N Engl J Med* 321, 1696 (1%)

### Other

Ageusia (<0.3%)
Dysgeusia
Hypesthesia
Parosmia (<0.3%)
Stomatitis
Xerostomia (1.6%)

## RISEDRONATE

**Trade name:** Actonel (Procter & Gamble)
**Indications:** Paget's disease of bone, postmenopausal osteoporosis
**Category:** Biphosphonate bone resorption inhibitor
**Half-life:** terminal: 220 hours

### *Reactions*

#### Skin

Ecchymoses (4.3%)
Edema
Flu-like syndrome (sic) (9.8%)
Peripheral edema (8.2%)
Pruritus (3.0%)
Rash (sic) (11.5%)

#### Other

Glossitis (<1%)
Myalgia (6.6%)
Paresthesias (2.1%)
Tendon disorder (sic) (3.0%)
Tooth disorder (sic) (2.1%)

## RISPERIDONE

**Trade name:** Risperdal (Janssen)
**Indications:** Psychotic disorders
**Category:** Antipsychotic
**Half-life:** 3–30 hours
**Clinically important, potentially hazardous interactions with:** clozapine

### *Reactions*

#### Skin

Acne (<1%)
Allergic reactions (sic) (<1%)
(1998): Terao T+, *J Clin Psychiatry* 59, 82
Angioedema
(2001): Kores Plesnicar B+, *Eur Psychiatry* 16(8), 506
(1995): Cooney C+, *BMJ* 311, 1204
Bullous eruption (<1%)
Bullous pemphigoid
(1996): Wijeratne C+, *Am J Psychiatry* 153, 735
Dermatitis (sic)
Diaphoresis (<1%)
Edema
(2001): Ravasia S, *Can J Psychiatry* 46(5), 453
(1996): Baldassano CF+, *J Clin Psychiatry* 57, 422 (generalized)
Exfoliative dermatitis (0.1–1%)
Flushing (<1%)
(2001): Masi G+, *J Child Neurol* 16(6), 395
Furunculosis (<1%)
Hyperkeratosis (sic) (<1%)
Hypohidrosis (<1%)
Lichenoid eruption (<1%)
Peripheral edema
(2001): Hwang JP+, *J Clin Psychopharmacol* 21(6), 583 (16.4%)
Photosensitivity (1–10%)
(1998): Almond DS+, *Postgrad Med J* 74, 252
Pigmentation (1%)
Pruritus (<1%)
Psoriasis (<1%)
Purpura (<1%)
Rash (sic) (5%)
Seborrhea
Skin irritation (sic)
(2002): McCracken JT+, *N Engl J Med* 347(5), 314 (22%)
Ulceration (<1%)
Urticaria (<0.1%)
Warts (<1%)
Xerosis (2%)

#### Hair

Hair – alopecia (<1%)
(2000): Mercke Y+, *Ann Clin Psychiatry* 12, 35
Hair – hypertrichosis (<1%)

#### Other

Anaphylactoid reactions
Dysgeusia (<1%)
Dysphagia
(2001): Nair S+, *Gen Hosp Psychiatry* 23(4), 231
Galactorrhea (1–10%)
(2001): Gupta S+, *J Am Acad Dermatol* 40(5), 504
(1998): Popli A+, *Ann Clin Psychiatry* 10, 31
Gingivitis (<1%)
Gynecomastia (1–10%)
(1999): Benazzi F, *Pharmacopsychiatry* 32, 41
Hypesthesia (<1%)
Mastodynia (<1%)
Muscle rigidity
(2002): McCracken JT+, *N Engl J Med* 347(5), 314 (10%)
Myalgia (<1%)
Neuroleptic malignant syndrome
(2002): Aboraya A+, *W V Med J* 98(2), 63 (with olanzapine)
Paresthesias (<1%)
Parkinsonism
(2001): Takahashi H+, *Clin Neuropharmacol* 24(6), 358
Priapism (1–10%)
(2002): Freudenreich O, *J Clin Psychiatry* 63(3), 249 (with citalopram)
(2001): Compton MT+, *J Clin Psychiatry* 62(5), 363 (passim)
Rhabdomyolysis
(2002): Giner V+, *J Intern Med* 251(2), 177 (with cerivastatin)
(1996): Meltzer HY+, *Neuropsychopharmacology* 15(4), 395
Sialopenia (5%)
Sialorrhea (2%)
(2001): Gajwani P+, *Psychosomatics* 42(3), 276
Stomatitis (<1%)
Stuttering
(2001): Lee HJ+, *J Clin Psychopharmacol* 21(1), 115
Thrombophlebitis (<1%)
Tinnitus
Tongue edema (<1%)
Tongue pigmentation (<1%)
Tremors
(2002): McCracken JT+, *N Engl J Med* 347(5), 314 (14%)
Xerostomia (1–10%)
(2002): McCracken JT+, *N Engl J Med* 347(5), 314 (18%)
(2001): Hodge CH+, *Vet Hum Toxicol* 43(6), 339 (2 cases)
(2001): Mullen J+, *Clin Ther* 23(11), 1839 (6.9%)

## RITODRINE

**Trade names:** Pre-Par; Yutopar (AstraZeneca)
**Indications:** Preterm labor
**Category:** Tocolytic (uterine relaxant); adrenergic agonist
**Half-life:** 1.3–12 hours

### *Reactions*

#### Skin

Chills (3–10%)
Diaphoresis (1–3%)
(1978): Hauser GA, *Ther Umsch* (German) 35, 422 (3–14%)
Erythema (10–15%)
Erythema multiforme
(1988): Beitner O+, *Drug Intell Clin Pharm* 22, 724
Exanthems
Pustular eruption (in a pregnant woman with psoriasis)
(1998): D'Incan M+, *J Eur Acad Dermatol Venereol* 11, 91
Rash (sic) (1–3%)
(2001): Yamada T+, *Arch Gynecol Obstet* 264(4), 218
Urticaria
Vasculitis
(1991): Bosnyak S+, *Am J Obstet Gyn* 165, 427

#### Other

Anaphylactoid reactions (1–3%)
Tremors (>10%)

## RITONAVIR

**Trade name:** Norvir (Abbott)
**Indications:** HIV infection
**Category:** Antiretroviral; protease inhibitor*
**Half-life:** 3–5 hours
**Clinically important, potentially hazardous interactions with:** alfentanil, alprazolam, amiodarone, bepridil, bupropion, chlordiazepoxide, clozapine, cyclosporine, diazepam, dihydroergotamine, ergot alkaloids, estazolam, fentanyl, flecainide, flurazepam, halazepam, ketoconazole, meperidine, methysergide, midazolam, nifedipine, oral contraceptives, phenytoin, pimozide, piroxicam, propafenone, propoxyphene, quazepam, quinidine, rifabutin, rifampin, rifapentine, saquinavir, sildenafil, simvastatin, **St John's wort**, triazolam, zolpidem

### *Reactions*

#### Skin

Acne (<2%)
Allergic reactions (sic) (<2%)
Angioedema
Bullous eruption (<2%)
Cheilitis (<2%)
(2000): Bonfanti P+, *J Acquir Immune Defic Syndr* 23(3), 236
Contact dermatitis (<2%)
Diaphoresis (1–10%)
Ecchymoses (<2%)
Eczema (sic) (<2%)
Edema
Exanthems (<2%)
(1997): Bachmeyer C+, *Dermatology* 195, 301 (2 HIV patients)
Facial edema (<2%)
Folliculitis (<2%)
Granulomas
(2002): Kawsar M+, *Int J STD AIDS* 13(4), 273
Peripheral edema (<2%)
Photosensitivity (<2%)
Pruritus (<2%)
Psoriasis (<2%)
Rash (sic) (1–10%)
Seborrhea (<2%)
Stevens–Johnson syndrome
Urticaria (<2%)
Xerosis (<2%)

#### Nails

Nails – ingrown toenails
(2001): James CW+, *Ann Pharmacother* 35(7), 881 (with indinavir)

#### Other

Ageusia (<2%)
Anaphylactoid reactions
Dysgeusia (10.3%)
Gingivitis (<2%)
Gynecomastia
(2001): Manfredi R+, *Ann Pharmacother* 35(4), 438
(2000): Bonfanti P+, *J Acquir Immune Defic Syndr* 23(3), 236
Hyperesthesia (<2%)
Lipodystrophy
(2002): Reid S, *Can Adv Drug Reaction Newsletter* 12, 5
(2001): van der Valk M+, *AIDS* 15(7), 847
Myalgia (1–10%)
Oral candidiasis (<2%)
Oral ulceration (<2%)
Paresthesias (2.6%)
(2001): Scully C+, *Oral Dis* 7(4), 205 (circumoral) (passim)
Parosmia (<2%)
Perioral parasthesias
(2001): McMahon D+, *Antivir Ther* 6(2), 105
Thrombophlebitis
(2000): Bonfanti P+, *J Acquir Immune Defic Syndr* 23(3), 236
Xerostomia (<2%)

***Note:** Protease inhibitors cause dyslipidemia which includes elevated triglycerides and cholesterol and redistribution of body fat centrally to produce the so-called "protease paunch," breast enlargement, facial atrophy, and "buffalo hump"

## RITUXIMAB

**Trade name:** Rituxan (IDEC)
**Indications:** Non-Hodgkin's lymphoma
**Category:** Monoclonal antibody; antineoplastic
**Half-life:** 60 hours (after first infusion)

### *Reactions*

#### Skin

Angioedema (>10%)
Chills (10%)
Diaphoresis
Exanthems (10%)
Flushing (<5%)
Peripheral edema
Pruritus (10%)
Rash (sic) (10%)
Urticaria (10%)

### Other
Cytomegalovirus infection (reactivation)
(2001): Suzan F+, *N Engl J Med* 345, 1000
Death
(2001): Huhn D+, *Blood* 98(5), 1326
(2001): Suzan F+, *N Engl J Med* 345(13), 1000
Infusion-site reactions (sic)
(2001): Stasi R+, *Blood* 98(4), 952
(2001): Wood AM, *Am J Health Syst Pharm* 58(3), 215
Injection-site reactions (sic)
Myalgia (7%)
Serum sickness
(2001): D'Arcy CA+, *Arthritis Rheum* 44, 1717

## RIVASTIGMINE

**Trade name:** Exelon (Novartis)
**Indications:** Alzheimer's disease and dementia
**Category:** Acetylcholinesterase inhibitor; cholinergic agent
**Half-life:** 1–2 hours
**Clinically important, potentially hazardous interactions with:** galantamine

#### *Reactions*

### Skin
Allergy (sic) (~1%)
Bullous eruption (~1%)
Cellulitis (~1%)
Clammy skin (~1%)
Contact dermatitis (~1%)
Diaphoresis (10%)
Edema (~1%)
Exanthems (~1%)
(2001): Monastero R+, *Am J Med* 111(7), 583
Exfoliative dermatitis (~1%)
Facial edema (~1%)
Flushing (~1%)
Herpes simplex (~1%)
Hot flashes (~1%)
Infections (sic) (~2%)
Periorbital edema (~1%)
Peripheral edema (~2%)
Psoriasis (~1%)
Purpura (~1%)
Rash (sic) (~2%)
Ulceration (~1%)
Urticaria (~1%)

### Hair
Hair – alopecia (~1%)

### Other
Ageusia (~1%)
Dysgeusia (~1%)
Foetor ex ore (halitosis) (~1%)
Gingivitis (~1%)
Glossitis (~1%)
Hypesthesia (~1%)
Mastodynia (~1%)
Myalgia (20%)
Paresthesias (~1%)
Sialorrhea (~1%)
Thrombophlebitis (<2%)
Tremors (4%)
Ulcerative stomatitis (~1%)
Vaginitis (~1%)
Xerostomia (~1%)

## RIZATRIPTAN

**Synonym:** MK462
**Trade name:** Maxalt (Merck)
**Indications:** Migraine
**Category:** Antimigraine; serotonin agonist
**Half-life:** 2–3 hours
**Clinically important, potentially hazardous interactions with:** dihydroergotamine, ergot-containing drugs, isocarboxazid, MAO inhibitors, methysergide, naratriptan, phenelzine, sibutramine, sumatriptan, tranylcypromine, zolmitriptan

#### *Reactions*

### Skin
Chills (<1%)
Diaphoresis (<1%)
Facial edema (<1%)
Flushing (1–10%)
Hot flashes (1–10%)
Pruritus (<1%)

### Other
Hypesthesia
Myalgia (<1%)
Paresthesias
Tongue edema
Xerostomia (<5%)

## ROFECOXIB

**Trade name:** Vioxx (Merck)
**Indications:** Osteoarthritis, acute pain
**Category:** Nonsteroidal anti-inflammatory (Cox-2 inhibitor); analgesic
**Half-life:** 17 hours
**Clinically important, potentially hazardous interactions with:** anisindione, anticoagulants, dicumarol, lithium, methotrexate, warfarin

#### *Reactions*

### Skin
Abrasion (<2%)
Allergy (sic) (<2%)
Angioedema
(2001): Kelkar PS+, *J Rheumatol* 28(11), 2553
(2000): Medicines Control Agency and Committee on Safety of Medicines Reports (5 cases)
Atopic dermatitis (<2%)
Basal cell carcinoma (<2%)
Bullous eruption (<2%)
Cellulitis (<2%)
Contact dermatitis (<2%)
Diaphoresis (<2%)
Edema (3.7%)

(2000): Medicines Control Agency and Committee on Safety of Medicines Reports (101 cases)
Erythema (<2%)
(2000): Wright WL, Castro Valley, CA (from Internet) (observation) (after the second day)
Exanthems
(2000): Blumenthal HL, Beachwood, OH (personal case) (observation)
Fixed eruption
(2002): Nederost ST+, *Cutis* 70, 125
(2001): Kaur C+, *Dermatology* 203(4), 351 (with sulfonamides)
(2000): Conners RC, Greenwich, CT (personal communication)
Flu-like syndrome (sic) (2.9%)
Flushing (<2%)
Fungal infection (<2%)
Granuloma annulare
(2000): Rotman H, Houston, TX (personal communication) (observation)
Herpes simplex (<2%)
Herpes zoster (<2%)
Peripheral edema (6%)
(2001): Litt JZ, Beachwood, OH (2 personal cases)
(2000): Litt JZ, Beachwood, OH (personal case)
Photosensitivity
(2001): Klein AD, Statesboro, GA (from Internet) (observation)
(2000): Valentine M, Everett, WA (from Internet) (observation)
(1999): Gregg LJ, Tulsa, OK (from Internet) (observation)
Phototoxicity
(2001): Klein AD, Statesboro, GA (from Internet) (observation)
Pruritus (<2%)
Purpura
(2001): Litt JZ, Beachwood, OH (personal case)
(2000): Litt JZ, Beachwood, OH (personal case)
Rash (sic) (<2%)
Urticaria (<2%)
(2002): Nettis E+, *Ann Allergy Asthma* 88(3), 331
(2001): Kelkar PS+, *J Rheumatol* 28(11), 2553
(2000): Wright WL, Castro Valley, CA (from Internet) (2 observations) (after the second day)
Xerosis (<2%)

### Hair

Hair – alopecia (<2%)

### Nails

Nails – disorder (sic) (<2%)

### Other

Aphthous stomatitis (<2%)
Death
(2001): Weaver J+, *Am J Gastroenterol* 96(12), 3449
Hypesthesia (<2%)
Myalgia (<2%)
Oral ulceration (<2%)
Paresthesias (<2%)
Tendinitis (<2%)
Tinnitus
(2001): Litt JZ, Beachwood, OH (personal case)
Xerostomia (<2%)

# ROPINIROLE

**Trade name:** Requip (GSK)
**Indications:** Parkinsonism
**Category:** Antiparkinsonian; dopamine agonist
**Half-life:** ~6 hours

## *Reactions*

### Skin

Balanoposthitis (<1%)
Basal cell carcinoma (>1%)
Cellulitis (<1%)
Dermatitis (sic) (<1%)
Diaphoresis (6%)
Eczema (sic) (<1%)
Edema (<1%)
Exanthems (<1%)
Flushing (3%)
Fungal dermatitis (sic) (<1%)
Furunculosis (<1%)
Herpes simplex (<1%)
Herpes zoster (<1%)
Hyperkeratosis (<1%)
Hypertrophy (sic) (<1%)
Peripheral edema (<1%)
Photosensitivity (<1%)
Pigmentation (<1%)
Pruritus (<1%)
Psoriasis (<1%)
Purpura (<1%)
Rash (sic) (>1%)
Ulceration (<1%)
Urticaria (<1%)
Viral infection

### Hair

Hair – alopecia (<1%)

### Other

Gingivitis (>1%)
Glossitis (<1%)
Gynecomastia (<1%)
Hypesthesia (4%)
Mastitis (<1%)
Paresthesias (5%)
Peyronie's disease (<1%)
Sialorrhea (>1%)
Stomatitis (<1%)
Thrombophlebitis (<1%)
Tongue edema (<1%)
Tremors (6%)
Ulcerative stomatitis (<1%)
Vaginal candidiasis (<1%)
Xerostomia (5%)

# ROSIGLITAZONE

**Trade name:** Avandia (GSK)
**Indications:** Type 2 diabetes
**Category:** Thiazolidinedione antidiabetic
**Half-life:** 3.5 hours

## *Reactions*

### Skin

Edema (4.8%)
(2001): Werner AL+, *Pharmacotherapy* 21(9), 1082

Exanthems
(1999): Rehbein HM, Jacksonville, FL (from Internet) (observation)

Exfoliative dermatitis
(2000): Vinson RP, El Paso, TX (from Internet) (observation)

# SACCHARIN

**Trade names:** Saccharin; Sweet 'n Low
**Indications:** Sugar substitute
**Category:** Sulfonamide* sweetening agent
**Half-life:** no data

### *Reactions*

#### Skin

Dermatitis (sic)
(1989): Birbeck J, *N Z Med J* 102, 24
(1972): Gordon H, *Am J Obstet Gynecol* 15, 1145
(1972): Gordon H, *Cutis* 10, 77
Exanthems
(1965): Boros E, *JAMA* 194, 571
(1965): Fujita H+, *Acta Derm* 60, 303
Fixed eruption
(1956): Stritzler C+, *Arch Dermatol* 74, 433
Notalgia paresthetica
(1986): Fishman HC, *J Am Acad Dermatol* 15, 1304
Photosensitivity
(1972): Gordon H, *Cutis* 10, 77
(1972): Taub SJ, *Eye Ear Nose Throat Mon* 51, 405
(1961): Kennedy B+, *J Louisiana Med Soc* 113, 365
Pruritus
(1989): Birbeck J, *N Z Med J* 102, 24
(1972): Gordon H, *Cutis* 10, 77
(1965): Boros E, *JAMA* 194, 571
Sensitivity (sic)
(1966): Kingsley HJ, *Cent Afr J Med* 12, 243
Urticaria
(1989): Birbeck J, *N Z Med J* 102, 24
(1974): Miller R+, *J Allergy Clin Immunol* 53, 240
(1972): Gordon H, *Cutis* 10, 77
(1956): Stritzler C+, *Arch Dermatol* 74, 433
(1955): Stritzler C+, *New York J Med* 55, 3479

#### Other

Dysgeusia
(1965): Boros E, *JAMA* 194, 571

***Note:** Saccharin is a sulfonamide and can be absorbed systemically. Sulfonamides can produce severe, possibly fatal, reactions such as toxic epidermal necrolysis and Stevens–Johnson syndrome

# SALMETEROL

**Trade name:** Serevent (GSK)
**Other common trade names:** *Salmeter; Serobid; Zantirel*
**Indications:** Asthma
**Category:** Sympathomimetic bronchodilator; adrenergic agonist
**Half-life:** 3–4 hours

### *Reactions*

#### Skin

Angioedema
Eczematoid eruption (sic)
(1997): Leal GB, Fortaleza, Brazil (from Internet) (observation)
Exanthems
Infections (sic) (12%)
(2000): Beeh KM+, *Pneumologie* (German) 54, 225 (2.7%)
Pruritus
Rash (sic) (1–3%)
(1994): D'Alonzo GE+, *JAMA* 271, 1412
(1991): Hatton MQ+, *Lancet* 337, 1169
Urticaria (1–3%)
(1991): Hatton MQF+, *Lancet* 337, 1169

#### Other

Hypersensitivity (<1%)
Myalgia (1–3%)
Oral candidiasis
(2002): Beeh KM+, *Pneumologie* 56(2), 91
Paresthesias
Trembling
Tremors (1–10)
(2001): Shrewsbury S+, *Ann Allergy Asthma Immunol* 87(6), 465 (5.7%)
(2000): Beeh KM+, *Pneumologie* (German) 54, 225

# SALSALATE

**Synonyms:** disalicylic acid; salicylic acid
**Trade names:** Disalcid (3M); Mono-Gesic (Schwarz); Salflex (Carnrick); Salsitab (Upsher Smith)
**Other common trade names:** *Argesic-SA; Artha-G; Atisuril; Disalgesic; Marthritic; Nobegyl; Salgesic; Salina; Umbradol*
**Indications:** Arthritis
**Category:** Nonsteroidal anti-inflammatory (NSAID); salicylate; analgesic
**Half-life:** 7–8 hours
**Clinically important, potentially hazardous interactions with:** methotrexate

### *Reactions*

#### Skin

Angioedema
Dermatitis (sic)
Exanthems
Lichenoid eruption
(2001): Powell MI+, *J Am Acad Dermatol* 45, 616
Pruritus
Purpura
Rash (sic) (1–10%)
Urticaria
(1986): Chudwin DS+, *Ann Allergy* 57, 133

#### Nails

Nails – onychoschizia
(2001): Powell MI+, *J Am Acad Dermatol* 45, 616

#### Other

Anaphylactoid reactions (1–10%)
Tinnitus

## SAQUINAVIR

**Trade names:** Fortovase (Roche); Invirase (Roche)
**Indications:** Advanced HIV infection
**Category:** Antiretroviral; protease inhibitor*
**Half-life:** 12 hours
**Clinically important, potentially hazardous interactions with:** alprazolam, clindamycin, dihydroergotamine, ergot derivatives, fentanyl, **garlic**, ketoconazole, methysergide, midazolam, phenytoin, pimozide, rifampin, ritonavir, sildenafil, **St John's wort**

### *Reactions*

**Skin**

Acne (<2%)
Bullous eruption
Candidiasis (<2%)
Cheilitis (<2%)
Dermatitis (sic) (<2%)
Diaphoresis (<2%)
Eczema (sic) (<2%)
Erythema (<2%)
Erythema multiforme
(1998): Garat H+, *Ann Dermatol Venereol* (French) 125, 42
Exanthems (<2%)
Fixed eruption
(2000): Smith KJ+, *Cutis* 66, 29 (2 cases)
Folliculitis (<2%)
Furunculosis
Guillain–Barré syndrome
Herpes simplex (<2%)
Herpes zoster (<2%)
Papulovesicular lesions
(2000): Smith KJ+, *Cutis* 66, 29 (2 cases)
Photosensitivity (<2%)
(1997): Winter AJ+, *Genitourin Med* 73, 323
Pigmentary changes (<2%)
(2000): Smith KJ+, *Cutis* 66, 29 (2 cases)
Pruritus
(2000): Smith KJ+, *Cutis* 66, 29 (2 cases)
Psoriasis
(2000): Bonfanti P+, *J Acquir Immune Defic Syndr* 23(3), 236
Rash (sic) (1.3%)
Seborrheic dermatitis (<2%)
Stevens–Johnson syndrome
Ulceration (<2%)
Urticaria (<2%)
Warts (<2%)
Xerosis (<2%)
(2000): Bonfanti P+, *J Acquir Immune Defic Syndr* 23(3), 236

**Hair**

Hair – alopecia
Hair – changes (sic) (<2%)

**Other**

Dysesthesia (<2%)
Dysgeusia (<2%)
Gingivitis (<2%)
Glossitis (<2%)
Gynecomastia
(2000): Bonfanti P+, *J Acquir Immune Defic Syndr* 23(3), 236
(1999): Donovan B+, *Int J STD AIDS* 10, 49
HAART (tendon xanthomata)
(2001): Leung N+, *Diabetes* 50(Suppl.2), 452
Hyperesthesia (<2%)
Lingual lesions (sic)
(1998): Ruscin JM+, *Ann Pharmacother* 32, 1248
Lipodystrophy
(2002): Reid S, *Can Adv Drug Reaction Newsletter* 12, 5
Oral ulceration (2.5%)
Paresthesias (2.6%)
Perioral parasthesias
(2001): McMahon D+, *Antivir Ther* 6(2), 105
Stomatitis (<2%)
Xerostomia (<2%)

***Note:** Protease inhibitors cause dyslipidemia which includes elevated triglycerides and cholesterol and redistribution of body fat centrally to produce the so-called "protease paunch," breast enlargement, facial atrophy, and "buffalo hump"

## SARGRAMOSTIN

(See GRANULOCYTE COLONY-STIMULATING FACTOR [GCSF])

## SAW PALMETTO

**Scientific names:** *Sabal serrulata; Serenoa repens; Serenoa serrulata*
**Other common names:** American Dwarf Palm Tree; Cabbage Palm; Ju-Zhong; Palmier Nain; Sabal; Sabal Fructus; Saw Palmetto Berry
**Family:** Arecaceae; Palmae
**Purported indications:** Benign prostatic hyperplasia, diuretic, sedative, anti-inflammatory, antiseptic
**Other uses:** Prostate cancer (in combination with seven other herbs – PC-Specs), aphrodisiac, hair growth, colds, coughs, sore throat, asthma, chronic bronchitis, migraines, cancer
**Clinically important, potentially hazardous interactions with:** oral contraceptives

### *Reactions*

**Skin**

None

## SCOPOLAMINE

**Trade names:** Isopto Hyoscine Ophthalmic*; Scopase; Transderm-Scop Patch (Novartis)
**Other common trade names:** *Scopace; Scopoderm-TTS; Transdermal-V*
**Indications:** Nausea and vomiting, excess salivation
**Category:** Anticholinergic; antispasmodic
**Half-life:** 8 hours
**Clinically important, potentially hazardous interactions with:** anticholinergics, arbutamine

### *Reactions*

**Skin**

Contact allergy (sic)
(2001): Decraene T+, *Contact Dermatitis* 45(5), 309

Contact dermatitis
(1989): Gordon CR+, *BMJ* 298, 1220
Dermatitis (sic) (transdermal patch and ophthalmic)
(1990): Hogan DJ+, *J Am Acad Dermatol* 22, 811
(1989): Holdiness MR, *Contact Dermatitis* 20, 3
(1988): van der Willigen AH+, *J Am Acad Dermatol* 18, 146
(1985): Clissold SP+, *Drugs* 29, 189
(1985): Trozak DJ, *J Am Acad Dermatol* 13, 247
(1984): Fisher AA, *Cutis* 34, 526
Edema (<1%) (ophthalmic)
Erythema
Erythema multiforme
(1986): Fisher AA, *Cutis* 37, 158; 262
(1979): Guill MA+, *Arch Dermatol* 115, 742
Exanthems
(1985): Clissold SP+, *Drugs* 29, 189 (transdermal patch)
Fixed eruption
(1981): Kanwar AJ+, *Dermatologica* 162, 378
Flushing
Hypohidrosis (>10%)
Photosensitivity (1–10%)
Rash (sic) (<1%)
Urticaria
Xerosis (>10%)

### Other

Anaphylactoid reactions
(1995): Manhart AR+, *J Toxicol Clin Toxicol* 33, 189 (fatal)
(1994): Watanabe F+, *J Toxicol Clin Toxicol* 32, 593 (fatal)
Death
Injection-site irritation (>10%)
Oral mucosal lesions
(1985): Clissold SP+, *Drugs* 29, 189 (transdermal patch) (>5%)
Xerostomia (>60%)
(2002): Kranke P+, *Anesth Analg* 95(1), 133
(1985): Clissold SP+, *Drugs* 29, 189 (transdermal patch) (66%)
(1981): Price NM+, *Clin Pharmacol Ther* 29, 414

***Note:** Systemic adverse effects have been reported following ophthalmic administration

## SECOBARBITAL

**Synonym:** quinalbarbitone
**Trade name:** Seconal (Lilly)
**Other common trade names:** *Immenoctal; Novo-Secobarb; Secanal*
**Indications:** Insomnia
**Category:** Short-acting barbiturate; hypnotic-sedative
**Half-life:** 15–40 hours
**Clinically important, potentially hazardous interactions with: alcohol**, anticoagulants, antihistamines, brompheniramine, buclizine, chlorpheniramine, dicumarol, ethanolamine, imatinib, warfarin

### *Reactions*

### Skin

Angioedema (<1%)
Exanthems
Exfoliative dermatitis (<1%)
Purpura
Rash (sic) (<1%)
Stevens–Johnson syndrome (<1%)
Urticaria

### Other

Hypersensitivity
Injection-site pain (>10%)
Rhabdomyolysis
(1990): Larpin R+, *Presse Med* 19(30), 1403
Serum sickness
Thrombophlebitis (<1%)

## SECRETIN

**Trade name:** Secretin-Ferring (Ferring)
**Indications:** Diagnosis of gastrinoma (Zollinger–Ellison syndrome)
**Category:** Gastrointestinal peptide hormone
**Half-life:** no data

### *Reactions*

### Skin

Allergic reactions (sic)
Urticaria
(1975): Baenkler HW+, *BMJ* 2, 747

### Other

Injection-site reactions (sic)
(1975): Baenkler HW+, *BMJ* 2, 747

## SELEGILINE

**Synonyms:** deprenyl; L-deprenyl
**Trade name:** Eldepryl (Somerset)
**Other common trade names:** *Apo-Selegiline; Carbex; Eldeprine; Jumex; Movergan; Novo-Selegiline; Plurimen*
**Indications:** Parkinsonism
**Category:** Monoamine oxidase (MAO) inhibitor; antiparkinsonian
**Half-life:** 9 minutes
**Clinically important, potentially hazardous interactions with:** carbodopa, citalopram, doxepin, ephedrine, fluoxetine, fluvoxamine, levodopa, meperidine, nefazodone, oral contraceptives, paroxetine, sertraline, venlafaxine

### *Reactions*

### Skin

Diaphoresis
Peripheral edema
Photosensitivity
Rash (sic)

### Hair

Hair – alopecia
Hair – hypertrichosis (facial)

### Other

Bruxism (1–10%)
Dysgeusia
Paresthesias
Tinnitus
Tremors
Xerostomia (>10%)
(1988): Golbe LI+, *Clin Neuropharmacol* 11, 45

## SENNA

**Scientific names:** *Cassia acutifolia; Cassia angustifolia; Cassia obtusifloia; Cassia senna; Cassia tora; Senna alexandrina; Senna obtusifolia; Senna tora*
**Other common names:** Agiolax; Agoral (Numark); Alesandrian; Black-Draught (Monticello); Ex-Lax (Novartis); Fletcher's Castoria (Mentholatum); Gentlax ; Glysennid; Goldline Senna; Herbal Trim Tea; Laci Le Beau Corp; Manevac; PMS-Sennosides; Prodiem Plus (Novartis); Riva-Senna; Senexon; Senna Lax; Senna-Gen; Sennatab; Senokot (Purdue Frederick); Senolax; Super Dieter's Tea; X-Prep
**Family:** Caesalpiniaceae (Fabaceae)
**Purported indications:** Anthraquinone stimulant laxative, cathartic, cholagogue, purgative

Part used: Leaves and/or seed pods

### *Reactions*

#### Skin

Adverse effects (sic)
(1996): Sykes NP, *J Pain Symptom Manage* 11(6), 363
(1993): Passmore AP+, *Pharmacology* 47, 249
(1988): Jagjivan B+, *Br J Radiol* 61(729), 853
Allergic reactions (sic)
(1991): Marks GB+, *Am Rev Respir Dis* 144(5), 1065
Contact dermatitis
(2001): Leventhal JM+, *Pediatrics* 107(1), 178
Edema
Pruritus
Rash (sic)
Rhinoconjuntivitis (occupational exposure)
Side effects (sic)
(1977): Perkin JM, *Curr Med Res* 4(8), 540

#### Other

Arthopathy (from abuse)
(1988): Fichter M+, *Nervenarzt* (German) 59(4), 244
(1981): Armstrong RD+, *Br Med J* (Clin Res Ed) 282(6279), 1836
Death (from abuse)
Finger clubbing (from abuse) (reversible)
(1980): Malmquist J+, *Postgrad Med J* 56(662), 862
(1978): Prior J+, *Lancet* 2(8096), 947
(1975): Silk DB+, *Gastroenterology* 68, 790

**Note:** Prolonged or excessive laxative use can lead to electrolyte and fluid disturbances, development of carthartic colon, and possible increased risk of colorectal cancer. Treatment should be limited to 8 to 10 days

## SERTRALINE

**Trade name:** Zoloft (Pfizer)
**Other common trade name:** *Atruline*
**Indications:** Depression, panic disorders, obsessive compulsive disorders
**Category:** Selective serotonin reuptake inhibitor (SSRI); antidepressant
**Half-life:** 24–26 hours
**Clinically important, potentially hazardous interactions with:** amphetamines, clarithromycin, dextroamphetamine, diethylpropion, erythromycin, isocarboxazid, linezolid, MAO inhibitors, mazindol, methamphetamine, metoclopramide, phendimetrazine, phenelzine, phentermine, phenylpropolamine, pseudoephedrine, selegiline, sibutramine, **St John's wort**, sumatriptan, sympathomimetics, tranylcypromine, trazodone, troleandromycin

### *Reactions*

#### Skin

Acne (<1%)
Allergic reactions (sic)
(1991): Guthrie SK, *Drug Intell Clin Pharm* 25, 952
Angioedema
(1994): Gales BJ+, *Am J Hosp Pharm* 51, 118
Balanoposthitis (<1%)
Bullous eruption (<1%)
Cutaneous reactions (sic)
(1998): Beauquier B+, *Encephale* (French) 24, 62
Dermatitis (sic) (<1%)
Diaphoresis (8.4%)
(2002): Fisher AA+, *Ann Pharmacother* 36(1), 67
(2000): Henney JE, *JAMA* 283, 596
(1991): Guthrie SK, *Drug Intell Clin Pharm* 25, 952
(1990): Reimherr FW+, *J Clin Psychiatry* 51, 18
(1988): Doogan DP+, *J Clin Psychiatry* 49, 46
Discoloration (sic) (<1%)
Edema (<1%)
Erythema
Erythema multiforme (<1%)
(1994): Gales BJ+, *Am J Hosp Pharm* 51, 118
Exanthems (<1%)
(2000): Fernandes B+, *Contact Dermatitis* 42, 287
(2000): Kittay SA, (from Internet) (observation)
(1999): Blumenthal HL, Beachwood, OH (personal case) (observation)
(1998): Litt JZ, Beachwood, OH (personal case) (observation)
Fixed eruption
(1997): Sawada KY, Wheat Ridge, CO (from Internet) (observation)
Flushing (2.2%)
Lupus erythematosus
(1998): Hill VA+, *J R Army Med Corps* 144, 109
Periorbital edema (<1%)
Photosensitivity (<1%)
Pruritus (<1%)
(1999): Blumenthal HL, Beachwood, OH (personal case) (observation)
Purpura (<1%)
Rash (sic) (2.1%)
Stevens–Johnson syndrome
(1999): Jan V+, *Acta Derm Venereol* 79, 401
Urticaria (<1%)
Xerosis (<1%)

### Hair

Hair – abnormal texture (sic) (<1%)
Hair – alopecia (<1%)
(1996): Bourgeois JA, *J Clin Psychopharmacol* 16, 91
Hair – hirsutism (<1%)

### Other

Aphthous stomatitis (<1%)
Bromhidrosis (<1%)
Bruxism (<1%)
Death
(2001): Fartoux-Heymann L+, *J Hepatol* 35(5), 683
(2001): Gillespie JA, *Ann Pharmacother* 35(12), 1671
(2001): Hoehns JD+, *Ann Pharmacother* 35(7), 862 (with clozapine)
Dysgeusia
Foetor ex ore (halitosis) (<1%)
Galactorrhea
(1993): Bronzo MR+, *Am J Psychiatry* 150, 1269
Gingival hyperplasia (<1%)
Glossitis (<1%)
Gynecomastia (<1%)
Hyperesthesia (<1%)
Hypesthesia (2%)
Paresthesias (2%)
Priapism
(1998): Rand EH, *J Clin Psychiatry* 59, 538
Serotonin syndrome
(2002): Fisher AA+, *Ann Pharmacother* 36(1), 67
(2000): Vandermegel X+, *Rev Med Brux* (French) 21(3), 161 (with metoclopramide)
Sialorrhea (<1%)
Stomatitis (<1%)
Tinnitus
Tongue edema (<1%)
Tongue ulceration (<1%)
Tremors (1–10%)
(2002): No Author, *Prescrire Int* 11(59), 69
Vaginitis (atrophic)
Xerostomia (16.3%)
(2000): Brady K+, *JAMA* 283, 1837
(1992): Berman H+, *Hosp Community Psychiatry* 43, 671
(1991): Guthrie SK, *Drug Intell Clin Pharm* 25, 952
(1990): Reimherr FW+, *J Clin Psychiatry* 51, 18
(1988): Doogan DP+, *J Clin Psychiatry* 49, 46

***Note:** These medications, along with sertraline, may precipitate the serotonin syndrome consisting of restlessness, confusion, agitation, myoclonus, hyperreflexia, diarrhea, diaphoresis, shivering, tremor, fever, and mental changes

## SIBERIAN GINSENG

**Scientific names:** *Acanthopanax senticosus; Eleutherococcus senticosus*
**Other common names:** Devil's root; Touch-me-not
**Family:** Araliaceae
**Category:** Adaptogen; anti-toxic; anti-radiation; anti-viral (RNA viruses); immunoprotector; immunoregulator
**Purported indications:** Alzheimer's disease, anaphylaxis, arthritis, colds, depression, fatigue, flu, impotence, infertility, menopause, multiple sclerosis, perimenopause, PMS, stress
**Clinically important, potentially hazardous interactions with:** antihypertensives, digoxin

#### *Reactions*

### Other

Headache
Mastalgia

**Note:** Eleutherococcus may prevent biotransformation of some drugs to less toxic compounds

## SIBUTRAMINE

**Trade name:** Meridia (Abbott)
**Indications:** Obesity
**Category:** Obesity management; anorexiant
**Half-life:** 1.1 hours
**Clinically important, potentially hazardous interactions with:** dextromethorphan, dihydroergotamine, ergot, fluoxetine, fluvoxamine, isocarboxazid, linezolid, lithium, MAO inhibitors, meperidine, methysergide, naratriptan, nefazodone, paroxetine, phenelzine, rizatriptan, sertraline, sumatriptan, tranylcypromine, **tryptophan**, venlafaxine, verapamil, zolmitriptan

#### *Reactions*

### Skin

Acne (1.0%)
Allergic reactions (sic) (1.5%)
Diaphoresis (2.5%)
Ecchymoses (0.7%)
Edema (2%)
Flu-like syndrome (sic) (1–10%)
Herpes simplex (1.3%)
Peripheral edema (>1%)
Pruritus (>1%)
Rash (sic) (3.8%)

### Other

Death
(2002): London, *Reuters Health Information* 3-26-02 (2 cases)
Dysgeusia (2.2%)
Myalgia (1.9%)
Paresthesias (2.0%)
Tooth disorder (sic)
Vaginal candidiasis (1.2%)
Xerostomia (17.2%)
(2001): Scheen AJ, *Rev Med Liege* 56(9), 656

# SILDENAFIL

**Trade name:** Viagra (Pfizer)
**Indications:** Erectile dysfunction
**Category:** Phosphodiesterase (type 5) enzyme inhibitor
**Half-life:** 4 hours
**Clinically important, potentially hazardous interactions with:** amprenavir, amyl nitrate, erythromycin, indinavir, isosorbide dinitrate, isosorbide mononitrate, itraconazole, ketoconazole, nelfinavir, nitrates, nitroglycerin, ritonavir, saquinavir

### *Reactions*

## Skin

Allergic reactions (sic) (<2%)
Contact dermatitis (<2%)
Diaphoresis (<2%)
Edema (<2%)
Exfoliative dermatitis (<2%)
(2002): Smith JG, Mobile, AL (from Internet) (observation)
Facial edema (<2%)
Fixed eruption (urticarial)
(1998): Reed BR, Denver, CO (from Internet) (observation)
Flushing (10%)
(2002): Fink HA+, *Arch Intern Med* 162(12), 1349 (12%)
(2002): Lim PH+, *Ann N Y Acad Sci* 962, 378
(2001): Chen KK+, *Int J Impot Res* 13(4), 221 (25%)
(2001): Rosenkranz S+, *Dtsch Med Wochenschr* 126(41), 1144
(2001): Steers W+, *Int J Impot Res* 13(5), 261
Genital edema (<2%)
Herpes simplex (<2%)
Lichenoid eruption
(2000): Goldman BD, *Cutis* 66, 282
Peripheral edema (<2%)
Photosensitivity (<2%)
Pruritus (<2%)
Rash (sic) (2%)
Ulceration (<2%)
Urticaria (<2%)

## Other

Death
(2002): Dumestre-Toulet V+, *Forensic Sci Int* 126(1), 71
Dyschromatopsia (3%) (blue-green vision)
(1998): Craig D+, *Cleveland Clinic Foundation* 52, 963 (11%)
Gingivitis (<2%)
Glossitis (<2%)
Gynecomastia (<2%)
Hypesthesia (<2%)
Myalgia (<2%)
Paresthesias (<2%)
Photophobia (<2%)
Priapism
(2000): Sur RL+, *Urology* 55, 950
Stomatitis (<2%)
Xerostomia (<2%)

# SIMVASTATIN

**Trade name:** Zocor (Merck)
**Other common trade names:** *Denan; Lipex; Liponorm; Lodales; Simovil; Sivastin; Zocord*
**Indications:** Hypercholesterolemia
**Category:** Antihyperlipidemic (cholesterol-lowering); HMG-CoA reductase inhibitor
**Half-life:** 1.9 hours
**Clinically important, potentially hazardous interactions with:** azithromycin, bosentan, clarithromycin, cyclosporine, diltiazem, erythromycin, gemfibrozil, imatinib, itraconazole, ritonavir, tacrolimus, verapamil

### *Reactions*

## Skin

Actinic dermatitis (sic)
(1998): Granados MT+, *Contact Dermatitis* 38, 294
Angioedema
Ankle edema
(1991): Borland Y+, *Nephron* 57, 365
Cheilitis
(1998): Mehregan DR+, *Cutis* 62, 197
Dermatomyositis
(1994): Khattak FH+, *Br J Rheumatol* 32(2), 199
Diaphoresis
(1991): Scott RS+, *N Z Med J* 104, 493
Eczema (sic)
(1995): Proksch E, *Hautarzt* (German) 46, 76
(1991): Steyn K+, *S Afr Med J* 79, 639
Eczematous eruption (generalized)
(1993): Feldmann R+, *Dermatology* 186, 272
(1993): Krasovec M+, *Dermatology* 186, 248
Eosinophilic fasciitis
(2001): Choquet-Kastylevsky G+, *Arch Intern Med* 161(11), 1456
Erythema multiforme
Erythematous scaly plaques
(1993): Feldmann R+, *Dermatology* 186, 272
Exanthems
(1991): McDowell IF+, *Br J Clin Pharmacol* 31, 340
Flushing
Lichen planus
(1991): Steyn K+, *S Afr Med J* 79, 639
Lichenoid eruption
(1994): Roger D+, *Clin Exp Dermatol* 19, 88
Lupus erythematosus
(1998): Hanson J+, *Lancet* 352, 1070
(1998): Khosia R+, *South Med J* 91, 873
(1992): Bannwarth B+, *Arch Intern Med* 152, 1093
Petechiae
(1997): Horiuchi Y+, *J Dermatol* 24, 549
Photosensitivity
(1995): Morimoto K+, *Contact Dermatitis* 33, 274
(1991): Brocard JJ+, *Schweiz Med Wochenschr* (German) 121, 977
Pruritus
(1993): Feldmann R+, *Dermatology* 186, 272
(1991): Steyn K+, *S Afr Med J* 79, 639
Purpura
(1998): Koduri PR, *Lancet* 352, 2020
(1991): Steyn K+, *S Afr Med J* 79, 639
Pustular eruption
Radiation recall
(1995): Abadir R+, *Clin Oncol R Coll Radiol* 7, 325
Rash (sic) (1–10%)

(2001): Coverman M, *The Schoch Letter* 51, 23 (with atorvastatin)
(1993): Feldmann R+, *Dermatology* 186, 272
(1990): Ziegler O+, *Cardiology* 77 (Suppl 4), 50
Rosacea
(1991): Brocard JJ+, *Schweiz Med Wochenschr* (German) 121, 977
Stevens–Johnson syndrome
Thrombocytopenic purpura
(1998): McCarthy LJ+, *Lancet* 352, 1284
Toxic epidermal necrolysis
Urticaria
Vasculitis

### Hair

Hair – alopecia
(1999): Litt JZ, Beachwood, OH (personal case) (observation)
(1998): Robb-Nicholson C, *Harv Womens Health Watch* 5, 8 (anecdote)
(1997): Shelley WB+, *Cutis* 60, 20 (observation)
(1995): Litt JZ, Beachwood, OH (personal case) (observation)
(1994): Litt JZ, Beachwood, OH (personal case) (observation)

### Other

Anaphylactoid reactions
Death
(2001): Federman DG+, *South Med J* 94(10), 1023
Dysgeusia (<1%)
(1991): Saito Y+, *Arterioscler Thromb* 11, 816
Gynecomastia
Hypersensitivity
Myalgia (1.6%)
(2002): Litt JZ, Beachwood, OH (personal observation)
(2001): Litt JZ, Beachwood, OH (personal case)
(2001): Rehbein H, Jacksonville, FL (from Internet) (observation)
Myopathy (1–10%)
(2002): Udawat H+, *J Assoc Physicians India* 50, 439
(1995): Garnett WR, *Am J Health Syst Pharm* 52(15), 1639
(1994): al-Jubouri MA+, *BMJ* 308, 588
(1991): Deslypere JP+, *Ann Intern Med* 114, 342
(1990): Bilheimer DW, *Cardiology* 77 (Suppl 4), 58
Paresthesias
Porphyria cutanea tarda
(1994): Perrot JL+, *Ann Dermatol Venereol* (French) 121, 817
Rhabdomyolysis
(2001): Borrego FJ+, *Nefrologia* 21(3), 309
(2001): Federman DG+, *South Med J* 94(10), 1023 (with gemfibrozil)
(2001): Kanathur N+, *Tenn Med* 94(9), 339 (with diltiazem)
(2001): Lee AJ, *Ann Pharmacother* 35(1), 26 (with clarithromycin)
(2001): Peces R+, *Nephron* 89(1), 117 (with diltiazem)
(2001): Reed BR, Denver, CO (from internet) (observation)
(2001): Stirling CM+, *Nephrol Dial Transplant* 16(4), 873
(2000): Al Shohaib, *Am J Nephrol* 20(3), 212
(2000): Davidson MH, *Curr Atheroscler Rep* 2(1), 14
(2000): Kusus M+, *Am J Med Sci* 320(6), 394 (with cyclosporine, digoxin and verapamil)
(2000): Oldemeyer JB+, *Cardiology* 94(2), 127 (with gemfibrozil)
(1999): Bottorff M, *Atherosclerosis* 147(Suppl 1), S23
(1999): Corsini A+, *Pharmacol Ther* 84, 413 (with either cyclosporine, mibefradil or nefazodone)
(1996): Ballantyne CM+, *Am J Cardiol* 78(5), 532
(1995): Farmer JA+, *Baillieres Clin Endocrinol Metab* 9(4), 825
(1995): Garnett WR, *Am J Health Syst Pharm* 52(15), 1639 (with either cyclosporine, erythromycin, gemfibrozil or niacin)
(1995): Meier C+, *Schweiz Med Wochenschr* 125(27), 1342 (with cyclosporine)
(1992): Blaison G+, *Rev Med Interne* 13(1), 61 (with cyclosporine)
Tendinopathy
(2001): Chazerain P+, *Joint Bone Spine* 68(5), 430

# SIROLIMUS

**Synonym:** Rapamycin
**Trade name:** Rapamune (Wyeth-Ayerst)
**Indications:** Prophylaxis of organ rejection in renal transplants
**Category:** Immunosuppressant
**Half-life:** 62 hours
**Clinically important, potentially hazardous interactions with:** voriconazole

## *Reactions*

### Skin

Abscess (3–20%)
Acne (20–31%)
(2001): Reitamo S+, *Br J Dermatol* 145(3), 438 (13%) (with cyclosporine)
(2000): Vasquez EM, *Am J Health Syst Pharm* 57, 437
Cellulitis (3–20%)
Chills (3–20%)
Dermatitis (sic)
Dermatitis herpetiformis (aggravation)
(2002): Gladstone GC, Worcester, MA (personal correspondence)
Diaphoresis (3–20%)
Ecchymoses (3–20%)
Edema (16–24%)
Eyelid edema
(2001): Mohaupt MG+, *Transplantation* 72(1), 162 (40%)
Facial edema (3–20%)
Flu-like syndrome (sic) (3–20%)
Fungal dermatitis (3–20%)
Hot flashes
(2001): Reitamo S+, *Br J Dermatol* 145(3), 438 (12%) (with cyclosporine)
Hypertrophy (3–20%)
Infections (sic)
Peripheral edema (54–64%)
Pruritus (3–20%)
(2002): Gladstone GC, Worcester, MA (personal correspondence)
Purpura (3–20%)
Rash (sic) (10–20%)
(2000): Vasquez EM, *Am J Health Syst Pharm* 57, 437
Scrotal edema
Ulceration (3–20%)
Upper respiratory infection (20–26%)

### Hair

Hair – hirsutism (3–20%)

### Other

Aphthous stomatitis
(2001): Reitamo S+, *Br J Dermatol* 145(3), 438 (9%) (with cyclosporin)
Arthralgia (25–31%)
(2000): Vasquez EM, *Am J Health Syst Pharm* 57, 437
Depression (3–20%)
Dysgeusia
(1999): Watson CJ+, *Transplantation* 67, 505
Gingival hyperplasia (3–20%)
Gingivitis (3–20%)
Hypesthesia (3–20%)
Myalgia (3–20%)
Oral candidiasis (3–20%)
Oral ulceration (3–20%)

Paresthesias (3–20%)
Stomatitis (3–20%)
Thrombophlebitis (3–20%)
Tinnitus (3–20%)
Tremors (21–31%)
(1999): Groth CG+, *Transplantation* 67, 1036

# SMALLPOX VACCINE

**Trade name:** Dryvax (Wyeth)
**Indications:** Prevention of smallpox (variola)
**Category:** Vaccine
**Half-life:** ~5 years
**Clinically important, potentially hazardous interactions with:** corticosteroids

### *Reactions*

## Skin

Acne vaccinatum
(1971): Schmitt BS+, *Pediatrics* 48(5), 815
Allergic reactions (sic)
(1967): De Carlo M+, *Arch Ital Sci Med Trop Parassitol* 48(1), 51
(1965): Keller W, *Monatsschr Kinderheilkd* 113(6), 394
Basal cell carcinoma
(1988): Ribeiro R+, *Med Cutan Ibero Lat Am* 16(2), 137
(1970): Riley KA, *Arch Dermatiol* 101, 416
(1968): Marmelzat W, *Arch Dermatol* 97, 400 (at vaccination scar) (5 cases)
(1968): Zelickson AS, *Arch Dermatol* 98(1), 35 (at vaccination site)
Bullous eruption
(1971): Martin J+, *Schweiz Med Wochensch* 101, 1446
(1963): Weber G+, *Dtsch Med Wochenschr* 88, 1878
Carcinoma
(1980): Gecht ML, *JAMA* 244(15), 1675
(1968): Bazex A+, *Bull Soc Fr Dermatol Syphiligr* 75(6), 743 (in scar)
Chills
(2002): Frey SE+, *N Engl J Med* 346, 1265
Cutaneous side effects (sic) (0.01%)
(1973): Patrone P+, *Archo Ital Dermatol Venereol* 38, 34
Eczema vaccinatum
(1974): Kage K+, *Rinsho Byori* 22 (10 Suppl), 353
(1972): Heitmann HJ, *Fortschr Med* 90(14), 530
(1971): Cherniaeva TV, *Vopr Okhr Materin Det* 16(8), 82
(1970): Gol'dshtein LM+, *Pediatriia* 49(11), 77
(1970): Grosfeld JC+, *Dermatologica* 141(1), 1
(1970): Hicks R+, *Ann Allergy* 28(10), 491
(1969): Castrow FF+, *Tex Med* 65(2), 48
(1969): Fierens F, *Arch Belg Dermatol Syphiligr* 25(3), 367
(1968): Hoede N+, *Med Welt* 4, 268
(1968): Piriatinskaia RG, *Vestn Dermatol Venerol* 42(8), 73
(1967): Gomez-Orozco L+, *Alergia* 14(4), 123
(1967): Kubiska E+, *Med Welt* 40, 2336
(1966): Tidstrom B, *Ugeskr Laeger* 128(1), 18
Erythema multiforme
(1975): Goldstein JA+, *Pediatrics* 55(3), 342
(1973): Patrone P+, *Archo Ital Dermatol Venereol* 38, 34
(1971): Martin J+, *Schweiz Med Wochensch* 101, 1446
(1970): Coskey RJ+, *Cutis* 6, 761
(1969): Loeffler A+, *Dermatologica* 138 (Suppl), 1
(1969): Scott EG+, *J Miss State Med Assoc* 10(2), 41
(1963): Weber G+, *Dtsch Med Wochenschr* 88, 1878
Erythema nodosum
(1971): Mattheis H, *Dermatologica* 142, 340
Exanthems
(1975): Goldstein JA+, *Pediatrics* 55(3), 342
(1973): Patrone P+, *Archo Ital Dermatol Venereol* 38, 34
(1971): Martin J+, *Schweiz Med Wochenschr* 101, 1446
(1971): Mattheis H, *Dermatologica* 142, 340
(1965): Cherry JD+, *J Pediatr* 67(4), 679
(1963): Weber G+, *Dtsch Med Wochenschr* 88, 1878
Exfoliative dermatitis
(1963): Weber G+, *Dtsch Med Wochenschr* 88, 1878
Herpes simplex
(1982): Mintz L, *JAMA* 247(19), 2704 (recurrent) (at site)
(1973): Patrone P+, *Archo Ital Dermatol Venereol* 38, 34
Histiocytoma, malignant fibrous
(1981): Slater DN+, *Br J Dermatol* 105(2), 215
Jadassohn-Borst epithelioma
(1972): Porter E+, *Br J Dermatol* 86, 177
Kaposi's varicelliform eruption
(1970): Proenca N+, *An Bras Dermatol* 45(4), 353
Keratoacanthoma
(1974): Haider S, *Br J Dermatol* 90(6), 689 (in vaccination site)
Lichen vaccinatus
(1963): Weber G+, *Dtsch Med Wochenschr* 88, 1878
Lupus erythematosus (Discoid)
(1987): Lupton GP, *J Am Acad Dermatol* 17, 688 (in vaccination scar)
Lymphadenitis
(1972): Charlebois G+, *Union Med Can* 101(8), 1587
(1968): Hartsock RJ, *Cancer* 21(4), 632
Melanoma
(1973): de Oreo G, *Int J Dermatol* 12, 217 (15 cases)
(1968): Marmelzat W, *Arch Dermatol* 97, 400 (in vaccination scar) (6 cases)
Photosensitivity
(1970): Coskey RJ+, *Cutis* 6, 761
(1969): Pace BF+, *Cutis* 5, 850
Pigmentation
(1978): Helman J, *S Afr Med J* 53(12), 430 (in scars)
Purpura
(1981): Burke PJ+, *Pa Med* 84(9), 49
(1971): Monuiko O+, *Pediatr Pol* 45, 919
(1971): Wong KY, *Hawaii Med J* 30(5), 388 (anaphylactoid)
(1970): Coskey RJ+, *Cutis* 6, 761
(1969): Casteles-Van Daele M, *N Engl J Med* 280(14), 781
(1969): Feyling T+, *Tidsskr Nor Laegeforen* 89(10), 725
(1969): Lane JM, *N Engl J Med* 280(14), 781
(1969): Wasser S+, *Kinderarztl Prax* 37(7), 299
(1968): Jiminez EL+, *N Engl J Med* 279(21), 1171
(1965): Hofele U, *Arch Kinderheilkd* 173(2), 175
(1963): Weber G+, *Dtsch Med Wochenschr* 88, 1878
Pustular vaccina
(1967): Epshtein AB+, *Gig Tr Prof Zabol* 11(4), 53 (occupational)
Pyogenic granuloma
(1974): Zayid I+, *Br J Dermatol* 90(3), 293
Rash (sic)
(2002): Frey SE+, *N Engl J Med* 346, 1265 (site other than vaccination site)
(1978): Lakotkina EA+, *Pediatriia* 12, 49
Scar
(1968): Kumar LR+, *Indian J Pediatr* 35(245), 283 (pigmented & hairy)
Stevens–Johnson syndrome
(1975): Goldstein JA+, *Pediatrics* 55(3), 342
Toxic epidermal necrolysis
(1978): Kacprzyk-Bergman I+, *Pediatr Pol* 63, 393 (patient had a rubeola infection)
(1971): Martin J+, *Schweiz Med Wochenschr* 101(40), 1446
(1970): Czarnecki L+, *Pol Tyg Lek* 25(26), 982
(1969): Debenedetti L, *Minerva Pediatr* 21(45), 2136

(1968): Kushner PG+, *J Am Osteopath Assoc* 67(10), 1134
Urticaria
(1975): Goldstein JA+, *Pediatrics* 55(3), 342
(1973): Patrone P+, *Archo Ital Dermatol* 38, 34
(1970): Coskey RJ+, *Cutis* 6, 761
(1963): Weber G+, *Dtsch Med Wochenschr* 88, 1878
(1955): Alexander HL, *Reactions with Drug Therapy* Philadelphia, Saunders
Vaccinia
(1979): Datta KK+, *Indian J Public Health* 23(2), 106 (generalized)
(1978): Pasternak J+, *Rev Inst Med Trop Sao Paulo* 20(6), 359 (progressive & fatal)
(1977): Robinson MJ+, *Aust Paediatr* 13(2), 125
(1977): Verret JL+, *Ann Dermatol Venereol* 104(3), 251
(1976): Beliaev NV, *Vestn Dermatol Venerol* 2, 63 (ulcerative)
(1975): Goldstein JA+, *Pediatrics* 55(3), 342 (generalizes)
(1974): Kulesza MO, *J Obstet Gynaecol Br Commonw* 81(3), 251
(1974): Russell G, *Tandlaegebladet* 78(2), 59 (oral)
(1972): Meyer A, *Dtsch Med Wochenschr* 97(28), 1073
(1968): Aitkens GH+, *Med J Aust* 2(4), 173 (fetal)
(1967): Abrassart C+, *Rev Med Liege* 22(1), 6
(1966): Green DM+, *Lancet* 1(7450), 1296 (generalized)
(1965): Chatterjee SN+, *Bull Calcutta Sch Trop Med* 13(4), 136 (generalized)
Vaccinia, accidental (face, eyelids, nose, mouth, genitalia & rectum)
(1980): Kanra G+, *Cutis* 26, 267 (vulva from 7–month-old daughter's vaccination)
(1976): Haim S, *Cutis* 17(2), 308 (vulva from heteroinoculation)
(1971): Polk LD, *Clin Pediatr* 10, 486
(1969): Andreev VC+, *Dermatol Int* 8(1), 5
(1969): Jelinek JE, *Arch Dermatol* 99(4), 504 (eye)
(1953): Berkowitz J, *Am J Surg* 86, 549
Vaccinia gangrenosum
(1973): Raff MJ, *J Ky Med Assoc* 71(2), 92
(1967): Van Rooyen CE+, *Can Med Assoc J* 97(4), 160
(1966): Hansson O+, *Acta Pediatr Scand* 55(3), 264
Vaccinia maculata
(1988): Landthaler M+, *Hautarzt* 39, 322
Vacinia necrosum
(1982): *MMWR Morb Mortality Wkly Rep* 31(36), 501
(1981): Funk EA+, *South Med J* 74(3), 383
(1977): Turkel SB+, *Cancer* 40(1), 226
(1972): Freed ER+, *Am J Med* 52(3), 411
(1970): Neff JM+, *JAMA* 213(1), 123
(1968): Colon VF+, *Geriatrics* 23(12), 81
Zoster
(1974): Verbov J, *Br J Dermatol* 90(1), 110
(1973): Patrone P+, *Archo Ital Dermatol Venerol* 38, 34

### Other

Death
(1979): Du Mont GC+, *BMJ* 1(6175), 1398 (3 cases)
(1979): Frongillo RF, *Ann Sclavo* 21(6), 856
(1977): Feery BJ, *Med J Aust* 2(6), 180
(1970): Lane JM+, *JAMA* 212(3), 441
(1966): Ehrengut W+, *Dtsch Med Wochenschr* 91(52), 2339
Injection-site pain
(2002): Frey SE+, *N Engl J Med* 346, 1265
Kerato-uveitis
(1994): Lee SF+, *Am J Opthalmol* 117(4), 480 (autoinoculation)
Myalgia
(2002): Frey SE+, *N Engl J Med* 346, 1265
Tumors
(1971): Mattheis H, *Dermatologica* 142, 340
(1968): Marmelzat W, *Arch Dermatol* 97, 400 (in vaccination scar) (24 cases) (malignant)
(1968): Reed WB+, *Arch Dermatol* 98, 132 (malignant)

# SODIUM CROMOGLYCATE

(See CROMOLYN)

# SOTALOL

**Trade name:** Betapace (Berlex)
**Other common trade names:** *Beta-Cardone; Betades; Cardol; Sotacor; Sotacor; Sotahexal; Sotalex*
**Indications:** Ventricular arrhythmias
**Category:** Beta-adrenergic blocker; antiarrhythmic class III
**Half-life:** 7–18 hours
**Clinically important, potentially hazardous interactions with:** arsenic, ciprofloxacin, enoxacin, gatifloxacin, lomefloxacin, moxifloxacin, norfloxacin, ofloxacin, quinolones, sparfloxacin

## *Reactions*

### Skin

Cold extremities (sic)
Cutaneous thickening (sic)
Diaphoresis (<1%)
(1995): Schmutz JL+, *Dermatology* 190, 86
Edema (5%)
Exanthems
Lichenoid eruption
(1994): O'Brien TJ+, *Australas J Dermatol* 35, 93
Peripheral edema
Photosensitivity (<1%)
Pruritus (1–10%)
Psoriasis
(1988): Heng MCY+, *Int J Dermatol* 27, 619
(1986): Czernielewski J+, *Lancet* 1, 808
(1984): Arntzen N+, *Acta Derm Venereol* (Stockh) 64, 346
Rash (sic) (3%)
Raynaud's phenomenon (<1%)
Scleroderma
(1988): Ahmad N+, *Scott Med J* 33, 210
(1979): Bonnetblanc JM+, *Ann Dermatol Venereol* (French) 106, 927
(1979): Michel JP+, *Lancet* 1, 54
Skin irritation (sic)
Urticaria
Vasculitis
(1998): Rustmann WC+, *J Am Acad Dermatol* 38, 111

### Hair

Hair – alopecia (<1%)

### Other

Dysgeusia
Injection-site extravasation (<1%)
Myalgia (<1%)
Myopathy
(1979): Forfar JC+, *BMJ* 2, 1331
Paresthesias (3%)
Phlebitis (<1%)
Xerostomia (<1%)

# SPARFLOXACIN

**Trade name:** Zagam (Bertek)
**Other common trade names:** *Spara; Sparlox; Torospar*
**Indications:** Community-acquired pneumonia
**Category:** Quinolone antibiotic
**Half-life:** 16–30 hours
**Clinically important, potentially hazardous interactions with:** amiodarone, amitriptyline, amoxapine, arsenic, bepridil, bretylium, calcium, chlorpromazine, clomipramine, desipramine, disopyramide, doxepin, erythromycin, fluphenazine, imipramine, iron salts, magnesium, mesoridazine, nortriptyline, pentamidine, perphenazine, phenothiazines, pimozide, procainamide, prochlorperazine, promazine, promethazine, protriptyline, quinidine, sotalol, sucralfate, thioridazine, tricyclic antidepressants, trifluoperazine, trimipramine, zinc salts

### *Reactions*

## Skin

Acne (<1%)
Allergic reactions (sic) (<1%)
Angioedema (<1%)
Bullous eruption (<1%)
Cellulitis (<1%)
Contact dermatitis (<1%)
Diaphoresis (<1%)
Ecchymoses (<1%)
Edema (<1%)
Erythema nodosum
Exanthems (<1%)
Exfoliative dermatitis (<1%)
Facial edema (<1%)
Fixed eruption
(2001): Sharma R, Aligarh, INdia (from Internet) (observation) (recurrence with ciprofloxacin)
Furunculosis (<1%)
Herpes simplex (<1%)
Lichenoid eruption
(1998): Hamanaka H+, *J Am Acad Dermatol* 38, 945
Peripheral edema (<1%)
Petechiae (<1%)
Photosensitivity (3.6%)
(2000): Schentag JJ, *Clin Ther* 22, 372
(1999): Hamanaka H, *J Dermatol Sci* 21, 27
(1999): Lipsky BA+, *Clin Ther* 21, 148
(1998): Hamanaka H+, *J Am Acad Dermatol* 38, 945
(1997): Burrow WH, Jackson, MS (from Internet) (observation)
(1996): Tokura Y+, *Arch Dermatol Res* 288, 45
(1995): Hamanaka H+, *Jpn J Dermatol* 105, 601
(1995): Hiramoto T+, *Rinsho Dermatol* (Japanese) 37, 1681
Phototoxicity (7.9%)
(2000): Pierfitte C+, *Br J Clin Pharmacol* 49, 609
(1999): Blondeau JM, *Clin Ther* 21, 6
(1996): Tokura Y+, *Arch Dermatol Res* 288, 45
Pigmentation (<1%)
Pruritus (3.3%)
Purpura
Pustular eruption (<1%)
Rash (sic) (1.1%)
Stevens–Johnson syndrome
Toxic epidermal necrolysis
Urticaria (<1%)
Vasculitis
Xerosis (<1%)

## Hair

Hair – alopecia (<1%)

## Other

Anaphylactoid reactions (<1%)
Anosmia
Dysgeusia (1.4%)
(1999): Lipsky BA+, *Clin Ther* 21, 148
Gingivitis (<1%)
Hyperesthesia (<1%)
Hypersensitivity
Hypesthesia (<1%)
Mastodynia (<1%)
Myalgia (<1%)
Oral candidiasis (<1%)
Oral ulceration (<1%)
Paresthesias (<1%)
Serum sickness
Stomatitis (<1%)
Tendon rupture
Tongue disorder (<1%)
Vaginal candidiasis (2.8%)
Vaginitis (<1%)
Xerostomia (1.4%)

# SPECTINOMYCIN

**Trade name:** Trobicin (Pharmacia & Upjohn)
**Other common trade name:** *Spectam*
**Indications:** Gonorrhea
**Category:** Antibiotic
**Half-life:** 1–3 hours

### *Reactions*

## Skin

Chills
Contact dermatitis
(1994): Dal-Monte A+, *Contact Dermatitis* 31, 204 (occupational)
(1991): Vilaplana J+, *Contact Dermatitis* 24, 225
Exanthems
Pruritus (<1%)
(1974): Bogden C+, *Schweiz Med Wochenschr* (German) 104, 46
Rash (sic) (<1%)
Urticaria (<1%)
(1971): *Med Lett* 13, 105

## Other

Anaphylactoid reactions
(1977): Raab W, *Z Hautkr* (German) 9, 14
Hypersensitivity
(1977): Raab W, *Z Hautkr* (German) 9, 14
Injection-site induration
Injection-site pain (<1%)
Oral mucosal lesions

# SPIRONOLACTONE

**Trade names:** Aldactazide (Searle); Aldactone (Searle)
**Other common trade names:** *Aldopur; Almatol; Diram; Merabis; Novo-Spiroton; Osiren; Spiroctan; Tensin*
**Indications:** Hyperaldosteronism, hirsutism, hypertension
**Category:** Potassium-sparing antihypertensive; diuretic
**Half-life:** 78–84 minutes
**Clinically important, potentially hazardous interactions with:** ACE inhibitors, **alcohol**, amiloride, barbiturates, benazepril, captopril, cyclosporine, enalapril, fosinopril, lisinopril, mitotane, moexipril, narcotics, NSAIDs, potassium chloride, potassium iodide, quinapril, ramipril, trandolapril, triamterene

Aldactazide is spironolactone and hydrochlorothiazide

## *Reactions*

### Skin

Bullous pemphigoid
(2002): Modeste AB+, *Ann Dermatol Venereol* 129(1), 56
Chills
Chloasma
(1988): Hughes BR+, *Br J Dermatol* 118, 687
Contact dermatitis
(1996): Corazza M+, *Contact Dermatitis* 35, 365
(1994): Aguirre A+, *Contact Dermatitis* 30, 312
(1994): Balato N+, *Contact Dermatitis* 31, 203
(1994): Fernandez-Vozmediano JM+, *Contact Dermatitis* 30, 118
(1993): Vincenzi C+, *Contact Dermatitis* 29, 277 (from anti-acne cream)
(1984): Klijn J, *Contact Dermatitis* 10, 105
Cutaneous side effects (sic)
(1973): Almeyda J+, *Br J Dermatol* 88, 313
Diaphoresis
Eczematous eruption (sic)
(1994): Balato N+, *Contact Dermatitis* 31, 203
(1994): Fernandez-Vozmediano JM+, *Contact Dermatitis* 30, 118
Erythema
Erythema annulare centrifugum
(1987): Carsuzaa F+, *Ann Dermatol Venereol* (French) 114, 375
Erythema multiforme
(1986): Greenberger PA+, *N Engl Reg Allergy Proc* 7, 343
Exanthems
(1994): Gupta AK+, *Dermatol* 189, 402
(1988): Hughes BR+, *Br J Dermatol* 118, 687 (9.3%)
(1986): Wathen CG+, *Lancet* 1, 919
(1979): Uddin MS+, *Cutis* 24, 198 (passim)
(1977): Ferguson RK+, *Clin Pharmacol Ther* 21, 62 (1–5%)
(1973): Greenblatt DJ+, *JAMA* 225, 40 (0.5%)
Facial edema
(1998): Lubbos HG+, *Arch Dermatol* 134, 1163
Flushing (<1%)
Graft-versus-host reaction
(1998): Jappe U+, *Hautarzt* (German) 49, 126 (passim)
Lichen planus
(1978): Downham TF, *JAMA* 240, 1138
Lichenoid eruption
(1998): Clark C+, *Clin Exp Dermatol* 23, 43
(1994): Schon MP+, *Acta Derm Venereol* 74, 476
Lupus erythematosus
(2002): Boye T+, *World Congress Dermatol* Poster, 0088
(1987): Leroy D+, *Ann Dermatol Venereol* (French) 114, 1237
Melasma
(2000): Shaw JC, *J Am Acad Dermatol* 43, 498
(1979): Uddin MS+, *Cutis* 24, 198
Necrotizing angiitis
Pemphigoid
(1997): Grange F+, *Ann Dermatol Venereol* (French) 124, 700
Pemphigus
(2002): Karam A+, *World Congress Dermatol* Poster, 0328
Photosensitivity
Pigmentation
(1988): Hughes BR+, *Br J Dermatol* 118, 687 (chloasma-like)
(1988): Hughes BR, *Dermatology Times* June, 10 (chloasma-like)
(1983): Luderschmidt C, *Dtsch Med Wochenschr* (German) 108, 1922
(1975): Davies DL+, *Drugs* 9, 214
Pruritus
(1988): Hughes BR, *Dermatology Times* June, 10
(1986): Wathen CG+, *Lancet* 1, 919
Purpura
Rash (sic) (1–10%)
(1988): Hughes BR, *Dermatology Times* June, 10
(1973): Greenblatt DJ+, *JAMA* 225, 40
Raynaud's phenomenon
(1975): Davies DL+, *Drugs* 9, 214
Urticaria
(1988): Helfer EL+, *J Clin Endocrinol Metab* 66, 208
(1979): Uddin MS+, *Cutis* 24, 198 (passim)
Vasculitis
(1984): Phillips GWL+, *BMJ* 288, 368
Xerosis
(2000): Shaw JC, *J Am Acad Dermatol* 43, 498
(1988): Hughes BR+, *Br J Dermatol* 118, 687 (40%)
(1988): Hughes BR, *Dermatology Times* June, 10

### Hair

Hair – alopecia
(1988): Helfer EL+, *J Clin Endocrinol Metab* 66, 208
(1975): Davies DL+, *Drugs* 9, 214
Hair – hirsutism

### Other

Acute intermittent porphyria
Ageusia
Anaphylactoid reactions
Gynecomastia (<1%)
(2001): Yamamoto S, *Intern Med* 40(6), 550
(2000): Hugues FC+, *Ann Med Interne (Paris)* (French) 151, 10 (passim)
(1994): Dove F, *Hosp Pract Off Ed* 29, 27
(1994): *BMJ* 308, 503
(1993): Thompson DF+, *Pharmacotherapy* 13, 37
(1988): Hughes BR+, *Br J Dermatol* 118, 687
(1977): Rose LI+, *Ann Intern Med* 87, 398
(1976): Loriaux DL, *Ann Intern Med* 85, 630
(1973): Greenblatt DJ+, *JAMA* 225, 40 (passim)
(1965): Clark E, *JAMA* 193, 163
(1963): Mann NM, *JAMA* 190, 160
Mastodynia
(2000): Shaw JC, *J Am Acad Dermatol* 43, 498
Oral lichen planus
(1990): Lamey PJ+, *Oral Surg Oral Med Oral Pathol* 70, 184
Paresthesias
Xerostomia

# ST JOHN'S WORT

**Scientific name:** *Hypericum perforatum*
**Other common names:** Amber; Demon Chaser; Fuga Daemonum; Goatweed; Hardhay; Hypereikon; Hypericum; Johns Wort; Klamath Weed; Rosin Rose; SJW; Tipton Weed
**Family:** Hypericaceae
**Purported indications:** Depression, dysthymic disorder, fatigue, insomnia, loss of appetite, anxiety, obsessive-compulsive disorders, mood disturbances, migraine headaches, neuralgia, fibrositis, sciatica, palpitations, exhaustion, headache, muscle pain
**Other uses:** Cancer, vitiligo, HIV/AIDS, diuretic, bruises, abrasions, muscle pain, first degree burns, hemorrhoids, neuralgia
**Clinically important, potentially hazardous interactions with:** amprenavir, bosentan, cyclosporine, fluoxetine, imatinib, indinavir, midazolam, nelfinavir, ritonavir, saquinavir, sertraline

### *Reactions*

## Skin

Allergic reactions (sic)
(1994): Woelk H+, *J Geriatr Psychiatry Neurol* 7 (Suppl 1), S34
Irritation (sic)
Photosensitivity
(1999): Gulick RM+, *Ann Intern Med* 130, 510
(1997): Brockmoller J+, *Pharmacopsychiatry* 30, 94
(1997): Golsch S+, *Hautarzt* (German) 48, 249
Pruritus
(1997): Golsch S+, *Hautarzt* 48, 249

## Hair

Hair – alopecia
(2001): Parker V+, *Can J Psychiatry* 46(1), 77

## Other

Hypersensitivity
Paresthesias
(1998): Ernst E+, *Eur J Clin Pharmacol* 54, 589
Serotonin syndrome
(2001): Parker V+, *Can J Psychiatry* 46(1), 77
(2000): Brown TM, *Am J Emerg Med* 18, 231
Xerostomia
(1997): *Med Lett Drugs Ther* 39, 107

**Note:** St. John's wort is a natural source of flavoring in Europe. Although not indigenous to Australia, and long considered a weed, St. John's wort is now grown there as a cash crop and produces 20% of the world's supply. The flowers of St. John's wort can have the brightest appearance on June 24, the birthday of St. John the Baptist

# STANOZOLOL

**Trade name:** Winstrol (Sanofi)
**Other common trade names:** *Menabol; Stromba*
**Indications:** Hereditary angioedema
**Category:** Anabolic steroid; androgen
**Half-life:** no data
**Clinically important, potentially hazardous interactions with:** anticoagulants, warfarin

### *Reactions*

## Skin

Acne (>10%)
(1995): Helfman T+, *J Am Acad Dermatol* 32, 254
Chills (1–10%)
Edema
Exanthems
Folliculitis
(1995): Helfman T+, *J Am Acad Dermatol* 32, 254
Pigmentation (1–10%)
Rosacea
(1995): Helfman T+, *J Am Acad Dermatol* 32, 254
Seborrheic dermatitis
(1995): Helfman T+, *J Am Acad Dermatol* 32, 254
Urticaria

## Hair

Hair – alopecia (in women)
Hair – hirsutism (in women)
(1995): Helfman T+, *J Am Acad Dermatol* 32, 254
(1987): Sheffer AL+, *J Allergy Clin Immunol* 80, 855

## Other

Gynecomastia (>10%)
(1995): Helfman T+, *J Am Acad Dermatol* 32, 254
Priapism (>10%)

# STAVUDINE

**Synonym:** d4T
**Trade name:** Zerit (Bristol-Myers Squibb)
**Indications:** Human immunodeficiency virus (HIV)
**Category:** Antiretroviral; nucleoside reverse transcriptase inhibitor (NRTI)
**Half-life:** 1.44 hours

### *Reactions*

## Skin

Allergic reactions (sic) (9%)
Buffalo hump
Chills (50%)
Diaphoresis (19%)
Neutrophilic eccrine hidradenitis
(1998): Krischer J+, *J Dermatol* 25, 199
Rash (sic) (~40%)

## Other

Death
(2001): Hwang SW+, *Singapore Med J* 42(6), 247 (2 cases) (with didanosine)
Gynecomastia
(2001): Aquilina C+, *Int J STD AIDS* 12(7), 481 (with didanosine)
(2001): Manfredi R+, *Ann Pharmacother* 35(4), 438 (with didanosine)
(2001): Manfredi R+, *Ann Pharmacother* 35(4), 438 (with lamivudine) (3 cases)
(1998): Melbourne KM+, *Ann Pharmacother* 32, 1108
HAART (tendon xanthomata)
(2001): Leung N+, *Diabetes* 50(Suppl.2), 452
Lipoatrophy
(2001): Lichtenstein KA+, *AIDS* 15(11), 1389
Lipodystrophy
(2002): Reid S, *Can Adv Drug Reaction Newsletter* 12, 5
(2001): Aquilina C+, *Int J STD AIDS* 12(7), 481 (with didanosine)
(2001): Arpadi SM+, *J Acquir Immune Defic Syndr* 27(1), 30
(2001): Bogner JR+, *J Acquir Immune Defic Syndr* 27(3), 237
(2001): van der Valk M+, *AIDS* 15(7), 847
(1999): Ruel M+, *Ann Med Interne (Paris)* (French) 150, 269
Myalgia (32%)
(2000): Miller KD+, *Ann Intern Med* 133, 192
Paresthesias

# STREPTOKINASE

**Trade names:** Kabikinase (Pharmacia & Upjohn); Streptase (AstraZeneca)
**Indications:** Pulmonary embolism, acute myocardial infarction
**Category:** Thrombolytic
**Half-life:** 83 minutes
**Clinically important, potentially hazardous interactions with:** bivalirudin

### *Reactions*

## Skin

Allergic reactions (sic) (4.4%)
(2001): Toquero J+, *Rev Esp Cardiol* 54(10), 1225
(1998): Stephens MB+, *Postgrad Med* 103, 89
(1997): Cannas S+, *G Ital Cardiol* (Italian) 27, 278
Angiitis
(1988): Sorber WA+, *Cutis* 42, 57
Angioedema (>10%)
(1994): Cooper JP+, *Postgrad Med J* 70, 592
Cutaneous bleeding
(1990): Goa KL+, *Drugs* 39, 693 (3.6%)
Diaphoresis (1–10%)
Ecchymoses
Exanthems (1–5%)
(1990): Goa KL+, *Drugs* 39, 693
(1976): Kohner GM+, *BMJ* 1, 550
Flushing (<1%)
Periorbital edema (>10%)
Pruritus (1–10%)
Purpura
Rash (sic) (1–10%)
Urticaria (1–5%)
(1990): Goa KL+, *Drugs* 39, 693
Vasculitis
(1994): Penswick J+, *BMJ* 309, 378
(1991): Patel A+, *J Am Acad Dermatol* 24, 652
(1988): Davidson JR+, *Clin Exp Rheumatol* 6, 381
(1988): Ong AC+, *Int J Cardiology* 21, 71
(1986): Manoharan A+, *Aust N Z J Med* 16, 815
(1985): Thompson RF+, *Clin Pharm* 4, 383

## Other

Anaphylactoid reactions (<1%)
(1993): Hohage H+, *Wien Klin Wochenschr* (German) 105, 176
Back pain
(2002): Pinheiro RF+, *Arq Bras Cardiol* 78(2), 230 (infusion)
Injection-site bleeding
(1990): Goa KL+, *Drugs* 39, 693 (3%)
Injection-site phlebitis
Serum sickness
(1995): Creamer JD+, *Clin Exp Dermatol* 20, 468
(1994): Proctor BD+, *N Engl J Med* 330, 576
(1991): Patel A+, *J Am Acad Dermatol* 24, 652
(1984): Alexopoulos D+, *Eur Heart J* 5, 1010
(1982): Totty WG+, *Am J Roentgenol* 138, 143
Stomatitis (following local application)
Tongue edema (with hemorrhagic swelling)

# STREPTOMYCIN

**Trade name:** Streptomycin (Pfizer)
**Indications:** Tuberculosis
**Category:** Aminoglycoside antibiotic; tuberculostatic
**Half-life:** 2–5 hours
**Clinically important, potentially hazardous interactions with:** aldesleukin, aminoglycosides, atracurium, bumetanide, doxacurium, ethacrynic acid, furosemide, methoxyflurane, non-depolarizing muscle relaxants, pancuronium, polypeptide antibiotics, rocuronium, succinylcholine, torsemide, vecuronium

### *Reactions*

## Skin

Acute generalized exanthematous pustulosis (AGEP)
(1995): Moreau A+, *Int J Dermatol* 34, 263 (passim)
Allergic reactions (sic)
(1961): Chakravarty S+, *Acta Tuberc Pneumol Scand* 41, 144 (11%)
(1947): Steiner K+, *Arch Dermatol* 56, 511 (18%)
Angioedema (<1%)
(1959): Bereston ES, *J Invest Dermatol* 33, 427
Bullous eruption (<1%)
Cheilitis (2%)
(1949): Cohen AC+, *Arch Dermatol* 60, 373
Contact dermatitis
(1988): Holdiness MR, *Contact Dermatitis* 15, 282
(1983): Fisher AA, *Cutis* 32, 314
Eczematous eruption (sic)
(1958): Wilson HT, *BMJ* 1, 1378
Edema
Erythema multiforme (<1%)
(1988): Hira SK+, *J Am Acad Dermatol* 19, 451 (in AIDS patient)
(1985): Holdiness MR, *Int J Dermatol* 24, 280 (1–5%)
(1985): Ting HC+, *Int J Dermatol* 24, 587
(1947): Steiner K+, *Arch Dermatol* 56, 511
Erythema nodosum (<1%)
Exanthems (>5%)
(1968): Sarkany I, *Proc R Soc Med* 61, 891
(1966): Smith JW+, *Ann Intern Med* 65, 629
(1961): Gupta SK, *Indian J Dermatol* 6, 115
(1960): Heijer A+, *Acta Derm Venereol* (Stockh) 40, 35
(1955): Yow EM, *Ann Intern Med* 43, 323 (10%)
(1949): Bunn PA+, *Streptomycin* Williams and Wilkins, Baltimore, 524
(1949): Cohen AC+, *Arch Dermatol* 60, 373 (11%)
(1948): Keefer CS+, *The Therapeutic Value of Streptomycin* Edwards, Ann Arbor
(1947): Steiner K+, *Arch Dermatol* 56, 511
Exfoliative dermatitis
(1992): Matsuzawa Y+, *Kekkaku* (Japanese) 67, 413
(1986): Sehgal VN+, *Dermatologica* 173, 278
(1985): Holdiness MR, *Int J Dermatol* 24, 280
(1973): Nicolis GD+, *Arch Dermatol* 108, 788
(1972): Kauppinen K, *Acta Derm Venereol* (Stockh) 52, 68
(1969): Agrawal R, *BMJ* 4, 540
(1965): McQueen A, *N Z Med J* 64, 663
(1961): Gupta SK, *Indian J Dermatol* 6, 115
(1959): Bereston ES, *J Invest Dermatol* 33, 427
(1949): Bunn PA+, *Streptomycin* Williams and Wilkins, Baltimore, 524
(1949): Cohen AC+, *Arch Dermatol* 60, 373
(1948): Coombs FC+, *N Y State J Med* 48, 2024
Fixed eruption (<1%)
Follicular pustular eruption (sic)
(1981): Kushimoto H+, *Arch Dermatol* 117, 444

Lichenoid eruption
(1958): Renkin A, *Arch Belg Dermatol Syph* (French) 14, 185
Lupus erythematosus
(1993): Toyoshima M+, *Kekkaku* (Japanese) 68, 319
(1986): Layer P+, *Dtsch Med Wochenschr* (German) 111, 1603
(1980): Agarwal MB+, *J Postgrad Med* 26, 263
(1959): Popkhristov P+, *Surv Med* (Sofia) 10, 81
Photosensitivity
(1971): Girard JP, *Helv Med Acta* 36, 3
Pruritus (<1%)
(1972): Levantine A+, *Br J Dermatol* 86, 651
Purpura
(1969): Peterkin GAG+, *Practitioner* 202, 117
(1965): Horowitz HI+, *Semin Hematol* 2, 287
(1955): Yow EM, *Ann Intern Med* 43, 323 (10%)
(1949): Bunn PA+, *Streptomycin* Williams and Wilkins, Baltimore, 524
Pustular eruption
(1981): Kushimoto H+, *Arch Dermatol* 117, 444
Rash (sic) (<1%)
Stevens–Johnson syndrome
(1988): Hira SK+, *J Am Acad Dermatol* 19, 451 (in AIDS patient)
(1985): Holdiness MR, *Int J Dermatol* 24, 280
(1982): Sarkar SK+, *Tubercle* 63, 137
Systemic eczematous contact dermatitis
Toxic epidermal necrolysis
(1994): *Drug Facts and Comparisons*, 1926
(1988): Fesenko IP+, *Vrach Delo* (Russian) April, 93
(1980): Jain VK+, *Indian J Chest Dis Allied Sci* 22, 73
(1979): Frontera-Izquierdo P+, *An Esp Pediatr* (Spanish) 12, 703
(1979): Odinokova VA+, *Arkh Patol* (Russian) 41, 37
(1974): Ruiz-Maldonado R+, *Bol Med Hosp Infant Mex* (Spanish) 31, 1201
(1973): Sehgal VN+, *Indian J Chest Dis* 15, 57
(1967): Lowney ED+, *Arch Dermatol* 95, 359
Toxic erythema (sic)
(1981): Kushimoto H+, *Arch Dermatol* 117, 444
Urticaria
(1961): Gupta SK, *Indian J Dermatol* 6, 115
(1960): Heijer A+, *Acta Derm Venereol* (Stockh) 40, 35
(1949): Bunn PA+, *Streptomycin* Williams and Wilkins, Baltimore, 524
(1949): Cohen AC+, *Arch Dermatol* 60, 373 (11%)
Vasculitis
(1971): Girard JP, *Helv Med Acta* 36, 3
(1949): Bunn PA+, *Streptomycin* Williams and Wilkins, Baltimore, 524

### Hair

Hair – hypertrichosis
(1992): Shelley WB+, *Advanced Dermatologic Diagnosis* WB Saunders, 725 (passim)

### Other

Anaphylactoid reactions
(1969): Levene GM+, *Trans St Johns Hosp Dermatol Soc* 55, 184
Black tongue
(1954): No Author, *Lancet* 2, 179
Embolia cutis medicamentosa (Nicolau syndrome)
(1972): Labouche F+, *Bull Soc Fr Dermatol Syphiligr* (French) 79, 559
Glossitis (2%)
(1949): Cohen AC+, *Arch Dermatol* 60, 373
Injection-site granuloma
Injection-site reactions (sic)
Oral mucosal eruption
(1972): Levantine A+, *Br J Dermatol* 86, 651
(1964): Dummett CO, *J Oral Ther Pharmacol* 1, 106
Oral ulceration
Paresthesias (<1%)
Stomatitis
(1964): Dummett CO, *J Oral Ther Pharmacol* 1, 106
(1948): Beham H+, *JAMA* 138, 495
Tinnitus
Tremors (<1%)

# STREPTOZOCIN

**Trade name:** Zanosar (Pharmacia & Upjohn)
**Indications:** Carcinoma of the pancreas, carcinoid tumor, Hodgkin's disease
**Category:** Antineoplastic
**Half-life:** 35 minutes
**Clinically important, potentially hazardous interactions with:** aldesleukin

## *Reactions*

### Skin

Edema
Exanthems
(1978): Levine N+, *Cancer Treat Rev* 5, 67
Pruritus
(1978): Levine N+, *Cancer Treat Rev* 5, 67
Purpura
Toxic epidermal necrolysis
(1975): Hadida E+, *Bull Soc Fr Dermatol Syphiligr* (French) 81, 76

### Other

Injection-site erythema
Injection-site necrosis
(1987): Dufresne RG, *Cutis* 39, 197
Injection-site pain (1–10%)

# SUCCINYLCHOLINE

**Synonym:** suxamethonium
**Trade name:** Anectine (GSK)
**Indications:** Skeletal muscle relaxation during general anesthesia
**Category:** Skeletal muscle relaxant; cholinergic
**Half-life:** no data
**Clinically important, potentially hazardous interactions with:** amikacin, aminoglycosides, galantamine, gentamicin, kanamycin, neomycin, paromomycin, streptomycin, tobramycin, vancomycin

## *Reactions*

### Skin

Contact dermatitis
(1996): Delgado J+, *Contact Dermatitis* 35, 120
Erythema (<1%)
(1975): Fisher MMcD, *Anaesth Intensive Care* 3, 180
Exanthems
Flushing
Pruritus (<1%)
Rash (sic) (<1%)
Urticaria

### Other

Anaphylactoid reactions
(1999): Porter JM+, *Ir J Med Sci* 168, 99

(1999): Villas Martinez F+, *J Investig Allergol Clin Immunol* 9, 126
(1998): Tresch K+, *Ann Fr Anesth Reanim* (French) 17, 1181
(1990): Moneret-Vautrin DA+, *Br J Anaesth* 64(6), 743
(1981): Moneret-Vautrin DA+, *Clin Allergy* 11, 175 (13 cases)
(1975): Mandappa JM+, *Br J Anaesth* 47, 523 (2 cases)

Hypersensitivity
(1983): Yamaya R+, *Masui* (Japanese) 32, 1464

Myalgia (<1%)
(1996): van den Berg AA+, *Anaesth Intensive Care* 24, 116

Myopathy
(1990): Shoji S, *Nippon Rinsho* (Japanese) 48, 1517

Rhabdomyolysis
(2001): Gronert GA, *Anesthesiology* 94(3), 523
(2000): Le Puura+, *Acta Anaesthesiol Belg* 51(1), 51
(2000): Matthews JM, *Anesth Analg* 91(6), 1552
(2000): Shaaban MJ+, *Middle East J Anesthesiology* 15(6), 681
(1996): Fiacchino F, *Anesthesiology* 84(2), 480
(1996): Pedrozzi NE+, *Pediatr Neurol* 15(3), 254 (2 cases)
(1996): Perret D+, *Ann Fr Anesth Reanim* 15(8), 1193
(1996): Takamatsu F+, *Masui* 45(11), 1406
(1995): Friedman S+, *Anesth Analg* 81(2), 422
(1994): Sullivan M+, *Can J Anaesth* 41(6), 497
(1993): Bhave CG+, *J Postgrad Med* 39(3), 157
(1992): Bakshi KK, *J Assoc Physicians India* 40(8), 549
(1991): Gokhale YA+, *J Assoc Physicians India* 39(12), 968
(1987): Lee SC+, *J Oral Maxillofac Surg* 45(9), 789 (with enflurane)
(1987): Lee SC+, *Ma Zui Xue Za Zhi* 25(2), 97
(1985): Hawker F+, *Anaesth Intensive Care* 13(2), 208
(1985): Sodano R+, *Minerva Anestesiol* 51(3), 109
(1984): Blumberg A+, *Schweiz Med Wochenschr* 114(30), 1068 (2 cases)
(1984): Hool GJ+, *Anaesth Intensive Care* 12(4), 360
(1981): Lewandowski KB, *Br J Anaesth* 53(9), 981
(1979): Bomholt A, *Ugeskr Laeger* 141(14), 925
(1978): Gibbs JM, *Anaesth Intensive Care* 6(2), 141
(1976): Moore WE+, *Anesth Analg* 55(5), 680 (with halothane)

Sialorrhea (1–10%)

# SUCRALFATE

**Trade name:** Carafate (Aventis)
**Other common trade names:** *Antepsin; Sucrabest; Sulcrate; Ulcar; Ulcogant; Ulcyte; Urbal*
**Indications:** Duodenal ulcer
**Category:** Antiulcer; gastric mucosa protectant
**Half-life:** no data
**Clinically important, potentially hazardous interactions with:** ciprofloxacin, clorazepate, ketoconazole, lansoprazole, lomefloxacin, phenytoin, sparfloxacin, tetracycline

### *Reactions*

## Skin

Angioedema
Exanthems
(1984): Brogden RN+, *Drugs* 17, 233
Facial edema
Pruritus (<0.5%)
Rash (sic) (<0.5%)
Urticaria

## Other

Xerostomia (<1%)

# SUFENTANIL

**Trade name:** Sufenta (Taylor)
**Indications:** Epidural and general anesthesia
**Category:** Narcotic analgesic
**Half-life:** 152 minutes
**Clinically important, potentially hazardous interactions with:** cimetidine

### *Reactions*

## Skin

Chills
Cold clammy skin (<1%)
Erythema
Pruritus (25%)
Rash (sic) (<1%)
Urticaria (<1%)

## Other

Dysesthesia (<1%)

# SULFACETAMIDE

**Trade names:** Ak-Sulf; Albucid; Antebor; Bleph-10 (Allergan); Cetamide; Cetasil; Colirio Sulfacetamido Kriya; Covosulf; Dansemid; Dayto-Sulf; Diosulf; I-Sulfacet; Infa-Sulf; Isopto Cetamid (Alcon); Klaron (Dermik); Lersa; Novacet; Ocu-Sul; Ocu-Sulf; Ophthacet; Optamide; Optin; Optisol; Ovace (Healthpoint); Plexion (Medicis); Prontamid; Sebizon; Sodium Sulamyd (Schering); Sodium Sulfacetamide; Spectro-Sulf; Spersacet; Storz-Sulf; Sulf-10; Sulfac; Sulfacel-15; Sulfacet Sodium; Sulfacet-R (Dermik); Sulfair; Sulfamide; Sulfex; Sulphacalre; Sulster; Sulten-10
**Indications:** Infectious conjunctivitis, acne vulgaris, seborrheic dermatitis
**Category:** Ophthalmic; sulfonamide antibiotic – topical lotion; ointment; anti-acne lotion
**Half-life:** 7–13 hours
**Clinically important, potentially hazardous interactions with:** anticoagulants, cyclosporine, silver salts

### *Reactions*

## Skin

Allergic reactions (sic)
(2002): Smith JG, Mobile, AL (from Internet) (observations 2 cases) (Klaron & Sulfacet-R)
(2000): Blumenthal HL, Beachwood, OH (personal case) (observation) (Novacet Lotion)
Edema
Erythema
Erythema multiforme
(1985): Genvert GI+, *Am J Ophthalmol* 99(4), 465 (topical)
Exfoliative dermatitis (1–10%)
Infections (sic)
Lupus erythematosus – dermatomyositis (sic)
(1979): Mackie BS+, *Australas J Dermatol* 20(1), 49 (eye-drops)
Photosensitivity
Pruritus
Stevens–Johnson syndrome (1–10%)
(1977): Rubin Z, *Arch Dermatol* 113(2), 235 (ophthalmic)

(1976): Gottschalk HR+, *Arch Dermatol* 112(4), 513 (ophthalmic) (previous bullous eruption to a sulfonamide)
Toxic epidermal necrolysis (1–10%)

### Other
Death
Hypersensitivity
Occular irritation
Ocular burning
Ocular stinging

## SULFADIAZINE

**Trade name:** Microsulfon
**Other common trade name:** *Coptin*
**Indications:** Various infections caused by susceptible organisms
**Category:** Sulfonamide* antibiotic
**Half-life:** 17 hours
**Clinically important, potentially hazardous interactions with:** anticoagulants, cyclosporine, methotrexate

### *Reactions*

### Skin
Allergy (sic)
(1991): de la Hoz Caballer B+, *J Allergy Clin Immunol* 88, 137
Argyria
(2002): Maitre S+, *Ann Dermatol Venereol* 129(2), 217 (topical silver sulfadiazine)
(2001): Thomas K+, *BJOG* 108(8), 890
(1992): Fraser-Moodie A, *Burns* 18, 74 (from silver sulfadiazine)
(1992): Payne CM+, *Lancet* 340, 126 (from silver sulfadiazine)
Chills
Erythema multiforme
(1983): Lockhart SP+, *Burns Incl Therm Inj* 10, 9
Exanthems
(1984): Finland M+, *JAMA* 251, 1467
Exfoliative dermatitis
Fixed eruption
(1991): Thankappen TP+, *Int J Dermatol* 30, 867 (12.4%)
Lupus erythematosus
Periorbital edema
Photosensitivity (>10%)
Pigmentation
(1985): Dupuis LL+, *J Am Acad Dermatol* 12, 1112
Pruritus (>10%)
Purpura
Rash (sic) (>10%)
Stevens–Johnson syndrome (1–10%)
(1999): Carrion-Carrion C+, *Ann Pharmacother* 33, 379 (fatal) (in AIDS patient)
(1965): Sharma R+, *J Assoc Physicians India* 13, 727
Toxic epidermal necrolysis (1–10%)
(1993): Correia O+, *Dermatology* 186, 32
Urticaria

### Other
Anaphylactoid reactions
(2001): Stephens R+, *Br J Anaesth* 87(2), 306 (with chlorhexidine)
Death
Hypersensitivity
(2001): Morand JJ+, *Ann Dermatol Venereol* 128(12), 1351
(1987): Volckaert A+, *Acta Clin Belg* 42, 381
(1985): Jia XM, *Chung Hua Cheng Hsing Shao Shang Wai Ko Tsa Chih* (Chinese) 1, 232
Serum sickness (<1%)
Stomatitis
Tinnitus

***Note:** Sulfadiazine is a sulfonamide and can be absorbed systemically. Sulfonamides can produce severe, possibly fatal, reactions such as toxic epidermal necrolysis and Stevens–Johnson syndrome

## SULFADOXINE

**Trade name:** Fansidar (Roche)
**Other common trade names:** *Cryodoxin; Malocide; Methipox*
**Indications:** Malaria
**Category:** Sulfonamide* antimalarial; folic acid antagonist
**Half-life:** 5–8 days

Fansidar is sulfadoxine and pyrimethamine (this combination is almost always prescribed)

### *Reactions*

### Skin
Bullous eruption
(1985): Hernborg A, *Lancet* 1, 1072
Erythema multiforme (<1%)
(1993): Sturchler D+, *Drug Saf* 8, 160
(1989): Ortel B+, *Dermatologica* 178, 39
(1986): Miller KD+, *Am J Trop Med Hyg* 35, 451
Exanthems
(1987): Groth H+, *Schweiz Rundsch Med Prax* (German) 76, 570
Exfoliative dermatitis
(1987): Elsas T+, *Tidsskr Nor Laegeforen* (Norwegian) 107, 1231
(1987): Zitelli BJ+, *Ann Intern Med* 106, 393
(1986): Langtry JA+, *Br Med J Clin Res Ed* 292, 1107
Lupus erythematosus
Necrosis (<1%)
Periorbital edema
Photosensitivity (>10%)
(1989): Ortel B+, *Dermatologica* 178, 39
(1985): Hernborg A, *Lancet* 1, 1072 (passim)
Pruritus
(1987): Groth H+, *Schweiz Rundsch Med Prax* (German) 76, 570
Purpura
(1985): Hernborg A, *Lancet* 1, 1072 (passim)
Pustular eruption
Rash (sic) (<1%)
Stevens–Johnson syndrome (1–10%)
(1993): Sturchler D+, *Drug Saf* 8, 160
(1990): Thiel HJ+, *Klin Monatsbl Augenheilkd* (German) 197, 142
(1989): Ortel B+, *Dermatologica* 178, 39
(1989): Phillips-Howard PA+, *Lancet* 2, 803
(1987): Hellgren U+, *Br Med J Clin Res Ed* 295, 365
(1987): Lenox-Smith I, *J Infect* 14, 90 (fatal)
(1986): Bamber MG+, *J Infect* 13, 31 (fatal)
(1986): Gascon-Brustenga J+, *Med Clin (Barc)* (Spanish) 87, 821
(1986): Jeffrey RF, *Postgrad Med J* 62, 893
(1986): Miller KD+, *Am J Trop Med Hyg* 35, 451
(1986): Steffen R+, *Lancet* 1, 610
(1985): Adams SJ+, *Postgrad Med J* 61, 263
(1985): Clareus BW+, *Lakartidningen* (Swedish) 82, 4211
(1985): Hernborg A, *Lancet* 2, 1072
(1985): Navin TR+, *Lancet* 1, 1332
(1983): Ligthelm RJ+, *Ned Tijdschr Geneeskd* (Dutch) 127, 1735
(1982): Aberer W+, *Hautarzt* (German) 33, 484

(1982): Hornstein OP+, *N Engl J Med* 307, 1529
(1982): Olsen VV+, *Lancet* 2, 994
Toxic epidermal necrolysis
(2000): Moussala M+, *J Fr Ophtalmol* (French) 23, 229
(1998): Moussala M+, *J Fr Ophtalmol* (French) 21, 72
(1998): Schmidt-Westhausen A+, *Oral Dis* 4, 90
(1993): Correia O+, *Dermatology* 186, 32
(1993): Sturchler D+, *Drug Saf* 8, 160
(1991): Kimura S+, *Jpn J Med* 30, 553
(1990): Ward DJ+, *Burns* 16, 97
(1989): Caumes E+, *Presse Med* (French) 18, 1708 (fatal)
(1988): No Author, *JAMA* 260, 2193 (fatal)
(1988): No Author, *Morb Mortal Wkly Rep* 37, 571 (fatal)
(1988): Raviglione MC+, *Arch Intern Med* 148, 2863 (fatal)
(1986): Miller KD+, *Am J Trop Med Hyg* 35, 451
(1984): Chan HL, *J Am Acad Dermatol* 10, 973
(1983): Ghinelli F+, *Acta Biomed Ateneo Parmense* (Italian) 54, 363
Urticaria

## Other

Ageusia
Anaphylactoid reactions
Death
Glossitis (>10%)
Hypersensitivity (>10%)
Oral lichenoid eruption
(1989): Zain RB, *Southeast Asian J Trop Med Public Health* 20, 253
Oral ulceration
(1985): Hernborg A, *Lancet* 1, 1072
Stomatitis
(1985): Hernborg A, *Lancet* 1, 1072 (passim)
Tinnitus
Tremors (>10%)
Urogenital ulceration
(1985): Hernborg A, *Lancet* 1, 1072

***Note:** Sulfadoxine is a sulfonamide and can be absorbed systemically. Sulfonamides can produce severe, possibly fatal, reactions such as toxic epidermal necrolysis and Stevens–Johnson syndrome

# SULFAMETHOXAZOLE

**Trade names:** Bactrim (Roche); Septra (Monarch)
**Other common trade names:** *Sinomin; Urobak*
**Indications:** Various infections caused by susceptible organisms
**Category:** Antibacterial and antiprotozoal sulfonamide*
**Half-life:** 7–12 hours
**Clinically important, potentially hazardous interactions with:** anticoagulants, cyclosporine, methotrexate, warfarin

**Note:** Sulfamethoxazole is commonly used in conjunction with trimethoprim (see co-trimoxazole)

### *Reactions*

## Skin

Acute febrile neutrophilic dermatosis (Sweet's syndrome)
(1996): Walker DC+, *J Am Acad Dermatol* 34, 918
(1989): Cobb MW, *J Am Acad Dermatol* 21, 339 (passim)
(1986): Su WPD+, *Cutis* 37, 167
Acute generalized exanthematous pustulosis (AGEP)
(1995): Moreau A+, *Int J Dermatol* 34, 263 (passim)
Angioedema
(1988): Fihn SD+, *Ann Intern Med* 108, 350 (1–5%)
Bullous eruption
(1989): Caumes E+, *Presse Med* (French) 18, 1708
Cutaneous side effects (sic)
(1994): Roudier C+, *Arch Dermatol* 130, 1383 (48% in AIDS patients)
(1971): Koch-Weser J+, *Arch Intern Med* 128, 399 (2.1%)
Dermatitis (sic)
(1989): Atahan IL+, *Br J Radiol* 62, 1107 (at previously irradiated area)
(1987): Vukelja SJ+, *Cancer Treat Rep* 71, 668 (at previously irradiated area)
(1984): Shelley WB+, *J Am Acad Dermatol* 11, 53 (at site of previous sunburn)
(1971): Cotterill JA+, *Br J Dermatol* 84, 366
Erythema multiforme
(1997): Rieder MJ+, *Pediatr Infect Dis J* 16, 1028 (70% in children with HIV)
(1991): Tilden ME+, *Arch Ophthalmol* 109, 67
(1990): Chan HL+, *Arch Dermatol* 126, 43
(1989): Alanko K+, *Acta Derm Venereol* (Stockh) 69, 223
(1988): Hira SK+, *J Am Acad Dermatol* 19, 451
(1988): Platt R+, *J Infect Dis* 158, 474
(1987): Penmetcha M, *BMJ* 295, 556
(1987): Schöpf E, *Infection* 15 (Suppl 5P), S254
(1985): Heer M+, *Gastroenterology* 88, 1954
(1982): Brettle RP+, *J Infect* 4, 149
(1979): Beck MH+, *Clin Exp Dermatol* 4, 201
(1978): Assaad D+, *Can Med Assoc J* 118, 154
(1978): Azinge NO+, *J Allergy Clin Immunol* 62, 125
(1975): Bernstein LS, *Can Med Assoc J* 112 (Suppl), 96
(1971): Koch-Weser J+, *Arch Intern Med* 128, 399 (0.15%)
Erythema nodosum
(1974): Delaney TJ+, *Br J Dermatol* 90, 205
(1971): Koch-Weser J+, *Arch Intern Med* 128, 399
Erythroderma
(1979): Kennedy C+, *BMJ* 1, 1356
Exanthems
(1998): Hattori N+, *J Dermatol* 25, 269
(1997): Caumes E+, *Arch Dermatol* 133, 465
(1995): Hertl M+, *Br J Dermatol* 132, 215
(1995): Wolkenstein P+, *Arch Dermatol* 131, 544
(1994): Litt JZ, Beachwood, OH (personal case) (observation)
(1993): Agarwal BR+, *Indian Pediatr* 30, 1026
(1993): Litt JZ, Beachwood, OH (personal case) (observation)
(1993): Malnick SDH+, *Ann Pharmacotherapy* 27, 1139
(1990): Medina I+, *N Engl J Med* 323, 776 (47% in AIDS patients)
(1988): DeRaeve L+, *Br J Dermatol* 119, 521 (in AIDS patient)
(1988): Fihn SD+, *Ann Intern Med* 108, 350 (1–5%)
(1988): Sattler FR+, *Ann Intern Med* 109, 280 (44% in AIDS patients)
(1988): Weinke T+, *Dtsch Med Wochenschr* (German) 113, 1129 (25% in AIDS patients)
(1987): Goa KL+, *Drugs* 33, 242 (65% in AIDS patients)
(1987): Schöpf E, *Infection* 15 (Suppl 5P), S254
(1986): Sonntag MR+, *Schweiz Med Wochenschr* (German) 116, 142
(1985): DeHovitz JA+, *Ann Intern Med* 103, 479
(1985): Maayan S+, *Arch Intern Med* 145, 1607
(1984): Gordon FM+, *Ann Intern Med* 100, 495 (51% in AIDS patients)
(1984): Kovacs JA+, *Ann Intern Med* 100, 663 (29% in AIDS patients)
(1983): Mitsuyasu R+, *N Engl J Med* 308, 1535 (69% in AIDS patients.)
(1982): Goetz MB+, *JAMA* 247, 3118
(1980): Fennell RS+, *Clin Pediatr* 19, 124
(1979): Abengowe CU, *Curr Med Res Opin* 5, 749 (3.2%)
(1977): Taylor B+, *BMJ* 2, 552 (12%)
(1976): Arndt KA+, *JAMA* 235, 918 (5.9%)
(1976): Gower PE+, *BMJ* 1, 684 (>5%)

(1975): Bernstein LS, *Can Med Assoc J* 112 (Suppl), 96 (1.9%)
(1975): Gleckman RA, *JAMA* 233, 427 (0.84%)
(1975): Sallam MA+, *Curr Med Res Opin* 3, 229 (3.4%)
(1972): Halpern GM, *BMJ* 1, 691
(1971): Koch-Weser J+, *Arch Intern Med* 128, 399 (1%)

Exfoliative dermatitis
(1990): Ponte CD+, *Drug Intell Clin Pharm* 24, 140 (feet)
(1975): Bernstein LS, *Can Med Assoc J* 112 (Suppl), 96
(1971): Koch-Weser J+, *Arch Intern Med* 128, 399

Fixed eruption
(1997): Gruber F+, *Clin Exp Dermatol* 22, 144
(1996): Sharma VK+, *J Dermatol* 23, 530
(1995): Wolkenstein P+, *Arch Dermatol* 131, 544
(1993): Oleaga JM+, *Contact Dermatitis* 29, 155
(1993): Ramam M+, *Indian Pediatr* 30, 110 (in an infant)
(1992): Lim JT+, *Ann Acad Med Singapore* 21, 408
(1991): Jain VK+, *Ann Dent* 50, 9 (oral mucous membrane)
(1991): Smoller BR+, *J Cutan Pathol* 18, 13
(1990): Gaffoor PMA+, *Cutis* 45, 242 (genitalia)
(1989): Basomba A+, *J Allergy Clin Immunol* 84, 409
(1989): Bharija SC+, *Australas J Dermatol* 30, 43
(1989): Gupta R, *Indian J Dermatol* 55, 181 (in an infant)
(1989): Varsano I+, *Dermatologica* 178, 232
(1988): Baird BJ+, *Int J Dermatol* 27, 170 (bullous and generalized)
(1988): Bharija SC+, *Dermatologica* 176, 108 (in an infant)
(1987): Amir J+, *Drug Intell Clin Pharm* 21, 41
(1987): Hughes BR+, *Br J Dermatol* 116, 241
(1987): Van Voorhees A+, *Am J Dermatopathol* 9, 528
(1986): Kanwar AJ+, *Dermatologica* 172, 230
(1985): Gomez B+, *Allergol Immunopathol Madr* (Spanish) 13, 87
(1984): Pandhi RK+, *Sex Transm Dis* 11, 164
(1982): Gibson JR, *BMJ* 284, 1529
(1980): Talbot MD, *Practitioner* 224, 823
(1978): Verbov J, *Arch Dermatol* 114, 963
(1972): Aoyama H+, *Jpn J Dermatol* 82, 16

Flushing
(1984): Jick SS+, *Lancet* 2, 631

Lichenoid eruption
(1994): Berger TG+, *Arch Dermatol* 130, 609

Linear IgA bullous dermatosis
(1994): Kuechle MK+, *J Am Acad Dermatol* 30, 187

Lupus erythematosus
(1985): Stratton MA, *Clin Pharm* 4, 657
(1975): Grennan DM+, *BMJ* 4, 385

Mucocutaneous syndrome
(1982): Brettle RP+, *J Infect* 4, 149

Photosensitivity (>10%)
(1994): Berger TG+, *Arch Dermatol* 130, 609 (in HIV-infected) (4 cases)
(1994): Shelley WB+, *Cutis* 53, 162 (observation)
(1987): Schöpf E, *Infection* 15 (Suppl 5P), S254
(1986): Chandler MJ, *J Infect Dis* 153, 1001

Pruritus (>10%)
(1997): Caumes E+, *Arch Dermatol* 133, 465
(1997): Thaler D, Monona, WI (from internet) (observation)
(1996): Litt JZ, Beachwood, OH (personal case) (observation)
(1990): Medina I+, *N Engl J Med* 323, 776 (1–5%)
(1987): Colebunders R+, *Ann Intern Med* 107, 599 (4% in AIDS patients)
(1986): Sher MR, *J Allergy Clin Immunol* 77, 133
(1984): Kramer BS+, *Cancer* 53, 329
(1975): Gleckman RA, *JAMA* 233, 427 (0.84%)
(1971): Koch-Weser J+, *Arch Intern Med* 128, 399 (0.15%)

Pruritus vulvae
(1981): *Modern Medicine* 49, 111

Psoriasis
(1979): Kennedy C+, *BMJ* 1, 1356

Purpura
(1993): Kaufman DW+, *Blood* 82, 2714
(1989): Saxena SK, *J Assoc Physicians India* 37, 479
(1971): Koch-Weser J+, *Arch Intern Med* 128, 399

Pustular eruption
(1994): Spencer JM+, *Br J Dermatol* 130, 514
(1990): Guy C+, *Nouv Dermatol* (French) 9, 540
(1989): Grattan CEH, *Dermatologica* 179, 57 (passim)
(1986): Macdonald KJS+, *BMJ* 293, 1279
(1978): Braun-Falco O+, *Hautarzt* (German) 29, 371
(1977): Knudsen L+, *Ugeskr Laeger* (Danish) 139, 1007

Radiation recall
(1990): Leslie MD+, *Br J Radiol* 63, 661
(1987): Vukelja SJ+, *Cancer Treat Rep* 71, 668 (at previously irradiated area)
(1984): Shelley WB+, *J Am Acad Dermatol* 11, 53 (at site of previous sunburn)

Rash (sic) (>10%)
(1995): Williams JW+, *JAMA* 273, 1015
(1993): Malnick SD+, *Ann Pharmacother* 27, 1139

Stevens–Johnson syndrome (1–10%)
(1997): Douglas R+, *Clin Infect Dis* 25, 1480
(1997): Rieder MJ+, *Pediatr Infect Dis J* 16, 1028 (10% in children with HIV)
(1996): Caumes E, *Rev Mal Respir* (French) 13, 101
(1996): McCarty J, Fort Worth, TX (from Internet) (observation)
(1995): Kuper K+, *Ophthalmologe* (German) 92, 823
(1995): Sharma VK+, *Pediatr Dermatol* 12, 178
(1995): Wolkenstein P+, *Arch Dermatol* 131, 544
(1994): Shelley WB+, *Cutis* 53, 159 (observation)
(1993): Litt JZ, Beachwood, OH (personal case) (observation)
(1990): Chan HL+, *Arch Dermatol* 126, 43
(1988): Platt R+, *J Infect Dis* 158, 474
(1985): Heer M+, *Gastroenterology* 88, 1954
(1982): Brettle RP+, *J Infect* 4, 149
(1979): Beck MH+, *Clin Exp Dermatol* 4, 201
(1978): Azinge NO+, *J Allergy Clin Immunol* 62, 125
(1978): Kikuchi S+, *Lancet* 2, 580
(1978): Thorpe JA+, *Lancet* 1, 276 (fatal)
(1975): Bernstein LS, *Can Med Assoc J* 112 (Suppl), 96
(1970): Shaw DJ+, *Johns Hopkins Med J* 126, 130

Toxic epidermal necrolysis (1–10%)
(2002): Nassif A+, *J Invest Dermatol* 118(4), 728
(2001): See S+, *Ann Pharmacother* 35(6), 694
(2000): Moussala M+, *J Fr Ophtalmol* (French) 23, 229
(1996): Caumes E, *Rev Mal Respir* 13, 101
(1996): Rehbein H, Jacksonville, FL (from Internet) (observation)
(1995): Sharma VK+, *Pediatr Dermatol* 12, 178
(1995): Wolkenstein P+, *Arch Dermatol* 131, 544 (7 cases)
(1993): Correia O+, *Dermatology* 186, 32
(1990): Chan HL+, *Arch Dermatol* 126, 43
(1990): Kobza Black A+, *Br J Dermatol* 123, 277
(1990): Roujeau JC+, *Arch Dermatol* 126, 37
(1990): Ward DJ+, *Burns* 16, 97
(1989): Carmichael AJ+, *Lancet* 2, 808
(1989): Whittington RM, *Lancet* 2, 574
(1988): De Raeve L+, *Br J Dermatol* 119, 521 (passim)
(1987): Guillaume JC+, *Arch Dermatol* 123, 1166
(1987): Schöpf E, *Infection* 15 (Suppl 5P), S254
(1986): Miller KD+, *Am J Trop Med Hyg* 33, 451
(1986): Revuz J, *J Dermatol Paris* 153
(1986): Roman O+, *Rev Pediatr Obstet Ginecol Pediatr* (Romanian) 35, 261
(1984): Fong PH+, *Singapore Med J* 25, 184
(1984): Westly ED+, *Arch Dermatol* 120, 721
(1983): Petersen P+, *Ugeskr Laeger* (Danish) 145, 3345
(1982): Ortiz JE+, *Ann Plast Surg* 9, 249
(1978): Assaad D+, *Can Med Assoc J* 118, 154
(1978): Petricevic I+, *Lijec Vjesn* (Serbo-Croatian-Roman) 100, 596
(1975): Bernstein LS, *Can Med Assoc J* 112 (Suppl), 96

(1973): Beyvin AJ+, *Anesth Analg Paris* (French) 30, 767
(1972): Chanial G+, *J Med Lyon* (French) 53, 859
(1971): Chanial G+, *Bull Soc Fr Dermatol Syphiligr* (French) 78, 565

Urticaria
(1994): Blumenthal HL, Beachwood, OH (personal case) (observation)
(1993): Litt JZ, Beachwood, OH (personal case) (observation)
(1991): Greenberger PA, *JAMA* 265, 458
(1987): Schöpf E, *Infection* 15 (Suppl 5P), S254
(1985): Goolamali SK, *Postgrad Med J* 61, 925
(1985): Maayan S+, *Arch Intern Med* 145, 1607
(1984): Kramer BS+, *Cancer* 53, 329
(1981): Abi-Mansur P+, *Am J Gastroenterol* 76, 356
(1971): Koch-Weser J+, *Arch Intern Med* 128, 399

Vasculitis (<1%)
(1989): Verne-Pignatelli J+, *Postgrad Med J* 65, 51
(1987): Schöpf E, *Infection* 15 (Suppl 5P), S254
(1978): Braun-Falco O+, *Hautarzt* (German) 29, 371
(1978): Coquin Y+, *Nouv Presse Med* (French) 7, 3145
(1976): Wåhlin A+, *Lancet* 2, 1415
(1971): Koch-Weser J+, *Arch Intern Med* 128, 399

Vulvovaginitis
(1985): Wong ES+, *Ann Intern Med* 102, 302

## Other

Anaphylactoid reactions
(1988): Arnold PA+, *Drug Intell Clin Pharm* 22, 43
(1985): Gossius G+, *Scand J Infect Dis* 16, 373

Aphthous stomatitis
(1981): *J Antimicrob Chemother* 7, 179

Black tongue
(1993): Blumenthal HL, Beachwood, OH (personal case) (observation)

Death

Dysgeusia
(1988): Fischl MA+, *JAMA* 259, 1185

Glossitis

Hypersensitivity
(1998): Chen D, Chicagi, IL (from Internet) (observation)
(1997): Hicks ME+, *Ann Pharmacother* 31, 1259
(1993): Marinac JS+, *Clin Infect Dis* 16, 178
(1993): Martin GJ+, *Clin Infect Dis* 16, 175
(1993): Mathelier-Fusade P+, *Presse Med* (French) 22, 1363
(1993): Mehta J+, *J Assoc Physicians India* 41, 235

Oral mucosal eruption
(1991): Tilden ME+, *Arch Ophthalmol* 109, 67
(1988): Fihn SD+, *Ann Intern Med* 108, 350 (1–5%)

Oral ulceration
(1987): Hughes WT+, *N Engl J Med* 316, 1627
(1981): Orenstein WA+, *Am J Med Sci* 282, 27

Pseudolymphoma
(1978): Laugier P+, *Z Hautkr* (German) 53, 353

Serum sickness (<1%)
(1988): Platt R+, *J Infect Dis* 158, 474

Stomatitis

Tongue ulceration
(1981): *J Antimicrob Chemother* 7, 179

***Note:** Sulfamethoxazole is a sulfonamide and can be absorbed systemically. Sulfonamides can produce severe, possibly fatal, reactions such as toxic epidermal necrolysis and Stevens–Johnson syndrome

# SULFASALAZINE

**Synonym:** salicylazosulfapyridine
**Trade name:** Azulfidine (Pharmacia & Upjohn)
**Other common trade names:** *Colo-Pleon; Salazopyrin; Salisulf; Saridine; SAS-500; Sulfazine; Ulcol*
**Indications:** Inflammatory bowel disease, ulcerative colitis, rheumatoid arthritis
**Category:** Sulfonamide*
**Half-life:** 5–10 hours
**Clinically important, potentially hazardous interactions with:** cholestyramine, methotrexate

### *Reactions*

## Skin

Acute generalized exanthematous pustulosis (AGEP)
(1999): Kawaguchi M+, *J Dermatol* 26, 359
(1998): Mitchell D, Thomasville, GA (from Internet) (observation)
(1993): Marce S+, *Presse Med* (French) 22, 271
(1993): Wainwright NJ+, *Drug Saf* 9, 437

Angioedema
(1990): Donovan S+, *Br J Rheumatol* 29, 201
(1990): Petterson T+, *Br J Rheumatol* 29, 239

Bullous eruption

Bullous pemphigoid
(1970): Bean SF+, *Arch Dermatol* 102, 205

Cheilitis
(1986): Farr M+, *Drugs* 32 (Suppl 1), 49

Cutaneous side effects (sic)
(1986): Amos RS+, *BMJ* 293, 420 (5.5%)

Dermatitis (sic)
(2001): Lau G+, *Forensic Sci Int* 122(2), 79
(1989): Challier P+, *Presse Med* (French) 18, 778

Diaphoresis
(1986): Farr M+, *Drugs* 32 (Suppl 1), 49

Eczematous eruption (sic)
(1947): Sulzberger MB+, *J Allergy* 18, 92

Erythema multiforme
(1987): Penmetcha M, *BMJ* 295, 556
(1986): Garcia e Silva L, *Acta Med Port* (Portuguese) 7, 71
(1985): Heer M+, *Gastroenterology* 88, 1954
(1985): Hernborg A, *Lancet* 2, 1072
(1985): Huff JC, *Dermatol Clin* 3, 141
(1982): Hornstein OP+, *N Engl J Med* 307, 1529
(1979): Beck MH+, *Clin Exp Dermatol* 4, 201
(1966): Cameron HA+, *BMJ* 2, 1174

Erythema nodosum
(1986): Areias E+, *Ann Dermatol Venereol* (French) 113, 197
(1971): Koch-Weser J+, *Arch Intern Med* 128, 399

Erythroderma
(1984): Sala F+, *Cronica Dermatol* (Italian) 15, 209

Exanthems
(1995): Wolkenstein P+, *Arch Dermatol* 131, 544
(1994): Akahoshi K+, *J Gastroenterol* 29, 772
(1992): Bodokh I+, *Presse Med* (French) 21, 630
(1991): Hertzberger-ten-Cate R+, *Clin Exp Rheumatol* 9, 85
(1990): Donovan S+, *Br J Rheumatol* 29, 201 (4.1%)
(1990): Gupta AK+, *Arch Dermatol* 126, 487 (23%)
(1990): Petterson T+, *Br J Rheumatol* 29, 239
(1989): Alanko K+, *Acta Derm Venereol* (Stockh) 69, 223
(1989): Gremse DA+, *J Pediatr Gastroenterol Nutr* 9, 261
(1988): Williams HJ+, *Arthritis Rheum* 31, 702 (7%)
(1986): Farr M+, *Drugs* 32 (Suppl 1), 49
(1986): Poland GA+, *Am J Med* 81, 707
(1985): Maayan S+, *Arch Intern Med* 145, 1607

(1984): Iwatsuki K+, *Arch Dermatol* 120, 964
(1984): Peppercorn MA, *Ann Intern Med* 101, 377
(1984): Purdy BH+, *Ann Intern Med* 100, 512
(1982): Goetz MB+, *JAMA* 247, 3118
(1980): Fennell RS+, *Clin Pediatr* 19, 124
(1976): Arndt KA+, *JAMA* 235, 918 (2%)
(1973): Das KM+, *N Engl J Med* 289, 491 (2%)
(1972): Halpern GM, *BMJ* 1, 691
(1968): Baron JH+, *Lancet* 1, 1094
(1962): Truelove SC+, *BMJ* 2, 1708 (3%)

Exfoliative dermatitis
(1990): Donovan S+, *Br J Rheumatol* 29, 201
(1984): Sala F+, *Cronica Dermatol* (Italian) 15, 209
(1978): Mihas AA+, *JAMA* 239, 2590
(1975): Bernstein LS, *Can Med Assoc J* 112, 96S
(1971): Koch-Weser J+, *Arch Intern Med* 128, 399

Fixed eruption
(1996): Kawada A+, *Contact Dermatitis* 34, 155
(1988): Bharija SC+, *Dermatologica* 176, 108
(1987): Hughes BR+, *Br J Dermatol* 116, 241
(1987): Kanwar AJ+, *Dermatologica* 174, 104
(1986): Kanwar AJ+, *Dermatologica* 172, 230
(1982): Gibson JR, *BMJ* 284, 1529
(1980): Talbot MD, *Practitioner* 224, 823

Flushing
(2000): Jung JH+, *Clin Exp Rheumatol* 18, 245
(1984): Jick SS+, *Lancet* 2, 631

Lichen planus
(1995): Kaplan S+, *J Rheumatol* 22, 191
(1991): Alstead EM+, *J Clin Gastroenterol* 13, 335

Lupus erythematosus
(2002): Angelova I+, *World Congress Dermatol* Poster, 0083 (patient has psoriasis)
(1997): Gunnarsson I+, *Br J Rheumatol* 36, 1089
(1996): Khattak FH+, *Br J Rheumatol* 35, 104
(1995): Veale DJ+, *Br J Rheumatol* 34, 383
(1994): Borg AA+, *Clin Rheumatol* 13, 522
(1994): Bray VJ+, *J Rheumatol* 21, 2157
(1994): Caulier M+, *J Rheumatol* 21, 750
(1994): Fritzler MJ, *Lupus* 3, 455
(1994): Mongey AB+, *Br J Rheumatol* 33, 789
(1994): Walker EM+, *Br J Rheumatol* 33, 175
(1993): Siam AR+, *J Rheumatol* 20, 207
(1993): Wildhagen K+, *Clin Rheumatol* 12, 265
(1992): Skaer TL, *Clin Ther* 14, 496
(1991): Alarcon-Segovia D+, *Baillieres Clin Rheumatol* 5, 1
(1989): Deboever G+, *Am J Gastroenterol* 84, 85
(1989): Sugimoto M+, *Nippon Naika Gakkai Zasshi* (Japanese) 78, 583
(1988): Clementz GL+, *Am J Med* 84, 535
(1987): Hobbs RN+, *Ann Rheum Dis* 46, 408
(1985): Lovisetto P+, *Recenti Prog Med* (Italian) 76, 110
(1985): Stratton MA, *Clin Pharm* 4, 657
(1983): Vanheule BA+, *Eur J Pediatr* 140, 66
(1982): Carr-Locke DL, *Am J Gastroenterol* 77, 614
(1980): Crisp AJ+, *J R Soc Med* 73, 60
(1980): Rouleau L+, *Union Med Can* (French) 109, 1326
(1979): Weiller PJ+, *Ann Med Interne Paris* (French) 130, 665
(1978): Jaup BH, *Dtsch Med Wochenschr* (German) 103, 1211
(1977): Griffiths ID+, *BMJ* 2, 1188
(1969): Alarcon-Segovia D, *Mayo Clin Proc* 44, 664
(1966): Cohen P+, *JAMA* 197, 817

Necrosis
(1988): Krakamp B+, *Med Klin* (German) 83, 611

Periorbital edema

Photosensitivity (>10%)
(1999): Bouyssou-Gauthier ML, *Dermatology* 198, 388
(1994): Shelley WB+, *Cutis* 53, 240 (observation)
(1986): Amos RS+, *BMJ* 293, 420 (1–5%)
(1986): Chandler MJ, *J Infect Dis* 153, 1001

Pigmentation
(1992): Gabazza EC+, *Am J Gastroenterol* 87, 1654 (orange-yellow)
(1970): Morse MO+, *Arch Dermatol* 102, 112
(1968): Yell J+, *BMJ* 4, 452

Pruritus (>10%)
(1993): Gran JT+, *Scand J Rheumatol* 22, 229
(1990): Donovan S+, *Br J Rheumatol* 29, 201
(1990): Peppercorn MA, *Ann Intern Med* 112, 50 (1–5%)
(1987): Colebunders R+, *Ann Intern Med* 107, 599
(1986): Farr M+, *Drugs* 32 (Suppl 1), 49
(1986): Sher MR, *J Allergy Clin Immunol* 77, 133
(1984): Kramer BS+, *Cancer* 53, 329

Pruritus vulvae
(1981): *Modern Medicine* 49, 111

Psoriasis
(1991): Bliddal H+, *Clin Rheumatol* 10, 178

Purpura
(1989): Gremse DA+, *J Pediatr Gastroenterol Nutr* 9, 261

Pustular eruption
(1994): Gallais V+, *Ann Dermatol Venereol* (French) 121, 11
(1976): Lindgren S+, *Acta Derm Venereol* (Stockh) 56, 139

Rash (sic) (>10%)
(2000): Jung JH+, *Clin Exp Rheumatol* 18, 245
(1999): Besnard M+, *Arch Pediatr* 6, 643
(1994): McCarthy C+, *Ir J Med Sci* 163, 238
(1993): Koski JM, *Clin Exp Dermatol* 11, 169
(1992): Brooks H+, *Clin Rheumatol* 11, 566
(1992): Giaffer MH+, *Aliment Pharmacol Ther* 6, 51 (10 cases))
(1989): Gyssens IC+, *Ned Tijdschr Geneeskd* (Dutch) 133, 1608
(1989): Scott DL+, *J Rheumatol* Suppl 16, 17
(1986): Bax DE+, *Ann Rheum Dis* 45, 139
(1984): Farr M+, *Clin Rheumatol* 3, 473
(1984): Purdy BH+, *Ann Intern Med* 100, 512
(1978): Mihas AA+, *JAMA* 239, 2590

Raynaud's phenomenon
(1984): Peppercorn MA, *Ann Intern Med* 101, 377
(1980): Reid J+, *Postgraduate Med J* 56, 106

Skin reactions (sic)
(1993): Gran JT+, *Scand J Rheumatol* 22, 229

Stevens–Johnson syndrome (<1%)
(2001): Martin L+, *Rev Pneumol Clin* 57(4), 297
(1966): Cameron HA+, *BMJ* 2, 1174

Toxic epidermal necrolysis (1–10%)
(2001): Martin L+, *Rev Pneumol Clin* 57(4), 297
(1995): Jullien D+, *Arthritis Rheum* 38, 573
(1987): Guillaume JC+, *Arch Dermatol* 123, 1166
(1985): Curley RK+, *Br Med J Clin Res Ed* 290, 471 (fatal)
(1985): Heng MCY, *Br J Dermatol* 113, 597
(1984): Peppercorn MA, *Ann Intern Med* 101, 377
(1981): Hensen E, *Tijdschr Ziekenverpl* (Dutch) 34, 563
(1981): Hensen EJ+, *Lancet* 2, 151
(1980): Maddocks JL+, *J R Soc Med* 73, 587
(1976): Varkonyi V+, *Orv Hetil* (Hungarian) 117, 971
(1975): Bernstein LS, *Can Med Assoc J* 112, 96S

Urticaria (<3%)
(2002): Liss WA, Pleasanton, WA (from Internet) (observation)
(2000): Jung JH+, *Clin Exp Rheumatol* 18, 245
(1989): Alanko K+, *Acta Derm Venereol* (Stockh) 69, 223
(1986): Amos RS+, *BMJ* 293, 420 (1–5%)
(1986): Farr M+, *Drugs* 32 (Suppl 1), 49
(1985): Maayan S+, *Arch Intern Med* 145, 1607
(1984): Kramer BS+, *Cancer* 53, 329
(1984): Peppercorn MA, *Ann Intern Med* 101, 377
(1984): Purdy BH+, *Ann Intern Med* 100, 512
(1981): Abi-Mansur P+, *Am J Gastroenterol* 76, 356
(1971): Koch-Weser J+, *Arch Intern Med* 128, 399

Vasculitis
(1971): Koch-Weser J+, *Arch Intern Med* 128, 399

(1965): McCombs RP, *JAMA* 194, 1059
Vulvovaginitis
(1985): Wong ES+, *Ann Intern Med* 102, 302
Xerosis
(1990): Donovan S+, *Br J Rheumatol* 29, 201

### Hair

Hair – alopecia
(1988): Fich A+, *J Clin Gastroenterol* 10, 466
(1987): Codeluppi P+, *Dig Dis Sci* 32, 221
(1986): Breen EG+, *BMJ* 292, 802
(1986): Farr M+, *Drugs* 32 (Suppl 1), 49
(1983): Taffet SL+, *Dig Dis Sci* 28, 833
(1981): Attar A+, *Gastroenterology* 80, 1102

### Other

Anaphylactoid reactions
(1990): Donovan S+, *Br J Rheumatol* 29, 201
(1988): Arnold PA+, *Drug Intell Clin Pharm* 22, 43
(1985): Gossius G+, *Scand J Infect Dis* 16, 373
Aphthous stomatitis
(1981): *J Antimicrob Chemother* 7, 179
Death
(2001): Lau G+, *Forensic Sci Int* 122(2), 79
DRESS syndrome
(2001): Descamps V+, *Arch Dermatol* 137, 301
(2001): Queyrel V+, *Rev Med Interne* 22(6), 582
(1998): Tohyama M+, *Arch Dermatol* 134, 1113
Dysgeusia
(1991): Marcus RW, *J Rheumatol* 18, 634
Glossitis
Hypersensitivity (1–5%)
(1998): Tohyama M+, *Arch Dermatol* 134, 1113
(1997): Otero S+, *Gastroenterol Hepatol* (Spanish) 20, 446
(1995): Tolia V, *Am J Gastroenterol* 87, 1029
(1992): Leroux JL+, *Clin Exp Rheumatol* 10, 427
(1987): Ackerman Z+, *Postgrad Med J* 63, 55
(1984): Korelitz BI+, *J Clin Gastroenterol* 6, 27
(1978): Mihas AA+, *JAMA* 289, 2590
(1978): Sotolongo RP+, *Gastroenterology* 75, 95
Hypogeusia
Lymphoproliferative disease
(1989): Lafeuillade A+, *Presse Med* (French) 18, 1709
Mononucleosis
(1984): Iwatsuki K+, *Arch Dermatol* 120, 964
Mucocutaneous side effects (sic)
(1990): Donovan S+, *Br J Rheumatol* 29, 201 (6.3%)
(1986): Farr M+, *Drugs* 32 (Suppl 1), 49 (5.5%)
Myalgia
Myopathy
(1994): Norden DK+, *Am J Gastroenterology* 89, 801
Oral mucosal eruption
(1990): Petterson T+, *Br J Rheumatol* 29, 239
(1986): Amos RS+, *BMJ* 293, 420 (0.3%)
(1984): Iwatsuki K+, *Arch Dermatol* 120, 964
(1966): Cameron HA+, *BMJ* 2, 1174
Oral ulceration
(1987): Hughes WT+, *N Engl J Med* 316, 1627
(1986): Farr M+, *Drugs* 32 (Suppl 1), 49
(1981): Orenstein WA+, *Am J Med Sci* 282, 27
Pseudolymphoma
(1994): Gallais V+, *Ann Dermatol Venereol* (French) 121, 11
(1975): Delage C+, *Union Med Can* (French) 104, 579
Serum sickness (<1%)
(1992): Brooks H+, *Clin Rheumatol* 11, 566
(1990): Petterson T+, *Br J Rheumatol* 29, 239
(1975): Delage C+, *Union Med Can* (French) 104, 579
Stomatitis
(1993): Gran JT+, *Scand J Rheumatol* 22, 229
Tongue ulceration
(1981): *J Antimicrob Chemother* 7, 179
Xerostomia
(1990): Donovan S+, *Br J Rheumatol* 29, 201

***Note:** Sulfasalazine is a sulfonamide and can be absorbed systemically. Sulfonamides can produce severe, possibly fatal, reactions such as toxic epidermal necrolysis and Stevens–Johnson syndrome

## SULFINPYRAZONE

**Trade name:** Anturane (Novartis)
**Other common trade names:** *Antazone; Antiran; Anturan; Anturano; Enturen; Falizal; Novopyrazone*
**Indications:** Gouty arthritis
**Category:** Antigout; antihyperuricemic sulfonamide*
**Half-life:** 2–7 hours
**Clinically important, potentially hazardous interactions with:** anisindione, anticoagulants, dicumarol, warfarin

#### *Reactions*

### Skin

Dermatitis (sic) (1–10%)
Edema
Exanthems (<3%)
Flushing (<1%)
Purpura
Rash (sic) (1–10%)

***Note:** Sulfinpyrazone is a sulfonamide and can be absorbed systemically. Sulfonamides can produce severe, possibly fatal, reactions such as toxic epidermal necrolysis and Stevens–Johnson syndrome

## SULFISOXAZOLE

**Trade name:** Pediazole (Ross)
**Other common trade names:** *Isoxazine; Novo-Soxazole; Oxazole; Sulfazin; Sulfazole; Sulizole; Thiazin; Urazole*
**Indications:** Various infections caused by susceptible organisms
**Category:** Urinary tract antibacterial and antiprotozoal sulfonamide*
**Half-life:** 3–7 hours
**Clinically important, potentially hazardous interactions with:** anticoagulants, cyclosporine, methotrexate, warfarin

#### *Reactions*

### Skin

Allergic reactions (sic)
(1971): Koch-Weser J+, *Arch Intern Med* 128, 399 (2.8%)
Angioedema (<1%)
(1971): Koch-Weser J+, *Arch Intern Med* 128, 399 (0.15%)
Bullous eruption (<1%)
(1966): Falk AB+, *Arch Dermatol* 94, 249
Cutaneous side effects (sic)
(1971): Koch-Weser J+, *Arch Intern Med* 128, 399 (2.1%)
Eczematous eruption (sic)
(1947): Sulzberger MB+, *J Allergy* 18, 92
Erythema multiforme (<1%)
(1987): Penmetcha M, *BMJ* 295, 556
(1985): Heer M+, *Gastroenterology* 88, 1954

(1985): Hernborg A, *Lancet* 2, 1072
(1979): Beck MH+, *Clin Exp Dermatol* 4, 201
(1975): Bernstein LS, *Can Med Assoc J* 112, 96S
(1971): Koch-Weser J+, *Arch Intern Med* 128, 399 (0.15%)
(1970): Shaw DJ+, *Johns Hopkins Med J* 126, 130

Erythema nodosum
(1971): Koch-Weser J+, *Arch Intern Med* 128, 399

Exanthems (1–5%)
(1985): Maayan S+, *Arch Intern Med* 145, 1607
(1982): Goetz MB+, *JAMA* 247, 3118
(1980): Fennell RS+, *Clin Pediatr* 19, 124
(1976): Arndt KA+, *JAMA* 235, 918 (1.7%)
(1972): Halpern GM, *BMJ* 1, 691
(1972): Kauppinen K, *Acta Derm Venereol* (Stockh) 52 (Suppl), 68
(1971): Koch-Weser J+, *Arch Intern Med* 128, 399 (1%)
(1967): Lehr D, *Ann N Y Acad Sci* 69, 417 (2%)
(1956): Davis JB, *JAMA* 161, 228

Exfoliative dermatitis
(1975): Bernstein LS, *Can Med Assoc J* 112, 96S
(1971): Koch-Weser J+, *Arch Intern Med* 128, 399

Fixed eruption (<1%)
(1988): Bharija SC+, *Dermatologica* 176, 108
(1987): Hughes BR+, *Br J Dermatol* 116, 241
(1986): Kanwar AJ+, *Dermatologica* 172, 230
(1982): Gibson JR, *BMJ* 284, 1529
(1980): Talbot MD, *Practitioner* 224, 823
(1968): Sarkany I, *Proc R Soc Med* 61, 891

Flushing
(1984): Jick SS+, *Lancet* 2, 631

Linear IgA bullous dermatosis
(1981): Safai B+, *J Am Acad Dermatol* 4, 435

Lupus erythematosus
(1975): Grossman J+, *Am J Dis Child* 129, 123
(1966): Cohen P+, *JAMA* 197, 817

Periorbital edema

Photoreactions

Photosensitivity (>10%)
(1986): Chandler MJ, *J Infect Dis* 153, 1001
(1981): Flach AJ+, *Arch Ophthalmol* 100, 1206 (from topical application)
(1981): Flach AJ+, *Arch Ophthalmol* 99, 609 (from topical application)
(1972): Kauppinen K, *Acta Derm Venereol* (Stockh) 52 (Suppl), 68

Phototoxicity
(1982): Flach AJ+, *Arch Ophthalmol* 100, 1286 (from topical application)

Pruritus (>10%)
(1987): Colebunders R+, *Ann Intern Med* 107, 599
(1986): Sher MR, *J Allergy Clin Immunol* 77, 133
(1984): Kramer BS+, *Cancer* 53, 329
(1971): Koch-Weser J+, *Arch Intern Med* 128, 399 (0.15%)

Pruritus vulvae
(1981): *Modern Medicine* 49, 111

Purpura
(1980): Miescher PA+, *Clin Haematol* 9, 505
(1977): Cimo PL+, *Am J Hematol* 2, 65
(1956): Green TW+, *JAMA* 161, 1563
(1951): Gale GL, *Can Med Assoc J* 64, 252

Pustular eruption

Rash (sic) (>10%)

Stevens–Johnson syndrome (1–10%)
(1983): Fischer PR+, *Am J Dis Child* 137, 914
(1970): Shaw DJ+, *Johns Hopkins Med J* 126, 130
(1956): Davis JB, *JAMA* 161, 228

Toxic epidermal necrolysis (1–10%)
(1995): Raymond F+, *Arch Pediatr* (French) 2, 494
(1990): Jacqz-Aigrain E+, *Lancet* 336, 1010
(1989): Alanko K+, *Acta Derm Venereol* (Stockh) 69, 223
(1975): Bernstein LS, *Can Med Assoc J* 112, 96S
(1972): Kauppinen K, *Acta Derm Venereol* (Stockh) 52 (Suppl), 68

Urticaria
(1985): Maayan S+, *Arch Intern Med* 145, 1607
(1984): Kramer BS+, *Cancer* 53, 329
(1981): Abi-Mansur P+, *Am J Gastroenterol* 76, 356
(1971): Koch-Weser J+, *Arch Intern Med* 128, 399 (0.04%)

Vasculitis (<1%)
(1971): Koch-Weser J+, *Arch Intern Med* 128, 399
(1967): Lee DK+, *JAMA* 200, 720
(1965): McCombs RP, *JAMA* 194, 1059

Vulvovaginitis
(1985): Wong ES+, *Ann Intern Med* 102, 302

## Hair

Hair – alopecia
(1975): Grossman J+, *Am J Dis Child* 129, 123

## Other

Anaphylactoid reactions
(1988): Arnold PA+, *Drug Intell Clin Pharm* 22, 43
(1985): Gossius G+, *Scand J Infect Dis* 16, 373

Aphthous stomatitis
(1981): *J Antimicrob Chemother* 7, 179

Dysgeusia
(1988): Fischl MA+, *JAMA* 259, 1185

Glossitis

Hypersensitivity

Myalgia

Oral psoriasis (sic)
(1974): Yaffee HS, *Int J Dermatol* 13, 185

Oral ulceration
(1987): Hughes WT+, *N Engl J Med* 316, 1627
(1981): Orenstein WA+, *Am J Med Sci* 282, 27

Serum sickness (<1%)
(1969): Mukherjee DN, *J Indian Med Assoc* 52, 225

Stomatitis

Temporal arteritis
(1967): Lee DK+, *JAMA* 200, 720

Tinnitus

Tongue ulceration
(1981): *J Antimicrob Chemother* 7, 179

***Note:** Sulfisoxazole is a sulfonamide and can be absorbed systemically. Sulfonamides can produce severe, possibly fatal, reactions such as toxic epidermal necrolysis and Stevens–Johnson syndrome

# SULINDAC

**Trade name:** Clinoril (Merck)
**Other common trade names:** *Aflodac; Algocetil; APO-Sulin; Arthrocine; Mobilin; Novo-Sundac; Sulene; Sulic; Suloril*
**Indications:** Arthritis
**Category:** Nonsteroidal anti-inflammatory (NSAID); analgesic
**Half-life:** 7.8–16.4 hours
**Clinically important, potentially hazardous interactions with:** methotrexate, warfarin

### *Reactions*

## Skin

Angioedema (<1%)

Dermatitis (sic)
(1991): Renaut JJ, *Allerg Immunol Paris* (French) 23, 365

Diaphoresis

Ecchymoses (<1%)

Edema
Erythema
(1991): Renaut JJ, *Allerg Immunol Paris* (French) 23, 365
Erythema multiforme (<1%)
(1987): Jeanmougin M+, *Ann Dermatol Venereol* (French) 114, 1400
(1985): Bigby M+, *J Am Acad Dermatol* 12, 866
(1985): O'Brien WM+, *J Rheumatol* 12, 13
(1984): Stern RS+, *JAMA* 252, 1433
(1982): Park GD+, *Arch Intern Med* 142, 1292
(1981): Husain Z+, *J Rheumatol* 8, 176
(1981): Maguire FW, *Del Med J* 53, 193
(1980): Russell IJ, *Ann Intern Med* 92, 716
Exanthems (1–5%)
(1993): Litt JZ, Beachwood, OH (personal case) (observation)
(1991): Hyson CP+, *Arch Intern Med* 151, 387
(1987): Jeanmougin M+, *Ann Dermatol Venereol* (French) 114, 1400
(1985): Bigby M+, *J Am Acad Dermatol* 12, 866
(1984): Stern RS+, *JAMA* 252, 1433
(1982): Park GD+, *Arch Intern Med* 142, 1292
(1981): Dhand A+, *Gastroenterology* 80, 585
(1980): Russell IJ, *Ann Intern Med* 92, 716
(1979): Anderson R, *N Engl J Med* 300, 735
(1977): Calabro JJ+, *Clin Pharmacol Ther* 22, 358 (3%)
Exfoliative dermatitis (<1%)
Exfoliative erythroderma
(1984): Stern RS+, *JAMA* 252, 1433
Facial erythema
(1979): Anderson R, *N Engl J Med* 300, 735
Fixed eruption (<1%)
(1987): Jeanmougin M+, *Ann Dermatol Venereol* (French) 114, 1400
(1986): Bruce DR+, *Cutis* 38, 323
(1985): Bigby M+, *J Am Acad Dermatol* 12, 866
(1984): Aram H, *Int J Dermatol* 23, 421
(1984): Stern RS+, *JAMA* 252, 1433
Hot flashes (<1%)
Jaundice
(1979): Wolfe PB, *Ann Intern Med* 91, 656
Lichen planus
(1983): Hamburger J+, *BMJ* 287, 1258
Pernio
(1981): Reinertsen JL, *Arthritis Rheum* 24, 1215
Photosensitivity (<1%)
(1987): Jeanmougin M+, *Ann Dermatol Venereol* (French) 114, 1400
(1984): Stern RS+, *JAMA* 252, 1433
Phototoxicity
Pruritus (1–10%)
(1987): Jeanmougin M+, *Ann Dermatol Venereol* (French) 114, 1400
(1985): Bigby M+, *J Am Acad Dermatol* 12, 866
(1984): Stern RS+, *JAMA* 252, 1433
(1982): Park GD+, *Arch Intern Med* 142, 1292
(1980): Russell IJ, *Ann Intern Med* 92, 716
Purpura (<1%)
(1987): Jeanmougin M+, *Ann Dermatol Venereol* (French) 114, 1400
(1984): Stern RS+, *JAMA* 252, 1433
Rash (sic) (>10%)
Raynaud's phenomenon
(1981): Reinertsen JL, *Arthritis Rheum* 24, 1215 (passim)
Skin pain (sic)
(1984): Stern RS+, *JAMA* 252, 1433
Stevens–Johnson syndrome (<1%)
(1993): Awaya N+, *Ryumachi* (Japanese) 33, 432
(1983): Klein SM+, *J Rheumatol* 10, 512
(1981): Husain Z+, *J Rheumatol* 8, 176
(1981): Maguire FW, *Del Med J* 53, 193
(1980): Levitt L+, *JAMA* 243, 1262
Toxic epidermal necrolysis (<1%)
(1990): Hovde O, *Tidsskr Nor Laegeforen* (Norwegian) 110, 2537
(1988): Small RE+, *Clin Pharm* 7, 766
(1987): Ikeda N+, *Z Rechtsmed* (German) 98, 141
(1987): Jeanmougin M+, *Ann Dermatol Venereol* (French) 114, 1400
(1986): Rodt SA+, *Tidsskr Nor Laegeforen* (Norwegian) 106, 2982
(1985): Bigby M+, *J Am Acad Dermatol* 12, 866
(1985): Chevrant-Breton JC, *Therapie* (French) 40, 67
(1985): Heng MCY, *Br J Dermatol* 113, 597
(1984): Stern RS+, *JAMA* 252, 1433
(1983): Klein SM+, *J Rheumatol* 10, 512
(1982): Park GD+, *Arch Intern Med* 142, 1292
(1980): Levitt L+, *JAMA* 243, 1262
(1980): Russell IJ, *Ann Intern Med* 92, 716
Urticaria (<1%)
(1987): Jeanmougin M+, *Ann Dermatol Venereol* (French) 114, 1400
(1985): Bigby M+, *J Am Acad Dermatol* 12, 866
(1984): Stern RS+, *JAMA* 252, 1433
(1981): Burrish G+, *Ann Emerg Med* 10, 154
Vasculitis (<1%)

## Hair

Hair – alopecia (<1%)

## Other

Ageusia (<1%)
Anaphylactoid reactions (<1%)
(1991): Hyson CP+, *Arch Intern Med* 151, 387
(1985): O'Brien WM+, *J Rheumatol* 12, 13
(1981): Burrish G+, *Ann Emerg Med* 10, 154
(1980): Smith F+, *JAMA* 244, 269
Aphthous stomatitis
Death
Dysesthesia
(1980): Russell IJ, *Ann Intern Med* 92, 716
Dysgeusia (<1%)
Glossitis (<1%)
Gynecomastia
(1983): Kapoor A, *JAMA* 250, 2284
Hypersensitivity (<1%) (potentially fatal)
Oral lichenoid eruption
(1983): Hamburger J+, *BMJ* 287, 1258
Oral mucosal eruption
(1985): Bigby M+, *J Am Acad Dermatol* 12, 866
(1977): Calabro JJ+, *Clin Pharmacol Ther* 22, 358 (3%)
Oral mucosal erythema
(1979): Anderson RJ, *N Engl J Med* 300, 735
Oral ulceration
Paresthesias (<1%)
Pseudolymphoma
(2000): Werth V, *Dermatology Times* 18
Rectal mucosal ulceration
(2002): Cruz-Correa M+, *Gastroenterology* 122(3), 641
Serum sickness
(1984): Stern RS+, *JAMA* 252, 1433
Stomatitis (<1%)
(1991): Renaut JJ, *Allerg Immunol Paris* (French) 23, 365
(1978): Brogden R+, *Drugs* 16, 97
Tinnitus
Xerostomia
(1980): Smith F+, *JAMA* 244, 269
(1978): Huskinson L+, *Ann Rheum Dis* 37, 89

# SUMATRIPTAN

**Trade name:** Imitrex (GSK)
**Other common trade name:** *Imigrane*
**Indications:** Migraine attacks
**Category:** Antimigraine; serotonin agonist
**Half-life:** 2.5 hours
**Clinically important, potentially hazardous interactions with:** citalopram, dihydroergotamine, ergot-containing drugs, fluoxetine, fluvoxamine, isocarboxazid, MAO inhibitors, methysergide, naratriptan, nefazodone, paroxetine, phenelzine, rizatriptan, sertraline, sibutramine, tranylcypromine, venlafaxine, zolmitriptan

## *Reactions*

### Skin

Angioedema
(1995): Dachs R+, *Am J Med* 99, 684
Burning (sic) (1–10%)
Diaphoresis (1.6%)
Erythema (<1%)
Exanthems
Flushing (6.6%)
Hot flashes (>10%)
Hot sensations
(1991): Multiple authors, *N Engl J Med* 325, 316
Photosensitivity (<1%)
Pruritus (<1%)
Rash (sic) (<1%)
Raynaud's phenomenon (<1%)
Sensitivity (sic)
(1994): Black P+, *N Z Med J* 107, 20
Urticaria
(1996): Pradalier A+, *Cephalalgia* 16, 280

### Other

Anaphylactoid reactions
Dysesthesia (<1%)
Dysgeusia (<1%)
(2001): Hershey AD+, *Headache* 41, 693
Glossodynia
Hyperesthesia (<1%)
Injection-site reactions (sic) (58%)
(1991): Multiple authors, *N Engl J Med* 325, 316 (10–20%)
Myalgia (1.8%)
Parageusia (<1%)
Paresthesias (13.5%)
Parosmia (<1%)
Xerostomia

## TACRINE

**Synonym:** THA
**Trade name:** Cognex (First Horizon)
**Indications:** Dementia of Alzheimer's disease
**Category:** Anticholinesterase; cholinergic
**Half-life:** 1.5–4 hours
**Clinically important, potentially hazardous interactions with:** fluvoxamine, galantamine

### *Reactions*

#### Skin
Acne (<1%)
Basal cell carcinoma
Bullous eruption
Cellulitis
Cyst (sic)
Dermatitis (sic) (<1%)
Desquamation (sic)
Diaphoresis
Eczema (sic)
Edema (<1%)
Exanthems (7%)
Facial edema (<1%)
Flushing (3%)
Furunculosis (<1%)
Herpes simplex (<1%)
Herpes zoster (<1%)
Melanoma (<1%)
Necrosis (<1%)
Peripheral edema (<1%)
Petechiae
Pruritus (7%)
Psoriasis (<1%)
Purpura (2%)
Rash (sic) (7%)
Seborrhea
Squamous cell carcinoma
Ulceration (<1%)
Urticaria (7%)
Xerosis (<1%)

#### Hair
Hair – alopecia (<1%)

#### Other
Dysgeusia (<1%)
Gingivitis (<1%)
Glossitis (<1%)
Myalgia (9%)
Paresthesias (<1%)
Parkinsonism
(1999): Cabeza-Alvarez CI+, *Neurologia* (Spanish) 14, 96
Sialorrhea (<1%)
Stomatitis (<1%)
Tremors (1–10%)
Xerostomia (<1%)

## TACROLIMUS

**Synonym:** FK506
**Trade names:** Prograf (Fujisawa); Protopic (Fujisawa)
**Indications:** Prophylaxis of organ rejection, atopic dermatitis (topical)
**Category:** Immunosuppressant; topical for atopic dermatitis
**Half-life:** ~8.7 hours
**Clinically important, potentially hazardous interactions with:** beta blockers, cyclosporine, danazol, erythromycin, **grapefruit juice**, HMG-CoA reductase inhibitors, ibuprofen, immunosuppressives, ketoconazole, lovastatin, mycophenolate, potassium, potassium-sparing diuretics, rifabutin, rifampin, rifapentine, simvastatin, **vaccines**

### *Reactions*

#### Skin
Burning
(2002): Rozycki TW+, *J Am Acad Dermatol* 46, 27
(2001): Goldman D, *J Am Acad Dermatol* 44, 995 (transient, localized)
(2000): Reitamo S+, *Arch Dermatol* 136, 999 (46.8%)
(1999): Ruzicka R+, *Arch Dermatol* 135, 574
(1998): Alaiti S+, *J Am Acad Dermatol* 38, 69
Connective tissue nevi (sic)
(1999): Reed BR, Denver, CO (from Internet) (observation) (confirmed by biopsies)
Diaphoresis (>3%)
Ecchymoses (>3%)
Edema (>10%)
Erythema
(2000): Reitamo S+, *Arch Dermatol* 136, 999 (12.3%)
Erythema (facial)
(2001): Bohannon JS, Midlothian, VA (from Internet) (observation) (from topical) (following wine)
Exanthems
(2001): Takamatsu Y+, *Bone Marrow Transplant* 28(4), 421 (with cyclosporine)
(2000): Reitamo S+, *Arch Dermatol* 136, 999 (4.1%)
Flushing
(2000): Reitamo S+, *Arch Dermatol* 136, 999
(1997): Sandborn WJ, *Am J Gastroenterol* 92, 876
Folliculitis
(2000): Reitamo S+, *Arch Dermatol* 136, 999 (10.8%)
Herpes simplex
(2000): Reitamo S+, *Arch Dermatol* 136, 999 (13%)
Infections (sic) (>10%)
Irritation
(2002): Rozycki TW+, *J Am Acad* 46(1), 27
Peripheral edema (26%)
Photosensitivity (>3%)
Pigmentation
(2002): Phillips R, Melbourne, AU (from Internet) (observation)
Pruritus (36%)
(2000): Emre S+, *Transpl Int* 13, 73
(2000): Reitamo S+, *Arch Dermatol* 136, 999 (25.3%)
Purpura
(1996): Nash RA+, *Blood* 88, 3634
Pustular eruption
(2000): Reitamo S+, *Arch Dermatol* 136, 999 (6.3%)
Rash (sic) (24%)
Squamous cell carcinoma
(2001): Otley CC+, *Arch Dermatol* 137, 459
Urticaria

(2001): Takamatsu Y+, *Bone Marrow Transplant* 28(4), 421 (with cyclosporine)

### Hair

Hair – alopecia (>3%)
(1999): Ushigome H+, *Transplant Proc* 31, 2885 (2 cases)
(1998): Shapiro R+, *Transplantation* 65, 1284
(1997): Talbot D+, *Transplantation* 64, 1631
Hair – growth (sic)
(1994): Yamamoto S+, *J Dermatol Sci* 7, S47
Hair – hirsutism

### Other

Anaphylactoid reactions (<1%)
(2001): Takamatsu Y+, *Bone Marrow Transplant* 28(4), 421 (with cyclosporine)
Application-site burning
(1997): Ruzicka T+, *N Engl J Med* 337, 816
Dysphagia (>3%)
(2001): Hernandez G+, *Oral Surg Oral Med Oral Pathol Oral Radiol Endod* 92(5), 526
Gingival hyperplasia
(2000): Schmutz J+, *Ann Dermatol Venereol* (French) 127, 646
(1998): Basile C+, *Nephrol Dial Transplant* 13, 2980
Hyperesthesia
Myalgia (>3%)
Oral candidiasis (>3%)
Oral ulceration
(2001): Hernandez G+, *Oral Surg Oral Med Oral Pathol Oral Radiol Endod* 92(5), 526
(2001): Macario-Barrel A+, *Ann Dermatol Venereol* 128(12), 1327
Paresthesias (40%)
(1997): Sandborn WJ, *Am J Gastroenterol* 92, 876
(1996): *Arch Dermatol* 132, 419
Tremors (>10%)

## TAMOXIFEN

**Trade name:** Nolvadex (AstraZeneca)
**Other common trade names:** *Apo-Tamox; Bilim; Istubol; Kessar; Mamofen; Novofen; Tamaxin; Tamofen; Tamoxan; Taxus; Valodex*
**Indications:** Advanced breast cancer
**Category:** Antiestrogen; antineoplastic estrogen receptor
**Half-life:** 7 days

#### *Reactions*

### Skin

Dermatomyositis
(1982): Harris AL+, *BMJ* 284, 1674
Diaphoresis
(1986): Buchanan RB+, *J Clin Oncology* 4, 1326
(1980): Pritchard KI+, *Cancer Treat Rep* 64, 787
Edema (3.8%)
(1986): Buchanan RB+, *J Clin Oncology* 4, 1326
(1978): Heel RC+, *Drugs* 16, 1 (2–6%)
Exanthems
(1999): Descamps V+, *Ann Dermatol Venereol* (French) 126, 716
(1980): Pritchard KI+, *Cancer Treat Rep* 64, 787
(1978): Heel RC+, *Drugs* 16, 1 (3.6%)
Flushing (>10%)
(1999): Drayton G, Los Angeles, CA (from Internet) (observation)
(1992): Shelley WB+, *Advanced Dermatologic Diagnosis* WB Saunders, 583 (passim)
(1989): Buckley MMT+, *Drugs* 37, 451 (10–20%)
(1986): Buchanan RB+, *J Clin Oncology* 4, 1326
(1981): Ingle JN+, *N Engl J Med* 304, 16 (29%)
(1980): Pritchard KI+, *Cancer Treat Rep* 64, 787
(1978): Heel RC+, *Drugs* 16, 1 (14%)
(1977): Kiang DT+, *Ann Intern Med* 87, 687 (21%)
(1973): Ward HWC, *BMJ* 1, 13 (12%)
Hot flashes
(2001): Vogel NE+, *Ned Tijdschr Geneeskd* 145(22), 1041
Peripheral edema
Pruritus
(1980): Pritchard KI+, *Cancer Treat Rep* 64, 787
Pruritus vulvae
(1980): Pritchard KI+, *Cancer Treat Rep* 64, 787
(1978): Heel RC+, *Drugs* 16, 1 (2–3%)
Purpura
(1978): Heel RC+, *Drugs* 16, 1
Radiation recall
(1999): Bostrom A+, *Acta Oncol* 38, 955
(1992): Parry BR, *Lancet* 340, 49
Rash (sic) (1–10%)
Urticaria
Vaginal pruritus
Vasculitis
(1994): Rzany B+, *J Am Acad Dermatol* 30, 509
(1990): Drago F+, *Ann Intern Med* 112, 965
Xerosis
(1978): Heel RC+, *Drugs* 16, 1 (7%)

### Hair

Hair – alopecia
(2001): Puglisi F+, *Ann Intern Med* 134(12), 1154 (total)
(1993): Litt JZ, Beachwood, OH (personal case) (observation)
(1980): Pritchard KI+, *Cancer Treat Rep* 64, 787
(1978): Heel RC+, *Drugs* 16, 1 (2%)
Hair – color change (sic)
(1995): Hampson JP+, *Br J Dermatol* 132, 483
Hair – hirsutism
(1980): Pritchard KI+, *Cancer Treat Rep* 64, 787
Hair – hypertrichosis

### Other

Depression
(2001): Day R+, *J Natl Cancer Inst* 93(21), 1615
Dysgeusia
Galactorrhea (1–10%)
Myopathy
(1982): Harris AL+, *BMJ* 284, 1674
Thrombophlebitis
(1996): Zimmet S, *The Schoch Letter* 46, 22 (#86) (observation)
Xerostomia
(1978): Heel RC+, *Drugs* 16, 1 (7%)

## TAMSULOSIN

**Trade name:** Flomax (Boehringer Ingelheim)
**Indications:** Benign prostatic hypertrophy
**Category:** Alpha-adrenergic blocking agent
**Half-life:** 9–13 hours

#### *Reactions*

### Skin

Angioedema
Eczematous eruption (sic)
(2000): Frederickson KS, Novalo, CA (from Internet) (observation)

Erythema multiforme
(1999): Reed BR, Denver, CO (from Internet) (observation)
Pruritus
Rash (sic)

### Other

Tooth disorder (sic)

# TARTRAZINE

**Synonyms:** Acid Yellow T; Acilan Yellow GG; Cake Yellow; Tartar Yellow S; Wool Yellow
**Trade names:** E102; FD&C yellow No.5
**Category:** A coal-tar derivative food colorant used in drinks; sweets; jams; cereals; snack foods; canned fish; packaged soups. Also used for coloring medications
**Half-life:** N/A

## *Reactions*

### Skin

Adverse reactions (sic)
(1986): Stevenson DD+, *J Allergy Clin Immunol* 78(1 Pt 2), 182
(1982): Rosenhall L, *Eur J Respir Dis* 63(5), 410
(1981): Neumann CJ+, *Am J Hosp Pharm* 38(6), 790, 792
Allergic reactions (sic)
(2000): Bhatia MS, *J Clin Psychiatry* 61(7), 473
(1989): Pollock I+, *BMJ* 299(6700), 649
(1988): McLean JD, *Can J Psychiatry* 33(4), 331
(1987): Pohl R+, *Am J Psychiatry* 144(2), 237 (in antidepressents)
(1982): MacCara ME, *Can Med Assoc J* 126(8), 910
(1979): Pellegrin A, *Ann Med Interne* (Paris) (French) 130(4), 211
(1977): Zlotlow MJ+, *Am J Clin Nutr* 30(7), 1023 (aspirin intolerance)
Angioedema
(1996): Jimenez-Aranda GS+, *Rev Alerg Mex* (Spanish) 43(6), 152
(1992): Novembre E+, *Pediatr Med Chir* (Italian) 14(1), 39 (passim)
(1989): Hong SP+, *Yonsei Med J* 30(4), 339
(1989): Montano Garcia ML+, *Rev Alerg Mex* (Spanish) 36(1), 15
(1989): Montano Garcia ML, *Rev Alerg Mex* (Spanish) 36(3), 107
(1985): Collins-Williams C, *J Asthma* 22(3), 139 (aspirin intolerance)
(1984): Diez Gomez ML+, *Allergol Immunopathol* (Madr) (Spanish) 12(3), 179
(1981): Alvarez Cuesta E+, *Allergol Immunopathol* (Madr) (Spanish) 9(1), 45
(1980): Makol GM+, *Ariz Med* 37(2), 79
(1978): Mikkelsen H+, *Arch Toxicol Suppl* Suppl 1, 141
Atopic dermatitis
(2001): Worm M+, *Clin Exp Allergy* 31(2), 265
(1992): Devlin J+, *Arch Dis Child* 67(6), 709
Contact dermatitis
(1990): Dipalma JR, *Am Fam Physician* 42(5), 1347
Edema
(1989): Pachor ML+, *Oral Surg Oral Med Oral Pathol* 67(4), 393
Fixed eruption
(1997): Orchard DC+, *Australas J Dermatol* 38(4), 212
Photosensitivity
(1978): Meneghini CL+, *Z Hautkr* (German) 53(10), 329
Pruritus
(1981): Alvarez Cuesta E+, *Allergol Immunopathol* (Madr) (Spanish) 9(1), 45
(1978): Neuman I+, *Clin Allergy* 8(1), 65
Purpura
(1999): Kalinke DU+, *Hautarzt* (German) 50(1), 47
(1993): Wuthrich B, *Ann Allergy* 71(4), 379
(1990): Dipalma JR, *Am Fam Physician* 42(5), 1347
(1985): Parodi G+, *Dermatologica* 171(1), 62
(1981): Alvarez Cuesta E+, *Allergol Immunopathol* (Madr) (Spanish) 9(1), 45
Rash (sic)
(1995): Thuvander A, *Lakartidningen* (Swedish) 92(4), 296
Urticaria (often related to aspirin intolerance)
(1996): Jimenez-Aranda GS+, *Rev Alerg Mex* (Spanish) 43(6), 152
(1993): Wuthrich B, *Ann Allergy* 71(4), 379
(1992): Novembre E+, *Pediatr Med Chir* (Italian) 14(1), 39
(1990): Dipalma JR, *Am Fam Physician* 42(5), 1347
(1989): Baumgardner DJ, *Postgrad Med* 85(6), 265
(1989): Hong SP+, *Yonsei Med J* 30(4), 339
(1989): Montano Garcia ML+, *Rev Alerg Mex* (Spanish) 36(1), 15
(1989): Montano Garcia ML, *Rev Alerg Mex* (Spanish) 36(3), 107
(1989): Wilson N+, *Clin Exp Allergy* 19(3), 267
(1987): Settipane GA, *N Engl Reg Allergy Proc* 8(1), 39 (aspirin intolerance)
(1986): Chudwin DS+, *Ann Allergy* 57(2), 133 (aspirin intolerance)
(1986): Simon RA, *N Engl Reg Allergy Proc* 7(6), 533
(1986): Warrington RJ+, *Clin Allergy* 16(6), 527
(1985): Collins-Williams C, *J Asthma* 22(3), 139 (aspirin intolerance)
(1985): Podell RN, *Postgrad Med* 78(8), 83, 87, 92
(1984): Diez Gomez ML+, *Allergol Immunopathol* (Madr) (Spanish) 12(3), 179
(1984): Royal College of Physicians and the British Nutrition Foundation, *J Royal College of Physicians of London* 18(2)
(1982): Ortolani C+, *Ann Allergy* 48(1), 50
(1982): Warin RP+, *Br Med J (Clin Res Ed)* 284(6327), 1443
(1981): Alvarez Cuesta E+, *Allergol Immunopathol* (Madr) (Spanish) 9(1), 45
(1981): Juhlin L, *Br J Dermatology* 104, 369
(1981): Wuthrich B+, *Schweiz Med Wochenschr* 111(39), 1445 (6.1%)
(1980): Makol GM+, *Ariz Med* 37(2), 79
(1980): Valverde E+, *Clin Allergy* 10(6), 691
(1979): Lindemayr H+, *Wien Klin Wochenschr* (German) 91(24), 817
(1978): Mikkelsen H+, *Arch Toxicol Suppl* 1, 141
(1978): Neuman I+, *Clin Allergy* 8(1), 65
(1977): Lockey SD Sr, *Ann Allergy* 38(3), 206 (aspirin intolerance)
(1977): Warin RP, *Hautarzt* (German) 28(10), 511
(1976): Settipane GA+, *J Allergy Clin Immunol* 57(6), 541 (aspirin intolerance)
(1975): Doeglas HM, *Br J Dermatol* 93(2), 135 (aspirin intolerance)
(1974): Noid HE+, *Arch Dermatology* 109, 866
(1972): Juhlin L+, *Allergy and Clin Immunol* 50, 92
Vasculitis
(1999): Kalinke DU+, *Hautarzt* (German) 50(1), 47
(1993): Wuthrich B, *Ann Allergy* 71(4), 379
(1990): Dipalma JR, *Am Fam Physician* 42(5), 1347

### Other

Anaphylactoid reactions
(1993): Wuthrich B, *Ann Allergy* 71(4), 379
(1989): Montano Garcia ML, *Rev Alerg Mex* (Spanish) 36(3), 107
(1981): Desmond RE+, *Ann Allergy* 46(2), 81
(1981): Schneiweiss F, *Ann Allergy* 46(5), 294
(1980): Kallos P+, *Med Hypotheses* 6(5), 487
(1978): Trautlein JJ+, *Ann Allergy* 41(1), 28
(1977): Morris SJ+, *Arch Intern Med* 137(9), 1222
Arthralgia
(1992): Novembre E+, *Pediatr Med Chir* (Italian) 14(1), 39
Asthenia
(1978): Neuman I+, *Clin Allergy* 8(1), 65
Depression

(1992): Novembre E+, *Pediatr Med Chir* (Italian) 14(1), 39
Gingival hypertrophy
(1989): Pachor ML+, *Oral Surg Oral Med Oral Pathol* 67(4), 393
Hypersensitivity
(1995): Sakakibara H+, *Nihon Kyobu Shikkan Gakkai Zasshi* (Japanese) 33, 106
(1995): Thuvander A, *Lakartidningen* (Swedish) 92(4), 296
(1980): Weliky N+, *Clin Allergy* 10(4), 375
(1979): Weliky N+, *Immunol Commun* 8(1), 65
(1978): Berglund F, *Arch Toxicol Suppl* 1, 33
(1978): Mikkelsen H+, *Arch Toxicol Suppl* 1, 141
(1976): Rosenhall L+, *Bull Int Union Tuberc* 51(1), 515 (aspirin intolerance)
(1976): Stenius BS+, *Clin Allergy* 6(2), 119 (aspirin intolerance)
(1975): Rosenhall L+, *Tubercle* 56(2), 168 (aspirin intolerance)
Paresthesias
(1981): Alvarez Cuesta E+, *Allergol Immunopathol* (Madr) (Spanish) 9(1), 45
Serum sickness
(1978): Wolfe MS+, *Am J Trop Med Hyg* 27(4), 762

**Note:** Tartrazine intolerance has been estimated to affect between 0.01% and 0.1% of the population. Adverse reactions are most common in people who are sensitive to aspirin. Banned in Norway and Austria

# TELMISARTAN

**Trade name:** Micardis (Boehringer Ingelheim)
**Indications:** Hypertension
**Category:** Angiotensin II receptor antagonist; antihypertensive
**Half-life:** 24 hours

### *Reactions*

## Skin
Allergic reactions (sic) (<1%)
Angioedema (>0.3%)
Dermatitis (sic) (>0.3%)
Diaphoresis (>0.3%)
Eczema (sic) (>0.3%)
Edema
(2001): Lacourciere Y+, *J Hum Hypertens* 15(11), 763
Flu-like syndrome (sic) (1%)
Flushing (>0.3%)
Fungal infection (sic) (>0.3%)
Leg edema (>0.3%)
Peripheral edema (1%)
Pruritus (>0.3%)
Rash (sic) (>0.3%)

## Other
Hypesthesia (>0.3%)
Myalgia (1%)
Paresthesias (>0.3%)
Xerostomia (>0.3%)

# TEMAZEPAM

**Trade name:** Temazepam
**Other common trade names:** *Apo-Temazepam; Cerepax; Euhypnos; Lenal; Levanxene; Normison; Nu-Temazepam; Planum*
**Indications:** Insomnia, anxiety
**Category:** Benzodiazepine sedative and hypnotic
**Half-life:** 8–15 hours
**Clinically important, potentially hazardous interactions with:** amprenavir, chlorpheniramine, clarithromycin, efavirenz, esomeprazole, imatinib, nelfinavir

### *Reactions*

## Skin
Bullous eruption
(1999): Verghese J+, *Acad Emerg Med* 6, 1071
Dermatitis (sic) (1–10%)
Diaphoresis (>10%)
Exanthems
Fixed eruption
(1988): Archer CB+, *Clin Exp Dermatol* 13, 336
Lichenoid eruption
(1986): Norris P+, *BMJ* 293, 510
Pruritus
Purpura
Rash (sic) (>10%)
Skin disorders (sic)
(1984): Stricker BH, *Ned Tijdschr Geneeskd* (Dutch) 128, 870
Urticaria

## Other
Anaphylactoid reactions
(1988): Mills PJ, *Anaesthesia* 43, 66
Dysgeusia
Paresthesias
Sialopenia (>10%)
Sialorrhea (1–10%)
Tremors (<1%)
Xerostomia (1.7%)

# TEMOZOLOMIDE

**Trade name:** Temodar (Schering)
**Indications:** Anaplastic astrocytoma
**Category:** Antineoplastic
**Half-life:** 1.8 hours

### *Reactions*

## Skin
Infections (sic)
Peripheral edema (11%)
Pruritus (8%)
Rash (sic) (8%)
Viral infection (sic) (11%)

## Other
Mastodynia (6%)
Myalgia (5%)
Paresthesias (9%)

# TENECTEPLASE

**Trade name:** TNKase (Genentech)
**Indications:** Acute myocardial infarction
**Category:** Thrombolytic; recombinant tissue plasminogen activator
**Half-life:** 90-130 minutes
**Clinically important, potentially hazardous interactions with:** bivalirudin

### *Reactions*

## Skin
Angioedema (<1%)
Ecchymoses
Hematomas (local) (12%)
Livedo reticularis (<1%)
Purple glove syndrome (<1% )
Purpura
Rash (sic) (<1%)
Urticaria (<1%)

## Other
Anaphylactoid reactions (<1%)
Gangrene (<1%)
Rhabdomyolysis (<1%)

# TENOFOVIR

**Synonyms:** PMPA; TDF
**Trade name:** Viread (Gilead)
**Indications:** Management of HIV Infections in combination with at least two other antiretroviral agents
**Category:** Antiretroviral agent; nucleotide reverse transcriptase inhibitor (NRTI)
**Half-life:** N/A
**Clinically important, potentially hazardous interactions with:** acycovir, cidofovir, didanosine, valganiciclovir

### *Reactions*

## Skin
Chills
Flu-like syndrome
Purpura
Rash (sic)

## Other
Pain (fingers or toes)
Paresthesias
Tremors

# TERAZOSIN

**Trade name:** Hytrin (Abbott)
**Other common trade names:** *Heitrin; Hitrin; Hytrine; Hytrinex; Itrin; Vicard*
**Indications:** Hypertension, benign prostatic hypertrophy
**Category:** Alpha$_1$-adrenergic blocking agent; antihypertensive
**Half-life:** 12 hours

### *Reactions*

## Skin
Diaphoresis (>1%)
Edema (1–10%)
Exanthems
(1998): Hernandez-Cano N+, *Lancet* 352, 202 (generalized)
(1998): Rosen R, (from Internet) (observation) (following PUVA)
Facial edema (>1%)
Flu-like syndrome (sic) (<1%)
Lichenoid eruption
(1993): Shelley WB+, *Cutis* 52, 88 (observation)
Peripheral edema (5.5%)
Phototoxicity
(1993): Shelley WB+, *Cutis* 52, 259 (observation)
Pruritus (>1%)
(1998): Hernandez-Cano N+, *Lancet* 352, 202
Rash (sic) (>1%)

## Other
Anaphylactoid reactions
Myalgia (>1%)
Paresthesias (2.9%)
Priapism (<1%)
(1998): Vaidyanathan S+, *Spinal Cord* 36, 805
Tinnitus
Xerostomia (1–10%)

# TERBINAFINE

**Trade name:** Lamisil (Novartis)
**Indications:** Fungal infections of the skin and nails
**Category:** Antifungal
**Half-life:** 22–26 hours

### *Reactions*

## Skin
Acute generalized exanthematous pustulosis (AGEP)
(2001): Rogalski C+, *Hautarzt* 52(5), 444
(2000): Hall AP+, *Australas J Dermatol* 41, 42
(1998): Condon CA+, *Br J Dermatol* 138, 709
(1997): Kempinaire A+, *J Am Acad Dermatol* 37, 653
(1996): Dupin N+, *Arch Dermatol* 132, 1253 (2 cases)
Allergic reactions (sic) (1–10%)
(1989): Savin R, *Clin Exp Dermatol* 14, 116
Angioedema
(1997): Hall M+, *Arch Dermatol* 133, 1213
Baboon syndrome
(2001): Weiss JM+, *Hautarzt* 52(12), 1104
Contact dermatitis (1–10%)
Cutaneous side effects (sic) (2.7%)
(1990): Villars V+, *J Dermatol Treat* 1, 33
Desquamation (sic)
(1995): Wachs F+, *Arch Dermatol* 131, 960 (passim)

Eczema (sic)
(1997): Hall M+, *Arch Dermatol* 133, 1213 (0.2%)
(1990): Villars V+, *J Dermatol Treat* 1, 33
Erythema multiforme
(1998): Gupta AK+, *Br J Dermatol* 138, 529 (5 patients)
(1997): Hall M+, *Arch Dermatol* 133, 1213
(1995): Todd P+, *Clin Exp Dermatol* 20, 247
(1995): Tramaloni S+, *Therapie* (French) 50, 594
(1994): Carstens J+, *Acta Derm Venereol* (Stockh) 74, 391
(1994): McGregor JM+, *Br J Dermatol* 131, 587
(1994): Rzany B+, *J Am Acad Dermatol* 30, 509
Erythroderma
(1998): Gupta AK+, *Br J Dermatol* 138, 529
(1996): Mitchell D, Charleston, SC (from Internet) (observation)
(1990): Villars V+, *J Dermatol Treat* 1, 33
Exanthems
(2001): Weiss JM+, *Hautarzt* 52(12), 1104
(1999): Valentine MC, Everett, WA (from Internet) (observation)
(1997): Sidhu JS, Malaysia (from Internet) (observation)
(1995): Hofmann H+, *Arch Dermatol* 131, 919
(1995): Wachs F+, *Arch Dermatol* 131, 960 (passim)
(1990): Villars V+, *J Dermatol Treat* 1, 33
Fixed eruption
(1995): Munn SE+, *Br J Dermatol* 133, 815
Lichenoid reaction
(2002): McCarty JR, Fort Worth, TX (from Internet) (observaion) (3 cases)
Lupus erythematosus
(2001): Bonsmann G+, *J Am Acad Dermatol* 44, 925 (subacute cutaneous) (4 cases)
(2001): Callen JP, *Arch Dermatol* 137, 1196
(2000): Callen JP, *Skin & Allergy News* March, 23 (subacute)
(2000): Gruchalla RS, *Lancet* 356, 1505
(2000): Reed BR, Denver, CO (personal communication) (from a meeting presented by Callen JP, Louisville, KY) (4 cases)
(1999): *Ann Dermatol Venereol* (French) 126, 463
(1999): Poster Exhibit #239, AAD Meeting, March 1999 (reported by ED and WB Shelley) (3 patients)
(1998): Brooke R+, *Br J Dermatol* 139, 1132
(1998): Holmes S+, *Br J Dermatol* 139, 1133
(1998): Murphy M+, *Br J Dermatol* 138, 708
(1997): Crowson AN+, *Hum Pathol* 28, 67 (subacute cutaneous)
Peripheral edema
(1997): Hall M+, *Arch Dermatol* 133, 1213
Photosensitivity
(1998): Litt JZ, Beachwood, OH (personal case) (observation)
(1997): Sidhu JS, Malaysia (from Internet) (observation)
Pityriasis rosea
(1998): Gupta AK+, *Br J Dermatol* 138, 529
Pruritus (2.8%)
(2001): Chambers WM+, *Eur J Gastroenterol Hepatol* 13, 1115
(1998): Litt JZ, Beachwood, OH (personal case) (observation)
(1997): Hall M+, *Arch Dermatol* 133, 1213 (0.3%)
(1995): Wachs F+, *Arch Dermatol* 131, 960 (passim)
(1990): Villars V+, *J Dermatol Treat* 1, 33
Psoriasis
(1998): Gupta AK+, *Br J Dermatol* 138, 529 (2 patients)
(1997): Gupta AK+, *J Am Acad Dermatol* 36, 858
(1995): Wachs F+, *Arch Dermatol* 131, 960 (erythema annulare centrifugum-like [sic])
Pustular eruption
(1999): Bennett ML+, *Int J Dermatol* 38, 596
Pustular psoriasis
(2000): Le Guyadec T+, *Ann Dermatol Venereol* (French) 127, 279
(1998): Papa CA+, *J Am Acad Dermatol* 39, 115
(1998): Wilson NJ+, *Br J Dermatol* 139, 168
(1995): Gupta AK+, unpublished findings
Rash (sic) (5.6%)
(1995): Haroon TS+, *Br J Dermatol* 135, 86
Stevens–Johnson syndrome
(1999): Rosen R, (from Internet) (observation)
(1994): Rzany B+, *J Am Acad Dermatol* 30, 509
Toxic epidermal necrolysis
(1996): White SI+, *Br J Dermatol* 134, 188
(1994): Carstens J+, *Acta Derm Venereol* (Stockh) 74, 391
(1993): Beutler M+, *BMJ* 307, 26
Toxicoderma
(1997): Hall M+, *Arch Dermatol* 133, 1213
Urticaria (1.1%)
(1998): Gupta AK+, *Br J Dermatol* 138, 529
(1998): Rademaker M+, *New Zealand Adverse Drug Reactions Committee*, April, 1998 (from Internet)
(1997): Billon S, *The Schoch Letter* 47, 32 (observation)
(1997): Hall M+, *Arch Dermatol* 133, 1213 (0.3%)
(1995): Wachs F+, *Arch Dermatol* 131, 960 (passim)
(1990): Savin RC, *J Am Acad Dermatol* 23, 807
(1990): Villars V+, *J Dermatol Treat* 1, 33

## Hair

Hair – alopecia (1–10%)
(2001): Richert B+, *Br J Dermatol* 145(5), 842
Hair – alopecia areata
(1990): Del Palacio Hernanz A+, *Clin Exp Dermatol* 15, 210

## Nails

Nails – onychocryptosis
(2000): Weaver TD+, *Cutis* 66, 211
(1995): Arenas R+, *Int J Dermatol* 34, 138

## Other

Ageusia
(2000): Schmutz JL+, *Ann Dermatol Venereol* (French) 127, 341 (persistent)
(1999): Private Patient Query (from Internet)
(1999): Villota Hoyos R+, *Aten Primaria* (Spanish) 23, 102
(1998): Bong JL+, *Br J Dermatol* 139, 747
(1997): Hall M+, *Arch Dermatol* 133, 1213 (0.3%)
(1995): Haroon TS+, *Br J Dermatol* 135, 86
(1995): Martinez-Yelamos S+, *Med Clin (Barc)* (Spanish) 105, 276
(1994): Cribier B+, *Ann Dermatol Venereol* (French) 121, 15
(1993): Stricker BHC, *Ned Tijdschr Geneeskd* 137, 617
(1992): Back D, *Lancet* 340, 252
(1992): Juhlin L, *Lancet* 339, 1483
(1992): Ottervanger JP+, *Lancet* 340, 728
(1992): Stricker BHC, *Ned Tijdschr Geneeskd* 136, 2438
Anaphylactoid reactions
Anosmia
(1993): Beutler M+, *BMJ* 307, 26
Aphthous stomatitis
(1998): Litt JZ, Beachwood, OH (personal case) (observation)
Depression
(2001): Richert B+, *Br J Dermatol* 145(5), 842
Dyschromatopsia (green vision)
(1996): Gupta AK+, *Arch Dermatol* 132, 845
Dysgeusia (2.8%) (metallic taste)
(2001): Lemont H+, *J Am Podiatr Med Assoc* 91(10), 540
(2000): Duxbury AJ+, *Br Dent J* 188, 295 ("persistent")
(2000): Marmelzat J, Los Angeles, CA (from Internet) (observation)
(1999): Marmelzat J, Los Angeles, CA (from Internet) (observation) (lasted for 6 months)
(1997): Danby FW, Kingston, Ontario (from Internet) (observation)
(1997): Hall M+, *Arch Dermatol* 133, 1213 (0.4%)
(1997): Marmelzat J, Los Angeles, CA (from Internet) (observation)
(1997): Sidhu JS, Malaysia (from Internet) (observation)

(1993): Beutler M+, *BMJ* 307, 26
(1992): Ottervanger JP+, *Lancet* 340, 728
Gingivitis
(1998): Gupta AK+, *J Am Acad Dermatol* 38, 765
Hypersensitivity*
(1998): Gupta AK+, *Australas J Dermatol* 39, 171
(1998): Schlienger RG+, *Epilepsia* 39, S3 (passim)
(1997): Gupta AK+, *J Am Acad Dermatol* 36, 1018
(1996): Gupta AK+, London, Ontario (observation)
(1996): Marmelzat J, Los Angeles, CA (from Internet) (observation)
(1996): Uhleman J, St. Charles, MO (from Internet) (observation)
Hypogeusia
(1992): Ottervanger JP+, *Lancet* 340, 728
Hyposmia
(1999): Villota Hoyos R+, *Aten Primaria* (Spanish) 23, 102
Parosmia
(1997): Hall M+, *Arch Dermatol* 133, 1213 (0.02%)
Parotid gland swelling
(1998): Torrens JK+, *BMJ* 316, 440
Serum sickness
(1995): Kruczynski K+, *Can J Clin Pharmacol* 2, 1
Stomatitis
(1998): Gupta AK+, *J Am Acad Dermatol* 38, 765
Tongue pigmentation
(1992): Ottervanger JP+, *Lancet* 340, 728

***Note:** The antiepileptic drug hypersensitivity syndrome is a severe, occasionally fatal, disorder characterized by any or all of the following: pruritic exanthems, toxic epidermal necrolysis, Stevens–Johnson syndrome, exfoliative dermatitis, fever, hepatic abnormalities, eosinophilia, and renal failure

# TERBUTALINE

**Trade names:** Brethaire (Novartis); Brethine (Novartis); Bricanyl (Aventis)
**Other common trade names:** *Ataline; Brothine; Bucaril; Butaline; Convon; Respirol; Vacanyl*
**Indications:** Bronchospasm
**Category:** Beta$_2$-adrenergic bronchodilator; sympathomimetic; tocolytic
**Half-life:** 11–16 hours
**Clinically important, potentially hazardous interactions with:** beta-blockers, epinephrine, propranolol, sympathomimetics

### *Reactions*

## Skin
Contact dermatitis (irritant)
(1988): Eedy DJ+, *Postgrad Med J* 64, 306
Diaphoresis (1–10%)
Exanthems
(1996): Drugge R, Stamford, CT (from Internet) (observation)
Flushing
Pruritus
(1996): Drugge R, Stamford, CT (from Internet) (observation)
Urticaria
Vasculitis
(1988): Enat R+, *Ann Allergy* 61, 275

## Other
Dysgeusia (1–10%)
Oral ulceration
(1987): High S, *BMJ* 294, 375
Rhabdomyolysis
(1989): Blake PG+, *Nephron* 53(1), 76
Xerostomia (1–10%)

# TERCONAZOLE

**Synonym:** triaconazole
**Trade name:** Terazol (Ortho-McNeil)
**Other common trade names:** *Fungistat; Gyno-Terazol; Tercospor*
**Indications:** Vulvovaginal candidiasis
**Category:** Antifungal
**Half-life:** no data

### *Reactions*

## Skin
Chills
Pruritus (2.3%)
Toxic epidermal necrolysis
(1998): Searles GE+, *J Cutan Med Surg* 3, 85 (from vaginal suppository)

## Other
Vulvovaginal burning (1–10%)

# TERFENADINE*

**Other common trade names:** *Alergist; Allerplus; Cyater; Ferdin; Teldane; Teldanex; Triludan*
**Category:** H$_1$-receptor antihistamine
**Half-life:** 16–22 hours
**Clinically important, potentially hazardous interactions with:** erythromycin

### *Reactions*

## Skin
Angioedema (<1%)
(1986): Stricker BHC+, *BMJ* 293, 536
Atopic dermatitis (exacerbation)
(1986): Goodfield MJD+, *BMJ* 293, 1103
Cutaneous side effects (sic)
(1995): McClintock AD+, *N Z Med J* 108, 208
Diaphoresis
Exanthems
(1986): Stricker BHC+, *BMJ* 293, 536
Exfoliation (sic)
(1986): Stricker BHC+, *BMJ* 293, 536
Fixed eruption
(1994): Gani F+, *Ann Allergy* 72, 76
Flushing
Lupus erythematosus
Photosensitivity (<1%)
(1994): Berger TG+, *Arch Dermatol* 130, 609 (in HIV-infected) (2 cases)
(1994): Shelley WB+, *Cutis* 53, 121 (observation)
(1986): Fenton D+, *BMJ* 293, 823
(1986): Stricker BHC+, *BMJ* 293, 536
Pruritus
Psoriasis (exacerbation)
(1990): Navaratnam AE+, *Clin Exp Dermatol* 15, 78

(1988): Harrison PV+, *Clin Exp Dermatol* 13, 275
Purpura
Rash (sic) (<1%)
Urticaria
(1986): Stricker BHC+, *BMJ* 293, 536

### Hair

Hair – alopecia
(1993): Shelley WB+, *Cutis* 52, 81 (observation)
(1992): Frazier CA, *N C Med J* 53, 390
(1985): Jones SK+, *BMJ* 291, 940

### Other

Anaphylactoid reactions
Galactorrhea
Gynecomastia
Myalgia (<1%)
Oral mucosal eruption
(1990): McTavish D+, *Drugs* 39, 552
Paresthesias (<1%)
Pseudolymphoma
(1995): Magro CM+, *J Am Acad Dermatol* 32, 419
Stomatitis
Xerostomia (1–10%)
(1990): McTavish D+, *Drugs* 39, 552

***Note:** Terfenadine has been withdrawn in the USA

## TESTOSTERONE

**Trade names:** Andro-L.A; Androderm (Watson); AndroGel; Androgel; Andronaq; Delatest; Delatestryl (BTG); depAndro; Duratest; Histerone; Testoderm (Alza)
**Other common trade names:** *Malogen; Testandro; Testex; Testopel*
**Indications:** Androgen replacement, hypogonadism, postpartum breast pain
**Category:** Androgen
**Half-life:** 10–100 minutes
**Clinically important, potentially hazardous interactions with:** anisindione, anticoagulants, cyclosporine, dicumarol, warfarin

### *Reactions*

### Skin

Acne (>10%)
(1998): Kwon PS+, *Arch Dermatol* 134, 376
(1995): Tabata N+, *J Am Acad Dermatol* 33, 676 (infantile)
(1992): Fyrand O+, *Acta Derm Venereol* 72, 148
(1990): Fuchs E+, *J Am Acad Dermatol* 23, 125
(1989): Fyrand O+, *Tidsskr Nor Laegeforen* (Norwegian) 109, 239
(1989): Hartmann AA+, *Monatsschr Kinderheilkd* (German) 137, 466
(1989): Heydenreich G, *Arch Dermatol* 125, 571 (fulminans)
(1989): Scott MJ+, *Cutis* 44, 30
(1989): von Muhlendahl KE+, *Dtsch Med Wochenschr* (German) 114, 712
(1988): Traupe H+, *Arch Dermatol* 124, 414 (fulminans)
(1987): Kiraly CL+, *Am J Dermatopathol* 9, 515
(1984): Lamb DR, *Am J Sports Med* 12, 31
(1965): Kennedy BJ, *J Am Geriatr Soc* 13, 230
(1965): Rook A, *Br J Dermatol* 77, 115
Contact dermatitis (4%)
(1998): Buckley DA+, *Contact Dermatitis* 39, 91 (from patch)
(1989): Holdiness MR, *Contact Dermatitis* 20, 3 (from patch)
Edema (1–10%)
Exanthems
(2001): McGriff NJ+, *Pharmacotherapy* 21(11), 1425
Flushing (1–10%)
(1965): Kennedy BJ, *J Am Geriatr Soc* 13, 230
Folliculitis
(1998): Kwon PS+, *Arch Dermatol* 134, 376
Furunculosis
(1989): Scott MJ+, *Cutis* 44, 30
Lichenoid eruption
(1989): Aihara M+, *J Dermatol* (Tokio) 16, 330
Lupus erythematosus
(1978): Robinson HM, *Z Haut* (German) 53, 349
Peripheral edema
Pruritus
(2001): McGriff NJ+, *Pharmacotherapy* 21(11), 1425
Psoriasis
(1990): O'Driscoll JB+, *Clin Exp Dermatol* 15, 68
Rash (sic) (2%)
Seborrhea (sic) (<1%)
Seborrheic dermatitis
(1989): Scott MJ+, *Cutis* 44, 30
Striae
(1989): Scott MJ+, *Cutis* 44, 30
Urticaria

### Hair

Hair – alopecia (<1%)
(1989): Scott MJ+, *Cutis* 44, 30
(1965): Kennedy BJ, *J Am Geriatr Soc* 13, 230
Hair – hirsutism (1–10%)
(1994): Castillo-Ceballos A+, *Med Clin (Barc)* (Spanish) 102, 78
(1991): Bates GW+, *Clin Obstet Gynecol* 34, 848
(1991): No Author, *Obstet Gynecol* 78, 474
(1991): Parker LU+, *Cleve Clin J Med* 58, 43
(1991): Urman B+, *Obstet Gynecol* 77, 595
(1989): Scott MJ+, *Cutis* 44, 30
(1974): Baron J, *Zentralbl Gynakol* (German) 96, 129
(1971): Fusi S+, *Folia Endocrinol* (Italian) 24, 412
(1965): Kennedy BJ, *J Am Geriatr Soc* 13, 230

### Other

Anaphylactoid reactions (<1%)
Application-site bullae (12%)
Application-site burning (3%)
Application-site erythema (7%)
Application-site induration (3%)
Application-site pruritus (37%)
Application-site vesicles (6%)
Gynecomastia (<1%)
Hypersensitivity (<1%)
Injection-site pain
Injection-site tenderness
(2002): Amory JK+, *J Androl* 23(1), 84
Mastodynia (>10%)
Paresthesias (<1%)
Priapism (>10%)
(2001): Madrid Garcia+, *Arch Esp Urol* 54(7), 703
Stomatitis

# TETRACYCLINE

**Trade names:** Achromycin V (Lederle); Ala-Tet (Del-Ray); Panmycin (Pharmacia & Upjohn); Robitet (Robins); Sumycin (Bristol-Myers Squibb)
**Other common trade names:** *Apo-Tetra; Economycin; Florocycline; Steclin; Teflin; Teline; Tetramig; Topicycline* (Topical); *Zorbenal-G*
**Indications:** Various infections caused by susceptible organisms
**Category:** Antibiotic
**Half-life:** 6–11 hours
**Clinically important, potentially hazardous interactions with:** acitretin, aluminum hydroxide, amoxicillin, ampicillin, antacids, bacampicillin, bismuth, calcium, cholestyramine, cloxacillin, corticosteroids, **dairy products**, didanosine, digoxin, **food**, iron, isotretinoin, methotrexate, methoxyflurane, mezlocillin, nafcillin, oxacillin, penicillins, retinoids, sucralfate, vitamin A, zinc

## *Reactions*

### Skin

Acne
(1971): Bean SF, *Br J Dermatol* 85, 585
(1969): Weary PE+, *Arch Dermatol* 100, 179
Angioedema
(1997): Shapiro LE+, *Arch Dermatol* 133, 1224
(1978): Jolly HW+, *Arch Dermatol* 114, 1485
Bullous eruption
(1971): Benazeraf C+, *Bull Soc Fr Dermatol Syphiligr* (French) 78, 19
Candidiasis
(1970): Lehner T+, *Br J Dermatol* 83, 161 (oral)
(1965): Clendenning WE, *Arch Dermatol* 91, 628
Cheilitis
(1978): Jolly HW+, *Arch Dermatol* 114, 1485
Dermatitis (sic)
(1970): Chilvers AS+, *Lancet* 1, 402 (leg)
Diaphoresis
Eczematous eruption (sic)
Erythema multiforme
(1988): Lewis-Jones MS+, *Clin Exp Dermatol* 13, 245
(1987): Curley RK+, *Clin Exp Dermatol* 12, 124
(1987): Leroy D+, *Photodermatol* 4, 52 (photodistributed)
(1987): Shoji A+, *Arch Dermatol* 123, 18
(1983): Albengres E+, *Therapie* (French) 38, 577
(1968): Bianchine JR+, *Am Med J* 44, 390
(1965): Clendenning WE, *Arch Dermatol* 91, 628
Exanthems
(1993): Chaffins ML+, *J Am Acad Dermatol* 28, 988
(1979): Patriarca G+, *Boll Ist Sieroter Milan* (Italian) 57, 805 (fixed)
(1978): Jolly HW+, *Arch Dermatol* 114, 1485
Exfoliative dermatitis (<1%)
(1978): Jolly HW+, *Arch Dermatol* 114, 1485
(1972): Kauppinen K, *Acta Derm Venereol* (Stockh) 52 (Suppl),68
Fixed eruption
(1998): Leal G, Fortaleza, Brazil (from Internet) (observation) (pulsating)
(1998): Mahboob A+, *Int J Dermatol* 37, 833
(1994): Bielan B, *Dermatol Nurs* 6, 198
(1991): Thankappen TP+, *Int J Dermatol* 30, 867 (15.9%)
(1990): Gaffoor PMA+, *Cutis* 45, 242
(1988): Chan HL+, *Ann Acad Med Singapore* 17, 514
(1986): Sehgal VH+, *Genitourin Med* 62, 56 (genital)
(1985): Chan HL+, *J Am Acad Dermatol* 13, 302
(1985): Dodds PR+, *J Urol* 133, 1044 (balanitis)
(1985): Kauppinen K+, *Br J Dermatol* 112, 575
(1985): Pandhi RK+, *Australas J Dermatol* 26, 88
(1984): Chan HL, *Int J Dermatol* 23, 607
(1984): Kanwar AJ+, *J Dermatol* 11, 383
(1984): Pandhi RK+, *Sex Transm Dis* 11, 164 (male genitalia)
(1982): Kanwar AJ+, *Dermatologica* 164, 115
(1981): Bhargava NC+, *Int J Dermatol* 20, 435
(1981): Fiumara NJ+, *Sex Transm Dis* 8, 258
(1981): Fiumara NJ+, *Sex Transm Dis* 8, 23 (penile)
(1979): Pasricha JS, *Br J Dermatol* 100, 183
(1979): Pasricha JS, *Br J Dermatol* 101, 361
(1979): Patriarca G+, *Boll Ist Sieroter Milan* (Italian) 57, 805
(1978): Jolly HW+, *Arch Dermatol* 114, 1485
(1978): Parish LC+, *Acta Derm Venereol* (Stockh) 58, 545 (pulsating)
(1976): Epstein JH+, *Arch Dermatol* 112, 661 (porphyria-like)
(1976): Farkas J, *Dermatol Monatsschr* (German) 162, 250
(1974): Brown ST, *JAMA* 227, 801 (balanitis)
(1974): Sehgal VN, *Dermatologica* 148, 120
(1973): Armati RP, *Australas J Dermatol* 14, 75
(1971): Csonka GW+, *Br J Ven Dis* 47, 42 (balanitis)
(1970): Brodin MB, *Arch Dermatol* 101, 621
(1970): Delaney TJ, *Br J Dermatol* 83, 357
(1970): Duricic S, *Med Arh* (Serbo-Croatian-Roman) 24, 143
(1970): Savin JA, *Br J Dermatol* 83, 546
(1970): Tarnowski WM, *Acta Derm Venereol* (Stockh) 50, 117
(1970): Tarnowski WM, *Arch Dermatol* 102, 234
(1969): Kandil E, *Dermatologica* 139, 37
(1969): Minkin W+, *Arch Dermatol* 100, 749
(1963): Reiner E+, *Arch Dermatol* 88, 465
(1962): Post CF+, *Arch Dermatol* 86, 678
(1961): Welsh AL+, *Arch Dermatol* 84, 1004
(1952): Dougherty JW, *Arch Dermatol* 65, 485
(1950): Peck SM+, *JAMA* 142, 1137
Lichenoid eruption
(1974): Maibach HI+, *Arch Dermatol* 109, 97
(1974): Tay C, *Asian J Med* 10, 223
(1971): Almeyda J+, *Br J Dermatol* 85, 604
Lupus erythematosus
(1999): Sturkenboom MCJM+, *Arch Int Med* 159, 493
(1985): Stratton MA, *Clin Pharm* 4, 657
(1964): Sulkowski SR+, *JAMA* 189, 152
(1959): Domz CA+, *Ann Intern Med* 50, 1217
Lymphoepithelioma
(1973): Sadoff L+, *Lancet* 1, 675
Photosensitivity (1–10%)
(1997): Shapiro LE+, *Arch Dermatol* 133, 1224
(1993): Wainwright NJ+, *Drug Saf* 9, 437
(1989): Rosen C, *Semin Dermatol* 8, 149
(1977): Epstein E, *Arch Dermatol* 113, 236
(1975): Breit R, *Munch Med Wochenschr* (German) 117, 23
(1969): Levene G+, *Br J Dermatol* 81, 712
(1969): Moller H, *Lakartidningen* (Swedish) 66, 1446
(1967): Ippen H, *Z Haut Geschlechtskr* (German) 42, 47
(1967): Tarsitani F+, *Policlinico Prat* (Italian) 74, 329
(1966): Cullen SI+, *Arch Dermatol* 93, 77
(1965): Clendenning WE, *Arch Dermatol* 91, 628
Phototoxicity
(2002): Sorkin M, Denver, CO (from Internet) (observation)
(1980): Stern RS+, *Arch Dermatol* 116, 1269
(1975): Breit R, *Munch Med Wochenschr* (German) 117, 23
Pigmentation
(2001): Dereure O, *Am J Clin Dermatol* 2(4), 253
(1983): White SW+, *Arch Dermatol* 119, 1
(1981): Brothers DM+, *Ophthalmology* 88, 1212 (conjunctival)
(1981): Granstein RD+, *J Am Acad Dermatol* 5, 1 (blue-black)
Pruritus (<1%)
(1995): Nowakowski J+, *J Am Acad Dermatol* 32, 223
Pruritus ani

Psoriasis (exacerbation)
(1990): Bergner T+, *J Am Acad Dermatol* 23, 770
(1988): Tsankov N+, *J Am Acad Dermatol* 19, 629
Purpura
(1965): Horowitz HI+, *Semin Hematol* 2, 287
Pustular eruption
(1973): Thomsen K+, *Br J Dermatol* 89, 293 (palms and soles)
Rash (sic)
(1997): Shapiro LE+, *Arch Dermatol* 133, 1224
Stevens–Johnson syndrome
(1997): Shoji T+, *J Am Acad Dermatol* 37, 337
(1993): Leenutaphong V+, *Int J Dermatol* 32, 428
(1985): Burge SM+, *J Am Acad Dermatol* 13, 665
(1968): Bianchine JR+, *Am Med J* 44, 390
Sunburn (exaggerated)
(1965): Clendenning WE, *Arch Dermatol* 91, 628
Toxic epidermal necrolysis
(1993): Leenutaphong V+, *Int J Dermatol* 32, 428
(1989): Davies MG+, *BMJ* 298, 1523
(1988): Gimova EK+, *Sov Med* (Russian) 6, 119
(1987): Curley RK+, *Clin Exp Dermatol* 12, 124
(1985): Burge SM+, *J Am Acad Dermatol* 13, 665
(1985): Tatnall FM+, *Br J Dermatol* 113, 629
(1984): Chan HL, *J Am Acad Dermatol* 10, 973
(1979): Izmailov GA+, *Khirurgiia Mosk* (Russian) September 102
(1974): Maibach HI+, *Arch Dermatol* 109, 97
(1970): Ocheret'ko MP, *Pediatriia* (Russian) 49, 86
(1967): Lowney ED+, *Arch Dermatol* 95, 359
(1966): Messaritakis J, *Ann Paediatr* 207, 236
(1959): Evans C, *BMJ* 2, 827
Urticaria
(1997): Shapiro LE+, *Arch Dermatol* 133, 1224
(1978): Jolly HW+, *Arch Dermatol* 114, 1485
(1977): McLundie S, *Ann Allergy* 38, 71
Vasculitis
(1960): Calnan CD+, *Trans A Rep St John's Hosp Derm Soc* (London) 44, 69
Warts (flat)
(1975): Gould WM, *Arch Dermatol* 111, 930

### Nails

Nails – discoloration (<1%)
(1980): Hendricks AA, *Arch Dermatol* 116, 438 (yellow lunulae)
Nails – onycholysis
(1979): Kanwar AJ+, *Cutis* 23, 657
(1976): Sanders CV+, *South Med J* 69, 1090
(1974): Merrill RH, *South Med J* 67, 677
(1972): Kestel JL, *Arch Dermatol* 106, 766
(1965): Clendenning WE, *Arch Dermatol* 91, 628
Nails – photo-onycholysis
(2002): Rudolph RI, Wyomissing, PA (from Internet) (observation)
(1987): Baran R+, *J Am Acad Dermatol* 17, 1012
(1983): Ibsen HH+, *Acta Derm Venereol* 63, 555
(1978): Hatch DJ+, *J Am Podiatry Assoc* 68, 172
(1978): Lasser AE+, *Pediatrics* 61, 98
(1977): Rothstein MS, *Arch Dermatol* 113, 520
(1973): Verma KC+, *Indian J Dermatol* 18, 23
(1971): Frank SB+, *Arch Dermatol* 103, 520

### Other

Anaphylactoid reactions (<1%)
(1965): Clendenning WE, *Arch Dermatol* 91, 628
Black tongue
(1954): Annotations, *Lancet* 2, 179
Fixed intraoral eruption
(1982): Murray VK+, *J Periodontology* 53, 267
Gingivitis
Glossitis
(1978): Jolly HW+, *Arch Dermatol* 114, 1485
Granulomas
(1979): Hagedorn M+, *Dermatologica* 158, 93 (multiple and pyogenic)
Hypersensitivity (<1%)
(1997): Shapiro LE+, *Arch Dermatol* 133, 1224
(1972): No Author, *Tidsskr Nor Laegeforen* (Norwegian) 92, 1478
Mucocutaneous febrile syndrome
(1972): *Tidsskr Nor Laegeforen* (Norwegian) 92, 175
Mucous membrane pigmentation
Oral ulceration
Paresthesias (<1%)
(1996): Sorkin M, *The Schoch Letter* 45 (5), 18 (observation)
(1994): Blanchard L,, *The Schoch Letter* 44, 6 (observation)
Porphyria cutanea tarda
(1992): Shelley WB+, *Advanced Dermatologic Diagnosis* WB Saunders, 414 (passim)
Pseudoporphyria
(1976): Epstein JH+, *Arch Dermatol* 112, 661
Pseudotumor cerebri
(1999): Quinn AG+, *J Aapos* 3, 53
(1998): Noll K, La Crosse, WI (from Internet) (observation)
(1995): Lee AG, *Cutis* 55, 165
(1986): Pierog SH+, *J Adolesc Health Care* 7, 139
(1981): Steigleder GK, *Z Haut* 56, 839
(1978): Stuart BH+, *J Pediatr* 92, 679
Serum sickness
(1997): Shapiro LE+, *Arch Dermatol* 133, 1224
Thrombophlebitis (<1%)
Tinnitus
Tongue pigmentation
Tooth discoloration (commonly in under 8-year-olds) (>10%)
(2002): Kugel G+, *Compend Contin Educ Dent* 23(1A), 29
(2001): Fukuta Y+, *J Oral Sci* 43(3), 213
(1998): Livingston HM+, *Ann Pharmacother* 32, 607
(1994): Hofmann H, *Hautarzt* (German) 45, 803
(1979): Jackson R, *Cutis* 23, 613
(1974): Moffitt JM+, *J Am Dent Ass* 88, 547
(1971): Grossman ER+, *Pediatrics* 47, 567
(1970): Conchie JM+, *Can Med Ass J* 103, 351
(1968): *Med Lett<D 10, 76*
(1964): Stewart DJ, *Br J Dermatol* 76, 374
(1962): Wallman IS+, *Lancet* 1, 827 (>5%)
Vaginitis
(1977): Hall JH+, *Cutis* 20, 97
(1972): Gilgor RS, *N C Med J* 33, 331
(1972): Litt IF, *Pediatrics* 49, 637

## THALIDOMIDE

**Trade names:** Contergan; Distaval; Kevadon; Thalidomid (Celgene)
**Indications:** Graft-versus-host reactions, recalcitrant aphthous stomatitis
**Category:** Immunosuppressant; treatment for graft-versus-host disease and nodose leprosy
**Half-life:** 8.7 hours

### *Reactions*

### Skin

Bullous eruption
(1975): Sheskin J, *Hautarzt* (German) 26, 1 (5%)
Burning
(1989): Gutierrez-Rodriguez O+, *J Rheumatol* 16, 158

Dermatitis (sic)
(1971): Waters MFR, *Lepr Rev* 42, 26
Diaphoresis
(1978): Smithells RW, *Lancet* 1, 1042
Edema
(2000): Oliver SJ+, *Clin Immunol* 97(2), 109
(1997): Duran McKinster C, *Skin and Allergy News* August, 37
(1996): Tseng S+, *J Am Acad Dermatol* 35, 969 (passim)
(1989): Grinspan D+, *J Am Acad Dermatol* 20, 1060
(1984): Gutierrez-Rodriguez O, *Arthritis Rheum* 27, 1118
Erythema
(1989): Gutierrez-Rodriguez O+, *J Rheumatol* 16, 158
Erythema nodosum
(2000): Gardener-Merwin JM+, *Ann Rheum Dis* 53, 828
(1988): Viraben R+, *Dermatologica* 176, 107
Erythroderma
(1996): Tseng S+, *J Am Acad Dermatol* 35, 969 (passim)
(1994): Bielsa I+, *Dermatology* (Basel) 189, 178
Exanthems
(2000): Camisa C+, *Arch Dermatol* 136, 1442
(1999): Burrow WH, Jackson, MS (from Internet) (observation)
(1991): Williams I+, *Lancet* 337, 436 (37% in AIDS patients)
Exfoliative dermatitis
(1996): Tseng S+, *J Am Acad Dermatol* 35, 969 (passim)
(1988): Salafia A+, *Int J Lepr Other Mycobact Dis* 56, 625
Facial erythema
(1989): Gutierrez-Rodriguez O+, *J Rheumatol* 16, 158
(1975): Sheskin J, *Hautarzt* (German) 26, 1 (1–5%)
Pedal edema
(2000): Bahl S+, *Skin and Aging,* May, 41
Peripheral edema
(2000): Camisa C+, *Arch Dermatol* 136, 1442
(2000): Gardener-Merwin JM+, *Ann Rheum Dis* 53, 828
Pruritus
(1996): Tseng S+, *J Am Acad Dermatol* 35, 969 (passim)
(1989): Gutierrez-Rodriguez O+, *J Rheumatol* 16, 158
Purpura
(1996): Tseng S+, *J Am Acad Dermatol* 35, 969 (passim)
Pustuloderma
(1999): Rua-Figuero I+, *Lupus* 8, 248
Rash (sic)
(2002): Steins MB+, *Blood* 99(3), 834
(2002): Tosi P+, *Haematologica* 87(4), 408 (11%)
(2001): Rajkumar SV, *Oncology (Huntingt)* 15(7), 867
(2001): Singhal S+, *BioDrugs* 15(3), 163 (30%)
(2000): Gardener-Merwin JM+, *Ann Rheum Dis* 53, 828
(2000): Oliver SJ+, *Clin Immunol* 97(2), 109
(2000): Rajkumar SV, *Oncology (Huntingt)* 14(12), 11
(1997): Haslett P+, *Infect Med* 14, 393
(1997): Jacobson JM+, *New Engl J Med* 336, 1487 (>50%)
(1993): Holm AL+, *Arch Dermatol* 129, 1548 (passim)
(1986): Hamza MH, *Clin Rheumatol* 5, 365
Red palms
(1996): Tseng S+, *J Am Acad Dermatol* 35, 969 (passim)
Shakes (sic)
(1999): Duong DJ, *Arch Dermatol* 135, 1079
Stevens–Johnson syndrome
(2001): Clark TE+, *Drug Saf* 24(2), 87
Toxic epidermal necrolysis
(2001): Diggle GE, *Int J Clin Pract* 55(9), 627
(2000): Rajkumar SV+, *N Engl J Med* 343(13), 972
(1999): Horowitz SB+, *Pharmacotherapy* 19, 1177
Toxic pustuloderma
(1997): Darvay A+, *Clin Exp Dermatol* 22, 297
Ulceration
(2001): Schlossberg H+, *Bone Marrow Transplant* 27, 229 (serious)
Urticaria
(1975): Sheskin J, *Hautarzt* (German) 26, 1 (3%)
Vasculitis
(1996): Tseng S+, *J Am Acad Dermatol* 35, 969 (passim)
Xerosis
(2002): Bariol C+, *J Gastroenterol Hepatol* 17(2), 135
(2000): Bahl S+, *Skin and Aging* May, 41
(2000): Oliver SJ+, *Clin Immunol* 97(2), 109
(1989): Gutierrez-Rodriguez O+, *J Rheumatol* 16, 158

### Hair

Hair – alopecia
(1989): Gutierrez-Rodriguez O+, *J Rheumatol* 16, 158

### Nails

Nails – brittle
(1996): Tseng S+, *J Am Acad Dermatol* 35, 969 (passim)

### Other

Death
(2001): Diggle GE, *Int J Clin* 55(9), 627
Dysesthesia
(1989): Grinspan D+, *J Am Acad Dermatol* 20, 1060
Galactorrhea
(1996): Tseng S+, *J Am Acad Dermatol* 35, 969 (passim)
Gynecomastia
(2002): Pulik M+, *Am J Hematol* 70(3), 265
Hypesthesia
(2000): Bahl S+, *Skin and Aging,* May, 41
Paresthesias
(2000): Bahl S+, *Skin and Aging,* May, 41
(2000): Ordi-Ros J+, *J Rheumatol* 27, 1429
(1999): Duong DJ, *Arch Dermatol* 135, 1079
(1998): Lee JB+, *J Am Acad Dermatol* 39, 835
Xerostomia
(2002): Bariol C+, *J Gastroenterol Hepatol* 17(2), 135
(2000): Bahl S+, *Skin and Aging* May, 41
(1999): Monastirli A+, *Skin Pharmacol Appl Skin Physiol* 12(6), 305
(1996): Tseng S+, *J Am Acad Dermatol* 35, 969 (passim)
(1994): Gardener-Merwin JM+, *Ann Rheum Dis* 53, 828
(1989): Grinspan D+, *J Am Acad Dermatol* 20, 1060
(1989): Gutierrez-Rodriguez O+, *J Rheumatol* 16, 158

# THEOPHYLLINE

(See AMINOPHYLLINE)

**Clinically important, potentially hazardous interactions with:** charcoal, cimetidine, ciprofloxacin, clorazepate, erythromycin, halothane, oral contraceptives, **tobacco**

## *Reactions*

### Other

Rhabdomyolysis
(2001): Teweleit S+, *Med Klin* 96(1), 40
(2000): Iwano J+, *J Med Invest* 47(1), 9
(1999): Shimada N+, *Nippon Jinzo Gakkai Shi* 41(4), 460 (with clarithromycin)

# THIABENDAZOLE

**Synonym:** tiabendazole
**Trade name:** Mintezol (Merck)
**Other common trade name:** *Triasox*
**Indications:** Various infections caused by susceptible helminths
**Category:** Anthelmintic
**Half-life:** 1.2 hours

### *Reactions*

**Skin**

Angioedema
Contact dermatitis
(1994): Mancuso G, *Contact Dermatitis* 31, 207
(1993): Izu R+, *Contact Dermatitis* 28, 243 (photoaggravated)
(1968): De Irureta-Goyena A, *Arch Dermatol* 97, 348
Erythema multiforme (<1%)
(1988): Humphreys F+, *Br J Dermatol* 118, 855
(1988): Kardaun SH+, *Br J Dermatol* 118, 545
Exanthems (>5%)
(1982): Sanchez del Rio J+, *Actas Dermosifiliogr* (Spanish) 73, 125
(1977): Casado-Jiminez M+, *Actas Dermosifiliogr* (Spanish) 68, 675
(1976): Marron-Gasca J+, *Actas Dermosifiliogr* (Spanish) 67, 701
(1965): Bowen J+, *Arch Dermatol* 91, 425
Fixed eruption (<1%)
(1976): Marron-Gasca J+, *Actas Dermosifiliogr* (Spanish) 67, 701
Flushing
Jarisch–Herxheimer reaction
Perianal rash
Pruritus (<1%)
(1965): Bowen J+, *Arch Dermatol* 91, 425
Psoriasis (exacerbation)
Rash (sic) (1–10%)
Sjøgren's syndrome
(1995): Bion E+, *J Hepatol* 23, 672
(1979): Fink AI+, *Ophthalmology* 86, 1892
Stevens–Johnson syndrome (1–10%)
Toxic epidermal necrolysis (<1%)
(1993): Correia O+, *Dermatology* 186, 32
(1976): Robinson HM+, *Arch Dermatol* 112, 1757
Urticaria (1–5%)
(1970): Tanowitz HB+, *J Trop Med Hyg* 73, 141

**Other**

Anaphylactoid reactions
Dry mucous membranes (sic)
Hypersensitivity (<1%)
Paresthesias
Tinnitus
Xanthopsia (<1%)
Xerostomia
(1979): Fink AI+, *Ophthalmology* 86, 1892

# THIAMINE

**Synonym:** vitamin $B_1$
**Trade names:** Betalin; Thiamilate
**Other common trade names:** *Actamin; Beneuril; Betabion; Betamin; Betaxin; Bewon; Biamine; Thiamilate; Tiamina; Vitantial*
**Indications:** Thiamine deficiency
**Category:** Water-soluble vitamin; nutritional supplement
**Half-life:** no data

### *Reactions*

**Skin**

Allergic reactions (sic)
(1969): Zheltakov MM+, *Vestn Dermatol Venerol* (Russian) 43, 62
Angioedema (<1%)
Contact dermatitis
(1989): Ingemann-Larsen A+, *Contact Dermatitis* 20, 387
(1958): Hjorth N, *J Invest Dermatol* 30, 261
Diaphoresis
Eczematous eruption (sic)
(1958): Hjorth N, *J Invest Dermatol* 30, 261
Exanthems
(1980): Kolz R+, *Hautarzt* (German) 31, 657
Pruritus (<1%)
Purpura
(1989): Nishioka K+, *J Dermatol* 16, 220
(1980): Nishioka K+, *Clin Exp Dermatol* 5, 213
Rash (sic) (<1%)
Systemic eczematous contact dermatitis
Urticaria
Vasculitis
(1989): Nishioka K+, *J Dermatol* 16, 220

**Other**

Anaphylactoid reactions
(2000): Johri S+, *Am J Emerg Med* 18(5), 642
(1998): Morinville V+, *Schweiz Med Wochenschr* 128, 1743
(1997): Fernandez M+, *Allergy* 52, 958
Foetor ex ore (halitosis)
Injection-site reactions (sic)
Paresthesias (<1%)

# THIMEROSAL

**Trade names:** Aeroaid; Mersol; Merthiolate
**Other common trade names:** *Curativ; Merseptyl; Topicaldermo; Vitaseptol*
**Indications:** Antiseptic, bacteriostatic, fungistatic
**Category:** Topical organomercurial antiseptic used in cosmetics; ophthalmic and otolaryngologic medications; vaccines
**Half-life:** N/A

### *Reactions*

**Skin**

Allergic dermatitis
(2000): Kiec-Swierczynska M+, *Int J Occup Med Environ Health* 13(3), 179
(1999): Lebrec H+, *Cell Biol Toxicol* 15(1), 57
(1999): McKenna KE, *Contact Dermatitis* 40(3), 158
(1995): Aberer W+, *Contact Dermatitis* 32(6), 367
(1995): Schafer T+, *Contact Dermatitis* 32(2), 114
Allergic reactions (sic)

(2001): Suneja T+, *J Am Acad Dermatol* 45(1), 23
(2000): Kiec-Swierczynska M+, *Int J Occup Med Environ Health* 13(3), 179
(1997): Rees S+, *Br Dent J* 183, 395 (in health care workersr)
(1997): Wray D, *Br Dent J* 183, 316 (in health care workers)
(1995): Barbaud A+, *Ann Dermatol Venereol* 122(3), 129
(1993): Pirker C+, *Contact Dermatitis* 29(3), 152
(1992): Wonk WK+, *Contact Dermatitis* 26(3), 195

Atopic dermatitis
(1999): Patrizi A+, *Contact Dermatitis* 40(2), 94
(1998): Romaguera C+, *Contact Dermatitis* 39(6), 277

Cheilitis
(1999): Kanthraj GR+, *Contact Dermatitis* 40(5), 285

Contact allergy (sic)
(2001): Trujillo MJ+, *Allergol Immunopathol* (Madr) 29(4), 133 (with piroxicam)

Contact dermatitis
(2001): Suneja T+, *J Am Acad Dermatol* 45(1), 23
(2000): Schafer MP+, *Contact Dermatitis* 43(3), 150
(2000): Westphal GA+, *Int Arch Occup Environ Health* 73(6), 384
(1999): Sertoli A+, *Am J Contact Dermat* 10(1), 18
(1999): Wolfe, S, Statesville, NC (from Internet) (observation) (eyelids)
(1998): Ramsay HM+, *Contact Dermatitis* 39(4), 205
(1998): Romaguera C+, *Contact Dermatitis* 39(6), 277
(1998): Santucci B+, *Contact Dermatitis* 38(6), 325
(1997): Luka RE+, *J Allergy Clin Immunol* 100(1), 138
(1995): Zenarola P+, *Contact Dermatitis* 32(2), 107 (systemic)
(1994): Meding B+, *Contact Dermatitis* 30(3), 129
(1994): Wantke F+, *Contact Dermatitis* 30(2), 115
(1994): Zemstov A+, *Contact Dermatitis* 30(1), 57 (bullous)
(1991): Oritz FJ+, *Contact Dermatitis* 25(3), 203
(1990): de Groot AC+, *Contact Dermatitis* 23(3), 168 (eyelids, from contact lens fluid)
(1990): Landa A+, *Contact Dermatitis* 22(5), 290
(1990): Wekkeli M+, *Contact Dermatitis* 22(5), 295
(1989): Seidenari S+, *G Ital Dermatol Venereol* 124(7–8), 335
(1987): Bardazzi F+, *Contact Dermatitis* 16(5), 298
(1987): Smith JM+, *Practitioner* 231, 579
(1987): Tosti A+, *G Ital Dermatol Venereol* 122(10), 543
(1986): Melino M+, *Contact Dermatitis* 14(2), 125
(1986): Novak M+, *Contact Dermatitis* 15(5), 309 (in infants)
(1985): Fisher AA, *Cutis* 36(3), 209
(1985): Whittington CV, *Contact Dermatitis* 13(3), 186 (eye cream)
(1984): Miller JR, *West J Med* 140(5), 791 (contact lens solution)
(1984): Stolman LP+, *N Engl J Med* 311(23), 1521 (contact lens)
(1982): Rietschel RL+, *Arch Dermatol* 118(3), 147 (contact lens)
(1981): Fisher AA, *Cutis* 27(6), 580 (merthiolate)
(1980): Miranda A+, *Actas Dermatosifiliogr* 71(7–8), 301
(1980): Moller H, *Int J Dermatol* 19(1), 29
(1980): Sertoli A+, *Contact Dermatitis* 6(4), 292 (soft contact lens)
(1979): WIlkinson DS, *Contact Dermatitis* 5(1), 58
(1978): Moriearty PL+, *Contact Dermatitis* 4(4), 185
(1978): Novak M+, *Cesk Dermatol* (Czech) 53(5), 313
(1976): Hannuksela M+, *Contact Dermatitis* 2(2), 105
(1975): *Contact Dermatitis* 1(5), 277

Dermatitis (sic)
(1986): Tosti A+, *Contact Dermatitis* 15, 187
(1977): Moeller H, *Acta Derm Venereol* (Stockh) 57(6), 509 (3.7%)

Eczema
(1999): Patrizi A+, *Contact Dermatitis* 40(2), 94
(1998): Romaguera C+, *Contact Dermatitis* 39(6), 277

Lichen planus
(2001): Scalf LA+, *Am J Contact Dermat* 12(3), 146

Lichenoid reaction
(1984): Lindemayr H+, *Hautarzt* 35, 192

Photoallergic reaction
(1993): de la Cuadra J, *Ann Dermatol Venereol* 120(1), 37 (with piroxicam)
(1991): de Castro JL+, *Contact Dermatitis* 24(3), 187 (with piroxicam)
(1989): de la Cuadra J+, *Contact Dermatitis* 21(5), 349 (with piroxicam)

Photodermatitis
(2001): Trujillo MJ+, *Allergol Immunopathol* (Madr) 29(4), 133 (with piroxicam)

Systemic reactions (sic)
(1986): Tosti A+, *Contact Dermatitis* 15(3), 187

Urticaria
(1987): Lohiya G+, *West J Med* 147(3), 341
(1984): Lindemayr H+, *Hautarzt* 35, 192

### Other

Conjunctivitis (allergic contact)
(1998): *Allergy* 53(3):333
(1988): Tosti A+, *Contact Dermatitis* 18(5), 268 (eye drops)
(1980): van Ketel WG+, *Contact Dermatitis* 6(5), 321 (soft contact lens)
(1978): Pedersen NB, *Contact Dermatitis* 4(3), 165 (soft contact lens)

Hypersensitivity (local)
(2001): Ball LK+, *Pediatrics* 107(5):1147
(2001): van't Veen AJ, *Drugs* 61(5), 565
(1994): van't Veen AJ+, *Contact Dermatitis* 31(5), 293
(1991): Aberer W, *Contact Dermatitis* 24(1), 6
(1991): Noel I+, *Lancet* 338(8768), 705 (in hepatitis B vaccine)
(1991): Osawa J+, *Contact Dermatitis* 24(3), 178
(1990): Rietschel RL+, *Dermatol Clin* 8(1), 161
(1989): Tosti A+, *Contact Dermatitis* 20(3), 173
(1980): Forstrom L+, *Contact Dermatitis* 6(4), 241
(1975): Maibach H, *Contact Dermatitis* 1(4), 221

Injection-site pain
(1984): Lindemayr H+, *Hautarzt* 35, 192
(1978): Wienert V+, *Z Haut* 53(13), 459

Injection-site urticaria
(1988): Bork K, *Cutaneous Side Effects Of Drugs* WB Saunders, 114

# THIOGUANINE

**Synonyms:** TG; 6-TG; 6-thioguanine; tioguanine
**Trade name:** Thioguanine (GSK)
**Other common trade name:** *Lanvis*
**Indications:** Leukemias
**Category:** Antineoplastic; antimetabolite
**Half-life:** 11 hours
**Clinically important, potentially hazardous interactions with:** aldesleukin, **vaccines**

## *Reactions*

### Skin

Cutaneous malignancies (sic)
(1997): Zackheim HS+, *J Am Acad Dermatol* 30, 452 (nonmelanoma)

Exanthems
(1988): Zimm S+, *J Clin Oncol* 6, 696

Painful red hands
(1988): Shall L+, *Br J Dermatol* 119, 249

Petechiae

Photosensitivity (<1%)
(1988): Zimm S+, *J Clin Oncol* 6, 696

Pruritus

(1999): Silvis NG+, *Arch Dermatol* 135, 433
Psoriasis
(1999): Silvis NG+, *Arch Dermatol* 135, 433
Purpura
Rash (sic) (1–10%)

### Hair

Hair – alopecia
(1999): Murphy FP+, *Arch Dermatol* 135, 1495
(1988): Zimm S+, *J Clin Oncol* 6, 696

### Other

Oral mucosal lesions
Stomatitis (1–10%)
Xerostomia
(1999): Silvis NG+, *Arch Dermatol* 135, 433

## THIOPENTAL

**Trade name:** Thiopental (Baxter)
**Other common trade names:** *Anesthal; Hypnostan; Intraval; Nesdonal; Sodipental; Trapanal*
**Indications:** Induction of anesthesia
**Category:** Barbiturate anesthetic; anticonvulsant; sedative
**Half-life:** 3–12 hours
**Clinically important, potentially hazardous interactions with:** ethanol, ethanolamine

#### *Reactions*

### Skin

Angioedema
(1975): Brown TP, *Anaesth Intensive Care* 3, 257
(1972): Almeyda J+, *Br J Dermatol* 86, 313
(1971): Fox GS+, *Anesthesiology* 35, 655
(1957): Hayward JR+, *J Oral Surg* 15, 61
Bullous eruption
(1987): Saiag P+, *Ann Dermatol Venereol* (French) 114, 1440
(1977): Evans JM+, *BMJ* 2, 735
Erythema (<1%)
Erythema multiforme
(1947): Hunter AR, *Lancet* 1, 47
(1946): Peterkin GAG, *BMJ* 2, 52
Exanthems
(1987): Boittiaux P+, *Ann Fr Anesth Reanim* (French) 6, 324 (3.3%)
(1971): Fox GS+, *Anesthesiology* 35, 655
(1946): Peterkin GAG, *BMJ* 2, 52
Exfoliative dermatitis
Fixed eruption
(1995): Bremang JA+, *Can J Anaesth* 42, 628
(1990): Desmeules H, *Anesth Analg* 70, 216 (non-pigmenting)
(1987): Saiag P+, *Ann Dermatol Venereol* (French) 114, 1440
Hypopigmentation
(1979): Coote N+, *Anaesthesia* 34, 336
Pruritus (<1%)
Purpura
(1972): Almeyda J+, *Br J Dermatol* 86, 313
(1946): Peterkin GAG, *BMJ* 2, 52
Rash (sic)
Shivering
(1987): Boittiaux P+, *Ann Fr Anesth Reanim* (French) 6, 324 (27%)
Stevens–Johnson syndrome
(1946): Peterkin GAG, *BMJ* 2, 52
Toxic epidermal necrolysis
(1987): Saiag P+, *Ann Dermatol Venereol* (French) 114, 1440
Urticaria
(1972): Almeyda J+, *Br J Dermatol* 86, 313
(1972): Barjenbruch KP+, *Anesth Analg* 51, 113
(1957): Hayward JR+, *J Oral Surg* 15, 61
(1946): Peterkin GAG, *BMJ* 2, 52

### Other

Anaphylactoid reactions (<1%)
(2001): Garvey LH+, *Acta Anaesthesiol Scand* 45(10), 1204
(1993): Seymour DG, *JAMA* 270, 2503 (letter)
(1992): Breathnach SM+, *Adverse Drug Reactions and the Skin* Blackwell, Oxford, 193 (passim)
(1988): Cheema AL+, *J Allergy Clin Immunol* 81, 220
(1975): Brown TP, *Anaesth Intensive Care* 3, 257
(1973): Kelly AJ+, *Anaesth Intensive Care* 1, 332
(1972): Barjenbruch KP+, *Anesth Analg* 51, 113
(1971): Davis J, *Br J Anaesth* 43, 1191
(1971): Sargent NW, *Br J Anaesth* 43, 591
Injection-site necrosis
Injection-site pain (>10%)
Injection-site phlebitis
(1981): Clark RSJ, *Drugs* 22,26 (6%)
Porphyria
(1993): Harrison GG+, *Anaesthesia* 48, 1008–1010
(1976): Panica D+, *Folia Med Plovdiv* 18, 161
(1975): Mees DE+, *South Med J* 68, 29
(1966): Eales L, *Anesthesiology* 27, 703
Rhabdomyolysis
(1990): Larpin R+, *Presse Med* 19(30), 1403
Thrombophlebitis (<1%)
Twitching (<1%)

## THIORIDAZINE

**Trade name:** Mellaril (Novartis)
**Other common trade names:** *Aldazine; Apo-Thioridazine; Calmaril; Dazine; Melleril; Ridazin; Thinin; Thioril*
**Indications:** Psychotic disorders
**Category:** Phenothiazine antipsychotic
**Half-life:** 21–25 hours
**Clinically important, potentially hazardous interactions with:** antihistamines, arsenic, chlorpheniramine, dofetilide, epinephrine, piperazine, quinolones, sparfloxacin

#### *Reactions*

### Skin

Acanthosis nigricans
(1979): Arnold HL+, *J Am Acad Dermatol* 1, 93
Angioedema (<1%)
(1964): Welsh AL, *Med Clin North Am* 48, 459
Dermatitis (sic)
(1968): Wolpert A+, *Clin Pharmacol Ther* 9, 456
Erythema multiforme
(1985): Rees TD, *J Periodontol* 56, 480
Exanthems
(1974): Rothstein E, *N Engl J Med* 290, 521
Exfoliative dermatitis
Hypohidrosis (>10%)
Lupus erythematosus
(1971): Fabius AJM+, *Acta Rheumatol Scand* 17, 137
Peripheral edema
Photoreactions
(1987): Röhrborn W+, *Contact Dermatitis* 17, 241
(1976): Suhonen R, *Contact Dermatitis* 2, 179

Photosensitivity (1–10%)
Phototoxicity
(1967): Satanove A+, *JAMA* 200, 209
(1960): Barsa JA+, *Am J Psychiatry* 116, 1028
Pigmentation (<1%) (blue-gray)
(1970): Ayd FJ, *Int Drug Ther Newsletter* 5, 24
(1969): Berger H, *Arch Dermatol* 100, 487
Purpura
Rash (sic) (1–10%)
(1981): Georgotas A+, *Psychopharmacology* 73, 292
(1969): Doyle JA+, *Curr Ther Res* 11, 429
(1960): May RH+, *J Nerv Mental Dis* 130, 230
Seborrhea
Toxic epidermal necrolysis
(1987): Harnar TJ+, *J Burn Care Rehabil* 8, 554
Urticaria
Xerosis

### Hair

Hair – alopecia
Hair – hypertrichosis
(1979): Phillips P+, *JAMA* 241, 920

### Other

Anaphylactoid reactions
Death
(2001): Glassman AH+, *Am J Psychiatry* 158(11), 1774
(2000): Timell AM, *Ann Clin Psychiatry* 12(3), 147 (4 cases)
Galactorrhea (<1%)
Gynecomastia
Hypersensitivity
Lymphoproliferative disease
(1992): Aguilar JL+, *Arch Dermatol* 128, 121
Mastodynia (1–10%)
Oral mucosal eruption
(1985): Rees TD, *J Periodontol* 56, 480
Paresthesias
Parkinsonism (>10%)
Parotitis
(1974): Rothstein E, *N Engl J Med* 290, 521
Porphyria
(1985): Kamal S+, *Union Med Can* (French) 114, 330
Priapism (<1%)
(2001): Compton MT+, *Clin Psychiatry* 62(5), 363 (passim)
Pseudolymphoma
(1988): Kardaun SH+, *Br J Dermatol* 118, 545
Tremors
Xerostomia
(1981): Georgotas A+, *Psychopharmacology* 73, 292

## THIOTEPA

**Synonym:** TSPA
**Trade name:** Thioplex (Immunex)
**Indications:** Breast, ovarian and bladder carcinomas
**Category:** Antineoplastic
**Half-life:** 109 minutes
**Clinically important, potentially hazardous interactions with:** aldesleukin

#### *Reactions*

### Skin

Allergic reactions (sic) (1–10%)
Angioedema
(1992): Breathnach SM+, *Adverse Drug Reactions and the Skin* Blackwell, Oxford, 292 (passim)
(1987): Lee M+, *J Urol* 138, 143
(1985): Levine N+, *Cancer Treat Rev* 5, 67
(1981): Weiss RB+, *Ann Intern Med* 94, 66
(1969): Veenema RJ+, *J Urol* 101, 711
Bruising
Ecchymoses
Eccrine squamous syringometaplasia
(1997): Valks R+, *Arch Dermatol* 133, 873
Leucoderma
(1979): Harben DJ+, *Arch Dermatol* 115, 973 (passim)
(1976): Rosai J+, *Hum Pathol* 7, 83
(1969): Berkow JW+, *Arch Ophthalmol* 82, 415 (periorbital)
(1966): Reed RJ+, *Arch Dermatol* 94, 396
Pigmentation (1–10%)
(1992): Breathnach SM+, *Adverse Drug Reactions and the Skin* Blackwell, Oxford, 292 (passim)
(1989): Horn TD+, *Arch Dermatol* 125, 524
(1974): Hornblass A+, *Ann Ophthalmol* 6, 1155
(1969): Howitt D+, *Am J Ophthalmol* 68, 473
Pruritus (1–10%)
(1992): Breathnach SM+, *Adverse Drug Reactions and the Skin* Blackwell, Oxford, 292 (passim)
(1987): Lee M+, *J Urol* 138, 143
(1985): Levine N+, *Cancer Treat Rev* 5, 67
(1981): Weiss RB+, *Ann Intern Med* 94, 66
(1969): Veenema RJ+, *J Urol* 101, 711
Rash (sic) (1–10%)
Urticaria
(1992): Breathnach SM+, *Adverse Drug Reactions and the Skin* Blackwell, Oxford, 292 (passim)
(1987): Lee M+, *J Urol* 138, 143
(1985): Levine N+, *Cancer Treat Rev* 5, 67
(1981): Weiss RB+, *Ann Intern Med* 94, 66
(1977): Greenspan E+, *JAMA* 237, 2288 (3.8%)
(1969): Veenema RJ+, *J Urol* 101, 711

### Hair

Hair – alopecia (1–10%)
(1966): Clavert W, *BMJ* 2, 831

### Other

Anaphylactoid reactions (<1%)
Injection-site pain (>10%)
Stomatitis (<1%)

## THIOTHIXENE

**Synonym:** tiotixene
**Trade name:** Navane (Pfizer)
**Other common trade name:** *Orbinamon*
**Indications:** Psychotic disorders
**Category:** Antipsychotic
**Half-life:** >24 hours

#### *Reactions*

### Skin

Diaphoresis
(1968): Wolpert A+, *Clin Pharmacol Ther* 9, 456 (14%)
Exanthems
(1994): Shelley WB+, *Cutis* 54, 71 (observation)
(1968): Wolpert A+, *Clin Pharmacol Ther* 9, 456 (14%)
Hypohidrosis (>10%)
Palmar erythema
(1982): Matsuoka LY, *J Am Acad Dermatol* 7, 405

Peripheral edema
Photosensitivity (1–10%)
(1970): *Med Lett* 12, 104
(1966): Gallant DM+, *Am J Psychiatry* 123, 345
Pigmentation (blue-gray) (<1%)
Pruritus
Rash (sic) (1–10%)
Raynaud's phenomenon
(1991): McCance-Katz EF, *J Clin Psychiatry* 52, 89
Seborrheic dermatitis
(1984): Binder RL+, *J Clin Psychiatry* 45, 125
(1983): Binder RL+, *Arch Dermatol* 119, 473
Sensitivity (sic)
(1982): Matsuoka LY, *J Am Acad Dermatol* 7, 405
Telangiectases
(1982): Matsuoka LY, *J Am Acad Dermatol* 7, 405
Urticaria

### Hair
Hair – alopecia

### Other
Anaphylactoid reactions
Black tongue
(2000): Heymann WR, *Cutis* 66, 25
Dysgeusia
(2000): Heymann WR, *Cutis* 66, 25
Galactorrhea (<1%)
Gynecomastia
Mastodynia (1–10%)
Paresthesias
Parkinsonism (>10%)
Priapism (<1%)
Sialorrhea
Xerostomia
(2000): Heymann WR, *Cutis* 66, 25
(1987): Sarai K+, *Pharmacopsychiatry* 20, 38

## TIAGABINE

**Trade name:** Gabitril (Abbott)
**Indications:** Partial seizures
**Category:** Anticonvulsant
**Half-life:** 7–9 hours

#### *Reactions*

### Skin
Acne (>1%)
Allergic reactions (sic) (<1%)
Carcinoma (sic) (<1%)
Contact dermatitis (<1%)
Diaphoresis (<1%)
Ecchymoses (>1%)
Eczema (sic) (<1%)
Edema (<1%)
Exanthems (<1%)
Exfoliative dermatitis (<1%)
Facial edema (<1%)
Furunculosis (<1%)
Herpes simplex (<1%)
Herpes zoster (<1%)
Neoplasms (benign) (<1%)
Nodules (sic) (<1%)
Peripheral edema (<1%)
Petechiae (<1%)
Photosensitivity (<1%)
Pigmentation (<1%)
Pruritus (2%)
Psoriasis (<1%)
Rash (sic) (5%)
Stevens–Johnson syndrome
Ulcerations (<1%)
Urticaria (<1%)
Vesiculobullous eruption (<1%)
Xerosis (<1%)

### Hair
Hair – alopecia (<1%)
Hair – hirsutism (<1%)

### Other
Ageusia (<1%)
Depression
(2001): Kalvianen R, *Epilepsia* 42(Suppl 3), 46
Dysgeusia (<1%)
Foetor ex ore (halitosis) (<1%)
Gingival hyperplasia (<1%)
Gingivitis (<1%)
Glossitis (<1%)
Gynecomastia (<1%)
Mastodynia (<1%)
Myalgia (>1%)
Oral ulceration (2%)
Paresthesias (4%)
Parosmia (<1%)
Sialorrhea (<1%)
Stomatitis (<1%)
Thrombophlebitis (<1%)
Tremors (>1%)
(2001): Kalvianen R, *Epilepsia* 42(Suppl 3), 43
(2000): Fakhoury T+, *Seizure* 9, 431 (31%)
Ulcerative stomatitis (<1%)
Vaginitis (<1%)
Xerostomia (>1%)

## TICARCILLIN

**Trade name:** Ticar (GSK)
**Indications:** Various infections caused by susceptible organisms
**Category:** Penicillinase-sensitive penicillin antibiotic
**Half-life:** 1.0–1.2 hours
**Clinically important, potentially hazardous interactions with:** anticoagulants, cyclosporine, demeclocycline, doxycycline, methotrexate, minocycline, oxytetracycline, tetracyclines

#### *Reactions*

### Skin
Allergic reactions (sic)
(1994): Pleasants RA+, *Chest* 106, 1124 (in patients with cystic fibrosis)
Angioedema
Bullous eruption
Ecchymoses
Erythema multiforme
Erythema nodosum
Exanthems

(1980): Brogden RN+, *Drugs* 20, 325 (1%)
Exfoliative dermatitis
Hematomas
Jarisch–Herxheimer reaction (<1%)
Pruritus
Purpura
Rash (sic) (<1%)
Stevens–Johnson syndrome
Toxic epidermal necrolysis
Urticaria
Vasculitis

### Other

Anaphylactoid reactions (<1%)
Black tongue
Dysgeusia
Glossitis
Glossodynia
Hypersensitivity (<1%)
Injection-site pain
(1980): Brogden RN+, *Drugs* 20, 325
Injection-site phlebitis
(1980): Brogden RN+, *Drugs* 20, 325
Oral candidiasis
Serum sickness
Stomatitis
Stomatodynia
Thrombophlebitis (<1%)
Vaginitis
Xerostomia

## TICLOPIDINE

**Trade name:** Ticlid (Roche)
**Other common trade names:** *Anagregal; Panaldine; Ticlidil; Ticlodix; Ticlodone; Tiklid; Tiklyd*
**Indications:** To reduce risk of thrombotic stroke
**Category:** Antithrombotic; platelet aggregation inhibitor
**Half-life:** 24 hours
**Clinically important, potentially hazardous interactions with:** alteplase, fondaparinux

### *Reactions*

### Skin

Acute generalized exanthematous pustulosis (AGEP)
(2000): Cannavò SP+, *Br J Dermatol* 142, 577
Angioedema (<1%)
(1999): Chassany O+, *Presse Med* (French) 28, 18
Cutaneous bleeding (sic)
(1990): McTavish D+, *Drugs* 40, 238 (1–5%)
(1984): Stiegler H+, *Dtsch Med Wochenschr* (German) 109, 1240 (4.4%)
Cutaneous side effects (sic)
(1984): Stiegler H+, *Dtsch Med Wochenschr* (German) 109, 1240 (8%)
Dermatitis (sic)
(1998): Ceylan C+, *Am J Hematol* 59, 260
Diaphoresis
(1984): Stiegler H+, *Dtsch Med Wochenschr* (German) 109, 1240 (1.7%)
Ecchymoses (<1%)
Erythema
(1990): McTavish D+, *Drugs* 40, 238
Erythema multiforme (<1%)
(1999): Yosipovitch G+, *J Am Acad Dermatol* 41, 473
Erythema nodosum (<1%)
Erythromelalgia
(1999): Yosipovitch G+, *J Am Acad Dermatol* 41, 473
Exanthems (1–11.9%)
(2000): Prost C+, *Presse Med* (French) 29, 303
(1999): Yosipovitch G+, *J Am Acad Dermatol* 41, 473
(1997): Litt JZ, Beachwood, OH (personal case) (observation)
(1990): McTavish D+, *Drugs* 40, 238 (7%)
(1989): Hass WK+, *N Engl J Med* 321, 501 (11.9%)
(1987): Saltiel E+, *Drugs* 34, 222 (1–5%)
Exfoliative dermatitis (<1%)
Facial erythema
(1999): Yosipovitch G+, *J Am Acad Dermatol* 41, 473
Fixed eruption
(2001): Garcia CM+, *Contact Dermatitis* 44, 40
(1999): Yosipovitch G+, *J Am Acad Dermatol* 41, 473
Hematomas
(1984): Stiegler H+, *Dtsch Med Wochenschr* (German) 109, 1240 (2.7%)
Lupus erythematosus (positive ANA) (<1%)
Petechiae
(1984): Stiegler H+, *Dtsch Med Wochenschr* (German) 109, 1240 (1.7%)
Phenytoin toxicity (sic)
(1998): Klaasen SL, *Ann Pharmacother* 32, 1295
Pruritus (1.3%)
(1999): Yosipovitch G+, *J Am Acad Dermatol* 41, 473
(1990): McTavish D+, *Drugs* 40, 238
(1987): Saltiel E+, *Drugs* 34, 222
Purpura (2.2%)
(2000): Chemnitz JM+, *Med Klin* (German) 95, 96
(2000): Tsai HM+, *Ann Intern Med* 132, 794
Rash (sic) (5.1%)
(1999): Quinn MJ+, *Circulation* 100, 1667
(1999): Whetsel TR+, *Pharmacotherapy* 19, 228
Stevens–Johnson syndrome (<1%)
Thrombocytopenic purpura (2.2%)
(2001): Medina PJ+, *Curr Opin Hematol* 8(5), 286
(2001): Naseer N+, *Heart Dis* 3(4), 221
(2001): Yang CW+, *Ren Fail* 23(6), 851 (2 cases)
(2000): Tsai H-M+, *Ann Intern Med* 132, 794
(1999): Bennett CL+, *Ann Intern Med* 159, 2524
(1999): Chen DK+, *Arch Intern Med* 159, 311
(1999): Elangovan L, *Arch Int Med* 159, 1624
(1999): Mauro M+, *Blood* 94, 1–646a
(1999): Steinhubl SR+, *JAMA* 281, 806
(1998): Bennett CL+, *Ann Intern Med* 128, 541
(1998): Bennett CL+, *Lancet* 352, 1036
(1998): Jamar S+, *Acta Cardiol* 53, 285
(1998): Mukamal KJ+, *Ann Intern Med* 129, 837
(1998): Muszkat M+, *Pharmacotherapy* 18, 1352
(1997): Kupfer Y+, *N Engl J Med* 337, 1245
(1996): Wysowski DK+, *JAMA* 276, 952
(1991): Page Y+, *Lancet* 337, 774
(1990): McTavish D+, *Drugs* 40, 238 (1–5%)
(1990): Takishita S+, *N Engl J Med* 323, 1487
(1989): Hass WK+, *N Engl J Med* 321, 501 (4%)
(1984): Stiegler H+, *Dtsch Med Wochenschr* (German) 109, 1240 (1–5%)
(1982): de Fraiture WH+, *Ned Tijdschr Geneeskd* (Dutch) 126, 1051
Toxic erythroderma (sic)
(1999): Hsi DH+, *N Engl J Med* 340, 1212
Urticaria (<1%)
(1999): Yosipovitch G+, *J Am Acad Dermatol* 41, 473
(1990): McTavish D+, *Drugs* 40, 238
(1989): Hass WK+, *N Engl J Med* 321, 501 (2%)

(1987): Saltiel E+, *Drugs* 34, 222 (1–5%)
Vasculitis (<1%)
(2001): Pintor E+, *Rev Esp Cardiol* 54(1), 114

### Other

Serum sickness
Tinnitus

## TIMOLOL

**Trade names:** Blocadren (Merck); CoSopt (Merck); Timolide (Merck); Timoptic (ophthalmic) (Merck)
**Other common trade names:** *Apo-Timol; Aquanil; Dispatim; Nu-Timolol; Tenopt; Tiloptic; Timacor; Timoptol*
**Indications:** Hypertension
**Category:** Beta-adrenergic blocker; antihypertensive
**Half-life:** 2–2.7 hours
**Clinically important, potentially hazardous interactions with:** clonidine, epinephrine, ergot, verapamil

CoSopt is timolol and dorzolamide; Timolide is timolol and hydrochlorothiazide. Dorzolamide and hydrocholorothiazide are sulfonamides and can be absorbed systemically. Sulfonamides can produce severe, possibly fatal, reactions such as toxic epidermal necrolysis and Stevens–Johnson syndrome

### *Reactions*

### Skin

Angioedema
Burning (from ophthalmic)
Contact dermatitis (eyedrops)
(2001): Holdiness MR, *Am J Contact Dermat* 12(4), 217
(2000): Quiralte J+, *Contact Dermatitis* 42, 245
(1995): Koch P, *Contact Dermatitis* 33, 140
(1993): Corazza M+, *Contact Dermatitis* 28, 188
(1993): O'Donnell BF+, *Contact Dermatitis* 28, 121
(1991): Cameli N+, *Contact Dermatitis* 25, 129
(1991): Kubota K+, *Br J Clin Pharmacol* 31, 471
(1988): Kanzaki T+, *Contact Dermatitis* 19, 388
(1986): Fernandez-Vozmediano JM+, *Contact Dermatitis* 14, 252
(1986): Romaguera C+, *Contact Dermatitis* 14, 248
Dermatitis (sic)
(1998): Lewis B, Colorado Springs, CO (from Internet) (observation) (glans penis)
Diaphoresis
Eczematous eruption (sic)
(1991): Cameli N+, *Contact Dermatitis* 25, 129
(1979): van Joost T, *Br J Dermatol* 101, 171
Edema (0.6%)
Erythema multiforme
Erythroderma
(1997): Shelley WB+, *J Am Acad Dermatol* 37, 799
(1993): Shelley WB+, *Cutis* 51, 330 (observation)
Exanthems
Exfoliative dermatitis
Hyperkeratosis (palms and soles)
Lichenoid eruption
(1978): Savage RL+, *BMJ* 1, 987
Lupus erythematosus
(1994): Cohen MG, *J Rheumatol* 21, 578
(1992): Zamber RW+, *J Rheumatol* 19, 977
Ocular allergy
(1998): LeBlanc RP, *Ophthalmology* 105, 1960
(1996): Schuman JS, *Surv Ophthalmol* 41, S27
Ocular burning
(1998): LeBlanc RP, *Ophthalmology* 105, 1960
(1997): Schuman JS+, *Arch Ophthalmol* 115, 847 (41.9%)
(1996): Schuman JS, *Surv Ophthalmol* 41, S27
Ocular stinging
(1998): LeBlanc RP, *Ophthalmology* 105, 1960
(1997): Schuman JS+, *Arch Ophthalmol* 115, 847 (41.9%)
(1996): Schuman JS, *Surv Ophthalmol* 41, S27
Pemphigoid
(1987): Fiore PM+, *Arch Ophthalmol* 105, 1660
Photosensitivity
Pigmentation
Pityriasis rubra pilaris
(1978): Finlay AY+, *BMJ* 1, 987
Pruritus (1–5%)
(1996): Lazarov A+, *Cutis* 58, 363 (from eye drops)
Psoriasis
(1992): Germain ML+, *Therapie* (French) 47, 447
(1989): Puig L+, *Am J Ophthalmol* 108, 455
(1987): Savola J+, *BMJ* 295, 637 (also aggravation of psoriasis)
(1986): Czernielewski J+, *Lancet* 1, 808
(1984): Arntzen N+, *Acta Derm Venereol* (Stockh) 64, 346
Purpura
Rash (sic) (1–10%)
Raynaud's phenomenon
(1984): Eliasson K+, *Acta Med Scand* 215, 333
(1976): Marshall AJ+, *BMJ* 1, 1498
Stinging (from ophthalmic)
Toxic epidermal necrolysis
Urticaria
Xerosis

### Hair

Hair – alopecia (also from Timoptic eye drops) (1–10%)
(1990): Fraunfelder FT+, *JAMA* 263, 1493

### Nails

Nails – dystrophy
Nails – onycholysis
Nails – pigmentation
(1981): Feiler-Ofry V, *Ophthalmologica* (Basel) 182, 153

### Other

Anaphylactoid reactions
Digital necrosis
(1989): Dompmartin A+, *Ann Dermatol Venereol* (French) 115, 593
Dysgeusia
Myalgia
Ocular pemphigoid
(1992): Shelley WB+, *Advanced Dermatologic Diagnosis* WB Saunders, 554 (passim)
Oculo-mucocutaneous syndrome
(1982): Cocco G+, *Curr Ther Res* 31, 362
Oral lichenoid eruption
Paresthesias (<1%)
Peyronie's disease
(1979): Pryor JP+, *Lancet* 1, 331
Tinnitus
Xerostomia
(1998): LeBlanc RP, *Ophthalmology* 105, 1960
(1997): Schuman JS+, *Arch Ophthalmol* 115, 847 (19.4%)
(1996): Schuman JS, *Surv Ophthalmol* 41, S27

**Note:** Cutaneous side effects of beta-receptor blockaders are clinically polymorphous. They apparently appear after several months of continuous therapy. Atypical psoriasiform, lichen planus-like, and eczematous chronic rashes are mainly observed. (1983): Hödl St, *Z Hautkr* (German) 1:58, 17

# TINZAPARIN

**Trade name:** Innohep (DuPont)
**Indications:** Acute symptomatic deep vein thrombosis
**Category:** Low molecular weight heparin; anticoagulant; thrombolytic
**Half-life:** 3-4 hours
**Clinically important, potentially hazardous interactions with:** butabarbital

### *Reactions*

**Skin**

Abscess (<1%)
Allergic reactions (sic)
Angioedema (<1%)
Bullous eruption (1–10%)
Cellulitis (<1%)
Ecchymoses
Epidermal necrosis (sic) (1%)
Exanthems (<1%)
Infections (sic)
Necrosis
Neoplasms (sic)
Pruritus (1–10%)
Purpura (<1%)
(1996): Simpson HK+, *Haemostasis* 26, 90
Rash (sic) (1%)
Urticaria (<1%)

**Other**

Anaphylactoid reactions (In sulfite-sensitive people)
Hypersensitivity
Injection-site hematoma (16%)
Injection-site pain
Phlebitis
Priapism (<1%)
Thrombophlebitis

# TIOPRONIN

**Trade name:** Thiola (Mission)
**Other common trade names:** *Acadione; Captimer*
**Indications:** Cystinuria
**Category:** Antiurolithic
**Half-life:** no data

### *Reactions*

**Skin**

Angioedema
(1988): Sigaud M+, *Rev Rhum Mal Osteoartic* (French) 55, 467 (14.5%)
Bullous pemphigoid
(1988): Nakajima H+, *Nippon Hifuka Gakkai Zasshi* (Japanese) 98, 803
Contact dermatitis
(1995): Romano A+, *Contact Dermatitis* 33, 269
Cutaneous side effects (sic)
(1988): Sigaud M+, *Rev Rhum Mal Osteoartic* (French) 55, 467 (27.5%)
Ecchymoses
Edema
Elastosis perforans serpiginosa
Erythema
(1990): Sany J+, *Rev Rhum Mal Osteoartic* (French) 57, 105
Erythema multiforme
(1988): Nakajima H+, *Nippon Hifuka Gakkai Zasshi* (Japanese) 98, 803
Exanthems
(1988): Sigaud M+, *Rev Rhum Mal Osteoartic* (French) 55, 467 (14.5%)
(1984): Shichiri M+, *Arch Intern Med* 144, 89
Lichenoid eruption
(1994): Pierard E+, *J Am Acad Dermatol* 31, 665
(1990): Kurumaji Y+, *J Dermatol* (Tokio) 17, 176
(1988): Kawabe Y+, *J Dermatol* (Tokio) 15, 434 (bullous)
Lupus erythematosus
(1986): Katayama I+, *J Dermatol* (Tokio) 13, 151
Pemphigus
(1994): Verdier-Sevrain S+, *Br J Dermatol* 130, 238
(1990): Meuhier L+, *Ann Dermatol Venereol* (French) 117, 959
(1990): Sany J+, *Rev Rhum Mal Osteoartic* (French) 57, 105
(1988): Sigaud M+, *Rev Rhum Mal Osteoartic* (French) 55, 467 (5.8%)
(1987): Enjolras O+, *Ann Dermatol Venereol* (French) 114, 25
Pemphigus erythematosus
(1982): Alinovi A+, *Acta Derm Venereol* (Stockh) 62, 452
Pemphigus foliaceus
(1983): Lucky PA+, *J Am Acad Dermatol* 8, 667
Photosensitivity
(1988): Sigaud M+, *Rev Rhum Mal Osteoartic* (French) 55, 467 (1.5%)
Pityriasis rosea
(1990): Sany J+, *Rev Rhum Mal Osteoartic* (French) 57, 105
(1988): Sigaud M+, *Rev Rhum Mal Osteoartic* (French) 55, 467 (5.8%)
Pruritus
Rash (sic)
Toxic epidermal necrolysis
Urticaria
Wrinkling (sic)

**Hair**

Hair – alopecia
(1990): Sany J+, *Rev Rhum Mal Osteoartic* (French) 57, 105
Hair – hypertrichosis
(1993): Arnaud M+, *Joint Bone Spine Dis* 60, 548

**Other**

Ageusia
(1989): Mordini M+, *Minerva Med* 80(9), 1019
Hypogeusia
Mucocutaneous side effects (sic)
(1990): Sany J+, *Rev Rhum Mal Osteoartic* (French) 57, 105 (32.8%)
Myopathy
(1988): Menkes CJ+, *Presse Med* (French) 17, 1156
Oral mucosal lesions
(1988): Sigaud M+, *Rev Rhum Mal Osteoartic* (French) 55, 467 (4.4%)
(1984): Shichiri M+, *Arch Intern Med* 144, 89
Oral ulceration
(2000): Madinier I+, *Ann Med Interne (Paris)* (French) 151, 248
Parageusia
Parosmia
Polymyositis
(1999): Cacoub B+, *Presse Med* (French) 28, 911
Stomatitis
(1990): Sany J+, *Rev Rhum Mal Osteoartic* (French) 57, 105
(1988): Sigaud M+, *Rev Rhum Mal Osteoartic* (French) 55, 467
Xerostomia

# TIROFIBAN

**Trade name:** Aggrastat (Merck)
**Indications:** Acute coronary syndrome
**Category:** Antiplatelet
**Half-life:** 2 hours
**Clinically important, potentially hazardous interactions with:** aspirin, fondaparinux, heparin, NSAIDs

### *Reactions*

**Skin**
Bleeding (sic)
Diaphoresis (2%)
Edema (2%)
Rash (sic) (<1%)
Urticaria (<1%)

**Other**
Leg pain (3%)

# TIZANIDINE

**Trade name:** Zanaflex (Athena)
**Other common trade names:** *Sirdalud; Ternalax; Ternelin*
**Indications:** Muscle spasticity, multiple sclerosis
**Category:** Alpha$_2$-adrenergic agonist
**Half-life:** 2.5 hours

### *Reactions*

**Skin**
Acne (<1%)
Allergic reactions (sic) (<1%)
Candidiasis (<1%)
Cellulitis (<1%)
Diaphoresis (>1%)
Ecchymoses (<1%)
Edema (<1%)
Exanthems (<1%)
Exfoliative dermatitis (<1%)
Herpes simplex (<1%)
Herpes zoster (<1%)
Petechiae (<1%)
Pruritus (1–10%)
Purpura (<1%)
Rash (sic) (1–10%)
Ulceration (>1%)
Urticaria (<1%)
Xerosis (<1%)

**Hair**
Hair – alopecia (<1%)

**Other**
Paresthesias (>1%)
Tremors (1–10%)
Vaginal candidiasis (<1%)
Xerostomia (49%)

# TOBRAMYCIN

**Trade names:** Nebcin (Lilly); TOBI (Pathogenesis); TobraDex (Alcon)
**Other common trade names:** *AKTob Ophthalmic; Oftalmotrisol-T; Tobra*
**Indications:** Various serious infections caused by susceptible organisms, superficial ocular infections
**Category:** Aminoglycoside antibiotic
**Half-life:** 2–3 hours
**Clinically important, potentially hazardous interactions with:** aldesleukin, aminoglycosides, atracurium, bumetanide, doxacurium, ethacrynic acid, furosemide, neuromuscular blockers, pancuronium, polypeptide antibiotics, rocuronium, succinylcholine, torsemide, vecuronium

TobraDex is tobramycin and dexamethasone

### *Reactions*

**Skin**
Contact dermatitis (from ophthalmic preparations) (<1%)
(1998): Litt JZ, Beachwood, OH (personal case) (observation)
(1995): Caraffini S+, *Contact Dermatitis* 32, 186
(1990): Menendez-Ramos F+, *Contact Dermatitis* 22, 305
Contact dermatitis (eyelids)
(2002): Litt JZ, Beachwood, OH (personal observation) (eyedrops)
Contact dermatitis
(2002): Litt JZ, Beachwood, OH (personal observation) (eyedrops)
Cutaneous side effects (sic)
(1976): Brogden RN+, *Drugs* 12, 166 (<1%)
Eczematous eruption (sic)
Erythema multiforme
(1983): Ansel J+, *Arch Dermatol* 119, 1006
Exanthems
(2002): Spigarelli MG+, *Pediatr Pulmonol* 33(4), 311
(1991): Karp S+, *Cutis* 47, 331
(1976): Brogden RN+, *Drugs* 12, 166
Exfoliative dermatitis
(1991): Karp S+, *Cutis* 47, 331
Eyelid edema (from ophthalmic preparations) (<1%)
Pruritus (<1%)
(1976): Brogden RN+, *Drugs* 12, 166
Purpura
Radiation recall
(2001): Krishnan RS+, *J Am Acad Dermatol* 44, 1045 (ultraviolet) (with piperacillin & ciprofloxacin)
Rash (sic) (<1%)
(2002): Spigarelli MG+, *Pediatr Pulmonol* 33(4), 311
Urticaria

**Other**
Hypersensitivity
(2002): Spigarelli MG+, *Pediatr Pulmonol* 33(4), 311
(1995): Schretlen-Doherty JS+, *Ann Pharmacother* 29, 704
Injection-site pain
Paresthesias (<1%)
Sialorrhea
Tinnitus
Tremors (<1%)

## TOCAINIDE

**Trade name:** Tonocard (AstraZeneca)
**Indications:** Ventricular arrhythmias
**Category:** Antiarrhythmic class I B
**Half-life:** 11–14 hours

### *Reactions*

#### Skin

Allergic reactions (sic)
(1987): Arrowsmith JB+, *Ann Intern Med* 107, 693
(1985): Coulter DM+, *N Z Med J* 98, 553
Clammy skin
Diaphoresis (<1%)
Erythema multiforme (<1%)
Exanthems
(1988): Dunn JM+, *Drug Intell Clin Pharm* 22, 142
Exfoliative dermatitis (<1%)
Lupus erythematosus (<1%)
(1994): Gelfand MS+, *South Med J* 87, 839
(1988): Oliphant LD+, *Chest* 94, 427
Pallor (<1%)
Pruritus (<1%)
Rash (sic) (0.5–8.4%)
Stevens–Johnson syndrome (<1%)
Vasculitis (<1%)

#### Hair

Hair – alopecia (<1%)

#### Other

Dysgeusia (8.4%)
Gingival bleeding
(1988): Dunn JM+, *Drug Intell Clin Pharm* 22, 142
Hypersensitivity (<1%)
Myalgia (<1%)
Paresthesias (3.5–9%)
Parosmia (<1%)
Stomatitis (<1%)
Tinnitus
Xerostomia (<1%)

## TOLAZAMIDE

**Trade name:** Tolinase (Pharmacia & Upjohn)
**Other common trade names:** *Diabewas; Diadutos; Norglycin; Tolanase; Tolisan*
**Indications:** Non-insulin dependent diabetes type II
**Category:** First generation sulfonylurea* hypoglycemic
**Half-life:** 7 hours
**Clinically important, potentially hazardous interactions with:** phenylbutazones

### *Reactions*

#### Skin

Dermatitis (sic)
(1966): Beidleman P+, *J Fla Med Assoc* 53, 191
Diaphoresis
Eczematous eruption (sic)
(1985): Frosch PJ+, *Contact Dermatitis* 13, 272
Erythema (0.4%)
Exanthems (0.4%)
Lichenoid eruption
(1990): Franz CB+, *J Am Acad Dermatol* 22, 128
(1984): Barnett JH+, *Cutis* 34, 542
Lupus erythematosus
Photosensitivity (1–10%)
Pruritus (0.4%)
Purpura
Rash (sic) (1–10%)
Urticaria (1–10%)

#### Other

Acute intermittent porphyria
Dysgeusia
Paresthesias
Porphyria cutanea tarda
Tongue ulceration
(1984): Barnett JH+, *Cutis* 34, 542

***Note:** Tolazamide is a sulfonamide and can be absorbed systemically. Sulfonamides can produce severe, possibly fatal, reactions such as toxic epidermal necrolysis and Stevens–Johnson syndrome

## TOLAZOLINE

**Trade name:** Priscoline (Novartis)
**Indications:** Pulmonary hypertension in the newborn
**Category:** Alpha-adrenergic blocking agent; peripheral vasodilator; antihypertensive (of the newborn)
**Half-life:** 3–10 hours (neonates)

### *Reactions*

#### Skin

Contact dermatitis
(1985): Frosch PJ+, *Contact Dermatitis* 13, 272
Edema
Exanthems
(1989): Cambazard F+, *Ann Dermatol Venereol* (French) 116, 499
Flushing
(1972): Coffman JD+, *Ann Intern Med* 76, 35 (66%)
Rash (sic)
Urticaria

#### Other

Injection-site burning (>10%)

## TOLBUTAMIDE

**Trade name:** Orinase (Pharmacia & Upjohn)
**Other common trade names:** *Abemin; Aglycid; Diaben; Diatol; Dolipol; Mobenol; Novo-Butamid; Orabet; Rastinon*
**Indications:** Non-insulin dependent diabetes type II
**Category:** First generation sulfonylurea* hypoglycemic
**Half-life:** 4–25 hours
**Clinically important, potentially hazardous interactions with:** phenylbutazones

### *Reactions*

#### Skin

Allergic reactions (sic)
(1965): Bernhard H, *Diabetes* 14, 59 (0.8%)
Bullous eruption (<1%)

Bullous pemphigoid
(1975): Glander HJ+, *Derm Monatsschr* (German) 161, 455
Contact dermatitis
(1982): Fisher AA, *Cutis* 29, 551 (systemic)
Cutaneous side effects (sic)
(1967): McKiddie MT+, *Scott Med J* 12, 6 (1.65%)
(1965): Ferguson BD, *Med Clin North Am* 49, 929 (0.35%)
(1959): O'Donovan CJ, *Curr Ther Res* 1, 69 (1.1%)
Erythema (1.1%)
Erythema multiforme (<1%)
Exanthems (1–5%)
(1972): Kuokkanen K, *Acta Allergol* 27, 407
(1971): Harris EL, *BMJ* 3, 29 (1–5%)
(1969): *Postgrad Med* 45, 211
Fixed eruption (<1%)
Flushing
(1981): Capretti L+, *BMJ* 283, 1361
(1966): Cohen P+, *JAMA* 197, 817
(1966): Muller SA, *Proc Staff Meet Mayo Clin* 41, 689
Lichenoid eruption
(1963): Hurlbut WB, *Arch Dermatol* 88, 105
Photoreactions
Photosensitivity (1–10%)
(1984): Kar PK+, *J Indian Med Assoc* 82, 289
(1978): Meneghini CL+, *Z Haut* (German) 53, 329
Poikiloderma
(1965): Esteves J+, *Hautarzt* (German) 16, 281
Pruritus (1.1%)
Purpura
(1965): Horowitz HI+, *Semin Hematol* 2, 287
(1959): Bradley RF, *Ann N Y Acad Sci* 82, 513
Rash (sic) (1–10%)
Toxic epidermal necrolysis (<1%)
Urticaria (1–10%)
(1960): Boshell BR, *N Engl J Med* 262, 80

### Other

Acute intermittent porphyria
Disulfiram-type reaction
Dysgeusia
Hypersensitivity (<1%)
Injection-site thrombophlebitis (<1%)
Oral lichenoid eruption
Paresthesias
Porphyria
(1968): De Matteis F, *Semin Hematol* 5, 409
Porphyria cutanea tarda
(1960): Rook A+, *BMJ* 1, 860
Thrombophlebitis (<1%)

***Note:** Tolbutamide is a sulfonamide and can be absorbed systemically. Sulfonamides can produce severe, possibly fatal, reactions such as toxic epidermal necrolysis and Stevens–Johnson syndrome

## TOLCAPONE

**Trade name:** Tasmar (Roche)
**Indications:** Parkinsonism
**Category:** Antiparkinsonian adjunct
**Half-life:** 2–3 hours

#### *Reactions*

### Skin

Allergic reactions (sic) (<1%)
Burning (sic) (2%)
Cellulitis (<1%)
Diaphoresis (7%)
Eczema (sic) (<1%)
Edema (<1%)
Erythema multiforme (<1%)
Facial edema (<1%)
Fungal infection (sic) (<1%)
Furunculosis (<1%)
Herpes simplex (<1%)
Herpes zoster (<1%)
Pigmentation (<1%)
Pruritus (<1%)
Rash (sic) (<1%)
Seborrhea (<1%)
Urticaria (<1%)
Vitiligo
(1999): Sabate M+, *Ann Pharmacother* 33, 1228 (with levodopa)

### Hair

Hair – alopecia (1%)

### Other

Hypesthesia (<1%)
Myalgia (<1%)
Oral ulceration (<1%)
Paresthesias (3%)
Parosmia (<1%)
Sialorrhea (<1%)
Tongue disorder (<1%)
Tooth disorder (<1%)
Tumors (sic) (1%)
Twitching (<1%)
Vaginitis (<1%)
Xerostomia (5%)

## TOLMETIN

**Trade name:** Tolectin (Ortho-McNeil)
**Other common trade names:** *Donison; Midocil; Novo-Tolmetin; Reutol; Safitex*
**Indications:** Arthritis
**Category:** Nonsteroidal anti-inflammatory (NSAID); analgesic
**Half-life:** 1–2 hours
**Clinically important, potentially hazardous interactions with:** methotrexate

#### *Reactions*

### Skin

Angioedema (<1%)
(1994): Shapiro N, *J Oral Maxillofac Surg* 52, 626
(1985): Ponte CD+, *Drug Intell Clin Pharm* 19, 479
Bullous eruption
Diaphoresis
Edema (3–9%)
Erythema multiforme (<1%)
Exanthems
(1985): Bigby M+, *J Am Acad Dermatol* 12, 866
(1984): Stern RS+, *JAMA* 252, 1433
(1981): Reimer GW, *S Afr Med J* 60, 843
(1977): Aylward M+, *Curr Res Med Opin* 4, 695 (9%)
Hot flashes (<1%)
Photodermatitis

(1993): Shelley WB+, *Cutis* 52, 201 (observation)
Pruritus (1–10%)
(1985): Bigby M+, *J Am Acad Dermatol* 12, 866
(1981): Reimer GW, *S Afr Med J* 60, 843
(1978): Restivo C+, *JAMA* 240, 246
Purpura
(1984): Stern RS+, *JAMA* 252, 1433
Rash (sic) (>10%)
Stevens–Johnson syndrome (<1%)
Toxic epidermal necrolysis (<1%)
(1992): Breathnach SM+, *Adverse Drug Reactions and the Skin* Blackwell, Oxford, 191 (passim)
(1985): Bigby M+, *J Am Acad Dermatol* 12, 866
(1984): Stern RS+, *JAMA* 252, 1433
Urticaria (1–5%)
(1985): Bigby M+, *J Am Acad Dermatol* 12, 866
(1985): Ponte CD+, *Drug Intell Clin Pharm* 19, 479
(1984): Stern RS+, *JAMA* 252, 1433
(1980): Ahmad S, *N Engl J Med* 303, 1417
(1978): Restivo C+, *JAMA* 240, 246

### Other

Anaphylactoid reactions
(1985): Bretza JA+, *Western J Med* 143, 55
(1985): O'Brien WM, *J Rheumatol* 12, 13
(1983): Paulus HE, *Arthritis Rheum* 26, 1397
(1982): Rossi AC+, *N Engl J Med* 307, 499
(1980): Ahmad S, *N Engl J Med* 303, 1417
(1980): McCall CY+, *JAMA* 243, 1263
(1978): Restivo C+, *JAMA* 240, 246
Aphthous stomatitis
Dysgeusia
Gingival ulceration
Glossitis (<1%)
Gynecomastia
Myalgia
Oral ulceration
Serum sickness (<1%)
Stomatitis (<1%)
Tinnitus
Xerostomia

## TOLTERODINE

**Trade name:** Detrol (Pharmacia & Upjohn)
**Indications:** Urinary incontinence
**Category:** Muscarinic antagonist for overactive bladder; anticholinergic
**Half-life:** 2–4 hours

***Reactions***

### Skin

Erythema (1.9%)
Flu-like syndrome (sic) (4.4%)
Fungal infection (sic) (1.1%)
Pruritus (1.3%)
Rash (sic) (1.9%)
Upper respiratory infection (sic) (5.9%)
Xerosis (1.7%)

### Other

Paresthesias (1.1%)
Xerostomia (40%)
(2001): Crandall C, *J Womens Health Gend Based Med* 10(8), 735
(2001): Harvey MA+, *Am J Obstet Gynecol* 185(1), 56
(2001): Malone-Lee J+, *J Urol* 165(5), 1452 (37%)
(2001): Olsson B+, *Clin Pharmacokinet* 40(3), 227
(2001): Van Kerrebroeck+, *Urology* 57(3), 414
(1999): Drutz HP+, *Int Urogynecol J Pelvic Floor Dysfunct* 10, 283
(1999): Millard R+, *J Urol* 161, 1551
(1999): Ruscin JM+, *Ann Pharmacother* 33, 1073
(1997): Appell RA, *Urology* 50, 90
(1997): Jonas U+, *World J Urol* 15, 144 (9%)

## TOPIRAMATE

**Trade name:** Topamax (Ortho-McNeil)
**Indications:** Partial onset seizures
**Category:** Anticonvulsant
**Half-life:** 21 hours

***Reactions***

### Skin

Acne (>1%)
Basal cell carcinoma (<1%)
Dermatitis (sic) (<1%)
Diaphoresis (1.8%)
Eczema (sic) (<1%)
Edema (1.8%)
Exanthems (<1%)
Facial edema (<1%)
Flu-like syndrome (sic) (1–10%)
Flushing (<1%)
Folliculitis (<1%)
Hot flashes (1–10%)
Hypohidrosis (<1%)
(2001): Arcas J+, *Epilepsia* 42(10), 1363
Photosensitivity (<1%)
Pigmentation (<1%)
Pruritus (1.8%)
Purpura (<1%)
Rash (sic) (4.4%)
Seborrhea (<1%)
Urticaria (<1%)
Xerosis (<1%)

### Hair

Hair – abnormal texture (<1%)
Hair – alopecia (>1%)

### Nails

Nails – disorder (sic) (<1%)

### Other

Ageusia (<1%)
Bromhidrosis (1.8%)
Depression
(2001): Klufas A+, *Am J Psychiatry* 158(10), 1736
Dysgeusia (>1%)
(2001): Storey JR+, *Headache* 41(10), 968
Foetor ex ore (halitosis)
Gingival hyperplasia (<1%)
Gingivitis (1.8%)
Gynecomastia (8.3%)
Hyperesthesia (<1%)
Hypesthesia (2.7%)
Mastodynia (3–9%)
Myalgia (1.8%)
Paresthesias (15%)

(2002): Appolinario JC+, *Can J Psychiatry* 47(3), 271
(2002): Silberstein SD, *Headache* 42(1), 85
(2001): Chengappa KN+, *Bipolar Disord* 3(5), 215
(2001): Ghaemi SN+, *Ann Clin Psychiatry* 13(4), 185
(2001): Storey JR+, *Headache* 41(10), 968
(1999): Glauser TA, *Epilepsia* 40, S71
Parosmia (<1%)
Sialorrhea
(2001): Buck ML, *Pediatr Pharmacol* 7 (4–5%)
Stomatitis (<1%)
Tongue edema (<1%)
Tremors (>10%)
Vaginitis
Xerostomia (2.7%)

## TOPOTECAN

**Synonyms:** hycamptamine; SKF 104864; TOPO; TPT
**Trade name:** Hycamtin (GSK)
**Indications:** Metastatic ovarian carcinoma
**Category:** Antineoplastic antibiotic
**Half-life:** 3 hours

### *Reactions*

#### Skin
Erythema (<1%)
Neutrophilic eccrine hidradenitis
(2002): Marini M+, *J Dermatolog Treat* 13(1), 35
Purpura (<1%)
Scleroderma
(2002): Ene-Stroescu D+, *Arthritis Rheum* 46(3), 844

#### Hair
Hair – alopecia (59%)
(2001): Clarke-Pearson DL+, *J Clin Oncol* 19(19), 3967
(2001): Gore M+, *Br J Cancer* 84(8), 1043
(2001): Mobus V+, *Anticancer Res* 21(5), 3551
(1999): Ormrod D+, *Drugs* 58, 533

#### Other
Death
(2001): Seiter K+, *Leuk Lymphoma* 42(5), 963
Mucositis
(2001): Seiter K+, *Leuk Lymphoma* 42(5), 963
Paresthesias (9%)
Stomatitis (24%)

## TOREMIFENE

**Trade name:** Fareston (Schering)
**Indications:** Metastatic breast cancer
**Category:** Antineoplastic; antiestrogen
**Half-life:** ~5 days

### *Reactions*

#### Skin
Dermatitis (sic)
Diaphoresis (20%)
(1997): Wiseman LR+, *Drugs* 54, 141
(1990): Valavaara R+, *J Steroid Biochem* 36, 229
Edema (5%)
(1997): Wiseman LR+, *Drugs* 54, 141
Hot flashes (35%)
(1997): Wiseman LR+, *Drugs* 54, 141
Pigmentation
Pruritus

#### Other
Galactorrhea (1–10%)
Priapism (1–10%)
Thrombophlebitis (1%)
Vaginal discharge (13%)
(1997): Wiseman LR+, *Drugs* 54, 141

## TORSEMIDE

**Trade name:** Demadex (Roche)
**Other common trade name:** *Unat*
**Indications:** Edema
**Category:** A sulfonylurea* loop diuretic; antihypertensive
**Half-life:** 2–4 hours
**Clinically important, potentially hazardous interactions with:** amikacin, aminoglycosides, gentamicin, kanamycin, neomycin, streptomycin, tobramycin

### *Reactions*

#### Skin
Angioedema
Edema (1.1%)
Exanthems
Lichenoid eruption
(1997): Byrd DR+, *Mayo Clin Proc* 72, 930 (photosensitive)
Photosensitivity (1–10%)
Pruritus
Purpura
(1998): Sanfelix Genoves J+, *Aten Primaria* (Spanish) 21, 252
Rash (sic) (<1%)
Stevens–Johnson syndrome
(1997): Billon S, *The Schoch Letter* 47, 32 (observation)
Urticaria (1–10%)
Vasculitis
(1998): Palop-Larrea V+, *Lancet* 352, 1909
(1998): Sanfelix Genoves J+, *Aten Primaria* (Spanish) 21, 252

#### Other
Injection-site erythema (<1%)
Myalgia (1.6%)
Tinnitus
Xerostomia

***Note:** Torsemide is a sulfonamide and can be absorbed systemically. Sulfonamides can produce severe, possibly fatal, reactions such as toxic epidermal necrolysis and Stevens–Johnson syndrome

## TRAMADOL

**Trade names:** Ultracet; Ultram (Ortho-McNeil)
**Other common trade names:** *Contramal; Tadol; Tradol; Tramal; Tramed; Tramol; Tridol; Zipan*
**Indications:** Pain
**Category:** Centrally-acting synthetic analgesic
**Half-life:** 6–7 hours
**Clinically important, potentially hazardous interactions with:** citalopram, fluoxetine, fluvoxamine, MAO inhibitors, nefazodone, phenelzine, tranylcypromine, venlafaxine

### *Reactions*

#### Skin

Allergic reactions (sic) (<1%)
Angioedema
(1996): Kind B+, *Schweiz Med Wochenschr* (German) 85, 567
Diaphoresis (9%)
Exanthems
(1999): Ghislain PD+, *Ann Dermatol Venereol* (French) 126, 38
Pruritus (10%)
(2002): Finkel JC+, *Anesth Analg* 94(6), 1469 (7%)
(1999): Ghislain PD+, *Ann Dermatol Venereol* (French) 126, 38
Rash (sic) (1–5%)
(2002): Finkel JC+, *Anesth Analg* 94(6), 1469
Toxic dermatitis (sic)
(1999): Ghislain PD+, *Ann Dermatol Venereol* (French) 126, 38
Urticaria (<1%)

#### Other

Anaphylactoid reactions
(1999): Moore PA, *J Am Dent Assoc* 130, 1075
Death
(2001): Musshoff F+, *Forensic Sci Int* 116(2), 197
Dysgeusia (<1%)
Paresthesias (<1%)
Stomatitis
Tremors (5–10%)
Xerostomia (10%)

## TRANDOLAPRIL

**Trade names:** Mavik (Abbott); Tarka (Abbott)
**Other common trade names:** *Gopten; Odrik; Udrik*
**Indications:** Hypertension
**Category:** Angiotensin-converting enzyme (ACE) inhibitor; calcium channel blocker (with verapamil); antihypertensive
**Half-life:** 24 hours
**Clinically important, potentially hazardous interactions with:** amiloride, spironolactone, triamterene

Tarka is trandolapril and verapamil

### *Reactions*

#### Skin

Angioedema (0.15%)
(2001): Cohen EG+, *Ann Otol Rhinol Laryngol* 110(8), 701 (64 cases)
(1996): *Med Lett Drugs Ther* 38, 104
Edema (>3%)
Flushing (>3%)
Pemphigus (<1%)
Pemphigus foliaceus
(2000): Ong CS+, *Australas J Dermatol* 41(4), 242
Pruritus (>3%)
Rash (sic) (>10%)

#### Other

Cough
(2001): Adigun AQ+, *West Afr J Med* 20(1), 46–7
(2001): Lee SC+, *Hypertension* 38(2), 166
Hypesthesia (>3%)
Myalgia (>3%)
Paresthesias (>3%)
Rhabdomyolysis
(2000): Gokel Y+, *Am J Emerg Med* 18(6), 738 (with verapamil)
Xerostomia (>3%)

## TRANYLCYPROMINE

**Trade name:** Parnate (GSK)
**Other common trade name:** *Siciton*
**Indications:** Depression
**Category:** Monoamine oxidase (MAO) inhibitor; antidepressant and antimanic
**Half-life:** 2.5 hours
**Clinically important, potentially hazardous interactions with:** amitriptyline, amoxapine, amphetamines, bupropion, citalopram, clomipramine, cyproheptadine, desipramine, dextroamphetamine, dextromethorphan, diethylpropion, dopamine, doxepin, entacapone, ephedrine, epinephrine, fluoxetine, fluvoxamine, imipramine, levodopa, mazindol, meperidine, methamphetamine, nefazodone, nortriptyline, paroxetine, phendimetrazine, phentermine, phenylephrine, phenylpropanolamine, protriptyline, pseudoephedrine, rizatriptan, sertraline, sibutramine, sumatriptan, sympathomimetics, tramadol, tricyclic antidepressants, trimipramine, **tryptophan**, **tyramine-containing foods**, venlafaxine, zolmitriptan

### *Reactions*

#### Skin

Diaphoresis
(1963): Adams PH+, *Lancet* 2, 692
Edema (<1%)
Exanthems
Flushing
(1963): Adams PH+, *Lancet* 2, 692
Peripheral edema
Photosensitivity (<1%)
Pruritus
Rash (sic) (<1%)
Urticaria

#### Other

Acute intermittent porphyria
(1963): Adams PH+, *Lancet* 2, 692
Black tongue
Paresthesias
Priapism
Tinnitus
Tremors
Twitching
Xerostomia (<1%)

***Note:** Tyramine-containing foods include the following: aged cheeses, avocados, banana skins, bologna and other processed luncheon meats, chicken livers, chocolate, figs, canned pickled herring, meat extracts, pepperoni, raisins, raspberries, soy sauce, vermouth, sherry and red wines

## TRASTUZUMAB

**Trade name:** Herceptin (Genentech)
**Indications:** Metastatic breast cancer
**Category:** Monoclonal antibody
**Half-life:** 5.8 days

### *Reactions*

#### Skin

Acne (2%)
Acral erythrodysesthesia syndrome (hand–foot syndrome*)
(2000): Merimsky O+, *Isr Med Assoc* 2(10), 786
Allergic reactions (sic) (3%)
Angioedema (<1%)
Cellulitis (<1%)
Chills (32%)
(2002): McKeage K+, *Drugs* 62(1), 209
(2002): Vogel CL+, *J Clin Oncol* 20(3), 719
(2001): Cook-Bruns N, *Oncology* 61, 58
(2001): Vogel CL+, *Oncology* 61, 37
(2000): Treish I+, *Am J Health Syst Pharm* 57(22), 2063
(1999): Goldenberg MM, *Clin Ther* 21(2), 309
Diaphoresis
(1999): Dillman RO, *Cancer Metastasis Rev* 18(4), 465
Edema (8%)
Flu-like syndrome (10%)
(2001): *Prescrire Int* 10(54), 102 (40%)
(1999): Dillman RO, *Cancer Metastasis Rev* 18(4), 465
Herpes simplex (2%)
Herpes zoster (~1%)
Infections (sic) (20%)
(1999): Goldenberg MM, *Clin Ther* 21(2), 309
Peripheral edema (10%)
Rash (sic) (18%)
(2001): Vogel CL+, *Oncology* 61, 37
(1999): Dillman RO, *Cancer Metastasis Rev* 18(4), 465
Ulceration (~1%)

#### Other

Anaphylactoid reactions (<1%)
(2002): McKeage K+, *Drugs* 62(1), 209
Arthralgia (6%)
Back pain (22%)
Bone pain (7%)
Cough (26%)
(1999): Goldenberg MM, *Clin Ther* 21(2), 309
Death
(2002): McKeage K+, *Drugs* 62(1), 209
Depression (6%)
Infusion-site reactions (<1%)
(2002): Tokuda Y+, *Gan To Kagaku Ryoho* 29(4), 645
(2001): Cook-Bruns N, *Oncology* 61, 58
(2001): Smith IE, *Anticancer Drugs* 12, S3
(2001): Vogel CL+, *Oncology* 61, 37
(2000): Treish I+, *Am J Health Syst Pharm* 57(22), 2063
Myopathy (~1%)
Pain (47%)
(2002): Vogel CL+, *J Clin Oncol* 20(3), 719 (18%)
(1999): Goldenberg MM, *Clin Ther* 21(2), 309
Paresthesias (9%)
Stomatitis (<1%)

***Note:** Hand–foot syndrome is also known as Acral dysesthesia syndrome

## TRAVOPROST

**Trade name:** Travatan (Alcon)
**Indications:** Open-angle glaucoma, ocular hypertension
**Category:** Ophthalmic prostaglandin
**Half-life:** N/A

### *Reactions*

#### Skin

Blepharitis (1–4%)
Eyelid margin crusting (1–4%)
Infections (sic)
Ocular hyperemia (35–50%)
Ocular pain (5–10%)
(2001): Goldberg I+, *J Glaucoma* 10(5), 414
Ocular pruritus (5–10%)
(2001): Goldberg I+, *J Glaucoma* 10(5), 414
Pruritus
(2001): Goldberg I+, *J Glaucoma* 10(5), 414

#### Hair

Hair – eyelash growth

#### Other

Arthritis (1–5%)
Depression (1–5%)
Iris pigmentation (1–4%)
(2001): Goldberg I+, *J Glaucoma* 10(5), 414
(2001): Netland PA+, *Am J Ophthalmol* 132(4), 472 (5%)
Pain
(2001): Goldberg I+, *J Glaucoma* 10(5), 414
Tearing

## TRAZODONE

**Trade name:** Desyrel (Apothecon)
**Other common trade names:** *Alti-Trazodone; Bimaran; Deprax; Desirel; Molipaxin; Sideril; Taxagon; Trazalon*
**Indications:** Depression
**Category:** Heterocyclic antidepressant and antineuralgic
**Half-life:** 3–6 hours
**Clinically important, potentially hazardous interactions with:** citalopram, fluoxetine, fluvoxamine, linezolid, nefazodone, paroxetine, sertraline, venlafaxine

### *Reactions*

#### Skin

Diaphoresis (>1%)
Edema (1–10%)
Erythema multiforme
(1985): Ford HE+, *J Clin Psychiatry* 46, 294
Exanthems
(1988): Warnock JK+, *Am J Psychiatry* 145, 425
(1986): Rongioletti F+, *J Am Acad Dermatol* 14, 274
(1984): Cohen LE, *J Am Acad Dermatol* 10, 303
(1984): Cohen LE, *J Am Acad Dermatol* 11, 526
(1980): Al-Yassiri MM+, *Neuropharmacology* 19, 1191
(1979): Trapp GA+, *Psychopharmacol Bull* 15, 25
Exfoliative dermatitis
(1983): Chu AG+, *Ann Intern Med* 99, 128
Formication
(1987): Peabody CA, *J Clin Psychiatry* 48, 385

Photosensitivity
(1994): Berger TG+, *Arch Dermatol* 130, 609 (in HIV-infected)
(1986): Rongioletti F+, *J Am Acad Dermatol* 14, 274
Pruritus (<1%)
Psoriasis (exacerbation)
(1992): Breathnach SM+, *Adverse Drug Reactions and the Skin* Blackwell, Oxford, 197 (passim)
(1986): Barth JH+, *Br J Dermatol* 115, 629 (generalized and pustular)
Purpura
Rash (sic) (<1%)
(1985): Longstreth GF+, *J Am Acad Dermatol* 13, 149
Urticaria
(1988): Warnock JK+, *Am J Psychiatry* 145, 425
(1984): Cohen LE, *J Am Acad Dermatol* 10, 303
(1983): Fabre LF+, *J Clin Psychiatry* 44, 17
Vasculitis
(1984): Mann SC+, *J Am Acad Dermatol* 10, 669

## Hair

Hair – alopecia
(2000): Mercke Y+, *Ann Clin Psychiatry* 12, 35
(1988): Warnock JK+, *Am J Psychiatry* 145, 425

## Nails

Nails – leukonychia
(1985): Longstreth GF+, *J Am Acad Dermatol* 13, 149

## Other

Dysgeusia (>10%)
Galactorrhea
Gynecomastia
Hypersensitivity
Myalgia (1–10%)
Paresthesias (>1%)
Parkinsonism
(2002): Fukunishi I+, *Nephron* 90(2), 222
Priapism
(2001): Warner MD+, *Pharmacopsychiatry* 34(4), 128 (12%)
(2000): Correas Gomez MA+, *Actas Urol Esp* (Spanish) 24(10), 840
(1998): Myrick H+, *Ann Clin Psychiatry* 10, 81
(1994): Thavundayil JX+, *Neuropsychobiology* 30, 4
(1993): Pescatori ES+, *J Urol* 149, 1557
Serotonin syndrome
(2001): McCue RE+, *Am J Psychiatry* 158(12), 2088
Sialorrhea
Tremors (1–10%)
Xerostomia (>10%)
(1982): Rawls WN, *Drug Intell Clin Pharm* 16, 7

# TRETINOIN

**Synonym:** All-trans-retinoic acid
**Trade names:** Aberela; Acnavit; Aknemycin Plus (Hermal); ATRA; Atragen; Avita (Bertek); Avitoin; Dermojuventus; Relief; Renova (Johnson & Johnson); Retin-A Micro (Ortho); Retinoic Acid; Retinova; SolagJJ (Bristol-Myers Squibb); SteiVAA; Vesanoid (Roche); Vitinoin
**Other common trade names:** *A-Acido; Aberal; Acid A Vit; Acta; Airol; Alquingel; Alten; Avitcid; Cordes VAS; Derm A; Dermairol; Epi-Aberel; Eudyna; Stieva-A; Vitamin A Acid*
**Indications:** Acne vulgaris, skin aging, facial roughness, fine wrinkles, hyperpigmentation [T], acute promyelocytic leukemia (APL) [O]
**Category:** Retinoid
**Half-life:** 0.5–2 hours
**Clinically important, potentially hazardous interactions with:** aldesleukin, bexarotene

**Note:** [T] = Topical, [O] = Oral

### *Reactions*

## Skin

Acne (1%)
(1996): Shalita A+, *J Am Acad Dermatol* 34, 482
Acute febrile neutrophilic dermatosis (Sweet's syndrome)
(1999): Takada S+, *Int J Hematol* 70(1), 26
(1997): Hatake K+, *Int J Hematol* 66(1), 13
(1996): Christ E+, *Leukemia* 10(4), 731
Bullous eruption
(1998): Webster GF, *J Am Acad Dermatol* 39, S38–44
(1997): Cunliffe WJ+, *J Am Acad Dermatol* 36, S126–34
Burning (10–40%) ([O][T])
(2001): Vandana B+, *AAPS PharmSciTech* 2(3), Technical Note 4
(1998): Ellis CN+, *Br J Dermatol* 139 Suppl 52, 41
(1998): Webster GF, *J Am Acad Dermatol* 39, S38–44
(1997): Cunliffe WJ+, *J Am Acad Dermatol* 36, S126–34
(1997): Gilchrest B, *J Am Acad Dermatol* 36, S27–36
(1997): *Drug Information Handbook* Fifth Ed., American Pharmaceutical Association, Hudson, OH
(1996): Shalita A+, *J Am Acad Dermatol* 34, 482
(1996): Shroot B, *Presented at Dermatology Update '95* (Montreal, Canada)
(1995): Hall R, *Inpharma* December, 13
(1995): *Package Insert* Hoffman-LaRoche, Inc. (Nutley, NJ)
(1992): Olsen EA+, *J Am Acad Dermatol* 26, 215
(1991): Weinstein GD+, *Arch Dermatol* 127, 659
(1989): Goldfarb MT+, *J Am Acad Dermatol* 21, 645
(1989): Leyden JJ+, *J Am Acad Dermatol* 21, 638
(1988): Cohen BA+, *Pediatric Dermatology* 1, New York: Churchill Livingstone, 663
(1977): Muller SA+, *Arch Dermatol* 113(8), 1052
Carcinoma ([O])
Cellulitis (1–10%) ([O])
(1997): *Drug Information Handbook* Fifth Ed., American Pharmaceutical Association (Hudson, OH)
(1995): Gillis JC+, *Drugs* 50(5), 897
(1995): *Package insert* Hoffman-LaRoche, Inc. (Nutley, NJ)
Cheilitis (10%) ([O])
(1997): *Drug Information Handbook* Fifth Ed. (American Pharmaceutical Association, Hudson, OH)
(1995): *Package insert* (Hoffman-LaRoche, Inc., Nutley, NJ)
Crusting
(1998): Webster GF, *J Am Acad Dermatol* 39, S38–44
(1997): Cunliffe WJ+, *J Am Acad Dermatol* 36, S126–34
Cutaneous infection (sic) (16%) ([O])

(1991): Chen ZX+, *Blood* 78, 1413
Dermatitis (sic)
(1997): Gilchrest B, *J Am Acad Dermatol* 36, S27–36
(1992): Olsen EA+, *J Am Acad Dermatol* 26, 215
(1991): Weinstein GD+, *Arch Dermatol* 127, 659
(1989): Goldfarb MT+, *J Am Acad Dermatol* 21, 645
(1989): Leyden JJ+, *J Am Acad Dermatol* 21, 638
Desquamation (14%)
Diaphoresis (20%)
Dryness of lips & skin (49–100%) ([O])
(1998): Soignet SL+, *Leukema* 12(10), 1518
(1995): Dockx P+, *Br J Dermatol* 133(3), 426
(1995): Gillis JC+, *Drugs* 50(5), 897
(1992): Fenaux P+, *Blood* 80(9), 2176
(1991): Chen ZX+, *Blood* 78(6), 1413
(1988): Huang ME+, *Blood* 72(2), 567
Edema (29%) ([O])
(1997): *Drug Information Handbook* Fifth Ed. (American Pharmaceutical Association, Hudson, OH)
(1995): *Package insert* (Hoffman-LaRoche, Inc., Nutley, NJ)
Erythema (1–49%) ([O][T])
(2001): Vandana B+, *AAPS PharmSciTech* 2(3), Technical Note 4
(2000): Kreusch+, *Curr Med Res & Opinion* 16(1), 1
(1998): Ellis CN+, *Br J Dermatol* 139 Suppl 52, 41
(1998): Webster GF, *J Am Acad Dermatol* 39(2), S38–44
(1997): Cunliffe WJ+, *J Am Acad Dermatol* 36(6), S126–34
(1997): Gilchrest BA, *J Am Acad Dermatol* 36(3), S27–36
(1997): *Drug Information Handbook* Fifth Ed (American Pharaceutical Association, Hudson, OH)
(1996): Shalita A+, *J Am Acad Dermatol* 34(3), 482
(1996): Shroot B, Presented at Dermatology Update '95, Montreal, Canada
(1995): Hall R, *Inpharma* December, 13
(1995): *Package insert* Hoffman-LaRoche, Inc., Nutley, NJ
(1992): Olsen EA+, *J Am Acad Dermatol* 26(2), 215
(1991): Weinstein GD+, *Arch Dermatol* 127, 659
(1989): Goldfarb MT+, *J Am Acad Dermatol* 21, 645
(1989): Leyden JJ+, *J Am Acad Dermatol* 21, 638
(1988): Cohen BA+, *Pediatric Dermatology* 1. New York: Churchill Livingstone, 663
(1977): Muller SA+, *Arch Dermatol* 113(8), 1052
Erythema nodosum
Exfoliation (8.3%) ([O])
(1998): Webster GF, *J Am Acad Dermatol* 39, S38–44
(1997): Cunliffe WJ+, *J Am Acad Dermatol* 36, S126–34
(1988): Huang ME+, *Blood* 72(2), 567
Facial edema (1–10%) ([O])
(1997): *Drug Information Handbook* Fifth Ed. American Pharmaceutical Association, Hudson, OH
(1995): *Package insert* Hoffman-LaRoche, Inc., Nutley NJ
Flaking (23%) ([O])
Flushing
(1997): *Drug Information Handbook* Fifth Ed. American Pharmaceutical Association, Hudson, OH
(1996): Miller VA+, *Clin Cancer Res* 2(3), 471
(1995): *Package insert* Hoffman-LaRoche, Inc., Nutley, NJ
Hyperkeratosis (78%) ([O])
(1991): Chen ZX+, *Blood* 78, 1413
Hypopigmentation (5%)
(1998): Webster GF, *J Am Acad Dermatol* 39, S38–44
(1997): Cunliffe WJ+, *J Am Acad Dermatol* 36, S126–34
Infections (sic) (58%) ([O])
(1997): *Drug Information Handbook* Fifth Ed. American Pharaceutical Association, Hudson, OH
(1995): *Package insert* Hoffman-LaRoche, Inc,. Nutley, NJ
Irritation (5%)
(2001): Vandana B+, *AAPS PharmSciTech* 2(3), Technical Note 4
(1998): Cohen BA+, *Pediatric Dermatology* 1, New York: Churchill Livingstone, 663

(1997): Clucas A+, *J Am Acad Dermatol* 36, S116–8
Localized edema
(1998): Webster GF, *J Am Acad Dermatol* 39, S38–44
(1997): Cunliffe WJ+, *J Am Acad Dermatol* 36, S126–34
(1997): Gilchrest BA, *J Am Acad Dermatol* 36, S27–36
(1992): Olsen EA+, *J Am Acad Dermatol* 26, 215
(1991): Weinstein GD+, *Arch Dermatol* 127, 659
(1989): Goldfarb MT+, *J Am Acad Dermatol* 21, 645
(1989): Leyden JJ+, *J Am Acad Dermatol* 21, 638
Ocular pruritus (10%) ([O])
(1997): *Drug Information Handbook* Fifth Ed. American Pharmaceutical Association, Hudson, OH
(1995): *Package insert* Hoffman-LaRoche, Inc., Natley, NJ
Pain (37%) ([O])
(1997): *Drug Information Handbook* Fifth Ed. American Pharmaceutical Association, Hudson, OH
(1995): *Package insert* Hoffman-LaRoche, Inc., Nutley, NJ
Pallor (1–10%) ([O])
(1997): *Drug Information Handbook* Fifth Ed. American Pharmaceutical Association, Hudson, OH
(1995): *Package insert* Hoffman-LaRoche, Inc., Nutley, NJ
Palmar–plantar peeling (1–10%) ([O])
(1997): *Drug Information Handbook* Fifth Ed. American Pharmaceutical Association, Hudson, OH
(1995): *Package insert* Hoffman-LaRoche, Inc., Nutley, NJ
Photosensitivity (10%) ([O][T])
(1998): Webster GF, *J Am Acad Dermatol* 39, S38–44
(1997): Cunliffe WJ+, *J Am Acad Dermatol* 36, S126–34
(1997): *Drug Information Handbook* Fifth Ed. American Pharmaceutical Association, Hudson, OH
(1995): *Package insert* Hoffman-LaRoche, Inc., Nutley, NJ
Pigmentation (5%)
(1998): Webster GF, *J Am Acad Dermatol* 39, S38–44
(1997): Cunliffe WJ+, *J Am Acad Dermatol* 36, S126–34
Pruritus (10–40%) ([O][T])
(2001): Vandana B+, *AAPS PharmSciTech* 2(3), Technical Note 4
(2000): Kreusch+, *Curr Med Res & Opinion* 16(1), 1
(1998): Ellis CN+, *Br J Dermatol* 139 Suppl 52, 41
(1998): Webster GF, *J Am Acad Dermatol* 39, S38–44
(1997): Cunliffe WJ+, *J Am Acad Dermatol* 36, S126–34
(1997): *Drug Information Handbook* Fifth Ed. American Pharmaceutical Association, Hudson, OH
(1996): Shalita A+, *J Am Acad Dermatol* 34, 482
(1995): Gillis JC+, *Drugs* 50(5), 897
(1995): *Package insert* Hoffman-LaRoche, Inc., Nutley, NJ
(1988): Cohen BA+, *Pediatric Dermatology* 1, New York:Churchill Livingstone, 663
(1977): Muller SA+, *Arch Dermatol* 113(8), 1052
Rash (sic) (54%) ([O][T])
(1998): Webster GF, *J Am Acad Dermatol* 39, S38–44
(1997): Cunliffe WJ+, *J Am Acad Dermatol* 36, S126–34
(1997): *Drug Information Handbook* Fifth Ed American Pharmaceutical Association, Hudson, OH
(1995): *Package insert* Hoffman-LaRoche, Inc.,Nutley, NJ
(1991): Warrell RP+, *N Engl J Med* 324, 1385
Scaling (10–40%)
(2001): Vandana B+, *AAPS PharmSciTech* 2(3), Technical Note 4
(2000): Kreusch+, *Curr Med Res & Opinion* 16(1), 1
(1998): Ellis CN+, *Br J Dermatol* 139 Suppl 52, 41
(1997): Gilchrest BA, *J Am Acad Dermatol* 36, S27–36
(1996): Shalita A+, *J Am Acad Dermatol* 34, 482
(1996): Shroot B, *Presented ar Dermatology Update '95* Montreal, Canada
(1995): Hall R, *Inpharma* December, 13
(1992): Olsen EA+, *J Am Acad Dermatol* 26, 215
(1991): Weinstein GD+, *Arch Dermatol* 127, 659
(1989): Goldfarb MT+, *J Am Acad Dermatol* 21, 645
(1988): Cohen BA+, *Pediatric Dermatology* 1 New York: Chrurchill Livingstone, 663

Shivering (63%) ([O])
(1997): *Drug Information Handbook* Fifth Ed. American Pharmaceutical Association, Hudson, OH
(1995): *Package insert* Hoffman-LaRoche, Inc., Nutley, NJ
Skin irritation (sic) (1%)
(1996): Shalita A+, *J Am Acad Dermatol* 34, 482
Stinging (1–26%)
(1997): Gilchrest BA, *J Am Acad Dermatol* 36, S27–36
(1996): Shalita A+, *J Am Acad Dermatol* 34, 482
(1992): Olsen EA+, *J Am Acad Dermatol* 26, 215
(1991): Weinstein GD+, *Arch Dermatol* 127, 659
(1989): Goldfarb MT+, *J Am Acad Dermatol* 21, 645
(1989): Leyden JJ+, *J Am Acad Dermatol* 21, 638
Sunburn (1%)
(1996): Shalita A+, *J Am Acad Dermatol* 34, 482
Ulceration (penile)
(2000): Esser AC+, *J Am Acad Dermatol* 43(2 Pt 1), 316
(1995): Gillis JC+, *Drugs* 50, 897
Vesiculobullous eruption
Xerosis (77%)
(2000): Kreusch+, *Curr Med Res & Opinion* 16(1), 1
(1997): Gilchrest BA, *J Am Acad Dermatol* 36, S27
(1996): Shalita A+, *J Am Acad Dermatol* 34, 482
(1992): Olsen EA+, *J Am Acad Dermatol* 26, 215
(1991): Weinstein GD+, *Arch Dermatol* 127, 659
(1989): Leyden JJ+, *J Am Acad Dermatol* 21, 638

## Hair

Hair – alopecia (14%) ([O])
(1997): *Drug Information Handbook* Fifth Ed American Pharmaceutical Association, Hudson, OH
(1995): *Package insert* Hoffman-LaRoche, Inc., Nutley, NJ

## Other

Arthralgia (10%) ([O])
(1997): *Drug Information Handbook* American Pharmaceutical Association, Hudson, OH
(1995): Gillis JC+, *Drugs* 50, 897
(1995): *Package insert* Hoffman-LaRoche, Inc., Nutley, NJ
Bone or joint pain (77%) ([O])
(1995): Gillis JC+, *Drugs* 50, 897
(1992): Fenaux P+, *Blood* 80, 2176
(1988): Huang ME+, *Blood* 72, 567
Conjunctivitis (<1%) ([O])
(1997): *Drug Information Handbook* Fifth Ed. American Pharmaceutical Association, Hudson, OH
(1995): *Package insert* Hoffman-LaRoche, Inc., Nutley, NJ
Death ([O])
(1997): Fenaux P+, *N Engl J* 337, 1076
(1997): Larson RA+ In: Hall JB+, *Principles of Critical Care* Second Ed. New York, McGraw-Hill
(1995): *Package insert* Hoffman-LaRoche, Inc., Nutley, NJ
Depression (14%) ([O])
(1997): *Drug Information Handbook* Fifth Ed, American Pharmaceutical Association, Hudson, OH
(1995): *Package insert* Hoffman-LaRoche, Inc., Nutley, NJ
Dry eyes (1–10%) ([O])
(1997): *Drug Information Handbook* Fifth Ed. American Pharmaceutical Association, Hudson, OH
(1995): *Package insert* Hoffman-LaRoche, Inc., Nutley, NJ
Fever ([O])
(1997): Fenaux P+, *N Engl J Med* 337, 1076
(1997): Larson RA+ In: Halll JB+, *Principles of Critical Care* Second Ed., New York, McGraw
(1995): *Package insert* Hoffman-LaRoche, Inc., Nutley, NJ
Gingival bleeding (<1%) ([O])
(1997): *Drug Information Handbook* Fifth Ed. American Pharmaceutical Association, Hudson, OH
(1995): *Package insert* Hoffman-LaRoche, Inc., Nutley, NJ
Injection-site reactions (17%)
Myalgia (14%) ([O])
(1997): *Drug Information Handbook* Fifth Ed. American Pharmaceutical Association, Hudson, OH
(1995): *Package insert* Hoffman-LaRoche, Inc., Nutley, NJ
Myositis
Paresthesias (17%) ([O])
(1997): *Drug Information Handbook* Fifth Ed. American Pharmaceutical Association, Hudson, OH
(1995): *Package insert* Hoffman-LaRoche, Inc., Nutley, NJ
Phlebitis (11%)
Photophobia (1–10%) ([O])
(1997): *Drug Information Handbook* Fifth Ed. American Pharmaceutical Association, Hudson, OH
(1995): *Package insert* Hoffman-LaRoche, Inc., Nutley, NJ
Pseudotumor cerebri (<1%) ([O])
(1997): Tallman MS+, *N Engl J Med* 337, 1021
(1996): Visani G+, *Leuk Lymphoma* 23(5–6), 437
(1995): *Package insert* Hoffman-LaRoche, Inc., Nutley, NJ
(1994): *Drug Information Handbook* Fifth Ed. American Pharmaceutical Association, Hudson, OH
(1993): Mahmoud HH+, *Lancet* 342(8884), 1394
(1991): Warrell RP+, *N Engl J Med* 324, 1385
Retinoic Acid–APL (RA-APL) syndrome * (25%) ([O])
(1997): Fenaux P+, *N Engl J Med* 337, 1076
(1997): Sacchi S+, *Haematologica* 82(1), 106
(1997): Tallman MS+, *N Engl J Med* 337, 1021
(1995): Gillis JC+, *Drugs* 50, 897
(1995): *Package insert* Hoffman-LaRoche, Inc., Nutley, NJ
(1992): Fenaux P+, *Blood* 80, 2176
Tingling (26%)
Tremors (1–10%) ([O])
(1997): *Drug Information Handbook* Fifth Ed. American Pharmaceutical Association, Hudson, OH
(1995): *Package insert* Hoffman-LaRoche, Inc., Nutley, NJ
Xerostomia (10%) ([O])
(1997): *Drug Information Handbook* Fifth Ed American Pharmaceutical Association, Hudson, OH
(1995): *Package insert* Hoffman-LaRoche, Inc., Nutley, NJ

**Note:** Oral tretinoin can cause birth defects, and women should avoid Tretinoin when pregnant or trying to conceive. Avoid prolonged exposure to sunlight

***Note:** The RA-APL syndrome is characterized by fever, dyspnea, weight gain, pulmonary infiltrates and pleural effusions. Some patients have expired due to multiorgan failure

# TRIAMTERENE

**Trade names:** Dyazide (GSK); Dyrenium (GSK); Maxzide (Bertek)
**Other common trade names:** *Amterene; Diarrol; Diuteren; Dytac; Reviten; Suloton; Trian*
**Indications:** Edema
**Category:** Potassium-sparing diuretic; antihypertensive
**Half-life:** 1–2 hours
**Clinically important, potentially hazardous interactions with:** ACE inhibitors, benazepril, captopril, cyclosporine, enalapril, fosinopril, indomethacin, lisinopril, moexipril, potassium iodide, potassium salts, quinapril, ramipril, spironolactone, trandolapril

Dyazide is triamterene and hydrochlorothiazide*; Maxzide is triamterene and hydrochlorothiazide*

### *Reactions*

## Skin

Chills
Diaphoresis
(1979): Fan WJ+, *Pediatrics* 64, 698
Edema (1–10%)
Exanthems
Flushing (<1%)
Lupus erythematosus (with hydrochlorothiazide)
(1991): Wollenberg A+, *Hautarzt* (German) 42, 709
(1988): Darken M+, *J Am Acad Dermatol* 18, 38
Perleche
Photosensitivity
(1989): Rosen C, *Semin Dermatol* 8, 149
(1987): Fernandez de Corres L+, *Contact Dermatitis* 17, 114
Pruritus
Purpura
Rash (sic) (1–10%)
Urticaria
Vasculitis

## Other

Anaphylactoid reactions
Dysgeusia
(1999): Sorkin M, Denver, CO (from Internet) (observation)
Glossitis
Gynecomastia (<1%)
Paresthesias
Pseudoporphyria
(1990): Motley RJ, *BMJ* 300, 1468
Stomatodynia
(1999): Sorkin M, Denver, CO (from Internet) (observation)
Xerostomia
(1987): Fernandez de Corres L+, *Contact Dermatitis* 17, 114

***Note:** Hydrochlorothiazide is a sulfonamide and can be absorbed systemically. Sulfonamides can produce severe, possibly fatal, reactions such as toxic epidermal necrolysis and Stevens–Johnson syndrome

# TRIAZOLAM

**Trade name:** Halcion (Pharmacia & Upjohn)
**Other common trade names:** *Dumozolam; Novo-Triolam; Nu-Triazo; Nuctane; Somese; Somniton; Songar; Trialam*
**Indications:** Insomnia
**Category:** Benzodiazepine sedative-hypnotic
**Half-life:** 1.5–5.5 hours
**Clinically important, potentially hazardous interactions with:** clarithromycin, delavirdine, efavirenz, erythromycin, indinavir, itraconazole, ketoconazole, rifampin, ritonavir

### *Reactions*

## Skin

Dermatitis (sic) (1–10%)
(1984): Greenblatt DJ+, *J Clin Psychiatry* 45, 192
Diaphoresis (>10%)
(1983): Kroboth PD+, *Drug Intell Clin Pharm* 17, 495
(1979): van der Kroef C, *Lancet* 2, 526
Exanthems
Photosensitivity
(1984): Hussar DA, *Am Drug* 190, 109
Pruritus
(1983): Poeldinger W+, *Neuropsychobiology* 9, 135
(1981): Cobden I+, *Postgrad Med J* 57, 730
Purpura
Rash (sic) (>10%)
(1985): Jerram TC, *Side Effects Drugs Annu* 9, 39
Urticaria

## Hair

Hair – alopecia
Hair – hirsutism

## Other

Dysesthesia (<1%)
Dysgeusia (<1%)
(1979): van der Kroef C, *Lancet* 2, 526
(1978): Fabre LF Jr+, *J Clin Psychiatry* 39, 679
Gingivitis
Glossitis (<1%)
Glossodynia (<1%)
Paresthesias (<1%)
(1979): van der Kroef C, *Lancet* 2, 526
Sialopenia (>10%)
(1995): Loesche WJ+, *J Am Geriatr Soc* 43, 401
Sialorrhea (1–10%)
Stomatitis (<1%)
Tinnitus
Tremors (1–10%)
Xerostomia (>10%)
(1995): Loesche WJ+, *J Am Geriatr Soc* 43, 401
(1986): Hughes RRL+, *Br J Clin Pract* 40, 279
(1984): Greenblatt DJ+, *J Clin Psychiatry* 45, 192
(1983): Cohn JB, *J Clin Psychiatry* 44, 401

# TRICHLORMETHIAZIDE

**Trade names:** Metahydrin (Aventis); Naqua (Schering)
**Other common trade names:** *Anatran; Aquacot; Carvacron; Diurese; Doqua; Esmarin; Flute; Iopran; Niazide; Trichlon; Trichlorex*
**Indications:** Edema, hypertension
**Category:** Thiazide* diuretic; antihypertensive
**Half-life:** no data
**Clinically important, potentially hazardous interactions with:** digoxin, lithium

### *Reactions*

#### Skin
Exanthems
Lichenoid eruption (<1%)
Lupus erythematosus
(1978): Pereyo-Torellas N, *Arch Dermatol* 114, 1097
Photosensitivity (<1%)
Purpura
(1962): Loftus LR+, *JAMA* 180, 410
Rash (sic)
Urticaria
Vasculitis
(1962): Loftus LR+, *JAMA* 180, 410

#### Other
Anaphylactoid reactions
Paresthesias
Xerostomia

***Note:** Trichlormethiazide is a sulfonamide and can be absorbed systemically. Sulfonamides can produce severe, possibly fatal, reactions such as toxic epidermal necrolysis and Stevens–Johnson syndrome

# TRIENTINE

**Trade name:** Syprine (Merck)
**Indications:** Wilson's disease
**Category:** Chelating agent; antidote (copper toxicity)
**Half-life:** no data

### *Reactions*

#### Skin
Dermatitis (sic)
(1980): Rudzki E, *Contact Dermatitis* 6, 235
Desquamation
Lupus erythematosus (<1%)
Thickening (sic) (<1%)

#### Other
Aphthous stomatitis
Oral mucosal lesions

# TRIFLUOPERAZINE

**Trade name:** Stelazine (GSK)
**Other common trade names:** *Calmazine; Domilium; Flupazine; Fluzine; Nerolet; Psyrazine; Sedizine; Tfp*
**Indications:** Psychoses, anxiety
**Category:** Phenothiazine tranquilizer; anxiolytic; antipsychotic
**Half-life:** 10–20 hours
**Clinically important, potentially hazardous interactions with:** antihistamines, arsenic, chlorpheniramine, dofetilide, piperazine, quinolones, sparfloxacin

### *Reactions*

#### Skin
Angioedema
(1974): Panikarskii VG, *Vrach Delo* (Russian) February, 118
Contact dermatitis
Diaphoresis
Eczema (sic)
Erythema
Exanthems
Exfoliative dermatitis
Fixed eruption
(1987): Kanwar AJ+, *Br J Dermatol* 117, 798
Hypohidrosis
Lupus erythematosus
Peripheral edema
Photosensitivity (1–10%)
(1970): *Med Lett* 12, 104
Pigmentation (blue-gray) (<1%)
(1994): Buckley C+, *Clin Exp Dermatol* 19, 149
Pruritus
Purpura
Rash (sic) (1–10%)
Seborrhea
Urticaria
Xerosis

#### Other
Anaphylactoid reactions
Galactorrhea (<1%)
Gynecomastia
Mastodynia (1–10%)
Oral mucosal eruption
(1988): Ward DF+, *Postgrad Med* 84, 99
Parkinsonism (>10%)
Priapism (<1%)
Tongue edema
(1988): Ward DF+, *Postgrad Med* 84, 99
Tremors
Xerostomia

## TRIHEXYPHENIDYL

**Trade name:** Artane (Lederle)
**Other common trade names:** *Acamed; Aparkane; Bentex; Hexinal; Hipokinon; Parkines; Partane; Tridyl; Trihexy; Trihexyphen*
**Indications:** Parkinsonism
**Category:** Antidyskinetic; antiparkinsonian; anticholinergic
**Half-life:** 3–4 hours
**Clinically important, potentially hazardous interactions with:** anticholinergics, arbutamine

### *Reactions*

#### Skin
Chills
Diaphoresis
Flushing
Hypohidrosis (>10%)
Photosensitivity (1–10%)
Rash (sic) (<1%)
Spider angiomas
(1953): Holt CL, *N Engl J Med* 249, 318
Urticaria
Xerosis (>10%)

#### Other
Glossitis
Glossodynia
Paresthesias
Xerostomia (30–50%)

## TRIMEPRAZINE

**Trade name:** Temaril (Allergan)
**Other common trade names:** *Nedeltran; Panectyl; Theralene; Vallergan; Variargil*
**Indications:** Pruritus, urticaria
**Category:** Phenothiazine $H_1$-receptor antihistamine and sedative-hypnotic
**Duration of action:** 3–6 hours

### *Reactions*

#### Skin
Angioedema (<1%)
(1959): Wright W, *JAMA* 171, 1642
Dermatitis (sic)
Diaphoresis
Edema (<1%)
Exanthems
(1959): Wright W, *JAMA* 171, 1642
Lupus erythematosus
Peripheral edema
Photosensitivity (<1%)
Pruritus
(1959): Wright W, *JAMA* 171, 1642
Purpura
Rash (sic) (<1%)
Urticaria

#### Other
Anaphylactoid reactions
Gynecomastia
Myalgia (<1%)
Paresthesias (<1%)
Stomatitis
Tinnitus
Xerostomia (1–10%)
(1992): Chambers FA+, *Anaesthesia* 47, 585

## TRIMETHADIONE

**Trade name:** Tridione (Abbott)
**Other common trade name:** *Mino Aleviatin*
**Category:** Anticonvulsant
**Half-life:** no data

### *Reactions*

#### Skin
Acne
Bullous eruption
Erythema multiforme
(1992): Breathnach SM+, *Adverse Drug Reactions and the Skin* Blackwell, Oxford, 210 (passim)
(1972): Levantine A+, *Br J Dermatol* 87, 646
(1961): Rallison ML+, *Am J Dis Child* 101, 725
(1948): Kevin JC, *Lancet* 1, 267
Exanthems
(1972): Levantine A+, *Br J Dermatol* 87, 646
(1962): LeVan P+, *Arch Dermatol* 86, 254
(1948): Kevin JC, *Lancet* 1, 267
Exfoliative dermatitis
(1992): Breathnach SM+, *Adverse Drug Reactions and the Skin* Blackwell, Oxford, 210 (passim)
(1948): Kevin JC, *Lancet* 1, 267
Fixed eruption
Infections (sic)
(2002): Sarris AH+, *J Clin Oncol* 20(12), 2876 (3%)
Lupus erythematosus
(1993): Drory VE+, *Clin Neuropharmacol* 16, 19
(1976): Singsen BH+, *Pediatrics* 57, 529
(1973): Beernink DH+, *J Pediatr* 82, 113
(1962): LeVan P+, *Arch Dermatol* 86, 254
(1961): Rallison ML+, *Am J Dis Child* 101, 725
Petechiae
Photosensitivity
(1962): LeVan P+, *Arch Dermatol* 86, 254
Pruritus
(1961): Weingartner L, *Monatsschr Kinderheilkd* (German) 109, 517
Purpura
(1956): Wintrobe MM+, *Arch Intern Med* 98, 559
Stevens–Johnson syndrome
(1961): Rallison ML+, *Am J Dis Child* 101, 725
Urticaria
(1992): Breathnach SM+, *Adverse Drug Reactions and the Skin* Blackwell, Oxford, 210 (passim)
(1964): Beall GN, *Medicine* (Baltimore) 43, 131
(1948): Kevin JC, *Lancet* 1, 267
Vasculitis
(1993): Drory VE+, *Clin Neuropharmacol* 16, 19
(1986): Hannedouche T+, *Ann Med Interne Paris* (French) 137, 57

#### Hair
Hair – alopecia
(1960): Holowach J+, *N Engl J Med* 263, 1187

### Other

Acute intermittent porphyria
Gingivitis
Mucositis
(2002): Sarris AH+, *J Clin Oncol* 20(12), 2876 (4%)
Paresthesias

## TRIMETHOBENZAMIDE

**Trade names:** Arrestin; Benzacot; Bio-Gan; Navogan; Stemetic; T-Gene; Tebamide; Tegamide; Ticon; Tigan (Roberts); Triban; Tribenzagen; Trimazide
**Other common trade names:** *Anaus; Elen; Ibikin*
**Indications:** Prevention and treatment of nausea and vomiting
**Category:** Antiemetic
**Half-life:** no data

#### *Reactions*

### Skin

Allergic reactions (sic) (<1%)

### Other

Hypersensitivity (<1%)
Injection-site reactions (sic)
Parkinsonism

## TRIMETHOPRIM*

**Trade names:** Bactrim (Roche); Septra (Monarch)
**Other common trade names:** *Abaprim; Alprim; Bactin; Idotrim; Ipral; Lidaprim; Methoprim; Monotrim; Primosept; Syraprim; Tiempe; Triprim; Unitrim; Wellcprim*
**Indications:** Various urinary tract infections caused by susceptible organisms
**Category:** Antibiotic
**Half-life:** 8–10 hours
**Clinically important, potentially hazardous interactions with:** dofetilide, methotrexate

#### *Reactions*

### Skin

Erythema multiforme
Erythema nodosum
(1983): *Ugeskr Laeger* (Danish) 145, 1070
Exanthems
Exfoliative dermatitis (<1%)
Photosensitivity
Pruritus (1–10%)
Rash (sic) (2.9–6.7%)
Stevens–Johnson syndrome
Toxic epidermal necrolysis

### Other

Anaphylactoid reactions
Dysgeusia
Glossitis

***Note:** Although trimethoprim has been known to elicit occasional adverse reactions by itself, it is most commonly used in conjunction with sulfamethoxazole (co-trimoxazole). The trade names for this combination are: Bactrim; Cotrim; Septra. Please see co-trimoxazole for the specific reaction patterns and references

## TRIMETREXATE

**Trade name:** Neutrexin (US Bioscience)
**Indications:** *Pneumocystis carinii* pneumonia
**Category:** Antineoplastic; folate antagonist; antiprotozoal
**Half-life:** 15–17 hours

#### *Reactions*

### Skin

Angioedema
(1990): Grem JL+, *Drugs* 8, 211
Exanthems
(1987): Leiby J+, *Invest New Drugs* 5, 136
Fixed eruption
Flu-like syndrome (sic) (1–10%)
Flushing
(1990): Grem JL+, *Drugs* 8, 211
Photosensitivity
Pruritus (5.5%)
(1990): Grem JL+, *Drugs* 8, 211
Rash (sic) (1–10%)

### Other

Hypersensitivity (1–10%)
Oral mucosal lesions
(1987): Leiby J+, *Invest New Drugs* 5, 136
Stomatitis (1–10%)

## TRIMIPRAMINE

**Trade name:** Surmontil (Wyeth-Ayerst)
**Other common trade names:** *Apo-Trimip; Rhotrimine; Stangyl; Sumontil*
**Indications:** Major depression
**Category:** Tricyclic antidepressant; antineuralgic and antiulcer
**Half-life:** 20–26 hours
**Clinically important, potentially hazardous interactions with:** amprenavir, arbutamine, bupropion, clonidine, epinephrine, formoterol, guanethidine, isocarboxazid, linezolid, MAO inhibitors, phenelzine, quinolones, sparfloxacin, tranylcypromine

#### *Reactions*

### Skin

Allergic reactions (sic) (<1%)
Diaphoresis (1–10%)
Exanthems
Petechiae
Photosensitivity (<1%)
Pruritus
Purpura
Rash (sic)
Urticaria

### Hair

Hair – alopecia (<1%)

### Other

Dysgeusia (>10%)
Galactorrhea (<1%)
Glossitis
Gynecomastia (<1%)
Paresthesias

Parkinsonism (1–10%)
Seizures
(2001): Enns MW, *J Clin Psychiatry* 62(6), 476 (with bupropion)
Stomatitis
Tinnitus
Tremors
Xerostomia (>10%)

# TRIOXSALEN

**Trade name:** Trisoralen (ICN)
**Other common trade names:** *Neosoralen; Puvadin*
**Indications:** Vitiligo, hypopigmentation
**Category:** Repigmenting agent and antipsoriatic; psoralen
**Half-life:** ~2 hours

### *Reactions*

## Skin

Acne
(1978): Nielsen EB+, *Acta Derm Venereol* (Stockh) 58, 374
Bullous eruption (with UVA)
(1999): Chuan MT+, *J Formos Med Assoc* 98, 335
(1979): Abel EA+, *Arch Dermatol* 115, 988
(1977): Melski JW+, *J Invest Dermatol* 68, 328
(1976): Thomsen K+, *Br J Dermatol* 95, 568
Eczematous eruption (sic)
(1979): Saihan EM, *BMJ* 2, 20
Freckles
(1984): Kietzmann E+, *Dermatologica* 168, 306
(1983): Kanerva L+, *Dermatologica* 166, 281
Granuloma annulare
(1979): Dorval JC+, *Ann Dermatol Venereol* (French) 106, 79
Herpes simplex
(1982): Stüttgen G, *Int J Dermatol* 21, 198
Herpes zoster
(1982): Stüttgen G, *Int J Dermatol* 21, 198
(1977): Roenigk HH+, *Arch Dermatol* 113, 1667
Lupus erythematosus
(1985): Bruze M+, *Acta Derm Venereol* (Stockh) 65, 31
Melanoma
(1980): Forrest JB+, *J Surg Oncol* 13, 337
Pemphigoid
(1978): Robinson JK, *Br J Dermatol* 99, 709
Photoreactions
(1978): Plewig G+, *Arch Derm Res* 261, 201
(1977): Ljunggren B, *Contact Dermatitis* 3, 85
Photosensitivity
(1976): Jonelis FJ+, *Arch Dermatol* 112, 1036
Phototoxicity
(2001): Snellman E+, *Acta Derm Venereol* 81(3), 171
(1992): George SA+, *Br J Dermatol* 127, 444
(1979): Fischer T+, *Acta Derm Venereol* (Stockh) 59, 171
Pigmentation
(1989): Weiss E+, *Int J Dermatol* 28, 188
(1987): Bruce DR+, *J Am Acad Dermatol* 16, 1087
(1986): MacDonald KJS+, *Br J Dermatol* 114, 395
Porokeratosis (actinic)
(1988): Beiteke U+, *Photodermatology* 5, 274
(1985): Hazen PG+, *J Am Acad Dermatol* 12, 1077
(1980): Reymond JL, *Acta Derm Venereol* (Stockh) 60, 539
Pruritus (>10%)
(1999): Chuan MT+, *J Formos Med Assoc* 98, 335
Scleroderma
(1976): Duperrat B+, *Bull Soc Franc Dermatol Syphiligr* (French) 83, 79
Seborrheic dermatitis
(1983): Tegner E, *Acta Derm Venereol* (Stockh) Suppl 107, 5
Skin pain (sic)
(1987): Norris PG+, *Clin Exp Dermatol* 12, 403
(1983): Tegner E, *Acta Derm Venereol* (Stockh) Suppl 107, 5
Vasculitis
(1981): Barriere H+, *Presse Med* (French) 10, 37
Vitiligo
(1983): Tegner E, *Acta Derm Venereol* (Stockh) Suppl 107, 5
(1976): Duperrat B+, *Bull Soc Franc Dermatol Syphiligr* (French) 83, 79
Xerosis
(1999): Chuan MT+, *J Formos Med Assoc* 98, 335

## Hair

Hair – hypertrichosis
(1983): Rampen FHJ, *Br J Dermatol* 109, 657
(1967): Singh G+, *Br J Dermatol* 79, 501

## Nails

Nails – photo-onycholysis
(1987): Baran R+, *J Am Acad Dermatol* 17, 1012
Nails – pigmentation
(1990): Trattner A+, *Int J Dermatol* 29, 310
(1989): Weiss E+, *Int J Dermatol* 28, 188
(1986): MacDonald KJS+, *Br J Dermatol* 114, 395
(1982): Naik RPC+, *Int J Dermatol* 21, 275

## Other

Lymphoproliferative disease
(1989): Aschinoff R+, *J Am Acad Dermatol* 21, 1134
Tumors (sic)
(1995): Halder RM+, *Arch Dermatol* 131, 734
(1989): Hannuksela M+, *J Am Acad Dermatol* 21, 813
(1988): Gupta AK+, *J Am Acad Dermatol* 19, 67
(1987): Henseler T+, *J Am Acad Dermatol* 16, 108
(1986): Kahn JR+, *Clin Exp Dermatol* 11, 398

# TRIPELENNAMINE

**Trade name:** PBZ (Novartis)
**Other common trade names:** *Azaron; Pyribenzamine; Triplen*
**Indications:** Allergic rhinitis, urticaria
**Category:** $H_1$-receptor blocker antihistamine
**Half-life:** no data
**Clinically important, potentially hazardous interactions with: alcohol**, barbiturates, chloral hydrate, ethchlorvynol, paraldehyde, phenothiazines

### *Reactions*

## Skin

Angioedema (<1%)
(1951): Guiducci A+, *Arch Dermatol* 63, 263
Diaphoresis
Edema (<1%)
Fixed eruption
(1961): Welsh AL+, *Arch Dermatol* 84, 1004
Flushing
Lichenoid eruption
(1947): Epstein E, *JAMA* 134, 782
Lupus erythematosus
Peripheral edema
Photosensitivity (<1%)

Pityriasis rosea
(1947): Epstein E, *JAMA* 134, 782
Purpura
(1956): Wintrobe MM+, *Arch Intern Med* 98, 559
(1951): Uvitsky IH, *J Allergy* 22, 544
Rash (sic) (<1%)
Systemic eczematous contact dermatitis
Urticaria
(1949): London ID, *J Invest Dermatol* 13, 317

### Other

Anaphylactoid reactions
Myalgia (<1%)
Paresthesias (<1%)
Stomatitis
Tremors (<1%)
Xerostomia (1–10%)

## TRIPROLIDINE

**Trade names:** Actagen; Actidil; Actifed; Allerphed; Cenafed; Genac; Myidil; Trifed; Triofed; Triposed (Various pharmaceutical companies)*
**Other common trade name:** *Actidilon*
**Indications:** Allergic rhinitis
**Category:** $H_1$-receptor antihistamine; sympathomimetic
**Half-life:** no data

### *Reactions*

### Skin

Angioedema (<1%)
Diaphoresis (1–10%)
Edema (<1%)
Exanthems
Fixed eruption
(1968): Brownstein MH, *Arch Dermatol* 97, 115
Flushing
Lichenoid eruption
(1964): Alexander S, *BMJ* 2, 512
Photosensitivity (<1%)
Purpura
Rash (sic) (<1%)
Urticaria

### Other

Myalgia (<1%)
Paresthesias (<1%)
Xerostomia (1–10%)

***Note:** Most of the trade name drugs contain pseudoephedrine as well

## TRIPTORELIN

**Synonym:** Decapeptyl
**Trade name:** Trelstar (Debio Recherche Pharmaceutique SA)
**Indications:** Palliative treatment of advanced prostate carcinoma
**Category:** Luteinizing hormone-releasing hormone analog; antineoplastic
**Half-life:** 2.8-1.2 hours

### *Reactions*

### Skin

Angioedema (<1%)
Hot flashes (59%)
(1996): Choktanasiri W+, *Int J Gynaecol Obstet* 54, 237
(1994): Neskovic-Konstantinovic ZB+, *Oncology* 51, 95
(1994): Vercellini P+, *Fertil Steril* 62, 938
Pruritus (1%)
Vasculitis
(1993): Amichai B+, *Eur J Obstet Gynecol Reprod Biol* 52, 217

### Hair

Hair – alopecia
(1997): Kauschansky A+, *Acta Derm Venereol* 77, 333

### Other

Anaphylactoid reactions (<1%)
Hypersensitivity (<1%)
Injection-site pain (4%)
Leg pain (2%)

## TROLEANDOMYCIN

**Trade name:** TAO (Pfizer)
**Indications:** Various infections caused by susceptible organisms
**Category:** Macrolide antibiotic
**Half-life:** no data
**Clinically important, potentially hazardous interactions with:** carbamazepine, colchicine, cyclosporine, dihydroergotamine, ergot alkaloids, fluoxetine, fluvoxamine, methysergide, oral contraceptives, paroxetine, pimozide, sertaline, warfarin

### *Reactions*

### Skin

Angioedema
(1971): *Med Lett* 13, 55
Erythema multiforme
Exanthems
(1961): Saslaw S, *Med Clin North Am* 45, 839
(1960): Welsh AL+, *Antibiotic Med Clin Ther* 7, 179
Pruritus
(1971): *Med Lett* 13, 55
Rash (sic) (1–10%)
Urticaria (1–10%)
(1971): *Med Lett* 13, 55

### Other

Anaphylactoid reactions
Oral mucosal lesions
(1971): *Med Lett* 13, 55

# TROVAFLOXACIN*

**Trade name:** Trovan (Pfizer)
**Indications:** Various infections caused by susceptible organisms
**Category:** 4th generation fluoroquinolone antibiotic
**Half-life:** 9.5 hours

### *Reactions*

#### Skin
Acne
Allergic reactions (sic) (<1%)
Angioedema (<1%)
Balanoposthitis (<1%)
Candidiasis (<1%)
Cheilitis (<1%)
Dermatitis (sic) (<1%)
Diaphoresis (<1%)
Edema (<1%)
Erythema multiforme
Exanthems
(1999): Litt JZ, Beachwood, OH (personal case) (observation)
Exfoliation (<1%)
Facial edema (<1%)
Flushing (<1%)
Lichen planus
(1999): Smith KC, Niagara Falls, NY (from Internet) (observation)
Periorbital edema (<1%)
Peripheral edema (<1%)
Photosensitivity (0.03%)
(2000): Ferguson J+, *J Antimicrob Chemother* 45, 503
Phototoxicity
(2000): Traynor NJ+, *Toxicol Vitr* 14, 275
Pruritus (2%)
(1999): Litt JZ, Beachwood, OH (personal case) (observation)
(1998): Mayne JT+, *J Antimicrob Chemother* 39, 67
Pruritus ani (<1%)
Rash (sic) (2%)
Seborrhea (<1%)
Stevens–Johnson syndrome (<1%)
Toxic epidermal necrolysis
(1999): Matthews MR+, *Arch Intern Med* 159, 2225
Ulceration (<1%)
Urticaria (<1%)
Vasculitis

#### Other
Anaphylactoid reactions (<1%)
Dysgeusia (<1%)
Foetor ex ore (halitosis) (<1%)
Gingivitis (<1%)
Hypersensitivity
Injection-site edema (<1%)
Injection-site inflammation (<1%)
Injection-site pain (<1%)
Myalgia (<1%)
Paresthesias (<1%)
Serum sickness
Sialorrhea (<1%)
Stomatitis (<1%)
Tendon rupture
Thrombophlebitis (<1%)
Tongue disorder (<1%)
Tongue edema (<1%)
Vaginitis (<10%)
Xerostomia (<1%)

***Note:** Trovafloxacin has been withdrawn in the USA except for intravenous hospital use

# TRYPTOPHAN

**Scientific name:** *L-2-amino-3-(indole-3yl) propionic acid*
**Other common names:** L-trypt; L-tryptophan
**Family:** None
**Purported indications:** Insomnia, depression, myofascial pain, premenstrual syndrome
**Other uses:** Smoking cessation, bruxism
**Clinically important, potentially hazardous interactions with:** fluoxetine, isocarboxazid, meperidine, phenelzine, sibutramine, tranylcypromine

### *Reactions*

#### Skin
None

#### Other
Eosinophilia–myalgia syndrome
Parkinsonism

**Note:** Tryptophan is an essential amino acid. It is a precursor of serotonin and is also converted to nicotinic acid and nicotinamide

# TURMERIC

**Scientific names:** *Curcuma aromatica; Curcuma domestica; Curcuma longa; Curcuma xanthorrhiza*
**Other common names:** Calebin-A; Chiang Huang; Curcuma; Curcumin; E100; Haridra; Indian Saffron; Jiang Huang; Yellow Root; Yu Jin; Zedoary
**Family:** Zingiberaceae
**Purported indications:** Antiarthritic, antibacterial, antioxidant, anticarcinogen, anti-inflammatory, stimulant, carminative. Used in amenorrhea, angina, asthma colorectal cancer, delirium, diarrhea, dyspepsia, flatulence, hemorrhage, hepatitis, hypercholesterolemia, hypertension, jaundice, mania, menstrual disorders, ophthalmia, tendonitis. Topically for conjuctivitis, skin cancer, smallpox, chickenpox, leg ulcers
**Other uses:** Orange-yellow colour used in cheese, margarine, sweets, snack foods, cosmetics, essential oil in perfumes, culinary spice

### *Reactions*

#### Skin
Allergic contact dermatitis
(1993): Futrell JM+, *Cutis* 52(5), 288
(1987): Goh CL+, *Contact Dermatitis* 17(3), 186
Allergic reactions (sic) (rare)
Contact dermatitis
(1997): Hata M+, *Contact Dermatitis* 36(2), 107

**Note:** Persons with symptoms of gallstones or obstruction of bile passages should avoid turmeric

## UNOPROSTONE

**Synonym:** UF-021
**Trade name:** Rescula (Novartis)
**Indications:** Open-angle glaucoma
**Category:** Ophthalmic anti-glaucoma agent
**Half-life:** 14 minutes

### *Reactions*

#### Skin
Allergic reactions (sic) (1–10%)
Diaphoresis
Eyelid edema
Flu-like syndrome (6%)
Local irritation
(1999): Hejkal TW+, *Semin Ophthalmol* 14, 114
Ocular burning (10–25%)
Ocular pruritus (10–25%)
Ocular stinging (10–25%)
Shivering

#### Hair
Hair – Eyelash length decreased (7%)
Hair – Eyelashes increased in number
(1999): Hejkal TW+, *Semin Ophthalmol* 14, 114
Hair – Hypertrichosis (eyelashes) (10–14%)

#### Other
Iris pigmentation increased
(1999): Hejkal TW+, *Semin Ophthalmol* 14, 114
Myalgia
Ocular erythema
(2001): Aung T+, *Am J Ophthalmol* 131(5), 636
Paresthesias (tongue)
(1998): Stewart WC+, *J Glaucoma* 7, 388
(1996): Haria M+, *Drugs Aging* 9, 213
(1993): Azuma I+, *Jpn J Ophthalmol* 37, 514
Xerostomia
(1998): Stewart WC+, *J Glaucoma* 7, 388
(1996): Haria M+, *Drugs Aging* 9, 213
(1993): Azuma I+, *Jpn J Ophthalmol* 37, 514

## UROKINASE

**Trade name:** Abbokinase (Abbott)
**Other common trade name:** *Ukidan*
**Indications:** Acute myocardial infarction, coronary artery thrombosis, pulmonary embolism
**Category:** Thrombolytic enzyme
**Half-life:** 10–20 minutes
**Clinically important, potentially hazardous interactions with:** aspirin, bivalirudin, ibuprofen, indomethacin

### *Reactions*

#### Skin
Angioedema (>10%)
(2001): Pechlaner C+, *Blood Coagul Fibrinolysis* 12(6), 491
Bleeding (44%)
Bullous eruption (hemorrhagic)
(1995): Ejaz AA+, *Am J Nephrol* 15, 178
Chills
Diaphoresis (<1%)
Ecchymoses
Exanthems
Flushing
Periorbital edema (>10%)
Pruritus
Purpura
Rash (sic) (<1%)
Urticaria

#### Other
Anaphylactoid reactions (>10%)
(2001): Pechlaner C+, *Blood Coagul Fibrinolysis* 12(6), 491
Hypersensitivity
(2001): Pechlaner C+, *Blood Coagul Fibrinolysis* 12(6), 491
Injection-site phlebitis

## URSODIOL

**Trade names:** Actigall (Novartis); Urso (Axcan)
**Other common trade names:** *Arsacol; Cholit-Ursan; Destolit; Litanin; Ursochol; Ursolvan*
**Indications:** Cholelithiasis
**Category:** Gallstone dissolution agent
**Half-life:** 100 hours

### *Reactions*

#### Skin
Diaphoresis
Lichen planus
(1992): Ellul JP+, *Dig Dis Sci* 37, 628
Lichenoid eruption
(2002): Matsuzaki Y+, *Gastroenterology* 122(5), 1547
(2001): Horiuchi Y, *Gastroenterology* 121(2), 501
Pruritus (<1%)
Rash (sic) (<1%)
Urticaria
Xerosis

#### Hair
Hair – alopecia

#### Other
Dysgeusia (<1%) (metallic taste)
Myalgia
Stomatitis

# VALACYCLOVIR

**Trade name:** Valtrex (GSK)
**Indications:** Genital herpes, herpes simplex, herpes zoster
**Category:** antiviral
**Half-life:** 3 hours
**Clinically important, potentially hazardous interactions with:** immunosuppressives, meperidine

### *Reactions*

## Skin

Facial edema (3–5%)
(2000): Colin J+, *Ophthalmology* (107) 1507 (3–5%)
Periorbital edema (3–5%)
(2000): Colin J+, *Ophthalmology* 107, 1507 (3–5%)
Pruritus (generalized)
(2001): Vaughan TK, Tacoma, WA (from Internt) (observation)
Purpura
(2000): Rivaud E+, *Arch Intern Med* 160, 1705
Systemic contact dermatitis
(2001): Lammintausta K+, *Contact Dermatitis* 45(3), 181

# VALDECOXIB

**Trade name:** Bextra (Pharmacia/Pfizer)
**Indications:** Osteoarthritis, adult rheumatoid arthritis, dysmenorrhea
**Category:** Nonsteroidal anti-inflammatory (NSAID); COX-2 inhibitor
**Half-life:** 8–11 hours
**Clinically important, potentially hazardous interactions with:** aspirin, dextromethorphan, lithium, warfarin

### *Reactions*

## Skin

Acne (<2%)
Allergy (sic) (<2%)
Basal cell carcinoma
Candidiasis
Cellulitis (<2%)
Chills (<2%)
Contact dermatitis (<2%)
Dermatitis (sic)
Diaphoresis (<2%)
Ecchymoses (<2%)
Eczema (sic) (<2%)
Edema (<2%)
Exanthems (<2%)
Facial edema (<2%)
Flu-like syndrome (2%)
Hemangioma (<2%)
Hematomas (<2%)
Herpes simplex
Herpes zoster
Hot flashes (<2%)
Malignant melanoma
Periorbital edema (<2%)
Peripheral edema (2–3%)
Photosensitivity (<2%)
Pruritus (<2%)
Psoriasis (<2%)
Rash (sic) (1–2)
Ulceration (<2%)
Upper respiratory tract infection (6–7%)
Urticaria (<2%)
Xerosis (<2%)

## Hair

Hair – alopecia (<2%)

## Other

Arthralgia (<2%)
Back pain (2–3%)
Cough (<2%)
Depression (<2%)
Dysgeusia (<2%)
Foetor ex ore (halitosis) (<2%)
Hyperesthesia (<2%)
Lipoma (<2%)
Myalgia (2%)
Paresthesias (<2%)
Stomatitis (<2%)
Tendinitis (<2%)
Thrombophlebitis (<2%)
Tinnitus (2–10%)
Tooth disorder (sic)
Tremors (<2%)
Twitching (<2%)
Vaginal candidiasis
Xerostomia (<2%)

# VALERIAN

**Scientific names:** *Valeriana edulis; Valeriana jatamansii; Valeriana officinalis; Valeriana sitchensis; Valeriana wallichii*
**Other common names:** All-Heal; Amantilla; Baldrian; Common Valerian; Garden Heliotrope; Valariane; Valeriana
**Family:** Valerianaceae
**Purported indications:** Sedative–hypnotic, anxiolytic, depression, tremors, epilepsy, attention deficit hyperactivity disorder
**Other uses:** Rheumatic pain, nervous asthma, gastric spasms, colic, menstrual cramps, hot flashes. Bath additive for restlessness and sleep disorders. Used as flavoring in foods and beverages

### *Reactions*

## Skin

None

# VALGANCICLOVIR*

**Trade name:** Valcyte (Roche)
**Indications:** Cytomegalovirus retinitis (in patients with AIDS)
**Category:** Antiviral*
**Half-life:** 4 hours (In severe renal impairment up to 68%)

***Note:** Valganciclovir is rapidly converted to ganciclovir in the body

### *Reactions*

## Skin

Allergic reactions (sic) (<5%)

Infections (sic) (<5%)
Rash (sic)

### Other

Paresthesias (8%)
(2001): Curran M+, *Drugs* 61(8), 1145

# VALPROIC ACID

**Trade names:** Depakene (Abbott); Depakote (Abbott)
**Indications:** Seizures, migraine
**Category:** anticonvulsant
**Half-life:** 6-16 hours
**Clinically important, potentially hazardous interactions with:** aspirin, cholestyramine, ivermectin

## *Reactions*

### Skin

Acne
Allergic reactions (sic) (<5%)
Bullous eruption
(2001): Christ EA+ (poster at meeting of the American Federation for Medical Research)
Contact dermatitis
Diaphoresis
(2001): Hebert AA+, *J Clin Psychiatry* 62(suppl 14), 22
Ecchymoses (<5%)
(2001): Christ EA+ (poster at meeting of the American Federation for Medical Research)
(2000): Picart N+, *Presse Med* (French) 29, 648
(1983): Bruni J+, *Arch Neurol* 40, 135
(1978): Lewis JR, *JAMA* 240, 2190
Edema
Erythema multiforme (<1%)
(2001): Hebert AA+, *J Clin Psychiatry* 62(suppl 14), 22
(1990): Chan HL+, *Arch Dermatol* 126, 43
Exanthems (5%)
Facial edema (>5%)
Fixed eruption
(1997): Chan HL+, *J Am Acad Dermatol* 36, 259
Furunculosis (<5%)
Lupus erythematosus
(1996): Park-Matsumoto YC+, *J Neurol Sci* 143, 185
(1994): Fritzler MJ, *Lupus* 3, 455
(1993): Drory VE+, *Clin Neuropharmacol* 16, 19 (passim)
(1990): Bleck TP+, *Epilepsia* 31, 343
Morphea
(1980): Goihman-Yahr M+, *Arch Dermatol* 116, 621
Peripheral edema (<5%)
Petechiae (<5%)
(2001): Hebert AA+, *J Clin Psychiatry* 62(suppl 14), 22
Photosensitivity
(2001): Hebert AA+, *J Clin Psychiatry* 62(suppl a4), 22
Pruritus (>5%)
(2001): Hebert AA+, *J Clin Psychiatry* 62(suppl 14), 22
Psoriasis
Purpura
(1984): *Drugs Ther Bull* 22, 23
(1976): Winfield DA+, *BMJ* 2, 98
Rash (sic) (>5%)
(2002): Gallagher RM+, *J Am Osteopath Assoc* 102(2), 92
(1978): Lewis JR, *JAMA* 240, 2190
Scleroderma
(1980): Goihman-Yahr M+, *Arch Dermatol* 116, 621
Seborrhea
Stevens–Johnson syndrome
(1999): Rzany B+, *Lancet* 353, 2190
(1998): Tsai SJ+, *J Clin Psychopharmacol* 18, 420
Toxic epidermal necrolysis
(1999): Rzany B+, *Lancet* 353, 2190
(1991): Porteous DM+, *Arch Dermatol* 127, 740
Urticaria
Vasculitis
(1991): Kamper AM+, *Lancet* 1, 497

### Hair

Hair – alopecia (7%)
(2002): Gallagher RM+, *J Am Osteopath Assoc* 102(2), 92
(2001): Hebert AA+, *J Clin Psychiatry* 62(suppl 14), 22
(1998): Fetterman M (Miami FL) (from Internet) (observation)
(1996): McKinney PA+, *Ann Clin Psychiatry* 8, 183
(1996): Wallace SJ, *Drug Saf* 15, 378
(1995): Fatemi SH+, *Ann Pharmacother* 29, 1302
(1981): Herranz JL, *Dev Med Child Neurol* 23, 386
(1978): *Drug Ther Bull* 16, 77 (up to 10%)
(1978): Lewis JR, *JAMA* 240, 2190
(1977): Pinder RM+, *Drugs* 13, 81 (.5%)
(1976): Winfield DA+, *BMJ* 2, 981
(1975): Barnes SE+, *Dev Med Child Neurol* 17, 175
(1974): Jeavons PM+, *BMJ* 2, 584
Hair – curly
(1977): Jeavons PM+, *Lancet* 1, 359
Hair – depigmentation
(1981): Herranz JL+, *Dev Med Child Neurol* 23, 386
Hair – kinky
(2001): Caneppele S+, *Ann Dermatol Venereol* 128(2), 134
Hair – perming effect (sic)
(1988): Gupta AK, *Br J Clin Pract* 42, 75

### Other

Acute intermittent porphyria
(1989): Herrick AL+, *Br J Clin Pharmacol* 27, 491
(1980): Garcia-Merino JA+, *Lancet* 2, 856
Aplasia cutis congenita
Dysgeusia (<5%)
Galactorrhea
(1983): Kollipara S+, *J Pediatr* 103, 501
Gingival hyperplasia
(1997): Anderson HH+, *ASDC J Dent Child* 64, 294
(1991): Behari M, *J Neurol Neurosurg Psychiatry* 54, 279
Glossitis (<5%)
Gynecomastia
(1983): Kollipara S+, *J Pediatr* 103, 501
Hypersensitivity
(2000): Moore SJ+, *J Med Genet* 37, 489
(1994): Garcia-Bravo B+, *Contact Dermatitis* 30, 40
Hypesthesia
Myalgia (<5%)
Paresthesias (<5%)
Parkinsonism
(2002): Iijima M, *J Clin Psychiatry* 63(1), 75
Porphyria
(1991): Jalil P+, *Rev Med Chil* 119, 920
(1981): Doss M+, *Lancet* 2, 91
Pseudolymphoma
(2001): Cogrel O+, *Br J Dermatology* 144, 1235
Rhabdomyolysis
(2001): Kottlors M+, *Neuromuscul Disord* 11(8), 757
Seizures
(2001): Lerman-Sagie T+, *Epilepsia* 42(7), 941
Sialorrhea
Stomatitis (<5%)

Tinnitus
(2000): Reeves RR+, *South Med J* 93(10), 1030
Tremors
(2002): Gallagher RM+, *J Am Osteopath Assoc* 102(2), 92
(2002): Tohen M+, *Arch Gen Psychiatry* 59(1), 62 (with lithium)
Vaginitis (<5%)
Xerostomia (<5%)
(2002): Tohen M+, *Arch Gen Psychiatry* 59(1), 62 (with olanzapine)

# VALSARTAN

**Trade name:** Diovan (Novartis)
**Indications:** Hypertension
**Category:** angiotensin II antagonist; antihypertensive
**Half-life:** 9 hours

## *Reactions*

### Skin

Allergic reactions (sic) (>2%)
Angioedema (>2%)
(2000): de la Serna Higuera C, *Med Clin (Barc)* (Spanish) 114, 599
(1998): Frye Cb+, *Pharmacotherapy* 18, 866
Edema (>1%)
(2000): Prat H, *Rev Med Chil* (Spanish) 128, 475
(1996): Corea L+, *Clin Pharmacol Ther* 60, 341
Flushing
(2000): Prat H, *Rev Med Chil* (Spanish) 128, 475
Photosensitivity
(1998): Frye Cb+, *Pharmacotherapy* (18) 866
Pruritus (>2%)
Rash (sic) (>2%)
Urticaria
(2000): de la Serna Higuera C, *Med Clin (Barc)* (Spanish) 114, 599

### Nails

Nails – bed changes (sic)
Nails – pigmentation

### Other

Aphthous stomatitis (1–10%)
Arthralgia (1–10%)
Cough
(2000): Prat H, *Rev Med Chil* 128, 475
Death
(2001): Briggs GG+, *Ann Pharmacother* 35(7), 859
Dysgeusia (>10%)
Infusion-site extravasation (<1%)
Infusion-site phlebitis
Infusion-site reactions (sic)
Injection-site pain
Myalgia (10–29%)
Paresthesias (>2%)
Xerostomia (>10%)

# VANCOMYCIN

**Trade name:** Vancocin (Lilly)
**Other common trade names:** *Balcoran; Diatracin; Vanmicina*
**Indications:** Various infections caused by susceptible organisms
**Category:** Narrow-spectrum antibiotic
**Half-life:** 5–11 hours
**Clinically important, potentially hazardous interactions with:** succinylcholine

## *Reactions*

### Skin

Acute generalized exanthematous pustulosis (AGEP)
(1996): Sawhney RA+, *Int J Dermatol* 35, 826
(1995): Moreau A+, *Int J Dermatol* 34, 263 (passim)
(1991): Roujeau J-C+, *Arch Dermatol* 127, 1333
Allergic reactions (sic) (<5%)
(2001): Bernedo N+, *Contact Dermatitis* 45(1), 43
(1997): Kahata S+, *Bone Marrow Transplant* 20, 1001
(1992): Breathnach SM+, *Adverse Drug Reactions and the Skin* Blackwell, Oxford, 158 (passim)
Angioedema
(1989): Koestner B+, *Schweiz Med Wochenschr* (German) 119, 28
(1959): Rothenberg HJ, *JAMA* 171, 1102
Bullous eruption
(1996): Heald PW, *Skin and Allergy News* 27, 18
(1992): Carpenter S+, *J Am Acad Dermatol* 26, 45
(1990): Forrence EA+, *Drug Intell Clin Pharm* 24, 369
(1988): Baden LA+, *Arch Dermatol* 124, 1186
Chills (>10%)
Cutaneous reactions (sic)
(1997): Korman TM+, *J Antimicrob Chemother* 39, 371
Erythema multiforme
(2001): Hsu SI, *Pharmacotherapy* 21(10), 1233
(2000): Padial MA+, *Allergy* 55, 1201
(1992): Laurencin CT, *Ann Pharmacotherapy* 26, 1520
(1988): Gutfeld MB+, *Drug Intell Clin Pharm* 22, 881
Exanthems
(1991): McCullough JM+, *Drug Intell Clin Pharm* 25, 1326
(1991): Valero R+, *J Cardiothorac Vasc Anesth* 5, 574
(1988): Neal D+, *BMJ* 296, 137
(1988): Schlemmer B+, *N Engl J Med* 318, 1127
(1987): Lacouture PG+, *J Pediatr* 111, 615 (35%)
(1987): Longon P+, *Presse Med* (French) 16, 682
(1986): Davis RL+, *Ann Intern Med* 104, 285
(1986): Markman M+, *South Med J* 79, 382 (passim)
(1986): McElrath MJ+, *Lancet* 1, 47
(1985): Schifter S+, *Lancet* 2, 499 (8%)
(1984): Odio C+, *Am J Dis Child* 138, 17
(1984): Rimailho A+, *Presse Med* (French) 13, 567
(1960): Kirby WMM+, *N Engl J Med* 262, 49 (1–5%)
Exfoliative dermatitis
(1990): Forrence EA+, *Drug Intell Clin Pharm* 24, 369
(1988): Gutfeld MB+, *Drug Intell Clin Pharm* 22, 881
(1988): Neal D+, *BMJ* 296, 137
Flushing (1–10%)
Linear IgA bullous dermatosis
(2002): Cohen LM+, *J Am Acad Dermatol* 46(2), S32
(2002): Neughebauer BI+, *Am J Med Sci* 323(5), 273
(2001): Ahkami R+, *Cutis* 67, 423
(2001): Chang A+, *Arch Dermatol* 137, 815
(2001): Palmer RA+, *Br J Dermatol* 145(5), 816 (2 cases)
(2001): Wiadrowski TP+, *Austral J Dermatol* 42, 196 (with ciprofloxacin)
(2000): Klein PA+, *J Am Acad Dermatol* 42, 316

(1999): Nousari HC+, *Medicine* 78, 1
(1998): Bernstein EF+, *Ann Intern Med* 129, 508
(1998): Nousari HC+, *Ann Intern Med* 129, 507
(1997): Norland A, Minneapolis, American Academy of Dermatology Meeting (SF) (Gross and Microscopic)
(1996): Bitman LM+, *Arch Dermatol* 1289
(1996): Primka E+, *J Cutan Pathol* 58
(1996): Tranvan A+, *J Am Acad Dermatol* 865
(1996): Whitworth JM+, *J Am Acad Dermatol* 890
(1995): Geissmann C+, *J Am Acad Dermatol* 296
(1995): Richards S+, *Arch Dermatol* 1447
(1994): Kuechle MK+, *J Am Acad Dermatol* 187
(1994): Piketty C+, *Br J Dermatol* 130
(1992): Carpenter S+, *J Am Acad Dermatol* 45
(1988): Baden LA+, *Arch Dermatol* 1186

Lupus erythematosus
(1993): Ena J+, *JAMA* 269, 598
(1986): Markman M+, *South Med J* 79, 382

Photoallergic reaction
(2001): Zabawski E, Longview, TX (from Internet) (observation)

Pruritus
(1991): Killian AD+, *Ann Intern Med* 115, 410
(1991): McCullough JM+, *Drug Intell Clin Pharm* 25, 1326
(1989): Koestner B+, *Schweiz Med Wochenschr* (German) 119, 28
(1986): Davis RL+, *Ann Intern Med* 104, 285
(1959): Rothenberg HJ, *JAMA* 171, 1102

Purpura
(1998): Michael S+, *Scand J Rheumatol* 27, 233

Rash (sic)
(2001): Hsu SI, *Pharmacotherapy* 21(10), 1233
(1997): Reis AG+, *Rev Paul Med* 115, 1452
(1993): Ena J+, *JAMA* 269, 598
(1983): Farber BF+, *Antimicrob Agents Chemother* 23, 138
(1978): Hook EW+, *Am J Med* 65, 411
(1976): Arndt KA+, *JAMA* 235, 918 (10%)

Red man syndrome* (1–10%)
(2002): Cohen E+, *J Antimicrob Chemother* 49(1), 155 (10–14%)
(2001): Wazny LD+, *Ann Pharmacother* 35(11), 1458
(2000): Wood MJ, *J Chemother* 12, 21
(1999): Khurana C+, *Postgrad Med J* 75, 41
(1998): Polk RE, *Ann Pharmacother* 32, 840
(1996): Szymusiak-Mutnick BA+, *Am J Health Syst Pharm* 53, 2098
(1995): Lilley LL+, *Am J Nurs* 95, 14
(1994): Bergeron L+, *Ann Pharmacother* 28, 581
(1993): Ena J+, *JAMA* 269, 598
(1993): O'Sullivan TL+, *J Infect Dis* 168, 773
(1993): Polk RE+, *Antimicrob Agents Chemother* 37, 2139
(1992): Levy M+, *Harefuah* (Hebrew) 122, 36
(1992): Rengo C+, *Recenti Prog Med* (Italian) 83, 726
(1991): Killian AD+, *Ann Intern Med* 115, 410
(1991): Maccabruni A+, *Recenti Prog Med* (Italian) 82, 17
(1991): Valero R+, *J Cardiothorac Vasc Anesth* 5, 574
(1991): Wallace MR+, *J Infect Dis* 164, 1180
(1990): Bailie GR+, *Clin Pharm* 9, 671
(1990): Healey DP+, *Antimicrob Agents Chemother* 34, 550
(1990): Levy M+, *Pediatrics* 86, 572
(1990): No Author, *Lancet* 335, 1006
(1990): Sahai J+, *Antimicrob Agents Chemother* 34, 765
(1989): Pearson DA, *J Am Dent Assoc* 118, 59
(1989): Sahai J+, *J Infect Dis* 160, 876
(1988): Polk RE+, *J Infect Dis* 157, 502
(1988): Rubin M+, *Ann Intern Med* 108, 30 (3%)
(1987): Duro JC+, *Med Clin (Barc)* (Spanish) 89, 218
(1986): Daly BM+, *Drug Intell Clin Pharm* 20, 986
(1986): Davis RL+, *Ann Intern Med* 104, 285
(1986): Rolston KV+, *JAMA* 255, 2445
(1986): Wade TP+, *Arch Surg* 121, 859
(1985): Cole DR+, *Lancet* 2, 280
(1985): Garrelts JC+, *N Engl J Med* 312, 245
(1985): Holliman R, *Lancet* 1, 1399

Red neck syndrome (sic)
(1985): Ackerman BH+, *Ann Intern Med* 102, 723
(1985): Pau AK+, *N Engl J Med* 313, 756

Stevens–Johnson syndrome (<1%)
(1996): Alexander II+, *Allergy Asthma Proc* 17, 75
(1995): Patterson R+, *Allergy Proc* 16, 115
(1992): Laurencin CT+, *Ann Pharmacother* 26, 1520
(1990): Forrence EA+, *Drug Intell Clin Pharm* 24, 369

Toxic epidermal necrolysis
(2001): Hsu SI, *Pharmacotherapy* 21(10), 1233
(2000): Chan-Tack K, *Mo Med* 97, 131
(1992): Vidal C+, *Ann Allergy* 68, 345
(1990): Hannah BA+, *South Med J* 83, 720
(1985): Heng MCY, *Br J Dermatol* 113, 597

Urticaria
(1989): Koestner B+, *Schweiz Med Wochenschr* (German) 119, 28
(1988): Neal D+, *BMJ* 296, 137
(1987): Longon P+, *Presse Med* (French) 16, 682
(1986): Davis RL+, *Ann Intern Med* 104, 285
(1986): Markman M+, *South Med J* 79, 382 (passim)
(1960): Kirby WMM+, *N Engl J Med* 262, 49 (1–5%)
(1959): Rothenberg HJ, *JAMA* 171, 1102 (1–5%)

Vasculitis (<1%)
(1987): Rawlinson WD+, *Med J Australia* 147, 470
(1986): Markman M+, *South Med J* 79, 382

## Other

Anaphylactoid reactions
(2001): Wazny LD+, *Ann Pharmacother* 35(11), 1458
(2000): Chopra N+, *Ann Allergy Asthma Immunol* 84, 633
(1992): Breathnach SM+, *Adverse Drug Reactions and the Skin* Blackwell, Oxford, 158 (passim)
(1988): Rubin M+, *Ann Intern Med* 108, 30 (1 in 63 patients)
(1987): Longon P+, *Presse Med* (French) 16, 682
(1986): Markman M+, *Southern Med J* 79, 382 (passim)

Death
(2001): Hsu SI, *Pharmacotherapy* 21(10), 1233

Dysgeusia (>10%)

Hypersensitivity
(2001): Hsu SI, *Pharmacotherapy* 21(10), 1233
(1997): Marik PE+, *Pharmacotherapy* 17, 1341

Injection-site thrombophlebitis

Paresthesias

Phlebitis
(2002): Cohen E+, *J Antimicrob Chemother* 49(1), 155 (14–23%)
(1983): Farber BF+, *Antimicrob Agents Chemother* 23, 138
(1978): Hook EW+, *Am J Med* 65, 411

Priapism
(1998): Czachor JS+, *N Engl J Med* 338, 1701

Tinnitus

***Note:** The vancomycin-induced red man syndrome is characterized by pruritus, erythema and, in severe cases, angioedema, hypotension, and cardiovascular collapse

# VASOPRESSIN

**Synonyms:** ADH; antidiuretic hormone
**Trade name:** Pitressin (Parke-Davis)
**Other common trade name:** *Pressyn*
**Indications:** Diabetes insipidus
**Category:** Vasoconstrictor and antidiuretic pituitary hormone; vasopressor; antidiuretic
**Half-life:** 10–20 minutes

### *Reactions*

#### Skin
Allergic reactions (sic) (<1%)
Angioedema
Bullous eruption
(1997): Lin RY+, *Dermatology* 195, 271
(1991): Colemont LJ+, *J Clin Gastroenterol* 13, 91
(1986): Korenberg RJ+, *J Am Acad Dermatol* 15, 393
Diaphoresis (1–10%)
Ecchymoses
(1997): Lin RY+, *Dermatology* 195, 271
(1985): Thomas TK, *Am J Gastroenterol* 80, 704
Exanthems
Pallor (1–10%)
Purpura
(1996): Lemlich G+, *Cutis* 57, 330
(1985): Thomas TK, *Am J Gastroenterol* 80, 704
Rash (sic)
Urticaria (1–10%)

#### Hair
Hair – alopecia
(1994): Maceyko RD+, *J Am Acad Dermatol* 31, 111

#### Other
Anaphylactoid reactions
Death
(2001): Rizzo V+, *J Pediatr Endocrinol Metab* 14(7), 861
Gangrene
(1997): Lin RY+, *Dermatology* 195, 271
Infusion-site necrosis
(1997): Lin RY+, *Dermatology* 195, 271 (amber-like)
(1996): Lemlich G+, *Cutis* 57, 330
(1991): Colemont LJ+, *J Clin Gastroenterol* 13, 91
(1990): Stump DL+, *Drugs* 39, 38
(1986): Korenberg RJ+, *J Am Acad Dermatol* 15, 393
(1985): Thomas TK, *Am J Gastroenterol* 80, 704
Rhabdomyolysis
(1995): Hino A+, *Rinsho Shinkeigaku* 35(8), 911
(1993): de Cuenca Moron B+, *Rev Clin Esp* 192(2), 79
(1993): Pierce ST+, *Am J Gastroenterol* 88(3), 424
(1991): Moreno-Sanchez D+, *Gastroenterology* 101(2), 529
(1991): Moreno-Sanchez D+, *Rev Esp Enferm Dig* 79(2), 160
Trembling
Tremors (1–10%)

# VENLAFAXINE

**Trade name:** Effexor (Wyeth-Ayerst)
**Indications:** Depression
**Category:** Heterocyclic antidepressant; selective serotonin reuptake inhibitor (SSRI)
**Half-life:** 3–7 hours
**Clinically important, potentially hazardous interactions with:** isocarboxazid, linezolid, MAO inhibitors, metoclopramide, phenelzine, selegiline, sibutramine, sumatriptan, tramadol, tranylcypromine, trazodone

### *Reactions*

#### Skin
Acne (<1%)
Allergic reactions (sic) (<1%)
Candidiasis
Contact dermatitis
Diaphoresis (12%)
(2002): Fisher AA+, *Ann Pharmacother* 36(1), 67
(2000): Gelenberg AJ+, *JAMA* 283, 3082
(2000): Pierre JM+, *J Clin Psychopharmacol* 20, 269
Ecchymoses (<1%)
Eczema (sic) (<1%)
Edema (<1%)
Exanthems (<1%)
Exfoliative dermatitis (<1%)
Facial edema (<1%)
Flushing
(2001): Grady-Weliky TA+, *Am J Psychiatry* 158(8), 1330
Furunculosis (<1%)
Herpes simplex (<1%)
Herpes zoster (<1%)
Lichenoid eruption (<1%)
Peripheral edema
Photosensitivity (<1%)
Pruritus (1–10%)
Psoriasis (<1%)
Pustular eruption (<1%)
Rash (sic) (3%)
Urticaria (<1%)
Vesiculobullous eruption (<1%)
Xerosis (<1%)

#### Hair
Hair – alopecia (<1%)
(2001): Pitchot W+, *Am J Psych* 158, 1159
Hair – discoloration (<1%)
Hair – hirsutism (<1%)

#### Other
Ageusia (<1%)
Bromhidrosis (<1%)
Bruxism
(2000): Jaffee MS+, *Psychosomatics* 41(6), 535
Dysgeusia (2%)
Gingivitis (<1%)
Glossitis (<1%)
Gynecomastia (<1%)
Hyperesthesia (<1%)
Hypesthesia (>1%)
Mastodynia
(2000): Bhatia SC+, *J Clin Psychopharmacol* 20(5), 590
(1996): Bhatia SC+, *J Clin Psychiatry* 57, 423

Myalgia (>1%)
Oral ulceration (<1%)
Paresthesias (3%)
Parosmia (<1%)
Serotonin syndrome
(2002): Fisher AA+, *Ann Pharmacother* 36(1), 67
(2001): McCue RE+, *Am J Psychiatry* 158(12), 2088
Sialorrhea (<1%)
Stomatitis (<1%)
Thrombophlebitis (<1%)
Tinnitus
Tongue edema (<1%)
Tongue pigmentation (<1%)
Tremors (1–10%)
Vaginal candidiasis (<1%)
Vaginitis
Xerostomia (22%)
(2000): Gelenberg AJ+, *JAMA* 283, 3082

# VERAPAMIL

**Trade names:** Calan (Searle); Covera-HS (Pharmacia); Isoptin (Abbott); Tarka (Abbott); Verelan (Schwarz)
**Other common trade names:** *APO-Verap; Arpamyl LP; Azupamil; Berkatens; Chronovera; Cordilox; Geangin; Isoptine; Nu-Verap; Veraken*
**Indications:** Angina, hypertension
**Category:** Calcium channel blocker; antianginal; antihypertensive and antiarrhythmic
**Half-life:** 2–8 hours
**Clinically important, potentially hazardous interactions with:** acebutolol, amiodarone, aspirin, atenolol, atorvastatin, betaxolol, carbamazepine, carteolol, clonidine, dantrolene, digoxin, dofetilide, epirubicin, esmolol, lovastatin, metoprolol, **mistletoe**, nadolol, penbutolol, pindolol, propranolol, quinidine, sibutramine, simvastatin, timolol

Tarka is trandolapril and verapamil

### *Reactions*

## Skin

Acne
(1989): Stern R+, *Arch Intern Med* 149, 829
Acute febrile neutrophilic dermatosis (Sweet's syndrome)
(1998): Knowles S+, *J Am Acad Dermatol* 38, 201 (passim)
Angioedema
(1998): Knowles S+, *J Am Acad Dermatol* 38, 201 (passim)
(1989): Sadick NS+, *J Am Acad Dermatol* 21, 132
(1989): Stern R+, *Arch Intern Med* 149, 829
Ankle edema
Cutaneous side effects (sic)
(1993): Kitamura K+, *J Dermatol* 20, 279 (psoriasiform)
(1989): McTavish D+, *Drugs* 38, 19. (0.6%)
Dermatitis (sic)
Diaphoresis (<1%)
(1989): Stern R+, *Arch Intern Med* 149, 829
(1983): Lewis JG, *Drugs* 25, 196
Ecchymoses (<1%)
(1989): Sadick NS+, *J Am Acad Dermatol* 21, 132
Edema (1.9%)
Erythema multiforme (<1%)
(1991): Kürkçüoglu N+, *J Am Acad Dermatol* 24, 511
(1989): Lin AYF+, *Drug Intell Clin Pharm* 23, 987
(1989): Stern R+, *Arch Intern Med* 149, 829
(1987): Naito S+, *Skin Res* (Japanese) 29, 602
Erythema nodosum
(1998): Knowles S+, *J Am Acad Dermatol* 38, 201 (passim)
Exanthems
(1998): Knowles S+, *J Am Acad Dermatol* 38, 201 (passim)
(1989): McTavish D+, *Drugs* 38, 19
(1989): Sadick NS+, *J Am Acad Dermatol* 21, 132
(1989): Stern R+, *Arch Intern Med* 149, 829
(1983): Lewis JG, *Drugs* 25, 196 (3.2%)
(1982): Anon, *Lakartidningen* (Swedish) 79, 3822
(1980): Midtbo K+, *Curr Ther Res* 27, 830
Exfoliative dermatitis
(1998): Knowles S+, *J Am Acad Dermatol* 38, 201 (passim)
(1989): Stern R+, *Arch Intern Med* 149, 829
Flushing (1–7%)
(1992): Shelley WB+, *Advanced Dermatologic Diagnosis* WB Saunders, 583 (passim)
(1989): McTavish D+, *Drugs* 38, 19 (1–5.4%)
(1983): Lewis JG, *Drugs* 25, 196 (4–7%)
(1980): Raftos J, *Med J Aust* 2, 78
Hyperkeratosis (palms) (<1%)
(1989): Sadick NS+, *J Am Acad Dermatol* 21, 132
(1983): Major P, *Tidsskr Nor Laegeforen* (Norwegian), 103, 2061
Lichenoid eruption
Lupus erythematosus
(1998): Callen JP, Academy '98 Meeting (4 patients)
(1997): Crowson AN+, *Hum Pathol* 28, 67 (subacute cutaneous)
Peripheral edema (1–10%)
(2002): No author, *Medscape Primary Care 4*
Photosensitivity
(1994): Berger TG+, *Arch Dermatol* 130, 609 (in HIV-infected)
(1989): McTavish D+, *Drugs* 38, 19
(1983): Lewis JG, *Drugs* 25, 196
(1979): Anon, *Med J Aust* 2, 204
Prurigo (sic)
(1983): Lewis JG, *Drugs* 25, 196
Pruritus
(1998): Knowles S+, *J Am Acad Dermatol* 38, 201 (passim)
(1989): McTavish D+, *Drugs* 38, 19
(1989): Stern R+, *Arch Intern Med* 149, 829
(1988): Burgunder JM+, *Hepatogastroenterology* 35, 169
(1983): Lewis JG, *Drugs* 25, 196
(1982): Fischer Hansen J+, *Clin Exp Pharmacol Physiol* 6, 31
Purpura (<1%)
(1982): *Lakartidningen* (Swedish) 79, 3822
Rash (sic) (1.2%)
(1989): Stern R+, *Arch Intern Med* 149, 829
(1987): Johnson BF+, *Clin Pharmacol Ther* 42, 66
Stevens–Johnson syndrome (<1%)
(1998): Knowles S+, *J Am Acad Dermatol* 38, 201 (passim)
(1992): Gonski PN, *Med J Aust* 156, 672
(1989): Lin AYF+, *Drug Intell Clin Pharm* 23, 987
(1989): Stern R+, *Arch Intern Med* 149, 829
Urticaria (<1%)
(1998): Knowles S+, *J Am Acad Dermatol* 38, 201 (passim)
(1989): McTavish D+, *Drugs* 38, 19
(1989): Sadick NS+, *J Am Acad Dermatol* 21, 132
(1989): Stern R+, *Arch Intern Med* 149, 829
(1983): Lewis JG, *Drugs* 25, 196
Vasculitis (<1%)
(1989): Sadick NS+, *J Am Acad Dermatol* 21, 132
(1983): Lewis JG, *Drugs* 25, 196

## Hair

Hair – alopecia (<1%)
(1994): Litt JZ, Beachwood, OH (personal case) (observation)
(1991): Shelley WB+, *Cutis* 48, 364 (observation)
(1989): Sadick NS+, *J Am Acad Dermatol* 21, 132

(1989): Stern R+, *Arch Intern Med* 149, 829
(1981): Rosing DR+, *Am J Cardiol* 48, 545
(1980): Rosing DR+, *Chest* 78 (Suppl), 239
Hair – hypertrichosis
(1991): Sever PS, *Lancet* 338, 1215
Hair – pigmentation
(1991): Read GM, *Lancet* 338, 1520

### Nails

Nails – dystrophy
(1989): Stern R+, *Arch Intern Med* 149, 829

### Other

Erythromelalgia
(1992): Drenth JP+, *Br J Dermatol* 127, 292
Galactorrhea (<1%)
Gingival hyperplasia (19%)
(1995): Moghadam BKH+, *Cutis* 56, 46 (passim)
(1993): Steele RM+, *Arch Intern Med* 120, 663
(1989): Pernu HE+, *J Oral Pathol Med* 18, 422
(1987): Giustiniani S+, *Int J Cardiol* 15, 247
Gynecomastia (<1%)
(2000): Hugues FC+, *Ann Med Interne (Paris)* (French) 151, 10 (passim)
(1994): Deniel-Rosanas J, *Med Clin (Barc)* (Spanish) 102, 399
(1994): *BMJ* 308, 503
(1988): Tanner LA+, *Arch Intern Med* 148, 379
Paresthesias (<1%)
Parkinsonism
Rhabdomyolysis
(2000): Gokel Y+, *Am J Emerg Med* 18, 738 (with trandolapril)
Serum sickness
(1989): Pascual-Velasco F, *Med Clin (Barc)* (Spanish) 92, 719
Xerostomia (<1%)

## VERTEPORFIN

**Trade name:** Visudyne (Novartis)
**Indications:** wet form of age-related macular degeneration
**Category:** macular degeneration adjunct; photosensitizer
**Half-life:** 5-6 hours

#### *Reactions*

### Skin

Burning mouth (1–10%)
(1998): Mitchell D, Thomasville, GA (from Internet) (observation)
Cheilitis
(1998): Mitchell D, Thomasville, GA (from Internet) (observation)
Chills
Diaphoresis
Eczema (sic) (1–10%)
Erythema
Flu-like syndrome (1–10%)
Ocular pruritus
Pallor
Photosensitivity (<3%)
(2000): Scott LJ+, *Drugs Aging* 16, 139
Pigmentation
Pruritus
Purpura
Rash (sic)
Shivering
Ulceration
Urticaria
(1998): Mitchell D, Thomasville, GA (generalized) (from Internet) (observation)
Vesicular eruptions
(1998): Mitchell D, Thomasville, GA (from Internet) (observation)

### Other

Arthralgia (1–10%)
Hypesthesia (1–10%)
Infusion-related back pain
(2000): Scott LJ+, *Drugs Aging* 16, 139
Injection-site reactions (sic)
Paresthesias

## VIDARABINE

**Synonyms:** adenine arabinoside; ara-A
**Trade name:** Vira-A Ophthalmic (Parke-Davis)
**Other common trade names:** *Adena a Ungena; Arasena*
**Indications:** Herpetic keratoconjunctivitis
**Category:** Ophthalmic antiviral
**Half-life:** 3.3 hours
**Clinically important, potentially hazardous interactions with:** insulin

#### *Reactions*

### Skin

Ocular burning
Ocular erythema
Ocular pruritus
Pruritus
Rash (sic)

## VINBLASTINE

**Trade name:** Velban (Lilly)
**Indications:** Lymphomas, melanoma, carcinomas
**Category:** Antineoplastic
**Half-life:** initial phase: 3.7 minutes; terminal phase: 24.8 hours
**Clinically important, potentially hazardous interactions with:** aldesleukin, erythromycin, fluconazole, itraconazole, ketoconazole, miconazole

#### *Reactions*

### Skin

Acne
(1962): Falkson G+, *Br J Dermatol* 74, 229
Acral gangrene
(1998): Reiser M+, *Eur J Clin Microbiol Infect Dis* 17, 58
(1997): Hladunewich M+, *J Rheumatol* 24, 2371
Bullous eruption (<1%)
Cellulitis
(1983): Bronner AK+, *J Am Acad Dermatol* 9, 645
Dermatitis (sic) (1–10%)
Erythema
(1969): Lampkin BC, *Lancet* 1, 891
Erythema multiforme
(1991): Arias D+, *J Cutan Pathol* 18, 344
Exanthems
Photosensitivity (1–10%)

(1992): Breathnach SM+, *Adverse Drug Reactions and the Skin* Blackwell, Oxford, 302 (passim)
(1975): Breza TS+, *Arch Dermatol* 111, 1168
Phototoxicity
Pigmentation
(2001): Mutafoglu-Uysal K+, *Turk J Pediatr* 43(2), 172
(1997): Smith KJ+, *J Am Acad Dermatol* 36, 329
(1994): Cecchi R+, *Dermatology* 188, 244
Purpura
Radiation recall
(1992): Nemechek PM+, *Cancer* 70, 1605
Radiodermatitis (reactivation)
(1969): Lampkin BC, *Lancet* 1, 891
Rash (sic) (1–10%)
Raynaud's phenomenon (1–10%)
(1998): Reiser M+, *Eur J Clin Microbiol Infect Dis* 17, 58
(1997): Hladunewich M+, *J Rheumatol* 24, 2371
(1993): von Gunten CF+, *Cancer* 72, 2004
(1992): Doll DC+, *Semin Oncol* 19(5), 580
(1981): Harvey HA+, *Ann Intern Med* 94, 542
(1981): Vogelzang NJ+, *Ann Intern Med* 95, 288
(1978): Rothberg H, *Cancer Treat Rep* 62, 569
(1977): Teutsch C+, *Cancer Treat Rep* 61, 925
Urticaria

### Hair

Hair – alopecia (>10%)
(1992): Breathnach SM+, *Adverse Drug Reactions and the Skin* Blackwell, Oxford, 302 (passim)
Hair – changes (sic)
(1971): Kostanecki W+, *Z Haut Geschlechtskr* (German) 46, 704

### Other

Dysgeusia (>10%) (metallic taste)
Hypersensitivity
(2001): Mutafoglu-Uysal K+, *Turk J Pediatr* 43(2), 172
Injection-site extravasation
(2000): Kassner E, *J Pediatr Oncon Nurs* 17, 135
Injection-site necrosis
(1992): Misery L+, *Presse Med* (French) 21, 2153
(1991): Arias D+, *J Cutan Pathol* 18, 344
Injection-site pain
Myalgia (1–10%)
Oral mucosal lesions
(1978): Levine N+, *Cancer Treat Rev* 5, 67 (1–5%)
Paresthesias (1–10%)
Phlebitis
(1989): Kerker BJ+, *Semin Dermatol* 8, 173
Rhabdomyolysis
(1995): Anderlini P+, *Cancer* 76(4), 678
Stomatitis (>10%)
Ulceration due to extravasation
Vesiculation of mouth (sic)

## VINCRISTINE

**Trade names:** Oncovin (Lilly); Vincasar (Pharmacia & Upjohn)
**Indications:** Leukemias, lymphomas, neuroblastoma, Wilm's tumor
**Category:** Antineoplastic
**Half-life:** 24 hours
**Clinically important, potentially hazardous interactions with:** aldesleukin, fluconazole, itraconazole, ketoconazole, miconazole

### *Reactions*

### Skin

Acral erythema
(1995): Komamura H+, *J Dermatol* 22(2), 116 (with cyclosphamide, doxorubicin and G-CSF)
Actinic keratosis inflammation
(1987): Johnson TM+, *J Am Dermatol* 17(2 Pt 1), 192
Angioedema
(1984): Gassel WD+, *Oncology* 41, 403
Dermatitis herpetiformis
(1986): Gottlieb D+, *Med J Aust* 145, 241 (flare)
Edema
Erythroderma
(1989): Matsumoto N+, *Gan To Kagaku Ryoho* (Japanese) 16, 2297
(1984): Gassel WD+, *Oncology* 41, 403
Exanthems
(1984): Gassel WD+, *Oncology* 41, 403
(1978): Levine N+, *Cancer Treat Rev* 5, 67
(1972): Zanoni G+, *Blut* (German) 25, 20
Palmar–plantar erythema
(1990): Pagliuca A+, *Postgrad Med J* 66, 242
Pruritus
(1978): Levine N+, *CancerTreat Rev* 5, 67
Rash (sic) (1–10%)
Raynaud's phenomenon
(1998): Reiser M+, *Eur J Clin Microbiol Infect Dis* 17, 58
Serpentine supravenous hyperpigmentation (sic)
(2000): Marcoux D+, *J Am Acad Dermatol* 43, 540 (with dactinomycin)
Sjøgren's syndrome
(1989): Monno S+, *Jpn J Med* 28, 399
Urticaria

### Hair

Hair – alopecia (20–70%)
(1987): David J+, *Nurs Times* 83, 36
(1973): Levantine A+, *Br J Dermatol* 89, 549 (>5%)
(1971): Helson L+, *N Engl J Med* 284, 336
(1970): O'Brien R+, *N Engl J Med* 283, 1469
(1966): Simister JM, *BMJ* 2, 1138
(1964): Knock FE, *Med Clin North Am* 48, 501 (>5%)
(1963): Martin J+, *Lancet* 2, 1080 (47%)

### Nails

Nails – Beau's lines (transverse nail bands)
(1994): Ben-Dayan D+, *Acta Haematol* 91, 89
Nails – leukonychia
(1990): Bader-Meunier B+, *Ann Pediatr Paris* (French) 37, 337 (transverse)
Nails – Mees' lines
(1983): James WD+, *Arch Dermatol* 119, 334
(1982): Jeanmougin M+, *Ann Dermatol Venereol* (French) 109, 169
Nails – onychodermal band

(1993): Kowal-Vern A+, *Cutis* 52, 43 (plus erythema of proximal nail fold)

### Other

Anaphylactoid reactions
Dysgeusia (1–10%) (metallic taste)
Injection-site cellulitis (>10%)
(1983): BronnerAK+, *J Am Acad Dermatol* 9, 645
Injection-site extravasation
(2000): Kassner E, *J Pediatr Oncon Nurs* 17, 135
Injection-site necrosis (>10%)
Myalgia (1–10%)
Oral mucosal lesions (1–10%)
(1989): KerkerBJ+, *Semin Dermatol* 8, 173 (1–5%)
(1964): Knock FE, *Med Clin North Am* 48, 501
Oral ulceration (1–10%)
Paresthesias (1–10%)
Phlebitis (1–10%)
Stomatitis (<1%)

## VINORELBINE

**Trade name:** Navelbine (GSK)
**Indications:** Non-small cell lung cancer
**Category:** Antineoplastic
**Half-life:** 28–44 hours
**Clinically important, potentially hazardous interactions with:** aldesleukin

#### *Reactions*

### Skin

Acral erythrodysesthesia syndrome (hand–foot syndrome)
(1998): Hoff PM+, *Cancer* 82, 965
Angioedema
Erythema
Flushing
Pigmentation
(1994): Cecchi R+, *Dermatology* 188, 244
Pruritus
Rash (sic) (<5%)
Toxic epidermal necrolysis
(1992): Misery L+, *Presse Med* (French) 21, 2153

### Hair

Hair – alopecia (12%)
(1994): Gasparini G+, *J Clin Oncol* 12, 2094
(1989): Marty M+, *Nouv Rev Fr Hematol* (French) 31, 77

### Other

Anaphylactoid reactions
Dysgeusia (>10%) (metallic taste)
Extravasation
(2001): Bertelli G+, *Tumori* 87(2), 112
Hyperesthesia (1–10%)
Infusion-site pain
(2001): Long TD+, *Am J Clin Oncol* 24(4), 414
Injection-site irritation (1–10%)
Injection-site necrosis (1–10%)
Injection-site pain (1.6%)
Injection-site phlebitis
(1998): Sauter C+, *Schweiz Med Wochenschr* (German) 128, 343
(1989): Marty M+, *Nouv Rev Fr Hematol* (French) 31, 77 (12%)
Myalgia (<5%)
Paresthesias (1–10%)
Phlebitis (7%)
Stomatitis (>10%)
(1989): Marty M+, *Nouv Rev Fr Hematol* (French) 31, 77 (12%)

## VITAMIN A

**Trade names:** Aquasol A (AstraZeneca); Del-Vi-A (DelRay); Palmitate A
**Other common trade names:** *Acaren; Acon; Afaxin; Arovit; Avipur; Avitin; Axerol; Dolce; Vogan*
**Indications:** Vitamin A deficiency
**Category:** Nutritional fat-soluble vitamin supplement
**Half-life:** no data
**Clinically important, potentially hazardous interactions with:** acitretin, bexarotene, **fish oil supplements**, isotretinoin, minocycline, tetracycline, warfarin

#### *Reactions*

### Skin

Cheilitis
Contact dermatitis
(1996): Bazzano C+, *Contact Dermatitis* 35, 261
(1995): Heidenheim M+, *Contact Dermatitis* 33, 439
(1994): Manzano A+, *Contact Dermatitis* 31, 324
(1994): Sanz de Galdeano C+, *Contact Dermatitis* 30, 50
(1984): Blondeel A, *Contact Dermatitis* 11, 191
Dermatitis (sic) (dry, scaly and keratotic – mainly palms and soles)
(1971): Muenter MD+, *Am J Med* 50, 129
(1958): Oliver TK, *Am J Dis Child* 95, 57
Eczematous eruption (pellagra-like)
(1982): Hamann K+, *Hautarzt* (German) 33, 559
Erythema
(1992): Breathnach SM+, *Adverse Drug Reactions and the Skin* Blackwell, Oxford, 254 (passim)
Erythema multiforme (<1%)
(1971): Muenter MD+, *Am J Med* 50, 129
Exanthems
(1971): Muenter MD+, *Am J Med* 50, 129
Exfoliation (sic)
(1970): Nater P+, *Acta Derm Venereol* (Stockh) 50, 109
Exfoliative dermatitis
Fissuring
(1992): Breathnach SM+, *Adverse Drug Reactions and the Skin* Blackwell, Oxford, 254 (passim)
Hyperkeratosis
(1992): Breathnach SM+, *Adverse Drug Reactions and the Skin* Blackwell, Oxford, 254 (passim)
Perleche
(1971): Muenter MD+, *Am J Med* 50, 129
Photosensitivity
Pigmentation (yellow-orange)
(1971): Muenter MD+, *Am J Med* 50, 129
Pruritus (<1%)
(1992): Breathnach SM+, *Adverse Drug Reactions and the Skin* Blackwell, Oxford, 254 (passim)
(1971): Muenter MD+, *Am J Med* 50, 129
Stevens–Johnson syndrome
(1971): Muenter MD+, *Am J Med* 50, 129
Xerosis (1–10%)
(1975): Stüttgen G, *Acta Derm Venereol* (Stockh) 55 (Suppl 74), 174

### Hair

Hair – alopecia
(1992): Breathnach SM+, *Adverse Drug Reactions and the Skin* Blackwell, Oxford, 254 (passim)
(1979): Schmunes E, *Arch Dermatol* 115, 882
(1975): Stüttgen G, *Acta Derm Venereol* (Stockh) 55 (Suppl 74), 174
(1973): Levantine A+, *Br J Dermatol* 89, 549
(1972): Mausle R+, *Fortschr Med* (German) 90, 687
(1971): Muenter MD+, *Am J Med* 50, 129
(1970): Ippen H, *Dtsch Med Wochenschr* (German) 95, 1411
(1967): di Benedetto RJ, *JAMA* 201, 700
(1965): Rook A, *Br J Dermatol* 77, 115
(1960): Morrice G+, *JAMA* 173, 1802

### Other

Anaphylactoid reactions
Gingivitis
Hypersensitivity
(1995): Shelley WB+, *BMJ* 311, 232
Oral mucosal eruption
(1971): Muenter MD+, *Am J Med* 50, 129
(1964): Smith JH, *Oral Surg* 17 (Suppl 3), 305
Pseudotumor cerebri
Stomatodynia
Xerostomia
(1992): Breathnach SM+, *Adverse Drug Reactions and the Skin* Blackwell, Oxford, 254 (passim)

## VITAMIN $B_1$

(See THIAMINE)

## VITAMIN $B_{12}$

(See CYANOCOBALAMIN)

## VITAMIN $B_2$

(See RIBOFLAVIN)

## VITAMIN $B_3$

(See NIACINAMIDE)

## VITAMIN $B_5$

(See PANTOTHENIC ACID)

## VITAMIN $B_6$

(See PYRIDOXINE)

## VITAMIN $B_9$

(See FOLIC ACID)

## VITAMIN C

(See ASCORBIC ACID)

## VITAMIN D

(See ERGOCALCIFEROL)

## VITAMIN E

**Synonym:** alpha tocopherol
**Trade names:** Aquasol E; E-Vitamin Succinate; Eprolin; Pheryl-E; Vita Plus E; Vitec (Various pharmaceutical companies)
**Other common trade names:** *Bio E; Davitamon E; Detulin; E Perle; Ephynal; Optovit-E; Vita-E*
**Indications:** Vitamin E deficiency
**Category:** Fat-soluble vitamin
**Half-life:** no data
**Clinically important, potentially hazardous interactions with:** amprenavir, warfarin

#### *Reactions*

### Skin

Contact dermatitis (<1%)
(1997): Parsad D+, *Contact Dermatitis* 37, 294 (xanthomatous)
(1994): Manzano D+, *Contact Dermatitis* 31, 324
(1994): Perrenoud D+, *Dermatology* 189, 225
(1992): Garcia-Bravo B+, *Contact Dermatitis* 26, 280 (generalized)
(1991): de Groot AC+, *Contact Dermatitis* 25, 302
(1991): Fisher AA, *Cutis* 48, 272
(1986): Goldman MP+, *J Am Acad Dermatol* 14, 133
(1976): Roed-Petersen J+, *Br J Dermatol* 94, 233
(1975): Roed-Petersen J+, *Contact Dermatitis* 1, 391
(1975): Schorr WF, *Am Fam Physician* 12, 90
(1973): Aeling JL+, *Arch Dermatol* 108, 579
Dermatitis (sic)
(1991): Hunter D+, *Cutis* 47, 193
Erythema multiforme
(1994): Spreux A+, *Therapie* (French) 49, 460
(1986): Fisher AA, *Cutis* 37, 158 and 262 (topical administration)
(1984): Saperstein H+, *Arch Dermatol* 120, 906
Exanthems
Lupus erythematosus
(1995): Whittam J+, *Am J Clin Nutr* 62, 1025
Urticaria

### Hair

Hair – depigmentation (at injection sites)
(1972): Sehgal VN, *Dermatologica* 145, 56

### Other

Gingival bleeding
(1998): Liede KE+, *Ann Med* 30, 542
Gynecomastia
(1994): Roberts HJ, *Hosp Pract Off Ed* 29, 12
Sclerosing lipogranuloma
(1983): Foucar E+, *J Am Acad Dermatol* 9, 103
Thrombophlebitis
(1979): Roberts HS, *Angiology* 30, 169
Yellow spots on dental enamel

# VITAMIN K

(See PHYTONADIONE)

# VORICONAZOLE

**Synonym:** UK109496
**Trade name:** Vfend (Pfizer)
**Indications:** Invasive Aspergillosis
**Category:** Triazole antifungal
**Half-life:** 6–24 hours (dose dependent)
**Clinically important, potentially hazardous interactions with:** barbiturates, carbamazepine, ergot alkaloids, pimozide, quinidine, rifabutin, rifampin, sirolimus

### *Reactions*

## Skin

Allergic reactions (sic) (<1%)
Angioedema (<1%)
Cellulitis (<1%)
Cheilitis (<1%)
Chills (3.1%)
 (2002): Herbrecht R+, *N Engl J Med* 347(6), 408
Contact dermatitis (<1%)
Diaphoresis (<1%)
Ecchymoses (<1%)
Eczema (<1%)
Edema (<1%)
Erythema multiforme
Exfoliative dermatitis (<1%)
Facial edema (<1%)
Facial erythema
 (2001): Denning DW+, *Clin Exp Dermatol* 26(8), 648
Fixed eruption (<1%)
Flu-like syndrome (<1%)
Furunculosis (<1%)
Graft-versus-host syndrome (<1%)
Granulomas (<1%)
Guillain–Barré syndrome (<1%)
Herpes simplex (<1%)
Infections (sic) (<1%)
Lupus erythematosus (<1%)
Peripheral edema (1%)
Petechiae (<1%)
Photosensitivity (8.2%)
 (2002): Herbrecht R+, *N Engl J Med* 347(6), 408 (8.2%)
Pigmentation (<1%)
Pruritus (8.2%)
 (2002): Herbrecht R+, *N Engl J Med* 347(6), 408 (8.2%)
Psoriasis (<1%)
Purpura (<1%)
Rash (sic) (8.2%)
 (2002): Herbrecht R+, *N Engl J Med* 347(6), 408 (8.2%)
Scrotal edema (<1%)
Stevens–Johnson syndrome
Toxic epidermal necrolysis
Urticaria (<1%)
Xerosis (<1%)

## Hair

Hair – alopecia (<1%)

## Other

Ageusia (<1%)
Anaphylactoid reactions (<1%)
Arthralgia (<1%)
Arthritis (<1%)
Back pain (<1%)
Bone pain (<1%)
Depression (<1%)
Dysgeusia (<1%)
Gingival hemorrhage (<1%)
Gingival hyperplasia (<1%)
Gingivitis (<1%)
Glossitis (<1%)
Hyperesthesia (<1%)
Injection-site infection (sic) (<1%)
Injection-site inflammation (<1%)
Injection-site pain (<1%)
Myalgia (<1%)
Myopathy (<1%)
Oral ulceration (<1%)
Pain (<1%)
Paresthesias (<1%)
Phlebitis (<1%)
Stomatitis (<1%)
Thrombophlebitis (<1%)
Tongue edema (<1%)
Tremors (<1%)
Visual disturbances
 (2002): Herbrecht R+, *N Engl J Med* 347(6), 408 (44.8%)
 (2002): Walsh TJ+, *N Engl J Med* 346(4), 225
 (2001): Ally R+, *Clin Infect Dis* 33(9), 1447 (23%)
Xerostomia (1%)

# WARFARIN

**Trade name:** Coumadin (DuPont)
**Other common trade names:** *Aldocumar; Coumadine; Marevan; Waran; Warfilone*
**Indications:** Thromboembolic disease, pulmonary embolism
**Category:** Oral anticoagulant
**Half-life:** 1.5–2.5 days (highly variable)
**Clinically important, potentially hazardous interactions with:** amiodarone, amobarbital, antithyroid agents, aprobarbital, aspirin, azithromycin, barbiturates, bismuth, bivalirubin, bosentan, butabarbital, cimetidine, clarithromycin, clofibrate, clopidogrel, clorazepate, co-trimoxazole, cyclosporin, danazol, delavirdine, dirithromycin, disulfiram, erythromycin, fenofibrate, fluconazole, fluoxymesterone, gemfibrozil, **ginkgo biloba**, glucagon, imatinib, itraconazole, ketoconazole, levothyroxine, liothyronine, mephobarbital, methimazole, methyltestosterone, metronidazole, miconazole, nalidixic acid, Peg-interfeon alfa-2B, penicillin, pentobarbital, phenobarbital, phenylbutazone, phytonadione, pipericillin, primidone, propoxyphene, propylthiouracil, quinidine, quinine, rifampin, rifapentine, rofecoxib, salicylates, secobarbital, stanozolol, sulfamethoxazole, sulfinpyrazone, sulfisoxazole, sulfonamides, sulindac, testosterone, thyroid, troleandomycin, valdecoxib, vitamin A, vitamin E, zileuton

**Note:** Alternative remedies, including herbals, may potentially increase the risk of bleeding or potentiate the effects of warfarin therapy. Some of these include the following: angelica root, arnica flower, anise, asafetida, bogbean, borage seed oil, bromelain, dan shen, devil's claw, fenugreek, feverfew, garlic, ginger, ginkgo biloba, ginseng, horse chestnut, lovage root, meadowsweet, onion, parsley, passionflower herb, poplar, quassia, red clover, rue, turmeric and willow bark. Also coenzyme $Q_{10}$, dong quai, green tea, papain and vitamin E

## *Reactions*

### Skin

Abscess
(1997): Clayton BD, *J Geriatr Dermatology* 5, 314
Acral purpura
(1986): Stone MS+, *J Am Acad Dermatol* 14, 796
Angioedema (<1%)
Bullous eruption
(1993): Elis A+, *J Intern Med* 234, 615 (hemorrhagic)
(1986): Stone MS+, *J Am Acad Dermatol* 14, 796 (passim)
Dermatitis (sic)
(1992): Breathnach SM+, *Adverse Drug Reactions and the Skin* Blackwell, Oxford, 248 (passim)
(1991): Quintavalla R+, *Int Angiol* 10, 103
Ecchymoses
(2000): Juaneza MA+, *Am J Med Sci* 320(6), 388
(1988): Cole MS+, *Surgery* 103, 271 (passim)
Exanthems
(1993): Antony SJ+, *South Med J* 86, 1413
(1989): Kruis-de Vries MH+, *Dermatologica* 178, 109
(1988): Cole MS+, *Surgery* 103, 271 (passim)
(1978): Kwong P+, *JAMA* 239, 1884
(1968): Schiff BL+, *Arch Dermatol* 98, 136
(1960): Adams CW+, *Circulation* 22, 947
Exfoliative dermatitis
Hematomas
(1997): Clayton BD, *J Geriatr Dermatology* 5, 314
Hemorrhagic skin infarcts
(1989): Geoghegan+, *BMJ* 298, 902
(1988): Cole MS, *Surgery* 103, 271
(1980): Schleicher SM+, *Arch Dermatol* 116, 444
Lingual hemorrhage
(2000): Shojania KG, *Am J Med* 109, 77
Livedo reticularis
(1993): Park S+, *Arch Dermatol* 129, 775
Necrosis (>10%)
(2002): Francesconi Do Valle F+, *World Congress Dermatol* Poster, 0101 (2 cases)
(2000): Ad-El DD+, *Br J Plast Surg* 53(7), 624
(2000): Chan YC+, *Br J Surgery* 87, 266
(2000): Zimbelman J+, *J Pediatr* 137, 266
(1999): Gailine D+, *Am J Hematol* 60, 231
(1999): Martin FL, *Am J Nursing* 99, 53
(1999): Stewart AJ+, *Postgrad Med J* 75, 233
(1999): Yang Y+, *N Engl J Med* 340, 735
(1998): Essex DW+, *Am J Hematol* 57, 233
(1998): Gelwix TJ+, *Am J Emerg Med* 16, 541
(1998): Sallah S+, *Haemostasis* 28, 25
(1997): English JC+, *J Am Acad Dermatol* 37, 1 (passim)
(1997): Hermes B+, *Acta Derm Venereol* 77, 35
(1997): Sallah S+, *Thromb Haemost* 78, 785
(1997): Wynn SS+, *Haemostasis* 27, 246
(1996): Jillella AP+, *Am J Hematol* 52, 117
(1996): Makris M+, *Thromb Haemost* 75, 523
(1995): DeFranzo AJ+, *Ann Plast Surg* 34, 203
(1995): Hauben M, *N Engl J Med* 332, 959
(1995): Sternberg ML+, *Ann Emerg Med* 26, 94
(1994): Lewandowski K+, *Thromb Haemost* 69, 311
(1994): Soisson AP+, *Mil Med* 159, 252
(1993): Bauer KA, *Arch Dermatol* 129, 766
(1993): Colman RW+, *Am J Hematol* 43, 300
(1993): Eby CS, *Hematol Oncol Clin North Am* 7, 1291
(1993): Hiers CL, *J Ark Med Soc* 89, 443
(1993): LaPrade RF+, *Orthopedics* 16, 703
(1993): Locht H+, *J Intern Med* 233, 287
(1993): Schramm W+, *Arch Dermatol* 129, 753
(1993): Yates P+, *Clin Exp Dermatol* 18, 138
(1992): Anderson DR+, *Haemostasis* 22, 124
(1992): McKnight JT+, *Arch Fam Med* 1, 105
(1992): Sharafuddin MA+, *Arch Dermatol* 128, 105
(1992): Viegas GV, *J Am Podiatr Med Assoc* 82, 463
(1991): Berkompas DC, *Indiana Med* 84, 788
(1991): Brooks LW+, *J Am Osteopath Assoc* 91, 601
(1991): Humphries JE+, *Am J Hematol* 37, 197
(1991): Ritchie AJ+, *Ulster Med J* 60, 248
(1990): Comp PC+, *Semin Thromb Hemost* 16, 293
(1989): Barkley C+, *J Urology* 141, 946
(1989): Grimaudo V+, *BMJ* 289, 233
(1988): Cole MS+, *Surgery* 103, 271
(1988): Conlan MG+, *Am J Hematol* 29, 226
(1988): Dominic W+, *Burns Incl Therm Inj* 14, 139
(1988): Kandrotas RJ+, *Pharmacotherapy* 8, 351
(1988): Konrad P+, *Vasa*, 17, 208
(1987): Gladson CL+, *Arch Dermatol* 123, 1701
(1987): Haimovici H+, *J Vasc Surg* 5, 655
(1987): Norris PG, *Clin Exp Dermatol* 12, 370
(1986): Brennan M+, *J Tenn Med Assoc* 79, 210
(1986): Everett RN+, *Postgrad Med* 79, 97
(1986): Rowbotham B+, *Aust N Z J Med* 16, 513
(1986): Sjoberg A+, *Lakartidningen* (Swedish) 83, 4089
(1986): Zauber NP+, *Ann Intern Med* 104, 659
(1984): Franson TR+, *Arch Dermatol* 120, 927
(1984): McGehee WG+, *Ann Intern Med* 101, 59
(1984): Schwartz RA+, *Dermatologica* 168, 31 (linear localized)
(1984): Slutzki S+, *Int J Dermatol* 23, 117
(1983): Caldwell EH+, *Plast Reconstr Surg* 72, 231
(1983): Leath MC, *Tex Med* 79, 62
(1983): Papa MA+, *Harefuah* (Hebrew) 104, 504
(1982): Faraci PA, *Int J Dermatol* 21, 329

(1982): Torngren S+, *Acta Chir Scand* 148, 471
(1981): Horn JR+, *Am J Hosp Pharm* 38, 1763
(1980): Hislop IG+, *Aust N Z J Med* 10, 51
(1980): Schleicher SM+, *Arch Dermatol* 116, 444
(1979): Boss JM+, *Br J Dermatol* 100, 617
(1979): Jones RR+, *Br J Dermatol* 101, 561
(1978): Faraci PA+, *Surg Gynecol Obstet* 146, 695
(1978): Kirby JD+, *Br J Dermatol* 98, 707
(1976): Kirby JD+, *Br J Dermatol* 94, 97
(1976): Renick AM, *South Med J* 69, 775
(1975): Lacy JP+, *Ann Intern Med* 82, 381
(1971): Nalbandian RM+, *Obstet Gynecol* 38, 395
(1970): Martin CM+, *Calif Med* 113, 78
(1969): Korbitz BD+, *Am J Cardiol* 24, 420
(1969): Lipp H+, *Med J Aust* 2, 351
(1969): Vaughan ED+, *JAMA* 210, 2282 (genitalia)
(1954): Verhagen H, *Acta Med Scand* 148, 453

Pruritus (<1%)
(1978): Kwong P+, *JAMA* 239, 1884

Purplish erythema (sic) (feet and toes) (<1%)
(1998): Krahn MJ+, *Can J Cardiol* 14, 90 ("purple toes")
(1997): Sallah S+, *Thromb Haemost* 78, 785 ("purple toes")
(1994): Soisson AP+, *Mil Med* 159, 252
(1993): Park S+, *Arch Dermatol* 129, 775
(1982): Lebsack CS+, *Postgrad Med* 71, 81 ("purple toes")
(1981): Akle CA+, *J R Soc Med* 74, 219 (purple toe syndrome)
(1978): Kwong P+, *JAMA* 239, 1884
(1961): Feder W+, *Ann Intern Med* 55, 911

Purpura
(1988): Cole MS+, *Surgery* 103, 271 (passim)
(1978): Friedenberg WR+, *Arch Dermatol* 114, 578 (fulminans)

Rash (sic) (<1%)

Urticaria
(1988): Cole MS+, *Surgery* 103, 271 (passim)
(1986): Stone MS+, *J Am Acad Dermatol* 14, 796 (passim)
(1959): Sheps ES+, *Am J Cardiol* 3, 118

Vasculitis
(1998): Krahn MJ+, *Can J Cardiol* 14, 90
(1994): Tamir A+, *Acta Derm Venereol* 74, 138
(1982): Howitt AJ+, *Postgrad Med J* 58, 233
(1982): Tanay A+, *Dermatologica* 165, 178

Vesicular eruptions
(1986): Stone MS+, *J Am Acad Dermatol* 14, 796 (passim)

### Hair

Hair – alopecia (>10%)
(1995): Nagao T+, *Lancet* 346, 1004
(1989): Kruis-de Vries MH+, *Dermatologica* 178, 109 (passim)
(1988): Umlas J+, *Cutis* 42, 63
(1986): Stone MS+, *J Am Acad Dermatol* 14, 796 (passim)
(1969): Baker H+, *Br J Dermatol* 81, 236
(1957): Cornbleet T+, *Arch Dermatol* 75, 440

### Other

Gangrene
(1978): Hardisty CA, *Postgrad Med J* 54, 123
(1976): Shnider M+, *Can J Surg* 19, 64
(1973): Chua FS+, *J Thorac Cardiovasc Surg* 65, 238

Hypersensitivity
(1968): Schiff BL+, *Arch Dermatol* 98, 136

Oral ulceration (<1%)

Priapism
(2000): Zimbelman J+, *J Pediatr* 137, 266
(1997): Daryanani S+, *Clin Lab Haematol* 19, 213

# WILLOW BARK

**Scientific names:** *Salix alba; Salix fragilis; Salix purpurea*
**Other common names:** Basket Willow; Bay Willow; Brittle Willow; Crack Willow; Daphne Willow; Laurel Willow; Purple Osier; Violet Willow; White Willow; Willowbark
**Family:** Salicaceae
**Purported indications:** Colds, infections, headaches, pain, muscle and joint aches, influenza, gouty arthritis, ankylosing spondylitis, rheumatoid arthritis
**Other uses:** Diseases accompanied by fever, rheumatic ailments

## *Reactions*

### Skin

Rash (sic)

# YOHIMBINE

**Scientific name:** *Pausinystalia yohimbe*
**Trade names:** Actibane (Consolidated Midland); Aphrodyne (Star); Yocon (Palisades); Yohimex (Kramer); Yomax
**Family:**
**Purported indications:** Impotence, $alpha_2$-adrenergic blocker, orthostatic hypertension
**Half life:** 36 minutes
**Clinically important, potentially hazardous interactions with:** tricyclic antidepressants

### *Reactions*

---

## Skin

Diaphoresis
Exfoliative dermatitis
(1993): Sandler B+, *Urology* 41, 343
Flushing
Lupus erythematosus
(1993): Sandler B+, *Urology* 41, 343

# ZAFIRLUKAST

**Trade name:** Accolate (AstraZeneca)
**Indications:** Asthma
**Category:** Antiasthmatic; leukotriene receptor antagonist
**Half-life:** 10 hours
**Clinically important, potentially hazardous interactions with:** CYP3A4 substrates, **high protein foods**

### *Reactions*

## Skin

Allergic granulomatous angiitis (Churg–Strauss syndrome)
(1999): Green RL+, *Lancet* 353, 725 (2 cases)
(1999): Wechsler ME+, *Chest* 116, 266
(1999): Wechsler ME+, *Lancet* 353, 1970
(1998): Churg J+, *JAMA* 279, 1949
(1998): Holloway J+, *J Am Osteopath Assoc* 98, 275
(1998): Honsinger RW, *JAMA* 279, 1949
(1998): Katz RS+, *JAMA* 279, 1949
(1998): Knoell DL+, *Chest* 114, 332
(1998): Wechsler ME+, *JAMA* 279, 457
Lupus erythematosus
(1999): Finkel TH+, *J Allergy Clin Immunol* 103, 533

## Other

Cough
(2001): Spector SL, *Ann Allergy Asthma Immunol* 86(6 Suppl 1), 18
Myalgia (1.6%)

# ZALCITABINE

**Synonyms:** ddC; dideoxycytidine
**Trade name:** Hivid (Roche)
**Indications:** Advanced HIV disease
**Category:** Antiretroviral; nucleoside reverse transcriptase inhibitor (NRTI)
**Half-life:** 2.9 hours

### *Reactions*

## Skin

Acne (<1%)
Angioedema
(1988): Yarchoan R+, *Lancet* 1, 76 (5%)
Ankle edema
(1989): Jeffries DJ, *J Antimicrob Chemother* 23, 29
Bullous eruption (<1%)
Cutaneous side effects (sic)
(1991): Yarchoan R+, *Blood* 78, 859
(1990): Broder S+, *Am J Med* 88, 31S
Dermatitis (sic) (<1%)
Diaphoresis (<1%)
Edema (<1%)
(1991): Pluda JM+, *Hematol Oncol Clin North Am* 5, 229
(1991): Yarchoan R+, *Blood* 78, 859
(1989): McNeely MC+, *J Am Acad Dermatol* 21, 1213 (70%) (dose-related)
Erythema multiforme
(1995): Wardropper AG+, *Int J STD AIDS* 6, 450
Erythroderma
(1989): McNeely MC+, *J Am Acad Dermatol* 21, 1213 (10%)
Exanthems (1–66%)
(1991): Fischl MA, *Recent Advances in Antiretroviral Therapy*, New York, Triclinica Communications
(1991): Merigan TC, *Am J Med* 90, 8S
(1991): Pluda JM+, *Hematol Oncol Clin North Am* 5, 229
(1990): Pizzo PA+, *J Pediatr* 117, 799
(1989): McNeely MC+, *J Am Acad Dermatol* 21, 1213 (40%)
(1989): Merigan TC+, *Ann Intern Med* 110, 189 (66%)
(1989): Yarchoan R+, *N Engl J Med* 321, 726 (1–5%)
(1988): Yarchoan R+, *Lancet* 1, 76 (65%)
(1987): Richman DD+, *N Engl J Med* 317, 192 (1–5%)
Exfoliative dermatitis (<1%)
Flushing (<1%)
Folliculitis
Granuloma annulare
(2001): Peñas PF+, *Arch Dermatol* 137, 964
Photosensitivity (<1%)
Pruritus (3–5%)
Rash (sic) (2–11%)
(1990): Bozzette SA+, *Am J Med* 88, 24S
(1989): Jeffries DJ, *J Antimicrob Chemother* 23, 29
Urticaria (3.4%)
(1992): Roche Laboratories Monograph
Xerosis (<1%)

## Hair

Hair – alopecia

## Nails

Nails – changes (sic)
(1989): Jeffries DJ, *J Antimicrob Chemother* 23, 29

## Other

Ageusia (<1%)
Anaphylactoid reactions
(1992): Roche Laboratories Monograph
Aphthous stomatitis
(1991): Fischl MA, *Recent Advances in Antiretroviral Therapy*. New York, Triclinica Communications
(1991): Merigan TC, *Am J Med* 90, 8S
(1991): Pluda JM+, *Hematol Oncol Clin North Am* 5, 229
(1989): Jeffries DJ, *J Antimicrob Chemother* 23, 29
(1989): Yarchoan R+, *N Engl J Med* 321, 726
(1988): Yarchoan R+, *Lancet* 1, 76
Dysgeusia (<1%)
Gingivitis (<1%)
Glossitis (<1%)
Glossodynia (<1%)
Myalgia (1–6%)
Myopathy (<1%)
Oral mucosal lesions (40–73%)
(1991): Fischl MA, *Recent Advances in Antiretroviral Therapy*. New York, Triclinica Communications
(1989): Merigan TC+, *Ann Intern Med* 110, 189 (73%)
(1988): Yarchoan R+, *Lancet* 1, 76 (40%)
Oral ulceration (3–64%)
(1990): Bozzette SA+, *Am J Med* 88, 24S
(1990): Pizzo PA+, *J Pediatr* 117, 799 (painful)
(1989): McNeely MC+, *J Am Acad Dermatol* 21, 1213 (64%)
Paresthesias
Parosmia (<1%)
Penile edema (<1%)
Stomatitis (3%)
(1991): Yarchoan R+, *Blood* 78, 859
Tinnitus
Tongue disorder (sic) (<1%)
Xerostomia (<1%)

## ZALEPLON

**Trade name:** Sonata (Wyeth-Ayerst)
**Indications:** Insomnia
**Category:** Nonbenzodiazepine hypnotic and sedative
**Half-life:** 1 hour

### *Reactions*

#### Skin

Acne (<1%)
Cheilitis (<1%)
Chills (<1%)
Contact dermatitis (<1%)
Diaphoresis (<1%)
Ecchymoses (<1%)
Eczema (<1%)
Edema (<1%)
Exanthems (<1%)
Facial edema (<1%)
Peripheral edema (1–10%)
Photosensitivity (1–10%)
Pigmentation (<1%)
Pruritus (<1%)
Psoriasis (<1%)
Purpura (<1%)
Pustular eruption (<1%)
Rash (sic) (<1%)
Vesiculobullous eruption (<1%)
Xerosis (<1%)

#### Hair

Hair – alopecia (<1%)

#### Other

Ageusia (<1%)
Aphthous stomatitis (<1%)
Gingival hemorrhage (<1%)
Gingivitis (<1%)
Glossitis (<1%)
Hyperesthesia (<1%)
Hypesthesia (2%)
Mastodynia (<1%)
Myalgia (5%)
Oral ulceration (<1%)
Paresthesias (3%)
Parosmia (2%)
Sialorrhea (<1%)
Stomatitis (<1%)
Thrombophlebitis (<1%)
Tongue discoloration (<1%)
Tremors (1–10%)
Vaginitis (<1%)
Xerostomia (1–10%)

## ZANAMIVIR

**Trade name:** Relenza (GSK)
**Indications:** Influenza A and B
**Category:** Inhibitor of viral neuranimidase (by oral inhalation)
**Half-life:** 2.5–5.1 hours

### *Reactions*

#### Skin

Infections (sic) (2%)
Urticaria (<1.5%)

#### Other

Myalgia (<1.5%)

## ZIDOVUDINE

**Synonyms:** azidothymidine; AZT; compound S
**Trade names:** Combivir (GSK); Retrovir (GSK)
**Other common trade names:** *Novo-AZT; Retrovis*
**Indications:** HIV infection
**Category:** Antiretroviral; nucleoside reverse transcriptase inhibitor (NRTI)
**Half-life:** 1 hour
**Clinically important, potentially hazardous interactions with:** clarithromycin, ganciclovir, Peg-interfeon alfa-2B, ribavirin

### *Reactions*

#### Skin

Acne (<5%)
(1988): McEvoy GK, *Am Hosp Formulary Service: Drug Info* 392
Blue vitiligo (sic)
(1994): Ivker R+, *J Am Acad Dermatol* 30, 829
Bullous eruption
(1989): Caumes E+, *Presse Med* (French) 18, 1708 (fatal in AIDS)
Diaphoresis (5–19%)
(1988): McEvoy GK, *Am Hosp Formulary Service: Drug Info* 392
Ecchymoses
(1992): Breathnach SM+, *Adverse Drug Reactions and the Skin* Blackwell, Oxford, 172 (passim)
Edema of lip (<5%)
(1988): McEvoy GK, *Am Hosp Formulary Service: Drug Info* 392
Erythema multiforme
(1989): Langtry HD+, *Drugs* 37, 408
(1989): Yarchoan R+, *N Engl J Med* 321, 726
Erythroderma
(1996): Duque S+, *J Allergy Clin Immunol* 98, 234
Exanthems
(1990): Petty BG+, *Lancet* 335, 1044 (1–5%) (in AIDS patients)
(1989): Gelman K+, *AIDS* 3, 555 (>5%)
(1989): Langtry HD+, *Drugs* 37, 408
(1987): Richman DD+, *N Engl J Med* 317, 192
Heightened cutaneous reactions to mosquito bites (sic)
(1988): Diven DG+, *Arch Intern Med* 148, 2296
Neutrophilic eccrine hidradenitis
(1990): Smith KJ+, *J Am Acad Dermatol* 23, 945
Pigmentation
(1993): Hermanns-Le T+, *Ann Pathol* (French) 13, 328
(1992): Baudo F+, *Eur J Dermatol* 2, 448
(1992): Hill DA+, *Hosp Pract Off Ed* 27, 29
(1991): Poizot-Martin I+, *Presse Med* (French) 20, 632
(1991): Tal A+, *Cutis* 48, 153

(1990): Greenberg RG+, *J Am Acad Dermatol* 22, 327
(1989): Bendick C+, *Arch Dermatol* 125, 1285 (palms and soles)
(1989): Merenich JA+, *Am J Med* 86, 469
(1989): Valencia ME+, *Med Clin (Barc)* (Spanish) 92, 357

Pruritus
(1989): Gelman K+, *AIDS* 3, 555 (>5%)
(1988): McEvoy GK, *Am Hosp Formulary Service: Drug Info* 392

Purpura

Rash (sic) (17%)
(1996): Henry K+, *Ann Intern Med* 124, 855
(1987): Richman DD+, *N Engl J Med* 317, 192

Stevens–Johnson syndrome
(1989): Langtry HD+, *Drugs* 37, 408
(1989): Yarchoan R+, *N Engl J Med* 321, 726

Toxic epidermal necrolysis
(1996): Murri R+, *Clin Infect Dis* 23, 640

Urticaria (<5%)
(1990): McKinley GF+, *Lancet* 336, 384
(1988): McEvoy GK, *Am Hosp Formulary Service: Drug Info* 392

Vasculitis
(1992): Torres RA+, *Arch Intern Med* 152, 850
(1990): Lee MH+, *Int Conf AIDS* 6, 360 (leukocytoclastic)

### Hair

Hair – alopecia
(1996): Geletko SM+, *Pharmacotherapy* 16, 69

Hair – hypertrichosis (eyelashes)
(1991): Klutman NE+, *N Engl J Med* 324, 1896
(1991): Sahai J+, *AIDS* 5, 1395

### Nails

Nails – blue lunulae
(1990): Don PC+, *Ann Intern Med* 112, 145 (30–67%)

Nails – paronychia
(1999): Russo F+, *J Am Acad Dermatol* 40, 322

Nails – pigmentation (42%)
(1992): Rahav G+, *Scand J Infect Dis* 24, 557
(1991): Sahai J+, *AIDS* 5, 1395
(1990): Don PC+, *Ann Intern Med* 112, 145 (42%)
(1990): Greenberg RG+, *J Am Acad Dermatol* 22, 327
(1990): Poizot-Martin I+, *Int Conf AIDS* 6, 357
(1990): Ramos C+, *Rev Clin Esp* (Spanish) 187, 94
(1989): Anders KH+, *J Am Acad Dermatol* 21, 792
(1989): Bendick C+, *Arch Dermatol* 125, 1285
(1989): Depaoli MA+, *G Ital Dermatol Venereol* (Italian) 124, 71
(1989): Dupon M+, *Scand J Infect Dis* 21, 237
(1989): Fisher CA+, *Cutis* 43, 552
(1989): Groark SP+, *J Am Acad Dermatol* 21, 1032
(1989): Langtry HD+, *Drugs* 37, 408
(1989): Merenich JA+, *Am J Med* 86, 469
(1989): Yarchoan R+, *N Engl J Med* 321, 726
(1988): Azon-Masoliver A+, *Arch Dermatol* 124, 1570
(1988): Gonzalez-Lahoz JM+, *Rev Clin Esp* (Spanish) 183, 278 (bluish)
(1988): Vaiopoulos G+, *Ann Intern Med* 108, 777
(1987): Furth PA+, *Ann Intern Med* 107, 350

Nails – pigmented bands
(1991): Tadini G+, *Arch Dermatol* 127, 267
(1990): Grau-Massanes M+, *J Am Acad Dermatol* 22, 687
(1990): Tosti A+, *Dermatologica* 180, 217 (longitudinal)
(1989): Bendick C+, *Z Hautkr* (German) 64, 91
(1989): Valencia ME+, *Rev Clin Esp* (Spanish) 185, 167 (blue striae)

### Other

Bromhidrosis (<5%)
(1988): McEvoy GK, *Am Hosp Formulary Service: Drug Info* 392

Death

Dysgeusia (5–19%)
(1988): McEvoy GK, *Am Hosp Formulary Service: Drug Info* 392
(1987): Richman DD+, *N Engl J Med* 317, 192

Foetor ex ore (halitosis)

Gingival bleeding

Hypersensitivity

Lipodystrophy
(2001): Bogner JR+, *J Acquir Immune Defic Syndr* 27(3), 237

Myopathy (<1%)
(1993): Simpson DM+, *Neurology* 43, 971
(1989): Gertner E+, *Am J Medicine* 86, 814
(1988): Helbert M+, *Lancet* 2, 689

Oral lichenoid eruption
(2001): Scully C+, *Oral Dis* 7(4), 205 (passim)
(1993): Ficarra G+, *Oral Surg Oral Med Oral Pathol* 76, 460

Oral mucosal eruption
(1989): Gelman K+, *AIDS* 3, 555 (>5%)

Oral mucosal pigmentation
(1991): Poizot-Martin I+, *Presse Med* (French) 20, 632
(1991): Tadini G+, *Arch Dermatol* 127, 267
(1990): Ficarra G+, *Oral Surg Oral Med Oral Pathol* 70, 748
(1990): Grau-Massanes M+, *J Am Acad Dermatol* 22, 687
(1990): Greenberg RG+, *J Am Acad Dermatol* 22, 327
(1990): Poizot-Martin I+, *Int Conf AIDS* 6, 357
(1989): Merenich JA+, *Am J Med* 86, 469

Oral ulceration (<5%)
(1988): McEvoy GK, *Am Hosp Formulary Service: Drug Info* 392

Paresthesias (<8%)
(1988): McEvoy GK, *Am Hosp Formulary Service: Drug Info* 392

Polymyositis
(1988): Bessen LJ+, *N Engl J Med* 318, 708 (4 patients)

Porphyria cutanea tarda
(1988): Ong EL+, *Postgrad Med J* 64, 956

Tongue edema (<5%)
(1988): McEvoy GK, *Am Hosp Formulary Service: Drug Info* 392

Tongue pigmentation
(1991): Tadini G+, *Arch Dermatol* 127, 267
(1991): Tal A+, *Cutis* 48, 153
(1990): Grau-Massanes M+, *J Am Acad Dermatol* 22, 687
(1990): Greenberg RG+, *J Am Acad Dermatol* 22, 327

Tongue ulceration
(1993): Schwander S+, *Med Klin* (German) 88, 60

## ZILEUTON

**Trade name:** Zyflo (Abbott)
**Indications:** Asthma
**Category:** Antiasthmatic bronchodilator; leukotriene receptor inhibitor
**Half-life:** 2.5 hours
**Clinically important, potentially hazardous interactions with:** anisindione, anticoagulants, dicumarol, pimozide, warfarin

### *Reactions*

### Skin

Allergic granulomatous angiitis (Churg–Strauss syndrome)
(2000): Dellaripa PF+, *Mayo Clin Proc* 75(6), 643

Eosinophilic fasciitis
(2000): Dellaripa PF+, *Mayo Clin Proc* 75(6), 643

Erythema nodosum
(2000): Dellaripa PF+, *Mayo Clin Proc* 75, 643

Morphea
(2000): Dellaripa PF+, *Mayo Clin Proc* 75(6), 643

Pruritus (>1%)

Scleroderma
(2000): Dellaripa PF+, *Mayo Clin Proc* 75(6), 643

### Other

Cough
(2001): Spector SL, *Ann Allergy Asthma Immunol* 86(6 Suppl 1), 18
Myalgia (3.2%)
Paresthesias (1%)
Vaginitis (>1%)

## ZIPRASIDONE

**Synonym:** Zeldox
**Trade name:** Geodon (Pfizer)
**Indications:** Schizophrenia
**Category:** Antipsychotic (benzothiazolylpiperazine); serotonin & dopamine antagonist
**Half-life:** 4-5 hours

#### *Reactions*

### Skin

Chills (<1%)
Contact dermatitis
Ecchymoses (<1%)
Eczema (<1%)
Exanthems (<1%)
Exfoliative dermatitis (<1%)
Facial edema (<1%)
Fungal dermatitis (sic) (2%)
Peripheral edema (<1%)
Photosensitivity (<1%)
Rash (sic) (4%)
Upper respiratory infection (8%)
Urticaria (5%)
Vesiculobullous eruption (<1%)

### Hair

Hair – alopecia (<1%)

### Other

Gingival hemorrhage (<1%)
Gynecomastia (<1%)
Hypesthesia (<1%)
Myalgia (1%)
Myopathy (<1%)
Paresthesias (<1%)
Priapism
Sialorrhea
Thrombophlebitis (<1%)
Tinnitus (<1%)
Tongue edema (<1%)
Tremors (<1%)
Xerostomia (4%)

## ZOLEDRONIC ACID

**Trade name:** Zometa (Novartis)
**Indications:** Hyperclacemia of malignancy, Paget's disease
**Category:** Biphosphonate (bone resorption inhibitor)
**Half-life:** 7 days

#### *Reactions*

### Skin

Candidiasis
Flu-like syndrome (1–10%)
(2001): Berenson JR+, *Clin Cancer Res* 7(3), 478
Upper respiratory infection
(2001): Berenson JR+, *Clin Cancer Res* (10%)

### Other

Arthralgia
Myalgia
Skeletal pain (1–10%)
(2001): Berenson JR+, *Cancer* 91(1), 144
(2001): Berenson JR+, *Cancer* 91(7), 1191
(2001): Berenson JR+, *Clin Cancer Res* 7(3), 478
(2001): Rosen LS+, *Cancer J* 7(5), 377

## ZOLMITRIPTAN

**Trade name:** Zomig (AstraZeneca)
**Indications:** Migraine attacks
**Category:** Antimigraine; serotonin agonist
**Half-life:** 3 hours
**Clinically important, potentially hazardous interactions with:** dihydroergotamine, ergot, isocarboxazid, MAO inhibitors, methysergide, naratriptan, phenelzine, rizatriptan, sibutramine, sumatriptan, tranylcypromine

#### *Reactions*

### Skin

Allergy (sic) (<1%)
Diaphoresis (2%)
Ecchymoses (<1%)
Edema (<1%)
Facial edema (<1%)
Flushing
Hot flashes (>10%)
Photosensitivity (<1%)
Pruritus (<1%)
Rash (sic) (<1%)
Urticaria (<1%)

### Other

Hyperesthesia (<1%)
Hypesthesia (2%)
Myalgia (2%)
Paresthesias (11%)
(1998): Multiple Authors, *Headache* 38, 173 (11%)
Parosmia (<1%)
Serotonin syndrome
(2001): Lucas C+, *Cephalalgia* 21, 421
Thrombophlebitis (<1%)
Tongue edema (<1%)
Twitching (<1%)
Xerostomia (3%)
(1997): Edmeads JG+, *Cephalalgia* 17, 41

# ZOLPIDEM

**Trade name:** Ambien (Searle)
**Other common trade names:** *Niotal; Stilnoct; Stilnox*
**Indications:** Insomnia
**Category:** Nonbenzodiazepine sedative-hypnotic
**Half-life:** 2.6 hours
**Clinically important, potentially hazardous interactions with:** antihistamines, azatadine, azelastine, brompheniramine, buclizine, chlorpheniramine, clemastine, dexchlorpheniramine, meclizine, ritonavir

## *Reactions*

### Skin

Acne (<1%)
Allergic reactions (sic) (4%)
Bullous eruption (<1%)
Dermatitis (sic) (<1%)
Diaphoresis (<1%)
Edema (<1%)
Facial edema (<1%)
Flushing (<1%)
Furunculosis (<1%)
Herpes simplex (<1%)
Herpes zoster (<1%)
Hot flashes (<1%)
Periorbital edema (<1%)
Photosensitivity (<1%)
Pruritus
(1994): Litt JZ, Beachwood, OH (personal case) (observation)
Purpura (<1%)
Rash (sic) (2%)
Urticaria (<1%)

### Other

Anaphylactoid reactions (<1%)
Dysgeusia (<1%)
Hypesthesia (<1%)
Injection-site inflammation (<1%)
Mastodynia (<1%)
Myalgia (7%)
Paresthesias (<1%)
Tinnitus
Tremors (<1%)
Vaginitis (<1%)
Xerostomia (3%)

# ZONISAMIDE

**Trade name:** Zonegran (Elan Pharma)
**Indications:** Epilepsy
**Category:** Anticonvulsant; sulfonamide*
**Half-life:** 63 hours

## *Reactions*

### Skin

Acne (<1%)
Allergic reactions (sic) (<1%)
Diaphoresis (<1%)
Ecchymoses (2%)
Eczema (<1%)
Edema (<1%)
Exanthems (<1%)
Facial edema (<1%)
Lupus erythematosus (<1%)
Peripheral edema (<1%)
Petechiae (<1%)
Pruritus (<1%)
Purpura (2%)
Pustular eruption (<1%)
Rash (sic) (3%)
Stevens–Johnson syndrome
(1985): Wilensky AJ+, *Epilepsia* 26, 212
Toxic epidermal necrolysis
Urticaria (<1%)
Vesiculobullous eruption (<1%)
Xerosis (<1%)

### Hair

Hair – alopecia (<1%)
Hair – hirsutism (<1%)

### Other

Dysgeusia (2%)
Gingival hyperplasia (<1%)
Gingivitis (<1%)
Glossitis (<1%)
Gynecomastia (<1%)
(1998): Ikeda A+, *J Neurol Neurosurg Psychiatry* 65, 803
Hyperesthesia (<1%)
Hyperpyrexia
(1997): Shimizu T+, *Brain Dev* 19, 366
Hypersensitivity
Myalgia (<1%)
Oligohydrosis
(1999): Isumi H+, *No To Hattatsu* (Japanese) 31, 468
(1997): Shimizu T+, *Brain Dev* 19, 366
(1996): Okumura A+, *No To Hattatsu* (Japanese) 28, 44
Oral ulceration (<1%)
Paresthesias (4%)
Parosmia (<1%)
Stomatitis (<1%)
Thrombophlebitis (<1%)
Tremors (<1%)
(1992): Taira T, *No To Shinkei* (Japanese) 44, 61
Ulcerative stomatitis (<1%)
Xerostomia (2%)

***Note:** Zonisamide is a sulfonamide and can be absorbed systemically. Sulfonamides can produce severe, possibly fatal, reactions such as toxic epidermal necrolysis and Stevens–Johnson syndrome

# DRUGS RESPONSIBLE FOR 102 COMMON REACTION PATTERNS

**Acanthosis Nigricans**
- Azathioprine
- Corticosteroids
- Diethylstilbestrol
- Estrogens
- Gemfibrozil
- Heroin
- Lithium
- Mechlorethamine
- Methsuximide
- Methyltestosterone
- Niacin
- Niacinamide
- Oral contraceptives
- Thioridazine

**Acneform Lesions**
- Acyclovir
- Alosetron
- Alprazolam
- Amitriptyline
- Amobarbital
- Amoxapine
- Androstenedione
- Atorvastatin
- Azathioprine
- Basiliximab
- Betaxolol
- Bexarotene
- Bisoprolol
- Botulinum toxin (A & B)
- Bupropion
- Buspirone
- Butabarbital
- Cabergoline
- Carbamazepine
- Carteolol
- Cefamandole
- Cefpodoxime
- Ceftazidime
- Cetirizine
- Chloral hydrate
- Chlorotrianisene
- Cidofovir
- Cimetidine
- Ciprofloxacin
- Clofazimine
- Clomiphene
- Clomipramine
- Corticosteroids
- Creatine
- Cyanocobalamin
- Cyclosporine
- Dactinomycin
- Danazol
- Dantrolene
- Deferoxamine
- Demeclocycline
- Desipramine
- Diazepam
- Diethylstilbestrol
- Diltiazem
- Disulfiram
- Eflornithine
- Epoetin alfa
- Erythromycin
- Esmolol
- Esomeprazole
- Estazolam
- Estrogens
- Ethambutol
- Ethionamide
- Famotidine
- Felbamate
- Fenoprofen
- Fexofenadine
- Fluconazole
- Fluoxetine
- Fluoxymesterone
- Fluvoxamine
- Folic acid
- Foscarnet
- Fosphenytoin
- Gabapentin
- Ganciclovir
- Gold and gold compounds
- Granulocyte colony-stimulating factor (GCSF)
- Haloperidol
- Halothane
- Heroin
- Imipramine
- Interferons, alfa-2
- Isoniazid
- Isotretinoin
- Lamotrigine
- Lansoprazole
- Leflunomide
- Leuprolide
- Levothyroxine
- Lithium
- Maprotiline
- MDMA
- Medroxyprogesterone
- Mephenytoin
- Mesalamine
- Methotrexate
- Methoxsalen
- Methyltestosterone
- Minoxidil
- Mirtazapine
- Mycophenolate
- Nabumetone
- Nafarelin
- Naltrexone
- Naratriptan
- Nefazodone
- Nimodipine
- Nisoldipine
- Nizatidine
- Nortriptyline
- Olsalazine
- Oral contraceptives
- Oxcarbazepine
- Pantoprazole
- Paramethadione
- Paroxetine
- Pentobarbital
- Pentostatin
- Pergolide
- Phenobarbital
- Phenytoin
- Potassium iodide
- Primidone
- Progestins
- Propafenone
- Propranolol
- Propylthiouracil
- Protriptyline
- Psoralens
- Pyrazinamide
- Pyridoxine
- Quinidine
- Quinine
- Ramipril
- Riboflavin
- Rifampin
- Rifapentine
- Risperidone
- Ritonavir
- Saquinavir
- Sertraline
- Sibutramine
- Sirolimus
- Sparfloxacin
- Stanozolol
- Tacrine
- Testosterone
- Tetracycline
- Tiagabine
- Tizanidine
- Topiramate
- Trastuzumab
- Tretinoin
- Trimethadione
- Trioxsalen
- Trovafloxacin
- Valdecoxib
- Valproic acid
- Venlafaxine
- Verapamil
- Vinblastine
- Zalcitabine
- Zaleplon
- Zidovudine
- Zolpidem
- Zonisamide

**Acral Erythema**
- Bleomycin
- Capecitabine
- Cisplatin
- Cyclophosphamide
- Cytarabine
- Didanosine
- Doxorubicin
- Fluorouracil
- Granulocyte colony-stimulating factor (GCSF)
- Hydroxyurea
- Idarubicin
- Lomustine
- Mercaptopurine
- Methotrexate
- Mitotane
- Paclitaxel
- Quinine
- Vincristine

**Acute Febrile Neutrophilic Dermatosis (Sweet's syndrome)**
- Arnica
- Celecoxib
- Clofazimine
- Co-trimoxazole
- Cytarabine
- Furosemide
- Gabapentin
- Glucagon
- Granulocyte colony-stimulating factor (GCSF)
- Hydralazine
- Hydroxyurea
- Minocycline
- Nitrofurantoin
- Oral contraceptives
- Sulfamethoxazole
- Tretinoin
- Verapamil

**Acute Generalized Exanthematous Pustulosis (AGEP)**
- Acetaminophen
- Acetazolamide
- Allopurinol
- Amoxapine
- Amoxicillin
- Ampicillin
- Aspirin
- Bacampicillin
- Carbamazepine
- Cefaclor
- Cefazolin
- Cefuroxime
- Cephalexin
- Cephradine
- Chloramphenicol
- Chloroquine
- Clindamycin
- Clozapine
- Co-trimoxazole
- Codeine
- Corticosteroids
- Diltiazem
- Doxycycline
- Erythromycin
- Fluconazole
- Furosemide
- Galantamine
- Hydrochlorothiazide
- Hydroxychloroquine
- Imipenem/cilastatin
- Isoniazid
- Itraconazole
- Lamotrigine
- Lansoprazole
- Methoxsalen
- Metronidazole

Mexiletine
Minocycline
Nifedipine
Nimodipine
Nystatin
Penicillins
Phenobarbital
Phenytoin
Progestins
Protease inhibitors
Pyrimethamine
Quinidine
Ranitidine
Streptomycin
Sulfamethoxazole
Sulfasalazine
Terbinafine
Ticlopidine
Vancomycin

**Ageusia**

Acarbose
Acetazolamide
Amitriptyline
Aspirin
Atorvastatin
Azelastine
Benazepril
Betaxolol
Captopril
Cetirizine
Cisplatin
Clidinium
Clomipramine
Clopidogrel
Cocaine
Cyclobenzaprine
Diazoxide
Dicyclomine
Enalapril
Etidronate
Feverfew
Fluoxetine
Fluvoxamine
Fosinopril
Hyoscyamine
Indomethacin
Interferons, alfa-2
Isotretinoin
Levodopa
Losartan
Methantheline
Methimazole
Mirtazapine
Nefazodone
Paroxetine
Penicillamine
Pentamidine
Phenytoin
Propantheline
Propylthiouracil
Ramipril
Rifabutin
Rimantadine
Ritonavir
Rivastigmine
Spironolactone
Sulfadoxine
Sulindac
Terbinafine
Tiagabine
Tiopronin
Topiramate
Venlafaxine
Voriconazole
Zalcitabine
Zaleplon

**Anaphylactoid Reactions**

Abacavir
Abciximab
Acetaminophen
Acetazolamide
Acyclovir
Alemtuzumab
Aloe vera (gel, juice, leaf)
Alteplase
Amiloride
Aminocaproic acid
Aminoglutethimide
Amitriptyline
Amoxicillin
Amphotericin B
Ampicillin
Anistreplase
Anthrax vaccine
Aprotinin
Asparaginase
Aspartame
Aspirin
Atenolol
Azathioprine
Azithromycin
Aztreonam
Bacampicillin
Basiliximab
Benactyzine
Bendroflumethiazide
Betaxolol
Bisoprolol
Bleomycin
Botulinum toxin (A & B)
Bromocriptine
Bupropion
Butalbital
Caffeine
Calcitonin
Captopril
Carbenicillin
Carboplatin
Carisoprodol
Carteolol
Carvedilol
Caspofungin
Cefaclor
Cefadroxil
Cefamandole
Cefazolin
Cefdinir
Cefditoren
Cefepime
Cefixime
Cefmetazole
Cefonicid
Cefotaxime
Cefotetan
Cefoxitin
Cefpodoxime
Cefprozil
Ceftazidime
Ceftizoxime
Ceftriaxone
Cefuroxime
Celecoxib
Cephalexin
Cephalothin
Cephapirin
Cephradine
Cetirizine
Cetrorelix
Chamomile
Chloramphenicol
Chlorhexidine
Chlorothiazide
Chlorpromazine
Chlorzoxazone
Cimetidine
Cinoxacin
Ciprofloxacin
Cisatracurium
Cisplatin
Clarithromycin
Clemastine
Clidinium
Clindamycin
Cloxacillin
Co-trimoxazole
Codeine
Colchicine
Corticosteroids
Creatine
Cromolyn
Cyanocobalamin
Cyclobenzaprine
Cyclophosphamide
Cyclosporine
Cyproheptadine
Cytarabine
Dacarbazine
Dactinomycin
Dalteparin
Dantrolene
Daunorubicin
Deferoxamine
Demeclocycline
Denileukin
Desloratadine
Dexchlorpheniramine
Dextromethorphan
Diazepam
Diclofenac
Dicloxacillin
Dicyclomine
Didanosine
Diflunisal
Dimenhydrinate
Diphenhydramine
Diphenoxylate
Dipyridamole
Dirithromycin
Dolasetron
Domperidone
Doxorubicin
Doxycycline
Echinacea
Edrophonium
Enalapril
Enoxaparin
Epirubicin
Epoetin alfa
Eptifibatide
Ertapenem
Erythromycin
Ethambutol
Ethanolamine
Etoposide
Felbamate
Fenoprofen
Fentanyl
Fluconazole
Flucytosine
Fluorouracil
Fluoxetine
Fluoxymesterone
Fluphenazine
Flurbiprofen
Fluvastatin
Fluvoxamine
Folic acid
Formoterol
Fosfomycin
Fosinopril
Furosemide
Ganciclovir
Garlic
Gatifloxacin
Gemcitabine
Gemfibrozil
Gentamicin
Gold and gold compounds
Goserelin
Granisetron
Granulocyte colony-stimulating factor (GCSF)
Griseofulvin
Heparin
Hepatitis B vaccine
Horse chestnut – seed
Hyoscyamine
Ibritumomab
Ibuprofen
Ifosfamide
Indapamide
Indomethacin
Infliximab
Insulin
Interferon beta 1-a
Ipodate
Ipratropium
Isoetharine
Itraconazole
Ketoconazole
Ketoprofen
Ketorolac
Labetalol
Lamivudine
Lamotrigine
Lansoprazole
Leflunomide
Leucovorin
Levamisole
Levofloxacin
Lidocaine
Lincomycin
Lisinopril
Loratadine
Losartan
Marihuana
Mechlorethamine
Medroxyprogesterone
Mefenamic acid
Meloxicam

Melphalan
Meprobamate
Mesoridazine
Metaxalone
Methantheline
Methicillin
Methocarbamol
Methohexital
Methotrexate
Methoxsalen
Methyclothiazide
Methyltestosterone
Metolazone
Mezlocillin
Miconazole
Midazolam
Minocycline
Minoxidil
Misoprostol
Mistletoe
Moexipril
Moxifloxacin
Nabumetone
Nafcillin
Nalidixic acid
Naproxen
Neomycin
Niacin
Nitrofurantoin
Nitroglycerin
Norfloxacin
Octreotide
Ofloxacin
Omeprazole
Ondansetron
Orphenadrine
Oxacillin
Oxaprozin
Oxytetracycline
Paclitaxel
Palivizumab
Pancuronium
Pantoprazole
PEG-interferon alfa-2b
Penicillins
Pentostatin
Perindopril
Perphenazine
Phenazopyridine
Phytonadione
Piperacillin
Piroxicam
Pravastatin
Prazosin
Probenecid
Prochlorperazine
Progestins
Promethazine
Propantheline
Propofol
Propranolol
Protamine
Psoralens
Pyrilamine
Pyrimethamine
Quinupristin/dalfopristin
Ramipril
Ranitidine
Repaglinide
Reteplase
Riboflavin
Rifampin
Risperidone
Ritodrine
Ritonavir
Salsalate
Scopolamine
Simvastatin
Sparfloxacin
Spectinomycin
Spironolactone
Streptokinase
Streptomycin
Succinylcholine
Sulfadiazine
Sulfadoxine
Sulfamethoxazole
Sulfasalazine
Sulfisoxazole
Sulindac
Sumatriptan
Tacrolimus
Tartrazine
Temazepam
Tenecteplase
Terazosin
Terbinafine
Testosterone
Tetracycline
Thiabendazole
Thiamine
Thiopental
Thioridazine
Thiotepa
Thiothixene
Ticarcillin
Timolol
Tinzaparin
Tolmetin
Tramadol
Trastuzumab
Triamterene
Trichlormethiazide
Trifluoperazine
Trimeprazine
Trimethoprim
Tripelennamine
Triptorelin
Troleandomycin
Trovafloxacin
Urokinase
Vancomycin
Vasopressin
Vincristine
Vinorelbine
Vitamin A
Voriconazole
Zalcitabine
Zolpidem

**Angioedema**

Acetaminophen
Albuterol
Aldesleukin
Alemtuzumab
Allopurinol
Alteplase
Aminoglutethimide
Aminosalicylate sodium
Amiodarone
Amitriptyline
Amobarbital
Amoxicillin
Amphotericin B
Ampicillin
Anistreplase
Anthrax vaccine
Aprobarbital
Aprotinin
Ascorbic acid
Asparaginase
Aspartame
Aspirin
Azatadine
Azathioprine
Azithromycin
Aztreonam
Bacampicillin
Benactyzine
Benazepril
Betaxolol
Bismuth
Bisoprolol
Bleomycin
Brompheniramine
Bupropion
Butabarbital
Caffeine
Candesartan
Captopril
Carbamazepine
Carbenicillin
Carisoprodol
Carteolol
Carvedilol
Cefaclor
Cefadroxil
Cefepime
Cefoxitin
Cefprozil
Ceftazidime
Ceftriaxone
Cefuroxime
Celecoxib
Cephalexin
Cetirizine
Chloral hydrate
Chlorambucil
Chloramphenicol
Chlordiazepoxide
Chloroquine
Chlorpheniramine
Chlorpromazine
Chlorpropamide
Chlorzoxazone
Cimetidine
Cinoxacin
Ciprofloxacin
Cisplatin
Clemastine
Clonazepam
Clonidine
Cloxacillin
Co-trimoxazole
Cocaine
Codeine
Colchicine
Corticosteroids
Cromolyn
Cyanocobalamin
Cyclamate
Cyclobenzaprine
Cyclophosphamide
Cyclosporine
Cyproheptadine
Dacarbazine
Danazol
Daunorubicin
Deferoxamine
Delavirdine
Demeclocycline
Desipramine
Dexchlorpheniramine
Diazepam
Diclofenac
Dicloxacillin
Dicumarol
Diethylstilbestrol
Diflunisal
Digoxin
Diltiazem
Dimenhydrinate
Diphenhydramine
Diphenoxylate
Dipyridamole
Disopyramide
Docetaxel
Dofetilide
Doxorubicin
Doxycycline
Echinacea
Enalapril
Epoetin alfa
Eprosartan
Esomeprazole
Estrogens
Ethambutol
Etidronate
Etodolac
Famotidine
Fenoprofen
Feverfew
Finasteride
Fluconazole
Fluorouracil
Fluoxetine
Fluphenazine
Flurbiprofen
Fluvastatin
Fluvoxamine
Formoterol
Fosfomycin
Fosinopril
Gatifloxacin
Gemfibrozil
Glucagon
Glyburide
Gold and gold compounds
Griseofulvin
Halothane
Heparin
Hepatitis B vaccine
Heroin
Hydralazine
Hydroxychloroquine
Hydroxyzine
Ibritumomab
Ibuprofen
Imipenem/cilastatin
Imipramine
Indapamide

Indomethacin
Insulin
Interferons, alfa-2
Isoniazid
Itraconazole
Ketoconazole
Ketoprofen
Ketorolac
Labetalol
Lamivudine
Lamotrigine
Levamisole
Levothyroxine
Lidocaine
Lincomycin
Lisinopril
Lithium
Loratadine
Losartan
Mebendazole
Mechlorethamine
Meclizine
Meclofenamate
Medroxyprogesterone
Mefenamic acid
Meloxicam
Melphalan
Meperidine
Mephenytoin
Mephobarbital
Meprobamate
Mesna
Mesoridazine
Methadone
Methicillin
Methohexital
Methylphenidate
Metoclopramide
Metoprolol
Metronidazole
Mezlocillin
Miconazole
Midazolam
Minocycline
Mitomycin
Mitotane
Moexipril
Montelukast
Nabumetone
Nafcillin
Nalidixic acid
Naloxone
Naproxen
Neomycin
Nifedipine
Nisoldipine
Nitrofurantoin
Nitroglycerin
Norfloxacin
Ofloxacin
Olmesartan
Omeprazole
Ondansetron
Oral contraceptives
Oxacillin
Oxaprozin
Oxcarbazepine
Oxytetracycline
Paclitaxel
Pamidronate
Pantoprazole
Paroxetine
PEG-interferon alfa-2b
Penicillins
Pentagastrin
Pentobarbital
Pentoxifylline
Perindopril
Perphenazine
Phenelzine
Phenindamine
Phenobarbital
Phenolphthalein
Phenytoin
Piperacillin
Piroxicam
Potassium iodide
Pravastatin
Prazosin
Primaquine
Procainamide
Procarbazine
Progestins
Promethazine
Propranolol
Propylthiouracil
Protamine
Protriptyline
Pseudoephedrine
Pyrilamine
Pyrimethamine
Quetiapine
Quinapril
Quinestrol
Quinidine
Quinine
Ramipril
Ranitidine
Riboflavin
Rifampin
Risperidone
Ritonavir
Rituximab
Rofecoxib
Salmeterol
Salsalate
Secobarbital
Sertraline
Simvastatin
Sparfloxacin
Streptokinase
Streptomycin
Sucralfate
Sulfamethoxazole
Sulfasalazine
Sulfisoxazole
Sulindac
Sumatriptan
Tamsulosin
Tartrazine
Telmisartan
Tenecteplase
Terbinafine
Tetracycline
Thiabendazole
Thiamine
Thiopental
Thioridazine
Thiotepa
Ticarcillin
Ticlopidine
Timolol
Tinzaparin
Tiopronin
Tolmetin
Torsemide
Tramadol
Trandolapril
Trastuzumab
Trifluoperazine
Trimeprazine
Trimetrexate
Tripelennamine
Triprolidine
Triptorelin
Troleandomycin
Trovafloxacin
Urokinase
Valsartan
Vancomycin
Vasopressin
Verapamil
Vincristine
Vinorelbine
Voriconazole
Warfarin
Zalcitabine

**Anosmia**

Acetazolamide
Ciprofloxacin
Cocaine
Cromolyn
Doxycycline
Enalapril
Ganciclovir
Interferons, alfa-2
Methazolamide
Minoxidil
Paroxetine
Pentamidine
Sparfloxacin
Terbinafine

**Aphthous Stomatitis**

Aldesleukin
Anagrelide
Asparaginase
Aspirin
Azathioprine
Azelastine
Aztreonam
Captopril
Cidofovir
Co-trimoxazole
Cyclosporine
Delavirdine
Diclofenac
Diflunisal
Doxepin
Fenoprofen
Fluoxetine
Flurbiprofen
Gold and gold compounds
Hepatitis B vaccine
Ibuprofen
Imiquimod
Indinavir
Indomethacin
Interferons, alfa-2
Ketoprofen
Ketorolac
Losartan
Meclofenamate
Midodrine
Mirtazapine
Naproxen
Olanzapine
Pantoprazole
Paroxetine
Penicillamine
Piroxicam
Rofecoxib
Sertraline
Sirolimus
Sulfamethoxazole
Sulfasalazine
Sulfisoxazole
Sulindac
Terbinafine
Tolmetin
Trientine
Valsartan
Zalcitabine
Zaleplon

**Black Hairy Tongue (Lingua Villosa Nigra)**

Amitriptyline
Amoxapine
Amoxicillin
Ampicillin
Bacampicillin
Benztropine
Carbenicillin
Chloramphenicol
Clarithromycin
Clomipramine
Clonazepam
Cloxacillin
Co-trimoxazole
Cocaine
Corticosteroids
Desipramine
Dicloxacillin
Fluoxetine
Griseofulvin
Imipramine
Isocarboxazid
Lansoprazole
Maprotiline
Methicillin
Methyldopa
Mezlocillin
Minocycline
Nafcillin
Nortriptyline
Oxacillin
Oxytetracycline
Penicillins
Phenelzine
Protriptyline
Streptomycin
Sulfamethoxazole
Tetracycline
Thiothixene
Ticarcillin
Tranylcypromine

**Bullous Eruptions**

Acetazolamide
Acitretin
Aldesleukin
Alemtuzumab

Alitretinoin
Aminocaproic acid
Aminosalicylate sodium
Amitriptyline
Amobarbital
Ampicillin
Argatroban
Arsenic
Aspirin
Atropine sulfate
Benactyzine
Bleomycin
Bumetanide
Buspirone
Busulfan
Butabarbital
Butalbital
Caffeine
Captopril
Carbamazepine
Carbenicillin
Cetirizine
Cevimeline
Chloral hydrate
Chloramphenicol
Chlorothiazide
Chlorpromazine
Chlorpropamide
Ciprofloxacin
Clopidogrel
Co-trimoxazole
Cocaine
Codeine
Colchicine
Corticosteroids
Cyanocobalamin
Cyclamate
Cyclosporine
Cytarabine
Dalteparin
Dapsone
Demeclocycline
Denileukin
Dextromethorphan
Diazepam
Diclofenac
Dicloxacillin
Dicumarol
Diethylstilbestrol
Diflunisal
Digoxin
Dirithromycin
Disulfiram
Ephedrine
Estrogens
Ethambutol
Ethchlorvynol
Ethotoin
Etodolac
Felbamate
Fenoprofen
Fluconazole
Fluorouracil
Fluoxetine
Flutamide
Fluvoxamine
Fondaparinux
Fosphenytoin
Frovatriptan
Furosemide
Ganciclovir
Garlic
Glyburide
Gold and gold compounds
Granulocyte colony-stimulating factor (GCSF)
Griseofulvin
Henna
Hydralazine
Hydrochlorothiazide
Hydroxychloroquine
Ibuprofen
Ibutilide
Idarubicin
Imipramine
Imiquimod
Indapamide
Indomethacin
Insulin
Interferons, alfa-2
Isoniazid
Ivermectin
Ketoprofen
Lamotrigine
Leflunomide
Lidocaine
Lindane
Lisinopril
Lithium
Mechlorethamine
Meclofenamate
Meloxicam
Mephenytoin
Meprobamate
Methicillin
Methotrexate
Methoxsalen
Mezlocillin
Miconazole
Minoxidil
Mitomycin
Mycophenolate
Nabumetone
Nafcillin
Nalidixic acid
Naproxen
Neomycin
Nifedipine
Nitrofurantoin
Norfloxacin
Ofloxacin
Omeprazole
Oral contraceptives
Oxacillin
Penicillamine
Pentamidine
Pentobarbital
Pentostatin
Phenobarbital
Phenolphthalein
Phenytoin
Piperacillin
Piroxicam
Promethazine
Propranolol
Pyridoxine
Pyrimethamine
Quinapril
Quinethazone
Quinidine
Quinine
Reserpine
Rifampin
Risperidone
Ritonavir
Rivastigmine
Rofecoxib
Saquinavir
Sertraline
Smallpox vaccine
Sparfloxacin
Streptomycin
Sulfadoxine
Sulfamethoxazole
Sulfasalazine
Sulfisoxazole
Tacrine
Temazepam
Testosterone
Tetracycline
Thalidomide
Thiopental
Ticarcillin
Tinzaparin
Tolbutamide
Tolmetin
Tretinoin
Trimethadione
Trioxsalen
Urokinase
Valproic acid
Vancomycin
Vasopressin
Vinblastine
Warfarin
Zalcitabine
Zidovudine
Zolpidem

**Bullous Pemphigoid**

Aldesleukin
Amoxicillin
Ampicillin
Bumetanide
Captopril
Cephalexin
Chloroquine
Ciprofloxacin
Dactinomycin
Enalapril
Fosinopril
Furosemide
Gold and gold compounds
Hepatitis B vaccine
Ibuprofen
Ivermectin
Mefenamic acid
Methoxsalen
Nadolol
Omeprazole
Penicillamine
Penicillins
Potassium iodide
Psoralens
Risperidone
Spironolactone
Sulfasalazine
Tiopronin
Tolbutamide

**Candidiasis**

Ampicillin
Basiliximab
Cefaclor
Cefadroxil
Cefdinir
Cefepime
Cefixime
Cefmetazole
Cefonicid
Cefoperazone
Cefotaxime
Cefotetan
Cefoxitin
Cefpodoxime
Cefprozil
Ceftazidime
Ceftibuten
Ceftizoxime
Ceftriaxone
Cefuroxime
Celecoxib
Cephalothin
Cephapirin
Chlorotrianisene
Ciprofloxacin
Danazol
Demeclocycline
Diazoxide
Eletriptan
Ertapenem
Esomeprazole
Fluoxetine
Gatifloxacin
Griseofulvin
Heroin
Imipenem/cilastatin
Infliximab
Interferons, alfa-2
Lansoprazole
Levofloxacin
Linezolid
Loracarbef
Methotrexate
Metronidazole
Minocycline
Moxifloxacin
Ofloxacin
Olanzapine
Oral contraceptives
Pamidronate
Paroxetine
Pentostatin
Piperacillin
Quetiapine
Quinupristin/dalfopristin
Riluzole
Saquinavir
Tetracycline
Tizanidine
Trovafloxacin
Valdecoxib
Venlafaxine
Zoledronic acid

**Cheilitis**

Acitretin
Atorvastatin
Bexarotene
Busulfan
Clofazimine
Clomipramine
Cyanocobalamin

Dactinomycin
Eflornithine
Frovatriptan
Gatifloxacin
Gold and gold compounds
Indinavir
Isotretinoin
Lithium
Methoxsalen
Methyldopa
Propolis
Propranolol
Psoralens
Ritonavir
Saquinavir
Simvastatin
Streptomycin
Sulfasalazine
Tetracycline
Thimerosal
Tretinoin
Trovafloxacin
Verteporfin
Vitamin A
Voriconazole
Zaleplon

**Chills**

Abacavir
Acitretin
Albuterol
Alemtuzumab
Allopurinol
Almotriptan
Amifostine
Amphotericin B
Anagrelide
Anastrozole
Anisindione
Anistreplase
Anthrax vaccine
Asparaginase
Azathioprine
Bexarotene
Bleomycin
Caffeine
Caspofungin
Ceftriaxone
Cidofovir
Cilostazol
Dantrolene
Daunorubicin
Denileukin
Dexchlorpheniramine
Dextroamphetamine
Didanosine
Dolasetron
Droperidol
Eletriptan
Enoxacin
Ertapenem
Estazolam
Ethacrynic acid
Ethambutol
Fludarabine
Fosphenytoin
Ganciclovir
Gatifloxacin
Gemtuzumab
Goserelin
Heparin
Hepatitis B vaccine
Hydralazine
Ibritumomab
Infliximab
Interferon beta 1-a
Interferons, alfa-2
Irbesartan
Irinotecan
Ketoconazole
Lamivudine
Levalbuterol
Lomefloxacin
MDMA
Metolazone
Miconazole
Midodrine
Mifepristone
Mirtazapine
Mistletoe
Mitoxantrone
Modafinil
Moxifloxacin
Naltrexone
Nifedipine
Nisoldipine
Nitrofurantoin
Ofloxacin
Ondansetron
Pergolide
Perindopril
Pilocarpine
Procainamide
Promethazine
Rabeprazole
Riluzole
Ritodrine
Rituximab
Rizatriptan
Sirolimus
Smallpox vaccine
Spectinomycin
Spironolactone
Stanozolol
Stavudine
Sufentanil
Sulfadiazine
Tenofovir
Terconazole
Trastuzumab
Triamterene
Trihexyphenidyl
Urokinase
Valdecoxib
Vancomycin
Verteporfin
Voriconazole
Zaleplon
Ziprasidone

**Contact Dermatitis**

Acetaminophen
Acyclovir
Albendazole
Albuterol
Aloe vera (gel, juice, leaf)
Amantadine
Aminocaproic acid
Aminolevulinic acid
Aminophylline
Amoxicillin
Amphotericin B
Ampicillin
Amyl nitrite
Apraclonidine
Arnica
Arsenic
Atorvastatin
Atropine sulfate
Azathioprine
Azelastine
Azithromycin
Bacampicillin
Bendroflumethiazide
Betaxolol
Biperiden
Bismuth
Bloodroot
Bumetanide
Captopril
Carbamazepine
Carmustine
Carteolol
Cefazolin
Cephalexin
Chamomile
Chloramphenicol
Chlorhexidine
Chloroquine
Chlorpheniramine
Chlorpromazine
Chlorpropamide
Cisplatin
Clindamycin
Clomipramine
Clonidine
Clotrimazole
Cloxacillin
Codeine
Corticosteroids
Cromolyn
Cyanocobalamin
Cyclophosphamide
Cyproheptadine
Daunorubicin
Dexchlorpheniramine
Diazepam
Diclofenac
Diphenhydramine
Disulfiram
Docusate
Dorzolamide
Doxepin
Doxorubicin
Eflornithine
Ephedrine
Epinephrine
Epoetin alfa
Erythromycin
Estrogens
Ethambutol
Ethanolamine
Famotidine
Feverfew
Fluorouracil
Fluoxetine
Fluoxymesterone
Fluphenazine
Flurbiprofen
Furazolidone
Garlic
Gentamicin
Ginger
Ginkgo biloba
Gold and gold compounds
Haloperidol
Henna
Heparin
Heroin
Horse chestnut – flower
Hydroxychloroquine
Hydroxyzine
Ibuprofen
Ibutilide
Indinavir
Indomethacin
Insulin
Interferon beta 1-a
Interferons, alfa-2
Ipratropium
Isoniazid
Ketoconazole
Ketoprofen
Labetalol
Lamivudine
Lansoprazole
Lavender
Levobetaxolol
Levobunolol
Licorice
Lidocaine
Lincomycin
Lindane
Mechlorethamine
Mesoridazine
Methoxsalen
Methyltestosterone
Metronidazole
Mezlocillin
Miconazole
Minoxidil
Mitomycin
Neomycin
Niacin
Nicotine
Nitrofurantoin
Nitroglycerin
Nizatidine
Norfloxacin
Nystatin
Olanzapine
Omeprazole
Oxcarbazepine
Oxytetracycline
Pantoprazole
Paroxetine
Penicillamine
Penicillins
Pentostatin
Perphenazine
Phenoxybenzamine
Phenylephrine
Phytonadione
Pilocarpine
Piroxicam
Promethazine
Propantheline
Propolis
Propranolol
Pseudoephedrine
Psoralens
Pyridoxine

Quinacrine
Quinidine
Quinine
Ranitidine
Rifampin
Ritonavir
Rivastigmine
Rofecoxib
Scopolamine
Senna
Sildenafil
Sparfloxacin
Spectinomycin
Spironolactone
Streptomycin
Succinylcholine
Tartrazine
Terbinafine
Terbutaline
Testosterone
Thiabendazole
Thiamine
Thimerosal
Tiagabine
Timolol
Tiopronin
Tobramycin
Tolazoline
Tolbutamide
Trifluoperazine
Turmeric
Valdecoxib
Valproic acid
Venlafaxine
Vitamin A
Vitamin E
Voriconazole
Zaleplon
Ziprasidone

**Dermatitis**

Acebutolol
Acetaminophen
Acitretin
Acyclovir
Aldesleukin
Almotriptan
Alprazolam
Altretamine
Amantadine
Amikacin
Aminocaproic acid
Aminophylline
Amitriptyline
Amlodipine
Amoxapine
Amyl nitrite
Anisindione
Apraclonidine
Arsenic
Aspartame
Atenolol
Baclofen
Benazepril
Beta-carotene
Bleomycin
Capecitabine
Captopril
Carbamazepine
Carmustine
Carteolol
Cefaclor
Ceftriaxone
Celecoxib
Cetirizine
Cevimeline
Chloral hydrate
Chloramphenicol
Chlordiazepoxide
Chlorhexidine
Chlorotrianisene
Chlorpheniramine
Chlorpromazine
Cimetidine
Citalopram
Clofibrate
Clomiphene
Clomipramine
Clonazepam
Clorazepate
Clozapine
Co-trimoxazole
Colchicine
Colestipol
Corticosteroids
Cromolyn
Cyclobenzaprine
Cycloserine
Cyproheptadine
Dacarbazine
Dactinomycin
Dantrolene
Deferoxamine
Delavirdine
Diazepam
Diclofenac
Dicloxacillin
Dicumarol
Diltiazem
Disopyramide
Docetaxel
Donepezil
Doxepin
Enalapril
Ephedrine
Ertapenem
Esomeprazole
Estazolam
Estrogens
Ethambutol
Etodolac
Famciclovir
Fluorouracil
Fluphenazine
Flurazepam
Fluvoxamine
Folic acid
Foscarnet
Gemcitabine
Gemfibrozil
Ginger
Gold and gold compounds
Guanethidine
Guanfacine
Heparin
Hydrochlorothiazide
Hydroxyurea
Ifosfamide
Indinavir
Interferons, alfa-2
Irbesartan
Isoxsuprine
Itraconazole
Ivermectin
Ketoprofen
Ketorolac
Leflunomide
Leuprolide
Levamisole
Levobetaxolol
Lithium
Loratadine
Lorazepam
Losartan
Loxapine
Mechlorethamine
Mefloquine
Meprobamate
Mercaptopurine
Metaxalone
Methotrexate
Methoxsalen
Misoprostol
Mistletoe
Mitomycin
Nadolol
Naproxen
Naratriptan
Nelfinavir
Neomycin
Nifedipine
Nystatin
Ofloxacin
Oral contraceptives
Orlistat
Oxazepam
Palivizumab
PEG-interferon alfa-2b
Penicillins
Pentazocine
Pentostatin
Phenindamine
Phenytoin
Pilocarpine
Piroxicam
Prazepam
Probenecid
Procainamide
Procarbazine
Progestins
Promazine
Promethazine
Propolis
Propylthiouracil
Protriptyline
Pseudoephedrine
Psoralens
Pyrazinamide
Pyrilamine
Pyrimethamine
Quazepam
Quinidine
Ramipril
Risperidone
Rofecoxib
Ropinirole
Saccharin
Salsalate
Saquinavir
Scopolamine
Sertraline
Simvastatin
Sirolimus
Sulfamethoxazole
Sulfasalazine
Sulfinpyrazone
Sulindac
Tacrine
Tartrazine
Telmisartan
Temazepam
Tetracycline
Thalidomide
Thimerosal
Thioridazine
Ticlopidine
Timolol
Tolazamide
Tolmetin
Topiramate
Toremifene
Tramadol
Tretinoin
Triazolam
Trientine
Trimeprazine
Trovafloxacin
Valacyclovir
Valdecoxib
Verapamil
Vinblastine
Vitamin A
Vitamin E
Warfarin
Zalcitabine
Ziprasidone
Zolpidem

**Dermatitis Herpetiformis (DH)**

Amitriptyline
Aspirin
Cyclophosphamide
Diclofenac
Doxorubicin
Flurbiprofen
Ibuprofen
Indomethacin
Interferons, alfa-2
Levothyroxine
Lithium
Mycophenolate
Oral contraceptives
Potassium iodide
Sirolimus
Vincristine

**Diaphoresis**

Acebutolol
Acetaminophen
Acetohexamide
Acitretin
Acyclovir
Albuterol
Allopurinol
Almotriptan
Alprazolam
Alprostadil
Amiloride
Aminophylline
Amiodarone
Amitriptyline
Amlodipine

Amoxapine
Amphotericin B
Amyl nitrite
Anastrozole
Anistreplase
Anthrax vaccine
Arbutamine
Asparaginase
Aspirin
Atenolol
Atorvastatin
Atovaquone
Azatadine
Aztreonam
Baclofen
Benazepril
Bendroflumethiazide
Bepridil
Betaxolol
Bethanechol
Bicalutamide
Biperiden
Bisacodyl
Bisoprolol
Black cohosh
Bretylium
Bumetanide
Bupropion
Buspirone
Butorphanol
Candesartan
Capecitabine
Carbamazepine
Carisoprodol
Carteolol
Carvedilol
Caspofungin
Cefamandole
Cefditoren
Cefpodoxime
Ceftazidime
Ceftriaxone
Celecoxib
Cetirizine
Cevimeline
Chlordiazepoxide
Chlorpheniramine
Cidofovir
Ciprofloxacin
Cisplatin
Citalopram
Cladribine
Clemastine
Clofibrate
Clomiphene
Clomipramine
Clonazepam
Clonidine
Clorazepate
Clozapine
Cocaine
Codeine
Corticosteroids
Cyclobenzaprine
Cyclophosphamide
Cyproheptadine
Danazol
Dantrolene
Delavirdine
Denileukin
Desipramine
Desmopressin
Dexchlorpheniramine
Dexmedetomidine
Dextroamphetamine
Diazepam
Diazoxide
Diclofenac
Didanosine
Diethylpropion
Diflunisal
Digoxin
Diltiazem
Dimenhydrinate
Diphenhydramine
Diphenoxylate
Dipyridamole
Dirithromycin
Disulfiram
Docusate
Dofetilide
Dolasetron
Domperidone
Donepezil
Doxapram
Doxazosin
Doxepin
Dronabinol
Droperidol
Edrophonium
Eletriptan
Enalapril
Enoxacin
Entacapone
Ephedrine
Epinephrine
Eprosartan
Ertapenem
Esmolol
Esomeprazole
Estazolam
Ethambutol
Ethchlorvynol
Etodolac
Etoposide
Exemestane
Felbamate
Felodipine
Fenoprofen
Fentanyl
Flecainide
Flumazenil
Fluoxetine
Fluphenazine
Flurazepam
Flurbiprofen
Flutamide
Fluvoxamine
Foscarnet
Fosinopril
Frovatriptan
Fulvestrant
Furosemide
Ganciclovir
Gatifloxacin
Gemcitabine
Glimepiride
Goserelin
Granulocyte colony-stimulating factor (GCSF)
Guanfacine
Haloperidol
Hawthorn (fruit, leaf, flower extract)
Hepatitis B vaccine
Hydralazine
Hydrochlorothiazide
Hydrocodone
Hydromorphone
Hydroxyzine
Ibritumomab
Ibuprofen
Imipenem/cilastatin
Imipramine
Indapamide
Indinavir
Indomethacin
Insulin
Interferon beta 1-a
Interferons, alfa-2
Irinotecan
Isocarboxazid
Isoproterenol
Isosorbide dinitrate
Isosorbide mononitrate
Isotretinoin
Isradipine
Ketoprofen
Ketorolac
Labetalol
Lamotrigine
Lansoprazole
Leflunomide
Letrozole
Leuprolide
Levalbuterol
Levodopa
Levofloxacin
Levothyroxine
Liothyronine
Lisinopril
Lomefloxacin
Loratadine
Lorazepam
Losartan
Loxapine
Maprotiline
Mazindol
MDMA
Medroxyprogesterone
Mefenamic acid
Meperidine
Mesalamine
Methadone
Methamphetamine
Methylphenidate
Metoclopramide
Metoprolol
Mexiletine
Milk thistle
Mirtazapine
Misoprostol
Mitoxantrone
Modafinil
Moexipril
Moricizine
Morphine
Moxifloxacin
Mycophenolate
Nabumetone
Nadolol
Naloxone
Naltrexone
Naproxen
Naratriptan
Nelfinavir
Nesiritide
Nicotine
Nifedipine
Nimodipine
Nisoldipine
Nitroglycerin
Nizatidine
Norfloxacin
Nortriptyline
Octreotide
Ofloxacin
Olanzapine
Omeprazole
Oxaprozin
Oxazepam
Oxcarbazepine
Oxycodone
Pantoprazole
Papaverine
Paroxetine
PEG-interferon alfa-2b
Penbutolol
Penicillins
Pentagastrin
Pentazocine
Pentostatin
Pentoxifylline
Pergolide
Perindopril
Perphenazine
Phendimetrazine
Phenelzine
Phenindamine
Phenolphthalein
Phentermine
Phytonadione
Pilocarpine
Pimozide
Pindolol
Piroxicam
Potassium iodide
Pramipexole
Prazepam
Praziquantel
Prazosin
Procarbazine
Prochlorperazine
Progestins
Promethazine
Propafenone
Propantheline
Propoxyphene
Propranolol
Protriptyline
Pseudoephedrine
Pyrilamine
Quazepam
Quetiapine
Quinapril
Quinine
Quinupristin/dalfopristin
Rabeprazole
Raloxifene
Ramipril

Rapacuronium
Rifampin
Risperidone
Ritodrine
Ritonavir
Rituximab
Rivastigmine
Rizatriptan
Rofecoxib
Ropinirole
Saquinavir
Selegiline
Sertraline
Sibutramine
Sildenafil
Simvastatin
Sirolimus
Sotalol
Sparfloxacin
Spironolactone
Stavudine
Streptokinase
Sulfasalazine
Sulindac
Sumatriptan
Tacrine
Tacrolimus
Tamoxifen
Telmisartan
Temazepam
Terazosin
Terbutaline
Tetracycline
Thalidomide
Thiamine
Thiothixene
Tiagabine
Ticlopidine
Timolol
Tirofiban
Tizanidine
Tocainide
Tolazamide
Tolcapone
Tolmetin
Topiramate
Toremifene
Tramadol
Tranylcypromine
Trastuzumab
Trazodone
Tretinoin
Triamterene
Triazolam
Trifluoperazine
Trihexyphenidyl
Trimeprazine
Trimipramine
Tripelennamine
Triprolidine
Trovafloxacin
Unoprostone
Urokinase
Ursodiol
Valdecoxib
Valproic acid
Vasopressin
Venlafaxine
Verapamil
Verteporfin
Voriconazole
Yohimbine
Zalcitabine
Zaleplon
Zidovudine
Zolmitriptan
Zolpidem
Zonisamide

**Dysgeusia**

Acebutolol
Acetaminophen
Acetazolamide
Acyclovir
Albuterol
Aldesleukin
Alemtuzumab
Alendronate
Allopurinol
Almotriptan
Alosetron
Alprazolam
Amifostine
Amiloride
Amiodarone
Amitriptyline
Amlodipine
Amoxapine
Amoxicillin
Amprenavir
Apraclonidine
Arbutamine
Arsenic
Aspirin
Atorvastatin
Atovaquone
Atropine sulfate
Azelastine
Aztreonam
Bacampicillin
Baclofen
Benazepril
Benzthiazide
Benztropine
Bepridil
Betaxolol
Bismuth
Bisoprolol
Botulinum toxin (A & B)
Brimonidine
Bromocriptine
Bupropion
Buspirone
Busulfan
Butorphanol
Calcitonin
Captopril
Carbamazepine
Carbenicillin
Carteolol
Cefaclor
Cefamandole
Cefditoren
Cefmetazole
Cefpodoxime
Ceftazidime
Ceftibuten
Ceftriaxone
Celecoxib
Cetirizine
Cevimeline
Chloral hydrate
Chlorhexidine
Chlormezanone
Chlorothiazide
Cholestyramine
Cidofovir
Cinoxacin
Ciprofloxacin
Citalopram
Clarithromycin
Clidinium
Clindamycin
Clofazimine
Clofibrate
Clomipramine
Clonazepam
Clonidine
Clotrimazole
Clozapine
Co-trimoxazole
Codeine
Cromolyn
Cyclobenzaprine
Cyproheptadine
Dacarbazine
Dantrolene
Delavirdine
Desipramine
Dextroamphetamine
Diazoxide
Diclofenac
Dicloxacillin
Dicyclomine
Diethylpropion
Dihydroergotamine
Dihydrotachysterol
Diltiazem
Dipyridamole
Dirithromycin
Disulfiram
Docusate
Dolasetron
Donepezil
Dorzolamide
Doxazosin
Doxepin
Doxycycline
Efavirenz
Eletriptan
Enalapril
Enoxacin
Entacapone
Ergocalciferol
Ertapenem
Esmolol
Esomeprazole
Estazolam
Ethchlorvynol
Ethionamide
Etidronate
Etoposide
Famotidine
Felbamate
Fenoprofen
Fentanyl
Flecainide
Fluconazole
Fludarabine
Fluorouracil
Fluoxetine
Flurazepam
Flurbiprofen
Fluvastatin
Fluvoxamine
Foscarnet
Fosinopril
Fosphenytoin
Frovatriptan
Ganciclovir
Gatifloxacin
Gemcitabine
Gemfibrozil
Glyburide
Glycopyrrolate
Gold and gold compounds
Granisetron
Griseofulvin
Guanabenz
Guanfacine
Hydrochlorothiazide
Hydroflumethiazide
Hydromorphone
Hydroxychloroquine
Hyoscyamine
Imipenem/cilastatin
Imipramine
Indinavir
Interferons, alfa-2
Ipratropium
Irinotecan
Isotretinoin
Ketoprofen
Ketorolac
Labetalol
Lamotrigine
Lansoprazole
Leflunomide
Leuprolide
Levamisole
Levobetaxolol
Levodopa
Levofloxacin
Linezolid
Lisinopril
Lithium
Lomefloxacin
Loratadine
Losartan
Lovastatin
Maprotiline
Mazindol
Mechlorethamine
Meclofenamate
Meloxicam
Mesalamine
Mesna
Metformin
Methamphetamine
Methantheline
Methazolamide
Methicillin
Methimazole
Methocarbamol
Methotrexate
Methyclothiazide
Metolazone
Metoprolol
Metronidazole
Mexiletine
Mezlocillin

Midazolam
Minoxidil
Mirtazapine
Modafinil
Moexipril
Moricizine
Moxifloxacin
Nadolol
Nafcillin
Naratriptan
Nefazodone
Nicotine
Nifedipine
Nisoldipine
Norfloxacin
Nortriptyline
Ofloxacin
Olanzapine
Olopatadine
Omeprazole
Ondansetron
Oxacillin
Oxaprozin
Oxcarbazepine
Pamidronate
Pantoprazole
Paroxetine
PEG-interferon alfa-2b
Penbutolol
Penicillamine
Penicillins
Pentamidine
Pentazocine
Pentostatin
Pentoxifylline
Pergolide
Perindopril
Phendimetrazine
Phentermine
Phytonadione
Pilocarpine
Pimozide
Pindolol
Pirbuterol
Plicamycin
Potassium iodide
Pramipexole
Pravastatin
Procainamide
Propafenone
Propantheline
Propofol
Propranolol
Propylthiouracil
Protriptyline
Pyrimethamine
Quazepam
Quinapril
Quinidine
Ramipril
Ranitidine
Ribavirin
Rifabutin
Riluzole
Rimantadine
Risperidone
Ritonavir
Rivastigmine
Saccharin
Saquinavir
Selegiline
Sertraline
Sibutramine
Simvastatin
Sirolimus
Sotalol
Sparfloxacin
Sulfamethoxazole
Sulfasalazine
Sulfisoxazole
Sulindac
Sumatriptan
Tacrine
Tamoxifen
Temazepam
Terbinafine
Terbutaline
Thiothixene
Tiagabine
Ticarcillin
Timolol
Tocainide
Tolazamide
Tolbutamide
Tolmetin
Topiramate
Tramadol
Trazodone
Triamterene
Triazolam
Trimethoprim
Trimipramine
Trovafloxacin
Ursodiol
Valdecoxib
Valproic acid
Valsartan
Vancomycin
Venlafaxine
Vinblastine
Vincristine
Vinorelbine
Voriconazole
Zalcitabine
Zidovudine
Zolpidem
Zonisamide

**Ecchymoses**

Allopurinol
Alprostadil
Alteplase
Amiodarone
Amoxicillin
Anagrelide
Anisindione
Anistreplase
Atorvastatin
Bacampicillin
Benactyzine
Beta-carotene
Botulinum toxin (A & B)
Bupropion
Buspirone
Caffeine
Carbenicillin
Celecoxib
Chlorzoxazone
Cholestyramine
Cilostazol
Cloxacillin
Corticosteroids
Delavirdine
Denileukin
Desipramine
Dicloxacillin
Dicumarol
Diethylpropion
Diltiazem
Donepezil
Enoxaparin
Etodolac
Etoposide
Fluvoxamine
Fosphenytoin
Gatifloxacin
Gemtuzumab
Heparin
Hepatitis B vaccine
Ibritumomab
Indomethacin
Interferon beta 1-a
Interferons, alfa-2
Irbesartan
Lamotrigine
Latanoprost
Leuprolide
Levetiracetam
Lindane
Losartan
Meprobamate
Mesalamine
Methicillin
Methotrexate
Mezlocillin
Mitoxantrone
Modafinil
Nafcillin
Naproxen
Nefazodone
Nisoldipine
Ofloxacin
Olanzapine
Oxacillin
Oxaprozin
Pantoprazole
Paroxetine
Penicillamine
Pentosan
Pentostatin
Perindopril
Piperacillin
Piroxicam
Plicamycin
Rabeprazole
Reteplase
Risedronate
Ritonavir
Sibutramine
Sirolimus
Sparfloxacin
Streptokinase
Sulindac
Tacrolimus
Tenecteplase
Thiotepa
Tiagabine
Ticarcillin
Ticlopidine
Tinzaparin
Tiopronin
Tizanidine
Urokinase
Valdecoxib
Valproic acid
Vasopressin
Venlafaxine
Verapamil
Voriconazole
Warfarin
Zaleplon
Zidovudine
Ziprasidone
Zolmitriptan
Zonisamide

**Eczema**

Acetohexamide
Aldesleukin
Amantadine
Aminocaproic acid
Aminosalicylate sodium
Ascorbic acid
Atorvastatin
Azelastine
Bisoprolol
Carbamazepine
Cevimeline
Chloral hydrate
Chloramphenicol
Citalopram
Clindamycin
Clonidine
Clopidogrel
Clozapine
Corticosteroids
Cromolyn
Cyanocobalamin
Diazepam
Diclofenac
Dimenhydrinate
Diphenhydramine
Disulfiram
Doxazosin
Efavirenz
Eprosartan
Erythromycin
Esmolol
Estrogens
Ethionamide
Fluorouracil
Fluoxetine
Fluphenazine
Flurbiprofen
Gemfibrozil
Gentamicin
Glipizide
Glyburide
Gold and gold compounds
Heparin
Hydralazine
Hydrochlorothiazide
Ibuprofen
Indomethacin
Interferons, alfa-2
Isoniazid
Isotretinoin
Kanamycin
Ketoconazole
Ketoprofen
Labetalol
Lamotrigine

Latanoprost
Leflunomide
Lidocaine
Lindane
Lithium
Lomefloxacin
Meprobamate
Mesalamine
Mesoridazine
Metformin
Methenamine
Methoxsalen
Methyldopa
Metoprolol
Minoxidil
Nadolol
Nefazodone
Neomycin
Nitrofurantoin
Nitroglycerin
Nystatin
Olanzapine
Omeprazole
Oral contraceptives
Oxcarbazepine
Palivizumab
Pantoprazole
Paroxetine
Penicillins
Pentostatin
Perphenazine
Phytonadione
Pindolol
Potassium iodide
Pravastatin
Procainamide
Prochlorperazine
Promethazine
Propranolol
Pseudoephedrine
Psoralens
Quinidine
Quinine
Ranitidine
Riluzole
Ritonavir
Ropinirole
Salmeterol
Saquinavir
Simvastatin
Spironolactone
Streptomycin
Sulfasalazine
Sulfisoxazole
Tacrine
Tamsulosin
Telmisartan
Terbinafine
Tetracycline
Thiamine
Thimerosal
Tiagabine
Timolol
Tobramycin
Tolazamide
Tolcapone
Topiramate
Trifluoperazine
Trioxsalen
Tripelennamine
Valdecoxib
Venlafaxine
Verteporfin
Vitamin A
Voriconazole
Zaleplon
Ziprasidone
Zonisamide

**Edema**

Abacavir
Acebutolol
Acetaminophen
Acitretin
Acyclovir
Aldesleukin
Alemtuzumab
Alitretinoin
Allopurinol
Alprazolam
Alprostadil
Amantadine
Aminocaproic acid
Aminolevulinic acid
Amiodarone
Amitriptyline
Amlodipine
Amoxapine
Amoxicillin
Amyl nitrite
Anagrelide
Anthrax vaccine
Apraclonidine
Asparaginase
Atenolol
Atorvastatin
Atracurium
Atropine sulfate
Azatadine
Azithromycin
Bacampicillin
Baclofen
Basiliximab
Benactyzine
Benazepril
Bendroflumethiazide
Bepridil
Betaxolol
Bexarotene
Bicalutamide
Bisoprolol
Bosentan
Botulinum toxin (A & B)
Brimonidine
Bromocriptine
Bumetanide
Bupropion
Buspirone
Butorphanol
Butterbur
Cabergoline
Caffeine
Calcitonin
Candesartan
Capecitabine
Carbamazepine
Carbenicillin
Carboplatin
Carisoprodol
Carteolol
Carvedilol
Caspofungin
Cefaclor
Cefamandole
Cefdinir
Cefmetazole
Cefonicid
Cefpodoxime
Ceftazidime
Ceftizoxime
Celecoxib
Cetirizine
Cetrorelix
Cevimeline
Chlorambucil
Chlordiazepoxide
Chlorhexidine
Chlormezanone
Chlorotrianisene
Chlorpropamide
Chlortetracycline
Cholestyramine
Chondroitin
Cidofovir
Cilostazol
Cinoxacin
Ciprofloxacin
Cisplatin
Citalopram
Cladribine
Clemastine
Clindamycin
Clofazimine
Clomiphene
Clomipramine
Clonazepam
Clonidine
Clopidogrel
Clotrimazole
Clozapine
Codeine
Colestipol
Corticosteroids
Cromolyn
Cyclobenzaprine
Cyclosporine
Cyproheptadine
Cytarabine
Dalteparin
Danaparoid
Danazol
Deferoxamine
Delavirdine
Denileukin
Desipramine
Desmopressin
Dexchlorpheniramine
Diazoxide
Diclofenac
Diethylstilbestrol
Diflunisal
Dihydroergotamine
Diltiazem
Dimenhydrinate
Diphenhydramine
Dipyridamole
Dirithromycin
Disopyramide
Docetaxel
Dofetilide
Dolasetron
Domperidone
Donepezil
Dorzolamide
Doxazosin
Doxepin
Doxercalciferol
Eflornithine
Eletriptan
Enalapril
Enoxacin
Enoxaparin
Ephedrine
Epoetin alfa
Eprosartan
Ertapenem
Esmolol
Esomeprazole
Estazolam
Estramustine
Estrogens
Ethosuximide
Etodolac
Etoposide
Exemestane
Famotidine
Felbamate
Felodipine
Fentanyl
Flecainide
Fludarabine
Fluorouracil
Fluoxetine
Fluoxymesterone
Fluphenazine
Flurbiprofen
Flutamide
Fluvoxamine
Fondaparinux
Foscarnet
Fosinopril
Fosphenytoin
Fulvestrant
Gabapentin
Galantamine
Ganciclovir
Gatifloxacin
Gemcitabine
Gentamicin
Ginseng
Glimepiride
Glipizide
Glyburide
Goserelin
Guanabenz
Guanfacine
Henna
Hepatitis B vaccine
Heroin
Hydralazine
Hydrocodone
Hydroxyurea
Hydroxyzine
Ibuprofen
Imatinib
Imipramine
Imiquimod
Indinavir
Indomethacin
Infliximab
Insulin

Interferon beta 1-a
Interferons, alfa-2
Irbesartan
Irinotecan
Isoproterenol
Isosorbide dinitrate
Isosorbide mononitrate
Isotretinoin
Isradipine
Itraconazole
Ivermectin
Kanamycin
Ketoprofen
Ketorolac
Labetalol
Lamotrigine
Lansoprazole
Latanoprost
Leuprolide
Levamisole
Levofloxacin
Licorice
Lidocaine
Lisinopril
Lithium
Lomefloxacin
Losartan
Loxapine
Maprotiline
Mazindol
Meclofenamate
Medroxyprogesterone
Mefenamic acid
Meloxicam
Melphalan
Mephenytoin
Mercaptopurine
Mesalamine
Mesoridazine
Methadone
Methenamine
Methimazole
Methohexital
Methoxsalen
Methyldopa
Methylphenidate
Methyltestosterone
Metolazone
Metoprolol
Mexiletine
Minoxidil
Mirtazapine
Mistletoe
Mitomycin
Mitoxantrone
Modafinil
Molindone
Moricizine
Morphine
Moxifloxacin
Mycophenolate
Nabumetone
Nadolol
Nafarelin
Naltrexone
Naproxen
Naratriptan
Nefazodone
Nicardipine
Nicotine
Nifedipine
Nimodipine
Nisoldipine
Nitroglycerin
Nizatidine
Norfloxacin
Nortriptyline
Nystatin
Octreotide
Ofloxacin
Olanzapine
Olmesartan
Olopatadine
Omeprazole
Oral contraceptives
Orlistat
Oxaprozin
Oxazepam
Oxcarbazepine
Paclitaxel
Palivizumab
Pamidronate
Pancuronium
Pantoprazole
Paroxetine
Penbutolol
Penicillamine
Pentamidine
Pentazocine
Pentostatin
Pentoxifylline
Pergolide
Perindopril
Phenazopyridine
Phenelzine
Phenobarbital
Pilocarpine
Pimozide
Pindolol
Pioglitazone
Piperacillin
Pirbuterol
Piroxicam
Pramipexole
Prazepam
Praziquantel
Prazosin
Procarbazine
Progestins
Promazine
Propafenone
Propofol
Propoxyphene
Propranolol
Propylthiouracil
Protriptyline
Psoralens
Quetiapine
Quinapril
Quinestrol
Quinine
Quinupristin/dalfopristin
Rabeprazole
Raloxifene
Ramipril
Rapacuronium
Reserpine
Rifampin
Riluzole
Rimantadine
Risedronate
Risperidone
Ritonavir
Rivastigmine
Rizatriptan
Rofecoxib
Ropinirole
Rosiglitazone
Scopolamine
Senna
Sertraline
Sibutramine
Sildenafil
Simvastatin
Sirolimus
Sotalol
Sparfloxacin
Spironolactone
Stanozolol
Streptokinase
Streptomycin
Streptozocin
Sucralfate
Sulfacetamide
Sulfinpyrazone
Sulindac
Tacrine
Tacrolimus
Tamoxifen
Tartrazine
Telmisartan
Terazosin
Testosterone
Thalidomide
Tiagabine
Timolol
Tiopronin
Tirofiban
Tizanidine
Tobramycin
Tolazoline
Tolcapone
Tolmetin
Topiramate
Toremifene
Torsemide
Trandolapril
Tranylcypromine
Trastuzumab
Trazodone
Tretinoin
Triamterene
Trifluoperazine
Trimeprazine
Tripelennamine
Triprolidine
Trovafloxacin
Unoprostone
Valacyclovir
Valdecoxib
Valproic acid
Valsartan
Venlafaxine
Verapamil
Vincristine
Voriconazole
Zalcitabine
Zaleplon
Zidovudine
Ziprasidone
Zolmitriptan
Zolpidem
Zonisamide

**Erythema**

Acarbose
Acetaminophen
Acetohexamide
Acitretin
Acyclovir
Albuterol
Aldesleukin
Alendronate
Allopurinol
Almotriptan
Aminocaproic acid
Aminoglutethimide
Aminolevulinic acid
Amiodarone
Amitriptyline
Amobarbital
Amphotericin B
Anisindione
Anthrax vaccine
Aprotinin
Arsenic
Ascorbic acid
Asparaginase
Atracurium
Atropine sulfate
Azithromycin
Betaxolol
Bexarotene
Bimatoprost
Bismuth
Bleomycin
Brimonidine
Busulfan
Butterbur
Capecitabine
Carbamazepine
Carboplatin
Carmustine
Caspofungin
Cefadroxil
Cefamandole
Cefonicid
Ceftazidime
Cetrorelix
Chloral hydrate
Chlorambucil
Chloramphenicol
Chlorotrianisene
Chlortetracycline
Cisplatin
Cladribine
Clomiphene
Clomipramine
Clonidine
Clotrimazole
Clozapine
Corticosteroids
Cromolyn
Cyclophosphamide
Cyclosporine
Cyproheptadine
Cytarabine
Dacarbazine
Dactinomycin
Dantrolene
Dapsone

Daunorubicin
Deferoxamine
Delavirdine
Desipramine
Desmopressin
Diclofenac
Dicumarol
Diethylpropion
Diltiazem
Dobutamine
Docetaxel
Domperidone
Donepezil
Doxapram
Doxepin
Doxorubicin
Eflornithine
Enalapril
Enoxaparin
Epirubicin
Ertapenem
Esmolol
Etanercept
Etoposide
Felodipine
Fentanyl
Fluorouracil
Fluphenazine
Flutamide
Folic acid
Formoterol
Furosemide
Gatifloxacin
Gentamicin
Ginkgo biloba
Glimepiride
Glipizide
Glyburide
Granulocyte colony-stimulating factor (GCSF)
Henna
Heparin
Hepatitis B vaccine
Heroin
Hydroxyurea
Idarubicin
Imipenem/cilastatin
Imipramine
Imiquimod
Interferon beta 1-a
Interferons, alfa-2
Irbesartan
Kanamycin
Ketamine
Lamotrigine
Latanoprost
Leucovorin
Levobunolol
Levofloxacin
Lincomycin
Lindane
Lisinopril
Lithium
Losartan
Lovastatin
Maprotiline
Mefloquine
Meperidine
Meprobamate
Mercaptopurine
Mesalamine
Mesna
Mesoridazine
Metformin
Methohexital
Methotrexate
Methoxsalen
Metronidazole
Miconazole
Minoxidil
Mistletoe
Mitomycin
Mitoxantrone
Modafinil
Nabumetone
Naratriptan
Nelfinavir
Niacin
Nicotine
Nifedipine
Nitroglycerin
Norfloxacin
Nortriptyline
Octreotide
Omeprazole
Ondansetron
Oral contraceptives
Oxaprozin
Paclitaxel
Palivizumab
Pancuronium
Penicillins
Pentamidine
Pentostatin
Perindopril
Perphenazine
Phenindamine
Phytonadione
Piroxicam
Plicamycin
Prochlorperazine
Propofol
Propranolol
Protriptyline
Pseudoephedrine
Psoralens
Quinacrine
Quinestrol
Quinine
Ramipril
Rapacuronium
Rifampin
Ritodrine
Rofecoxib
Saquinavir
Scopolamine
Sertraline
Simvastatin
Spironolactone
Streptomycin
Streptozocin
Succinylcholine
Sufentanil
Sulfacetamide
Sulindac
Sumatriptan
Tacrolimus
Testosterone
Thalidomide
Thiopental
Thiothixene
Ticlopidine
Tiopronin
Tolazamide
Tolbutamide
Tolterodine
Topotecan
Torsemide
Tretinoin
Trifluoperazine
Unoprostone
Verteporfin
Vidarabine
Vinblastine
Vincristine
Vinorelbine
Vitamin A
Voriconazole
Warfarin

**Erythema Annulare Centrifugum (EAC)**

Amitriptyline
Ampicillin
Chloroquine
Cimetidine
Gold and gold compounds
Hydrochlorothiazide
Hydroxychloroquine
Levamisole
Penicillins
Phenolphthalein
Piroxicam
Spironolactone

**Erythema Multiforme**

Acarbose
Acebutolol
Acetaminophen
Acetazolamide
Alendronate
Allopurinol
Amantadine
Aminosalicylate sodium
Amiodarone
Amlodipine
Amoxapine
Amoxicillin
Amphotericin B
Ampicillin
Anisindione
Arsenic
Aspirin
Atenolol
Atovaquone
Atropine sulfate
Azathioprine
Aztreonam
Bacampicillin
Benactyzine
Botulinum toxin (A & B)
Bumetanide
Bupropion
Busulfan
Butabarbital
Butalbital
Carbamazepine
Carbenicillin
Carisoprodol
Cefaclor
Cefadroxil
Cefamandole
Cefazolin
Cefdinir
Cefditoren
Cefepime
Cefixime
Cefonicid
Cefoperazone
Cefotaxime
Cefotetan
Cefpodoxime
Cefprozil
Ceftazidime
Ceftriaxone
Cefuroxime
Celecoxib
Cephalexin
Cephalothin
Cephapirin
Cephradine
Chloral hydrate
Chlorambucil
Chloramphenicol
Chlordiazepoxide
Chlormezanone
Chloroquine
Chlorothiazide
Chlorotrianisene
Chlorpromazine
Chlorpropamide
Chlorthalidone
Chlorzoxazone
Cimetidine
Cinoxacin
Ciprofloxacin
Clindamycin
Clofibrate
Clomiphene
Clonazepam
Cloxacillin
Clozapine
Co-trimoxazole
Codeine
Corticosteroids
Cyclophosphamide
Dactinomycin
Danazol
Dapsone
Deferoxamine
Delavirdine
Diclofenac
Dicloxacillin
Didanosine
Diethylpropion
Diethylstilbestrol
Diflunisal
Diltiazem
Dipyridamole
Doxycycline
Enalapril
Enoxacin
Erythromycin
Estrogens
Ethambutol
Ethosuximide
Etodolac
Etoposide
Famotidine
Fenoprofen
Fluconazole
Fluorouracil

Fluoxetine
Flurbiprofen
Fluvastatin
Fosphenytoin
Furazolidone
Furosemide
Gemfibrozil
Glucagon
Gold and gold compounds
Griseofulvin
Henna
Hepatitis B vaccine
Hydrochlorothiazide
Hydrocodone
Hydroxychloroquine
Hydroxyurea
Hydroxyzine
Ibuprofen
Imipenem/cilastatin
Indapamide
Indinavir
Indomethacin
Isoniazid
Isotretinoin
Itraconazole
Ketoprofen
Lamotrigine
Levamisole
Levofloxacin
Lidocaine
Lincomycin
Lithium
Loracarbef
Loratadine
Lorazepam
Lovastatin
Maprotiline
Mechlorethamine
Meclofenamate
Mefenamic acid
Mefloquine
Meloxicam
Mephenytoin
Meprobamate
Methenamine
Methicillin
Methotrexate
Methsuximide
Methyclothiazide
Methyldopa
Methylphenidate
Metoprolol
Mezlocillin
Midodrine
Minocycline
Minoxidil
Mitomycin
Mitotane
Nabumetone
Nadolol
Nafcillin
Nalidixic acid
Naproxen
Neomycin
Nifedipine
Nitrofurantoin
Nitroglycerin
Norfloxacin
Nystatin
Ofloxacin
Omeprazole
Oral contraceptives
Oxacillin
Oxaprozin
Oxazepam
Oxcarbazepine
Oxybutynin
Pantoprazole
Paramethadione
Paroxetine
Penicillamine
Penicillins
Pentobarbital
Phenobarbital
Phenolphthalein
Phensuximide
Phenytoin
Pindolol
Piroxicam
Pravastatin
Primidone
Probenecid
Progestins
Promethazine
Propranolol
Pyrazinamide
Pyrimethamine
Quinidine
Quinine
Ramipril
Ranitidine
Ribavirin
Rifampin
Ritodrine
Saquinavir
Scopolamine
Sertraline
Simvastatin
Smallpox vaccine
Spironolactone
Streptomycin
Sulfacetamide
Sulfadiazine
Sulfadoxine
Sulfamethoxazole
Sulfasalazine
Sulfisoxazole
Sulindac
Tamsulosin
Terbinafine
Tetracycline
Thiabendazole
Thiopental
Thioridazine
Ticarcillin
Ticlopidine
Timolol
Tiopronin
Tobramycin
Tocainide
Tolbutamide
Tolcapone
Tolmetin
Trazodone
Trimethadione
Trimethoprim
Troleandomycin
Trovafloxacin
Valproic acid
Vancomycin
Verapamil
Vinblastine
Vitamin A
Vitamin E
Voriconazole
Zalcitabine
Zidovudine

**Erythema Nodosum**

Acetaminophen
Acyclovir
Aldesleukin
Amiodarone
Arsenic
Aspirin
Azathioprine
Busulfan
Carbamazepine
Carbenicillin
Cefdinir
Chlordiazepoxide
Chlorotrianisene
Chlorpropamide
Ciprofloxacin
Clomiphene
Co-trimoxazole
Codeine
Colchicine
Dapsone
Diclofenac
Dicloxacillin
Diethylstilbestrol
Disopyramide
Echinacea
Enoxacin
Estrogens
Fluoxetine
Furosemide
Glucagon
Gold and gold compounds
Granulocyte colony-stimulating factor (GCSF)
Hepatitis B vaccine
Hydralazine
Hydroxychloroquine
Ibuprofen
Indomethacin
Interferons, alfa-2
Isotretinoin
Levofloxacin
Loperamide
Meclofenamate
Medroxyprogesterone
Meprobamate
Mesalamine
Methicillin
Methimazole
Methyldopa
Mezlocillin
Minocycline
Montelukast
Naproxen
Nifedipine
Nitrofurantoin
Ofloxacin
Omeprazole
Oral contraceptives
Oxacillin
Paroxetine
Penicillamine
Penicillins
Piperacillin
Progestins
Propylthiouracil
Smallpox vaccine
Sparfloxacin
Streptomycin
Sulfamethoxazole
Sulfasalazine
Sulfisoxazole
Thalidomide
Ticarcillin
Ticlopidine
Tretinoin
Trimethoprim
Verapamil
Zileuton

**Erythroderma**

Abacavir
Acitretin
Aldesleukin
Amitriptyline
Aspirin
Captopril
Carbamazepine
Chloroquine
Cimetidine
Ciprofloxacin
Clindamycin
Clofazimine
Co-trimoxazole
Colchicine
Cytarabine
Dapsone
Dicloxacillin
Diflunisal
Hydroxychloroquine
Lansoprazole
Meclofenamate
Methotrexate
Minocycline
Minoxidil
Nitroglycerin
Nystatin
Omeprazole
Pentostatin
Phenobarbital
Phenytoin
Piroxicam
Propolis
Sulfamethoxazole
Sulfasalazine
Terbinafine
Thalidomide
Timolol
Vincristine
Zalcitabine
Zidovudine

**Exanthems**

Abacavir
Acebutolol
Acetaminophen
Acetazolamide
Acetohexamide
Acitretin
Acyclovir
Albuterol
Aldesleukin
Alendronate
Allopurinol
Alprazolam

Altretamine
Amantadine
Amikacin
Amiloride
Aminocaproic acid
Aminoglutethimide
Aminophylline
Aminosalicylate sodium
Amiodarone
Amitriptyline
Amlodipine
Amobarbital
Amoxapine
Amoxicillin
Amphotericin B
Ampicillin
Amprenavir
Anisindione
Anistreplase
Aprobarbital
Aprotinin
Arsenic
Asparaginase
Aspartame
Aspirin
Atenolol
Atorvastatin
Atovaquone
Atropine sulfate
Azatadine
Azathioprine
Azelastine
Azithromycin
Aztreonam
Bacampicillin
Baclofen
Benactyzine
Benazepril
Bendroflumethiazide
Benztropine
Betaxolol
Bexarotene
Bicalutamide
Biperiden
Bisacodyl
Bismuth
Bisoprolol
Bleomycin
Bromocriptine
Brompheniramine
Bumetanide
Bupropion
Buspirone
Busulfan
Butabarbital
Butalbital
Butorphanol
Calcitonin
Candesartan
Captopril
Carbamazepine
Carbenicillin
Carboplatin
Carisoprodol
Carmustine
Carteolol
Carvedilol
Cefaclor
Cefadroxil
Cefamandole
Cefazolin
Cefdinir
Cefepime
Cefoperazone
Cefotaxime
Cefotetan
Cefoxitin
Cefprozil
Ceftazidime
Ceftriaxone
Cefuroxime
Celecoxib
Cephalexin
Cephalothin
Cephradine
Cetirizine
Cevimeline
Chloral hydrate
Chlorambucil
Chloramphenicol
Chlordiazepoxide
Chlormezanone
Chloroquine
Chlorothiazide
Chlorpromazine
Chlorpropamide
Chlorthalidone
Chlorzoxazone
Cholestyramine
Cimetidine
Ciprofloxacin
Cisplatin
Citalopram
Cladribine
Clarithromycin
Clemastine
Clindamycin
Clofazimine
Clofibrate
Clomiphene
Clomipramine
Clonazepam
Clonidine
Clopidogrel
Clorazepate
Cloxacillin
Clozapine
Co-trimoxazole
Codeine
Colchicine
Colestipol
Corticosteroids
Cromolyn
Cyanocobalamin
Cyclamate
Cyclophosphamide
Cycloserine
Cyclosporine
Cyclothiazide
Cyproheptadine
Cytarabine
Dacarbazine
Dactinomycin
Dalteparin
Danazol
Dantrolene
Dapsone
Daunorubicin
Deferoxamine
Delavirdine
Demeclocycline
Denileukin
Desipramine
Diazepam
Diazoxide
Diclofenac
Dicloxacillin
Dicumarol
Dicyclomine
Didanosine
Diethylpropion
Diethylstilbestrol
Diflunisal
Digoxin
Dihydrotachysterol
Diltiazem
Dimenhydrinate
Diphenhydramine
Dipyridamole
Disopyramide
Disulfiram
Docetaxel
Docusate
Dopamine
Doxazosin
Doxepin
Doxorubicin
Doxycycline
Efavirenz
Eletriptan
Enalapril
Enoxacin
Enoxaparin
Ephedrine
Epinephrine
Epoetin alfa
Eprosartan
Erythromycin
Esomeprazole
Estramustine
Estrogens
Etanercept
Ethacrynic acid
Ethambutol
Ethionamide
Ethosuximide
Etidronate
Etodolac
Etoposide
Famotidine
Felodipine
Fenofibrate
Fenoprofen
Fentanyl
Flavoxate
Flecainide
Fluconazole
Flucytosine
Fludarabine
Fluorouracil
Fluoxetine
Fluoxymesterone
Fluphenazine
Flurazepam
Flurbiprofen
Flutamide
Fluvoxamine
Folic acid
Foscarnet
Fosfomycin
Fosphenytoin
Furazolidone
Furosemide
Gabapentin
Ganciclovir
Gatifloxacin
Gemcitabine
Gemfibrozil
Gentamicin
Ginkgo biloba
Glimepiride
Glipizide
Glucagon
Glyburide
Gold and gold compounds
Granisetron
Granulocyte colony-stimulating factor (GCSF)
Griseofulvin
Guanethidine
Guanfacine
Haloperidol
Halothane
Heparin
Heroin
Hydralazine
Hydrochlorothiazide
Hydrocodone
Hydromorphone
Hydroxychloroquine
Hydroxyurea
Hydroxyzine
Ibuprofen
Idarubicin
Imipenem/cilastatin
Imipramine
Indapamide
Indinavir
Indomethacin
Insulin
Interferon beta 1-a
Interferons, alfa-2
Ipodate
Ipratropium
Isocarboxazid
Isoniazid
Isotretinoin
Isradipine
Itraconazole
Ivermectin
Kanamycin
Ketamine
Ketoconazole
Ketoprofen
Ketorolac
Labetalol
Lamivudine
Lamotrigine
Lansoprazole
Letrozole
Leuprolide
Levamisole
Levodopa
Levofloxacin
Lidocaine
Lincomycin
Lisinopril
Lithium
Lomefloxacin
Loperamide

Loratadine
Lorazepam
Losartan
Lovastatin
Loxapine
Maprotiline
Marihuana
Mazindol
Mebendazole
Mechlorethamine
Meclizine
Meclofenamate
Medroxyprogesterone
Mefenamic acid
Mefloquine
Meloxicam
Melphalan
Mephenytoin
Mephobarbital
Meprobamate
Mercaptopurine
Mesalamine
Mesna
Metformin
Methadone
Methantheline
Methazolamide
Methenamine
Methicillin
Methimazole
Methocarbamol
Methohexital
Methotrexate
Methoxsalen
Methsuximide
Methyclothiazide
Methyldopa
Methylphenidate
Methyltestosterone
Methysergide
Metoclopramide
Metolazone
Metoprolol
Metronidazole
Mexiletine
Mezlocillin
Miconazole
Midazolam
Minocycline
Minoxidil
Misoprostol
Mitomycin
Mitotane
Moexipril
Moricizine
Morphine
Moxifloxacin
Nabumetone
Nadolol
Nafarelin
Nafcillin
Nalidixic acid
Naloxone
Naltrexone
Naproxen
Naratriptan
Nateglinide
Nefazodone
Nelfinavir
Neomycin
Nevirapine
Niacin
Nicardipine
Nifedipine
Nimodipine
Nisoldipine
Nitrofurantoin
Nitroglycerin
Nizatidine
Norfloxacin
Nortriptyline
Nystatin
Octreotide
Ofloxacin
Olanzapine
Olsalazine
Omeprazole
Ondansetron
Oral contraceptives
Orphenadrine
Oxacillin
Oxaprozin
Oxazepam
Oxcarbazepine
Oxytetracycline
Paclitaxel
Pamidronate
Pantoprazole
Pantothenic acid
Papaverine
Paramethadione
Paromomycin
Paroxetine
Pemoline
Penbutolol
Penicillamine
Penicillins
Pentagastrin
Pentamidine
Pentazocine
Pentobarbital
Pentostatin
Pentoxifylline
Pergolide
Perindopril
Perphenazine
Phenazopyridine
Phenelzine
Phenobarbital
Phenolphthalein
Phenytoin
Phytonadione
Pimozide
Pindolol
Piperacillin
Piroxicam
Plicamycin
Polythiazide
Potassium iodide
Pravastatin
Prazepam
Prazosin
Primaquine
Primidone
Probenecid
Procainamide
Procarbazine
Prochlorperazine
Progestins
Promazine
Promethazine
Propafenone
Propantheline
Propofol
Propoxyphene
Propranolol
Propylthiouracil
Protamine
Protriptyline
Pseudoephedrine
Pyrazinamide
Pyrimethamine
Quinacrine
Quinapril
Quinethazone
Quinidine
Quinine
Quinupristin/dalfopristin
Ramipril
Ranitidine
Rapacuronium
Reserpine
Ribavirin
Rifampin
Ritodrine
Ritonavir
Rituximab
Rivastigmine
Rofecoxib
Ropinirole
Rosiglitazone
Saccharin
Salmeterol
Salsalate
Saquinavir
Scopolamine
Secobarbital
Sertraline
Simvastatin
Smallpox vaccine
Sotalol
Sparfloxacin
Spectinomycin
Spironolactone
Stanozolol
Streptokinase
Streptomycin
Streptozocin
Succinylcholine
Sucralfate
Sulfadiazine
Sulfadoxine
Sulfamethoxazole
Sulfasalazine
Sulfinpyrazone
Sulfisoxazole
Sulindac
Sumatriptan
Tacrine
Tacrolimus
Tamoxifen
Temazepam
Terazosin
Terbinafine
Terbutaline
Testosterone
Tetracycline
Thalidomide
Thiabendazole
Thiamine
Thioguanine
Thiopental
Thioridazine
Thiothixene
Tiagabine
Ticarcillin
Ticlopidine
Timolol
Tinzaparin
Tiopronin
Tizanidine
Tobramycin
Tocainide
Tolazamide
Tolazoline
Tolbutamide
Tolmetin
Topiramate
Torsemide
Tramadol
Tranylcypromine
Trazodone
Triamterene
Triazolam
Trichlormethiazide
Trifluoperazine
Trimeprazine
Trimethadione
Trimethoprim
Trimetrexate
Trimipramine
Triprolidine
Troleandomycin
Trovafloxacin
Urokinase
Valdecoxib
Valproic acid
Vancomycin
Vasopressin
Venlafaxine
Verapamil
Vinblastine
Vincristine
Vitamin A
Vitamin E
Warfarin
Zalcitabine
Zaleplon
Zidovudine
Ziprasidone
Zonisamide

**Exfoliative Dermatitis**

Acebutolol
Acetaminophen
Acitretin
Aldesleukin
Alitretinoin
Allopurinol
Aminoglutethimide
Aminophylline
Aminosalicylate sodium
Amiodarone
Amitriptyline
Amobarbital
Amoxicillin
Amphotericin B
Ampicillin
Anisindione
Aprobarbital
Arsenic

Aspirin
Atropine sulfate
Aztreonam
Bacampicillin
Benactyzine
Bendroflumethiazide
Betaxolol
Bexarotene
Bismuth
Bisoprolol
Bumetanide
Bupropion
Butabarbital
Butalbital
Capecitabine
Captopril
Carbamazepine
Carbenicillin
Carteolol
Carvedilol
Cefdinir
Cefoxitin
Chlorambucil
Chloroquine
Chlorothiazide
Chlorpromazine
Chlorpropamide
Chlorthalidone
Cimetidine
Ciprofloxacin
Cisplatin
Clofazimine
Clofibrate
Cloxacillin
Co-trimoxazole
Codeine
Cromolyn
Cytarabine
Dapsone
Demeclocycline
Desipramine
Diazepam
Diclofenac
Dicloxacillin
Diethylstilbestrol
Diflunisal
Diltiazem
Doxorubicin
Doxycycline
Eletriptan
Enalapril
Enoxacin
Ephedrine
Epirubicin
Esmolol
Estrogens
Ethambutol
Ethosuximide
Etodolac
Fenoprofen
Fentanyl
Flecainide
Fluconazole
Fluoxetine
Fluphenazine
Flurbiprofen
Fluvoxamine
Fosinopril
Fosphenytoin
Furosemide
Ganciclovir
Gemfibrozil
Gentamicin
Gold and gold compounds
Granulocyte colony-stimulating factor (GCSF)
Griseofulvin
Guanfacine
Haloperidol
Hydrochlorothiazide
Hydroxychloroquine
Imipramine
Indomethacin
Isoniazid
Ketoconazole
Ketoprofen
Ketorolac
Labetalol
Levamisole
Levofloxacin
Lidocaine
Lincomycin
Lithium
Meclofenamate
Mefenamic acid
Mefloquine
Mephenytoin
Mephobarbital
Meprobamate
Mesoridazine
Methantheline
Methicillin
Methimazole
Methoxsalen
Methsuximide
Methylphenidate
Metolazone
Metoprolol
Mexiletine
Mezlocillin
Minocycline
Mirtazapine
Mitomycin
Nadolol
Nafcillin
Nalidixic acid
Naproxen
Nifedipine
Nisoldipine
Nitrofurantoin
Nitroglycerin
Nizatidine
Norfloxacin
Ofloxacin
Omeprazole
Oxacillin
Oxaprozin
Oxytetracycline
Paramethadione
Penicillamine
Penicillins
Pentobarbital
Pentostatin
Perphenazine
Phenobarbital
Phenolphthalein
Phenytoin
Pindolol
Piperacillin
Piroxicam
Primidone
Procarbazine
Prochlorperazine
Propranolol
Propylthiouracil
Pseudoephedrine
Pyrimethamine
Quinacrine
Quinapril
Quinidine
Quinine
Rifampin
Riluzole
Risperidone
Rivastigmine
Rosiglitazone
Secobarbital
Sildenafil
Smallpox vaccine
Sparfloxacin
Streptomycin
Sulfacetamide
Sulfadiazine
Sulfadoxine
Sulfamethoxazole
Sulfasalazine
Sulfisoxazole
Sulindac
Tetracycline
Thalidomide
Thiopental
Thioridazine
Tiagabine
Ticarcillin
Ticlopidine
Timolol
Tizanidine
Tobramycin
Tocainide
Trazodone
Trifluoperazine
Trimethadione
Trimethoprim
Vancomycin
Venlafaxine
Verapamil
Vitamin A
Voriconazole
Warfarin
Yohimbine
Zalcitabine
Ziprasidone

**Fixed Eruptions**

Acetaminophen
Acyclovir
Albendazole
Alendronate
Allopurinol
Aminosalicylate sodium
Amitriptyline
Amoxicillin
Amphotericin B
Ampicillin
Arsenic
Aspirin
Atenolol
Atropine sulfate
Azathioprine
Azithromycin
Bacampicillin
Benactyzine
Bisacodyl
Bismuth
Butabarbital
Butalbital
Cabergoline
Carbamazepine
Carisoprodol
Cefazolin
Cephalexin
Cetirizine
Chloral hydrate
Chloramphenicol
Chlordiazepoxide
Chlorhexidine
Chlormezanone
Chloroquine
Chlorothiazide
Chlorpromazine
Chlorpropamide
Cimetidine
Ciprofloxacin
Clarithromycin
Clindamycin
Co-trimoxazole
Codeine
Colchicine
Corticosteroids
Cyclosporine
Dacarbazine
Dapsone
Demeclocycline
Dextromethorphan
Diazepam
Diclofenac
Diflunisal
Dimenhydrinate
Diphenhydramine
Disulfiram
Docetaxel
Doxycycline
Ephedrine
Epinephrine
Erythromycin
Estrogens
Ethchlorvynol
Ethotoin
Etodolac
Fentanyl
Fluconazole
Flurbiprofen
Foscarnet
Ganciclovir
Gatifloxacin
Gold and gold compounds
Griseofulvin
Guanethidine
Heparin
Heroin
Hydralazine
Hydrochlorothiazide
Hydroxychloroquine
Hydroxyurea
Hydroxyzine
Ibuprofen
Imipramine
Indapamide
Indomethacin
Isotretinoin
Itraconazole

Ketoconazole
Lamotrigine
Levamisole
Lidocaine
Loratadine
Lorazepam
Meclofenamate
Mefenamic acid
Melatonin
Meprobamate
Mesna
Metaxalone
Methenamine
Methimazole
Methyldopa
Methylphenidate
Metronidazole
Minocycline
Moxifloxacin
Naproxen
Neomycin
Niacin
Nifedipine
Nitrofurantoin
Norfloxacin
Nystatin
Ofloxacin
Omeprazole
Ondansetron
Oral contraceptives
Orphenadrine
Oxaprozin
Oxazepam
Oxytetracycline
Paclitaxel
Papaverine
Penicillins
Pentobarbital
Phenobarbital
Phenolphthalein
Phenylpropanolamine
Phenytoin
Piroxicam
Procarbazine
Prochlorperazine
Promethazine
Propofol
Pseudoephedrine
Pyrazinamide
Pyridoxine
Pyrimethamine
Quinacrine
Quinidine
Quinine
Ranitidine
Rifampin
Rofecoxib
Saccharin
Saquinavir
Scopolamine
Sertraline
Sildenafil
Sparfloxacin
Streptomycin
Sulfadiazine
Sulfamethoxazole
Sulfasalazine
Sulfisoxazole
Sulindac
Tartrazine
Temazepam
Terbinafine
Tetracycline
Thiabendazole
Thiopental
Ticlopidine
Tolbutamide
Trifluoperazine
Trimethadione
Trimetrexate
Tripelennamine
Triprolidine
Valproic acid
Voriconazole

**Flushing**

Acetaminophen
Albuterol
Alemtuzumab
Alitretinoin
Alprostadil
Amifostine
Amiloride
Aminophylline
Amiodarone
Amitriptyline
Amlodipine
Amoxapine
Amphotericin B
Amyl nitrite
Anastrozole
Anistreplase
Arbutamine
Ascorbic acid
Asparaginase
Aspirin
Atracurium
Atropine sulfate
Azatadine
Azelastine
Baclofen
Benazepril
Betaxolol
Bethanechol
Biperiden
Bisoprolol
Bleomycin
Bosentan
Bretylium
Bromocriptine
Bupropion
Buspirone
Butorphanol
Calcitonin
Captopril
Carboplatin
Carisoprodol
Carmustine
Carteolol
Caspofungin
Cefaclor
Cefamandole
Cefoxitin
Cefpodoxime
Ceftazidime
Ceftriaxone
Cetirizine
Chloral hydrate
Chlormezanone
Chlorpropamide
Chlorzoxazone
Ciprofloxacin
Cisatracurium
Cisplatin
Clemastine
Clidinium
Clomiphene
Clomipramine
Co-trimoxazole
Codeine
Colchicine
Corticosteroids
Cromolyn
Cyclobenzaprine
Cyclophosphamide
Cyclosporine
Cyproheptadine
Dacarbazine
Danazol
Daunorubicin
Deferoxamine
Denileukin
Desipramine
Desmopressin
Diazepam
Diazoxide
Diclofenac
Dicyclomine
Diethylpropion
Diethylstilbestrol
Diflunisal
Diltiazem
Dimenhydrinate
Diphenoxylate
Dipyridamole
Disulfiram
Docetaxel
Dolasetron
Donepezil
Doxapram
Doxazosin
Doxepin
Doxorubicin
Dronabinol
Edrophonium
Efavirenz
Enalapril
Ephedra
Epinephrine
Epirubicin
Ertapenem
Esmolol
Esomeprazole
Estazolam
Estramustine
Estrogens
Etodolac
Etoposide
Famotidine
Felbamate
Felodipine
Fentanyl
Flecainide
Flumazenil
Fluoxetine
Fluoxymesterone
Flurazepam
Flurbiprofen
Fluvastatin
Folic acid
Foscarnet
Fosinopril
Frovatriptan
Furazolidone
Furosemide
Glipizide
Glyburide
Glycopyrrolate
Granulocyte colony-stimulating factor (GCSF)
Griseofulvin
Haloperidol
Hepatitis B vaccine
Hydralazine
Hydrocodone
Hydromorphone
Hydroxyzine
Hyoscyamine
Ibritumomab
Ibuprofen
Imipenem/cilastatin
Imipramine
Indapamide
Indinavir
Indomethacin
Insulin
Ipratropium
Irbesartan
Irinotecan
Isoniazid
Isoproterenol
Isosorbide dinitrate
Isosorbide mononitrate
Isotretinoin
Isradipine
Ketorolac
Labetalol
Lamotrigine
Leuprolide
Levodopa
Levothyroxine
Lisinopril
Lomefloxacin
Lomustine
Loratadine
Losartan
Maprotiline
MDMA
Medroxyprogesterone
Meperidine
Mesna
Mesoridazine
Methadone
Methantheline
Methocarbamol
Methyltestosterone
Methysergide
Metoclopramide
Metronidazole
Miconazole
Midodrine
Minoxidil
Mitotane
Moexipril
Morphine
Nafarelin
Nefazodone
Niacin
Nicardipine
Nicotine
Nifedipine

Nimodipine
Nisoldipine
Nitrofurantoin
Nitroglycerin
Nortriptyline
Octreotide
Ondansetron
Orphenadrine
Oxybutynin
Paclitaxel
Pancuronium
Papaverine
PEG-interferon alfa-2b
Penbutolol
Penicillamine
Pentagastrin
Pentazocine
Pentostatin
Pentoxifylline
Phendimetrazine
Phenindamine
Phentolamine
Phytonadione
Pilocarpine
Plicamycin
Pravastatin
Probenecid
Procainamide
Procarbazine
Progestins
Promethazine
Propafenone
Propofol
Propoxyphene
Propranolol
Protamine
Protriptyline
Pyrazinamide
Pyrilamine
Quinapril
Quinidine
Quinine
Ramipril
Rapacuronium
Reserpine
Rifampin
Risperidone
Rituximab
Rivastigmine
Rizatriptan
Rofecoxib
Ropinirole
Scopolamine
Sertraline
Sildenafil
Simvastatin
Spironolactone
Streptokinase
Succinylcholine
Sulfamethoxazole
Sulfasalazine
Sulfinpyrazone
Sulfisoxazole
Sumatriptan
Tacrine
Tacrolimus
Tamoxifen
Telmisartan
Terbutaline
Testosterone
Thiabendazole
Tolazoline
Tolbutamide
Topiramate
Trandolapril
Tranylcypromine
Tretinoin
Triamterene
Trihexyphenidyl
Trimetrexate
Tripelennamine
Triprolidine
Trovafloxacin
Urokinase
Valsartan
Vancomycin
Venlafaxine
Verapamil
Vinorelbine
Yohimbine
Zalcitabine
Zolmitriptan
Zolpidem

**Galactorrhea**

Alprazolam
Amitriptyline
Amoxapine
Buspirone
Chlordiazepoxide
Chlorpromazine
Cimetidine
Citalopram
Clomipramine
Cyclobenzaprine
Desipramine
Domperidone
Doxepin
Estrogens
Fluoxetine
Fluphenazine
Haloperidol
Imipramine
Isotretinoin
Loxapine
Maprotiline
Medroxyprogesterone
Mesoridazine
Methyldopa
Metoclopramide
Minocycline
Molindone
Nitrofurantoin
Nortriptyline
Octreotide
Olanzapine
Oral contraceptives
Paroxetine
Perphenazine
Pimozide
Prochlorperazine
Progestins
Promazine
Promethazine
Protriptyline
Risperidone
Sertraline
Tamoxifen
Thalidomide
Thioridazine
Thiothixene
Toremifene
Trazodone
Trifluoperazine
Trimipramine
Valproic acid
Verapamil

**Gingival Hyperplasia**

Amlodipine
Basiliximab
Cevimeline
Co-trimoxazole
Cyclosporine
Diltiazem
Erythromycin
Estrogens
Ethosuximide
Ethotoin
Felodipine
Fosphenytoin
Ganciclovir
Isradipine
Ketoconazole
Lamotrigine
Lithium
Mephenytoin
Methsuximide
Mycophenolate
Nicardipine
Nifedipine
Nisoldipine
Oral contraceptives
Oxcarbazepine
Phensuximide
Phenytoin
Primidone
Riluzole
Sertraline
Sirolimus
Tacrolimus
Tartrazine
Tiagabine
Topiramate
Valproic acid
Verapamil
Voriconazole
Zonisamide

**Glossitis**

Aldesleukin
Amitriptyline
Amoxapine
Amoxicillin
Ampicillin
Atorvastatin
Azelastine
Bacampicillin
Betaxolol
Bleomycin
Bupropion
Captopril
Carbamazepine
Carbenicillin
Cefaclor
Cefadroxil
Cefamandole
Cefpodoxime
Cefprozil
Ceftazidime
Ceftriaxone
Chloramphenicol
Chlorhexidine
Clarithromycin
Clomipramine
Cloxacillin
Co-trimoxazole
Cyclosporine
Demeclocycline
Dicloxacillin
Doxepin
Doxycycline
Enalapril
Estazolam
Etidronate
Etodolac
Felbamate
Fluoxetine
Fluvoxamine
Gabapentin
Gatifloxacin
Gold and gold compounds
Guanadrel
Guanethidine
Hydroxyurea
Imipenem/cilastatin
Imipramine
Lansoprazole
Lincomycin
Mefenamic acid
Mercaptopurine
Methicillin
Methotrexate
Metronidazole
Mezlocillin
Minocycline
Mirtazapine
Moxifloxacin
Nabumetone
Nafcillin
Nefazodone
Nisoldipine
Olanzapine
Oxacillin
Pantoprazole
Paroxetine
Penicillamine
Penicillins
Phenelzine
Pirbuterol
Protriptyline
Pyrimethamine
Quetiapine
Rabeprazole
Riluzole
Risedronate
Rivastigmine
Ropinirole
Saquinavir
Sertraline
Sildenafil
Streptomycin
Sulfadoxine
Sulfamethoxazole
Sulfasalazine
Sulfisoxazole
Sulindac
Tacrine
Tetracycline
Tiagabine
Ticarcillin
Tolmetin
Triamterene

Triazolam
Trihexyphenidyl
Trimethoprim
Trimipramine
Valproic acid
Venlafaxine
Voriconazole
Zalcitabine
Zaleplon
Zonisamide

**Gynecomastia**

Alprazolam
Amiloride
Amitriptyline
Amlodipine
Amoxapine
Amprenavir
Androstenedione
Arsenic
Atorvastatin
Bendroflumethiazide
Bicalutamide
Bupropion
Busulfan
Captopril
Carmustine
Chlordiazepoxide
Chlorotrianisene
Chlorpromazine
Cimetidine
Ciprofloxacin
Citalopram
Cladribine
Clofibrate
Clomiphene
Clomipramine
Clonidine
Cyclobenzaprine
Cyclosporine
Delavirdine
Desipramine
Diazepam
Didanosine
Diethylpropion
Diethylstilbestrol
Digoxin
Diltiazem
Disopyramide
Domperidone
Doxepin
Efavirenz
Enalapril
Estazolam
Estramustine
Estrogens
Ethionamide
Etodolac
Famotidine
Felodipine
Finasteride
Fluoxetine
Fluoxymesterone
Fluphenazine
Flutamide
Fluvastatin
Foscarnet
Fosinopril
Gabapentin
Goserelin
Griseofulvin
Guanabenz
Haloperidol
Ibuprofen
Imipramine
Indinavir
Indomethacin
Isoniazid
Isotretinoin
Itraconazole
Ketoconazole
Ketoprofen
Lamivudine
Lansoprazole
Latanoprost
Leuprolide
Loratadine
Lovastatin
Loxapine
Maprotiline
Medroxyprogesterone
Melphalan
Meprobamate
Mesoridazine
Methotrexate
Methyldopa
Methyltestosterone
Metoclopramide
Metronidazole
Minocycline
Minoxidil
Mirtazapine
Misoprostol
Molindone
Morphine
Nafarelin
Nefazodone
Nelfinavir
Nifedipine
Nisoldipine
Nizatidine
Nortriptyline
Octreotide
Omeprazole
Penicillamine
Pentostatin
Perphenazine
Phenytoin
Pimozide
Pravastatin
Procarbazine
Prochlorperazine
Progestins
Promazine
Promethazine
Protriptyline
Pyrilamine
Quinestrol
Rabeprazole
Ranitidine
Reserpine
Risperidone
Ritonavir
Ropinirole
Saquinavir
Sertraline
Sildenafil
Simvastatin
Spironolactone
Stanozolol
Stavudine
Sulindac
Testosterone
Thalidomide
Thioridazine
Thiothixene
Tiagabine
Tolmetin
Topiramate
Trazodone
Triamterene
Trifluoperazine
Trimeprazine
Trimipramine
Valproic acid
Venlafaxine
Verapamil
Vitamin E
Ziprasidone
Zonisamide

**Hair – Alopecia**

Acebutolol
Acetaminophen
Acetohexamide
Acitretin
Acyclovir
Albendazole
Aldesleukin
Alitretinoin
Allopurinol
Altretamine
Amantadine
Amiloride
Aminophylline
Aminosalicylate sodium
Amiodarone
Amitriptyline
Amlodipine
Amoxapine
Amphotericin B
Anagrelide
Anastrozole
Androstenedione
Anisindione
Anthrax vaccine
Arsenic
Asparaginase
Aspirin
Atenolol
Atorvastatin
Azathioprine
Balsalazide
Bendroflumethiazide
Betaxolol
Bexarotene
Bicalutamide
Bismuth
Bisoprolol
Bleomycin
Bromocriptine
Bupropion
Buspirone
Busulfan
Capecitabine
Captopril
Carbamazepine
Carboplatin
Carmustine
Carteolol
Carvedilol
Celecoxib
Cetirizine
Cevimeline
Chlorambucil
Chloramphenicol
Chlordiazepoxide
Chloroquine
Chlorothiazide
Chlorotrianisene
Chlorpropamide
Chlorthalidone
Chondroitin
Cidofovir
Cimetidine
Cisplatin
Citalopram
Clofibrate
Clomiphene
Clomipramine
Clonazepam
Clonidine
Colchicine
Corticosteroids
Cyclobenzaprine
Cyclophosphamide
Cyclosporine
Cytarabine
Dacarbazine
Dactinomycin
Dalteparin
Danazol
Daunorubicin
Delavirdine
Desipramine
Diazoxide
Diclofenac
Dicumarol
Didanosine
Diethylpropion
Diethylstilbestrol
Diflunisal
Digoxin
Diltiazem
Disopyramide
Docetaxel
Donepezil
Dopamine
Doxazosin
Doxepin
Doxorubicin
Efavirenz
Eflornithine
Eletriptan
Enalapril
Epinephrine
Epirubicin
Epoetin alfa
Esmolol
Estramustine
Estrogens
Ethambutol
Ethionamide
Ethosuximide
Etidronate
Etodolac
Etoposide
Exemestane
Famotidine
Felbamate
Fenofibrate
Fenoprofen

Finasteride
Flecainide
Fluconazole
Fludarabine
Fluorouracil
Fluoxetine
Fluoxymesterone
Flurbiprofen
Fluvastatin
Fluvoxamine
Foscarnet
Gabapentin
Ganciclovir
Gemcitabine
Gemfibrozil
Gentamicin
Gold and gold compounds
Granisetron
Granulocyte colony-stimulating factor (GCSF)
Guanethidine
Guanfacine
Haloperidol
Halothane
Heparin
Hepatitis B vaccine
Hydromorphone
Hydroxychloroquine
Hydroxyurea
Ibuprofen
Idarubicin
Ifosfamide
Imipramine
Indinavir
Indomethacin
Interferon beta 1-a
Interferons, alfa-2
Ipratropium
Irinotecan
Isoniazid
Isotretinoin
Itraconazole
Ketoconazole
Ketoprofen
Labetalol
Lamivudine
Lamotrigine
Lansoprazole
Leflunomide
Letrozole
Leucovorin
Leuprolide
Levamisole
Levobetaxolol
Levobunolol
Levodopa
Levothyroxine
Liothyronine
Lisinopril
Lithium
Lomustine
Loperamide
Loratadine
Lorazepam
Losartan
Lovastatin
Loxapine
Maprotiline
Mebendazole
Mechlorethamine
Meclofenamate
Medroxyprogesterone
Mefloquine
Melphalan
Mephenytoin
Mercaptopurine
Mesalamine
Mesoridazine
Metformin
Methimazole
Methotrexate
Methsuximide
Methyldopa
Methylphenidate
Methyltestosterone
Methysergide
Metoprolol
Mexiletine
Minocycline
Minoxidil
Misoprostol
Mitomycin
Mitotane
Mitoxantrone
Moexipril
Mycophenolate
Nabumetone
Nadolol
Nalidixic acid
Naltrexone
Naproxen
Naratriptan
Nefazodone
Neomycin
Nifedipine
Nimodipine
Nisoldipine
Nitrofurantoin
Nortriptyline
Octreotide
Olanzapine
Omeprazole
Ondansetron
Oral contraceptives
Oxaprozin
Oxcarbazepine
Paclitaxel
Pantoprazole
Paramethadione
Paroxetine
PEG-interferon alfa-2b
Penbutolol
Penicillamine
Penicillins
Pentosan
Pentostatin
Pergolide
Phensuximide
Phentermine
Phenytoin
Pindolol
Pirbuterol
Piroxicam
Pravastatin
Prazepam
Prazosin
Probenecid
Procarbazine
Progestins
Propafenone
Propranolol
Propylthiouracil
Protriptyline
Pyrimethamine
Quazepam
Quinacrine
Quinapril
Quinidine
Rabeprazole
Ramipril
Ranitidine
Ribavirin
Riluzole
Risperidone
Rivastigmine
Rofecoxib
Ropinirole
Saquinavir
Selegiline
Sertraline
Simvastatin
Sotalol
Sparfloxacin
Spironolactone
St John's wort
Stanozolol
Sulfasalazine
Sulfisoxazole
Sulindac
Tacrine
Tacrolimus
Tamoxifen
Terbinafine
Testosterone
Thalidomide
Thioguanine
Thioridazine
Thiotepa
Thiothixene
Tiagabine
Timolol
Tiopronin
Tizanidine
Tocainide
Tolcapone
Topiramate
Topotecan
Trazodone
Triazolam
Trimethadione
Trimipramine
Triptorelin
Ursodiol
Valdecoxib
Valproic acid
Vasopressin
Venlafaxine
Verapamil
Vinblastine
Vincristine
Vinorelbine
Vitamin A
Voriconazole
Warfarin
Zalcitabine
Zaleplon
Zidovudine
Ziprasidone
Zonisamide

**Hair – Alopecia Areata**

Clomipramine
Cyclosporine
Fluvoxamine
Haloperidol
Imipramine
Interferons, alfa-2
Lithium
Oral contraceptives
Propranolol
Terbinafine

**Hair – Hirsutism**

Acetazolamide
Aminoglutethimide
Androstenedione
Bupropion
Chlorotrianisene
Clonazepam
Corticosteroids
Danazol
Diethylstilbestrol
Diltiazem
Donepezil
Estrogens
Ethosuximide
Fluoxetine
Fluoxymesterone
Gemfibrozil
Isotretinoin
Lamotrigine
Lorazepam
Medroxyprogesterone
Methsuximide
Methyltestosterone
Minoxidil
Nafarelin
Olanzapine
Oral contraceptives
Penicillamine
Pergolide
Phensuximide
Phenytoin
Prazepam
Progestins
Quazepam
Sertraline
Sirolimus
Spironolactone
Stanozolol
Tacrolimus
Tamoxifen
Testosterone
Tiagabine
Triazolam
Venlafaxine
Zonisamide

**Hair – Hypertrichosis**

Amantadine
Amiodarone
Basiliximab
Betaxolol
Cetirizine
Citalopram
Clomiphene
Clomipramine
Corticosteroids
Cyclosporine
Diazoxide
Epoetin alfa
Interferons, alfa-2

Latanoprost
Methoxsalen
Minoxidil
Phenytoin
Psoralens
Risperidone
Selegiline
Streptomycin
Tamoxifen
Thioridazine
Tiopronin
Trioxsalen
Unoprostone
Verapamil
Zidovudine

**Herpes Simplex**

Aspirin
Azathioprine
Azelastine
Basiliximab
Butabarbital
Butalbital
Celecoxib
Chlorambucil
Cidofovir
Clonidine
Corticosteroids
Cyclosporine
Diazoxide
Eflornithine
Eprosartan
Fluoxetine
Flurbiprofen
Foscarnet
Gemtuzumab
Indinavir
Infliximab
Interferon beta 1-a
Interferons, alfa-2
Isotretinoin
Latanoprost
Leflunomide
Meperidine
Methotrexate
Methoxsalen
Mirtazapine
Modafinil
Mycophenolate
Naltrexone
Nisoldipine
Oral contraceptives
Pantoprazole
Pentobarbital
Pentostatin
Perindopril
Phenobarbital
Pimecrolimus
Psoralens
Ribavirin
Rivastigmine
Rofecoxib
Ropinirole
Saquinavir
Sibutramine
Sildenafil
Smallpox vaccine
Sparfloxacin
Tacrine
Tacrolimus
Tiagabine
Tizanidine
Tolcapone
Trastuzumab
Trioxsalen
Valdecoxib
Venlafaxine
Voriconazole
Zolpidem

**Herpes Zoster**

Acyclovir
Azathioprine
Basiliximab
Celecoxib
Chlorambucil
Corticosteroids
Cyclosporine
Cytarabine
Enalapril
Etanercept
Fluoxetine
Flurbiprofen
Gold and gold compounds
Griseofulvin
Hepatitis B vaccine
Indinavir
Interferon beta 1-a
Isoniazid
Mechlorethamine
Mercaptopurine
Methoxsalen
Naltrexone
Nisoldipine
Pantoprazole
Pentostatin
Procarbazine
Psoralens
Rabeprazole
Rofecoxib
Ropinirole
Saquinavir
Tacrine
Tiagabine
Tizanidine
Tolcapone
Trastuzumab
Trioxsalen
Valdecoxib
Venlafaxine
Zolpidem

**Hot Flashes**

Anastrozole
Anthrax vaccine
Arbutamine
Bicalutamide
Bupropion
Cabergoline
Cefmetazole
Celecoxib
Cevimeline
Citalopram
Clomiphene
Cyclosporine
Doxazosin
Efavirenz
Epirubicin
Eprosartan
Estramustine
Estrogens
Exemestane
Fenoprofen
Flumazenil
Fluoxetine
Flurbiprofen
Flutamide
Frovatriptan
Fulvestrant
Ganirelix
Goserelin
Granisetron
Hydrocodone
Ibuprofen
Indomethacin
Interferons, alfa-2
Ketoprofen
Lamotrigine
Letrozole
Leuprolide
Levodopa
Meclofenamate
Medroxyprogesterone
Mefenamic acid
Meloxicam
Mexiletine
Modafinil
Nabumetone
Nafarelin
Naltrexone
Naproxen
Oxcarbazepine
Oxybutynin
Piroxicam
Raloxifene
Rivastigmine
Rizatriptan
Sirolimus
Sulindac
Sumatriptan
Tamoxifen
Tolmetin
Topiramate
Toremifene
Triptorelin
Valdecoxib
Zolmitriptan
Zolpidem

**Hypersensitivity**

Abacavir
Acetaminophen
Acyclovir
Alendronate
Allopurinol
Aloe vera (gel, juice, leaf)
Alteplase
Aminophylline
Aminosalicylate sodium
Amitriptyline
Amobarbital
Amoxicillin
Ampicillin
Anisindione
Anistreplase
Anthrax vaccine
Aprotinin
Asparaginase
Aspirin
Azathioprine
Azithromycin
Aztreonam
Bacampicillin
Balsalazide
Basiliximab
Benazepril
Bismuth
Bleomycin
Bupropion
Butterbur
Calcitonin
Capecitabine
Carbamazepine
Carbenicillin
Carboplatin
Cefaclor
Cefadroxil
Cefamandole
Cefazolin
Cefepime
Cefixime
Cefmetazole
Cefonicid
Cefoperazone
Cefotaxime
Cefotetan
Cefpodoxime
Cefprozil
Ceftazidime
Ceftibuten
Ceftriaxone
Cefuroxime
Cephalexin
Cephapirin
Cephradine
Chamomile
Chloral hydrate
Chlorambucil
Chloramphenicol
Chlorhexidine
Chlorpheniramine
Chlorzoxazone
Cimetidine
Cinoxacin
Ciprofloxacin
Cisatracurium
Cisplatin
Clarithromycin
Clemastine
Clindamycin
Clopidogrel
Cloxacillin
Co-trimoxazole
Colchicine
Corticosteroids
Cromolyn
Cyanocobalamin
Cyclamate
Cyclophosphamide
Cyclosporine
Cytarabine
Dacarbazine
Dapsone
Denileukin
Desipramine
Desloratadine
Diazoxide
Diclofenac
Dicloxacillin
Dicumarol
Didanosine
Diflunisal
Diltiazem
Diphenhydramine

Dobutamine
Docetaxel
Domperidone
Doxycycline
Echinacea
Edrophonium
Efavirenz
Enoxacin
Enoxaparin
Ephedra
Epirubicin
Epoetin alfa
Ertapenem
Erythromycin
Ethambutol
Ethchlorvynol
Etidronate
Etoposide
Famciclovir
Flavoxate
Fluconazole
Fluoxetine
Fluoxymesterone
Flurbiprofen
Garlic
Gatifloxacin
Gentamicin
Glyburide
Gold and gold compounds
Goserelin
Granisetron
Haloperidol
Hawthorn (fruit, leaf, flower extract)
Henna
Heparin
Hepatitis B vaccine
Heroin
Hydralazine
Hydroxyzine
Ibritumomab
Ibuprofen
Imipenem/cilastatin
Inamrinone
Indomethacin
Infliximab
Insulin
Interferon beta 1-a
Interferons, alfa-2
Ipodate
Isoniazid
Kanamycin
Kava
Ketoconazole
Ketorolac
Labetalol
Lamotrigine
Lansoprazole
Leucovorin
Levalbuterol
Levobunolol
Levothyroxine
Lidocaine
Liothyronine
Lomefloxacin
Loperamide
Lovastatin
Meadowsweet
Mechlorethamine
Meclofenamate
Meloxicam
Melphalan
Meprobamate
Mesalamine
Methazolamide
Methicillin
Methyldopa
Methylphenidate
Methyltestosterone
Metronidazole
Mezlocillin
Minocycline
Nafarelin
Nafcillin
Naproxen
Nelfinavir
Neomycin
Nevirapine
Nicotine
Nisoldipine
Nitrofurantoin
Nystatin
Ofloxacin
Olanzapine
Ondansetron
Orphenadrine
Oxacillin
Oxcarbazepine
Oxytetracycline
Paclitaxel
Pamidronate
Pancuronium
PEG-interferon alfa-2b
Penicillamine
Penicillins
Pentagastrin
Pentobarbital
Phenobarbital
Phenylephrine
Phenytoin
Phytonadione
Pilocarpine
Piperacillin
Pravastatin
Primidone
Probenecid
Procarbazine
Promethazine
Propolis
Propylthiouracil
Protamine
Protease inhibitors
Pyrazinamide
Pyridoxine
Pyrimethamine
Quinapril
Quinethazone
Quinidine
Quinine
Ramipril
Ranitidine
Salmeterol
Secobarbital
Simvastatin
Sparfloxacin
Spectinomycin
St John's wort
Succinylcholine
Sulfacetamide
Sulfadiazine
Sulfadoxine
Sulfamethoxazole
Sulfasalazine
Sulfisoxazole
Sulindac
Tartrazine
Terbinafine
Testosterone
Tetracycline
Thiabendazole
Thimerosal
Thioridazine
Ticarcillin
Tinzaparin
Tobramycin
Tocainide
Tolbutamide
Trazodone
Trimethobenzamide
Trimetrexate
Triptorelin
Trovafloxacin
Urokinase
Valproic acid
Vancomycin
Vinblastine
Vitamin A
Warfarin
Zidovudine
Zonisamide

**Jarisch–Herxheimer Reaction**

Amoxicillin
Bacampicillin
Carbenicillin
Ceftriaxone
Cefuroxime
Cloxacillin
Dicloxacillin
Griseofulvin
Ketoconazole
Methicillin
Mezlocillin
Nafcillin
Oxacillin
Penicillins
Pentamidine
Piperacillin
Thiabendazole
Ticarcillin

**Kaposi's Sarcoma**

Aldesleukin
Aminocaproic acid
Azathioprine
Busulfan
Captopril
Chlorambucil
Corticosteroids
Cyclosporine
Heroin
Interferons, alfa-2

**Lichen Planus (LP)**

Allopurinol
Amitriptyline
Amlodipine
Arsenic
Aspirin
Captopril
Carbamazepine
Diflunisal
Doxazosin
Felbamate
Gemfibrozil
Glipizide
Gold and gold compounds
Hepatitis B vaccine
Hydroxyurea
Imipramine
Indomethacin
Interferons, alfa-2
Labetalol
Levamisole
Levobunolol
Lithium
Mesalamine
Methyldopa
Naproxen
Omeprazole
Penicillamine
Phenytoin
Prazosin
Procainamide
Psoralens
Quinidine
Quinine
Simvastatin
Spironolactone
Sulfasalazine
Sulindac
Thimerosal
Trovafloxacin
Ursodiol

**Lichenoid (Lichen Planus-like) Eruptions**

Acebutolol
Acetohexamide
Acyclovir
Aminosalicylate sodium
Amlodipine
Aspirin
Atenolol
Atorvastatin
Azathioprine
Captopril
Carbamazepine
Chloral hydrate
Chloroquine
Chlorothiazide
Chlorpromazine
Chlorpropamide
Co-trimoxazole
Colchicine
Cycloserine
Cyclosporine
Cyproheptadine
Dapsone
Demeclocycline
Diazoxide
Diclofenac
Diflunisal
Diltiazem
Doxazosin
Enalapril
Epoetin alfa
Ethambutol
Fluoxetine
Fluoxymesterone
Flurbiprofen
Furosemide
Glipizide
Glyburide

Gold and gold compounds
Granulocyte colony-stimulating factor (GCSF)
Griseofulvin
Hepatitis B vaccine
Hydrochlorothiazide
Hydroxychloroquine
Hydroxyurea
Ibuprofen
Indomethacin
Interferons, alfa-2
Isoniazid
Isotretinoin
Ketoconazole
Labetalol
Lansoprazole
Levamisole
Lisinopril
Lorazepam
Mercaptopurine
Mesalamine
Metformin
Methamphetamine
Methyldopa
Methyltestosterone
Metoprolol
Minocycline
Nadolol
Naproxen
Nifedipine
Omeprazole
Oral contraceptives
Pantoprazole
Penicillamine
Phenytoin
Pindolol
Piroxicam
Pravastatin
Prazosin
Propranolol
Propylthiouracil
Pyrimethamine
Quinacrine
Quinidine
Quinine
Ramipril
Ranitidine
Risperidone
Salsalate
Sildenafil
Simvastatin
Sotalol
Sparfloxacin
Spironolactone
Streptomycin
Sulfadoxine
Sulfamethoxazole
Sulindac
Temazepam
Terazosin
Testosterone
Tetracycline
Timolol
Tiopronin
Tolazamide
Tolbutamide
Torsemide
Trichlormethiazide
Tripelennamine
Triprolidine
Ursodiol
Venlafaxine
Verapamil
Zidovudine

**Linear Iga Bullous Dermatosis (LABD)**

Aldesleukin
Amiodarone
Ampicillin
Atorvastatin
Captopril
Carbamazepine
Cefamandole
Ceftriaxone
Ciprofloxacin
Co-trimoxazole
Cyclosporine
Diclofenac
Furosemide
Glyburide
Granulocyte colony-stimulating factor (GCSF)
Ibuprofen
Interferons, alfa-2
Lithium
Metronidazole
Naproxen
Penicillins
Phenytoin
Piroxicam
Rifampin
Sulfamethoxazole
Sulfisoxazole
Vancomycin

**Livedo Reticularis**

Amantadine
Anistreplase
Arsenic
Bromocriptine
Ciprofloxacin
Dihydrotachysterol
Diphenhydramine
Estrogens
Felbamate
Heparin
Ibuprofen
Minocycline
Quinidine
Tenecteplase
Warfarin

**Lupus Erythematosus**

Acebutolol
Acetazolamide
Albuterol
Allopurinol
Aminoglutethimide
Aminosalicylate sodium
Amiodarone
Amitriptyline
Amlodipine
Anthrax vaccine
Atenolol
Benazepril
Betaxolol
Bisoprolol
Butabarbital
Butalbital
Captopril
Carbamazepine
Carteolol
Chlorambucil
Chlordiazepoxide
Chlorothiazide
Chlorpromazine
Chlorpropamide
Chlorthalidone
Cimetidine
Clofibrate
Clonidine
Clozapine
Co-trimoxazole
Corticosteroids
Cyclophosphamide
Cyclosporine
Cyproheptadine
Danazol
Dapsone
Demeclocycline
Diclofenac
Diethylstilbestrol
Diltiazem
Disopyramide
Domperidone
Doxazosin
Doxycycline
Enalapril
Estrogens
Etanercept
Ethambutol
Ethionamide
Ethosuximide
Ethotoin
Felbamate
Fluoxetine
Fluoxymesterone
Fluphenazine
Flutamide
Fluvastatin
Fosphenytoin
Furosemide
Gemfibrozil
Gold and gold compounds
Griseofulvin
Guanethidine
Hepatitis B vaccine
Hydralazine
Hydrochlorothiazide
Hydroxyurea
Ibuprofen
Imipramine
Interferon beta 1-a
Interferons, alfa-2
Isoniazid
Labetalol
Lamotrigine
Leuprolide
Levodopa
Lidocaine
Lisinopril
Lithium
Lovastatin
Meclofenamate
Mephenytoin
Meprobamate
Mercaptopurine
Mesalamine
Mesoridazine
Methimazole
Methoxsalen
Methsuximide
Methyldopa
Methyltestosterone
Methysergide
Metoprolol
Mexiletine
Minocycline
Minoxidil
Nadolol
Nalidixic acid
Naproxen
Nifedipine
Nitrofurantoin
Olsalazine
Omeprazole
Oral contraceptives
Oxcarbazepine
Oxytetracycline
Pantoprazole
Paramethadione
Penicillamine
Penicillins
Pentobarbital
Perphenazine
Phenelzine
Phenindamine
Phenobarbital
Phenolphthalein
Phensuximide
Phenytoin
Pindolol
Piroxicam
Potassium iodide
Pravastatin
Prazosin
Primidone
Procainamide
Prochlorperazine
Promethazine
Propafenone
Propranolol
Propylthiouracil
Psoralens
Pyrilamine
Quinidine
Quinine
Ranitidine
Reserpine
Rifabutin
Rifampin
Sertraline
Simvastatin
Smallpox vaccine
Spironolactone
Streptomycin
Sulfadiazine
Sulfadoxine
Sulfamethoxazole
Sulfasalazine
Sulfisoxazole
Terbinafine
Testosterone
Tetracycline
Thioridazine
Ticlopidine
Timolol
Tiopronin
Tocainide
Tolazamide
Triamterene
Trichlormethiazide

Trientine
Trifluoperazine
Trimeprazine
Trimethadione
Trioxsalen
Tripelennamine
Valproic acid
Vancomycin
Verapamil
Vitamin E
Voriconazole
Yohimbine
Zafirlukast
Zonisamide

**Mastodynia**

Anastrozole
Azelastine
Aztreonam
Betaxolol
Bexarotene
Bicalutamide
Cabergoline
Celecoxib
Cetirizine
Chlorotrianisene
Chlorpromazine
Citalopram
Clomiphene
Clomipramine
Clozapine
Diethylstilbestrol
Dipyridamole
Doxazosin
Eletriptan
Estramustine
Estrogens
Fenoprofen
Finasteride
Fluoxetine
Fluoxymesterone
Fluphenazine
Fluvoxamine
Ganciclovir
Gatifloxacin
Ginseng
Goserelin
Haloperidol
Interferon beta 1-a
Lansoprazole
Leuprolide
Lisinopril
Loratadine
Medroxyprogesterone
Mesoridazine
Methyltestosterone
Metoclopramide
Minoxidil
Mirtazapine
Nafarelin
Nefazodone
Nitrofurantoin
Pantoprazole
Pergolide
Perphenazine
Prochlorperazine
Promazine
Promethazine
Quinestrol
Raloxifene
Riluzole
Risperidone
Rivastigmine
Sparfloxacin
Spironolactone
Temozolomide
Testosterone
Thioridazine
Thiothixene
Tiagabine
Topiramate
Trifluoperazine
Venlafaxine
Zaleplon
Zolpidem

**Melanoma**

Aminolevulinic acid
Arsenic
Clomiphene
Cyclosporine
Diazepam
Gemfibrozil
Interferons, alfa-2
Levodopa
Methotrexate
Oral contraceptives
Paroxetine
Psoralens
Smallpox vaccine
Tacrine
Trioxsalen

**Myalgia**

Abacavir
Abciximab
Acebutolol
Aldesleukin
Alemtuzumab
Alitretinoin
Allopurinol
Almotriptan
Aminocaproic acid
Aminoglutethimide
Amphotericin B
Anagrelide
Anastrozole
Anistreplase
Anthrax vaccine
Apraclonidine
Aspirin
Atorvastatin
Azatadine
Azathioprine
Azelastine
Aztreonam
Balsalazide
Basiliximab
Benazepril
Bepridil
Betaxolol
Bexarotene
Bicalutamide
Bisoprolol
Brompheniramine
Bupropion
Buspirone
Candesartan
Capecitabine
Captopril
Carteolol
Carvedilol
Caspofungin
Cefditoren
Cefonicid
Celecoxib
Cetirizine
Cevimeline
Chloroquine
Chlorpheniramine
Cidofovir
Cilostazol
Cimetidine
Citalopram
Cladribine
Clemastine
Clofibrate
Clomiphene
Clomipramine
Co-trimoxazole
Colchicine
Colesevelam
Creatine
Cromolyn
Cyclosporine
Cyproheptadine
Cytarabine
Dacarbazine
Dactinomycin
Dantrolene
Delavirdine
Denileukin
Desloratadine
Dexchlorpheniramine
Dicloxacillin
Didanosine
Diethylpropion
Dihydroergotamine
Dihydrotachysterol
Dimenhydrinate
Diphenhydramine
Dipyridamole
Dirithromycin
Docetaxel
Dolasetron
Doxazosin
Dronabinol
Efavirenz
Eletriptan
Enalapril
Enoxacin
Ephedra
Epirubicin
Epoetin alfa
Eprosartan
Ergocalciferol
Estazolam
Famotidine
Felbamate
Felodipine
Fenofibrate
Flecainide
Fludarabine
Fluoxetine
Fluvastatin
Fluvoxamine
Formoterol
Foscarnet
Fosfomycin
Fosinopril
Frovatriptan
Fulvestrant
Gabapentin
Ganciclovir
Gatifloxacin
Gemcitabine
Gemfibrozil
Glipizide
Glyburide
Granulocyte colony-stimulating factor (GCSF)
Guanethidine
Hepatitis B vaccine
Hydralazine
Hydroxyzine
Ibritumomab
Imatinib
Imiquimod
Indinavir
Infliximab
Interferon beta 1-a
Interferons, alfa-2
Isotretinoin
Itraconazole
Ivermectin
Ketoprofen
Ketorolac
Lamivudine
Lamotrigine
Lansoprazole
Latanoprost
Leflunomide
Leuprolide
Levalbuterol
Levamisole
Levofloxacin
Levothyroxine
Liothyronine
Lisinopril
Lomefloxacin
Loratadine
Losartan
Lovastatin
MDMA
Meclizine
Mefloquine
Mesalamine
Methimazole
Methotrexate
Methyldopa
Methysergide
Minocycline
Mirtazapine
Mitotane
Modafinil
Moexipril
Moxifloxacin
Mycophenolate
Nabumetone
Nafarelin
Naltrexone
Naproxen
Nebivolol
Nefazodone
Nelfinavir
Nevirapine
Nicardipine
Nicotine
Nifedipine
Nitrofurantoin
Nizatidine
Norfloxacin
Ofloxacin

Olanzapine
Olmesartan
Omeprazole
Orlistat
Paclitaxel
Pamidronate
Pancuronium
Pantoprazole
Paroxetine
PEG-interferon alfa-2b
Pentamidine
Pentostatin
Pergolide
Perindopril
Phentermine
Pilocarpine
Pimozide
Pindolol
Pioglitazone
Pramipexole
Pravastatin
Procainamide
Procarbazine
Promethazine
Propofol
Propranolol
Propylthiouracil
Pyrazinamide
Quetiapine
Quinapril
Quinidine
Quinupristin/dalfopristin
Rabeprazole
Raloxifene
Ranitidine
Rapacuronium
Ribavirin
Rifabutin
Rifampin
Risedronate
Risperidone
Ritonavir
Rituximab
Rivastigmine
Rizatriptan
Rofecoxib
Salmeterol
Sibutramine
Sildenafil
Simvastatin
Sirolimus
Smallpox vaccine
Sotalol
Sparfloxacin
Stavudine
Succinylcholine
Sulfasalazine
Sulfisoxazole
Sumatriptan
Tacrine
Tacrolimus
Telmisartan
Temozolomide
Terazosin
Tiagabine
Timolol
Tocainide
Tolcapone
Tolmetin
Topiramate
Torsemide
Trandolapril
Trazodone
Tretinoin
Trimeprazine
Tripelennamine
Triprolidine
Trovafloxacin
Unoprostone
Ursodiol
Valdecoxib
Valproic acid
Valsartan
Venlafaxine
Vinblastine
Vincristine
Vinorelbine
Voriconazole
Zafirlukast
Zalcitabine
Zaleplon
Zanamivir
Zileuton
Ziprasidone
Zoledronic acid
Zolmitriptan
Zolpidem
Zonisamide

**Nails – Onycholysis**

Acebutolol
Allopurinol
Atenolol
Bleomycin
Captopril
Chloramphenicol
Chlorpromazine
Clofazimine
Clorazepate
Cloxacillin
Demeclocycline
Diflunisal
Docetaxel
Doxorubicin
Doxycycline
Estrogens
Etoposide
Fluorouracil
Gold and gold compounds
Hydroxyurea
Ibuprofen
Indomethacin
Isoniazid
Isotretinoin
Ketoprofen
Methotrexate
Methoxsalen
Metoprolol
Minocycline
Mycophenolate
Nadolol
Nitrofurantoin
Norfloxacin
Ofloxacin
Oral contraceptives
Paclitaxel
Pindolol
Piroxicam
Propranolol
Psoralens
Quinine
Tetracycline
Timolol
Trioxsalen

**Nails – Pigmented**

Arsenic
Betaxolol
Bleomycin
Busulfan
Chloroquine
Chlorpromazine
Cyclophosphamide
Dacarbazine
Daunorubicin
Demeclocycline
Docetaxel
Doxorubicin
Epirubicin
Fluorouracil
Flurbiprofen
Gold and gold compounds
Hydroxychloroquine
Hydroxyurea
Idarubicin
Kava
Ketoconazole
Methotrexate
Methoxsalen
Minocycline
Oxytetracycline
Paclitaxel
Phenytoin
Psoralens
Quinacrine
Timolol
Trioxsalen
Valsartan
Zidovudine

**Neuroleptic Malignant Syndrome**

Donepezil
Haloperidol
Olanzapine
Quetiapine
Risperidone

**Oral Candidiasis**

Amoxicillin
Ampicillin
Atovaquone
Bacampicillin
Capecitabine
Carbenicillin
Cefaclor
Cefadroxil
Cefamandole
Cefazolin
Cefditoren
Cefepime
Cefpodoxime
Cefprozil
Ceftazidime
Ceftibuten
Ceftizoxime
Cefuroxime
Cephalexin
Cidofovir
Ciprofloxacin
Clarithromycin
Cloxacillin
Corticosteroids
Dicloxacillin
Ertapenem
Erythromycin
Gatifloxacin
Griseofulvin
Leflunomide
Linezolid
Mesalamine
Methicillin
Mezlocillin
Mirtazapine
Mycophenolate
Nafcillin
Nefazodone
Olanzapine
Omeprazole
Oxacillin
Palivizumab
Pantoprazole
Penicillins
Piperacillin
Quinupristin/dalfopristin
Riluzole
Ritonavir
Salmeterol
Sirolimus
Sparfloxacin
Tacrolimus
Ticarcillin

**Oral Ulceration**

Abacavir
Aldesleukin
Alendronate
Allopurinol
Alprazolam
Aminoglutethimide
Anisindione
Aspirin
Atorvastatin
Azathioprine
Aztreonam
Betaxolol
Bleomycin
Butabarbital
Butalbital
Capecitabine
Captopril
Carbamazepine
Cefadroxil
Cefditoren
Chloral hydrate
Chlorambucil
Chloramphenicol
Chloroquine
Chlorpromazine
Cidofovir
Cisplatin
Clofibrate
Clonazepam
Clorazepate
Co-trimoxazole
Codeine
Colesevelam
Cyclophosphamide
Cyclosporine
Cytarabine
Delavirdine
Diclofenac
Dicumarol
Diflunisal
Dirithromycin

Doxorubicin
Enalapril
Epirubicin
Ertapenem
Erythromycin
Estazolam
Ethionamide
Ethosuximide
Fenoprofen
Feverfew
Flavoxate
Fluconazole
Fluoxetine
Foscarnet
Ganciclovir
Gatifloxacin
Gold and gold compounds
Heroin
Hydralazine
Hydroxychloroquine
Hydroxyurea
Ibuprofen
Imipramine
Indomethacin
Ipratropium
Irinotecan
Isoniazid
Lamotrigine
Leflunomide
Levamisole
Lithium
Losartan
Meclofenamate
Mefenamic acid
Melphalan
Meprobamate
Mesalamine
Mesna
Methimazole
Methotrexate
Methsuximide
Methyldopa
Metronidazole
Minocycline
Mitomycin
Modafinil
Mycophenolate
Nabumetone
Naproxen
Nefazodone
Nelfinavir
Nisoldipine
Olanzapine
Paroxetine
Penicillamine
Penicillins
Pentobarbital
Pentosan
Phenobarbital
Phenolphthalein
Phensuximide
Phenytoin
Promethazine
Propolis
Propranolol
Propylthiouracil
Quazepam
Quetiapine
Quinidine
Quinine
Rabeprazole
Ritonavir
Rofecoxib
Saquinavir
Sirolimus
Sparfloxacin
Streptomycin
Sulfadoxine
Sulfamethoxazole
Sulfasalazine
Sulfisoxazole
Sulindac
Tacrolimus
Terbutaline
Tetracycline
Tiagabine
Tiopronin
Tolcapone
Tolmetin
Venlafaxine
Vincristine
Voriconazole
Warfarin
Zalcitabine
Zaleplon
Zidovudine
Zonisamide

**Paresthesias**

Abacavir
Acetazolamide
Acetohexamide
Acitretin
Acyclovir
Alitretinoin
Allopurinol
Almotriptan
Alprazolam
Altretamine
Amikacin
Amiloride
Amiodarone
Amitriptyline
Amlodipine
Amoxapine
Amphotericin B
Amprenavir
Anagrelide
Anastrozole
Anthrax vaccine
Apraclonidine
Arbutamine
Aspirin
Atorvastatin
Azatadine
Aztreonam
Baclofen
Basiliximab
Benactyzine
Benazepril
Bendroflumethiazide
Benzthiazide
Benztropine
Bepridil
Betaxolol
Bicalutamide
Biperiden
Bisoprolol
Bleomycin
Bromocriptine
Brompheniramine
Bupropion
Buspirone
Butorphanol
Cabergoline
Caffeine
Calcitonin
Candesartan
Capecitabine
Captopril
Carisoprodol
Carteolol
Carvedilol
Caspofungin
Cefaclor
Cefamandole
Cefotaxime
Cefpodoxime
Cefprozil
Ceftazidime
Ceftibuten
Ceftizoxime
Celecoxib
Cephapirin
Cetirizine
Cevimeline
Chloramphenicol
Chlordiazepoxide
Chlorothiazide
Chlorpheniramine
Chlorpropamide
Chlorthalidone
Cholestyramine
Cidofovir
Cilostazol
Cinoxacin
Ciprofloxacin
Citalopram
Clemastine
Clomipramine
Clonazepam
Clopidogrel
Clorazepate
Codeine
Cromolyn
Cyanocobalamin
Cyclamate
Cyclobenzaprine
Cycloserine
Cyclosporine
Cyclothiazide
Cyproheptadine
Dacarbazine
Danaparoid
Danazol
Delavirdine
Demeclocycline
Denileukin
Desipramine
Dexchlorpheniramine
Diazepam
Diazoxide
Diclofenac
Didanosine
Diflunisal
Dihydroergotamine
Diltiazem
Dimenhydrinate
Diphenhydramine
Diphenoxylate
Dipyridamole
Dirithromycin
Disopyramide
Disulfiram
Dobutamine
Docetaxel
Dofetilide
Dolasetron
Donepezil
Doxapram
Doxazosin
Doxepin
Doxycycline
Dronabinol
Echinacea
Efavirenz
Eflornithine
Eletriptan
Enalapril
Enoxacin
Epoetin alfa
Eprosartan
Ertapenem
Esmolol
Esomeprazole
Estazolam
Ethambutol
Ethchlorvynol
Etidronate
Etodolac
Etoposide
Exemestane
Famciclovir
Famotidine
Felbamate
Felodipine
Fenofibrate
Fentanyl
Flecainide
Fluconazole
Flucytosine
Fludarabine
Flumazenil
Fluorouracil
Fluoxetine
Fluoxymesterone
Flurazepam
Flurbiprofen
Flutamide
Fluvastatin
Fluvoxamine
Foscarnet
Fosfomycin
Fosinopril
Fosphenytoin
Frovatriptan
Fulvestrant
Furosemide
Gabapentin
Galantamine
Ganciclovir
Gatifloxacin
Gemcitabine
Gemfibrozil
Gentamicin
Glipizide
Glyburide
Griseofulvin
Guanadrel
Guanethidine
Guanfacine

Hepatitis B vaccine
Hydralazine
Hydrochlorothiazide
Hydroflumethiazide
Hydromorphone
Ibuprofen
Imipenem/cilastatin
Imipramine
Indapamide
Indinavir
Indomethacin
Infliximab
Insulin
Interferon beta 1-a
Interferons, alfa-2
Ipratropium
Irbesartan
Isoniazid
Isradipine
Kanamycin
Ketoconazole
Ketoprofen
Ketorolac
Labetalol
Lamivudine
Lamotrigine
Lansoprazole
Leflunomide
Leuprolide
Levalbuterol
Levamisole
Levetiracetam
Levodopa
Levofloxacin
Lidocaine
Lindane
Lisinopril
Lomefloxacin
Loratadine
Lorazepam
Losartan
Lovastatin
Loxapine
Mazindol
MDMA
Meclizine
Meclofenamate
Medroxyprogesterone
Meloxicam
Meprobamate
Mesalamine
Mesoridazine
Methazolamide
Methimazole
Methyclothiazide
Methyldopa
Methyltestosterone
Methysergide
Metoclopramide
Metolazone
Metoprolol
Metronidazole
Mexiletine
Midazolam
Midodrine
Minocycline
Minoxidil
Mirtazapine
Mitomycin
Modafinil
Moricizine
Moxifloxacin
Mycophenolate
Nabumetone
Nadolol
Nafarelin
Nalidixic acid
Naratriptan
Nebivolol
Nefazodone
Nelfinavir
Nesiritide
Nevirapine
Niacin
Niacinamide
Nicardipine
Nicotine
Nifedipine
Nisoldipine
Nitrofurantoin
Nizatidine
Norfloxacin
Nortriptyline
Ofloxacin
Omeprazole
Ondansetron
Orphenadrine
Oxazepam
Oxytetracycline
Paclitaxel
Pantoprazole
Paramethadione
Paroxetine
Penbutolol
Pentagastrin
Pentazocine
Pentostatin
Pentoxifylline
Pergolide
Perindopril
Phenylephrine
Phenytoin
Pindolol
Pirbuterol
Piroxicam
Polythiazide
Potassium iodide
Pramipexole
Pravastatin
Prazepam
Prazosin
Procarbazine
Promethazine
Propafenone
Propranolol
Propylthiouracil
Protriptyline
Pyridoxine
Pyrilamine
Quazepam
Quetiapine
Quinapril
Quinethazone
Quinupristin/dalfopristin
Rabeprazole
Ramipril
Repaglinide
Rifabutin
Riluzole
Risedronate
Risperidone
Ritonavir
Rivastigmine
Rizatriptan
Rofecoxib
Ropinirole
Salmeterol
Saquinavir
Selegiline
Sertraline
Sibutramine
Sildenafil
Simvastatin
Sirolimus
Sotalol
Sparfloxacin
Spironolactone
St John's wort
Stavudine
Streptomycin
Sulindac
Sumatriptan
Tacrine
Tacrolimus
Tartrazine
Telmisartan
Temazepam
Temozolomide
Tenofovir
Terazosin
Testosterone
Tetracycline
Thalidomide
Thiabendazole
Thiamine
Thioridazine
Thiothixene
Tiagabine
Timolol
Tizanidine
Tobramycin
Tocainide
Tolazamide
Tolbutamide
Tolcapone
Tolterodine
Topiramate
Topotecan
Tramadol
Trandolapril
Tranylcypromine
Trastuzumab
Trazodone
Tretinoin
Triamterene
Triazolam
Trichlormethiazide
Trihexyphenidyl
Trimeprazine
Trimethadione
Trimipramine
Tripelennamine
Triprolidine
Trovafloxacin
Unoprostone
Valdecoxib
Valganciclovir
Valproic acid
Valsartan
Vancomycin
Venlafaxine
Verapamil
Verteporfin
Vinblastine
Vincristine
Vinorelbine
Voriconazole
Zalcitabine
Zaleplon
Zidovudine
Zileuton
Ziprasidone
Zolmitriptan
Zolpidem
Zonisamide

**Parkinsonism**

Amitriptyline
Bupropion
Busulfan
Carboplatin
Cyclosporine
Diltiazem
Domperidone
Doxepin
Flucytosine
Fluphenazine
Haloperidol
Imipramine
Interferons, alfa-2
Kava
Lithium
Loxapine
Maprotiline
MDMA
Methyldopa
Metoclopramide
Nabumetone
Nortriptyline
Olanzapine
Pemoline
Perphenazine
Phenelzine
Prochlorperazine
Promazine
Promethazine
Protriptyline
Reserpine
Risperidone
Tacrine
Thioridazine
Thiothixene
Trazodone
Trifluoperazine
Trimethobenzamide
Trimipramine
Tryptophan
Valproic acid
Verapamil

**Parosmia**

Almotriptan
Alosetron
Aminophylline
Amiodarone
Amlodipine
Apraclonidine
Atorvastatin
Buspirone
Cetirizine
Cevimeline
Clarithromycin

Doxazosin
Efavirenz
Eletriptan
Esomeprazole
Fluoxetine
Flurbiprofen
Fluvoxamine
Gatifloxacin
Isotretinoin
Levamisole
Mirtazapine
Nifedipine
Ofloxacin
Propafenone
Rimantadine
Ritonavir
Sumatriptan
Terbinafine
Tiagabine
Tiopronin
Tocainide
Tolcapone
Topiramate
Venlafaxine
Zalcitabine
Zaleplon
Zolmitriptan
Zonisamide

**Periorbital Edema**

Acyclovir
Aspirin
Cabergoline
Carbamazepine
Cefmetazole
Chlorambucil
Clozapine
Creatine
Diltiazem
Donepezil
Ethosuximide
Famotidine
Foscarnet
Furosemide
Ibuprofen
Imatinib
Indomethacin
Methsuximide
Moricizine
Nifedipine
Omeprazole
Phensuximide
Phenylephrine
Pimozide
Rivastigmine
Sertraline
Streptokinase
Sulfadiazine
Sulfadoxine
Sulfasalazine
Sulfisoxazole
Trovafloxacin
Urokinase
Valacyclovir
Valdecoxib
Zolpidem

**Peripheral Edema**

Abciximab
Acyclovir
Aldesleukin
Alemtuzumab
Alendronate
Amantadine
Amlodipine
Anagrelide
Anastrozole
Basiliximab
Benazepril
Bepridil
Bexarotene
Bicalutamide
Bosentan
Botulinum toxin (A & B)
Bupropion
Cabergoline
Candesartan
Carteolol
Carvedilol
Cefditoren
Celecoxib
Cetrorelix
Cevimeline
Chlorotrianisene
Chlorpromazine
Chondroitin
Cilostazol
Clonidine
Cyproheptadine
Danaparoid
Delavirdine
Diclofenac
Diethylstilbestrol
Diflunisal
Diltiazem
Dirithromycin
Docetaxel
Dofetilide
Dolasetron
Doxazosin
Efavirenz
Eletriptan
Enoxaparin
Eprosartan
Esomeprazole
Estrogens
Etodolac
Exemestane
Felodipine
Fenoprofen
Fluoxetine
Fluphenazine
Flurbiprofen
Foscarnet
Fulvestrant
Gabapentin
Galantamine
Gatifloxacin
Gemcitabine
Gemtuzumab
Granulocyte colony-stimulating factor (GCSF)
Guanadrel
Guanethidine
Guanfacine
Heparin
Hydroxyurea
Ibritumomab
Imatinib
Indapamide
Indomethacin
Isocarboxazid
Isosorbide dinitrate
Isradipine
Itraconazole
Ivermectin
Ketoprofen
Labetalol
Lansoprazole
Leflunomide
Leuprolide
Lisinopril
Loratadine
Meclofenamate
Meprobamate
Mesalamine
Mesoridazine
Methyldopa
Methysergide
Metoprolol
Midazolam
Minoxidil
Mirtazapine
Moexipril
Molindone
Montelukast
Morphine
Moxifloxacin
Mycophenolate
Naproxen
Nefazodone
Nicardipine
Nifedipine
Nimodipine
Nisoldipine
Nitroglycerin
Olanzapine
Olmesartan
Omeprazole
Pantoprazole
Paroxetine
Penbutolol
Penicillamine
Pentostatin
Pergolide
Perphenazine
Phenelzine
Phentermine
Pindolol
Piroxicam
Pramipexole
Prochlorperazine
Propranolol
Quinapril
Quinestrol
Quinupristin/dalfopristin
Rabeprazole
Raloxifene
Rapacuronium
Reserpine
Rifapentine
Riluzole
Risedronate
Risperidone
Ritonavir
Rituximab
Rivastigmine
Rofecoxib
Ropinirole
Selegiline
Sibutramine
Sildenafil
Sirolimus
Sotalol
Sparfloxacin
Tacrine
Tacrolimus
Tamoxifen
Telmisartan
Temozolomide
Terazosin
Terbinafine
Testosterone
Thalidomide
Thioridazine
Thiothixene
Tiagabine
Tranylcypromine
Trastuzumab
Trifluoperazine
Trimeprazine
Tripelennamine
Trovafloxacin
Valdecoxib
Valproic acid
Venlafaxine
Verapamil
Voriconazole
Zaleplon
Ziprasidone
Zonisamide

**Petechiae**

Abciximab
Aldesleukin
Alendronate
Allopurinol
Amitriptyline
Amlodipine
Amoxapine
Amoxicillin
Anisindione
Aspirin
Atorvastatin
Aztreonam
Benactyzine
Carbamazepine
Chlorzoxazone
Cladribine
Clozapine
Cytarabine
Danazol
Delavirdine
Denileukin
Desipramine
Diltiazem
Fluconazole
Fludarabine
Fluoxetine
Gemcitabine
Gemfibrozil
Gemtuzumab
Griseofulvin
Heparin
Hepatitis B vaccine
Ibritumomab
Imatinib
Imipramine
Indomethacin
Interferon beta 1-a
Lamotrigine
Maprotiline
Melphalan

- Meprobamate
- Mercaptopurine
- Methyldopa
- Minocycline
- Mirtazapine
- Mitoxantrone
- Nisoldipine
- Nortriptyline
- Octreotide
- Ofloxacin
- Pentostatin
- Piroxicam
- Plicamycin
- Procarbazine
- Protriptyline
- Riluzole
- Simvastatin
- Sparfloxacin
- Tacrine
- Thioguanine
- Tiagabine
- Ticlopidine
- Tizanidine
- Trimethadione
- Trimipramine
- Valproic acid
- Voriconazole
- Zonisamide

**Peyronie's Disease**

- Acebutolol
- Atenolol
- Betaxolol
- Bisoprolol
- Carteolol
- Interferon beta 1-a
- Labetalol
- Methotrexate
- Metoprolol
- Nadolol
- Penbutolol
- Phenytoin
- Pindolol
- Propranolol
- Ropinirole
- Timolol

**Photosensitivity**

- Acetaminophen
- Acetazolamide
- Acetohexamide
- Acitretin
- Acyclovir
- Aldesleukin
- Alitretinoin
- Allopurinol
- Almotriptan
- Alprazolam
- Amantadine
- Amiloride
- Aminolevulinic acid
- Aminosalicylate sodium
- Amiodarone
- Amitriptyline
- Amobarbital
- Amoxapine
- Anagrelide
- Anthrax vaccine
- Arsenic
- Atenolol
- Atorvastatin
- Atropine sulfate
- Azatadine
- Azathioprine
- Azithromycin
- Benazepril
- Bendroflumethiazide
- Benzthiazide
- Benztropine
- Betaxolol
- Bexarotene
- Bisoprolol
- Brompheniramine
- Bumetanide
- Bupropion
- Butabarbital
- Butalbital
- Capecitabine
- Captopril
- Carbamazepine
- Carisoprodol
- Carteolol
- Carvedilol
- Cefazolin
- Ceftazidime
- Celecoxib
- Cetirizine
- Cevimeline
- Chlorambucil
- Chlordiazepoxide
- Chlorhexidine
- Chloroquine
- Chlorothiazide
- Chlorotrianisene
- Chlorpheniramine
- Chlorpromazine
- Chlorpropamide
- Chlortetracycline
- Chlorthalidone
- Cinoxacin
- Ciprofloxacin
- Citalopram
- Clemastine
- Clofazimine
- Clofibrate
- Clomipramine
- Clorazepate
- Clozapine
- Co-trimoxazole
- Cromolyn
- Cyclamate
- Cyclobenzaprine
- Cyclothiazide
- Cyproheptadine
- Dacarbazine
- Danazol
- Dantrolene
- Dapsone
- Demeclocycline
- Desipramine
- Dexchlorpheniramine
- Diazoxide
- Diclofenac
- Diflunisal
- Diltiazem
- Dimenhydrinate
- Diphenhydramine
- Disopyramide
- Docetaxel
- Doxepin
- Doxycycline
- Efavirenz
- Enalapril
- Enoxacin
- Epirubicin
- Epoetin alfa
- Estazolam
- Estrogens
- Ethacrynic acid
- Ethambutol
- Ethionamide
- Etodolac
- Felbamate
- Fenofibrate
- Flucytosine
- Fluorouracil
- Fluoxetine
- Fluphenazine
- Flurbiprofen
- Flutamide
- Fluvastatin
- Fluvoxamine
- Fosinopril
- Furazolidone
- Furosemide
- Ganciclovir
- Gatifloxacin
- Gentamicin
- Glimepiride
- Glipizide
- Glyburide
- Glycopyrrolate
- Gold and gold compounds
- Griseofulvin
- Haloperidol
- Henna
- Heroin
- Hydralazine
- Hydrochlorothiazide
- Hydroflumethiazide
- Hydroxychloroquine
- Hydroxyurea
- Hydroxyzine
- Hyoscyamine
- Ibuprofen
- Imipramine
- Indapamide
- Indomethacin
- Infliximab
- Interferon beta 1-a
- Interferons, alfa-2
- Isocarboxazid
- Isoniazid
- Isotretinoin
- Itraconazole
- Kanamycin
- Kava
- Ketoconazole
- Ketoprofen
- Ketotifen
- Lamotrigine
- Leuprolide
- Levofloxacin
- Lincomycin
- Lisinopril
- Lomefloxacin
- Loratadine
- Losartan
- Loxapine
- Maprotiline
- Meclizine
- Meclofenamate
- Medroxyprogesterone
- Mefenamic acid
- Melatonin
- Meloxicam
- Meprobamate
- Mercaptopurine
- Mesalamine
- Mesoridazine
- Metformin
- Methazolamide
- Methenamine
- Methotrexate
- Methoxsalen
- Methyclothiazide
- Methyldopa
- Methylphenidate
- Metolazone
- Minocycline
- Minoxidil
- Mirtazapine
- Mitomycin
- Moexipril
- Molindone
- Moxifloxacin
- Nabumetone
- Nalidixic acid
- Naproxen
- Naratriptan
- Nefazodone
- Nifedipine
- Nisoldipine
- Nitrofurantoin
- Norfloxacin
- Nortriptyline
- Ofloxacin
- Olanzapine
- Oral contraceptives
- Oxaprozin
- Oxcarbazepine
- Oxytetracycline
- Paclitaxel
- Pantoprazole
- Paroxetine
- Pentobarbital
- Pentosan
- Pentostatin
- Perphenazine
- Phenelzine
- Phenindamine
- Phenobarbital
- Pimozide
- Piroxicam
- Polythiazide
- Pravastatin
- Procarbazine
- Prochlorperazine
- Procyclidine
- Promazine
- Promethazine
- Propranolol
- Propylthiouracil
- Protriptyline
- Psoralens
- Pyridoxine
- Pyrilamine
- Pyrimethamine
- Quetiapine
- Quinacrine
- Quinapril
- Quinestrol

Quinethazone
Quinidine
Quinine
Rabeprazole
Ramipril
Ranitidine
Ribavirin
Riluzole
Risperidone
Ritonavir
Rofecoxib
Ropinirole
Saccharin
Saquinavir
Scopolamine
Selegiline
Sertraline
Sildenafil
Simvastatin
Smallpox vaccine
Sotalol
Sparfloxacin
Spironolactone
St John's wort
Streptomycin
Sulfacetamide
Sulfadiazine
Sulfadoxine
Sulfamethoxazole
Sulfasalazine
Sulfisoxazole
Sulindac
Sumatriptan
Tacrolimus
Tartrazine
Terbinafine
Tetracycline
Thioguanine
Thioridazine
Thiothixene
Tiagabine
Timolol
Tiopronin
Tolazamide
Tolbutamide
Topiramate
Torsemide
Tranylcypromine
Trazodone
Tretinoin
Triamterene
Triazolam
Trichlormethiazide
Trifluoperazine
Trihexyphenidyl
Trimeprazine
Trimethadione
Trimethoprim
Trimetrexate
Trimipramine
Trioxsalen
Tripelennamine
Triprolidine
Trovafloxacin
Valdecoxib
Valproic acid
Valsartan
Venlafaxine
Verapamil
Verteporfin
Vinblastine
Vitamin A
Voriconazole
Zalcitabine
Zaleplon
Ziprasidone
Zolmitriptan
Zolpidem

**Phototoxicity**

Acitretin
Alprazolam
Aspirin
Bendroflumethiazide
Captopril
Cefazolin
Cetirizine
Chlorpromazine
Ciprofloxacin
Demeclocycline
Docetaxel
Doxycycline
Enoxacin
Fenofibrate
Fluorouracil
Fluoxetine
Furosemide
Glipizide
Hydrochlorothiazide
Hydroxychloroquine
Itraconazole
Levofloxacin
Lomefloxacin
Methoxsalen
Minocycline
Nabumetone
Nalidixic acid
Naproxen
Norfloxacin
Nortriptyline
Ofloxacin
Oxaprozin
Pantoprazole
Prochlorperazine
Promazine
Propranolol
Protriptyline
Psoralens
Rofecoxib
Sparfloxacin
Sulfisoxazole
Sulindac
Terazosin
Tetracycline
Thioridazine
Trioxsalen
Trovafloxacin
Vinblastine

**Pigmentation**

Acebutolol
Alitretinoin
Aminolevulinic acid
Amiodarone
Amitriptyline
Amphotericin B
Arsenic
Azathioprine
Betaxolol
Bimatoprost
Bismuth
Bisoprolol
Bleomycin
Busulfan
Captopril
Carbamazepine
Carboplatin
Carmustine
Carteolol
Chlorhexidine
Chloroquine
Chlorotrianisene
Chlorpromazine
Cidofovir
Ciprofloxacin
Cisplatin
Citalopram
Clofazimine
Clomipramine
Clonazepam
Clonidine
Corticosteroids
Cyclobenzaprine
Cyclophosphamide
Cyclosporine
Dactinomycin
Dapsone
Daunorubicin
Deferoxamine
Demeclocycline
Desipramine
Diazepam
Dicumarol
Diethylstilbestrol
Diltiazem
Donepezil
Doxorubicin
Doxycycline
Eletriptan
Enoxacin
Epirubicin
Esmolol
Estramustine
Estrogens
Etodolac
Etoposide
Fluorouracil
Fluoxetine
Fluphenazine
Fluvoxamine
Foscarnet
Ganciclovir
Gold and gold compounds
Griseofulvin
Haloperidol
Henna
Heroin
Hydroxychloroquine
Hydroxyurea
Ifosfamide
Imipramine
Imiquimod
Indinavir
Insulin
Interferon beta 1-a
Irinotecan
Isotretinoin
Kava
Ketoconazole
Ketoprofen
Labetalol
Latanoprost
Leflunomide
Leuprolide
Lidocaine
Linezolid
Lomefloxacin
Loxapine
Mechlorethamine
Medroxyprogesterone
Mephenytoin
Mercaptopurine
Mesoridazine
Methamphetamine
Methimazole
Methotrexate
Methoxsalen
Methyldopa
Methysergide
Metoprolol
Minocycline
Minoxidil
Mitomycin
Mitotane
Mitoxantrone
Molindone
Niacin
Nisoldipine
Ofloxacin
Olanzapine
Oral contraceptives
Orphenadrine
Oxytetracycline
Pantoprazole
Paroxetine
Pentazocine
Pentostatin
Perphenazine
Phenazopyridine
Phenolphthalein
Phenytoin
Pimozide
Procarbazine
Prochlorperazine
Progestins
Promazine
Promethazine
Propranolol
Propylthiouracil
Psoralens
Pyrimethamine
Quinacrine
Quinestrol
Quinidine
Quinine
Rabeprazole
Rifabutin
Rifapentine
Risperidone
Ropinirole
Saquinavir
Smallpox vaccine
Sparfloxacin
Spironolactone
Stanozolol
Sulfadiazine
Sulfasalazine
Tacrolimus
Terbinafine
Tetracycline
Thioridazine
Thiotepa

Thiothixene
Tiagabine
Timolol
Tolcapone
Topiramate
Toremifene
Tretinoin
Trifluoperazine
Trioxsalen
Venlafaxine
Verteporfin
Vinblastine
Vincristine
Vinorelbine
Vitamin A
Voriconazole
Zaleplon
Zidovudine

**Pityriasis Rosea**

Acetaminophen
Ampicillin
Arsenic
Aspirin
Captopril
Clonidine
Codeine
Corticosteroids
Gold and gold compounds
Griseofulvin
Isotretinoin
Ketotifen
Meprobamate
Metronidazole
Mitomycin
Naproxen
Omeprazole
Penicillins
Terbinafine
Tiopronin
Tripelennamine

**Porphyria**

Amlodipine
Butabarbital
Butalbital
Carbamazepine
Chloral hydrate
Chlorambucil
Chloramphenicol
Chlordiazepoxide
Chlormezanone
Chloroquine
Chlorotrianisene
Chlorpropamide
Cimetidine
Cisplatin
Clonidine
Clorazepate
Cocaine
Cyclophosphamide
Danazol
Dapsone
Demeclocycline
Diazepam
Diclofenac
Dimenhydrinate
Estrogens
Ethchlorvynol
Ethosuximide
Flurazepam
Furosemide
Glipizide
Gold and gold compounds
Griseofulvin
Hydroxychloroquine
Indinavir
Isoniazid
Ketoprofen
Lamotrigine
Lidocaine
Meclofenamate
Meprobamate
Methyldopa
Metoclopramide
Metronidazole
Nalidixic acid
Nortriptyline
Ondansetron
Oral contraceptives
Pentobarbital
Phenobarbital
Phensuximide
Phenytoin
Primidone
Pyrazinamide
Quinestrol
Quinidine
Quinine
Ranitidine
Rifampin
Spironolactone
Thiopental
Thioridazine
Tolazamide
Tolbutamide
Tranylcypromine
Trimethadione
Valproic acid

**Priapism**

Alprostadil
Androstenedione
Anisindione
Bromocriptine
Bupropion
Chlorpromazine
Citalopram
Clozapine
Cocaine
Dicumarol
Fluoxetine
Fluoxymesterone
Fluphenazine
Fluvoxamine
Gabapentin
Guanethidine
Haloperidol
Heparin
Hydroxyzine
Labetalol
Levodopa
Loxapine
MDMA
Mesoridazine
Methyltestosterone
Nefazodone
Olanzapine
Oxcarbazepine
Papaverine
Paroxetine
Pergolide
Perphenazine
Phenelzine
Phenoxybenzamine
Phentolamine
Prazosin
Prochlorperazine
Promazine
Promethazine
Quetiapine
Risperidone
Sertraline
Sildenafil
Stanozolol
Terazosin
Testosterone
Thioridazine
Thiothixene
Tinzaparin
Toremifene
Tranylcypromine
Trazodone
Trifluoperazine
Vancomycin
Warfarin
Ziprasidone

**Pruritus**

Abacavir
Abciximab
Acebutolol
Acetaminophen
Acetazolamide
Acetohexamide
Acitretin
Acyclovir
Albendazole
Albuterol
Aldesleukin
Alendronate
Alfentanil
Alitretinoin
Allopurinol
Almotriptan
Alprazolam
Alprostadil
Altretamine
Amantadine
Amikacin
Amiloride
Aminocaproic acid
Aminoglutethimide
Aminolevulinic acid
Aminophylline
Aminosalicylate sodium
Amiodarone
Amitriptyline
Amlodipine
Amoxapine
Amoxicillin
Amphotericin B
Ampicillin
Amprenavir
Anagrelide
Anastrozole
Anthrax vaccine
Apraclonidine
Aprotinin
Arsenic
Asparaginase
Aspartame
Aspirin
Atenolol
Atorvastatin
Atovaquone
Atracurium
Atropine sulfate
Azithromycin
Aztreonam
Bacampicillin
Baclofen
Balsalazide
Basiliximab
Benactyzine
Benazepril
Bendroflumethiazide
Benztropine
Betaxolol
Bexarotene
Bicalutamide
Bimatoprost
Bismuth
Bisoprolol
Bleomycin
Bosentan
Botulinum toxin (A & B)
Brimonidine
Bumetanide
Bupropion
Buspirone
Butabarbital
Butalbital
Butorphanol
Butterbur
Cabergoline
Caffeine
Calcitonin
Capecitabine
Captopril
Carbamazepine
Carbenicillin
Carboplatin
Carisoprodol
Carteolol
Carvedilol
Caspofungin
Cefaclor
Cefadroxil
Cefamandole
Cefazolin
Cefdinir
Cefditoren
Cefepime
Cefixime
Cefmetazole
Cefonicid
Cefoperazone
Cefotaxime
Cefotetan
Cefoxitin
Cefpodoxime
Cefprozil
Ceftazidime
Ceftibuten
Ceftizoxime
Ceftriaxone
Cefuroxime
Celecoxib
Cephalexin
Cephalothin
Cephapirin
Cephradine
Cetirizine

Cetrorelix
Cevimeline
Chloral hydrate
Chlorambucil
Chloramphenicol
Chlordiazepoxide
Chlormezanone
Chloroquine
Chlorothiazide
Chlorpromazine
Chlorpropamide
Chlortetracycline
Chlorzoxazone
Cidofovir
Cilostazol
Cimetidine
Cinoxacin
Ciprofloxacin
Cisplatin
Citalopram
Cladribine
Clarithromycin
Clindamycin
Clofazimine
Clofibrate
Clomiphene
Clomipramine
Clonazepam
Clonidine
Clopidogrel
Clorazepate
Clotrimazole
Cloxacillin
Clozapine
Co-trimoxazole
Codeine
Colchicine
Corticosteroids
Cromolyn
Cyanocobalamin
Cyclamate
Cyclobenzaprine
Cyclophosphamide
Cycloserine
Cyclosporine
Cytarabine
Dactinomycin
Dalteparin
Dan-shen
Danaparoid
Danazol
Dantrolene
Dapsone
Daunorubicin
Deferoxamine
Delavirdine
Demeclocycline
Denileukin
Desipramine
Diazepam
Diazoxide
Diclofenac
Dicloxacillin
Dicumarol
Dicyclomine
Didanosine
Diethylpropion
Diethylstilbestrol
Diflunisal
Digoxin
Dihydroergotamine
Dihydrotachysterol
Diltiazem
Diphenhydramine
Diphenoxylate
Dipyridamole
Dirithromycin
Disopyramide
Dobutamine
Docetaxel
Dolasetron
Domperidone
Donepezil
Dopamine
Doxapram
Doxazosin
Doxepin
Doxercalciferol
Doxorubicin
Doxycycline
Efavirenz
Eflornithine
Eletriptan
Enalapril
Enoxacin
Enoxaparin
Epirubicin
Epoetin alfa
Eprosartan
Ergocalciferol
Ertapenem
Erythromycin
Esomeprazole
Estazolam
Estramustine
Estrogens
Etanercept
Ethambutol
Ethchlorvynol
Ethosuximide
Etidronate
Etodolac
Etoposide
Exemestane
Famciclovir
Famotidine
Felbamate
Felodipine
Fenofibrate
Fenoprofen
Fentanyl
Flecainide
Fluconazole
Flucytosine
Fluorouracil
Fluoxetine
Fluoxymesterone
Fluphenazine
Flurazepam
Flurbiprofen
Fluvastatin
Fluvoxamine
Folic acid
Fondaparinux
Formoterol
Foscarnet
Fosfomycin
Fosinopril
Fosphenytoin
Frovatriptan
Furazolidone
Furosemide
Gabapentin
Ganciclovir
Ganirelix
Gatifloxacin
Gemcitabine
Gemfibrozil
Gentamicin
Ginkgo biloba
Ginseng
Glimepiride
Glipizide
Glyburide
Gold and gold compounds
Granulocyte colony-stimulating factor (GCSF)
Griseofulvin
Guanabenz
Guanfacine
Haloperidol
Henna
Heparin
Hepatitis B vaccine
Heroin
Hydralazine
Hydrochlorothiazide
Hydrocodone
Hydromorphone
Hydroxychloroquine
Hydroxyurea
Ibritumomab
Ibuprofen
Imatinib
Imipenem/cilastatin
Imipramine
Imiquimod
Indapamide
Indinavir
Indomethacin
Infliximab
Insulin
Interferon beta 1-a
Interferons, alfa-2
Ipodate
Ipratropium
Irbesartan
Isocarboxazid
Isoniazid
Isoproterenol
Isosorbide mononitrate
Isotretinoin
Isradipine
Itraconazole
Ivermectin
Kanamycin
Kava
Ketamine
Ketoconazole
Ketoprofen
Ketorolac
Ketotifen
Labetalol
Lamivudine
Lamotrigine
Lansoprazole
Latanoprost
Leflunomide
Letrozole
Leucovorin
Leuprolide
Levalbuterol
Levamisole
Levobunolol
Levofloxacin
Levothyroxine
Lidocaine
Lincomycin
Lindane
Linezolid
Lisinopril
Lithium
Lomefloxacin
Loperamide
Loracarbef
Loratadine
Lorazepam
Losartan
Lovastatin
Loxapine
Maprotiline
Marihuana
Mebendazole
Mechlorethamine
Meclofenamate
Medroxyprogesterone
Mefenamic acid
Mefloquine
Meloxicam
Melphalan
Meperidine
Mephenytoin
Meprobamate
Mercaptopurine
Mesalamine
Mesna
Mesoridazine
Metaxalone
Metformin
Methadone
Methazolamide
Methenamine
Methicillin
Methimazole
Methocarbamol
Methotrexate
Methoxsalen
Methsuximide
Methyldopa
Methylphenidate
Methyltestosterone
Methysergide
Metolazone
Metoprolol
Metronidazole
Mexiletine
Mezlocillin
Miconazole
Midazolam
Midodrine
Minocycline
Minoxidil
Mirtazapine
Mistletoe
Mitomycin
Mitotane
Modafinil
Moexipril
Molindone
Moricizine

Morphine
Moxifloxacin
Mycophenolate
Nabumetone
Nadolol
Nafarelin
Nafcillin
Nalidixic acid
Naloxone
Naltrexone
Naproxen
Nefazodone
Nelfinavir
Neomycin
Nesiritide
Nevirapine
Niacin
Niacinamide
Nicotine
Nifedipine
Nimodipine
Nisoldipine
Nitrofurantoin
Nizatidine
Norfloxacin
Nortriptyline
Nystatin
Octreotide
Ofloxacin
Olanzapine
Olopatadine
Olsalazine
Omeprazole
Ondansetron
Oral contraceptives
Orphenadrine
Oxacillin
Oxaprozin
Oxazepam
Oxcarbazepine
Oxybutynin
Oxycodone
Oxytetracycline
Paclitaxel
Pancuronium
Pantoprazole
Pantothenic acid
Papaverine
Paramethadione
Paromomycin
Paroxetine
PEG-interferon alfa-2b
Penbutolol
Penicillamine
Penicillins
Pentagastrin
Pentamidine
Pentazocine
Pentobarbital
Pentosan
Pentostatin
Pentoxifylline
Pergolide
Perindopril
Perphenazine
Phenazopyridine
Phenelzine
Phenobarbital
Phenolphthalein
Phensuximide
Phenytoin
Pilocarpine
Pimecrolimus
Pimozide
Pindolol
Piperacillin
Pirbuterol
Piroxicam
Pramipexole
Pravastatin
Prazepam
Praziquantel
Prazosin
Primaquine
Probenecid
Procainamide
Procarbazine
Prochlorperazine
Progestins
Propafenone
Propofol
Propoxyphene
Propranolol
Propylthiouracil
Protriptyline
Psoralens
Pyrazinamide
Pyrimethamine
Quazepam
Quinacrine
Quinapril
Quinethazone
Quinidine
Quinine
Quinupristin/dalfopristin
Rabeprazole
Ramipril
Ranitidine
Rapacuronium
Reserpine
Ribavirin
Rifampin
Rifapentine
Riluzole
Risedronate
Risperidone
Ritonavir
Rituximab
Rizatriptan
Rofecoxib
Ropinirole
Saccharin
Salmeterol
Salsalate
Saquinavir
Senna
Sertraline
Sibutramine
Sildenafil
Simvastatin
Sirolimus
Sotalol
Sparfloxacin
Spectinomycin
Spironolactone
St John's wort
Streptokinase
Streptomycin
Streptozocin
Succinylcholine
Sucralfate
Sufentanil
Sulfacetamide
Sulfadiazine
Sulfadoxine
Sulfamethoxazole
Sulfasalazine
Sulfisoxazole
Sulindac
Sumatriptan
Tacrine
Tacrolimus
Tamoxifen
Tamsulosin
Tartrazine
Telmisartan
Temazepam
Temozolomide
Terazosin
Terbinafine
Terbutaline
Terconazole
Testosterone
Tetracycline
Thalidomide
Thiabendazole
Thiamine
Thioguanine
Thiopental
Thiotepa
Thiothixene
Tiagabine
Ticarcillin
Ticlopidine
Timolol
Tinzaparin
Tiopronin
Tizanidine
Tobramycin
Tocainide
Tolazamide
Tolbutamide
Tolcapone
Tolmetin
Tolterodine
Topiramate
Toremifene
Torsemide
Tramadol
Trandolapril
Tranylcypromine
Travoprost
Trazodone
Tretinoin
Triamterene
Triazolam
Trifluoperazine
Trimeprazine
Trimethadione
Trimethoprim
Trimetrexate
Trimipramine
Trioxsalen
Triptorelin
Troleandomycin
Trovafloxacin
Unoprostone
Urokinase
Ursodiol
Valacyclovir
Valdecoxib
Valproic acid
Valsartan
Vancomycin
Venlafaxine
Verapamil
Verteporfin
Vidarabine
Vincristine
Vinorelbine
Vitamin A
Voriconazole
Warfarin
Zalcitabine
Zaleplon
Zidovudine
Zileuton
Zolmitriptan
Zolpidem
Zonisamide

**Pseudolymphoma**

Alprazolam
Amitriptyline
Aspirin
Atenolol
Carbamazepine
Cefixime
Chlorpromazine
Cimetidine
Clarithromycin
Clonazepam
Clonidine
Co-trimoxazole
Cyclosporine
Desipramine
Diclofenac
Diflunisal
Diltiazem
Doxepin
Fluoxetine
Furosemide
Gemcitabine
Gemfibrozil
Gold and gold compounds
Ibuprofen
Indomethacin
Ketoprofen
Lamotrigine
Lithium
Lorazepam
Losartan
Methotrexate
Nabumetone
Naproxen
Nizatidine
Oxaprozin
Perphenazine
Phenytoin
Ranitidine
Sulfamethoxazole
Sulfasalazine
Sulindac
Thioridazine
Valproic acid

**Psoriasis**

Acebutolol
Acitretin
Aldesleukin
Amiodarone
Amoxicillin

Ampicillin
Arsenic
Aspirin
Atenolol
Betaxolol
Bisoprolol
Botulinum toxin (A & B)
Captopril
Carbamazepine
Carteolol
Carvedilol
Celecoxib
Chlorambucil
Chloroquine
Chlorthalidone
Cimetidine
Citalopram
Clarithromycin
Clomipramine
Clonidine
Co-trimoxazole
Cyclosporine
Diclofenac
Digoxin
Diltiazem
Dipyridamole
Doxycycline
Eletriptan
Enalapril
Esmolol
Flecainide
Fluoxetine
Fluoxymesterone
Foscarnet
Ganciclovir
Gemfibrozil
Glimepiride
Glipizide
Glyburide
Gold and gold compounds
Granulocyte colony-stimulating factor (GCSF)
Henna
Hydroxychloroquine
Hydroxyurea
Ibuprofen
Indomethacin
Infliximab
Interferons, alfa-2
Ketoprofen
Labetalol
Letrozole
Levamisole
Levobetaxolol
Lithium
Meclofenamate
Mefloquine
Mesalamine
Methotrexate
Methyltestosterone
Metoprolol
Modafinil
Nadolol
Omeprazole
Oral contraceptives
PEG-interferon alfa-2b
Penbutolol
Penicillamine
Pentostatin
Perindopril
Pindolol
Primaquine
Propranolol
Psoralens
Quinidine
Quinine
Rabeprazole
Ranitidine
Risperidone
Ritonavir
Rivastigmine
Ropinirole
Saquinavir
Sotalol
Sulfamethoxazole
Sulfasalazine
Sulfisoxazole
Tacrine
Terbinafine
Testosterone
Tetracycline
Thiabendazole
Thioguanine
Tiagabine
Timolol
Trazodone
Valdecoxib
Valproic acid
Venlafaxine
Voriconazole
Zaleplon

**Purpura**

Acetaminophen
Acetazolamide
Acitretin
Aldesleukin
Alemtuzumab
Allopurinol
Alprazolam
Alteplase
Amiloride
Aminocaproic acid
Aminoglutethimide
Aminosalicylate sodium
Amiodarone
Amitriptyline
Amlodipine
Amobarbital
Amoxapine
Amoxicillin
Amphotericin B
Ampicillin
Anistreplase
Aprobarbital
Arsenic
Aspartame
Aspirin
Atenolol
Azatadine
Azathioprine
Aztreonam
Bendroflumethiazide
Benzthiazide
Beta-carotene
Betaxolol
Bisoprolol
Botulinum toxin (A & B)
Bromocriptine
Bumetanide
Buspirone
Busulfan
Butabarbital
Butalbital
Caffeine
Capecitabine
Captopril
Carbamazepine
Carbenicillin
Carteolol
Carvedilol
Cefaclor
Cefamandole
Cefdinir
Cefmetazole
Cefonicid
Cefoxitin
Ceftriaxone
Cefuroxime
Cephalexin
Cephalothin
Cephradine
Cetirizine
Chloral hydrate
Chlorambucil
Chloramphenicol
Chlordiazepoxide
Chlorothiazide
Chlorpromazine
Chlorpropamide
Chlorthalidone
Cilostazol
Cimetidine
Ciprofloxacin
Citalopram
Cladribine
Clemastine
Clidinium
Clindamycin
Clofibrate
Clomiphene
Clomipramine
Clonazepam
Clopidogrel
Clorazepate
Clozapine
Co-trimoxazole
Colchicine
Corticosteroids
Cyclobenzaprine
Cyclophosphamide
Cyclosporine
Cyclothiazide
Cyproheptadine
Danaparoid
Danazol
Dapsone
Deferoxamine
Delavirdine
Demeclocycline
Denileukin
Desipramine
Diazepam
Diazoxide
Diclofenac
Dicloxacillin
Dicumarol
Didanosine
Diethylpropion
Diethylstilbestrol
Diflunisal
Digoxin
Diltiazem
Diphenhydramine
Dipyridamole
Disopyramide
Disulfiram
Dolasetron
Donepezil
Doxazosin
Doxepin
Doxorubicin
Doxycycline
Enalapril
Enoxacin
Enoxaparin
Entacapone
Ephedrine
Eprosartan
Esmolol
Estazolam
Estramustine
Estrogens
Ethacrynic acid
Ethambutol
Ethchlorvynol
Ethionamide
Ethosuximide
Ethotoin
Etodolac
Etoposide
Famotidine
Felbamate
Felodipine
Fenoprofen
Fentanyl
Fluconazole
Flucytosine
Fluoxetine
Fluoxymesterone
Fluphenazine
Flurazepam
Flurbiprofen
Fluvastatin
Fluvoxamine
Fondaparinux
Frovatriptan
Furosemide
Gabapentin
Galantamine
Ganciclovir
Gentamicin
Glipizide
Glyburide
Gold and gold compounds
Griseofulvin
Guanethidine
Guanfacine
Haloperidol
Heparin
Hepatitis B vaccine
Heroin
Horse chestnut – bark
Horse chestnut – flower
Horse chestnut – leaf
Horse chestnut – seed
Hydralazine
Hydrochlorothiazide
Hydroflumethiazide
Hydroxychloroquine
Hydroxyurea

Hydroxyzine
Ibritumomab
Ibuprofen
Imipramine
Indapamide
Indomethacin
Insulin
Interferons, alfa-2
Ipodate
Isoniazid
Itraconazole
Ketoconazole
Ketoprofen
Ketorolac
Labetalol
Leflunomide
Leuprolide
Levamisole
Levodopa
Levofloxacin
Lidocaine
Lincomycin
Lindane
Lisinopril
Lithium
Lomefloxacin
Loratadine
Lorazepam
Losartan
Lovastatin
Loxapine
Maprotiline
Mechlorethamine
Meclofenamate
Medroxyprogesterone
Mefenamic acid
Meloxicam
Melphalan
Mephenytoin
Mephobarbital
Meprobamate
Mercaptopurine
Metformin
Methadone
Methazolamide
Methicillin
Methimazole
Methotrexate
Methoxsalen
Methsuximide
Methyclothiazide
Methyldopa
Methylphenidate
Methyltestosterone
Metolazone
Metoprolol
Mexiletine
Miconazole
Minocycline
Mitomycin
Mitoxantrone
Nalidixic acid
Naltrexone
Naproxen
Naratriptan
Nifedipine
Nimodipine
Nitrofurantoin
Nitroglycerin
Nortriptyline
Octreotide
Ofloxacin
Omeprazole
Oral contraceptives
Oxaprozin
Oxazepam
Oxcarbazepine
Oxytetracycline
Paclitaxel
Paroxetine
PEG-interferon alfa-2b
Penbutolol
Penicillamine
Penicillins
Pentagastrin
Pentamidine
Pentobarbital
Pentosan
Pentostatin
Pentoxifylline
Perindopril
Perphenazine
Phenindamine
Phenobarbital
Phensuximide
Phentermine
Phenytoin
Pindolol
Piperacillin
Pirbuterol
Piroxicam
Plicamycin
Polythiazide
Potassium iodide
Pravastatin
Prazepam
Procainamide
Procarbazine
Prochlorperazine
Promazine
Promethazine
Propafenone
Propranolol
Propylthiouracil
Protriptyline
Pyrazinamide
Pyridoxine
Pyrilamine
Pyrimethamine
Quazepam
Quinethazone
Quinidine
Quinine
Rabeprazole
Ramipril
Ranitidine
Rapacuronium
Reserpine
Reteplase
Rifampin
Rifapentine
Riluzole
Risperidone
Rivastigmine
Rofecoxib
Ropinirole
Salsalate
Secobarbital
Sertraline
Simvastatin
Sirolimus
Smallpox vaccine
Sparfloxacin
Spironolactone
Streptokinase
Streptomycin
Streptozocin
Sulfadiazine
Sulfadoxine
Sulfamethoxazole
Sulfasalazine
Sulfinpyrazone
Sulfisoxazole
Sulindac
Tacrine
Tacrolimus
Tamoxifen
Tartrazine
Temazepam
Tenecteplase
Tenofovir
Tetracycline
Thalidomide
Thiamine
Thioguanine
Thiopental
Thioridazine
Ticarcillin
Ticlopidine
Timolol
Tinzaparin
Tizanidine
Tobramycin
Tolazamide
Tolbutamide
Tolmetin
Topiramate
Topotecan
Torsemide
Trazodone
Triamterene
Triazolam
Trichlormethiazide
Trifluoperazine
Trimeprazine
Trimethadione
Trimipramine
Tripelennamine
Triprolidine
Urokinase
Valacyclovir
Valproic acid
Vancomycin
Vasopressin
Verapamil
Verteporfin
Vinblastine
Voriconazole
Warfarin
Zaleplon
Zidovudine
Zolpidem
Zonisamide

**Pustular Eruption**

Acetazolamide
Allopurinol
Aminolevulinic acid
Amoxicillin
Ampicillin
Azithromycin
Bacampicillin
Bexarotene
Captopril
Carbamazepine
Cefaclor
Cefazolin
Cefoxitin
Cefuroxime
Cephalexin
Cephradine
Chloramphenicol
Chloroquine
Chlorpromazine
Clarithromycin
Clomipramine
Co-trimoxazole
Dactinomycin
Diltiazem
Disulfiram
Erythromycin
Felbamate
Fentanyl
Fluoxetine
Furosemide
Heroin
Hydroxychloroquine
Imipenem/cilastatin
Infliximab
Isoniazid
Ivermectin
Lithium
Lomefloxacin
Minocycline
Nadolol
Naproxen
Nisoldipine
Norfloxacin
Olanzapine
Oxytetracycline
Paclitaxel
Perindopril
Phenobarbital
Phenytoin
Pyrimethamine
Quinidine
Ranitidine
Ritodrine
Simvastatin
Sparfloxacin
Streptomycin
Sulfadoxine
Sulfamethoxazole
Sulfasalazine
Sulfisoxazole
Tacrolimus
Terbinafine
Tetracycline
Venlafaxine
Zaleplon
Zonisamide

**Pustular Psoriasis**

Acetazolamide
Aminoglutethimide
Amiodarone
Amoxicillin
Ampicillin
Aspirin
Atenolol
Chloroquine
Cimetidine

Corticosteroids
Cyclosporine
Diclofenac
Diltiazem
Doxorubicin
Hydroxychloroquine
Indomethacin
Lithium
Methicillin
Penicillins
Potassium iodide
Propranolol
Terbinafine

**Radiation Recall**

Bleomycin
Buspirone
Capecitabine
Ciprofloxacin
Co-trimoxazole
Codeine
Dactinomycin
Docetaxel
Doxorubicin
Epirubicin
Etoposide
Fluorouracil
Gemcitabine
Hydroxyurea
Idarubicin
Interferons, alfa-2
Mercaptopurine
Methotrexate
Paclitaxel
Piperacillin
Simvastatin
Sulfamethoxazole
Tamoxifen
Tobramycin
Vinblastine

**Rash**

Abacavir
Acarbose
Acebutolol
Acetaminophen
Acetazolamide
Acetohexamide
Acitretin
Acyclovir
Albendazole
Aldesleukin
Alendronate
Alfentanil
Alitretinoin
Allopurinol
Almotriptan
Alprazolam
Alprostadil
Alteplase
Altretamine
Amantadine
Amifostine
Amikacin
Amiloride
Aminocaproic acid
Aminoglutethimide
Aminophylline
Amiodarone
Amitriptyline
Amlodipine
Amobarbital
Amoxapine
Amoxicillin
Amphotericin B
Ampicillin
Amprenavir
Amyl nitrite
Anagrelide
Anastrozole
Anistreplase
Anthrax vaccine
Aprobarbital
Aprotinin
Arbutamine
Argatroban
Asparaginase
Aspartame
Aspirin
Atenolol
Atorvastatin
Atovaquone
Atropine sulfate
Azatadine
Azathioprine
Azithromycin
Aztreonam
Bacampicillin
Baclofen
Balsalazide
Basiliximab
Benazepril
Bendroflumethiazide
Benzthiazide
Benztropine
Bepridil
Betaxolol
Bexarotene
Bicalutamide
Biperiden
Bismuth
Bisoprolol
Botulinum toxin (A & B)
Bretylium
Bromocriptine
Brompheniramine
Bumetanide
Bupropion
Buspirone
Butabarbital
Butalbital
Butorphanol
Butterbur
Caffeine
Calcitonin
Candesartan
Captopril
Carbamazepine
Carbenicillin
Carboplatin
Carisoprodol
Carteolol
Carvedilol
Caspofungin
Cefaclor
Cefadroxil
Cefamandole
Cefazolin
Cefdinir
Cefditoren
Cefepime
Cefixime
Cefmetazole
Cefonicid
Cefoperazone
Cefotaxime
Cefotetan
Cefoxitin
Cefpodoxime
Cefprozil
Ceftazidime
Ceftibuten
Ceftizoxime
Ceftriaxone
Cefuroxime
Celecoxib
Cephalexin
Cephalothin
Cephapirin
Cephradine
Cetirizine
Cevimeline
Chloral hydrate
Chlorambucil
Chloramphenicol
Chlordiazepoxide
Chlorhexidine
Chlormezanone
Chlorothiazide
Chlorotrianisene
Chlorpromazine
Chlorpropamide
Chlortetracycline
Chlorthalidone
Chlorzoxazone
Cholestyramine
Cidofovir
Cilostazol
Cimetidine
Cinoxacin
Ciprofloxacin
Cisatracurium
Cisplatin
Citalopram
Cladribine
Clarithromycin
Clemastine
Clindamycin
Clofazimine
Clofibrate
Clomiphene
Clomipramine
Clonazepam
Clonidine
Clopidogrel
Clorazepate
Cloxacillin
Clozapine
Co-trimoxazole
Codeine
Colchicine
Creatine
Cromolyn
Cyclobenzaprine
Cyclophosphamide
Cycloserine
Cyclosporine
Cyclothiazide
Cyproheptadine
Cytarabine
Dacarbazine
Dalteparin
Danaparoid
Danazol
Dantrolene
Dapsone
Daunorubicin
Deferoxamine
Delavirdine
Denileukin
Desipramine
Desmopressin
Dexchlorpheniramine
Dextroamphetamine
Diazepam
Diazoxide
Diclofenac
Dicloxacillin
Dicumarol
Dicyclomine
Didanosine
Diethylpropion
Diethylstilbestrol
Diflunisal
Digoxin
Diltiazem
Dimenhydrinate
Diphenhydramine
Dipyridamole
Dirithromycin
Disopyramide
Disulfiram
Docetaxel
Docusate
Dofetilide
Dolasetron
Domperidone
Dorzolamide
Doxacurium
Doxazosin
Doxepin
Doxorubicin
Doxycycline
Edrophonium
Efavirenz
Eflornithine
Eletriptan
Enalapril
Enoxacin
Epirubicin
Epoetin alfa
Eprosartan
Ertapenem
Erythromycin
Esmolol
Estazolam
Estramustine
Estrogens
Etanercept
Ethacrynic acid
Ethambutol
Ethchlorvynol
Ethionamide
Ethosuximide
Ethotoin
Etidronate
Etodolac
Etoposide
Exemestane
Famotidine
Felbamate
Felodipine

Fenofibrate
Fenoprofen
Fentanyl
Finasteride
Flavoxate
Flecainide
Fluconazole
Flucytosine
Fludarabine
Flumazenil
Fluoxetine
Fluphenazine
Flurazepam
Flurbiprofen
Flutamide
Fluvastatin
Fluvoxamine
Folic acid
Fondaparinux
Formoterol
Foscarnet
Fosfomycin
Fosinopril
Fosphenytoin
Frovatriptan
Fulvestrant
Furazolidone
Furosemide
Gabapentin
Ganciclovir
Gatifloxacin
Gemcitabine
Gemfibrozil
Gemtuzumab
Gentamicin
Ginkgo biloba
Glimepiride
Glipizide
Glucagon
Glyburide
Glycopyrrolate
Gold and gold compounds
Goserelin
Granisetron
Granulocyte colony-stimulating factor (GCSF)
Griseofulvin
Guanabenz
Guanfacine
Haloperidol
Hawthorn (fruit, leaf, flower extract)
Henna
Heparin
Hepatitis B vaccine
Hydralazine
Hydrochlorothiazide
Hydrocodone
Hydroflumethiazide
Hydromorphone
Hydroxychloroquine
Hydroxyurea
Hydroxyzine
Hyoscyamine
Ibritumomab
Ibuprofen
Idarubicin
Imatinib
Imipenem/cilastatin
Imipramine
Indapamide
Indinavir
Indomethacin
Infliximab
Interferons, alfa-2
Ipodate
Ipratropium
Irbesartan
Irinotecan
Isocarboxazid
Isoniazid
Isoproterenol
Isosorbide
Isosorbide mononitrate
Isotretinoin
Isradipine
Itraconazole
Ivermectin
Kanamycin
Kava
Ketamine
Ketoconazole
Ketoprofen
Ketorolac
Ketotifen
Labetalol
Lamivudine
Lamotrigine
Lansoprazole
Latanoprost
Leflunomide
Letrozole
Leucovorin
Leuprolide
Levamisole
Levetiracetam
Levobetaxolol
Levobunolol
Levodopa
Levofloxacin
Levothyroxine
Lidocaine
Lincomycin
Linezolid
Liothyronine
Lisinopril
Lithium
Lomefloxacin
Lomustine
Loperamide
Loracarbef
Loratadine
Lorazepam
Losartan
Lovastatin
Loxapine
Maprotiline
Mazindol
MDMA
Meadowsweet
Mebendazole
Mechlorethamine
Meclizine
Meclofenamate
Medroxyprogesterone
Mefenamic acid
Mefloquine
Meloxicam
Melphalan
Meperidine
Mephobarbital
Meprobamate
Mercaptopurine
Mesalamine
Mesna
Mesoridazine
Metaxalone
Metformin
Methadone
Methamphetamine
Methazolamide
Methenamine
Methicillin
Methimazole
Methocarbamol
Methohexital
Methotrexate
Methoxsalen
Methsuximide
Methyclothiazide
Methyldopa
Methylphenidate
Methysergide
Metoclopramide
Metolazone
Metoprolol
Metronidazole
Mexiletine
Mezlocillin
Miconazole
Midazolam
Midodrine
Miglitol
Minocycline
Minoxidil
Mirtazapine
Misoprostol
Mitomycin
Mitotane
Mitoxantrone
Modafinil
Moexipril
Molindone
Montelukast
Moricizine
Morphine
Moxifloxacin
Mycophenolate
Nabumetone
Nadolol
Nafarelin
Nafcillin
Nalidixic acid
Naloxone
Naltrexone
Naproxen
Naratriptan
Nateglinide
Nefazodone
Nelfinavir
Neomycin
Nesiritide
Nevirapine
Niacin
Niacinamide
Nicardipine
Nicotine
Nifedipine
Nimodipine
Nisoldipine
Nitrofurantoin
Nitroglycerin
Nizatidine
Norfloxacin
Nortriptyline
Nystatin
Octreotide
Ofloxacin
Olanzapine
Olmesartan
Olsalazine
Omeprazole
Ondansetron
Orlistat
Orphenadrine
Oxacillin
Oxaprozin
Oxazepam
Oxcarbazepine
Oxybutynin
Oxycodone
Paclitaxel
Palivizumab
Pamidronate
Pancuronium
Pantoprazole
Papaverine
Paroxetine
PEG-interferon alfa-2b
Pemoline
Penbutolol
Penicillamine
Penicillins
Pentagastrin
Pentamidine
Pentazocine
Pentobarbital
Pentosan
Pentostatin
Pentoxifylline
Pergolide
Perindopril
Perphenazine
Phenazopyridine
Phenelzine
Phenindamine
Phenobarbital
Phensuximide
Phentermine
Phenytoin
Phytonadione
Pilocarpine
Pimozide
Pindolol
Piperacillin
Pirbuterol
Piroxicam
Polythiazide
Potassium iodide
Pramipexole
Pravastatin
Prazepam
Praziquantel
Prazosin
Primidone
Probenecid
Procainamide
Procarbazine
Prochlorperazine
Procyclidine

Progestins
Promazine
Promethazine
Propafenone
Propantheline
Propofol
Propoxyphene
Propranolol
Propylthiouracil
Protriptyline
Psoralens
Pyrazinamide
Pyrilamine
Pyrimethamine
Quazepam
Quetiapine
Quinapril
Quinestrol
Quinethazone
Quinidine
Quinine
Quinupristin/dalfopristin
Rabeprazole
Raloxifene
Ramipril
Ranitidine
Rapacuronium
Reserpine
Ribavirin
Rifabutin
Rifampin
Rifapentine
Rimantadine
Risedronate
Risperidone
Ritodrine
Ritonavir
Rituximab
Rivastigmine
Rofecoxib
Ropinirole
Salmeterol
Salsalate
Saquinavir
Scopolamine
Secobarbital
Selegiline
Senna
Sertraline
Sibutramine
Sildenafil
Simvastatin
Sirolimus
Smallpox vaccine
Sotalol
Sparfloxacin
Spectinomycin
Spironolactone
Stavudine
Streptokinase
Streptomycin
Succinylcholine
Sucralfate
Sufentanil
Sulfadiazine
Sulfadoxine
Sulfamethoxazole
Sulfasalazine
Sulfinpyrazone
Sulfisoxazole
Sulindac
Sumatriptan
Tacrine
Tacrolimus
Tamoxifen
Tamsulosin
Tartrazine
Telmisartan
Temazepam
Temozolomide
Tenecteplase
Tenofovir
Terazosin
Terbinafine
Testosterone
Tetracycline
Thalidomide
Thiabendazole
Thiamine
Thioguanine
Thiopental
Thioridazine
Thiotepa
Thiothixene
Tiagabine
Ticarcillin
Ticlopidine
Timolol
Tinzaparin
Tiopronin
Tirofiban
Tizanidine
Tobramycin
Tocainide
Tolazamide
Tolazoline
Tolbutamide
Tolcapone
Tolmetin
Tolterodine
Topiramate
Torsemide
Tramadol
Trandolapril
Tranylcypromine
Trastuzumab
Trazodone
Tretinoin
Triamterene
Triazolam
Trichlormethiazide
Trifluoperazine
Trihexyphenidyl
Trimeprazine
Trimethoprim
Trimetrexate
Trimipramine
Tripelennamine
Triprolidine
Troleandomycin
Trovafloxacin
Urokinase
Ursodiol
Valdecoxib
Valganciclovir
Valproic acid
Valsartan
Vancomycin
Vasopressin
Venlafaxine
Verapamil
Verteporfin
Vidarabine
Vinblastine
Vincristine
Vinorelbine
Voriconazole
Warfarin
Willow bark
Zalcitabine
Zaleplon
Zidovudine
Ziprasidone
Zolmitriptan
Zolpidem
Zonisamide

**Raynaud's Phenomenon**

Acebutolol
Amphotericin B
Arsenic
Atenolol
Azathioprine
Betaxolol
Bisoprolol
Bleomycin
Bromocriptine
Carteolol
Cisplatin
Clonidine
Cyclosporine
Dopamine
Doxorubicin
Estrogens
Ethosuximide
Fluoxetine
Gemfibrozil
Hepatitis B vaccine
Interferon beta 1-a
Interferons, alfa-2
Labetalol
Methysergide
Metoprolol
Minocycline
Nadolol
Octreotide
Phentermine
Pindolol
Propofol
Propranolol
Sotalol
Spironolactone
Sulfasalazine
Sulindac
Sumatriptan
Thiothixene
Timolol
Vinblastine
Vincristine

**Rhabdomyolysis**

Acetaminophen
Aldesleukin
Aminocaproic acid
Aminophylline
Amitriptyline
Amobarbital
Amphotericin B
Aprobarbital
Atorvastatin
Azathioprine
Bupropion
Butabarbital
Butalbital
Caffeine
Carbamazepine
Cisplatin
Clarithromycin
Clofibrate
Clozapine
Co-trimoxazole
Cocaine
Colchicine
Creatine
Cyclophosphamide
Cyclosporine
Dacarbazine
Danazol
Delavirdine
Dextroamphetamine
Diazepam
Diclofenac
Diltiazem
Diphenhydramine
Doxepin
Enflurane
Erythromycin
Fenofibrate
Fluoxetine
Fluphenazine
Fluvastatin
Gemfibrozil
Haloperidol
Halothane
Heroin
Ibuprofen
Interferon beta 1-a
Interferons, alfa-2
Isoniazid
Isotretinoin
Itraconazole
Lamivudine
Licorice
Lindane
Lithium
Lorazepam
Lovastatin
Loxapine
MDMA
Mephobarbital
Meprobamate
Methadone
Methamphetamine
Methohexital
Mirtazapine
Morphine
Naltrexone
Norfloxacin
Olanzapine
Pancuronium
Pemoline
Pentamidine
Pentobarbital
Perphenazine
Phenelzine
Phenobarbital
Phenylpropanolamine
Phenytoin
Pravastatin
Primidone
Protriptyline
Risperidone

Secobarbital
Simvastatin
Succinylcholine
Tenecteplase
Terbutaline
Theophylline
Thiopental
Trandolapril
Valproic acid
Vasopressin
Verapamil
Vinblastine

**Scleroderma**

Aldesleukin
Arsenic
Azathioprine
Bleomycin
Bromocriptine
Cocaine
Dapsone
Diethylpropion
Docetaxel
Estrogens
Fosinopril
Heparin
Hepatitis B vaccine
Lithium
Medroxyprogesterone
Melphalan
Mephenytoin
Methoxsalen
Methysergide
Metoprolol
Penicillamine
Pentazocine
Phenytoin
Phytonadione
Psoralens
Sotalol
Topotecan
Trioxsalen
Valproic acid
Zileuton

**Seborrhea**

Acitretin
Atorvastatin
Cetirizine
Clomipramine
Danazol
Delavirdine
Doxycycline
Fluoxetine
Fluoxymesterone
Fluphenazine
Flurbiprofen
Fluvoxamine
Foscarnet
Gemfibrozil
Indinavir
Interferon beta 1-a
Loxapine
Mesoridazine
Methyltestosterone
Minoxidil
Mirtazapine
Nafarelin
Naltrexone
Olanzapine
Oral contraceptives
Palivizumab
Pentostatin
Pergolide
Perphenazine
Prochlorperazine
Risperidone
Ritonavir
Tacrine
Testosterone
Thioridazine
Tolcapone
Topiramate
Trifluoperazine
Trovafloxacin
Valproic acid

**Seborrheic Dermatitis**

Buspirone
Chlorpromazine
Cimetidine
Ethionamide
Fluorouracil
Fluoxymesterone
Gold and gold compounds
Griseofulvin
Haloperidol
Interferons, alfa-2
Kava
Lithium
Methoxsalen
Methyldopa
Methyltestosterone
Psoralens
Saquinavir
Stanozolol
Testosterone
Thiothixene
Trioxsalen

**Serum Sickness**

Amobarbital
Amoxicillin
Ampicillin
Anistreplase
Aprobarbital
Asparaginase
Azathioprine
Bacampicillin
Bupropion
Carbamazepine
Carbenicillin
Cefaclor
Cefadroxil
Cefamandole
Cefazolin
Cefdinir
Cefditoren
Cefixime
Cefmetazole
Cefonicid
Cefoperazone
Cefotaxime
Cefotetan
Cefoxitin
Cefpodoxime
Cefprozil
Ceftazidime
Ceftibuten
Ceftizoxime
Ceftriaxone
Cefuroxime
Cephalexin
Cephalothin
Cephapirin
Cephradine
Ciprofloxacin
Cloxacillin
Co-trimoxazole
Cromolyn
Diclofenac
Dicloxacillin
Doxycycline
Fluoxetine
Furazolidone
Gatifloxacin
Griseofulvin
Hepatitis B vaccine
Heroin
Ibuprofen
Indomethacin
Ipodate
Isoniazid
Itraconazole
Lincomycin
Loracarbef
Meclofenamate
Mephobarbital
Mercaptopurine
Methicillin
Methimazole
Metronidazole
Mezlocillin
Minocycline
Nafcillin
Nizatidine
Ofloxacin
Oxacillin
Oxaprozin
Penicillamine
Penicillins
Pentoxifylline
Phenytoin
Piperacillin
Piroxicam
Potassium iodide
Propranolol
Rifampin
Rituximab
Secobarbital
Sparfloxacin
Streptokinase
Sulfadiazine
Sulfamethoxazole
Sulfasalazine
Sulfisoxazole
Sulindac
Tartrazine
Terbinafine
Tetracycline
Ticarcillin
Ticlopidine
Tolmetin
Trovafloxacin
Verapamil

**Sialorrhea**

Acitretin
Almotriptan
Alprazolam
Amiodarone
Amitriptyline
Amoxapine
Betaxolol
Bethanechol
Bupropion
Buspirone
Cetirizine
Cevimeline
Chlordiazepoxide
Citalopram
Clomipramine
Clonazepam
Clorazepate
Clozapine
Delavirdine
Diazepam
Diazoxide
Echinacea
Edrophonium
Eletriptan
Estazolam
Ethionamide
Etodolac
Fluoxetine
Fluphenazine
Flurazepam
Fluvoxamine
Frovatriptan
Gabapentin
Galantamine
Gentamicin
Guanabenz
Guanethidine
Guanfacine
Haloperidol
Ifosfamide
Imipenem/cilastatin
Irinotecan
Kanamycin
Ketamine
Ketoprofen
Lamotrigine
Levodopa
Lithium
Loratadine
Lorazepam
Maprotiline
Mefenamic acid
Mesoridazine
Methohexital
Midazolam
Mirtazapine
Modafinil
Molindone
Nabumetone
Nefazodone
Nicotine
Olanzapine
Oxazepam
Pancuronium
Pantoprazole
Paroxetine
Pentoxifylline
Perphenazine
Pilocarpine
Pimozide
Potassium iodide
Pramipexole
Prazepam
Prochlorperazine
Propofol
Quazepam
Quetiapine
Ramipril

Rapacuronium
Reserpine
Risperidone
Rivastigmine
Ropinirole
Sertraline
Succinylcholine
Tacrine
Temazepam
Thiothixene
Tiagabine
Tobramycin
Tolcapone
Topiramate
Trazodone
Triazolam
Trovafloxacin
Valproic acid
Venlafaxine
Zaleplon
Ziprasidone

**Stevens–Johnson Syndrome**

Acetaminophen
Acetazolamide
Acyclovir
Albendazole
Allopurinol
Aminophylline
Amiodarone
Amobarbital
Amoxicillin
Ampicillin
Amprenavir
Aprobarbital
Arsenic
Aspirin
Atropine sulfate
Azithromycin
Bacampicillin
Bleomycin
Bupropion
Butabarbital
Butalbital
Captopril
Carbamazepine
Carbenicillin
Carvedilol
Cefaclor
Cefadroxil
Cefamandole
Cefazolin
Cefdinir
Cefditoren
Cefepime
Cefixime
Cefmetazole
Cefonicid
Cefoperazone
Cefotaxime
Cefotetan
Cefoxitin
Cefpodoxime
Cefprozil
Ceftazidime
Ceftibuten
Ceftizoxime
Ceftriaxone
Cefuroxime
Celecoxib
Cephalexin
Cephalothin
Cephapirin
Cephradine
Chlorambucil
Chloramphenicol
Chlormezanone
Chloroquine
Chlorothiazide
Chlorpropamide
Chlorthalidone
Cimetidine
Cinoxacin
Ciprofloxacin
Cisplatin
Clarithromycin
Clindamycin
Clofibrate
Cloxacillin
Clozapine
Co-trimoxazole
Cyclophosphamide
Cycloserine
Danazol
Dapsone
Delavirdine
Demeclocycline
Diclofenac
Dicloxacillin
Didanosine
Diflunisal
Diltiazem
Dipyridamole
Doxycycline
Enalapril
Enoxacin
Erythromycin
Ethambutol
Ethosuximide
Etidronate
Etodolac
Etoposide
Felbamate
Fenoprofen
Fluconazole
Fluoxetine
Flurbiprofen
Fluvastatin
Fluvoxamine
Fosphenytoin
Furosemide
Gabapentin
Ganciclovir
Gatifloxacin
Ginseng
Griseofulvin
Hepatitis B vaccine
Hydrochlorothiazide
Hydrocodone
Hydroxychloroquine
Ibuprofen
Indapamide
Indinavir
Indomethacin
Isoniazid
Itraconazole
Ketoprofen
Ketorolac
Lamotrigine
Leflunomide
Levamisole
Levofloxacin
Lidocaine
Lincomycin
Lisinopril
Lomefloxacin
Loracarbef
Lorazepam
Lovastatin
Maprotiline
Mebendazole
Mechlorethamine
Meclofenamate
Mefenamic acid
Mefloquine
Meloxicam
Mephenytoin
Mephobarbital
Meprobamate
Methazolamide
Methicillin
Methotrexate
Methsuximide
Methyclothiazide
Methyldopa
Metolazone
Mexiletine
Mezlocillin
Minocycline
Minoxidil
Nabumetone
Nafcillin
Naproxen
Nevirapine
Nifedipine
Nitrofurantoin
Norfloxacin
Nystatin
Ofloxacin
Omeprazole
Oral contraceptives
Oxacillin
Oxaprozin
Oxcarbazepine
Pantoprazole
Penicillamine
Penicillins
Pentamidine
Pentobarbital
Phenobarbital
Phenolphthalein
Phensuximide
Phenytoin
Piperacillin
Piroxicam
Pravastatin
Promethazine
Propranolol
Pyrimethamine
Quinine
Ranitidine
Rifampin
Ritonavir
Saquinavir
Secobarbital
Sertraline
Simvastatin
Smallpox vaccine
Sparfloxacin
Streptomycin
Sulfacetamide
Sulfadiazine
Sulfadoxine
Sulfamethoxazole
Sulfasalazine
Sulfisoxazole
Sulindac
Terbinafine
Tetracycline
Thalidomide
Thiabendazole
Thiopental
Tiagabine
Ticarcillin
Ticlopidine
Tocainide
Tolmetin
Torsemide
Trimethadione
Trimethoprim
Trovafloxacin
Valproic acid
Vancomycin
Verapamil
Vitamin A
Voriconazole
Zidovudine
Zonisamide

**Stomatitis**

Acitretin
Aldesleukin
Alemtuzumab
Allopurinol
Amitriptyline
Amoxapine
Amoxicillin
Amphotericin B
Ampicillin
Anisindione
Arsenic
Atorvastatin
Azathioprine
Azelastine
Bacampicillin
Basiliximab
Benactyzine
Bismuth
Bleomycin
Botulinum toxin (A & B)
Bupropion
Busulfan
Capecitabine
Carbamazepine
Carbenicillin
Carboplatin
Carmustine
Cefdinir
Cefditoren
Celecoxib
Cetirizine
Cevimeline
Chloral hydrate
Chlorambucil
Chloramphenicol
Chlorhexidine
Chloroquine
Cidofovir
Ciprofloxacin
Citalopram
Clarithromycin
Clofibrate

Clomipramine
Cloxacillin
Co-trimoxazole
Corticosteroids
Cyclobenzaprine
Cyclophosphamide
Cyclosporine
Cytarabine
Dacarbazine
Dactinomycin
Daunorubicin
Delavirdine
Desipramine
Diclofenac
Dicloxacillin
Diflunisal
Docetaxel
Doxepin
Doxorubicin
Eletriptan
Enalapril
Enoxacin
Epirubicin
Ertapenem
Esomeprazole
Ethionamide
Etidronate
Etodolac
Etoposide
Fenoprofen
Fludarabine
Fluorouracil
Fluoxetine
Fluoxymesterone
Flurbiprofen
Fluvoxamine
Foscarnet
Frovatriptan
Furosemide
Gabapentin
Gatifloxacin
Gemcitabine
Gemtuzumab
Gentamicin
Ginkgo biloba
Gold and gold compounds
Granulocyte colony-stimulating factor (GCSF)
Griseofulvin
Hydroxychloroquine
Hydroxyurea
Ibuprofen
Idarubicin
Ifosfamide
Imipramine
Indomethacin
Interferons, alfa-2
Ipratropium
Irinotecan
Ketoprofen
Ketorolac
Lamotrigine
Lansoprazole
Leflunomide
Levamisole
Lidocaine
Lincomycin
Lithium
Lomustine
Loratadine
Lovastatin
Maprotiline
Meclofenamate
Meloxicam
Melphalan
Mephenytoin
Meprobamate
Mercaptopurine
Methenamine
Methicillin
Methotrexate
Methyltestosterone
Metronidazole
Mezlocillin
Mirtazapine
Mitomycin
Moxifloxacin
Nabumetone
Nafcillin
Naproxen
Nefazodone
Nevirapine
Nicotine
Norfloxacin
Nortriptyline
Olanzapine
Olsalazine
Oxacillin
Oxaprozin
Oxcarbazepine
Paclitaxel
Pamidronate
Pantoprazole
Paroxetine
Penicillamine
Penicillins
Pentostatin
Piroxicam
Plicamycin
Pravastatin
Procarbazine
Propolis
Protriptyline
Pyrilamine
Quetiapine
Quinupristin/dalfopristin
Rabeprazole
Rifampin
Riluzole
Rimantadine
Risperidone
Rivastigmine
Ropinirole
Saquinavir
Sertraline
Sildenafil
Sirolimus
Sparfloxacin
Streptokinase
Streptomycin
Sulfadiazine
Sulfadoxine
Sulfamethoxazole
Sulfasalazine
Sulfisoxazole
Sulindac
Tacrine
Terbinafine
Testosterone
Thioguanine
Thiotepa
Tiagabine
Ticarcillin
Tiopronin
Tocainide
Tolmetin
Topiramate
Topotecan
Tramadol
Trastuzumab
Triazolam
Trimeprazine
Trimetrexate
Trimipramine
Tripelennamine
Trovafloxacin
Ursodiol
Valdecoxib
Valproic acid
Venlafaxine
Vinblastine
Vincristine
Vinorelbine
Voriconazole
Zalcitabine
Zaleplon
Zonisamide

**Stomatodynia**
Alemtuzumab
Amoxicillin
Anisindione
Bacampicillin
Benztropine
Biperiden
Carbenicillin
Dicloxacillin
Erythromycin
Ethionamide
Garlic
Griseofulvin
Lithium
Methicillin
Mezlocillin
Nafcillin
Oxacillin
Piperacillin
Potassium iodide
Ticarcillin
Triamterene
Vitamin A

**Telangiectases**
Amlodipine
Carmustine
Corticosteroids
Estrogens
Felodipine
Hydroxychloroquine
Hydroxyurea
Interferons, alfa-2
Isocarboxazid
Isotretinoin
Lisinopril
Lithium
Methotrexate
Methysergide
Nifedipine
Oral contraceptives
Phenelzine
Progestins
Thiothixene

**Tendinitis**
Amlodipine
Celecoxib
Cevimeline
Ciprofloxacin
Eprosartan
Gatifloxacin
Indinavir
Levobetaxolol
Levofloxacin
Methotrexate
Minoxidil
Moxifloxacin
Norfloxacin
Orlistat
Risedronate
Rofecoxib
Valdecoxib

**Tendon Rupture**
Ciprofloxacin
Enoxacin
Gatifloxacin
Leflunomide
Levofloxacin
Lomefloxacin
Mirtazapine
Moxifloxacin
Norfloxacin
Ofloxacin
Sparfloxacin
Trovafloxacin

**Toxic Epidermal Necrolysis (TEN)**
Acebutolol
Acetaminophen
Acetazolamide
Aldesleukin
Allopurinol
Alprostadil
Aminosalicylate sodium
Amiodarone
Amobarbital
Amoxapine
Amoxicillin
Ampicillin
Asparaginase
Aspirin
Atenolol
Atorvastatin
Azathioprine
Aztreonam
Betaxolol
Butabarbital
Butalbital
Captopril
Carbamazepine
Carbenicillin
Cefaclor
Cefadroxil
Cefamandole
Cefazolin
Cefdinir
Cefditoren
Cefepime
Cefmetazole
Cefonicid
Cefoperazone
Cefotaxime
Cefotetan
Cefoxitin

Cefpodoxime
Cefprozil
Ceftazidime
Ceftibuten
Ceftizoxime
Ceftriaxone
Cefuroxime
Celecoxib
Cephalexin
Cephalothin
Cephapirin
Cephradine
Chlorambucil
Chloramphenicol
Chlormezanone
Chloroquine
Chlorothiazide
Chlorpromazine
Chlorpropamide
Chlorthalidone
Cimetidine
Cinoxacin
Ciprofloxacin
Cladribine
Clarithromycin
Clindamycin
Clofibrate
Co-trimoxazole
Codeine
Colchicine
Cyclophosphamide
Cyclosporine
Cytarabine
Dactinomycin
Dapsone
Deferoxamine
Demeclocycline
Dextroamphetamine
Diclofenac
Dicloxacillin
Diflunisal
Diltiazem
Diphenhydramine
Dipyridamole
Disulfiram
Docetaxel
Doxycycline
Enalapril
Enoxacin
Erythromycin
Ethambutol
Etidronate
Etodolac
Famotidine
Felbamate
Fenofibrate
Fenoprofen
Fluconazole
Fluoxetine
Fluphenazine
Flurbiprofen
Flutamide
Fluvastatin
Fluvoxamine
Foscarnet
Fosphenytoin
Furosemide
Gatifloxacin
Gentamicin
Gold and gold compounds
Griseofulvin
Heparin
Heroin
Hydrochlorothiazide
Hydrocodone
Hydroxychloroquine
Ibuprofen
Imipenem/cilastatin
Indapamide
Indomethacin
Isoniazid
Isotretinoin
Ketoprofen
Ketorolac
Lamotrigine
Leflunomide
Levofloxacin
Lisinopril
Lovastatin
Meclofenamate
Mefenamic acid
Mefloquine
Meloxicam
Meperidine
Mephenytoin
Meprobamate
Mercaptopurine
Methamphetamine
Methazolamide
Methicillin
Methotrexate
Methyldopa
Metolazone
Metoprolol
Metronidazole
Mezlocillin
Nabumetone
Nadolol
Nafcillin
Nalidixic acid
Naproxen
Neomycin
Nevirapine
Nifedipine
Nitrofurantoin
Norfloxacin
Ofloxacin
Omeprazole
Oxacillin
Oxaprozin
Oxazepam
Oxcarbazepine
Pantoprazole
Papaverine
Paroxetine
Penicillamine
Penicillins
Pentamidine
Pentazocine
Pentobarbital
Phenobarbital
Phenolphthalein
Phenytoin
Pindolol
Piperacillin
Piroxicam
Plicamycin
Pravastatin
Primidone
Procarbazine
Prochlorperazine
Promethazine
Propranolol
Pyridoxine
Pyrimethamine
Quinidine
Quinine
Ranitidine
Reserpine
Rifampin
Simvastatin
Smallpox vaccine
Sparfloxacin
Streptomycin
Streptozocin
Sulfacetamide
Sulfadiazine
Sulfadoxine
Sulfamethoxazole
Sulfasalazine
Sulfisoxazole
Sulindac
Terbinafine
Terconazole
Tetracycline
Thalidomide
Thiabendazole
Thiopental
Thioridazine
Ticarcillin
Timolol
Tiopronin
Tolbutamide
Tolmetin
Trimethoprim
Trovafloxacin
Valproic acid
Vancomycin
Vinorelbine
Voriconazole
Zidovudine
Zonisamide

**Urticaria**

Acarbose
Acebutolol
Acetaminophen
Acetazolamide
Acetohexamide
Acitretin
Acyclovir
Albendazole
Albuterol
Aldesleukin
Alemtuzumab
Alfentanil
Allopurinol
Alprazolam
Alprostadil
Alteplase
Amantadine
Amikacin
Amiloride
Aminocaproic acid
Aminoglutethimide
Aminophylline
Aminosalicylate sodium
Amiodarone
Amitriptyline
Amlodipine
Amobarbital
Amoxapine
Amoxicillin
Amphotericin B
Ampicillin
Anagrelide
Anisindione
Anistreplase
Anthrax vaccine
Aprobarbital
Aprotinin
Arsenic
Asparaginase
Aspartame
Aspirin
Atenolol
Atorvastatin
Atracurium
Atropine sulfate
Azatadine
Azathioprine
Azithromycin
Aztreonam
Bacampicillin
Baclofen
Benactyzine
Benazepril
Bendroflumethiazide
Benzthiazide
Benztropine
Betaxolol
Biperiden
Bisacodyl
Bisoprolol
Bleomycin
Botulinum toxin (A & B)
Bromocriptine
Bumetanide
Bupropion
Buspirone
Busulfan
Butabarbital
Butalbital
Butorphanol
Caffeine
Calcitonin
Captopril
Carbamazepine
Carbenicillin
Carboplatin
Carisoprodol
Cefaclor
Cefadroxil
Cefamandole
Cefazolin
Cefdinir
Cefditoren
Cefepime
Cefixime
Cefmetazole
Cefonicid
Cefoperazone
Cefotaxime
Cefotetan
Cefoxitin
Cefpodoxime
Cefprozil
Ceftazidime
Ceftibuten
Ceftizoxime
Ceftriaxone

Cefuroxime
Celecoxib
Cephalexin
Cephalothin
Cephapirin
Cephradine
Cetirizine
Chloral hydrate
Chlorambucil
Chloramphenicol
Chlordiazepoxide
Chlorhexidine
Chlormezanone
Chloroquine
Chlorothiazide
Chlorotrianisene
Chlorpromazine
Chlorpropamide
Chlorthalidone
Chlorzoxazone
Cholestyramine
Cidofovir
Cilostazol
Cimetidine
Cinoxacin
Ciprofloxacin
Cisplatin
Citalopram
Clarithromycin
Clemastine
Clidinium
Clindamycin
Clofazimine
Clofibrate
Clomiphene
Clomipramine
Clonazepam
Clonidine
Clopidogrel
Clorazepate
Clotrimazole
Cloxacillin
Clozapine
Co-trimoxazole
Cocaine
Codeine
Colchicine
Colestipol
Corticosteroids
Cromolyn
Cyanocobalamin
Cyclamate
Cyclobenzaprine
Cyclophosphamide
Cycloserine
Cyclosporine
Cyclothiazide
Cyproheptadine
Cytarabine
Dacarbazine
Dactinomycin
Danazol
Dantrolene
Dapsone
Daunorubicin
Deferoxamine
Delavirdine
Demeclocycline
Denileukin
Desipramine
Dexchlorpheniramine
Dextroamphetamine
Diazepam
Diazoxide
Diclofenac
Dicloxacillin
Dicumarol
Dicyclomine
Didanosine
Diethylpropion
Diethylstilbestrol
Diflunisal
Digoxin
Diltiazem
Dimenhydrinate
Diphenhydramine
Diphenoxylate
Dipyridamole
Dirithromycin
Disopyramide
Disulfiram
Docetaxel
Dolasetron
Domperidone
Donepezil
Dopamine
Doxacurium
Doxazosin
Doxepin
Doxorubicin
Doxycycline
Echinacea
Edrophonium
Efavirenz
Eletriptan
Enalapril
Enoxacin
Enoxaparin
Ephedrine
Epinephrine
Epirubicin
Epoetin alfa
Ertapenem
Erythromycin
Esmolol
Esomeprazole
Estazolam
Estramustine
Estrogens
Etanercept
Ethacrynic acid
Ethambutol
Ethchlorvynol
Ethionamide
Ethosuximide
Etidronate
Etodolac
Etoposide
Famotidine
Felbamate
Felodipine
Fenofibrate
Fenoprofen
Fentanyl
Finasteride
Flavoxate
Flecainide
Fluconazole
Flucytosine
Flumazenil
Fluorouracil
Fluoxetine
Fluoxymesterone
Fluphenazine
Flurazepam
Flurbiprofen
Flutamide
Fluvastatin
Fluvoxamine
Folic acid
Formoterol
Foscarnet
Fosinopril
Furazolidone
Furosemide
Gabapentin
Ganciclovir
Garlic
Gatifloxacin
Gemfibrozil
Gentamicin
Glimepiride
Glipizide
Glucagon
Glyburide
Glycopyrrolate
Gold and gold compounds
Goserelin
Granisetron
Granulocyte colony-stimulating factor (GCSF)
Griseofulvin
Guanethidine
Guanfacine
Haloperidol
Halothane
Henna
Heparin
Hepatitis B vaccine
Heroin
Hydralazine
Hydrochlorothiazide
Hydrocodone
Hydroflumethiazide
Hydromorphone
Hydroxychloroquine
Hydroxyurea
Hydroxyzine
Hyoscyamine
Ibritumomab
Ibuprofen
Idarubicin
Imipenem/cilastatin
Imipramine
Indapamide
Indinavir
Indomethacin
Infliximab
Insulin
Interferon beta 1-a
Interferons, alfa-2
Ipodate
Ipratropium
Irbesartan
Isoniazid
Isoproterenol
Isotretinoin
Isradipine
Itraconazole
Ivermectin
Kanamycin
Ketoconazole
Ketoprofen
Ketorolac
Labetalol
Lamivudine
Lamotrigine
Lansoprazole
Leflunomide
Leucovorin
Leuprolide
Levamisole
Levobunolol
Levodopa
Levofloxacin
Levothyroxine
Lidocaine
Lincomycin
Lindane
Liothyronine
Lisinopril
Lithium
Lomefloxacin
Loperamide
Loracarbef
Loratadine
Lorazepam
Losartan
Lovastatin
Loxapine
Maprotiline
Marihuana
Mazindol
Mebendazole
Mechlorethamine
Meclizine
Meclofenamate
Medroxyprogesterone
Mefenamic acid
Mefloquine
Meloxicam
Melphalan
Meperidine
Mephenytoin
Mephobarbital
Meprobamate
Mercaptopurine
Mesalamine
Mesna
Mesoridazine
Metaxalone
Metformin
Methadone
Methamphetamine
Methantheline
Methazolamide
Methenamine
Methicillin
Methimazole
Methocarbamol
Methohexital
Methotrexate
Methoxsalen
Methsuximide
Methyclothiazide
Methyldopa
Methylphenidate
Methyltestosterone
Methysergide
Metoclopramide

Metolazone
Metoprolol
Metronidazole
Mexiletine
Mezlocillin
Miconazole
Midazolam
Milk thistle
Minocycline
Minoxidil
Mitomycin
Mitotane
Mitoxantrone
Moexipril
Montelukast
Moricizine
Moxifloxacin
Nabumetone
Nadolol
Nafarelin
Nafcillin
Nalidixic acid
Naloxone
Naproxen
Naratriptan
Nefazodone
Nelfinavir
Neomycin
Niacin
Nicardipine
Nicotine
Nifedipine
Nisoldipine
Nitrofurantoin
Nitroglycerin
Nizatidine
Norfloxacin
Nortriptyline
Nystatin
Octreotide
Ofloxacin
Olanzapine
Olsalazine
Omeprazole
Ondansetron
Oral contraceptives
Orphenadrine
Oxacillin
Oxaprozin
Oxazepam
Oxybutynin
Oxycodone
Oxytetracycline
Paclitaxel
Pantoprazole
Pantothenic acid
Papaverine
Paroxetine
PEG-interferon alfa-2b
Penicillamine
Penicillins
Pentagastrin
Pentamidine
Pentazocine
Pentobarbital
Pentosan
Pentostatin
Pentoxifylline
Pergolide
Perphenazine
Phendimetrazine
Phenelzine
Phenindamine
Phenobarbital
Phenolphthalein
Phentermine
Phenytoin
Phytonadione
Pilocarpine
Pimozide
Pindolol
Piperacillin
Piroxicam
Polythiazide
Potassium iodide
Pravastatin
Prazepam
Praziquantel
Prazosin
Primaquine
Primidone
Probenecid
Procainamide
Procarbazine
Prochlorperazine
Procyclidine
Progestins
Promazine
Promethazine
Propafenone
Propantheline
Propofol
Propoxyphene
Propranolol
Propylthiouracil
Protamine
Protriptyline
Pseudoephedrine
Psoralens
Pyrazinamide
Pyrilamine
Pyrimethamine
Quazepam
Quinacrine
Quinapril
Quinestrol
Quinethazone
Quinidine
Quinine
Quinupristin/dalfopristin
Rabeprazole
Ramipril
Ranitidine
Rapacuronium
Reserpine
Ribavirin
Riboflavin
Rifabutin
Rifampin
Rifapentine
Risperidone
Ritodrine
Ritonavir
Rituximab
Rivastigmine
Rofecoxib
Ropinirole
Saccharin
Salmeterol
Salsalate
Saquinavir
Scopolamine
Secobarbital
Secretin
Sertraline
Sildenafil
Simvastatin
Smallpox vaccine
Sotalol
Sparfloxacin
Spectinomycin
Spironolactone
Stanozolol
Streptokinase
Streptomycin
Succinylcholine
Sucralfate
Sufentanil
Sulfadiazine
Sulfadoxine
Sulfamethoxazole
Sulfasalazine
Sulfisoxazole
Sulindac
Sumatriptan
Tacrine
Tacrolimus
Tamoxifen
Tartrazine
Temazepam
Tenecteplase
Terbinafine
Terbutaline
Testosterone
Tetracycline
Thalidomide
Thiabendazole
Thiamine
Thimerosal
Thiopental
Thioridazine
Thiotepa
Thiothixene
Tiagabine
Ticarcillin
Ticlopidine
Timolol
Tinzaparin
Tiopronin
Tirofiban
Tizanidine
Tobramycin
Tolazamide
Tolazoline
Tolbutamide
Tolcapone
Tolmetin
Topiramate
Torsemide
Tramadol
Tranylcypromine
Trazodone
Triamterene
Triazolam
Trichlormethiazide
Trifluoperazine
Trihexyphenidyl
Trimeprazine
Trimethadione
Trimipramine
Tripelennamine
Triprolidine
Troleandomycin
Trovafloxacin
Urokinase
Ursodiol
Valdecoxib
Valproic acid
Valsartan
Vancomycin
Vasopressin
Venlafaxine
Verapamil
Verteporfin
Vinblastine
Vincristine
Vitamin E
Voriconazole
Warfarin
Zalcitabine
Zanamivir
Zidovudine
Ziprasidone
Zolmitriptan
Zolpidem
Zonisamide

**Vaginal Candidiasis**

Acitretin
Ampicillin
Aztreonam
Botulinum toxin (A & B)
Cefamandole
Cefdinir
Cefditoren
Cefixime
Cefpodoxime
Ceftazidime
Celecoxib
Chlorotrianisene
Delavirdine
Diethylstilbestrol
Dirithromycin
Enoxacin
Ertapenem
Estrogens
Lamotrigine
Leflunomide
Lomefloxacin
Metronidazole
Norfloxacin
Paroxetine
Riluzole
Ropinirole
Sibutramine
Sparfloxacin
Tizanidine
Valdecoxib
Venlafaxine

**Vaginitis**

Acyclovir
Amitriptyline
Amoxapine
Amoxicillin
Azithromycin
Aztreonam
Bacampicillin
Bupropion
Carbenicillin
Cefaclor
Cefadroxil

Cefamandole
Cefazolin
Cefdinir
Cefditoren
Cefepime
Cefixime
Cefmetazole
Cefonicid
Cefotaxime
Cefpodoxime
Cefprozil
Ceftazidime
Ceftibuten
Ceftizoxime
Ceftriaxone
Cefuroxime
Celecoxib
Cephalexin
Cephapirin
Cephradine
Cetirizine
Cevimeline
Chlorotrianisene
Cilostazol
Ciprofloxacin
Clomipramine
Cloxacillin
Dicloxacillin
Dirithromycin
Donepezil
Doxycycline
Eletriptan
Enoxacin
Ertapenem
Esomeprazole
Fenofibrate
Fluvoxamine
Fosfomycin
Gatifloxacin
Gold and gold compounds
Imipramine
Interferon beta 1-a
Lamotrigine
Leuprolide
Levofloxacin
Lincomycin
Lomefloxacin
Loratadine
Medroxyprogesterone
Methicillin
Mezlocillin
Mifepristone
Mirtazapine
Moxifloxacin
Nafarelin
Nafcillin
Nefazodone
Nisoldipine
Nortriptyline
Nystatin
Octreotide
Ofloxacin
Olanzapine
Orlistat
Oxacillin
Oxcarbazepine
Pantoprazole
Paroxetine
Pentostatin
Perindopril
Piperacillin
Quinupristin/dalfopristin
Raloxifene
Rivastigmine
Sertraline
Sparfloxacin
Tetracycline
Tiagabine
Ticarcillin
Tolcapone
Topiramate
Trovafloxacin
Valproic acid
Venlafaxine
Zaleplon
Zileuton
Zolpidem

**Vasculitis**

Acebutolol
Acetaminophen
Acyclovir
Allopurinol
Amiloride
Aminosalicylate sodium
Amiodarone
Amitriptyline
Amlodipine
Amoxapine
Amoxicillin
Ampicillin
Anistreplase
Aspartame
Aspirin
Atenolol
Azathioprine
Bendroflumethiazide
Benzthiazide
Bexarotene
Bismuth
Bromocriptine
Bumetanide
Busulfan
Butabarbital
Butalbital
Captopril
Carbamazepine
Carbenicillin
Caspofungin
Cefdinir
Celecoxib
Cevimeline
Chloramphenicol
Chlordiazepoxide
Chloroquine
Chlorothiazide
Chlorpromazine
Chlorpropamide
Chlorthalidone
Cimetidine
Ciprofloxacin
Citalopram
Clarithromycin
Clindamycin
Clomipramine
Clorazepate
Clozapine
Co-trimoxazole
Cocaine
Colchicine
Corticosteroids
Cromolyn
Cyclophosphamide
Cyclosporine
Cyclothiazide
Cyproheptadine
Cytarabine
Dacarbazine
Delavirdine
Desipramine
Diazepam
Diclofenac
Dicloxacillin
Didanosine
Diflunisal
Digoxin
Diltiazem
Diphenhydramine
Disulfiram
Doxepin
Doxycycline
Efavirenz
Enalapril
Ephedrine
Erythromycin
Estrogens
Etanercept
Ethacrynic acid
Etodolac
Famotidine
Fluoxetine
Flurbiprofen
Fluvastatin
Fosinopril
Furosemide
Gatifloxacin
Gemcitabine
Gemfibrozil
Gentamicin
Ginkgo biloba
Glucagon
Glyburide
Gold and gold compounds
Granulocyte colony-stimulating factor (GCSF)
Griseofulvin
Guanethidine
Heparin
Hepatitis B vaccine
Heroin
Hydralazine
Hydrochlorothiazide
Hydroflumethiazide
Hydroxychloroquine
Hydroxyurea
Ibuprofen
Imipenem/cilastatin
Imipramine
Indapamide
Indinavir
Indomethacin
Insulin
Interferons, alfa-2
Isoniazid
Isotretinoin
Itraconazole
Ketoconazole
Leflunomide
Levamisole
Levofloxacin
Lisinopril
Lithium
Lomefloxacin
Lovastatin
Maprotiline
Meclofenamate
Mefenamic acid
Mefloquine
Meloxicam
Melphalan
Meprobamate
Mercaptopurine
Mesalamine
Metformin
Methazolamide
Methicillin
Methimazole
Methotrexate
Methoxsalen
Methyldopa
Methylphenidate
Metolazone
Metronidazole
Mezlocillin
Minocycline
Mitotane
Nabumetone
Nafcillin
Naproxen
Nelfinavir
Nicotine
Nifedipine
Nizatidine
Norfloxacin
Nortriptyline
Ofloxacin
Omeprazole
Oxacillin
Oxaprozin
Oxytetracycline
Paroxetine
Penicillamine
Penicillins
Pentamidine
Pentobarbital
Pergolide
Phenobarbital
Phenytoin
Phytonadione
Piperacillin
Piroxicam
Polythiazide
Potassium iodide
Pravastatin
Procainamide
Propylthiouracil
Protriptyline
Psoralens
Pyridoxine
Pyrimethamine
Quinapril
Quinethazone
Quinidine
Quinine
Ramipril
Ranitidine
Rifampin
Ritodrine
Simvastatin
Sotalol
Sparfloxacin

Spironolactone
Streptokinase
Streptomycin
Sulfamethoxazole
Sulfasalazine
Sulfisoxazole
Sulindac
Tamoxifen
Tartrazine
Terbutaline
Tetracycline
Thalidomide
Thiamine
Ticarcillin
Ticlopidine
Tocainide
Torsemide
Trazodone
Triamterene
Trichlormethiazide
Trimethadione
Trioxsalen
Triptorelin
Trovafloxacin
Valproic acid
Vancomycin
Verapamil
Warfarin
Zidovudine

**Vesicular Eruption**

Acyclovir
Aminolevulinic acid
Amoxicillin
Amphotericin B
Bexarotene
Carbenicillin
Carteolol
Clofibrate
Clonidine
Clotrimazole
Colchicine
Delavirdine
Denileukin
Dicloxacillin
Dicumarol
Enoxaparin
Estrogens
Etodolac
Fenoprofen
Gatifloxacin
Ginkgo biloba
Glyburide
Ibuprofen
Imiquimod
Letrozole
Lincomycin
Meclofenamate
Melphalan
Naproxen
Nefazodone
Olanzapine
Penicillamine
Penicillins
Piperacillin
Piroxicam
Propylthiouracil
Pyridoxine
Tiagabine
Tretinoin
Venlafaxine
Verteporfin
Vinblastine
Warfarin
Zaleplon
Ziprasidone
Zonisamide

**Xerosis**

Acebutolol
Acitretin
Aldesleukin
Alitretinoin
Alprazolam
Amiloride
Amlodipine
Amoxapine
Amphotericin B
Apraclonidine
Atenolol
Atorvastatin
Atropine sulfate
Benztropine
Betaxolol
Bexarotene
Bicalutamide
Bisoprolol
Bleomycin
Bupropion
Buspirone
Busulfan
Capecitabine
Captopril
Carteolol
Celecoxib
Cetirizine
Cevimeline
Chlorpromazine
Chlortetracycline
Cidofovir
Cilostazol
Cimetidine
Citalopram
Clindamycin
Clofazimine
Clofibrate
Clomipramine
Delavirdine
Desipramine
Dexmedetomidine
Diazoxide
Dicyclomine
Disopyramide
Docetaxel
Doxazosin
Eflornithine
Eletriptan
Estazolam
Estramustine
Famotidine
Fluorouracil
Fluoxetine
Fluphenazine
Flurbiprofen
Fluvastatin
Fluvoxamine
Foscarnet
Gemfibrozil
Glycopyrrolate
Gold and gold compounds
Hydroxyurea
Hyoscyamine
Imipramine
Indinavir
Interferons, alfa-2
Isotretinoin
Kava
Ketoconazole
Labetalol
Lamotrigine
Leflunomide
Leuprolide
Levamisole
Levobetaxolol
Levothyroxine
Liothyronine
Lithium
Loratadine
Losartan
Mechlorethamine
Medroxyprogesterone
Mesalamine
Mesoridazine
Methantheline
Methoxsalen
Metolazone
Metoprolol
Mexiletine
Midodrine
Minoxidil
Mirtazapine
Modafinil
Moricizine
Moxifloxacin
Nabumetone
Nadolol
Naratriptan
Nefazodone
Niacin
Nisoldipine
Nizatidine
Nortriptyline
Olanzapine
Omeprazole
Orlistat
Oxybutynin
Pantoprazole
Paroxetine
PEG-interferon alfa-2b
Penicillamine
Pentamidine
Pentostatin
Pergolide
Perindopril
Perphenazine
Pindolol
Prochlorperazine
Procyclidine
Promazine
Propantheline
Propranolol
Protriptyline
Quetiapine
Rabeprazole
Ranitidine
Risperidone
Ritonavir
Rofecoxib
Saquinavir
Scopolamine
Sertraline
Sparfloxacin
Spironolactone
Sulfasalazine
Tacrine
Tamoxifen
Thalidomide
Thioridazine
Tiagabine
Timolol
Tizanidine
Tolterodine
Topiramate
Tretinoin
Trifluoperazine
Trihexyphenidyl
Trioxsalen
Ursodiol
Valdecoxib
Venlafaxine
Vitamin A
Voriconazole
Zalcitabine
Zaleplon
Zonisamide

**Xerostomia**

Acebutolol
Acetazolamide
Acitretin
Albendazole
Albuterol
Aldesleukin
Almotriptan
Alprazolam
Alprostadil
Amantadine
Amifostine
Amiloride
Amitriptyline
Amlodipine
Amoxapine
Amoxicillin
Amphotericin B
Anastrozole
Apraclonidine
Arbutamine
Atropine sulfate
Azatadine
Azathioprine
Azelastine
Bacampicillin
Baclofen
Balsalazide
Benactyzine
Bendroflumethiazide
Benztropine
Bepridil
Betaxolol
Bexarotene
Bicalutamide
Biperiden
Bismuth
Bisoprolol
Botulinum toxin (A & B)
Brimonidine
Bromocriptine
Brompheniramine
Buclizine
Bumetanide
Bupropion
Buspirone
Butorphanol

Cabergoline
Captopril
Carbamazepine
Carbenicillin
Carisoprodol
Carteolol
Carvedilol
Cefditoren
Cefixime
Ceftibuten
Celecoxib
Cetirizine
Cevimeline
Chloramphenicol
Chlordiazepoxide
Chlormezanone
Chlorpheniramine
Chlorpromazine
Chlortetracycline
Cidofovir
Cimetidine
Ciprofloxacin
Citalopram
Clarithromycin
Clemastine
Clidinium
Clomipramine
Clonazepam
Clonidine
Clorazepate
Clozapine
Codeine
Cromolyn
Cyclobenzaprine
Cyproheptadine
Delavirdine
Desipramine
Desloratadine
Dexchlorpheniramine
Dextroamphetamine
Diazepam
Diazoxide
Diclofenac
Dicloxacillin
Dicyclomine
Didanosine
Diethylpropion
Diflunisal
Dihydroergotamine
Dihydrotachysterol
Diltiazem
Dimenhydrinate
Diphenhydramine
Diphenoxylate
Dirithromycin
Disopyramide
Donepezil
Doxazosin
Doxepin
Dronabinol
Efavirenz
Enalapril
Enoxacin
Entacapone
Ephedrine
Epinephrine
Eprosartan
Ergocalciferol
Esmolol
Esomeprazole
Estazolam
Ethacrynic acid
Ethionamide
Etodolac
Famotidine
Felbamate
Felodipine
Fenoprofen
Fentanyl
Flavoxate
Flecainide
Fluconazole
Flucytosine
Flumazenil
Fluoxetine
Fluphenazine
Flurazepam
Flurbiprofen
Fluvoxamine
Formoterol
Foscarnet
Fosfomycin
Fosinopril
Fosphenytoin
Frovatriptan
Furosemide
Gabapentin
Galantamine
Ganciclovir
Glycopyrrolate
Griseofulvin
Guanabenz
Guanadrel
Guanethidine
Guanfacine
Haloperidol
Hydrochlorothiazide
Hydrocodone
Hydromorphone
Hydroxyzine
Hyoscyamine
Ibuprofen
Imipramine
Indapamide
Indinavir
Indomethacin
Interferon beta 1-a
Interferons, alfa-2
Ipratropium
Isocarboxazid
Isoetharine
Isoniazid
Isoproterenol
Isosorbide dinitrate
Isotretinoin
Isradipine
Itraconazole
Ketoprofen
Ketorolac
Labetalol
Lamotrigine
Lansoprazole
Leflunomide
Levodopa
Levofloxacin
Lisinopril
Lithium
Lomefloxacin
Loperamide
Loratadine
Lorazepam
Losartan
Lovastatin
Loxapine
Maprotiline
Mazindol
MDMA
Mebendazole
Meclizine
Meclofenamate
Mefenamic acid
Meloxicam
Meperidine
Meprobamate
Mesoridazine
Methadone
Methamphetamine
Methantheline
Methazolamide
Methicillin
Methyldopa
Methylphenidate
Metoclopramide
Metolazone
Metronidazole
Mexiletine
Mezlocillin
Midodrine
Mirtazapine
Modafinil
Moexipril
Molindone
Moricizine
Morphine
Moxifloxacin
Nabumetone
Nadolol
Nafcillin
Naltrexone
Naproxen
Nefazodone
Niacin
Nicardipine
Nicotine
Nifedipine
Nisoldipine
Nitrofurantoin
Nitroglycerin
Nizatidine
Norfloxacin
Nortriptyline
Octreotide
Ofloxacin
Olanzapine
Omeprazole
Ondansetron
Orphenadrine
Oxacillin
Oxazepam
Oxcarbazepine
Oxybutynin
Oxycodone
Pantoprazole
Papaverine
Paroxetine
Penicillins
Pentamidine
Pentazocine
Pentoxifylline
Pergolide
Perindopril
Perphenazine
Phendimetrazine
Phenelzine
Phenindamine
Phenobarbital
Phenoxybenzamine
Phentermine
Phenylpropanolamine
Pimozide
Pirbuterol
Piroxicam
Pramipexole
Prazepam
Prazosin
Procarbazine
Prochlorperazine
Procyclidine
Promazine
Promethazine
Propafenone
Propantheline
Propofol
Propoxyphene
Propranolol
Protriptyline
Pseudoephedrine
Pyrilamine
Pyrimethamine
Quazepam
Quetiapine
Quinapril
Quinethazone
Rabeprazole
Ramipril
Reserpine
Riluzole
Rimantadine
Risperidone
Ritonavir
Rivastigmine
Rizatriptan
Rofecoxib
Ropinirole
Saquinavir
Scopolamine
Selegiline
Sertraline
Sibutramine
Sildenafil
Sotalol
Sparfloxacin
Spironolactone
St John's wort
Sucralfate
Sulfasalazine
Sulindac
Sumatriptan
Tacrine
Tamoxifen
Telmisartan
Temazepam
Terazosin
Terbutaline
Thalidomide
Thiabendazole
Thioguanine
Thioridazine
Thiothixene
Tiagabine

Ticarcillin
Timolol
Tiopronin
Tizanidine
Tocainide
Tolcapone
Tolmetin
Tolterodine
Topiramate
Torsemide
Tramadol
Trandolapril
Tranylcypromine
Trazodone
Tretinoin
Triamterene
Triazolam
Trichlormethiazide
Trifluoperazine
Trihexyphenidyl
Trimeprazine
Trimipramine
Tripelennamine
Triprolidine
Trovafloxacin
Unoprostone
Valdecoxib
Valproic acid
Valsartan
Venlafaxine
Verapamil
Vitamin A
Voriconazole
Zalcitabine
Zaleplon
Ziprasidone
Zolmitriptan
Zolpidem
Zonisamide

# DESCRIPTION OF THE 31 MOST COMMON REACTION PATTERNS

## Acanthosis nigricans

Acanthosis nigricans (AN) is a process characterized by a soft, velvety, brown or grayish-black thickening of the skin that is symmetrically distributed over the axillae, neck, inguinal areas and other body folds.

While most cases of AN are seen in obese and prepubertal children, it can occur as a marker for various endocrinopathies as well as in female patients with elevated testosterone levels, irregular menses, and hirsutism.

It is frequently a concomitant of an underlying malignant condition, principally an adenocarcinoma of the intestinal tract.

## Acneform lesions

Acneform eruptions are inflammatory follicular reactions that resemble acne vulgaris and that are manifested clinically as papules or pustules. They are monomorphic reactions, have a monomorphic appearance, and are found primarily on the upper parts of the body. Unlike acne vulgaris, there are rarely comedones present. Consider a drug-induced acneform eruption if:

- The onset is sudden
- There is a worsening of existing acne lesions
- The extent is considerable from the outset
- The appearance is monomorphic
- The localization is unusual for acne as, for example, when the distal extremities are involved
- The patient's age is unusual for regular acne
- There is an exposure to a potentially responsible drug.

The most common drugs responsible for acneform eruptions are: ACTH, androgenic hormones, anticonvulsants (hydantoin derivatives, phenobarbital, trimethadione), corticosteroids, danazol, disulfiram, halogens (bromides, chlorides, iodides), lithium, oral contraceptives, tuberculostatics (ethionamide, isoniazid, rifampin), vitamins $B_2$, $B_6$, and $B_{12}$.

## Acute generalized exanthematous pustulosis

Arising on the face or intertriginous areas, acute generalized exanthematous pustulosis (AGEP) is characterized by a rapidly evolving, widespread, scarlatiniform eruption covered with hundreds of small superficial pustules.

Often accompanied by a high fever, AGEP is most frequently associated with penicillin and macrolide antibiotics, and usually occurs within 24 hours of the drug exposure.

## Alopecia

Many drugs have been reported to occasion hair loss. Commonly appearing as a diffuse alopecia, it affects women more frequently than men and is limited in most instances to the scalp. Axillary and pubic hairs are rarely affected except with anticoagulants.

The hair loss from cytostatic agents, which is dose-dependent and begins about 2 weeks after the onset of therapy, is a result of the interruption of the anagen (growing) cycle of hair. With other drugs the hair loss does not begin until 2–5 months after the medication has been begun. With cholesterol-lowering drugs, diffuse alopecia is a result of interference with normal keratinization.

The scalp is normal and the drug-induced alopecia is almost always reversible within 1–3 months after the therapy has been discontinued. The regrown hair is frequently depigmented and occasionally more curly.

The most frequent offenders are cytostatic agents and anticoagulants, but hair loss can occur with a variety of common drugs, including hormones, anticonvulsants, amantadine, amiodarone, captopril, cholesterol-lowering drugs, cimetidine, colchicine, etretinate, isotretinoin, ketoconazole, heavy metals, lithium, penicillamine, valproic acid, and propranolol.

## Angioedema

Angioedema is a term applied to a variant of urticaria in which the subcutaneous tissues, rather than the dermis, are mainly involved.

Also known as Quincke's edema, giant urticaria, and angioneurotic edema, this acute, evanescent, skin-colored, circumscribed edema usually affects the most distensible tissues: the lips, eyelids, earlobes, and genitalia. It can also affect the mucous membranes of the tongue, mouth, and larynx.

Symptoms of angioedema, frequently unilateral, asymmetrical and non-pruritic, last for an hour or two but can persist for 2–5 days.

The etiological factors associated with angioedema are as varied as that of urticaria (which see).

## Aphthous stomatitis

Aphthous stomatitis – also known as canker sores – is a common disease of the oral mucous membranes.

Arising as tiny, discrete or grouped, papules or vesicles, these painful lesions develop into small (2–5 mm in diameter), round, shallow ulcerations having a grayish, yellow base surrounded by a thin red border.

Located predominantly over the labial and buccal mucosae, these aphthae heal without scarring in 10–14 days. Recurrences are common.

### Black hairy tongue (lingua villosa nigra)

Black hairy tongue (BHT) represents a benign hyperplasia of the filiform papillae of the anterior two-thirds of the tongue.

These papillary elongations, usually associated with black, brown, or yellow pigmentation attributed to the overgrowth of pigment-producing bacteria, may be as long as 2 cm.

Occurring only in adults, BHT has been associated with the administration of oral antibiotics, poor dental hygiene, and excessive smoking.

### Bullous eruptions

Bullous and vesicular drug eruptions are diseases in which blisters and vesicles occur as a complication of the administration of drugs. Blisters are a well-known manifestation of cutaneous reactions to drugs.

In many types of drug reactions, bullae and vesicles may be found in addition to other manifestations. Bullae are usually noted in erythema multiforme, Stevens–Johnson syndrome, toxic epidermal necrolysis, fixed eruptions when very intense, urticaria, vasculitis, porphyria cutanea tarda, and phototoxic reactions (from furosemide and nalidixic acid). Tense, thick-walled bullae can be seen in bromoderma and iododerma as well as in barbiturate overdosage.

Common drugs that cause bullous eruptions and bullous pemphigoid are: nadalol, penicillamine, piroxicam, psoralens, rifampin, clonidine, furosemide, diclofenac, mefenamic acid, bleomycin, and others.

### Erythema multiforme and Stevens–Johnson syndrome

Erythema multiforme is a relatively common, acute, self-limited, inflammatory reaction pattern that is often associated with a preceding herpes simplex or mycoplasma infection. Other causes are associated with connective tissue disease, physical agents, X-ray therapy, pregnancy and internal malignancies, to mention a few. In 50% of the cases, no cause can be found. In a recent prospective study of erythema multiforme, only 10% were drug related.

The eruption rapidly occurs over a period of 12 to 24 hours. In about half the cases there are prodromal symptoms of an upper respiratory infection accompanied by fever, malaise, and varying degrees of muscular and joint pains.

Clinically, bluish-red, well-demarcated, macular, papular, or urticarial lesions, as well as the classical 'iris' or 'target lesions', sometimes with central vesicles, bullae, or purpura, are distributed preferentially over the distal extremities, especially over the dorsa of the hands and extensor aspects of the forearms. Lesions tend to spread peripherally and may involve the palms and trunk as well as the mucous membranes of the mouth and genitalia. Central healing and overlapping lesions often lead to arciform, annular and gyrate patterns. Lesions appear over the course of a week or 10 days and resolve over the next 2 weeks.

The Stevens–Johnson syndrome (erythema multiforme major), a severe and occasionally fatal variety of erythema multiforme, has an abrupt onset and is accompanied by any or all of the following: fever, myalgia, malaise, headache, arthralgia, ocular involvement, with occasional bullae and erosions covering less than 10% of the body surface. Painful stomatitis is an early and conspicuous symptom. Hemorrhagic bullae may appear over the lips, mouth and genital mucous membranes. Patients are often acutely ill with high fever. The course from eruption to the healing of the lesions may extend up to 6 weeks.

The following drugs have been most often associated with erythema multiforme and Stevens–Johnson syndrome: allopurinol, lamotrigine phenytoin, barbiturates, carbamazepine, estrogens/progestins, gold, NSAIDs, penicillamine, sulfonamides, tetracycline, and tolbutamide.

### Erythema nodosum

Erythema nodosum is a cutaneous reaction pattern characterized by erythematous, tender or painful subcutaneous nodules commonly distributed over the anterior aspect of the lower legs, and occasionally elsewhere.

More common in young women, erythema nodosum is often associated with increased estrogen levels as occurs during pregnancy and with the ingestion of oral contraceptives. It is also an occasional manifestation of streptococcal infection, sarcoidosis, secondary syphilis, tuberculosis, certain deep fungal infections, Hodgkin's disease, leukemia, ulcerative colitis, and radiation therapy and is often preceded by fever, fatigue, arthralgia, vomiting, and diarrhea.

The incidence of erythema nodosum due to drugs is low and it is impossible to distinguish clinically between erythema nodosum due to drugs and that caused by other factors.

Some of the drugs that are known to occasion erythema nodosum are: antibiotics, estrogens, amiodarone, gold, NSAIDs, oral contraceptives, sulfonamides, and opiates.

### Exanthems

Exanthems, commonly resembling viral rashes, represent the most common type of cutaneous drug eruption. Described as maculopapular or morbilliform eruptions, these flat, barely raised, erythematous patches, from one to several millimeters in diameter, are usually bilateral and symmetrical. They commonly begin on the head and neck or upper torso and progress downward to the limbs. They may present or develop into confluent areas and may be accompanied by pruritus and a mild fever.

The exanthems caused by drugs can be classified as either:

- Morbilliform eruptions: fingernail-sized erythematous patches
- Scarlatiniform eruptions: punctate, pinpoint, or pinhead-sized lesions in erythematous areas that have a tendency to coalesce. Circumoral pallor and the subsequent appearance of scaling may also be noted.

Maculopapular drug eruptions usually fade with desquamation and, occasionally, postinflammatory hyperpigmentation, in about 2 weeks. They invariably recur on rechallenge.

Exanthems often have a sudden onset during the first 2 weeks of administration, except for semisynthetic penicillins that frequently develop after the first 2 weeks following the initial dose.

The drugs most commonly associated with exanthems are: amoxicillin, ampicillin, bleomycin, captopril, carbamazepine, chlorpromazine, co-trimoxazole, gold, nalidixic acid, naproxen, phenytoin, penicillamine, and piroxicam.

### Exfoliative dermatitis

Exfoliative dermatitis is a rare but serious reaction pattern that is characterized by erythema, pruritus and scaling over the entire body (erythroderma).

Drug-induced exfoliative dermatitis usually begins a few weeks or longer following the administration of a culpable drug. Beginning as erythematous, edematous patches, often on the face, it spreads to involve the entire integument. The skin becomes swollen and scarlet and may ooze a straw-colored fluid; this is followed in a few days by desquamation.

High fever, severe malaise and chills, along with enlargement of lymph nodes, often coexist with the cutaneous changes.

One of the most dangerous of all reaction patterns, exfoliative dermatitis can be accompanied by any or all of the following: hypothermia, fluid and electrolyte loss, cardiac failure, and gastrointestinal hemorrhage. Death may supervene if the drug is continued after the onset of the eruption. Secondary infection often complicates the course of the disease. Once the active dermatitis has receded, hyperpigmentation as well as loss of hair and nails may ensue. The following drugs, among others, can bring about exfoliative dermatitis: barbiturates, captopril, carbamazepine, cimetidine, furosemide, gold, isoniazid, lithium, nitrofurantoin, NSAIDs, penicillamine, phenytoin, pyrazolons, quinidine, streptomycin, sulfonamides, and thiazides.

### Fixed eruptions

A fixed eruption is an unusual hypersensitivity reaction characterized by one or more well demarcated erythematous plaques that recur at the same cutaneous (or mucosal) site or sites each time exposure to the offending agent occurs. The sizes of the lesions vary from a few millimeters to as much as 20 centimeters in diameter. Almost any drug that is ingested, injected, inhaled, or inserted into the body can trigger this skin reaction.

The eruption typically begins as a sharply marginated, solitary edematous papule or plaque – occasionally surmounted by a large bulla – which usually develops 30 minutes to 8 hours following the administration of a drug. If the offending agent is not promptly eliminated, the inflammation intensifies, producing a dusky red, violaceous or brown patch that may crust, desquamate, or blister within 7 to 10 days. The lesions are rarely pruritic. Favored sites are the hands, feet, face, and genitalia – especially the glans penis.

The reason for the specific localization of the skin lesions in a fixed drug eruption is unknown. The offending drug cannot be detected at the skin site. Certain drugs cause a fixed eruption at specific sites, for example, tetracycline and ampicillin often elicit a fixed eruption on the penis, whereas aspirin usually causes skin lesions on the face, limbs and trunk.

Common causes of fixed eruptions are: ampicillin, aspirin, barbiturates, dapsone, metronidazole, NSAIDs, oral contraceptives, phenolphthalein, phenytoin, quinine, sulfonamides, and tetracyclines.

### Gingival hyperplasia

Gingival hyperplasia, a common, undesirable, non-allergic drug reaction begins as a diffuse swelling of the interdental papillae.

Particularly prevalent with phenytoin therapy, gingival hyperplasia begins about 3 months after the onset of therapy, and occurs in 30 to 70% of patients receiving it. The severity of the reaction is dose-dependent and children and young adults are more frequently affected. The most severe cases are noted in young women.

In many cases, gingival hyperplasia is accompanied by painful and bleeding gums. There is often superimposed secondary bacterial gingivitis. This can be so extensive that the teeth of the maxilla and mandible are completely overgrown.

While it is characteristically a side effect of hydantoin derivatives, it may occur during the administration of phenobarbital, nifedipine, diltiazem and other medications.

### Lichenoid (lichen planus-like) eruptions

Lichenoid eruptions are so called because of their resemblance to lichen planus, a papulosquamous disorder that characteristically presents as multiple, discrete, violaceous, flat-topped papules, often polygonal in shape and which are extremely pruritic.

Not infrequently, lichenoid lesions appear weeks or months following exposure to the responsible drug. As a rule, the symptoms begin to recede a few weeks following the discontinuation of the drug.

Common drug causes of lichenoid eruptions are: antimalarials, beta-blockers, chlorpropamide, furosemide, gold, methyldopa, phenothiazines, quinidine, thiazides, and tolazamide.

### Lupus erythematosus

A reaction, clinically and pathologically resembling idiopathic systemic lupus erythematosus (SLE), has been reported in association with a large variety of drugs. There is some evidence that drug-induced SLE, invariably accompanied by a positive ANA reaction with 90% having antihistone antibodies, may have a genetically determined basis. These symptoms of SLE, a relatively benign form of lupus, recede within days or weeks following the discontinuation of the responsible drug. Skin lesions occur in about 20% of cases. Drugs cause fewer than 8% of all cases of systemic LE.

The following drugs have been commonly associated with inducing, aggravating or unmasking SLE: beta-blockers, carbamazepine, chlorpromazine, estrogens, griseofulvin, hydralazine, isoniazid (INH), lithium, methyldopa, minoxidil, oral contraceptives, penicillamine, phenytoin (diphenylhydantoin), procainamide, propylthiouracil, quinidine, and testosterone.

### Neuroleptic Malignant Syndrome (NMS)

NMS is a rare, potentially life-threatening neuroleptic-induced movement disorder characterized by fever, muscular rigidity, altered mental status, and autonomic dysfunction.

NMS is a result of complex neurochemical changes induced by neuroleptics, particularly haloperidol and trifluoperazine – during the initial stages of treatment.

Diagnostic criteria for NMS include administration of neuroleptics; hyperthermia (>38°C) (in 100% of patients); extreme muscle rigidity (90%), described as 'lead-pipe', is a core feature of NMS; and diaphoresis (60%). Other signs and symptoms include mental status change, tremor, tachycardia, incontinence, labile blood pressure, metabolic acidosis, CPK elevation, sialorrhea, and leukocytosis.

Almost all classes of drugs, primarily antipsychotics that induce dopamine-2 receptor blockade – dopamine agonists and levodopa – have been associated with NMS.

### Onycholysis

Onycholysis, the painless separation of the nail plate from the nail bed, is one of the most common nail disorders.

The unattached portion, which is white and opaque, usually begins at the free margin and proceeds proximally, causing part or most of the nail plate to become separated. The attached, healthy portion of the nail, by contrast, is pink and translucent.

### Pemphigus vulgaris

Pemphigus vulgaris (PV) is a rare, serious, acute or chronic, blistering disease involving the skin and mucous membranes.

Characterized by thin-walled, easily ruptured, flaccid bullae that are seen to arise on normal or erythematous skin and over mucous membranes, the lesions of PV appear initially in the mouth (in about 60% of the cases) and then spread, after weeks or months, to involve the axillae and groin, the scalp, face and neck. The lesions may become generalized.

Because of their fragile roofs, the bullae rupture leaving painful erosions and crusts may develop principally over the scalp.

### Photosensitivity

A photosensitive reaction is a chemically induced change in the skin that makes an individual unusually sensitive to electromagnetic radiation (light). On absorbing light of a specific wavelength, an oral, injected or topical drug may be chemically altered to produce a reaction ranging from macules and papules, vesicles and bullae, edema, urticaria, or an acute eczematous reaction.

Any eruption that is prominent on the face, the dorsa of the hands, the 'V' of the neck, and the presternal area should suggest an adverse reaction to light. The distribution is the key to the diagnosis.

Initially the eruption, which consists of erythema, edema, blisters, weeping and desquamation, involves the forehead, rims of the ears, the nose, the malar eminences and cheeks, the sides and back of the neck, the extensor surfaces of the forearms and the dorsa of the hands. These reactions commonly spare the shaded areas: those under the chin, under the nose, behind the ears and inside the fold of the upper eyelids. There is usually a sharp cut-off at the site of jewelry and at clothing margins. All light-exposed areas need not be affected equally.

There are two main types of photosensitive reactions: the phototoxic and the photoallergic reaction.

Phototoxic reactions, the most common type of drug-induced photosensitivity, resemble an exaggerated sunburn and occur within 5 to 20 hours after the skin has been exposed to a photosensitizing substance and light of the proper wavelength and intensity. It is not a form of allergy – prior sensitization is not required – and, theoretically, could occur in anyone given enough drug and light. Phototoxic reactions are dose-dependent both for drug and sunlight. Patients with phototoxicity reactions are commonly sensitive to ultraviolet A (UVA radiation), the so-called 'tanning rays' at 320–400 nm. Phototoxic reactions may cause onycholysis, as the nailbed is particularly susceptible because of its lack of melanin protection.

Patients with a true photoallergy (the interaction of drug, light and the immune system), a less common form of drug-induced photosensitivity, are often sensitive to UVB radiation, the so-called 'burning rays' at 290–320 nm. Photoallergic reactions, unlike phototoxic responses, represent an immunologic change and require a latent period of from 24 to 48 hours during which sensitization occurs. They are not dose-related.

If the photosensitizer acts internally, it is a photodrug reaction; if it acts externally, it is photocontact dermatitis.

Drugs that are likely to cause phototoxic reactions are: amiodarone, nalidixic acid, various NSAIDs, phenothiazines (especially chlorpromazine), and tetracyclines (particularly demeclocycline).

Photoallergic reactions may occur as a result of exposure to systemically-administered drugs such as griseofulvin, NSAIDs, phenothiazines, quinidine, sulfonamides, sulfonylureas, and thiazide diuretics as well as to external agents such as para-aminobenzoic acid (found in sunscreens), bithionol (used in soaps and cosmetics), paraphenylenediamine, and others.

## Pigmentation

Drug-induced pigmentation on the skin, hair, nails, and mucous membranes is a result of either melanin synthesis, increased lipofuscin synthesis, or post-inflammatory pigmentation.

Color changes, which can be localized or widespread, can also be a result of a deposition of bile pigments (jaundice), exogenous metal compounds, and direct deposition of elements such as carotene or quinacrine.

Post-inflammatory pigmentation can follow a variety of drug-induced inflammatory cutaneous reactions; fixed eruptions are known to leave a residual pigmentation that can persist for months.

The following is a partial list of those drugs that can cause various pigmentary changes: anticonvulsants, antimalarials, cytostatics, hormones, metals, tetracyclines, phenothiazine tranquilizers, psoralens, amiodarone, etc.

## Pityriasis rosea-like eruptions

Pityriasis rosea, commonly mistaken for ringworm, is a unique disorder that usually begins as a single, large, round or oval pinkish patch known as the 'mother' or 'herald' patch. The most common sites for this solitary lesion are the chest, the back, or the abdomen. This is followed in about 2 weeks by a blossoming of small, flat, round or oval, scaly patches of similar color, each with a central collarette scale, usually distributed in a Christmas tree pattern over the trunk and, to a lesser degree, the extremities. This eruption seldom itches and usually limits itself to areas from the neck to the knees.

While the etiology of idiopathic pityriasis rosea is unknown, we do know that various medications have been reported to give rise to this friendly disorder. These are: barbiturates, beta-blockers, bismuth, captopril, clonidine, gold, griseofulvin, isotretinoin, labetalol, meprobamate, metronidazole, penicillin, and tripelennamine.

In drug-induced pityriasis rosea, the 'herald patch' is usually absent, and the eruption will often not follow the classic pattern.

## Pruritus

Generalized itching, without any visible signs, is one of the least common adverse reactions to drugs. More frequently than not, drug-induced itching – moderate or severe – is fairly generalized.

For most drugs it is not known in what way they elicit pruritus; some drugs can cause itching directly or indirectly through cholestasis. Pruritus may develop by different pathogenetic mechanisms: allergic, pseudoallergic (histamine release), neurogenic, by vasodilatation, cholestatic effect, and others.

A partial list of those drugs that can cause pruritus are as follows: aspirin, NSAIDs, penicillins, sulfonamides, chloroquine, ACE inhibitors, amiodarone, nicotinic acid derivatives, lithium, bleomycin, tamoxifen, interferons, gold, penicillamine, methoxsalen, isotretinoin, etc.

## Psoriasis

Many drugs, as a result of their pharmacological action, have been implicated in the precipitation or exacerbation of psoriasis or psoriasiform eruptions.

Psoriasis is a common, chronic, papulosquamous disorder of unknown etiology with characteristic histopathological features and many biochemical, physiological, and immunological abnormalities.

Drugs that can precipitate psoriasis are, among others, beta-blockers and lithium. Drugs that are reported to aggravate psoriasis are antimalarials, beta-blockers, lithium, NSAIDs, quinidine, and photosensitizing drugs. The effect and extent of these drug-induced psoriatic eruptions are dose-dependent.

## Purpura

Purpura, a result of hemorrhage into the skin, can be divided into thrombocytopenic purpura and non-thrombocytopenic purpura (vascular purpura). Both thrombocytopenic and vascular purpura may be due to drugs, and most of the drugs producing purpura may do so by giving rise to vascular damage and thrombocytopenia. In both types of purpura, allergic or toxic (nonallergic) mechanisms may be involved.

Some drugs combine with platelets to form an antigen, stimulating formation of antibody to the platelet–drug combination. Thus, the drug appears to act as a hapten; subsequent antigen–antibody reaction causes platelet destruction leading to thrombocytopenia.

The purpuric lesions are usually more marked over the lower portions of the body, notably the legs and dorsal aspects of the feet in ambulatory patients.

Other drug-induced cutaneous reactions – erythema multiforme, erythema nodosum, fixed eruption, necrotizing vasculitis, and others – can have a prominent purpuric component.

A whole host of drugs can give rise to purpura, the most common being: NSAIDs, thiazide diuretics, phenothiazines, cytostatics, gold, penicillamine, hydantoins, thiouracils, and sulfonamides.

### Raynaud's phenomenon

Raynaud's phenomenon is the paroxysmal, cold-induced constriction of small arteries and arterioles of the fingers and, less often, the toes.

Occurring more frequently in women, Raynaud's phenomenon is characterized by blanching, pallor, and cyanosis. In severe cases, secondary changes may occur: thinning and ridging of the nails, telangiectases of the nail folds, and, in the later stages, sclerosis and atrophy of the digits.

### Rhabdomyolysis

Rhabdomyolysis is the breakdown of muscle fibers, the result of skeletal muscle injury, that leads to the release of potentially toxic intracellular contents into the plasma. The causes are diverse: muscle trauma from vigorous exercise, electrolyte imbalance, extensive thermal burns, crush injuries, infections, various toxins and drugs, and a host of other factors.

Rhabdomyolysis can result from direct muscle injury by myotoxic drugs such as cocaine, heroin and alcohol. About 10 to 40 percent of patients with rhabdomyolysis develop acute renal failure.

The classic triad of symptoms of rhabdomyolysis is muscle pain, weakness and dark urine. Most frequently, the involved muscle groups are those of the back and lower calves. The primary diagnostic indicator of this syndrome is significantly elevated serum creatine phosphokinase.

Some of the drugs that have been reported to cause rhabdomyolysis are salicylates, amphotericin, quinine, statin drugs, SSRIs, theophylline, amphetamines, and others.

### Toxic epidermal necrolysis (TEN)

Also known as Lyell's syndrome, toxic epidermal necrolysis is a rare, serious, acute exfoliative, bullous eruption of the skin and mucous membranes that usually develops as a reaction to diverse drugs. TEN can also be a result of a bacterial or viral infection and can develop after radiation therapy or vaccinations.

In the drug-induced form of TEN, a morbilliform eruption accompanied by large red, tender areas of the skin will develop shortly after the drug has been administered. This progresses rapidly to blistering, and a widespread exfoliation of the epidermis develops dramatically over a very short period accompanied by high fever. The hairy parts of the body are usually spared. The mucous membranes and eyes are often involved.

The clinical picture resembles an extensive second-degree burn; the patient is acutely ill. Fatigue, vomiting, diarrhea and angina are prodromal symptoms. In a few hours the condition becomes grave.

TEN is a medical emergency and unless the offending agent is discontinued immediately, the outcome may be fatal in the course of a few days.

Drugs that are the most common cause of TEN are: allopurinol, ampicillin, amoxicillin, carbamazepine, NSAIDs, phenobarbital, pentamidine, phenytoin (diphenylhydantoin), pyrazolones, and sulfonamides.

### Urticaria

Urticaria induced by drugs is, after exanthems, the second most common type of drug reaction. Urticaria, or hives, is a vascular reaction of the skin characterized by pruritic, erythematous wheals. These welts – or wheals – caused by localized edema, can vary in size from one millimeter in diameter to large palm-sized swellings, favor the covered areas (trunk, buttocks, chest), and are, more often than not, generalized. Urticaria usually develops within 36 hours following the administration of the responsible drug. Individual lesions rarely persist for more than 24 hours.

Urticaria may be the only symptom of drug sensitivity, or it may be a concomitant or followed by the manifestations of serum sickness. Urticaria may be accompanied by angioedema of the lips or eyelids. It may, on rare occasions, progress to anaphylactoid reactions or to anaphylaxis.

The following are the most common causes of drug-induced urticaria: antibiotics, notably penicillin (more commonly following parenteral administration than by ingestion), barbiturates, captopril, levamisole, NSAIDs, quinine, rifampin, sulfonamides, thiopental, and vancomycin.

### Vasculitis

Drug-induced cutaneous necrotizing vasculitis, a clinicopathologic process characterized by inflammation and necrosis of blood vessels, often presents with a variety of small, palpable purpuric lesions most frequently distributed over the lower extremities: urticaria-like lesions, small ulcerations, and occasional hemorrhagic vesicles and pustules. The basic process involves an immunologically mediated response to antigens that result in vessel wall damage.

Beginning as small macules and papules, they ultimately eventuate into purpuric lesions and, in the more severe cases, into hemorrhagic blisters and frank ulcerations. A polymorphonuclear infiltrate and fibrinoid changes in the small dermal vessels characterize the vasculitic reaction.

Drugs that are commonly associated with vasculitis are: ACE inhibitors, amiodarone, ampicillin, cimetidine, coumadin, furosemide, hydantoins, hydralazine, NSAIDs, pyrazolons, quinidine, sulfonamides, thiazides, and thiouracils.

## Xerostomia

Xerostomia is a dryness of the oral cavity that makes speaking, chewing and swallowing difficult.

Resulting from a partial or complete absence of saliva production, xerostomia can be caused by a variety of medications.

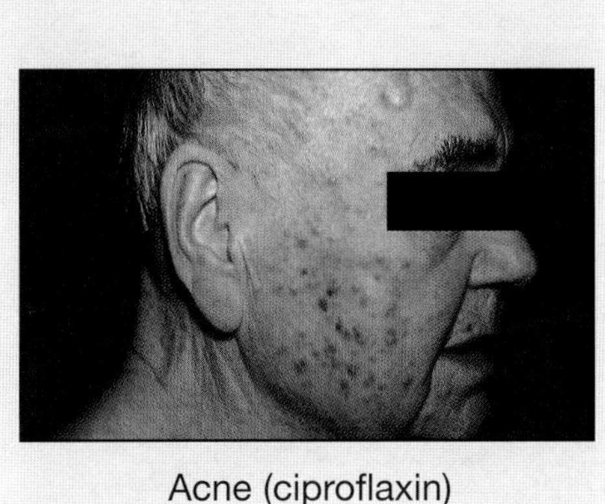

Acne (ciproflaxin)

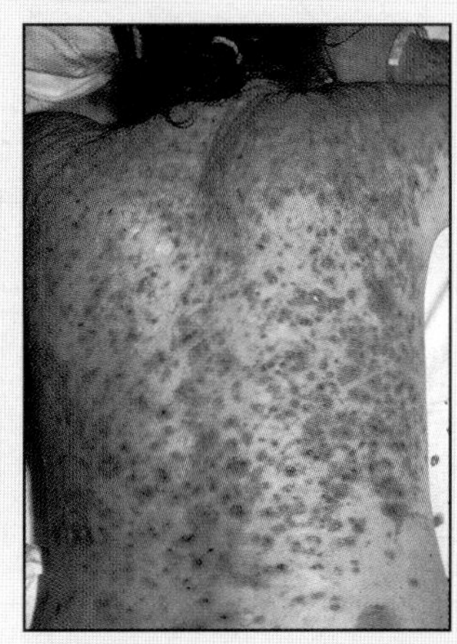

Acne fulminans

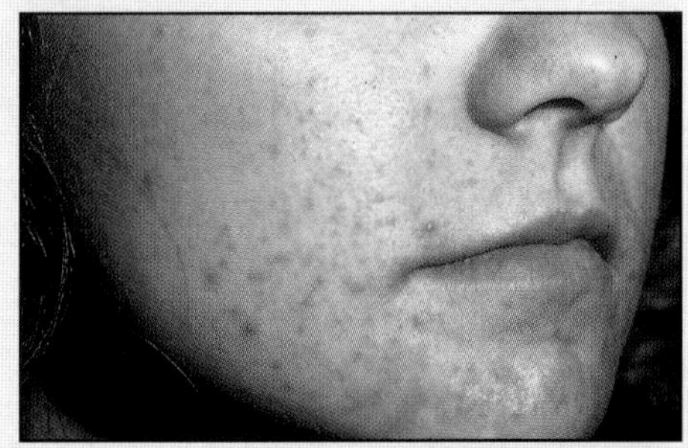

Acne (systemic corticosteroids)

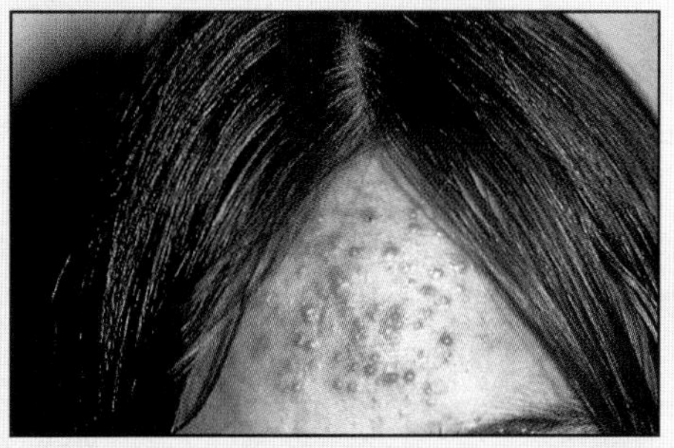

Acne (iodine)

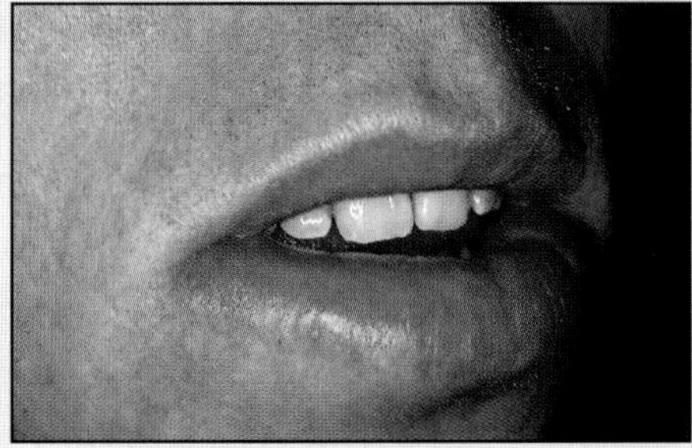

Angioedema

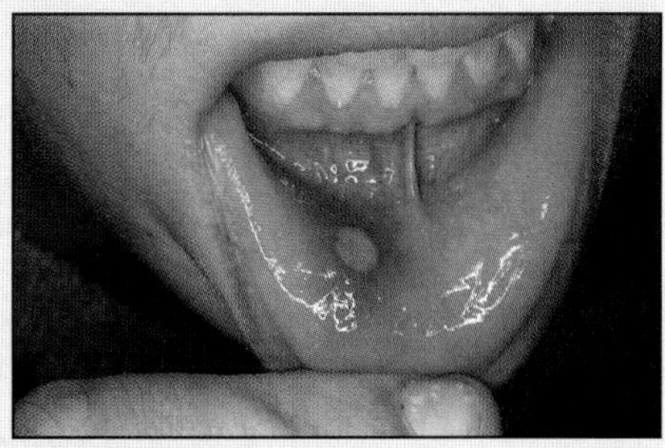

Aphthous stomatitis

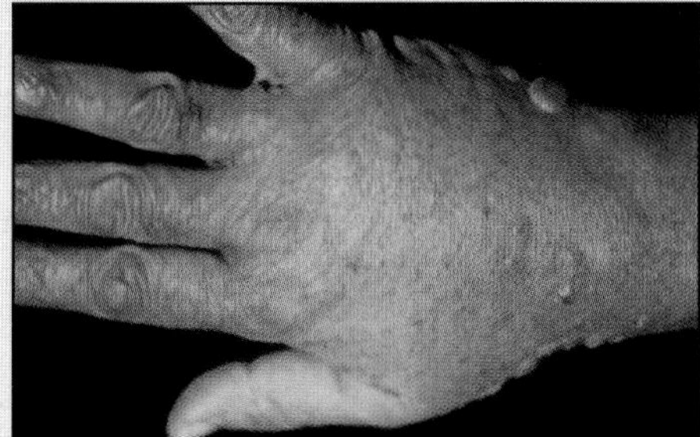

Bullous pemphigoid

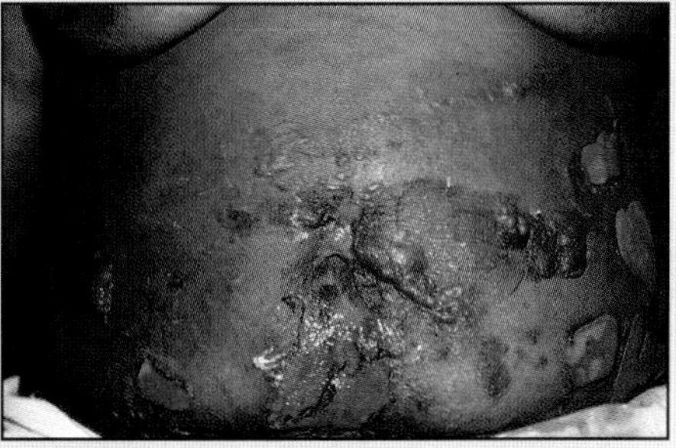

Bullous pemphigoid

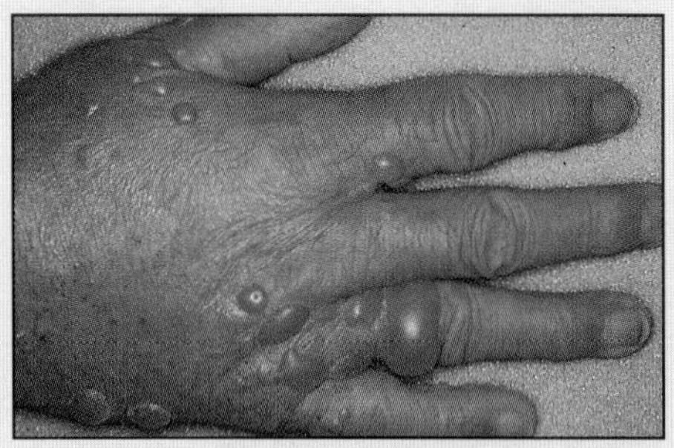

Bullous pemphigoid

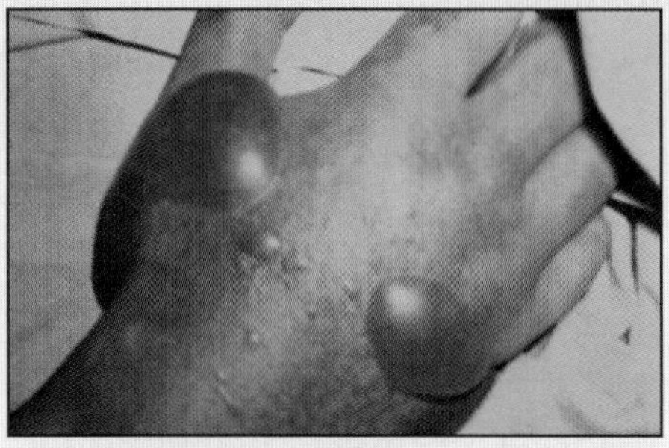

Bullous drug eruption

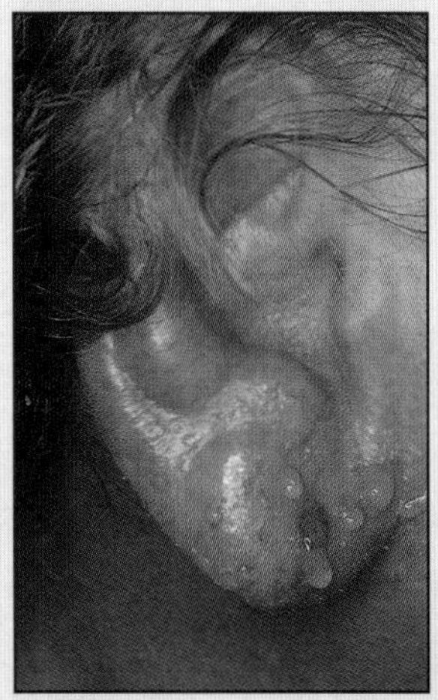

Contact (neomycin)

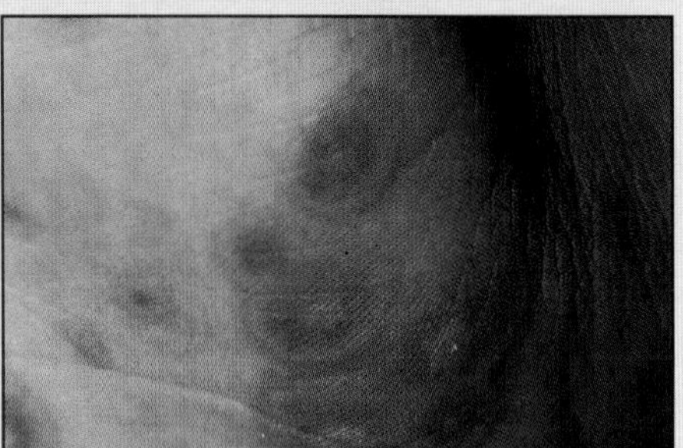

Erythema multiforme

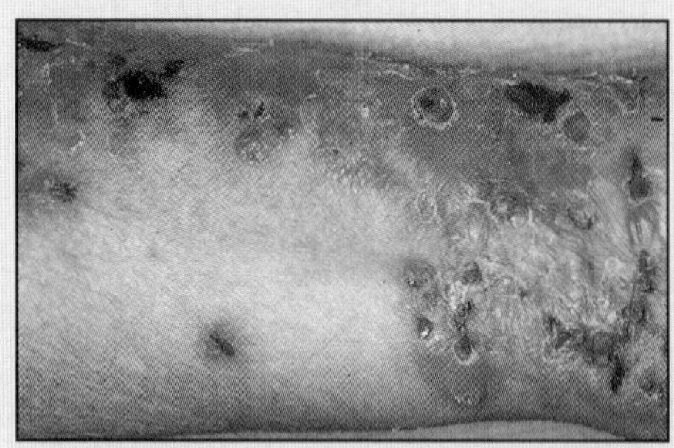

Bullous pemphigoid

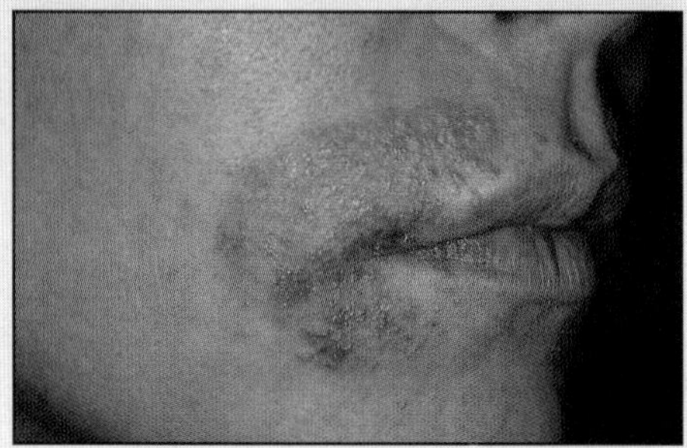

Contact (mycolog cream)

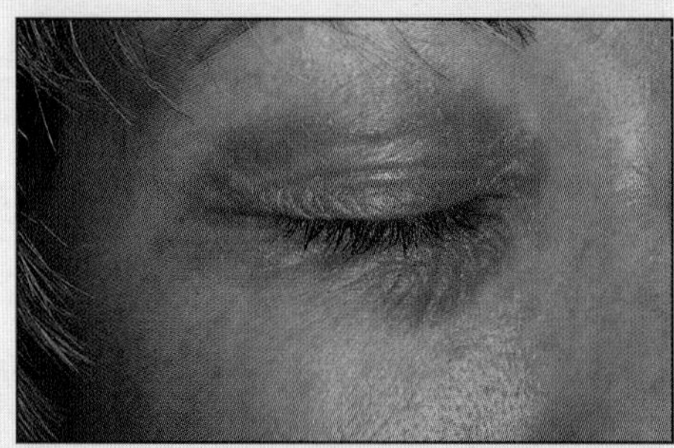

Contact (vitamin E cream)

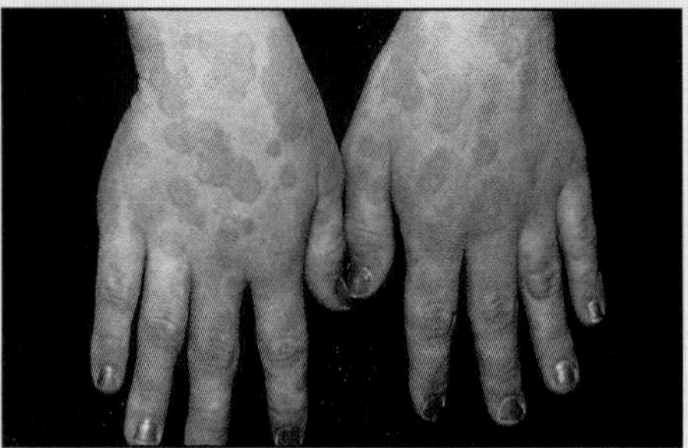

Erythema multiforme

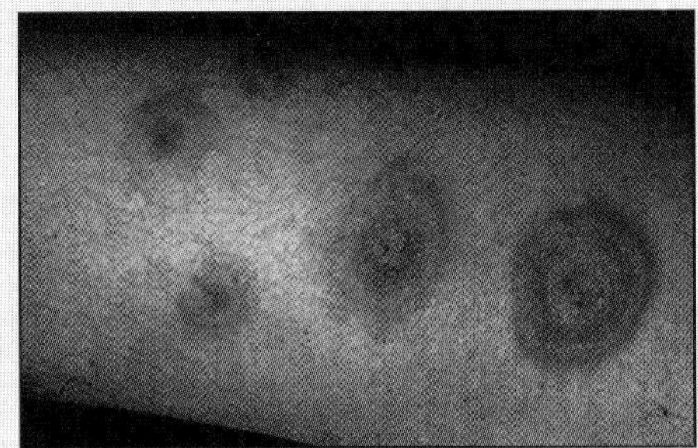
Erythema multiforme

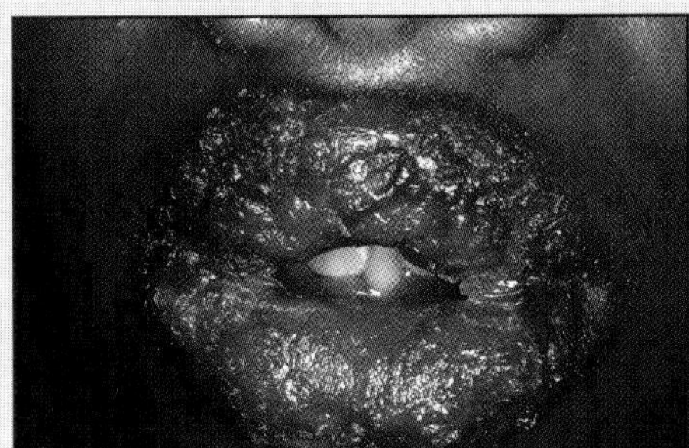
Erythema multiforme

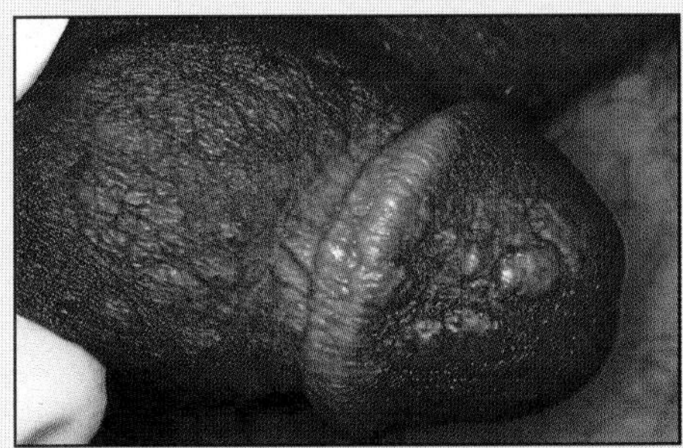
Erythema multiforme

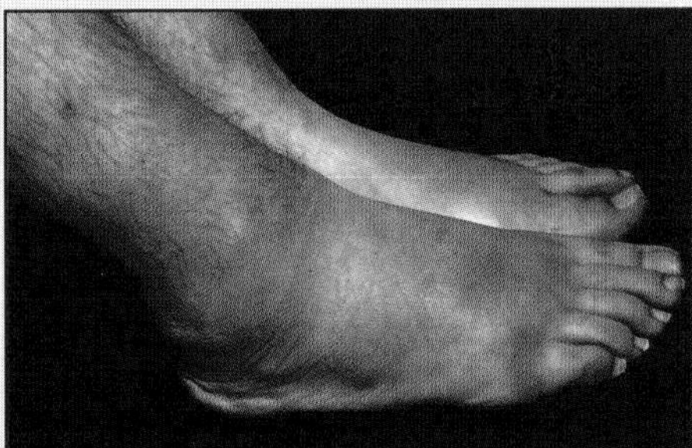
Erythema nodosum

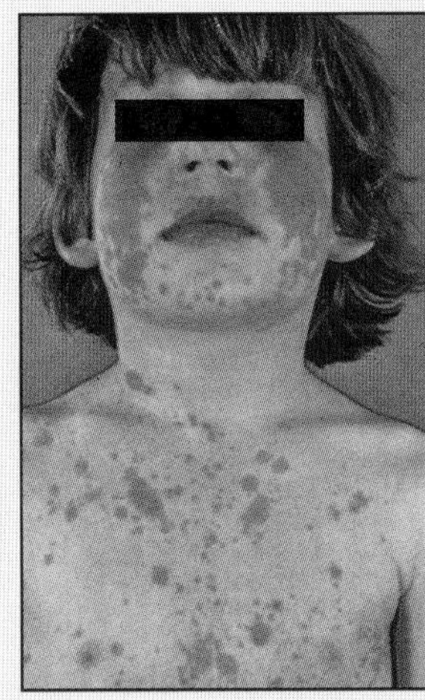
Erythema multiforme

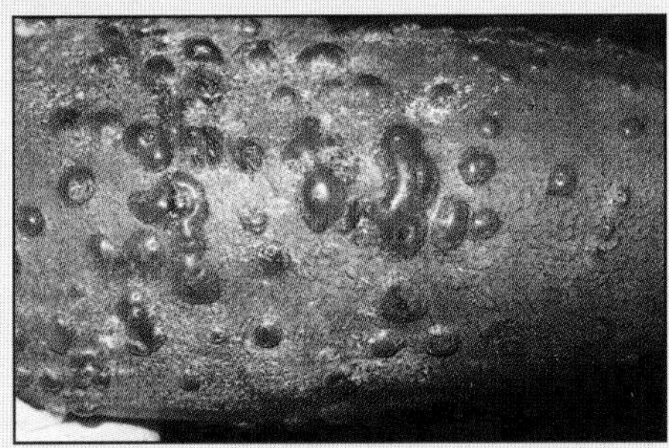
Erythema multiforme

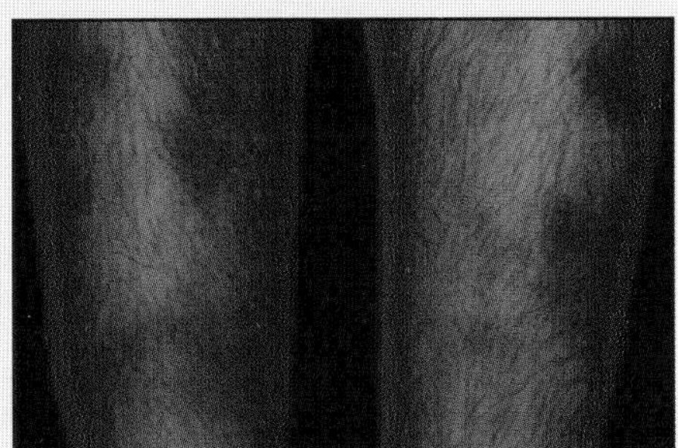
Erythema nodosum

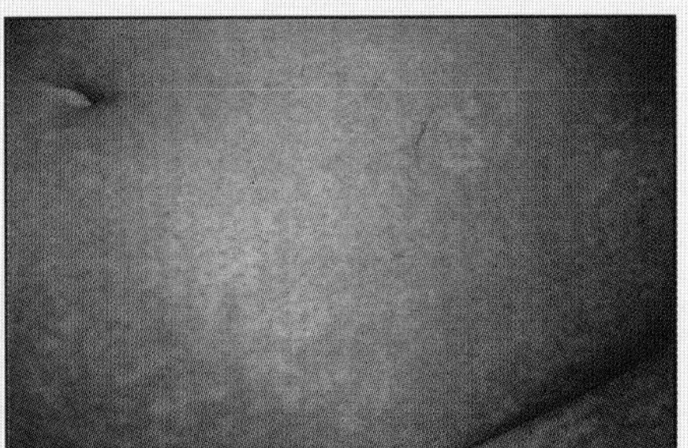
Erythroderma

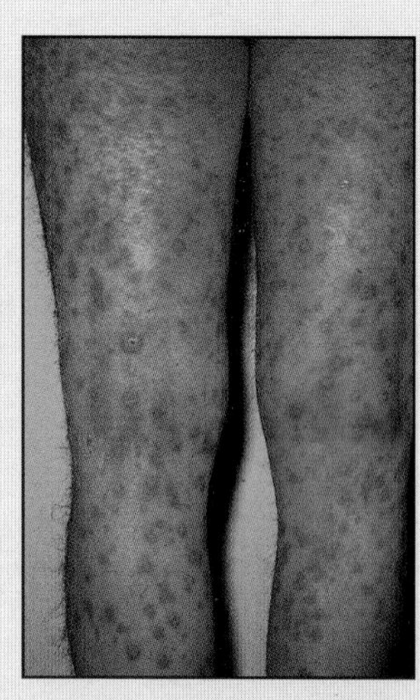

Exanthems (phenobarbital)

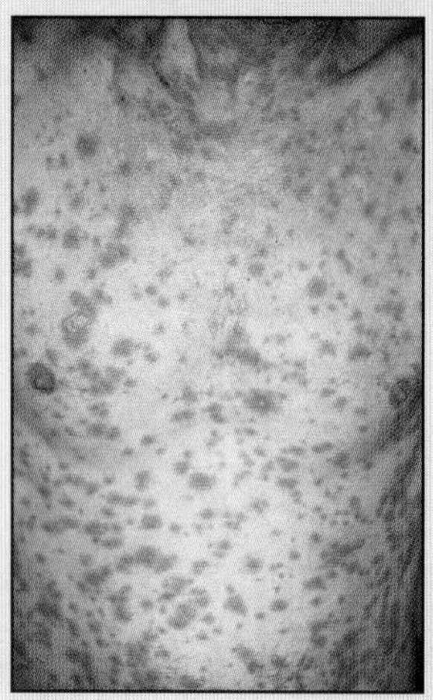

Exanthems (griseofulvin)

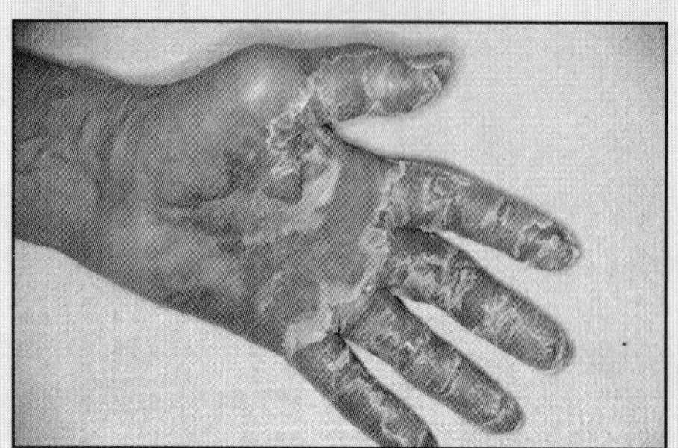

Exfoliative dermatitis

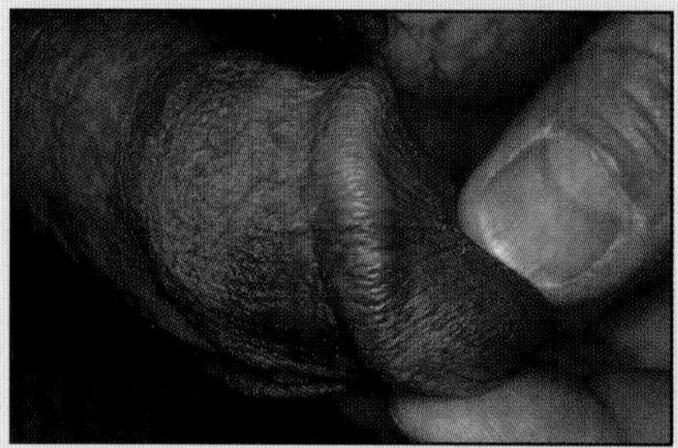

Fixed eruption

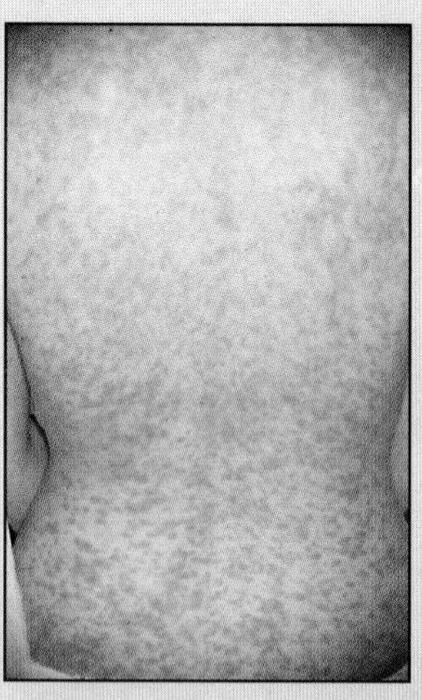

Exanthems (ampicillin)

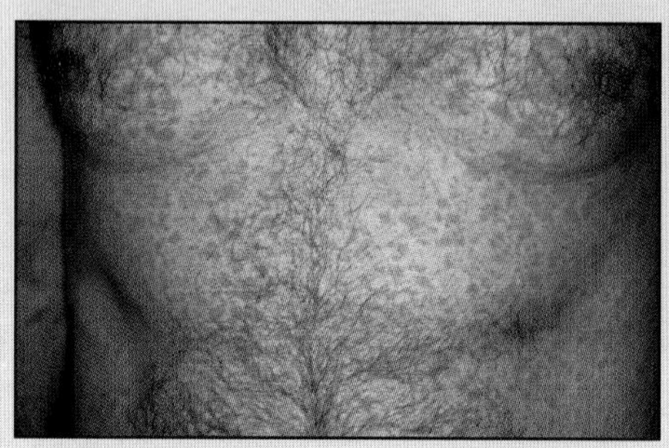

Exanthems (cotrimoxazole)

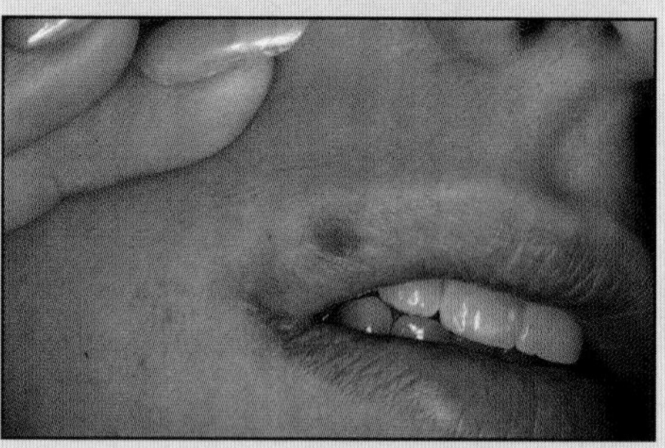

Fixed eruption

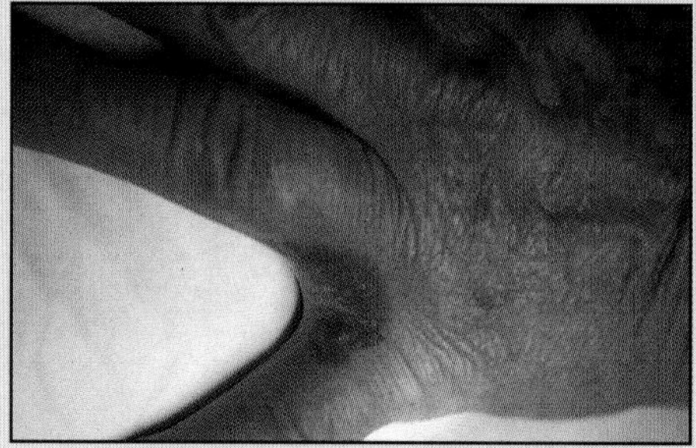

Fixed eruption

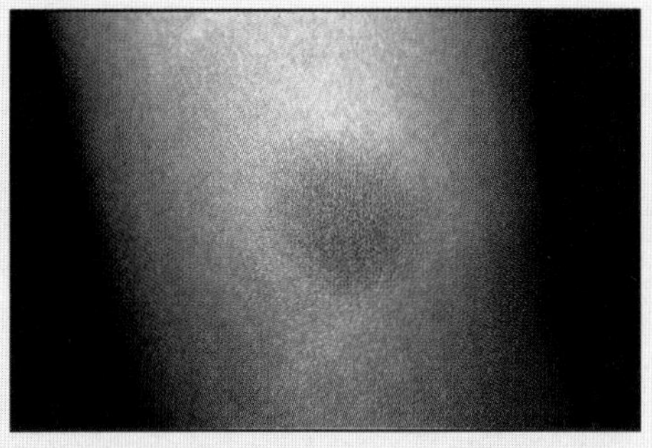

Fixed eruption (cyclophosphamide)

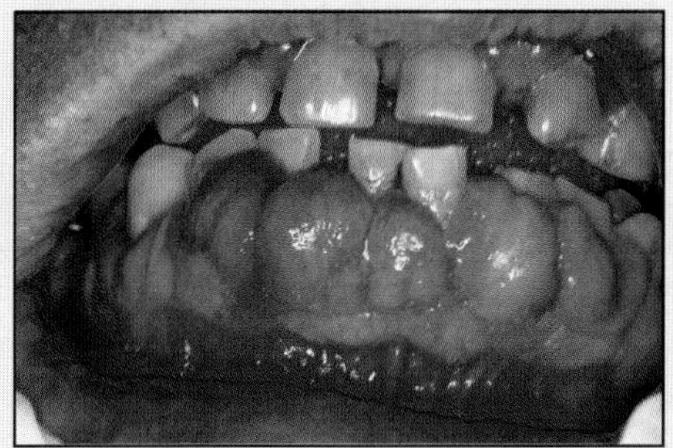

Gingival hyperplasia (verapamil)

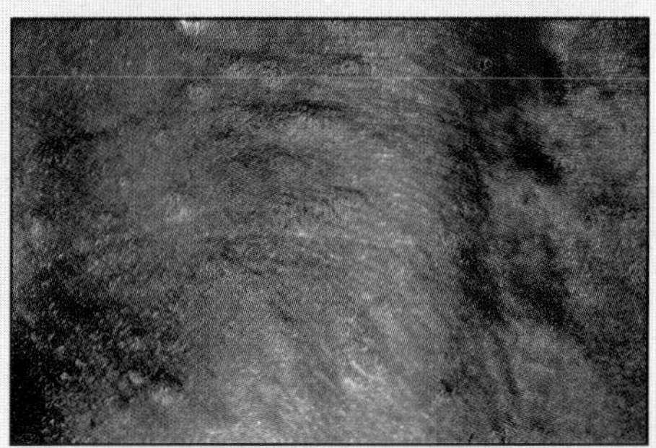

Lichenoid eruption

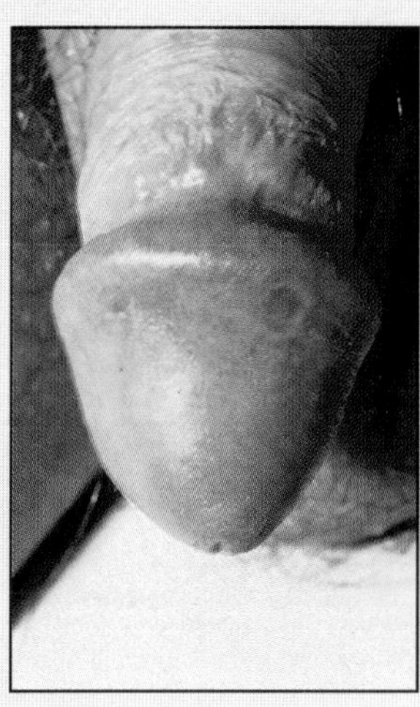

Lichen planus

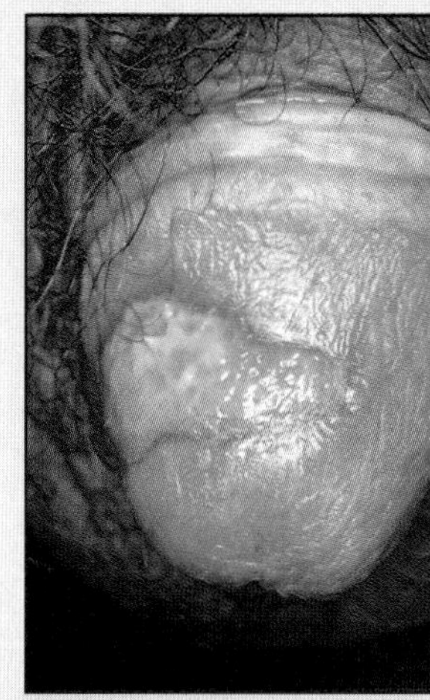

Fixed eruption

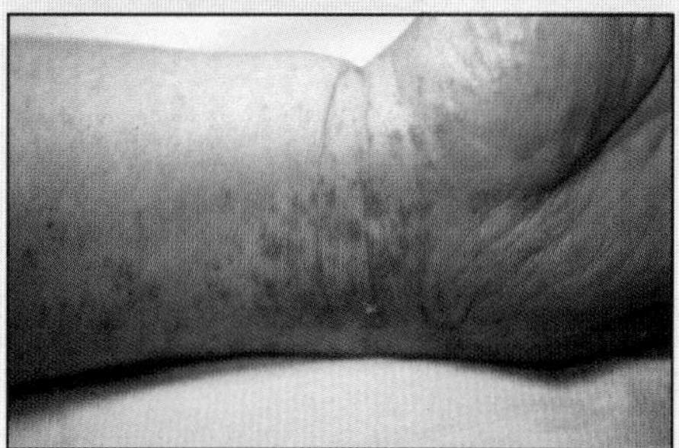

Lichenoid eruption

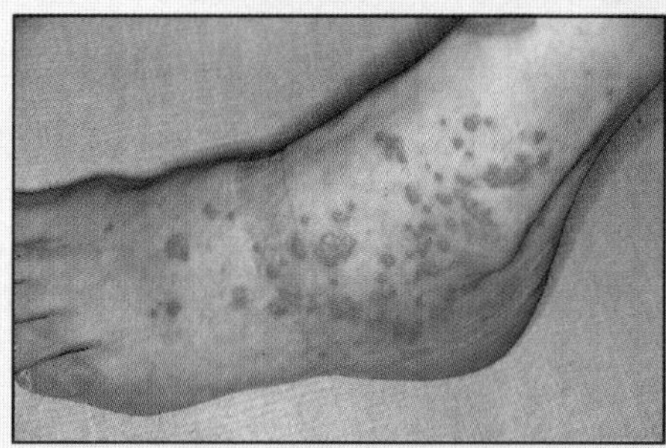

Lichenoid planus

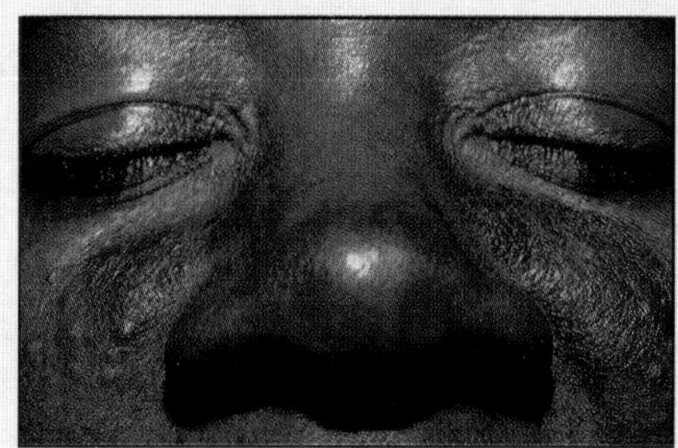

Lupus erythematosus

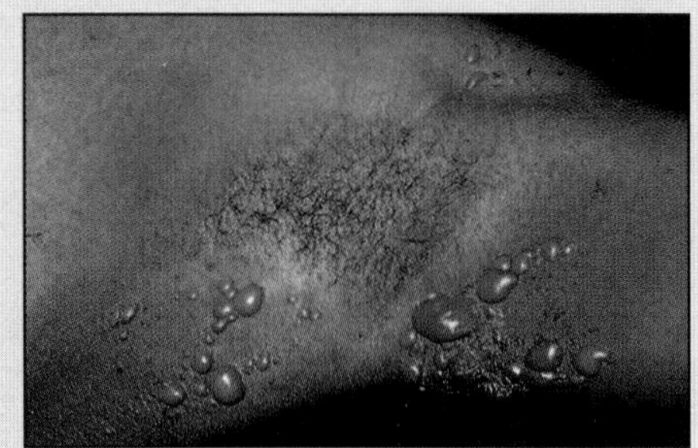

Bullous lupus erythematosus

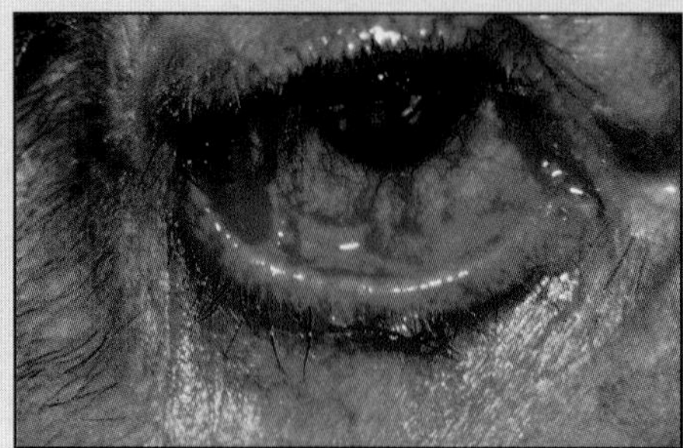

Cicatrical pemphigoid

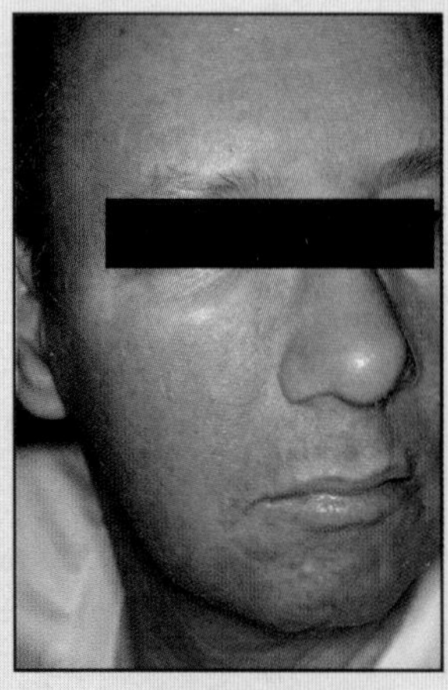

Photosensitivity

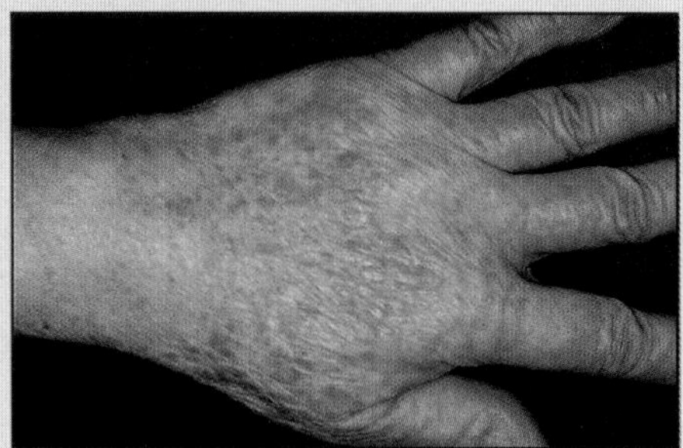

Photosensitivity (lichenoid)

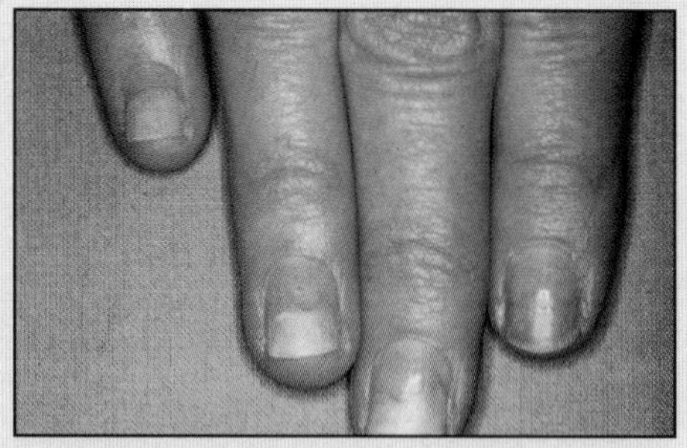

Photo-onycholysis (tetracycline)

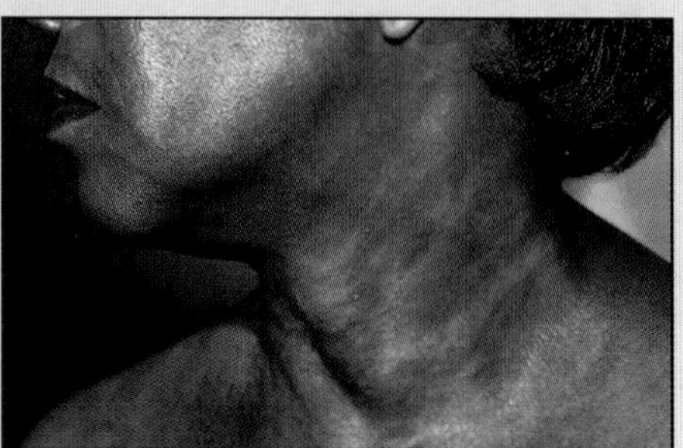

Photocontact dermatitis

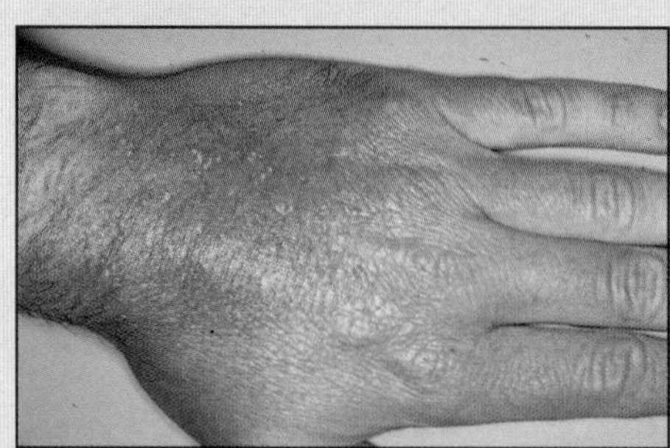

Photosensitivity

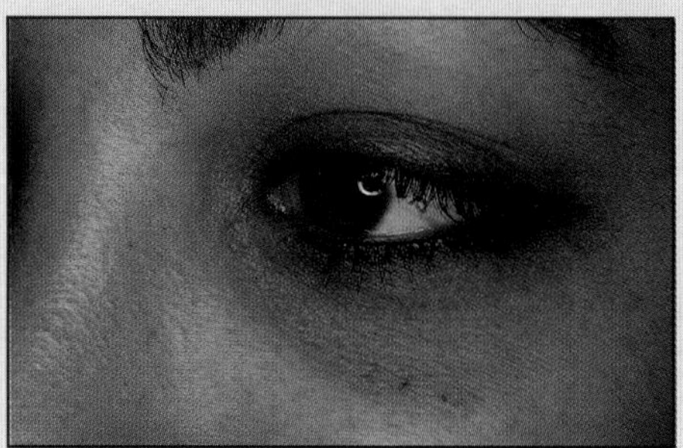

Pigmentation

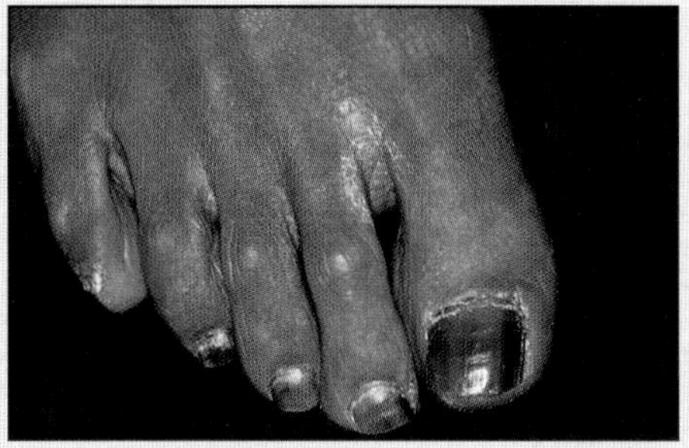
Pigmentation (zidovudine)

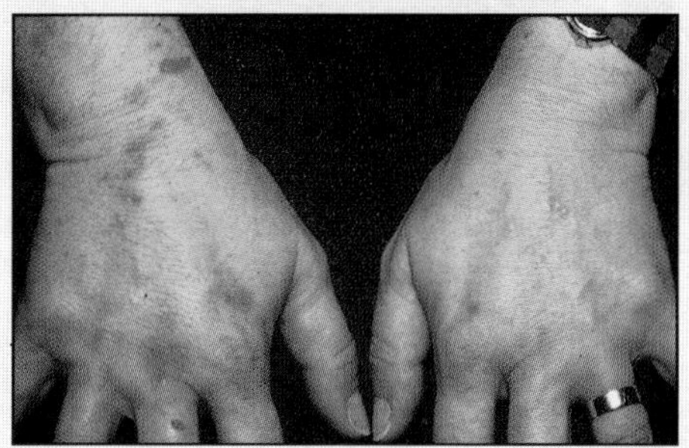
Porphyria (estrogens)

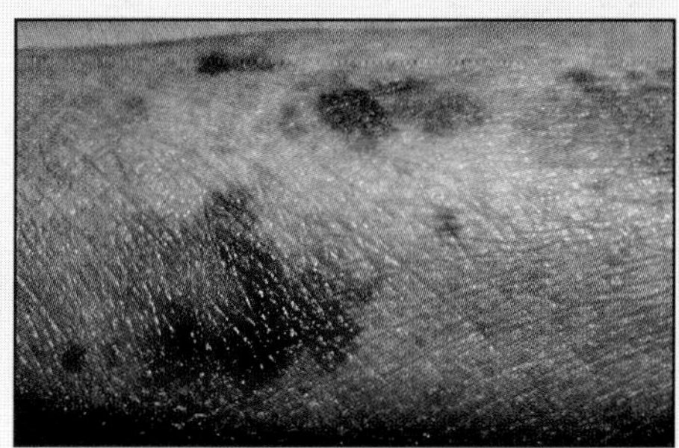
Purpura (aspirin)

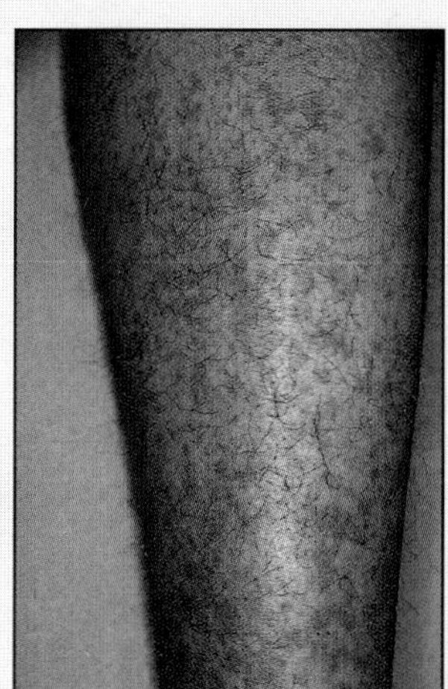
Purpura (naproxen)

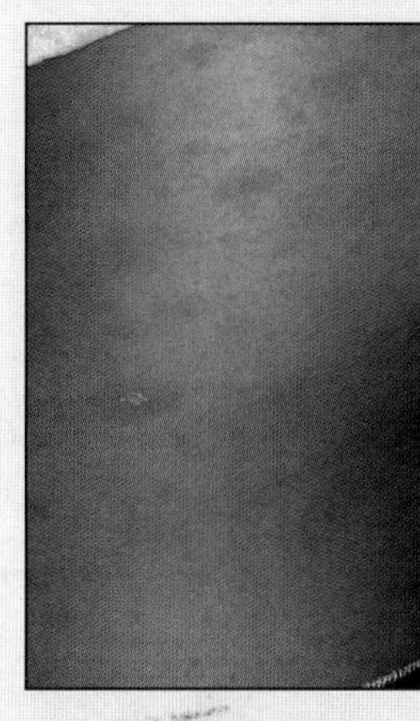
Pityriasis rosea

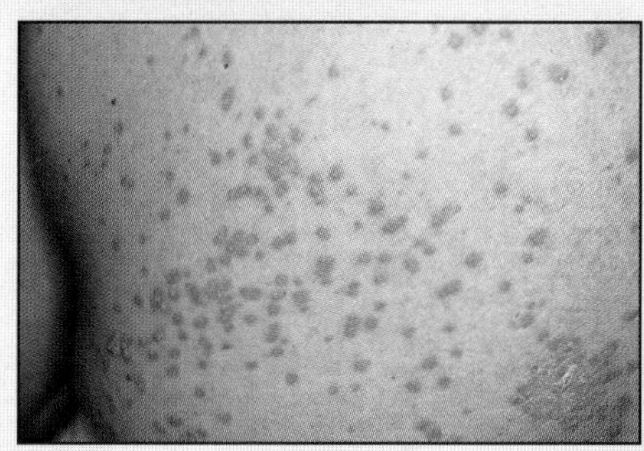
Psoriasis

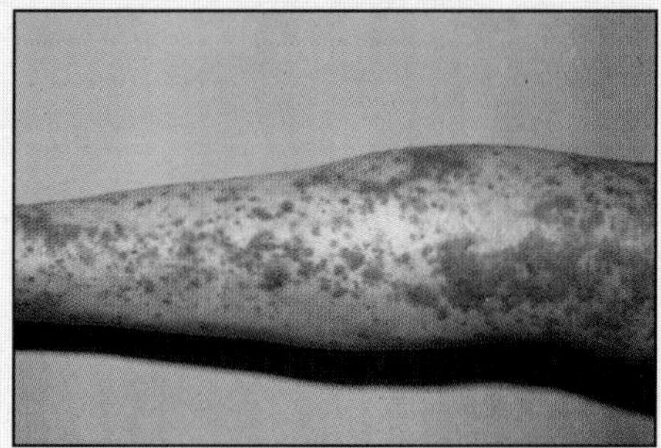
Purpura

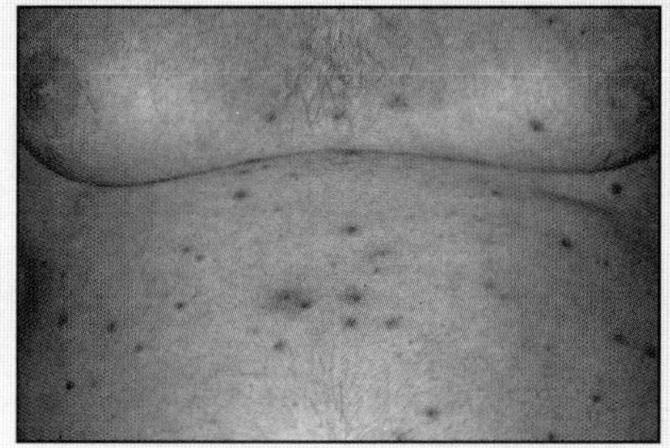
Pustular eruption (lithium)

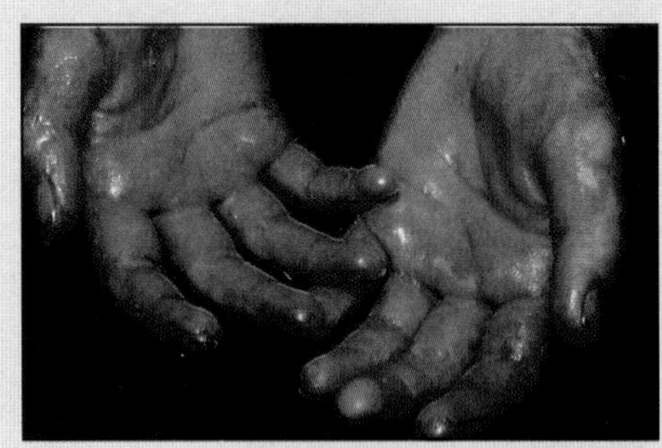
Stevens-Johnson Syndrome (dilantin)

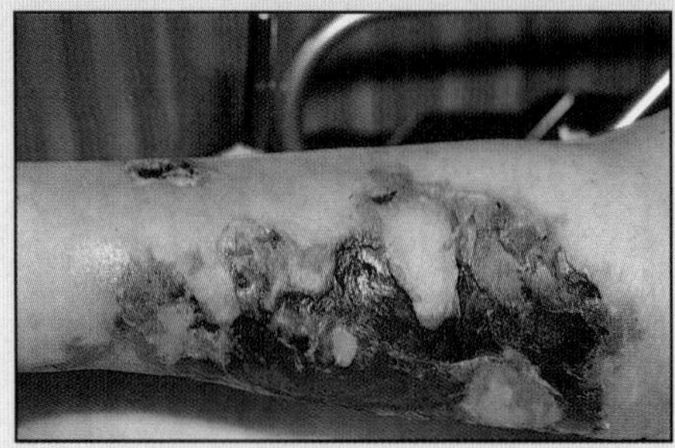
Necrosis

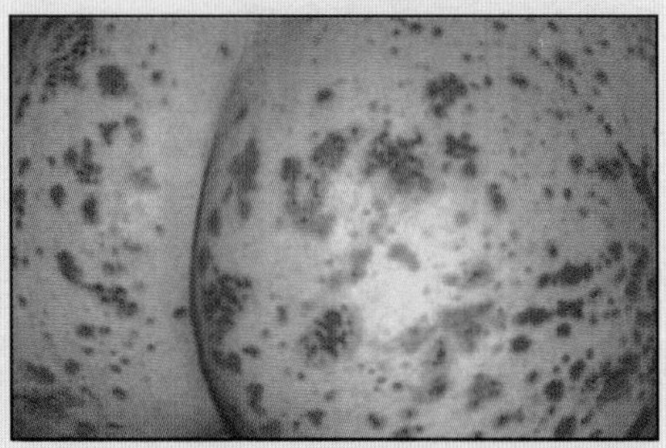
Vasculitis

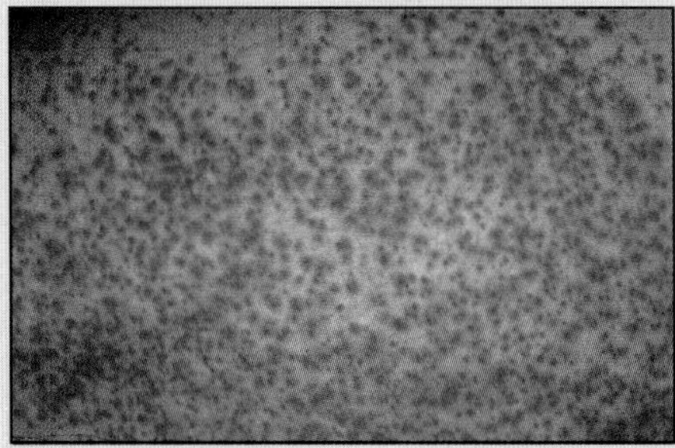
Leukocytoclastic vasculitis

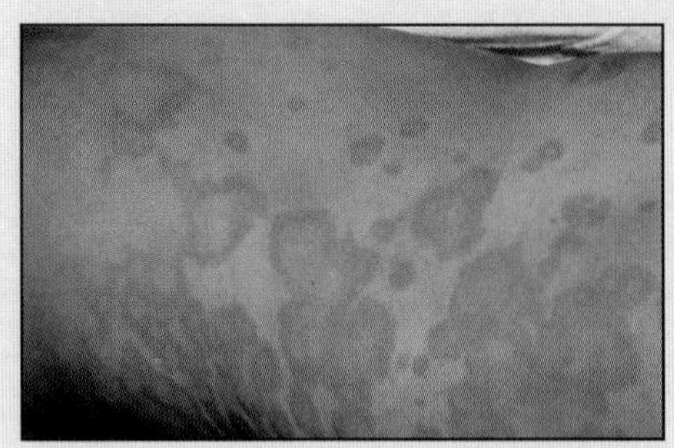
Urticaria

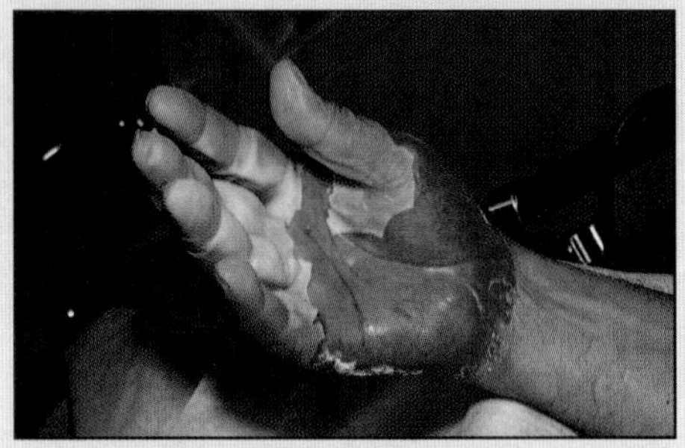
Toxic epidermal necrolysis

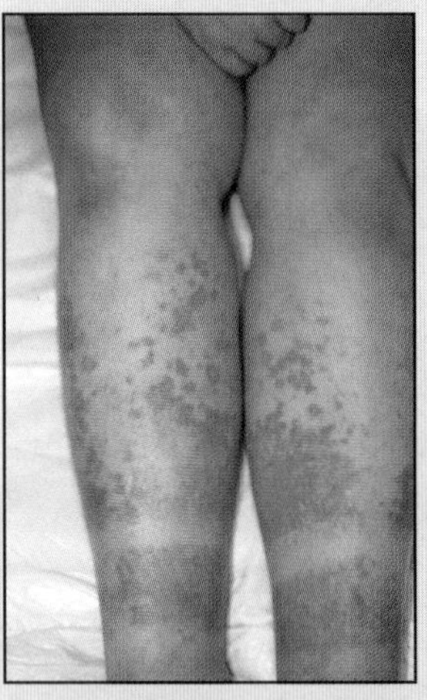
Vasculitis

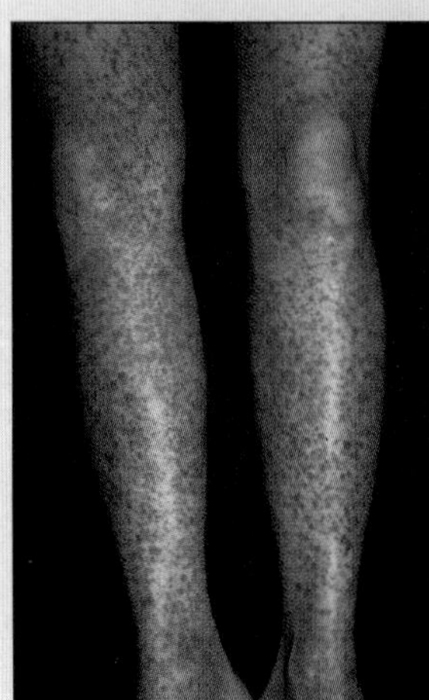
Vasculitis

*Litt's*

# DRUG ERUPTION REFERENCE MANUAL on CD-ROM

This CD-ROM allows users to search the whole database in a highly sophisticated and flexible way. Drugs can be searched by generic name or trade name – or searches can be made on the basis of reaction patterns. The CD-ROM also has the added capacity for multiple drug searching – the user may enter, for example, the names of all the drugs taken by a patient and it will identify if any of these are responsible for an adverse reaction. Results of all searches can be printed out.

**Instructions for installing**

To install Litt's DRUG ERUPTION REFERENCE MANUAL, double click on the file 'Setup'.

**Minimum System Requirements for CD Users**

**Windows**

- Intel-compatible computer
- Microsoft® Windows® 95, Windows 98, Windows 2000, or Windows NT® Pack 3.51 or later
- 8 MB of available RAM (16 MB recommended)
- 10 MB of available hard disk space
- CD-ROM drive

**Macintosh**

- MacOS-based computer
- MacOS software version 7.1 or later
- 8 MB of available RAM (16 MB recommended)
- 10 MB of available hard disk space
- CD-ROM drive
- 800 x 600 (SVGA) with 16 bit high color display (recommended)

**Technical support**

Technical support enquiries can be emailed from the Litt Drug Eruption Database website Help section support@drugeruptiondata.com.